The MIT Encyclopedia of
Communication Disorders

The MIT Encyclopedia of Communication Disorders

Edited by Raymond D. Kent

A Bradford Book
The MIT Press
Cambridge, Massachusetts
London, England

© 2004 Massachusetts Institute of Technology

This book was set in Times New Roman on 3B2 by Asco Typesetters, Hong Kong, and was printed and bound in the United States of America.

Library of Congress Cataloging-in-Publication Data

The MIT encyclopedia of communication disorders / edited by Raymond D. Kent.
    p.   cm.
  Includes bibliographical references and index.
  ISBN 0-262-11278-7 (cloth)
  1. Communicative disorders—Encyclopedias. I. Kent, Raymond D. II. Massachusetts Institute of Technology.
RC423.M56   2004
616.85′5′003—dc21

2003059941

Contents

Introduction

The MIT Encyclopedia of Communication Disorders (MITECD) is a comprehensive volume that presents essential information on communication sciences and disorders. The pertinent disorders are those that affect the production and comprehension of spoken language and include especially disorders of speech production and perception, language expression, language comprehension, voice, and hearing. Potential readers include clinical practitioners, students, and research specialists. Relatively few comprehensive books of similar design and purpose exist, so MITECD stands nearly alone as a resource for anyone interested in the broad field of communication disorders.

MITECD is organized into the four broad categories of Voice, Speech, Language, and Hearing. These categories represent the spectrum of topics that usually fall under the rubric of communication disorders (also known as speech-language pathology and audiology, among other names). For example, roughly these same categories were used by the National Institute on Deafness and Other Communication Disorders (NIDCD) in preparing its national strategic research plans over the past decade. The *Journal of Speech, Language, and Hearing Research*, one of the most comprehensive and influential periodicals in the field, uses the editorial categories of speech, language, and hearing. Although voice could be subsumed under speech, the two fields are large enough individually and sufficiently distinct that a separation is warranted. Voice is internationally recognized as a clinical and research specialty, and it is represented by journals dedicated to its domain (e.g., the *Journal of Voice*). The use of these four categories achieves a major categorization of knowledge but avoids a narrow fragmentation of the field at large. It is to be expected that the *Encyclopedia* would include cross-referencing within and across these four major categories. After all, they are integrated in the definitively human behavior of language, and disorders of communication frequently have wide-ranging effects on communication in its essential social, educational, and vocational roles.

In designing the content and structure of MITECD, it was decided that each of these major categories should be further subdivided into Basic Science, Disorders (nature and assessment), and Clinical Management (intervention issues). Although these categories are not always transparent in the entire collection of entries, they guided the delineation of chapters and the selection of contributors. These categories are defined as follows:

Basic Science entries pertain to matters such as normal anatomy and physiology, physics, psychology and psychophysics, and linguistics. These topics are the foundation for clinical description and interpretation, covering basic principles and terminology pertaining to the communication sciences. Care was taken to avoid substantive overlap with previous MIT publications, especially the *MIT Encyclopedia of the Cognitive Sciences* (MITECS).

The Disorders entries offer information on issues such as syndrome delineation, definition and characterization of specific disorders, and methods for the identification and assessment of disorders. As such, these chapters reflect contemporary nosology and nomenclature, as well as guidelines for clinical assessment and diagnosis.

The Clinical Management entries discuss various interventions including behavioral, pharmacological, surgical, and prosthetic (mechanical and electronic). There is a general, but not necessarily one-to-one, correspondence between chapters in the Disorders and Clinical Management categories. For example, it is possible that several types of disorder are related to one general chapter on clinical management. It is certainly the case that different management strategies are preferred by different clinicians. The chapters avoid dogmatic statements regarding interventions of choice.

Because the approach to communicative disorders can be quite different for children and adults, a further cross-cutting division was made such that for many topics separate chapters for children and adults are included. Although some disorders that are first diagnosed in childhood may persist in some form throughout adulthood (e.g, stuttering, specific language impairment, and hearing loss may be lifelong conditions for some individuals), many disorders can have an onset either in childhood or in adulthood and the timing of onset can have implications for both assessment and intervention. For instance, when a child experiences a significant loss of hearing, the sensory deficit may greatly impair the learning of speech and language. But when a loss of the same degree has an onset in adulthood, the problem is not in acquiring speech and language, but rather in maintaining communication skills. Certainly, it is often true that an understanding of a given disorder has common features in both the developmental and acquired forms, but commonality cannot be assumed as a general condition.

Many decisions were made during the preparation of this volume. Some were easy, but others were not. In the main, entries are uniform in length and number of references. However, in a few instances, two or more entries were combined into a single longer entry. Perhaps inevitably in a project with so many contributors, a small number of entries were dropped because of personal issues, such as illness, that interfered with timely preparation of an entry. Happily, contributors showed great enthusiasm for this project, and their entries reflect an assembled expertise that is high tribute to the science and clinical practice in communication disorders.

Raymond D. Kent

Acknowledgments

MITECD began as a promising idea in a conversation with Amy Brand, a previous editor with MIT Press. The idea was further developed, refined, elaborated, and refined again in many ensuing e-mail communications, and I thank Amy for her constant support and assistance through the early phases of the project. When she left MIT Press, Tom Stone, Senior Editor of Cognitive Sciences, Linguistics, and Bradford Books, stepped in to provide timely advice and attention. I also thank Margy Avery, Acquisitions Assistant, for her help in keeping this project on track. I am indebted to all of them.

Speech, voice, language, and hearing are vast domains individually, and several associated editors helped to select topics for inclusion in MITECD and to identify contributors with the necessary expertise. The associate editors and their fields of responsibility are as follows:

Fred H. Bess, Ph.D., Hearing Disorders in Children
Joseph R. Duffy, Ph.D., Speech Disorders in Adults
Steven D. Gray, M.D. (deceased), Voice Disorders in Children
Robert E. Hillman, Ph.D., Voice Disorders in Adults
Sandra Gordon-Salant, Ph.D., Hearing Disorders in Adults
Mabel L. Rice, Ph.D., Language Disorders in Children
Lawrence D. Shriberg, Ph.D., Speech Disorders in Children
David A. Swinney, Ph.D., and Lewis P. Shapiro, Ph.D., Language Disorders in Adults

The advice and cooperation of these individuals is gratefully acknowledged. Sadly, Dr. Steven D. Gray died within the past year. He was an extraordinary man, and although I knew him only briefly, I was deeply impressed by his passion for knowledge and life. He will be remembered as an excellent physician, creative scientist, and valued friend and colleague to many.

Dr. Houri Vorperian greatly facilitated this project through her inspired planning of a computer-based system for contributor communications and record management. Sara Stuntebeck and Sara Brost worked skillfully and accurately on a variety of tasks that went into different phases of MITECD. They offered vital help with communications, file management, proofreading, and the various and sundry tasks that stood between the initial conception of MITECD and the submission of a full manuscript.

P. M. Gordon and Associates took on the formidable task of assembling 200 entries into a volume that looks and reads like an encyclopedia. I thank Denise Bracken for exacting attention to the editing craft, creative solutions to unexpected problems, and forbearance through it all.

MITECD came to reality through the efforts of a large number of contributors—too many for me to acknowledge personally here. However, I draw the reader's attention to the list of contributors included in this volume. I feel a sense of community with all of them, because they believed in the project and worked toward its completion by preparing entries of high quality. I salute them not only for their contributions to MITECD but also for their many career contributions that define them as experts in the field. I am honored by their participation and their patient cooperation with the editorial process.

Raymond D. Kent

Part I: Voice

Acoustic Assessment of Voice

Acoustic assessment of voice in clinical applications is dominated by measures of fundamental frequency (f_0), cycle-to-cycle perturbations of period (jitter) and intensity (shimmer), and other measures of irregularity, such as noise-to-harmonics ratio (NHR). These measures are widely used, in part because of the availability of electronic and microcomputer-based instruments (e.g., Kay Elemetrics Computerized Speech Laboratory [CSL] or Multispeech, Real-Time Pitch, Multi-Dimensional Voice Program [MDVP], and other software/hardware systems), and in part because of long-term precedent for perturbation (Lieberman, 1961) and spectral noise measurements (Yanagihara, 1967). Absolute measures of vocal intensity are equally basic but require calibrations and associated instrumentation (Winholtz and Titze, 1997).

Independently, these basic acoustic descriptors—f_0, intensity, jitter, shimmer, and NHR—can provide some very basic characterizations of vocal health. The first two, f_0 and intensity, have very clear perceptual correlates—pitch and loudness, respectively—and should be assessed for both stability and variability and compared to age and sex norms (Kent, 1994; Baken and Orlikoff, 2000). Ideally, these tasks are recorded over headset microphones with direct digital acquisition at very high sampling rates (at least 48 kHz). The materials to be assessed should be obtained following standardized elicitation protocols that include sustained vowel phonations at habitual levels, levels spanning a client's vocal range in both f_0 and intensity, running speech, and speech tasks designed to elicit variation (Titze, 1995; Awan, 2001). Note, however, that not all measures will be appropriate for all tasks; perturbation statistics, for example, are usually valid only when extracted from sustained vowel phonations.

These basic descriptors are not in any way comprehensive of the range of available measures or the available signal properties and dimensions. Table 1 categorizes measures (Buder, 2000) based on primary basic signal representations from which measures are derived. Although these categories are intended to be exhaustive and mutually exclusive, some more modern algorithms process components through several types. (For more detail on the measurement types, see Buder, 2000, and Baken and Orlikoff, 2000.) Modern algorithmic approaches should be selected for (1) interpretability with respect to aerodynamic and physiological models of phonation and (2) the incorporation of multivariate measures to characterize vocal function.

Interdependence of Basic Measures. The interdependence between f_0 and intensity is mapped in a voice range profile, or phonetogram, which is an especially valuable assessment for the professional voice user (Coleman, 1993). Furthermore, the dependence of perturbations and signal-to-noise ratios on both f_0 and intensity is well known (Klingholz, 1990; Pabon, 1991).

Table 1. Outline of Traditional Acoustic Algorithm Types

f_0 statistics
    Short-term perturbations
    Long-term perturbations
Amplitude statistics
    Short-term perturbations
    Long-term perturbations
f_0/amplitude covariations
Waveform perturbations
Spectral measures
    Spectrographic measures
    Fourier and LPC spectra
    Long-term average spectra
    Cepstra
Inverse filter measures
    Radiated signal
    Flow-mask signals
Dynamic measures

This dependence is not often assessed rigorously, perhaps because of the time-consuming and strenuous nature of a full voice profile. However, an abbreviated or focused profiling in which samples related to habitual f_0 by a set number of semitones, or related to habitual intensity by a set number of decibels, could be standardized to control for this dependence efficiently. Finally, it should be understood that perturbations and NHR-type measures will usually covary for many reasons, the simplest ones being methodological (Hillenbrand, 1987): an increase in any one of the underlying phenomena detected by a single measure will also affect the other measures.

Periodicity as a Reference. The chief problem with nearly all acoustic assessments of voice is the determination of f_0. Most voice quality algorithms are based on the prior identification of the periodic component in the signal (based on glottal pulses in the time domain or harmonic structure in the frequency domain). Because phonation is ideally a nearly periodic process, it is logical to conceive of voice measures in terms of the degree to which a given sample deviates from pure periodicity. There are many conceptual problems with this simplification, however. At the physiological level, glottal morphology is multidimensional—superior-inferior asymmetry is a basic feature of the two-mass model (Ishizaka and Flanagan, 1972), and some anterior-posterior asymmetry is also inevitable—rendering it unlikely that a glottal pulse will be marked by a discrete or even a single instant of glottal closure. At the level of the signal, the deviations from periodicity may be either random or correlated, and in many cases they are so extreme as to preclude identification of a regular period. Finally, at the perceptual level, many factors related to deviations from a pure f_0 can contribute to pitch perception (Zwicker and Fastl, 1990).

At any or all of these levels, it becomes questionable to characterize deviations with pure periodicity as a reference. In acoustic assessment, the primary level of concern is the signal. The National Center for Voice and

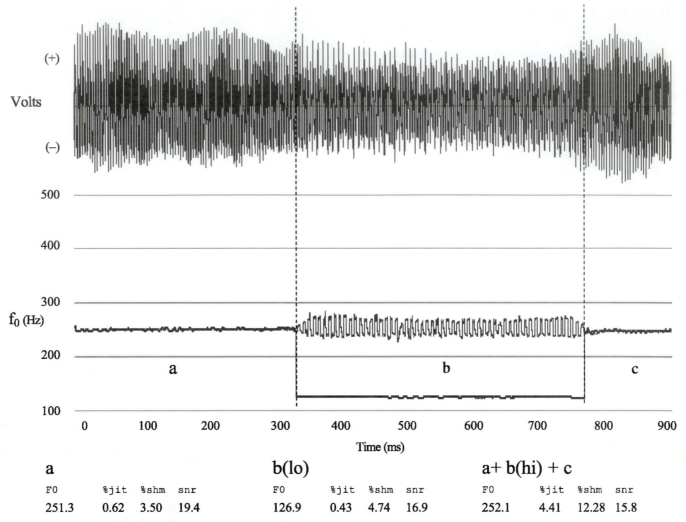

a				b(lo)				a+ b(hi) + c			
FO	%jit	%shm	snr	FO	%jit	%shm	snr	FO	%jit	%shm	snr
251.3	0.62	3.50	19.4	126.9	0.43	4.74	16.9	252.1	4.41	12.28	15.8

Figure 1. Approximately 900 ms of a sustained vowel phonation waveform (top panel) with two fundamental frequency analyses (bottom panel). Average f_0, %jitter, %shimmer, and SNR results for selected segments were from the "newjit" routine of TF32 program (Milenkovic, 2001).

Speech issued a summary statement (Titze, 1995) recommending a typology for categorizing deviations from periodicity in voices (see also Baken and Orlikoff, 2000, for further subtypes). This typology capitalizes on the categorical nature of dynamic states in nonlinear systems; all the major categories, including stable points, limit cycles, period-doubling/tripling/..., and chaos can be observed in voice signals (Herzel et al., 1994; Sataloff and Hawkshaw, 2001). As in most highly nonlinear dynamic systems, deviations from periodicity can be categorized on the basis of bifurcations, or sudden qualitative changes in vibratory pattern from one of these states to another.

Figure 1 displays a common form for one such bifurcation and illustrates the importance of accounting for its presence in the application of perturbation measures. In this sustained vowel phonation by a middle-aged woman with spasmodic dysphonia, a transition to subharmonics is clearly visible in segment *b* (similar patterns occur in individuals without dysphonias). Two f_0

extractions are presented for this segment, one at the targeted level of approximately 250 Hz and another which the tracker finds one octave below this; inspection of the waveform and a perceived biphonia both justify this 125-Hz analysis as a new fundamental frequency, although it can also be understood in this context as a subharmonic to the original fundamental. There is therefore some ambiguity as to which fundamental is valid during this episode, and an automatic analysis could plausibly identify either frequency. (Here the waveform-matching algorithm implemented in CSpeechSP [Milenkovic, 1997] does identify either frequency, depending on where in the waveform the algorithm is applied; initiating the algorithm within the subharmonic segment predisposes it to identify the lower fundamental.)

The acoustic measures of the segments displayed in Figure 1 reveal the nontrivial differences that result, depending on the basic glottal pulse form under consideration. When the pulses of segment *a* are considered, the perturbations around the base period associated with the high f_0 are low and normative; in segment b, perturbations around the longer periods of the lower f_0 are still low (jitter is improved, while shimmer and the signal-to-noise ratio show some degradation). However, when all segments are considered together to include the perturbations around the high f_0 tracked through segment b and into c, the perturbation statistics are all increased by an order of magnitude. Many important methodological and theoretical questions should be raised by such common scenarios in which we must consider not just voice typing, but the segment-by-segment validity of applying perturbation measures with a particular f_0 as reference. If, as is often assumed, jitter and shimmer are ascribed to "random" variations, then the correlated modulations of a strong subharmonic episode should be excluded. Alternatively, the perturbations might be analyzed with respect to the subharmonic f_0. In any case, assessment by means of perturbation statistics with no consideration of their underlying sources is unwise.

Perceptual, Aerodynamic, and Physiological Correlates of Acoustic Measures. Regarding perceptual voice rat-

ings, Gerratt and Kreiman (2000) have critiqued traditional assessments on several important methodological and theoretical points. However, these points may not apply to acoustic analysis if (1) acoustic analysis is validated on its own success and not exclusively in relation to the problematic perceptual classifications, and (2) acoustic analysis is thoroughly grounded for interpretation in some clear aerodynamic or physiological model of phonation. Gerratt and Kreiman also argue that clinical classification may not be derived along a continuum that is defined with reference to normal qualities, but again, this argument may need to be reversed for the acoustic domain. It is only by reference to a specific model that any assessment on acoustic grounds can be interpreted (though this does not preclude development of an independent model for a pathological phonatory mechanism). In clinical settings, acoustic voice assessment often serves to corroborate perceptual assessment. However, as guided by auditory experience and in conjunction with the ear and other instrumental assessments, careful acoustic analysis can be oriented to the identification of physiological status.

In attempting to draw safe and reasonably direct inferences from acoustic signal, aerodynamic models

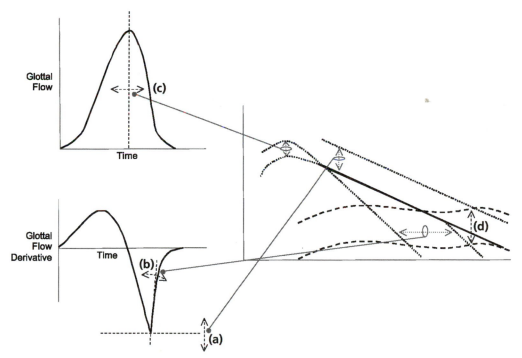

Figure 2. Spectral features associated with models of phonation, including the Liljencrants-Fant (LF) model of glottal flow and aperiodicity source models developed by Stevens. The LF model of glottal flow is shown at top left. At bottom left is the LF model of glottal flow derivative, showing the rate of change in flow. At right is a spectrum schematic showing four effects. These effects include three derived parameters of the LF model: **(a)** excitation strength (the maximum negative amplitude of the flow derivative, which is positively correlated with overall harmonic energy), **(b)** dynamic leakage or non-zero return phase following the point of maximum excitation (which is negatively correlated with high-frequency harmonic energy), and **(c)** pulse skewing (which is negatively correlated with low-frequency harmonic energy; this low-frequency region is also positively correlated with open quotient and peak volume velocity measures of the glottal flow waveform). The effect of turbulence due to high airflow through the glottis is schematized by **(d)**, indicating the associated appearance of high-frequency aperiodic energy in the spectrum. See VOICE ACOUSTICS for other graphical and quantitative associations between glottal status and spectral characteristics.

of glottal behavior present important links to the physiological domain. Attempts to recover the glottal flow waveform, either from a face mask-transduced flow recording (Rothenberg, 1973) or a microphone-transduced acoustic recording (Davis, 1975), have proved to be labor-intensive and prone to error (Ní Chasaide and Gobl, 1997). Rather than attempting to eliminate the effects of the vocal tract, it may be more fruitful to understand its in situ relationship with phonation, and infer, via the types of features displayed in Figure 2, the status of the glottis as a sound source. Interpretation of spectral features, such as the amplitudes of the first harmonics and at the formant frequencies, may be an effective alternative when guided by knowledge of glottal aerodynamics and acoustics (Hanson, 1997; Ní Chasaide and Gobl, 1997; Hanson and Chuang, 1999). Deep familiarity with acoustic mechanisms is essential for such interpretations (Titze, 1994; Stevens, 1998), as is a model with clear and meaningful parameters, such as the Liljencrants-Fant (LF) model (Fant, Liljencrants, and Lin, 1985). The parameters of the LF model have proved to be meaningful in acoustic studies (Gauffin & Sundberg, 1989) and useful in refined efforts at inverse filtering (Fröhlich, Michaelis, and Strube, 2001). Figure 2 summarizes selected parameters of the LF source model following Ní Chasaide and Gobl (1997) and the glottal turbulence source following Stevens (1998); see also VOICE ACOUSTICS for other approaches relating glottal status to spectral measures.

Other spectral-based measures implement similar model-based strategies by selecting spectral component ratios (e.g., the VTI and SPI parameters of MDVP). Sophisticated spectral noise characterizations control for perturbations and modulations (Murphy, 1999; Qi, Hillman, and Milstein, 1999), or employ curve-fitting and statistical models to produce more robust measures (Alku, Strik, and Vilkman, 1997; Michaelis, Fröhlich, and Strube, 1998; Schoentgen, Bensaid, and Bucella, 2000). A particularly valuable modern technique for detecting turbulence at the glottis, the glottal-to-noise-excitation ratio (Michaelis, Gramss, and Strube, 1997), has been especially successful in combination with other measures (Fröhlich et al., 2000). The use of acoustic techniques for voice will only improve with the inclusion of more knowledge-based measures in multivariate representations (Wolfe, Cornell, and Palmer, 1991; Callen et al., 2000; Wuyts et al., 2000).

—*Eugene H. Buder*

References

Alku, P., Strik, H., and Vilkman, E. (1997). Parabolic spectral parameter: A new method for quantification of the glottal flow. *Speech Communication, 22,* 67–79.

Awan, S. N. (2001). *The voice diagnostic profile: A practical guide to the diagnosis of voice disorders.* Gaithersburg, MD: Aspen.

Baken, R. J., and Orlikoff, R. F. (2000). *Clinical measurement of speech and voice.* San Diego, CA: Singular Publishing Group.

Buder, E. H. (2000). Acoustic analysis of voice quality: A tabulation of algorithms 1902–1990. In M. J. Ball (Ed.), *Voice quality measurement* (pp. 119–244). San Diego, CA: Singular Publishing Group.

Callen, D. E., Kent, R. D., Roy, N., and Tasko, S. M. (2000). The use of self-organizing maps for the classification of voice disorders. In M. J. Ball (Ed.), *Voice quality measurement* (pp. 103–116). San Diego, CA: Singular Publishing Group.

Coleman, R. F. (1993). Sources of variation in phonetograms. *Journal of Voice, 7,* 1–14.

Davis, S. B. (1975). Preliminary results using inverse filtering of speech for automatic evaluation of laryngeal pathology. *Journal of the Acoustical Society of America, 58,* SIII.

Fant, G., Liljencrants, J., and Lin, Q. (1985). A four-parameter model of glottal flow. *Speech Transmission Laboratory Quarterly Progress and Status Report, 4,* 1–13.

Fröhlich, M., Michaelis, D., and Strube, H. (2001). SIM-simultaneous inverse filtering and matching of a glottal flow model for acoustic speech signals. *Journal of the Acoustical Society of America, 110,* 479–488.

Fröhlich, M., Michaelis, D., Strube, H., and Kruse, E. (2000). Acoustic voice analysis by means of the hoarseness diagram. *Journal of Speech, Language, and Hearing Research, 43,* 706–720.

Gauffin, J., and Sundberg, J. (1989). Spectral correlates of glottal voice source waveform characteristics. *Journal of Speech and Hearing Research, 32,* 556–565.

Gerratt, B., and Kreiman, J. (2000). Theoretical and methodological development in the study of pathological voice quality. *Journal of Phonetics, 28,* 335–342.

Hanson, H. M. (1997). Glottal characteristics of female speakers: Acoustic correlates. *Journal of the Acoustical Society of America, 101,* 466–481.

Hanson, H. M., and Chuang, E. S. (1999). Glottal characteristics of male speakers: Acoustic correlates and comparison with female data. *Journal of the Acoustical Society of America, 106,* 1064–1077.

Herzel, H., Berry, D., Titze, I. R., and Saleh, M. (1994). Analysis of vocal disorders with methods from nonlinear dynamics. *Journal of Speech and Hearing Research, 37,* 1008–1019.

Hillenbrand, J. (1987). A methodological study of perturbation and additive noise in synthetically generated voice signals. *Journal of Speech and Hearing Research, 30,* 448–461.

Ishizaka, K., and Flanagan, J. L. (1972). Synthesis of voiced sounds from a two-mass model of the vocal cords. *Bell System Technical Journal, 51,* 1233–1268.

Kent, R. D. (1994). *Reference manual for communicative sciences and disorders: Speech and language.* Austin, TX: Pro-Ed.

Klingholz, F. (1990). Acoustic representation of speaking-voice quality. *Journal of Voice, 4,* 213–219.

Lieberman, P. (1961). Perturbations in vocal pitch. *Journal of the Acoustical Society of America, 33,* 597–603.

Michaelis, D., Fröhlich, M., and Strube, H. W. (1998). Selection and combination of acoustic features for the description of pathologic voices. *Journal of the Acoustical Society of America, 103,* 1628–1638.

Michaelis, D., Gramss, T., and Strube, H. W. (1997). Glottal to noise excitation ratio: A new measure for describing patholocial voices. *Acustica, 83,* 700–706.

Milenkovic, P. (1997). CSpeechSP [Computer software]. Madison, WI: University of Wisconsin–Madison.

Milenkovic, P. (2001). TF32 [Computer software]. Madison, WI: University of Wisconsin–Madison.

Murphy, P. J. (1999). Perturbation-free measurement of the harmonics-to-noise ratio in voice signals using pitch synchronous harmonic analysis. *Journal of the Acoustical Society of America, 105,* 2866–2881.

Ní Chasaide, A., and Gobl, C. (1997). Voice source variation. In J. Laver (Ed.), *The handbook of phonetic sciences* (pp. 427–461). Oxford, UK: Blackwell.

Pabon, J. P. H. (1991). Objective acoustic voice-quality parameters in the computer phonetogram. *Journal of Voice*, 5, 203–216.

Qi, Y., Hillman, R., and Milstein, C. (1999). The estimation of signal-to-noise ratio in continuous speech for disordered voices. *Journal of the Acoustical Society of America*, 105, 2532–2535.

Rothenberg, M. (1973). A new inverse-filtering technique for deriving the glottal air flow waveform during voicing. *Journal of the Acoustical Society of America*, 53, 1632–1645.

Sataloff, R. T., and Hawkshaw, M. (Eds.). (2001). *Chaos in medicine: Source readings*. San Diego, CA: Singular Publishing Group.

Schoentgen, J., Bensaid, M., and Bucella, F. (2000). Multivariate statistical analysis of flat vowel spectra with a view to characterizing dysphonic voices. *Journal of Speech, Language, and Hearing Research*, 43, 1493–1508.

Stevens, K. N. (1998). *Acoustic phonetics*. Cambridge, MA: MIT Press.

Titze, I. R. (1994). *Principles of voice production*. Englewood Cliffs, NJ: Prentice Hall.

Titze, I. R. (1995). *Workshop on acoustic voice analysis: Summary statement*. Iowa City, IA: National Center for Voice and Speech.

Winholtz, W. S., and Titze, I. R. (1997). Conversion of a head-mounted microphone signal into calibrated SPL units. *Journal of Voice*, 11, 417–421.

Wolfe, V., Cornell, R., and Palmer, C. (1991). Acoustic correlates of pathologic voice types. *Journal of Speech and Hearing Research*, 34, 509–516.

Wuyts, F. L., De Bodt, M. S., Molenberghs, G., Remacle, M., Heylen, L., Millet, B., et al. (2000). The Dysphonia Severity Index: An objective measure of vocal quality based on a multiparameter approach. *Journal of Speech, Language, and Hearing Research*, 43, 796–809.

Yanagihara, N. (1967). Significance of harmonic changes and noise components in hoarseness. *Journal of Speech and Hearing Research*, 10, 531–541.

Zwicker, E., and Fastl, H. (1990). *Psychoacoustics: Facts and models*. Heidelberg, Germany: Springer-Verlag.

Aerodynamic Assessment of Vocal Function

A number of methods have been used to quantitatively assess the air volumes, airflows, and air pressures involved in voice production. The methods have been mostly used in research to investigate mechanisms that underlie normal and disordered voice and speech production. The clinical use of aerodynamic measures to assess patients with voice disorders has been increasing (Colton and Casper, 1996; Hillman, Montgomery, and Zeitels, 1997; Hillman and Kobler, 2000).

Measurement of Air Volumes.   Respiratory research in human communication has focused primarily on the measurement of the air volumes that are typically expended during selected speech and singing tasks, and on specifying the ranges of lung inflation levels across which such tasks are normally performed (cf. Hixon, Goldman, and Mead, 1973; Watson and Hixon, 1985; Hoit and Hixon, 1987; Hoit et al., 1990). Air volumes are measured in standard metric units (liters, cubic centimeters, milliliters) and lung inflation levels are usually specified in terms of a percentage of the vital capacity or total lung volume.

Both direct and indirect methods have been used to measure air volumes expended during phonation. Direct measurement of orally displaced air volumes during phonatory tasks can be accomplished, to a limited extent, by means of a mouthpiece or face mask connected to a measurement device such as a spirometer (Beckett, 1971) or pneumotachograph (Isshiki, 1964). The use of a mouthpiece essentially limits speech production to sustained vowels, which are sufficient for assessing selected volumetric-based phonatory parameters. There are also concerns that face masks interfere with normal jaw movements and that the oral acoustic signal is degraded, so that auditory feedback is reduced or distorted and simultaneous acoustic analysis is limited. These limitations, which are inherent to the use of devices placed in or around the mouth to directly collect oral airflow, plus additional measurement-related restrictions (Hillman and Kobler, 2000) have helped motivate the development and application of indirect measurement approaches.

Most speech breathing research has been carried out using indirect approaches for estimating lung volumes by means of monitoring changes in body dimensions. The basic assumption underlying the indirect approaches is that changes in lung volume are reflected in proportional changes in body torso size. One relatively cumbersome but time-honored approach has been to place subjects in a sealed chamber called a body plethysmograph to allow estimation of the air volume displaced by the body during respiration (Draper, Ladefoged, and Whitteridge, 1959). More often used for speech breathing research are transducers (magnetometers: Hixon, Goldman, and Mead, 1973; inductance plethysmographs: Sperry, Hillman, and Perkell, 1994) that unobtrusively monitor changes in the dimensions of the rib cage and abdomen (referred to collectively as the chest wall) that account for the majority of respiratory-related changes in torso dimension (Mead et al., 1967). These approaches have been primarily employed to study respiratory function during continuous speech and singing tasks that include both voiced and voiceless sound production, as opposed to assessing air volume usage during phonatory tasks that involve only laryngeal production of voice (e.g., sustained vowels). There are also ongoing efforts to develop more accurate methods for non-invasively monitoring chest wall activity to capture finer details of how the three-dimensional geometry of the body is altered during respiration (see Cala et al., 1996).

Measurement of Airflow.   Airflow associated with phonation is usually specified in terms of volume velocity (i.e., volume of air displaced per unit of time). Volume velocity airflow rates for voice production are typically reported in metric units of volume displaced (liters or cubic centimeters) per second.

Estimates of average airflow rates can be obtained by simply dividing air volume estimates by the duration of the phonatory task. Average glottal airflow rates have usually been estimated during vowel phonation by using a mouthpiece or face mask to channel the oral air stream through a pneumotachograph (Isshiki, 1964). There has also been somewhat limited use of hot wire anemometer devices (mounted in a mouthpiece) to estimate average glottal airflow during sustained vowel phonation (Woo, Colton, and Shangold, 1987). Estimates of average glottal airflow rates can be obtained from the oral airflow during vowel production because the vocal tract is relatively nonconstricted, with no major sources of turbulent airflow between the glottis and the lips.

There have also been efforts to obtain estimates of the actual airflow waveform that is generated as the glottis rapidly opens and closes during flow-induced vibration of the vocal folds (the glottal volume velocity waveform). The glottal volume velocity waveform cannot be directly observed by measuring the oral airflow signal because the waveform is highly convoluted by the resonance activity (formants) of the vocal tract. Thus, recovery of the glottal volume velocity waveform requires methods that eliminate or correct for the influences of the vocal tract. This has typically been accomplished aerodynamically by processing the output of a fast-responding pneumotachograph (high-frequency response) using a technique called inverse filtering, in which the major resonances of the vocal tract are estimated and the oral airflow signal is processed (inverse filtered) to eliminate them (Rothenberg, 1977; Holmberg, Hillman, and Perkell, 1988).

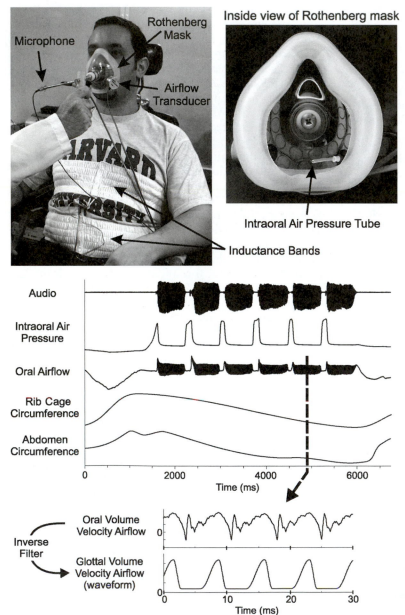

Figure 1. Instrumentation and resulting signals for simultaneous collection of oral airflow, intraoral air pressure, the acoustic signal, and chest wall (rib cage and abdomen) dimensions during production of the syllable string /pi-pi-pi/. Signals shown in the bottom panel are processed and measured to provide estimates of average glottal airflow rate, average subglottal air pressure, lung volume, and glottal waveform parameters.

Measurement of Air Pressure. Measurements of air pressures below (subglottal) and above (supraglottal) the vocal folds are of primary interest for characterizing the pressure differential that must be achieved to initiate and maintain vocal fold vibration during normal exhalatory phonation. In practice, air pressure measurements related specifically to voice production are typically acquired during vowel phonation when there are no vocal tract constrictions of sufficient magnitude to build up positive supraglottal pressures. Under these conditions, it is usually assumed that supraglottal pressure is essentially equal to atmospheric pressure and only subglottal pressure measurements are obtained. Air pressures associated with voice and speech production are usually specified in centimeters of water (cm H_2O).

Both direct and indirect methods have been used to measure subglottal air pressures during phonation. Direct measures of subglottal air pressure can be obtained by inserting a hypodermic needle into the subglottal airway through a puncture in the anterior neck at the cricothyroid space (Isshiki, 1964). The needle is connected to a pressure transducer by tubing. This method is very accurate but also very invasive. It is also possible to insert a very thin catheter through the posterior cartilaginous glottis (between the arytenoids) to sense subglottal air pressure during phonation, or to use an array of miniature transducers positioned directly above and below the glottis (Cranen and Boves, 1985). These methods cannot be tolerated by all subjects, and the heavy topical anesthetization of the larynx that is required can affect normal function.

Indirect estimates of tracheal (subglottal) air pressure can be obtained via the placement of an elongated balloon-like device into the esophagus (Liberman, 1968). The deflated esophageal balloon is attached to a catheter that is typically inserted transnasally and then swallowed into the esophagus to be positioned at the midthoracic level. The catheter is connected to a pressure transducer and the balloon is slightly inflated. Accurate use of this invasive method also requires simultaneous monitoring of lung volume.

Noninvasive, indirect estimates of subglottal air pressure can be obtained by measuring intraoral air pressure during specially constrained utterances (Smitheran and Hixon, 1981). This is usually done by sensing air pressure just behind the lips with a translabially placed catheter connected to a pressure transducer. These intraoral pressure measures are obtained as subjects produce strings of bilabial /p/ + vowel syllables (e.g., /pi-pi-pi-pi-pi/) at constant pitch and loudness. This method works because the vocal folds are abducted during /p/ production, thus allowing pressure to equilibrate throughout the airway, making intraoral pressure equal to subglottal pressure (Fig. 1).

Additional Derived Measures. There have been numerous attempts to extend the utility of aerodynamic measures by using them in the derivation of additional parameters aimed at better elucidating underlying mechanisms of vocal function. Such derived measures

usually take the form of ratios that relate aerodynamic parameters to each other, or that relate aerodynamic parameters to simultaneously obtained acoustic measures. Common examples include (1) airway (glottal) resistance (see Smitheran and Hixon, 1981), (2) vocal efficiency (Schutte, 1980; Holmberg, Hillman, and Perkell, 1988), and (3) measures that interrelate glottal volume velocity waveform parameters (Holmberg, Hillman, and Perkell, 1988).

Normative Data. As is the case for most measures of vocal function, there is not currently a set of normative data for aerodynamic measures that is universally accepted and applied in research and clinical work. Methods for collecting such data have not been standardized, and study samples have generally not been of sufficient size or appropriately stratified in terms of age and sex to ensure unbiased estimates of underlying aerodynamic phonatory parameters in the normal population. However, there are several sources in the literature that provide estimates of normative values for selected aerodynamic measures (Kent, 1994; Baken, 1996; Colton and Casper, 1996).

See also VOICE PRODUCTION: PHYSICS AND PHYSIOLOGY.

—*Robert E. Hillman*

References

Baken, R. J. (1996). *Clinical measurement of voice and speech.* San Diego, CA: Singular Publishing Group.

Beckett, R. L. (1971). The respirometer as a diagnostic and clinical tool in the speech clinic. *Journal of Speech and Hearing Disorders, 36,* 235–241.

Cala, S. J., Kenyon, C. M., Ferrigno, G., Carnevali, P., Aliverti, A., Pedotti, A., et al. (1996). Chest wall and lung volume estimation by optical reflectance motion analysis. *Journal of Applied Physiology, 81,* 2680–2689.

Colton, R. H., and Casper, J. K. (1996). *Understanding voice problems: A physiological perspective for diagnosis and treatment.* Baltimore: Williams and Wilkins.

Cranen, B., and Boves, L. (1985). Pressure measurements during speech production using semiconductor miniature pressure transducers: Impact on models for speech production. *Journal of the Acoustical Society of America, 77,* 1543–1551.

Draper, M., Ladefoged, P., and Whitteridge, P. (1959). Respiratory muscles in speech. *Journal of Speech and Hearing Research, 2,* 16–27.

Hillman, R. E., and Kobler, J. B. (2000). Aerodynamic measures of voice production. In R. Kent and M. Ball (Eds.), *The handbook of voice quality measurement,* San Diego, CA: Singular Publishing Group.

Hillman, R. E., Montgomery, W. M., and Zeitels, S. M. (1997). Current diagnostics and office practice: Use of objective measures of vocal function in the multidisciplinary management of voice disorders. *Current Opinion in Otolaryngology–Head and Neck Surgery, 5,* 172–175.

Hixon, T. J., Goldman, M. D., and Mead, J. (1973). Kinematics of the chest wall during speech production: Volume displacements of the rib cage, abdomen, and lung. *Journal of Speech and Hearing Research, 16,* 78–115.

Hoit, J. D., and Hixon, T. J. (1987). Age and speech breathing. *Journal of Speech and Hearing Research, 30,* 351–366.

Hoit, J. D., Hixon, T. J., Watson, P. J., and Morgan, W. J. (1990). Speech breathing in children and adolescents. *Journal of Speech and Hearing Research, 33*, 51–69.

Holmberg, E. B., Hillman, R. E., and Perkell, J. S. (1988). Glottal airflow and transglottal air pressure measurements for male and female speakers in soft, normal, and loud voice [published erratum appears in *Journal of the Acoustical Society of America*, 1989, 85(4), 1787]. *Journal of the Acoustical Society of America, 84*, 511–529.

Isshiki, N. (1964). Regulatory mechanisms of vocal intensity variation. *Journal of Speech and Hearing Research, 7*, 17–29.

Kent, R. D. (1994). *Reference manual for communicative sciences and disorders.* San Diego, CA: Singular Publishing Group.

Lieberman, P. (1968). Direct comparison of subglottal and esophageal pressure during speech. *Journal of the Acoustical Society of America, 43*, 1157–1164.

Mead, J., Peterson, N., Grimgy, N., and Mead, J. (1967). Pulmonary ventilation measured from body surface movements. *Science, 156*, 1383–1384.

Rothenberg, M. (1977). Measurement of airflow in speech. *Journal of Speech and Hearing Research, 20*, 155–176.

Schutte, H. (1980). *The efficiency of voice production.* Groningen, The Netherlands: Kemper.

Smitheran, J. R., and Hixon, T. J. (1981). A clinical method for estimating laryngeal airway resistance during vowel production. *Journal of Speech and Hearing Disorders, 46*, 138–146.

Sperry, E., Hillman, R. E., and Perkell, J. S. (1994). The use of an inductance plethysmograph to assess respiratory function in a patient with nodules. *Journal of Medical Speech-Language Pathology, 2*, 137–145.

Watson, P. J., and Hixon, T. J. (1985). Respiratory kinematics in classical (opera) singers. *Journal of Speech and Hearing Research, 28*, 104–122.

Woo, P., Colton, R. H., and Shangold, L. (1987). Phonatory airflow analysis in patients with laryngeal disease. *Annals of Otology, Rhinology, and Laryngology, 96*, 549–555.

Alaryngeal Voice and Speech Rehabilitation

Loss of the larynx due to disease or injury will result in numerous and significant changes that cross anatomical, physiological, psychological, social, psychosocial, and communication domains. Surgical removal of the larynx, or total laryngectomy, involves resectioning the entire framework of the larynx. Although total laryngectomy may occur in some instances due to traumatic injury, the majority of cases worldwide are the result of cancer. Approximately 75% of all laryngeal tumors arise from squamous epithelial tissue of the true vocal fold (Bailey, 1985). In some instances, and because of the location of many of these lesions, less aggressive approaches to medical intervention may be pursued. This may include radiation therapy or partial surgical resection, which seeks to conserve portions of the larynx, or the use of combined chemoradiation protocols (Hillman et al., 1998; Orlikoff et al., 1999). However, when malignant lesions are sufficiently large or when the location of the tumor threatens the lymphatic compartment of the larynx, total laryngectomy is often indicated for reasons of oncological safety (Doyle, 1994).

Effects of Total Laryngectomy

The two most prominent effects of total laryngectomy as a surgical procedure are change of the normal airway and loss of the normal voicing mechanism for verbal communication. Once the larynx is surgically removed from the top of the trachea, the trachea is brought forward to the anterior midline neck and sutured into place near the sternal notch. Thus, total laryngectomy necessitates that the airway be permanently separated from the upper aerodynamic (oral and pharyngeal) pathway. When the laryngectomy is completed, the tracheal airway will remain separate from the oral cavity, pharynx, and esophagus. Under these circumstances, not only is the primary structure for voice generation lost, but the intimate relationship between the pulmonary system and that of the structures of the upper airway, and consequently the vocal tract, is disrupted. Therefore, if verbal communication is to be acquired and used postlaryngectomy, an alternative method of creating an alaryngeal voice source must be achieved.

Methods of Postlaryngectomy Communication

Following laryngectomy, the most significant communicative component to be addressed via voice and speech rehabilitation is the lost voice source. Once the larynx is removed, some alternative method of providing a new, "alaryngeal" sound source is required. There are two general categories in which an alternative, alaryngeal voice source may be achieved. These categories are best described as intrinsic and extrinsic methods. The distinction between these two methods is contingent on the manner in which the alaryngeal voice source is achieved. Intrinsic alaryngeal methods imply that the alaryngeal voice source is found within the system; that is, alternative physical-anatomical structures are used to generate sound. In contrast, extrinsic methods of alaryngeal speech rely on the use of an external sound source, typically an electronic source, or what is termed the artificial larynx, or the electrolarynx. The fundamental differences between intrinsic and extrinsic methods of alaryngeal speech are discussed below.

Intrinsic Methods of Alaryngeal Speech

The two most prominent methods of intrinsic alaryngeal speech are esophageal speech (Diedrich, 1966; Doyle, 1994) and tracheoesophageal (TE) speech (Singer and Blom, 1980). While these two intrinsic methods of alaryngeal speech are dissimilar in some respects, both rely on generation of an alaryngeal voice source by creating oscillation of tissues in the area of the lower pharynx and upper esophagus. This vibratory structure is somewhat variable in regard to width, height, and location (Diedrich and Youngstrom, 1966; Damste, 1986); hence, the preferred term for this alaryngeal voicing source is the pharyngoesophageal (PE) segment. One muscle that comprises the PE segment is the cricopharyngeal muscle. Beyond the commonality in the use of the PE segment as a vicarious voicing source for both esophageal and TE methods of alaryngeal speech, the manner in which these methods are achieved does differ.

Esophageal Speech. For esophageal speech, the speaker must move air from the oral cavity across the tonically closed PE segment in order to insufflate the esophageal reservoir (located inferior to the PE segment). Two methods of insufflation may be utilized. These methods might be best described as being either direct or indirect approaches to insufflation. Direct methods require the individual speaker to actively manipulate air in the oral cavity to effect a change in pressure. When pressure build-up is achieved in the oral cavity via compression maneuvers, and when the pressure becomes of sufficient magnitude to overcome the muscular resistance of the PE segment, air will move across the segment (inferiorly) into the esophagus. This may be accomplished with nonspeech tasks (tongue maneuvers) or as a result of producing specific sounds (e.g., stop consonants).

In contrast, for the indirect (inhalation) method of air insufflation, the speaker indirectly creates a negative pressure in the esophageal reservoir via rapid inhalation through the tracheostoma. This results in a negative pressure in the esophagus relative to the normal atmospheric pressure within the oral cavity/vocal tract (Diedrich and Youngstrom, 1966; Diedrich, 1968; Doyle, 1994). Air then moves passively across the PE segment in order to equalize pressures between the pharynx and esophagus. Once insufflation occurs, this air can be used to generate PE segment vibration in the same manner following other methods of air insufflation. While a distinction between direct and indirect methods permits increased understanding of the physical requirements for esophageal voice production, many esophageal speakers who exhibit high levels of proficiency will often utilize both methods for insufflation. Regardless of which method of air insufflation is used, this air can then be forced back up across the PE segment, and as a result, the tissue of this sphincter will oscillate. This esophageal sound source can then be manipulated in the upper regions of the vocal tract into the sounds of speech.

The acquisition of esophageal speech is a complex process of skill building that must be achieved under the direction of an experienced instructor. Clinical emphasis typically involves tasks that address four skills believed to be fundamental to functional esophageal speech (Berlin, 1963): (1) the ability to phonate reliably on demand, (2) the ability to maintain a short latency between air insufflation and esophageal phonation, (3) the ability to maintain adequate duration of voicing, and (4) the ability to sustain voicing while articulating. These foundation skills have been shown to reflect those progressive abilities that have historically defined speech skills of "superior" esophageal speakers (Wepman et al., 1953; Snidecor, 1968). However, the successful acquisition of esophageal speech may be limited, for many reasons.

Regardless of which method of insufflation is used, esophageal speakers will exhibit limitations in the physical dimensions of speech. Specifically, fundamental frequency is reduced by about one octave (Curry and Snidecor, 1961), intensity is reduced by about 10 dB SPL from that of the normal speaker (Weinberg, Horii, and Smith, 1980), and the durational characteristics of speech are also reduced. Speech intelligibility is also decreased due to limits in the aerodynamic and voicing characteristics of esophageal speech. As it is not an abductory-adductory system, voiced-for-voiceless perceptual errors (e.g., perceptual identification of *b* for *p*) are common. This is a direct consequence of the esophageal speaker's inability to insufflate large or continuous volumes of air into the reservoir. Esophageal speakers must frequently reinsufflate the esophageal reservoir to maintain voicing. Because of this, it is not uncommon to see esophageal speakers exhibit pauses at unusual points in an utterance, which ultimately alters the normal rhythm of speech. Similarly, the prosodic contour of esophageal speech and associated features is often perceived to be abnormal. In contrast to esophageal speech, the TE method capitalizes on the individual's access to pulmonary air for esophageal insufflation, which offers several distinct advantages relative to esophageal speech.

Tracheoesophageal Speech. TE speech uses the same voicing source as traditional esophageal speech, the PE segment. However, in TE speech the speaker is able to access and use pulmonary air as a driving source. This is achieved by the surgical creation of a controlled midline puncture in the trachea, followed by insertion of a one-way TE puncture voice prosthesis (Singer and Blom, 1980), either at the time of laryngectomy or as a second procedure at some point following laryngectomy. Thus, TE speech is best described as a surgical-prosthetic method of voice restoration. Though widely used, TE voice restoration is not problem-free. Limitations in application must be considered, and complications may occur.

The design of the TE puncture voice prosthesis is such that when the tracheostoma is occluded, either by hand or via use of a complementary tracheostoma breathing valve, air is directed from the trachea through the prosthesis and into the esophageal reservoir. This access permits a variety of frequency, intensity, and durational variables to be altered in a fashion different from that of the traditional esophageal speaker (Robbins et al., 1984; Pauloski, 1998). Because the TE speaker has direct access to a pulmonary air source, his or her ability to modify the physical (frequency, intensity, and durational) characteristics of the signal in response to changes in the aerodynamic driving source, along with associated changes in prosodic elements of the speech signal (i.e., stress, intonation, juncture), is enhanced considerably. Such changes have a positive impact on auditory-perceptual judgments of this method of alaryngeal speech.

While the frequency of TE speech is still reduced from that of normal speech, the intensity is greater, and the durational capabilities meet or exceed those of normal speakers (Robbins et al., 1984). Finally, research into the influence of increased aerodynamic support in TE speakers relative to traditional esophageal speech on speech intelligibility has suggested that positive effects may be observed (Doyle, Danhauer, and Reed, 1988) despite continued voiced-for-voiceless perceptual errors. Clearly, the rapidity of speech reacquisition in addition to the relative increases in speech intelligibility and the changes in the overall physical character of TE speech offers considerable advantages from the perspective of communication rehabilitation.

Artificial Laryngeal Speech. Extrinsic methods of alaryngeal voice production are common. Although some pneumatic devices have been introduced, they are not widely used today. The most frequently used extrinsic method of producing alaryngeal speech uses an electronic artificial larynx, or electrolarynx. These devices provide an external energy (voice) source that is introduced either directly into the oral cavity (intraoral) or by placing a device directly on the tissues of the neck (transcervical). Whether the electrolaryngeal tone is introduced into the oral cavity directly or through transmission via tissues of the neck, the speaker is able to modulate the electrolaryngeal source into speech.

The electrolayrnx is generally easy to use. Speech can be acquired relatively quickly, and the device offers a reasonable method of functional communication to those who have undergone total laryngectomy (Doyle, 1994). Its major limitations have traditionally related to negative judgments of electrolaryngeal speech relative to the mechanical nature of many devices. Current research is seeking to modify the nature of the electronic sound source produced. The intelligibility of electrolaryngeal speech is relatively good, given the external nature of the alaryngeal voice source and the electronic character of sound production. A reduction in speech intelligibility is primarily observed for voiceless consonants (i.e., voiced-for-voiceless errors) due to the fact that the electrolarynx is a continuous sound source (Weiss and Basili, 1985).

Rehabilitative Considerations

All methods of alaryngeal speech, whether esophageal, TE, or electrolaryngeal, have distinct advantages and disadvantages. Advantages for esophageal speech include a nonmechanical and hands-free method of communication. For TE speech, pitch is near normal, loudness exceeds normal, and speech rate and prosody is near normal; for artificial larynx speech, it may be acquired quickly by most people and may be used in conditions of background noise. In contrast, disadvantages for esophageal speech include lowered pitch, loudness, and speech rate. For TE speech, it involves use and maintenance of a prosthetic device with associated costs; for artificial larynx speech, a mechanical quality is common and it requires the use of one hand. While "normal" speech cannot be restored with these methods, no matter how proficient the speaker's skills, all methods are viable postlaryngectomy communication options, and at least

one method can be used with a functional communicative outcome in most instances. Professionals who work with individuals who have undergone total laryngectomy must focus on identifying a method that meets each speaker's particular needs. Although clinical intervention must focus on making any given alaryngeal method as proficient as possible, the individual speaker's needs, as well as the relative strengths and weaknesses of each method, must be considered. In this way, use of a given method may be enhanced so that the individual may achieve the best level of social reentry following laryngectomy. Further, nothing prevents an individual from using multiple methods of alaryngeal speech, although one or another may be preferred in a given communication context or environment. But an important caveat is necessary: Just because a method of alaryngeal speech has been acquired and it has been deemed "proficient" at the clinical level (e.g., results in good speech intelligibility) and is "functional" for basic communication purposes, this does not imply that "rehabilitation" has been successfully achieved.

The reacquisition of verbal communication is without question a critical component of recovery and rehabilitation postlaryngectomy; however, it is only one dimension of the complex picture of a successful return to as normal a life as possible. All individuals who have undergone a laryngectomy will confront myriad restrictions in multiple domains, including anatomical, physiological, psychological, communicative, and social. As a result, postlaryngectomy rehabilitation efforts that address these areas may increase the likelihood of a successful postlaryngectomy outcome.

See also LARYNGECTOMY.

—*Philip C. Doyle and Tanya L. Eadie*

References

Bailey, B. J. (1985). Glottic carcinoma. In B. J. Bailey and H. F. Biller (Eds.), *Surgery of the larynx* (pp. 257–278). Philadelphia: Saunders.

Berlin, C. I. (1963). Clinical measurement of esophageal speech: I. Methodology and curves of skill acquisition. *Journal of Speech and Hearing Disorders, 28,* 42–51.

Curry, E. T., and Snidecor, J. C. (1961). Physical measurement and pitch perception in esophageal speech. *Laryngoscope, 71,* 415–424.

Damste, P. H. (1986). Some obstacles to learning esophageal speech. In R. L. Keith and F. L. Darley (Eds.), *Laryngectomee rehabilitation* (2nd ed., pp. 85–92). San Diego: College-Hill Press.

Diedrich, W. M. (1968). The mechanism of esophageal speech. *Annals of the New York Academy of the Sciences, 155,* 303–317.

Diedrich, W. M., and Youngstrom, K. A. (1966). *Alaryngeal speech.* Springfield, IL: Charles C. Thomas.

Doyle, P. C. (1994). *Foundations of voice and speech rehabilitation following laryngeal cancer.* San Diego, CA: Singular Publishing Group.

Doyle, P. C., Danhauer, J. L., and Reed, C. G. (1988). Listeners' perceptions of consonants produced by esophageal and tracheoesophageal talkers. *Journal of Speech and Hearing Disorders, 53,* 400–407.

Hillman, R. E., Walsh, M. J., Wolf, G. T., Fisher, S. G., and Hong, W. K. (1998). Functional outcomes following treatment for advanced laryngeal cancer. *Annals of Otology, Rhinology and Laryngology, 107,* 2–27.

Orlikoff, R. F., Kraus, D. S., Budnick, A. S., Pfister, D. G., and Zelefsky, M. J. (1999). Vocal function following successful chemoradiation treatment for advanced laryngeal cancer: Preliminary results. *Phonoscope, 2,* 67–77.

Pauloski, B. R. (1998). Acoustic and aerodynamic characteristics of tracheoesophageal voice. In E. D. Blom, M. I. Singer, and R. C. Hamaker (Eds.), *Tracheoesophageal voice restoration following total laryngectomy* (pp. 123–141). San Diego, CA: Singular Publishing Group.

Robbins, J., Fisher, H. B., Blom, E. D., and Singer, M. I. (1984). A comparative acoustic study of normal, esophageal, and tracheoesophageal speech production. *Journal of Speech and Hearing Disorders, 49,* 202–210.

Singer, M. I., and Blom, E. D. (1980). An endoscopic technique for restoration of voice after laryngectomy. *Annals of Otology, Rhinology, and Laryngology, 89,* 529–533.

Snidecor, J. C. (1968). *Speech rehabilitation of the laryngectomized.* Springfield, IL: Charles C. Thomas.

Weiss, M. S., and Basili, A. M. (1985). Electrolaryngeal speech produced by laryngectomized subjects: Perceptual characteristics. *Journal of Speech and Hearing Research, 28,* 294–300.

Wepman, J. M., MacGahan, J. A., Rickard, J. C., and Shelton, N. W. (1953). The objective measurement of progressive esophageal speech development. *Journal of Speech and Hearing Disorders, 18,* 247–251.

Further Readings

Andrews, J. C., Mickel, R. D., Monahan, G. P., Hanson, D. G., and Ward, P. H. (1987). Major complications following tracheoesophageal puncture for voice restoration. *Laryngoscope, 97,* 562–567.

Batsakis, J. G. (1979). *Tumors of the head and neck: Clinical and pathological considerations* (2nd ed.). Baltimore: Williams and Wilkins.

Blom, E. D., Singer, M. I., and Hamaker, R. C. (1982). Tracheostoma valve for postlaryngectomy voice rehabilitation. *Annals of Otology, Rhinology, and Laryngology, 91,* 576–578.

Doyle, P. C. (1997). Speech and voice rehabilitation of patients treated for head and neck cancer. *Current Opinion in Otolaryngology and Head and Neck Surgery, 5,* 161–168.

Doyle, P. C., and Keith, R. L. (Eds.). (2003). *Contemporary considerations in the treatment and rehabilitation of head and neck cancer: Voice, speech, and swallowing.* Austin, TX: Pro-Ed.

Gandour, J., and Weinberg, B. (1984). Production of intonation and contrastive contrasts in electrolaryngeal speech. *Journal of Speech and Hearing Research, 27,* 605–612.

Gates, G., Ryan, W. J., Cantu, E., and Hearne, E. (1982). Current status of laryngectomy rehabilitation: II. Causes of failure. *American Journal of Otolaryngology, 3,* 8–14.

Gates, G., Ryan, W. J., Cooper, J. C., Lawlis, G. F., Cantu, E., Hayashi, T., et al. (1982). Current status of laryngectomee rehabilitation: I. Results of therapy. *American Journal of Otolaryngology, 3,* 1–7.

Gates, G., Ryan, W. J., and Lauder, E. (1982). Current status of laryngectomee rehabilitation: IV. Attitudes about laryngectomee rehabilitation should change. *American Journal of Otolaryngology, 3,* 97–103.

Hamaker, R. C., Singer, M. I., and Blom, E. D. (1985). Primary voice restoration at laryngectomy. *Archives of Otolaryngology, 111,* 182–186.

Iverson-Thoburn, S. K., and Hayden, P. A. (2000). Alaryngeal speech utilization: A survey. *Journal of Medical Speech-Language Pathology, 8,* 85–99.

Pfister, D. G., Strong, E. W., Harrison, L. B., Haines, I. E., Pfister, D. A., Sessions, R., et al. (1991). Larynx preservation with combined chemotherapy and radiation therapy in advanced but respectable head and neck cancer. *Journal of Clinical Oncology, 9,* 850–859.

Reed, C. G. (1983). Surgical-prosthetic techniques for alaryngeal speech. *Communicative Disorders, 8,* 109–124.

Salmon, S. J. (1996/1997). Using an artificial larynx. In E. Lauder (Ed.), *Self-help for the laryngectomee* (pp. 31–33). San Antonio, TX: Lauder Enterprises.

Scarpino, J., and Weinberg, B. (1981). Junctural contrasts in esophageal and normal speech. *Journal of Speech and Hearing Research, 46,* 120–126.

Shanks, J. C. (1986). Essentials for alaryngeal speech: Psychology and physiology. In R. L. Keith and F. L. Darley (Eds.), *Laryngectomee rehabiliation* (pp. 337–349). San Diego, CA: College-Hill Press.

Shipp, T. (1967). Frequency, duration, and perceptual measures in relation to judgment of alaryngeal speech acceptability. *Journal of Speech and Hearing Research, 10,* 417–427.

Singer, M. I. (1988). The upper esophageal sphincter: Role in alaryngeal speech acquisition. *Head and Neck Surgery, Supplement II,* S118–S123.

Singer, M. I., Hamaker, R. C., Blom, E. D., and Yoshida, G. Y. (1989). Applications of the voice prosthesis during laryngectomy. *Annals of Otology, Rhinology, and Laryngology, 98,* 921–925.

Weinberg, B. (1982). Speech after laryngectomy: An overview and review of acoustic and temporal characteristics of esophageal speech. In A. Sekey (Ed.), *Electroacoustic analysis and enhancement of alaryngeal speech* (pp. 5–48). Springfield, IL: Charles C. Thomas.

Weinberg, B., Horii, Y., and Smith, B. E. (1980). Long-time spectral and intensity characteristics of esophageal speech. *Journal of the Acoustical Society of America, 67,* 1781–1784.

Williams, S., and Watson, J. B. (1985). Differences in speaking proficiencies in three laryngectomy groups. *Archives of Otolaryngology, 111,* 216–219.

Woodson, G. E., Rosen, C. A., Murry, T., Madasu, R., Wong, F., Hengested, A., et al. (1996). Assessing vocal function after chemoradiation for advanced laryngeal carcinoma. *Archives of Otolaryngology–Head and Neck Surgery, 122,* 858–864.

Anatomy of the Human Larynx

The larynx is an organ that sits in the hypopharynx, at the crossroads of the upper respiratory and upper digestive tracts. The larynx is intimately involved in respiration, deglution, and phonation. Although it is the primary sound generator of the peripheral speech mechanism, it must be viewed primarily as a respiratory organ. In this capacity it controls the flow of air into and out of the lower respiratory tract, prevents food from becoming lodged in the trachea or bronchi (which would threaten life and interfere with breathing), and, through the cough reflex, assists in dislodging material from the lower airway. The larynx also plays a central role in the development of the intrathoracic and intra-abdominal pressures needed for lifting, elimination of bodily wastes, and sound production.

Throughout life, the larynx undergoes maturational and involutional (aging) changes (Kahane, 1996), which influence its capacity as a sound source. Despite these naturally and slowly occurring structural changes, the larynx continues to function relatively flawlessly. This is a tribute to the elegance of its structure.

Regional Anatomical Relationships. The larynx is located in the midline of the neck. It lies in front of the vertebral column and between the hyoid bone above and the trachea below. In adults, it lies between the third and sixth cervical vertebrae. The root, or pharyngeal portion, of the tongue is interconnected with the epiglottis of the larynx by three fibroelastic bands, the glossoepiglottic folds. The lowermost portion of the pharynx, the hypopharynx, surrounds the posterior aspect of the larynx. Muscle fibers of the inferior pharyngeal constrictor attach to the posterolateral aspect of the thyroid and cricoid cartilages. The esophagus lies inferior and posterior to the larynx. It is a muscular tube that interconnects the pharynx and the stomach. Muscle fibers originating from the cricoid cartilage form part of the muscular valve, which opens to allow food to pass from the pharynx into the esophagus.

Cartilaginous Skeleton.   The larynx is composed of five major cartilages: thyroid, cricoid, one pair of arytenoids, and the epiglottis (Fig. 1). The hyoid bone, though intimately associated with the larynx, is not part of it. The cartilaginous components of the larynx are joined by ligaments and membranes. The *thyroid and cricoid cartilages* are composed of hyaline cartilage, which provides them with form and rigidity. They are interconnected by the cricothyroid joints and surround the laryngeal cavity. These cartilages support the soft tissues of the laryngeal cavity, thereby protecting this vital passageway for unencumbered movement of air into and out of the lower airway. The thyroid cartilage is composed of two quadrangular plates that are united at midline in an angle called the thyroid angle or laryngeal prominence. In the male, the junction of the laminae forms an acute angle, while in the female it is obtuse. This sexual dimorphism emerges after puberty. The cricoid cartilage is signet ring shaped and sits on top of the first ring of the trachea, ensuring continuity of the airway from the larynx into the trachea (the origin of the lower respiratory tract). The *epiglottis* is a flexible leaf-shaped cartilage whose deformability results from its elastic cartilage composition. During swallowing, the epiglottis closes over the entrance into the laryngeal cavity, thus preventing food and liquids from passing into the laryngeal cavity, which could obstruct the airway and interfere with breathing. The *arytenoid cartilages* are interconnected to the cricoid cartilage via the cricoarytenoid joint. These pyramid-shaped cartilages serve as points of

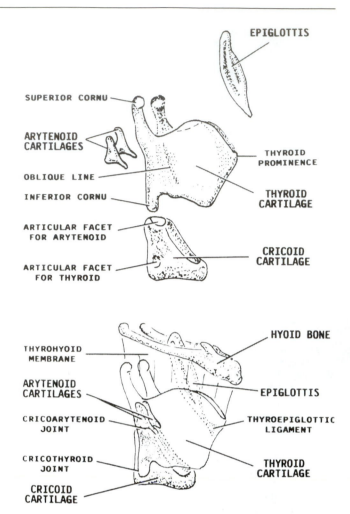

Figure 1. Laryngeal cartilages shown separately (top) and articulated (bottom) at the laryngeal joints. The hyoid bone is not part of the larynx but is attached to it by the thyrohyoid membrane. (From Orlikoff, R. F., and Kahane, J. C. [1996]. Structure and function of the larynx. In N. J. Lass [Ed.], *Principles of experimental phonetics*. St. Louis: Mosby. Reproduced with permission.)

attachment for the vocal folds, all but one pair of the intrinsic laryngeal muscles, and the vestibular folds.

The thyroid, cricoid and arytenoid cartilages are interconnected to each other by two movable joints, the cricothyroid and cricoarytenoid joints. The *cricothyroid joint* joins the thyroid and cricoid cartilages and allows the cricoid cartilage to rotate upward toward the cricoid (Stone and Nuttal, 1974). Since the vocal folds are attached anteriorly to the inside face of the thyroid cartilage and posteriorly to the arytenoid cartilages, which in turn are attached to the upper rim of the cricoid, this rotation effects lengthening and shortening of the vocal folds, with concomitant changes in tension. Such changes in tension are the principal method of changing the rate of vibration of the vocal folds. The *cricoarytenoid joint* joins the arytenoid cartilages to the superolateral rim of the cricoid. Rocking motions of the arytenoids on the upper rim of the cricoid cartilage allow

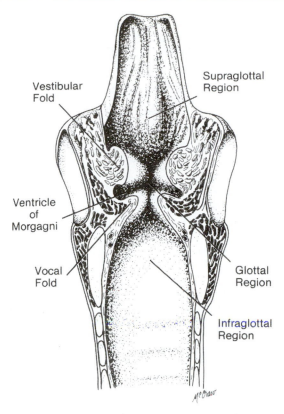

Figure 2. The laryngeal cavity, as viewed posteriorly. (From Kahane, J. C. [1988]. Anatomy and physiology of the organs of the peripheral speech mechanism. In N. J. Lass, L. L. McReynolds, J. L. Northern, and D. E. Yoder [Eds.], *Handbook of speech-language pathology and audiology*. Toronto: B. C. Decker. Reproduced with permission.)

the arytenoids and the attached vocal folds to be drawn away (abducted) from midline and brought toward (adducted) midline. The importance of these actions has been emphasized by von Leden and Moore (1961), as they are necessary for developing the transglottal impedances to airflow that are needed to initiate vocal fold vibration. The effect of such movements is to change the size and shape of the glottis, the space between the vocal folds, which is of importance in laryngeal articulation, producing devoicing and pauses, and facilitating modes of vocal atttack.

Laryngeal Cavity.   The laryngeal cartilages surround an irregularly shaped tube called the laryngeal cavity, which forms the interior of the larynx (Fig. 2). It extends from the laryngeal inlet (laryngeal aditus), through which it communicates with the hypopharynx, to the level of the inferior border of the cricoid cartilage. Here the laryngeal cavity is continuous with the lumen of the trachea. The walls of the laryngeal cavity are formed by fibroelastic tissues lined with epithelium. These fibroelastic tissues (quadrangular membrane and conus elasticus) restore the dimensions of the laryngeal cavity, which become altered through muscle activity, passive stretch from adjacent structures, and aeromechanical forces.

The laryngeal cavity is conventionally divided into three regions. The upper portion is a somewhat expanded supraglottal cavity or vestibule whose walls are reinforced by the quadrangular membrane. The middle region, called the glottal region, is bounded by the vocal folds; it is the narrowest portion. The lowest region, the infraglottal or subglottal region, is bounded by the conus elasticus. The area of primary laryngeal valving is the glottal region, where the shape and size of the *rima glottidis* or *glottis* (space between the vocal folds) is modified during respiration, vocalization, and sphincteric closure. The rima glottidis consists of an intramembranous portion, which is bordered by the soft tissues of the vocal folds, and an intracartilaginous portion, the posterior two-fifths of the rima glottidis, which is located between the vocal processes and the bases of the arytenoid cartilages. The anterior two-thirds of the glottis is an area of dynamic change occasioned by the positioning and aerodynamic displacement of the vocal folds. The overall dimensions of the intracartilaginous glottis remain relatively stable except during strenuous sphincteric valving.

The epithelium that lines the laryngeal cavity exhibits regional specializations. Stratified squamous epithelium covers surfaces subjected to contact, compressive, and vibratory forces. Typical respiratory epithelium (pseudostratified ciliated columnar epithelium with goblet cells) is plentiful in the laryngeal cavity and lines the supraglottis, ventricles, and nonvibrating portions of the vocal folds; it also provides filtration and moisturization of flowing air. The epithelium and immediately underlying connective tissue form the muscosa, which is supplied by an array of sensory receptors sensitive to pressure, chemical, and tactile stimuli, pain, and direction and velocity of airflow (Wyke and Kirchner, 1976). These receptors are innervated by sensory branches from the superior and recurrent laryngeal nerves. They are essential components of the exquisitely sensitive protective reflex mechanism within the larynx that includes initiating coughing, throat clearing, and sphincteric closure.

Laryngeal Muscles.   The larynx is acted upon by extrinsic and intrinsic laryngeal muscles (Tables 1 and 2). The *extrinsic laryngeal muscles* are attached at one end to the larynx and have one or more sites of attachment to a distant site (e.g., the sternum or hyoid bone). The suprahyoid and infrahyoid muscles attach to the hyoid bone and are generally considered extrinsic laryngeal muscles (Fig. 3). Although these muscles do not attach to the larynx, they influence laryngeal position in the neck through their action on the hyoid bone. The thyroid cartilage is connected to the hyoid bone by the hyothyroid membrane and ligaments. The larynx is moved through displacement of the hyoid bone. The suprahyoid and infrahyoid muscles also stabilize the hyoid bone, allowing other muscles in the neck to act directly on the laryngeal cartilages. The suprahyoid and infrahyoid muscles are innervated by a combination of cranial and spinal nerves. Cranial nerves V and VII

Table 1. Morphological Characteristics of the Suprahyoid and Infrahyoid Muscles

Muscles	Origin	Insertion	Function	Innervation
Suprahyoid Muscles				
Anterior digastric	Digastric fossa of mandible	Body of hyoid bone	Raises hyoid bone	Cranial nerve V
Posterior digastric	Mastoid notch of temporal bone	To hyoid bone via an intermediate tendon	Raises and retracts hyoid bone	Cranial nerve VII
Stylohyoid	Posterior border of styloid process	Body of hyoid	Raises hyoid bone	Cranial nerve VII
Mylohyoid	Mylohyoid line of mandible	Median raphe, extending from deep surface of mandible at midline to hyoid bone	Raises hyoid bone	Cranial nerve V
Geniohyoid	Inferior pair of genial tubercles of mandible	Anterior surface of body of hyoid bone	Raises hyoid bone and draws it forward	Cervical nerve I carried via descendens hypoglossi
Infrahyoid Muscles				
Sternohyoid	Deep surface of manubrium; medial end of clavical	Medial portion of inferior surface of body of hyoid bone	Depresses hyoid bone	Ansa cervicalis
Omohyoid	From upper border of scapula (inferior belly) into tendon issuing superior belly	Inferior aspect of body of hyoid bone	Depresses hyoid bone	Cervical nerves I–III carried by the ansa cervicalis
Sternothyroid	Posterior surface of manubrium; edge of first costal cartilage	Oblique line of thyroid cartilage	Lowers hyoid bone; stabilizes hyoid bone	Ansa cervicalis
Thyrohyoid	Oblique line of thyroid cartilage	Lower border of body and greater wing of hyoid bone	When larynx is stabilized, lowers hyoid bone; when hyoid is fixed, larynx is raised	Cervical nerve I, through descendens hypoglossi

Table 2. Morphological Characteristics of the Intrinsic Laryngeal Muscles

Muscle	Origin	Insertion	Function	Innervation
Cricothyroid	Lateral surface of cricoid cartilage arch; fibers divide into upper portion (pars recta) and lower portion (pars obliqua)	Pars recta fibers attach to anterior lateral half of inferior border of thyroid cartilage; pars obliqua fibers attach to anterior margin of inferior corner of thyroid cartilage	Rotational approximation of the cricoid and thyroid cartilages; lengthens and tenses vocal folds	External branch of superior laryngeal nerve (cranial nerve X)
Lateral cricoarytenoid	Upper border of arch of cricoid cartilage	Anterior aspect of muscular process of arytenoid cartilage	Adducts vocal folds; closes rima glottidis	Recurrent laryngeal nerve (cranial nerve X)
Posterior cricoarytenoid	Cricoid lamina	Muscular process of arytenoid cartilage	Abducts vocal folds; opens rima glottidis	Recurrent laryngeal nerve (cranial nerve X)
Interarytenoid				
Transverse fibers	Horizontally coursing fibers extending between the dorso-lateral ridges of each arytenoid cartilage	Dorsolateral ridge of opposite arytenoid cartilage	Approximates bases of arytenoid cartilages, assists vocal fold adduction	Recurrent laryngeal nerve (cranial nerve X)
Oblique fibers	Obliquely coursing fibers from base of one arytenoid cartilage	Inserts onto apex of opposite arytenoid cartilage	Same as transverse fibers	Recurrent laryngeal nerve (cranial nerve X)
Thyroarytenoid	Deep surface of thyroid cartilage at midline	Fovea oblonga of arytenoid cartilage; vocalis fibers attach close to vocal process; muscularis fibers attach more laterally	Adduction, tensor, relaxer of vocal folds (depending on what parts of muscles are active)	Recurrent laryngeal nerve (cranial nerve X)

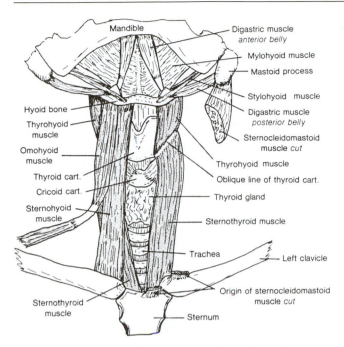

Figure 3. The extrinsic laryngeal muscles. (From Bateman, H. E., and Mason, R. M. [1984]. *Applied anatomy and physiology of the speech and hearing mechanism.* Springfield, IL: Charles C Thomas. Reproduced with permission.)

supply all of the suprahyoid muscles except the geniohyoid. All of the infrahyoid muscles are innervated by spinal nerves from the upper (cervical) portion of the spinal cord.

The suprahyoid and infrahyoid muscles have been implicated in fundamental frequency control under a construct proposed by Sonninen (1956), called the *external frame function.* Sonninen suggested that the extrinsic laryngeal muscles are involved in producing fundamental frequency changes by exerting forces on the laryngeal skeleton that effect length and tension changes in the vocal folds.

The designation of extrinsic laryngeal muscles adopted here is based on strict anatomical definition as well as on research data on the action of the extrinsic laryngeal muscles during speech and singing. One of the most convincing studies in this area was done by Shipp (1975), who showed that the sternothyroid and thyrohyoid muscles systematically change the vertical position of the larynx in the neck, particularly with changes in fundamental frequency. Shipp demonstrated that the sternothyroid lowers the larynx with decreasing pitch, while the thyrohyoid raises it.

The *intrinsic muscles* of the larynx (Fig. 4) are a collection of small muscles whose points of attachment are all in the larynx (to the laryngeal cartilages). The anatomical properties of the intrinsic laryngeal muscles are summarized in Table 2. The muscles can be categorized according to their effects on the shape of the rima glottidis, the positioning of the folds relative to midline, and the vibratory behavior of the vocal folds. Hirano and Kakita (1985) nicely summarized these behaviors (Table 3). Among the most important functional or

biomechanical outcomes of the actions of the intrinsic laryngeal muscles are (1) abduction and adduction of the vocal folds, (2) changing the position of the laryngeal cartilages relative to each other, (3) transiently changing the dimensions and physical properties of the vocal folds (i.e., length, tension, mass per unit area, compliance, and elasticity), and (4) modifying laryngeal airway resistance by changing the size or shape of the glottis.

The intrinsic laryngeal muscles are innervated by nerve fibers carried in the trunk of the *vagus nerve.* These branches are usually referred to as the superior and inferior laryngeal nerves. The cricothyroid muscle is innervated by the superior laryngeal nerve, while all other intrinsic laryngeal muscles are innervated by the inferior (recurrent) laryngeal nerve. Sensory fibers from these nerves supply the entire laryngeal cavity.

Histochemical studies of intrinsic laryngeal muscles (Matzelt and Vosteen, 1963; Rosenfield et al., 1982) have enabled us to appreciate the unique properties of the intrinsic muscles. The intrinsic laryngeal muscles contain, in varying proportions, fibers that control fine movements for prolonged periods (type 1 fibers) and fibers that develop tension rapidly within a muscle (type 2 fibers). In particular, laryngeal muscles differ from the standard morphological reference for striated muscles, the limb muscles, in several ways: (1) they typically have a smaller mean diameter of muscle fibers; (2) they are less regular in shape; (3) the muscle fibers are generally uniform in diameter across the various intrinsic muscles; (4) individual muscle fibers tend not to be uniform in their directionality within a fascicle but exhibit greater variability in the course of muscle fibers, owing to the tendency for fibers to intermingle in their longitudinal and transverse planes; and (5) laryngeal muscles have a greater investment of connective tissues.

Vocal Folds. The vocal folds are multilayered vibrators, not a single homogeneous band. Hirano (1974) showed that the vocal folds are composed of several layers of tissues, each with different physical properties and only 1.2 mm thick. The vocal fold consists of one layer of epithelium, three layers of connective tissue (lamina propria), and the vocalis fibers of the thyroarytenoid muscle (Fig. 5). Based on examination of ultra-high-speed films and biomechanical testing of the vocal folds, Hirano (1974) found that functionally, the epithelium and superficial layer of the lamina propria form the *cover,* which is the most mobile portion of the vocal fold. *Wavelike* mucosal disturbances travel along the surface during sound production. These movements are essential for developing the agitation and patterning of air molecules in transglottal airflow during voice production. The superficial layer of the lamina propria is composed of sparse amounts of loosely interwoven collagenous and elastic fibers. This area, also known as Reinke's space, is important clinically because it is the principal site of swelling or edema formation in the vocal folds following vocal abuse or in laryngitis. The intermediate and deep layers of the lamina propria are called the *transition.* The vocal ligament is formed from elastic and collagenous fibers in these layers. It provides

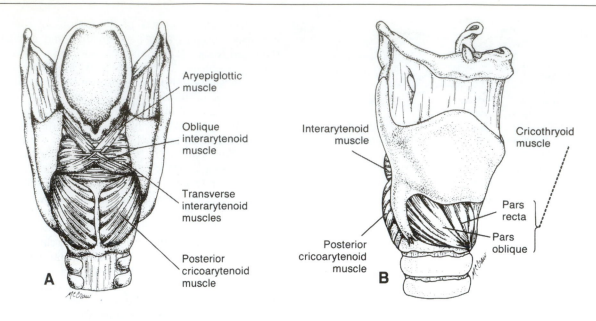

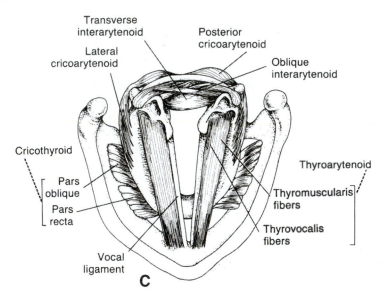

Figure 4. The intrinsic laryngeal muscles as shown in lateral (**A**), posterior (**B**), and superior (**C**) views. (From Kahane, J. C. [1988]. Anatomy and physiology of the organs of the peripheral speech mechanism. In N. J. Lass, L. L. McReynolds, J. L. Northern, and D. E. Yoder [Eds.], *Handbook of speech-language pathology and audiology*. Toronto: B. C. Decker. Reproduced with permission.)

Table 3. Actions of Intrinsic Laryngeal Muscles on Vocal Fold Position and Shape

Vocal Fold Parameter	CT	VOC	LCA	IA	PCA
Position	Paramedian	*Adduct*	*Adduct*	*Adduct*	*Adduct*
Level	Lower	Lower	*Lower*	0	*Elevate*
Length	*Elongate*	*Shorten*	Elongate	(Shorten)	*Elongate*
Thickness	*Thin*	*Thicken*	Thin	(Thicken)	Thin
Edge	*Sharpen*	*Round*	Sharpen	0	Round
Muscle (body)	*Stiffen*	*Stiffen*	Stiffen	(Slacken)	Stiffen
Mucosa (cover and transition)	*Stiffen*	*Slacken*	Stiffen	(Slacken)	Stiffen

Note: 0 indicates no effect; parentheses indicate slight effect; italics indicate marked effect; normal type indicates consistent, strong effect.

Abbreviations: CT, cricothyroid muscle; VOC, vocalis muscle; LCA, lateral cricoarytenoid muscle; IA, interarytenoid muscle; PCA, posterior cricoarytenoid muscle.

From Hirano, M., and Kakita, Y. (1985). Cover-body theory of vocal fold vibration. In R. G. Daniloff (Ed.), *Speech science: Recent advances.* San Diego, CA: College-Hill Press. Reproduced with permission.

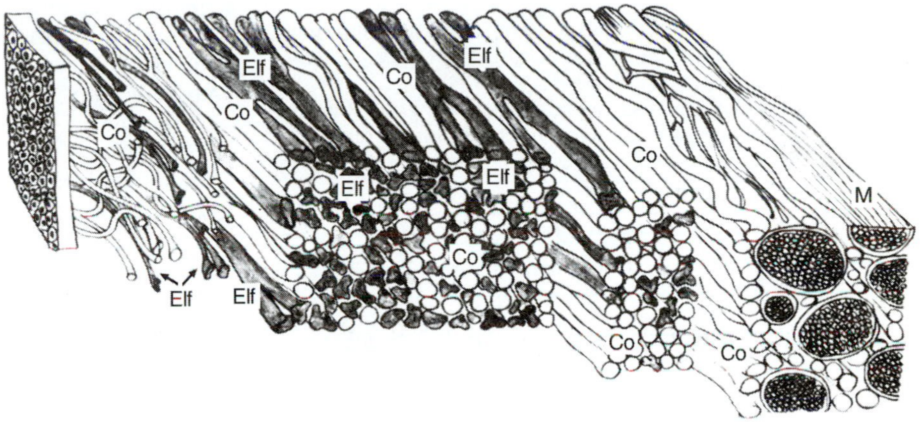

Figure 5. Schematic of the layered structure of the vocal folds. The leading edge of the vocal fold with its epithelium is at left. Co, collaginous fibers; Elf, elastic fibers; M, vocalis muscle fibers. (From Hirano, M. [1975]. Official report: Phonosurgery. Basic and clinical investigations. *Otologia* [Fukuoka], *21*, 239–440. Reproduced with permission.)

resiliency and longitudinal stability to the vocal folds during voice production. The transition is stiffer than the cover but more pliant than the vocalis muscle fibers, which form the *body* of the vocal folds. These muscle fibers are active in regulating fundamental frequency by influencing the tension in the vocal fold and the compliance and elasticity of the vibrating surface (cover).

See also VOICE PRODUCTION: PHYSICS AND PHYSIOLOGY.

—*Joel C. Kahane*

References

Faaborg-Andersen, K., and Sonninen, A. (1960). The function of the extrinsic laryngeal muscles at different pitch. *Acta Otolaryngologica, 51*, 89–93.

Hirano, M. (1974). Morphological structure of the vocal cord as a vibrator and its vartions. *Folia Phoniatrica, 26*, 89–94.

Hirano, M., and Kakita, Y. (1985). Cover-body theory of vocal fold vibration. In R. G. Danoloff (Ed.), *Speech science: Recent advances* (pp. 1–46). San Diego, CA: College-Hill Press.

Kahane, J. C. (1996). Life span changes in the larynx: An anatomical perspective. In W. S. Brown, B. P. Vinson, and M. A. Crary (Eds.), *Organic voice disorders* (pp. 89–111). San Diego, CA: Singular Publishing Group.

Matzelt, D., and Vosteen, K. H. (1963). Electroenoptische und enzymatische Untersuchungen an menschlicher Kehlkopfmuskulatur. *Archiv für Ohren-Nasen- und Kehlkopfheilkunde, 181*, 447–457.

Rosenfield, D. B., Miller, R. H., Sessions, R. B., and Patten, B. M. (1982). Morphologic and histochemical characteristics of laryngeal muscle. *Archives of Otolaryngology, 108*, 662–666.

Shipp, T. (1975). Vertical laryngeal positioning during continuous and discrete vocal frequency change. *Journal of Speech and Hearing Research, 18*, 707–718.

Sonninen, A. (1956). The role of the external laryngeal muscles in length-adjustment of the vocal cords in singing. *Archives of Otolaryngology (Stockholm), Supplement, 118*, 218–231.

Stone, R. E., and Nuttal, A. L. (1974). Relative movements of the thyroid and cricoid cartilages assisted by neural stimulation in dogs. *Acta Otolaryngologica, 78*, 135–140.

von Leden, H., and Moore, P. (1961). The mechanics of the cricoarytenoid joint. *Archives of Otolaryngology, 73*, 541–550.

Wyke, B. D., and Kirchner, J. A. (1976). Neurology of the larynx. In R. Hinchcliffe and D. Harrison (Eds.), *Scientific foundations of otolaryngology* (pp. 546–574). London: Heinemann.

Further Readings

Fink, B. (1975). *The human larynx*. New York: Raven Press.

Hast, M. H. (1970). The developmental anatomy of the larynx. *Otolaryngology Clinics of North America, 3,* 413–438.

Hirano, M. (1981). Structure of the vocal fold in normal and disease states anatomical and physical studies. In C. L. Ludlow and M. O. Hart (Eds.), *Proceedings of the Conference on the Assessment of Vocal Pathology* (ASHA Reports 11). Rockville, MD: American Speech-Language-Hearing Assoc.

Hirano, M., and Sato, K. (1993). *Histological color atlas of the human larynx*. San Diego, CA: Singular Publishing Group.

Kahane, J. C. (1998). Functional histology of the larynx and vocal folds. In C. W. Cummings, J. M. Frederickson, L. A. Harker, C. J. Krause, and D. E. Schuller (Eds.), *Otolaryngology Head and Neck Surgery* (pp. 1853–1868). St. Louis: Mosby.

Konig, W. F., and von Leden, H. (1961). The peripheral nervous system of the human larynx: I. The mucous membrane. *Archives of Otolaryngology, 74,* 1–14.

Negus, V. (1928). *The mechanism of the larynx*. St. Louis: Mosby.

Orlikoff, R. F., and Kahane, J. C. (1996). Structure and function of the larynx. In N. J. Lass (Ed.), *Principles of experimental phonetics*. St. Louis: Mosby.

Rossi, G., and Cortesina, G. (1965). Morphological study of the laryngeal muscles in man: Insertions and courses of muscle fibers, motor end-plates and proprioceptors. *Acta Otolaryngologica, 59,* 575–592.

Assessment of Functional Impact of Voice Disorders

Introduction

Voice disorders occur in approximately 6% of all adults and in as many as 12% of children. Within the adult group, specific professions report the presence of a voice problem that interferes with their employment. As many as 50% of teachers and 33% of secretaries complain of voice problems that restrict their ability to work or to function in a normal social environment (Smith et al., 1998). The restriction of work, or lifestyle, due to a voice disorder has gone virtually undocumented until recently. While voice scientists and clinicians have focused most of their energy, talent, and time on diagnosing and measuring the severity of voice disorders with various perceptual, acoustic, or physiological instruments, little attention has been given to the effects of a voice disorder on the daily needs of the patient. Over the past few years, interest has increased in determining the functional impact of the voice disorder due to the Internet in using patient-based outcome measures to establish efficacy of treatments and the desire to match treatment needs with patient's needs. This article reviews the evolution of the assessment of functional impact of voice disorders and selected applications of those assessments.

Assessment of the physiological consequences of voice disorders has evolved from a strong interest in the relationship of communication ability to global quality-of-life measurement. Hassan and Weymuller (1993), List et al. (1998), Picarillo (1994), and Murry et al. (1998) have all demonstrated that voice communication is an essential element in patients' perception of their quality of life following treatment for head and neck cancer. Patient-based assessment of voice handicap has been lacking in the area of noncancerous voice disorders. The developments and improvements of software for assessing acoustic objective measures of voice and relating measures of abnormal voices to normal voices have gone on for a number of years. However, objective measures primarily assess specific treatments and do not encompass functional outcomes from the patient's perspective. These measures do not necessarily discriminate the severity of handicap as it relates to specific professions. Objective test batteries are useful to quantify disease severity (Rosen, Lombard, and Murry, 2000), categorize acoustic/physiological profiles of the disease (Hartl et al., 2001), and measure changes that occur as a result of treatment (Dejonckere, 2000). A few objective and subjective measures are correlated with the diagnosis of the voice disorder (Wolfe, Fitch, and Martin, 1997), but until recently, none have been related to the patient's perception of the severity of his or her problem. This latter issue is important in all diseases and disorders when life is not threatened since it is ultimately the patient's perception of disease severity and his or her motivation to seek treatment that dictates the degree of treatment success.

Functional impact relates to the degree of handicap or disability. Accordingly, there are three levels of a disorder: impairment, disability, and handicap (World Health Organization, 1980). Handicap is the impact of the impairment of the disability on the social, environmental, or economic functioning of the individual. Treatment usually relates to the physical well-being of a patient, and it is this physical well-being that generally takes priority when attempting to assess the severity of the handicap. A more comprehensive approach might seek to address the patient's own impression of the severity of the disorder and how the disorder interferes with the individual's professional and personal lifestyle.

Measurement of functional impact is somewhat different from assessment of disease status in that it does not directly address treatment efficacy, but rather addresses the value of a particular treatment for a particular individual. This may be considered treatment effectiveness. Efficacy, on the other hand, looks at whether or not a treatment can produce an expected result based on previous studies. Functional impact relates to the degree of impact a disorder has on an individual patient, not necessarily to the severity of the disease.

Voice Disorders and Outcomes Research

Assessment of functional impact on the voice is barely beyond the infancy stage. Interest in the issues relating to functional use of the voice stems from the development of instruments to measure all aspects of vocal function related to the patient, the disease, and the treatment.

Moreover, there are certain parameters of voice disorders that cannot be easily measured in the voice laboratory, such as endurance, acceptance of a new voice, and vocal effectiveness.

The measurement of voice handicap must take into account issues such as "can the person teach in the classroom all day?" or "can a shop foreman talk loud enough to be heard over the noise of factory machines?" An outcome measure that takes into account the patient's ability to speak in the classroom or a factory will undoubtedly provide a more accurate assessment of voice handicap (although not necessarily an accurate assessment of the disease, recovery from disease, or quality of voice) than the acoustic measures obtained in the voice laboratory. Thus, patient-based measures of voice handicap provide significant information that cannot be obtained from biological and physiologic variables traditionally used in voice assessment models.

Voice handicap measures may measure an individual's perceived level of general health, an individual's quality of life, her ability to continue with her current employment versus opting for a change in employment, her satisfaction with treatment regardless of the disease state, or the cost of the treatment. Outcome of treatment for laryngeal cancer is typically measured using Kaplan-Myer curves (Adelstein et al., 1990). While this tool measures the disease-related status of the patient, it does not presume to assess overall patient satisfaction with treatment. Rather, the degree to which swallowing status improves and voice communication returns to normal are measured by instruments that generally focus on quality of life (McHorney et al., 1993).

Voice disorders are somewhat different than the treatment of a life threatening disease such as laryngeal cancer. Treatment that involves surgery, pharmacology, or voice therapy requires the patient's full cooperation throughout the course of treatment. The quality and accuracy of surgery or the level of voice therapy may not necessarily reflect the long-term outcome if the patient does not cooperate with the treatment procedure. Assessment of voice handicap involves the patient's ability to use his or her voice under normal circumstances of social and work-related speaking situations. The voice handicap will be reflected to the extent that the voice is usable in those situations.

Outcome Measures: General Health Versus Specific Disease

There are two primary ways to assess the handicap of a voice disorder. One is to look at the patient's overall well-being. The other is to compare his or her voice to normal voice measures. The first usually encompasses social factors as well as physical factors that are related to the specific disorder. One measure that has been used to look at the effect of disease on life is the Medical Outcomes Study (MOS), a 36-item short-form general health survey (McHorney et al., 1993). The 36-item short form, otherwise known as SF-36, measures eight areas of health that are commonly affected or changed by diseases and treatments: physical functioning, role

functioning, bodily pain, general health, vitality, social functioning, mental health, and health transition. The SF-36 has been used for a wide range of disease-specific topics once it was shown to be a valid measure of the degree of general health. The SF-36 is a pencil-and-paper test that has been used in numerous studies for assessing outcomes of treatment. In addition, because each scale has been determined to be a reliable and valid measure of health in and of itself, this assessment has been used to validate other assessments of quality of life and handicap that are disease specific. However, one of the difficulties with using such a test for a specific disease is that one or more of the subscales may not be important or appropriate. For example, when considering certain voice disorders, the subscale of the SF-36 known as bodily pain may not be quite appropriate. Thus, the SF-36 is not a direct assessment of voice handicap but rather a general measure of well-being.

The challenge to develop a specific scale related to a specific organ function such as a scale for voice disorders presents problems unlike the development of the SF-36 or other general quality-of-life scales.

Assessing Voice Handicap

Currently there are no federal regulations defining voice handicap, unlike the handicap measures associated with hearing loss, which is regulated by the Department of Labor. The task of measuring the severity of a voice disorder may be somewhat difficult because of the areas that are affected, namely emotional, physical, functional, economic, etc. Moreover, as already indicated, while measures such a perceptual judgments of voice characteristics, videostroboscopic visual perceptual findings, acoustic perceptual judgments, as well as physiological measures objectively obtained provide some input as to the severity of the voice compared to normal, these measures do not provide insight as to the degree of handicap and disability that a specific patient is experiencing. It should be noted, however, that there are handicap/disability measures developed for other aspects of communication, namely hearing loss and dizziness (Newman et al., 1990; Jacobson et al., 1994). These measures have been used to quantify functional outcome following various interventions in auditory function.

Development of the Voice Handicap Index

In 1997, Jacobson and her colleagues proposed a measure of voice handicap known as the Voice Handicap Index (VHI) (Jacobson et al., 1998). This patient self-assessment tool consists of ten items in each of three domains: emotional, physical, and functional aspects of voice disorders. The functional subscale includes statements that describe the impact of a person's voice on his daily activities. The emotional subscale indicates the patient's affective responses to the voice disorder. The items in the physical subscale are statements that relate to either the patient's perception of laryngeal discomfort or the voice output characteristics such as too low or too high a pitch. From an original 85-item list, a 30-item questionnaire using a five-point response scale from 0, indicating he "never" felt this about his voice problem to 4, where he "always" felt this to be the case, was finally obtained. This 30-item questionnaire was then assessed for test-retest stability in total as well as the three subscales, and was validated against the SF-36. A shift in the total score of 18 points or greater is required in order to be certain that a change is due to intervention and not to unexplained variability. The Voice Handicap Index was designed to assess all types of voice disorders, even those encountered by tracheoesophageal speakers. A detailed analysis of patient data using this test has recently been published (Benninger et al., 1998).

Since the VHI has been published, others have proposed similar tests of handicap. Hogikian (1999) and Glicklich (1999) have both demonstrated their assessment tools to have validity and reliability in assessing a patient's perception of the severity of a voice problem.

One of the additional uses of the VHI as suggested by Benninger and others is to assess measures after treatment (1998). Murry and Rosen (2001) evaluated the VHI in three groups of speakers to determine the relative severity of voice disorders in patients with muscular tension dysphonia (MTD), benign vocal fold lesions (polyps/cysts), and vocal fold paralysis prior to and following treatments. Figure 1 shows that subjects with vocal fold paralysis displayed the highest self-perception of handicap both before and after treatment. Subjects with benign vocal fold lesions demonstrated the lowest perception of handicap severity before and after treatment. It can be seen that in general, there was a 50% or greater improvement in the mean VHI for the combined groups. However, the patients with vocal fold paralysis initially began with the highest pretreatment VHI and remained with the highest VHI after treatment. Although the VHI scores following treatment were significantly lower, there still remained a measure of handicap in all subjects. Overall, in 81% of the patients, there was a perception of significantly reduced voice handicap,

either because of surgery, voice therapy, or a combination of both.

The same investigators examined the application of the VHI to a specific group of patients with voice disorders, singers (Murry and Rosen, 2000). Singers are unique in that they often complain of problems related only to their singing voice. Murry and Rosen examined 73 professional and 33 nonprofessional singers and compared them with a control group of 369 nonsingers.

The mean VHI score for the 106 singers was 34.7, compared with a mean of 53.2 for the 336 nonsingers. The VHI significantly separated singers from nonsingers in terms of severity. Moreover, the mean VHI score for the professional singers was significantly lower (31.0 vs. 43.2) than for the recreational singers. Although lower VHI scores were found in singers than in nonsingers, this does not imply that the VHI is not a useful instrument for assessing voice problems in singers. On the contrary, several questions were singled out as specifically sensitive to singers. The findings of this study should alert clinicians that the use of the VHI points to the specific needs as well as the seriousness of a singer's handicap. Although the quality of voice may be mildly disordered, the voice handicap may be significant.

Recently, Rosen and Murry (in press) presented reliability data on a revised 10-question VHI. The results suggest that a 10-question VHI produces is highly correlated with the original VHI. The 10-item questionnaire provides a quick, reliable assessment of the patient's perception of voice handicap.

Other measures of voice outcome have been proposed and studied. Recently, Gliklich, Glovsky, and Montgomery examined outcomes in patients with vocal fold paralysis (Hogikyan and Sethuraman, 1999). The instrument, which contains five questions, is known as the Voice Outcome Survey (VOS). Overall reliability of the VOS was related to the subscales of the SF-36 for a group of patients with unilateral vocal fold paralysis.

Additional work has been done by Hogikyan (1999). These authors presented a measure of voice-related quality of life (VR-QOL). They also found that this self-administered 10-question patient assessment of severity was related to changes in treatment. Their subjects consisted primarily of unilateral vocal fold paralysis patients and showed a significant change from pre- to post-treatment.

A recent addition to functional assessment is the Voice Activity and Participation Profile (VAPP). This tool assesses the effects voice disorders have on limiting and participating in activities which require use of the voice (Ma and Yiu, 2001). Activity limitation refers to constraints imposed on voice activities and participation restriction refers to a reduction or avoidance of voice activities. This 28-item tool examines five areas: self-perceived severity of the voice problem; effect on the job; effect on daily communication; effect on social communication; and effect on emotion. The VAPP has been found to be a reliable and valid assessment tool for assessing self-perceived voice severity as it relates to activity and participation in vocal activities.

Voice Handicapped Index: Change Following Treatment

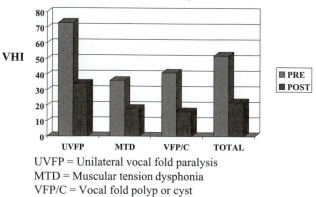

UVFP = Unilateral vocal fold paralysis
MTD = Muscular tension dysphonia
VFP/C = Vocal fold polyp or cyst

Figure 1. Pre- and post-treatment voice handicap scores for selected populations.

Summary

The study of functional voice assessment to identify the degree of handicap is novel for benign voice disorders. For many years, investigators have focused on acoustic and aerodynamic measures of voice production to assess change in voice following treatment. These measures, although extremely useful in understanding treatment efficacy, have not shed significant light on patients' perception of their disorder. Measures such as the VHI, VOS, and VR-QOL have demonstrated that regardless of age, sex, or disease type, the degree of handicap can be identified. Furthermore, treatment for these handicaps can also be assessed in terms of effectiveness for the patient. Patients' self-assessment of perceived severity also allows investigators to make valid comparisons of the impact of an intervention for patients who use their voices in different environments and the patients' perception of the treatment from a functional perspective. Assessment of voice based on a patient's perceived severity and the need to recover vocal function may be the most appropriate manner to assess severity of voice handicap.

—Thomas Murry and Clark A. Rosen

References

Adelstein, D. J., Sharon, V. M., Earle, A. S., et al. (1990). Long-term results after chemoradiotherapy of locally confined squamous cell head and neck cancer. *American Journal of Clinical Oncology, 13,* 440–447.

Benninger, M. S., Atiuja, A. S., Gardner, G., and Grywalski, C. (1998). Assessing outcomes for dysphonic patients. *Journal of Voice, 12,* 540–550.

Dejonckere, P. H. (2000). Perceptual and laboratory assessment of dysphonia. *Otolaryngology Clinics of North America, 33,* 33–34.

Glicklich, R. E., Glovsky, R. M., Montgomery, W. W. (1999). Validation of a voice outcome survey for unilateral vocal fold paralysis. *Otolaryngology–Head and Neck Surgery, 120,* 152–158.

Hartl, D. M., Hans, S., Vaissiere, J., Riquet, M., et al. (2001). Objective voice analysis after autologous fat injection for unilateral vocal fold paralysis. *Annals of Otology, Rhinology, and Laryngology, 110,* 229–235.

Hassan, S. J., and Weymuller, E. A. (1993). Assessment of quality of life in head and neck cancer patients. *Head and Neck Surgery, 15,* 485–494.

Hogikyan, N. D., and Sethuraman, G. (1999). Validation of an instrument to measure voice-related quality of life (V-RQOL). *Journal of Voice, 13,* 557–559.

Jacobson, B. H., Johnson, A., Grywalski, C., et al. (1998). The Voice Handicap Index (VHI): Development and validation. *Journal of Voice, 12,* 540–550.

Jacobson, G. P., Ramadan, N. M., Aggarwal, S., and Newman, C. W. (1994). The development of the Henry Ford Hospital Headache Disability Inventory (HDI). *Neurology, 44,* 837–842.

List, M. A., Ritter-Sterr, C., and Lansky, S. B. (1998). A performance status scale for head and neck patients. *Cancer, 66,* 564–569.

Ma, E. P., and Yiu, E. M. (2001). Voice activity and participation profile: Assessing the impact of voice disorders on daily activities. *Journal of Speech, Language, and Hearing Research, 44,* 511–524.

McHorney, C. A., Ware, J. E., Jr., Lu, J. F., and Sherbourne, C. D. (1993). The MOS 36-item short form health survey (SF-36): II. Psychometric and clinical tests of validity in measuring physical and medical health constructs. *Medical Care, 31,* 247–263.

Murry, T., Madassu, R., Martin, A., and Robbins, K. T. (1998). Acute and chronic changes in swallowing and quality of life following intraarterial chemoradiation for organ preservation in patients with advanced head and neck cancer. *Head and Neck Surgery, 20,* 31–37.

Murry, T., and Rosen, C. A. (2001). Occupational voice disorders and the voice handicap index. In P. Dejonckere (Ed.), *Occupational voice disorders: Care and cure* (pp. 113–128). The Hague, the Netherlands: Kugler Publications.

Murry, T., and Rosen, C. A. (2000). Voice Handicap Index results in singers. *Journal of Voice, 14,* 370–377.

Newman, C., Weinstein, B., Jacobson, G., and Hug, G. (1990). The hearing handicap inventory for adults: Psychometric adequacy and audiometric correlates. *Ear and Hearing, 11,* 430–433.

Picarillo, J. F. (1994). Outcome research and otolaryngology. *Otolaryngology–Head and Neck Surgery, 111,* 764–769.

Rosen, C. A., and Murry, T. (in press). The VHI 10: An outcome measure following voice disorder treatment. *Journal of Voice.*

Rosen, C., Lombard, L. E., and Murry, T. (2000). Acoustic, aerodynamic and videostroboscopic features of bilateral vocal fold lesions. *Annals of Otology Rhinology and Laryngology, 109,* 823–828.

Smith, E., Lemke, J., Taylor, M., Kirchner, L., and Hoffman, H. (1998). Frequency of voice problems among teachers and other occupations. *Journal of Voice, 12,* 480–488.

Wolfe, V., Fitch, J., and Martin, D. (1997). Acoustic measures of dysphonic severity across and within voice types. *Folia Phoniatrica, 49,* 292–299.

World Health Organization. (1980). *International Classification of Impairments, Disabilities and Handicaps: A manual of classification relating to the consequences of disease* (pp. 25–43). Geneva: World Health Organization.

Electroglottographic Assessment of Voice

A number of instruments can be used to help characterize the behavior of the glottis and vocal folds during phonation. The signals derived from these instruments are called *glottographic waveforms* or *glottograms* (Titze and Talkin, 1981). Among the more common glottograms are those that track change in glottal flow, via inverse filtering; glottal width, via kymography; glottal area, via photoglottography; and vocal fold movement, via ultrasonography (Baken and Orlikoff, 2000). Such signals can be used to obtain several different physiological measures, including the glottal open quotient and the maximum flow declination rate, both of which are highly valuable in the assessment of vocal function. Unfortunately, the routine application of these techniques has been hampered by the cumbersome and time-consuming way in which these signals must be acquired, conditioned, and analyzed. One glottographic method, *electroglottography* (EGG), has emerged as the most commonly used technique, for several reasons: (1) it is noninvasive, requiring no probe placement within the vocal tract; (2) it is easy to acquire, alone or in conjunction with other speech signals; and (3) it offers unique information about the mucoundulatory behavior of the vocal folds, which contemporary theory suggests is a critical element in the assessment of voice production.

Electroglottography (known as electrolaryngography in the United Kingdom) is a plethysmographic technique that entails fixing a pair of surface electrodes to each side of the neck at the thyroid lamina, approximating the level of the vocal folds. An imperceptible low-amplitude, high-frequency current is then passed between these electrodes. Because of their electrolyte content, tissue and body fluids are relatively good conductors of electricity, whereas air is a particularly poor conductor. When the vocal folds separate, the current path is forced to circumvent the glottal air space, decreasing effective voltage. Contact between the vocal folds affords a conduit through which current can take a more direct route across the neck. Electrical impedance is thus highest when the current path must completely bypass an open glottis and progressively decreases as greater contact between the vocal folds is achieved. In this way, the voltage across the neck is modulated by the contact of the vocal folds, forming the basis of the EGG signal. The glottal region, however, is quite small compared with the total region through which the current is flowing. In fact, most of the changes in transcervical impedance are due to strap muscle activity, laryngeal height variation induced by respiration and articulation, and pulsatile blood volume changes. Because increasing and decreasing vocal fold contact has a relatively small effect on the overall impedance, the *electroglottogram* is both high-pass filtered to remove the far slower nonphonatory impedance changes and amplified to boost the laryngeal contribution to the signal. The result is a waveform—sometimes designated *Lx*—that varies chiefly as a function of vocal fold contact area (Gilbert, Potter, and Hoodin, 1984).

First proposed by Fabre in 1957 as a means to assess laryngeal physiology, the clinical potential of EGG was recognized by the mid-1960s. Interest in EGG increased in the 1970s as the importance of mucosal wave dynamics for vocal fold vibration was confirmed, and accelerated greatly in the 1980s with the advent of personal computers and commercially available EGGs that were technologically superior to previous instruments. Today, EGG has a worldwide reputation as a useful tool to supplement the evaluation and treatment of vocal pathology. The clinical challenge, however, is that a valid and reliable EGG assessment demands a firm understanding of normal vocal fold vibratory behavior along with recognition of the specific capabilities and limitations of the technique.

Instead of a simple mediolateral oscillation, the vocal folds engage in a quite complex undulatory movement during phonation, such that their inferior margins approximate before the more superior margins make contact. Because EGG tracks effective medial contact area,

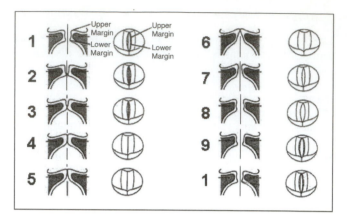

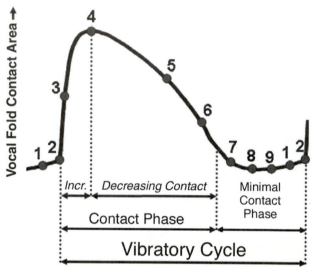

Figure 1. At the top is shown a schematic representation of a single cycle of vocal fold vibration viewed coronally (left) and superiorly (right) (after Hirano, 1981). Below it is a normal electroglottogram depicting relative vocal fold contact area. The numbered points on the trace correspond approximately to the points of the cycle depicted above. The contact phases of the vibratory cycle are shown beneath the electroglottogram.

the *pattern* of vocal fold vibration can be characterized quite well (Fig. 1). The contact pattern will vary as a consequence of several factors, including bilateral vocal fold mass and tension, medial compression, and the anatomy and orientation of the medial surfaces. Considerable research has been devoted to establishing the important features of the EGG and how they relate to specific aspects of vocal fold status and behavior. Despite these efforts, however, the contact area function is far from perfectly understood, especially in the face of pathology. Given the complexity of the "rolling and peeling" motion of the glottal margins and the myriad possibilities for abnormality of tissue structure or biomechanics, it is not surprising that efforts to formulate simple rules relating abnormal details to specific pathologies have not met with notable success. In short, the clinical value of EGG rests in documenting the vibratory *consequence* of pathology rather than in diagnosing the pathology itself.

Using multiple glottographic techniques, Baer, Löfqvist, and McGarr (1983) demonstrated that, for normal modal-register phonation, the "depth of closure" was very shallow just before glottal opening and quite deep soon after closure was initiated. Most important, they showed that the instant at which the glottis first appears occurs sometime *before* all contact is lost, and that the instant of glottal closure occurs sometime *after* the vocal folds first make contact. Thus, although the EGG is sensitive to the depth of contact, it cannot be used to determine the width, area, or shape of the glottis. For this reason, EGG is not a valid technique for the measurement of glottal open time or, therefore, the open quotient. Likewise, since EGG does not specify which parts of the vocal folds are in contact, it cannot be used to measure glottal closed time, nor can it, without additional evidence, be used to determine whether maximal vocal fold contact indeed represents complete obliteration of the glottal space. Identifying the exact moment when (and if) all medial contact is lost has also proved particularly problematic. Once the vocal folds do lose contact, however, it can no longer be assumed that the EGG signal conveys any information whatsoever about laryngeal behavior. During such intervals, the signal may vary solely as a function of the instrument's automatic gain control and filtering (Rothenberg, 1981).

Although the EGG provides useful information only about those parts of the vibratory cycle during which there is some vocal fold contact, these characteristics may provide important clinical insight, especially when paired with videostroboscopy and other data traces. EGG, with its ability to demonstrate contact change in both the horizontal and vertical planes, can quite effectively document the normal voice registers (Fig. 2) as well as abnormal and unstable modes of vibration (Fig. 3). However, to qualitatively assess EGG wave characteristics and to derive useful indices of vocal fold contact behavior, it may be best to view the EGG in terms of a *vibratory cycle* composed of a *contact phase* and a *minimal-contact phase* (see Fig. 1). The contact phase includes intervals of increasing and decreasing contact, whereas the peak represents maximal vocal fold contact and, presumably, maximal glottal closure. The minimal-contact phase is that portion of the EGG wave during which the vocal folds are *probably* not in contact. Much clinical misinterpretation can be avoided if no attempt is made to equate the vibratory contact phase with the glottal closed phase or the minimal-contact phase with the glottal open phase.

For the typical modal-register EGG, the contact phase is asymmetrical; that is, the increase in contact takes less time than the interval of decreasing contact. The degree of contact asymmetry is thought to vary not only as a consequence of vocal fold tension but also as a function of vertical mucosal convergence and dynamics (i.e., phasing; Titze, 1990). A dimensionless ratio, the *contact index* (CI), can be used to assess contact symmetry (Orlikoff, 1991). Defined as the difference between the increasing and decreasing contact durations divided by the duration of the contact phase, CI will vary be-

Pulse register

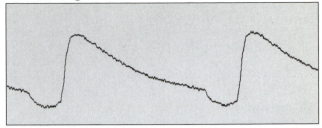

Modal register

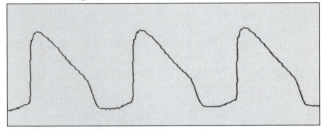

Falsetto register

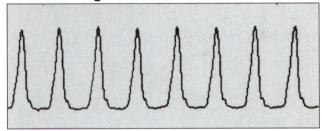

Figure 2. Typical electroglottograms obtained from a normal man prolonging phonation in the low-frequency pulse, moderate-frequency modal, and high-frequency falsetto voice registers.

tween −1 for a contact phase maximally skewed to the left and +1 for a contact phase maximally skewed to the right. For normal modal-register phonation, CI varies between −0.6 and −0.4 for both men and women, but, as can be seen in Figure 2, it is markedly different for other voice registers. Pulse-register EGGs typically have CIs in the vicinity of −0.8, whereas in falsetto it would not be uncommon to have a CI that approximates zero, indicating a symmetrical or nearly symmetrical contact phase.

Another EGG measure that is gaining some currency in the clinical literature is the *contact quotient* (CQ). Defined as the duration of the contact phase relative to the period of the entire vibratory cycle, there is evidence from both in vivo testing and mathematical modeling to suggest that CQ varies with the degree of medial compression of the vocal folds (see Fig. 3) along a hypoadducted "loose" (or "breathy") to a hyperadducted "tight" (or "pressed") phonatory continuum (Rothenberg and Mahshie, 1988; Titze, 1990). Under typical vocal circumstances, CQ is within the range of 40%– 60%, and despite the propensity for a posterior glottal

"Pressed" phonation

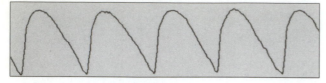

"Breathy" phonation

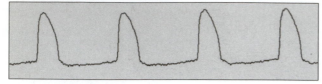

Diplophonic "creaky" phonation

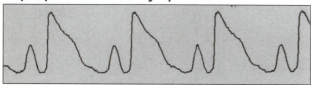

Irregular "chaotic" phonation

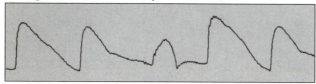

Figure 3. Electroglottograms representing different abnormal modes of vocal fold vibration.

chink in women, there does not seem to be a significant sex effect. This is probably due to the fact that EGG (and thus the CQ) is insensitive to glottal gaps that are not time varying. Unlike men, however, women tend to show an increase in CQ with vocal F0. It has been conjectured that this may be the result of greater medial compression employed by women at higher F0s that serves to diminish the posterior glottal gap. Nonetheless, a strong relationship between CQ and vocal intensity has been documented in both men and women, consistent with the known relationship between vocal power and the adductory presetting of the vocal folds. Because vocal intensity is also related to the rate of vocal fold contact (Kakita, 1988), there have been some preliminary attempts to derive useful EGG measures of the contact rise time.

Because EGG is relatively unaffected by vocal tract resonance and turbulence noise (Orlikoff, 1995), it allows evaluation of vocal fold behavior under conditions not well-suited to other voice assessment techniques. For this reason, and because the EGG waveshape is a relatively simple one, the EGG has found some success both as a trigger signal for laryngeal videostroboscopy and as a means to define and describe phonatory onset, offset,

intonation, voicing, and fluency characteristics. In fact, EGG has, for many, become the preferred means by which to measure vocal fundamental frequency and jitter.

In summary, EGG provides an innocuous, straightforward, and convenient way to assess vocal fold vibration through its ability to track the relative area of contact. Although it does not supply valid information about the opening and closing of the glottis, the technique affords a unique perspective on vocal fold behavior. When conservatively interpreted, and when combined with other tools of laryngeal evaluation, EGG can substantially further the clinician's understanding of the malfunctioning larynx and play an effective role in therapeutics as well.

See also ACOUSTIC ASSESSMENT OF VOICE.

—*Robert F. Orlikoff*

References

Baer, T., Löfqvist, A., and McGarr, N. S. (1983). Laryngeal vibrations: A comparison between high-speed filming and glottographic techniques. *Journal of the Acoustical Society of America, 73,* 1304–1308.

Baken, R. J., and Orlikoff, R. F. (2000). Laryngeal function. In *Clinical measurement of speech and voice* (2nd ed., pp. 394–451). San Diego, CA: Singular Publishing Group.

Fabre, P. (1957). Un procédé électrique percutané d'inscription de l'accolement glottique au cours de la phonation: Glottographie de haute fréquence. Premiers resultats. *Bulletin de l'Académie Nationale de Médecine, 141,* 66–69.

Gilbert, H. R., Potter, C. R., and Hoodin, R. (1984). Laryngograph as a measure of vocal fold contact area. *Journal of Speech and Hearing Research, 27,* 178–182.

Hirano, M. (1981). *Clinical examination of voice.* New York: Springer-Verlag.

Kakita, Y. (1988). Simultaneous observation of the vibratory pattern, sound pressure, and airflow signals using a physical model of the vocal folds. In O. Fujimura (Ed.), *Vocal physiology: Voice production, mechanisms, and functions* (pp. 207–218). New York: Raven Press.

Orlikoff, R. F. (1991). Assessment of the dynamics of vocal fold contact from the electroglottogram: Data from normal male subjects. *Journal of Speech and Hearing Research, 34,* 1066–1072.

Orlikoff, R. F. (1995). Vocal stability and vocal tract configuration: An acoustic and electroglottographic investigation. *Journal of Voice, 9,* 173–181.

Rothenberg, M. (1981). Some relations between glottal air flow and vocal fold contact area. *ASHA Reports, 11,* 88–96.

Rothenberg, M., and Mahshie, J. J. (1988). Monitoring vocal fold abduction through vocal fold contact area. *Journal of Speech and Hearing Research, 31,* 338–351.

Titze, I. R. (1990). Interpretation of the electroglottographic signal. *Journal of Voice, 4,* 1–9.

Titze, I. R., and Talkin, D. (1981). Simulation and interpretation of glottographic waveforms. *ASHA Reports, 11,* 48–55.

Further Readings

Abberton, E., and Fourcin, A. J. (1972). Laryngographic analysis and intonation. *British Journal of Disorders of Communication, 7,* 24–29.

Baken, R. J. (1992). Electroglottography. *Journal of Voice, 6,* 98–110.

Carlson, E. (1993). Accent method plus direct visual feedback of electroglottographic signals. In J. C. Stemple (Ed.), *Voice therapy: Clinical studies* (pp. 57–71). St. Louis: Mosby–Year Book.

Carlson, E. (1995). Electrolaryngography in the assessment and treatment of incomplete mutation (puberphonia) in adults. *European Journal of Disorders of Communication, 30,* 140–148.

Childers, D. G., Hicks, D. M., Moore, G. P., and Alsaka, Y. A. (1986). A model of vocal fold vibratory motion, contact area, and the electroglottogram. *Journal of the Acoustical Society of America, 80,* 1309–1320.

Childers, D. G., Hicks, D. M., Moore, G. P., Eskenazi, L., and Lalwani, A. L. (1990). Electroglottography and vocal fold physiology. *Journal of Speech and Hearing Research, 33,* 245–254.

Childers, D. G., and Krishnamurthy, A. K. (1985). A critical review of electroglottography. *CRC Critical Review of Biomedical Engineering, 12,* 131–161.

Colton, R. H., and Conture, E. G. (1990). Problems and pitfalls of electroglottography. *Journal of Voice, 4,* 10–24.

Cranen, B. (1991). Simultaneous modelling of EGG, PGG, and glottal flow. In J. Gauffin and B. Hammarberg (Eds.), *Vocal fold physiology: Acoustic, perceptual, and physiological aspects of voice mechanisms* (pp. 57–64). San Diego, CA: Singular Publishing Group.

Croatto, L., and Ferrero, F. E. (1979). L'esame elettroglottografico appliato ad alcuni casi di disodia. *Acta Phoniatrica Latina, 2,* 213–224.

Fourcin, A. J. (1981). Laryngographic assessment of phonatory function. *ASHA Reports, 11,* 116–127.

Gleeson, M. J., and Fourcin, A. J. (1983). Clinical analysis of laryngeal trauma secondary to intubation. *Journal of the Royal Society of Medicine, 76,* 928–932.

Gómez Gonzáles, J. L., and del Cañizo Alvarez, C. (1988). Nuevas tecnicas de exploración funcional laríngea: La electroglotografía. *Anales Oto-Rino-Otolaríngologica Ibero-Americana, 15,* 239–362.

Hacki, T. (1989). Klassifizierung von Glottisdysfunktionen mit Hilfe der Elecktroglottographie. *Folia Phoniatrica, 41,* 43–48.

Hertegård, S., and Gauffin, J. (1995). Glottal area and vibratory patterns studied with simultaneous stroboscopy, flow glottography, and electroglottography. *Journal of Speech and Hearing Research, 38,* 85–100.

Kitzing, P. (1990). Clinical applications of electroglottography. *Journal of Voice, 4,* 238–249.

Kitzing, P. (2000). Electroglottography. In A. Ferlito (Ed.), *Diseases of the larynx* (pp. 127–138). New York: Oxford University Press.

Motta, G., Cesari, U., Iengo, M., and Motta, G., Jr. (1990). Clinical application of electroglottography. *Folia Phoniatrica, 42,* 111–117.

Neil, W. F., Wechsler, E., and Robinson, J. M. (1977). Electrolaryngography in laryngeal disorders. *Clinical Otolaryngology, 2,* 33–40.

Nieto Altazarra, A., and Echarri San Martin, R. (1996). Electroglotografía. In R. García-Tapia Urrutia and I. Cobeta Marco (Eds.), *Diagnóstico y tratamiento de los transtornos de la voz* (pp. 163–169). Madrid, Spain: Editorial Garsi.

Orlikoff, R. F. (1998). Scrambled EGG: The uses and abuses of electroglottography. *Phonoscope, 1,* 37–53.

Roubeau, C., Chevrie-Muller, C., and Arabia-Guidet, C. (1987). Electroglottographic study of the changes of voice registers. *Folia Phoniatrica, 39,* 280–289.

Wechsler, E. (1977). A laryngographic study of voice disorders. *British Journal of Disorders of Communication, 12,* 9–22.

Functional Voice Disorders

The human voice is acutely responsive to changes in emotional state, and the larynx plays a prominent role as an instrument for the expression of intense emotions such as fear, anger, grief, and joy. Consequently, many regard the voice as a sensitive barometer of emotions and the larynx as the control valve that regulates the release of these emotions (Aronson, 1990). Furthermore, the voice is one of the most individual and characteristic expressions of a person—a "mirror of personality." Thus, when the voice becomes disordered, it is not uncommon for clinicians to suggest personality traits, psychological factors, or emotional or inhibitory processes as primary causal mechanisms. This is especially true in the case of *functional dysphonia* or *aphonia*, in which no visible structural or neurological laryngeal pathology exists to explain the partial or complete loss of voice.

Functional dysphonia, which may account for more than 10% of cases referred to multidisciplinary voice clinics, occurs predominantly in women, commonly follows upper respiratory infection symptoms, and varies in its response to treatment (Bridger and Epstein, 1983; Schalen and Andersson, 1992). The term *functional* implies a voice disturbance of physiological function rather than anatomical structure. In clinical circles, *functional* is usually contrasted with *organic* and often carries the added meaning of *psychogenic*. Stress, emotion, and psychological conflict are frequently presumed to cause or exacerbate functional symptoms.

Some confusion surrounds the diagnostic category of functional dysphonia because it includes an array of medically unexplained voice disorders: psychogenic, conversion, hysterical, tension-fatigue syndrome, hyperkinetic, muscle misuse, and muscle tension dysphonia. Although each diagnostic label implies some degree of etiologic heterogeneity, whether these disorders are qualitatively different and etiologically distinct remains unclear. When applied clinically, these various labels frequently reflect clinician supposition, bias, or preference. Voice disorder taxonomies have yet to be adequately operationalized; consequently, diagnostic categories often lack clear thresholds or discrete boundaries to determine patient inclusion or exclusion. To improve precision, some clinicians prefer the term *psychogenic voice disorder*, to put the emphasis on the psychological origins of the disorder. According to Aronson (1990), a psychogenic voice disorder is synonymous with a functional one but offers the clinician the advantage of stating confidently, after an exploration of its causes, that the voice disorder is a manifestation of one or more forms of psychological disequilibrium. At the purely phenomenological level there may be little difference between functional and psychogenic voice disorders. Therefore, in this discussion, the terms functional and psychogenic will be used synonymously, which reflects current trends in the clinical literature (nosological imprecision notwithstanding).

In clinical practice, "psychogenic voice disorder" should not be a default diagnosis for a voice problem of undetermined cause. Rather, at least three criteria should be met before such a diagnosis is offered: symptom psychogenicity, symptom incongruity, and symptom reversibility (Sapir, 1995). *Symptom psychogenicity* refers to the finding that the voice disorder is logically linked in time of onset, course, and severity to an identifiable psychological antecedent, such as a stressful life event or interpersonal conflict. Such information is acquired through a complete case history and psychosocial interview. *Symptom incongruity* refers to the observation that the vocal symptoms are physiologically incompatible with existing or suspected disease, are internally inconsistent, and are incongruent with other speech and language characteristics. An often cited example of symptom incongruity is complete aphonia (whispered speech) in a patient who has a normal throat clear, cough, laugh, or hum, whereby the presence of such normal nonspeech vocalization is at odds with assumptions regarding neural integrity and function of the laryngeal system. Finally, *symptom reversibility* refers to complete, sustained amelioration of the voice disorder with short-term voice therapy (usually one or two sessions) or through psychological abreaction. Furthermore, maintaining the voice improvement requires no compensatory effort on the part of the patient. In general, psychogenic dysphonia may be suspected when strong evidence exists for symptom incongruity and symptom psychogenicity, but it is confirmed only when there is unmistakable evidence of symptom reversibility.

A wide array of psychopathological processes contributing to voice symptom formation in functional dysphonia have been proposed. These mechanisms include, but are not limited to, conversion reaction, hysteria, hypochondriasis, anxiety, depression and various personality dispositions or emotional stresses or conflicts that induce laryngeal musculoskeletal tension. Roy and Bless (2000) provide a more complete exploration of the putative psychological and personality processes involved in functional dysphonia, as well as related research.

The dominant psychological explanation for dysphonia unaccounted for by pathological findings is the concept of conversion disorder. According to the *DSM-IV*, conversion disorder involves unexplained symptoms or deficits affecting voluntary motor or sensory function that suggest a neurological or other general medical condition (American Psychiatric Association, 1994). The conversion symptom represents an unconscious simulation of illness that ostensibly prevents conscious awareness of emotional conflict or stress, thereby displacing the mental conflict and reducing anxiety. When the laryngeal system is involved, the condition is referred to as conversion dysphonia or aphonia. In *aphonia*, patients lose their voice suddenly and completely and articulate in a whisper. The whisper may be pure, harsh, or sharp, with occasional high-pitched squeaklike traces of phonation. In *dysphonia*, phonation is preserved but disturbed in quality, pitch, or loudness. Myriad dysphonia types are encountered, including hoarseness (with or without strain), breathiness, and high-pitched falsetto, as well as voice and pitch breaks that vary in consistency and severity.

In conversion voice disorders, psychological factors are judged to be associated with the voice symptoms because conflicts or other stressors precede the onset or exacerbation of the dysphonia. In short, patients convert intrapsychic distress into a voice symptom. The voice loss, whether partial or complete, is also often interpreted to have symbolic meaning. Primary or secondary gains are thought to play an important role in maintaining and reinforcing the conversion disorder. Primary gain refers to anxiety alleviation accomplished by preventing the psychological conflict from entering conscious awareness. Secondary gain refers to the avoidance of an undesirable activity or responsibility and the extra attention or support conferred on the patient.

Butcher and colleagues (Butcher et al., 1987; Butcher, Elias, and Raven, 1993; Butcher, 1995) have argued that there is little research evidence that conversion disorder is the most common cause of functional voice loss. Butcher advised that the conversion label should be reserved for cases of aphonia in which lack of concern and motivation to improve the voice coexists with clear evidence of a temporally linked psychosocial stressor. In the place of conversion, Butcher (1995) offered two alternative models to account for psychogenic voice loss. Both models minimized the role of primary and secondary gain in maintaining the voice disorder. The first was a slightly reformulated psychoanalytic model that stated, "if predisposed by social and cultural bias as well as early learning experiences, and then exposed to interpersonal difficulties that stimulate internal conflict, particularly in situations involving conflict over self-expression or voicing feelings, intrapsychic conflict or stress becomes channeled into musculoskeletal tension, which physically inhibits voice production" (p. 472). The second model, based on cognitive-behavioral principles, stated that "life stresses and interpersonal problems in an individual predisposed to having difficulties expressing feelings or views would produce involuntary anxiety symptoms and musculoskeletal tension, which would center on and inhibit voice production" (p. 473). Both models clearly emphasized the inhibitory effects of excess laryngeal muscle tension on voice production, although through slightly different causal mechanisms.

Recently, Roy and Bless (2000) proposed a theory that links personality to the development of functional dysphonia. The "trait theory of functional dysphonia" shares Butcher's (1995) theme of inhibitory laryngeal behavior but attributes this muscularly inhibited voice production to specific personality types. In brief, the authors speculate that the combination of personality traits such as introversion and neuroticism (trait anxiety) and constraint leads to predictable and conditioned laryngeal inhibitory responses to certain environmental signals or cues. For instance, when undesirable punishing or frustrating outcomes have been paired with previous attempts to speak out, this can lead to muscularly inhibited voice. The authors contend that this conflict between laryngeal inhibition and activation (with origins in personality and nervous system functioning) results in elevated laryngeal tension states and can give rise to incomplete or disordered vocalization in a structurally and neurologically intact larynx.

As is apparent from the foregoing discussion, the exquisite sensitivity and prolonged hypercontraction of the intrinsic and extrinsic laryngeal muscles in response to stress, anxiety, depression, and inhibited emotional expression is frequently cited as the common denominator underlying the majority of functional voice problems. Nichol, Morrison, and Rammage (1993) proposed that excess muscle tension arises from overactivity of autonomic and voluntary nervous systems in individuals who are unduly aroused and anxious. They added that such overactivity leads to hypertonicity of the intrinsic and extrinsic laryngeal muscles, resulting in muscle tension dysphonias sometimes associated with adjustment or anxiety disorders, or with certain personality trait disturbances.

Finally, some researchers have noted that their "psychogenic dysphonia and aphonia" patients had an abnormally high number of reported allergy, asthma, or upper respiratory infection symptoms, suggesting a link between psychological factors and respiratory and phonatory disorders (Milutinovic, 1991; Schalen and Andersson, 1992). They have speculated that organic changes in the larynx, pharynx, and nose facilitate the appearance of a functional voice problem; that is, these changes direct the somatization of psychodynamic conflict. Likewise, Rammage, Nichol, and Morrison (1987) proposed that a relatively minor organic change such as edema, infection, or reflux laryngitis may trigger functional misuse, particularly if the individual is exceedingly anxious about his or her voice or health. In a similar vein, the same authors felt that anticipation of poor voice production in hypochondriacal, dependent, or obsessive-compulsive individuals leads to excessive vigilance over sensations arising from the throat (larynx) and respiratory system that may lead to altered voice production.

Research evidence to support the various psychological mechanisms offered to explain functional voice problems has seldom been provided. A complete review of the relevant findings and interpretations is provided in Roy et al. (1997). The empirical literature evaluating the functional dysphonia–psychology relationship is characterized by divergent results regarding the frequency and degree of specific personality traits (Aronson, Peterson, and Litin, 1966; Kinzl, Biebl, and Rauchegger, 1988; Gerritsma, 1991; Roy, Bless, and Heisey, 2000a, 2000b), conversion reaction (House and Andrews, 1987; Roy et al., 1997), and psychopathological symptoms such as depression and anxiety (Aronson, Peterson, and Litin, 1966; Pfau, 1975; House and Andrews, 1987; Gerritsma, 1991; Roy et al., 1997; White, Deary, and Wilson, 1997; Roy, Bless, and Heisey, 2000a, 2000b). Despite methodological differences, these studies have identified a general trend toward elevated levels of (1) state and trait anxiety, (2) depression, (3) somatic preoccupation or complaints, and (4) introversion in the functional dysphonia population. Patients have been described as inhibited, stress reactive, socially anxious, nonassertive, and with a tendency toward restraint (Friedl, Friedrich, and Egger, 1990; Gerritsma, 1991; Roy, Bless, and Heisey, 2000a, 2000b).

In conclusion, the larynx can be a site of neuromuscular tension arising from stress, emotional inhibition, fear or threat, communication breakdown, and certain personality types. This tension can produce severely disordered voice in the context of a structurally normal larynx. Although the precise mechanisms underlying and maintaining psychogenic voice problems remain unclear, the voice disorder is a powerful reminder of the intimate relationship between mind and body.

See also PSYCHOGENIC VOICE DISORDERS: DIRECT THERAPY.

—Nelson Roy

References

American Psychiatric Association. (1994). *Diagnostic and statistical manual of mental disorders—Fourth edition*. Washington, DC: American Psychiatric Press.

Aronson, A. E. (1990). *Clinical voice disorders: An interdisciplinary approach* (3rd ed.). New York: Thieme.

Aronson, A. E., Peterson, H. W., and Litin, E. M. (1966). Psychiatric symptomatology in functional dysphonia and aphonia. *Journal of Speech and Hearing Disorders, 31*, 115–127.

Bridger, M. M., and Epstein, R. (1983). Functional voice disorders: A review of 109 patients. *Journal of Laryngology and Otology, 97*, 1145–1148.

Butcher, P. (1995). Psychological processes in psychogenic voice disorder. *European Journal of Disorders of Communication, 30*, 467–474.

Butcher, P., Elias, A., Raven, R. (1993). *Psychogenic voice disorders and cognitive behaviour therapy*. San Diego, CA: Singular Publishing Group.

Butcher, P., Elias, A., Raven, R., Yeatman, J., and Littlejohns, D. (1987). Psychogenic voice disorder unresponsive to speech therapy: Psychological characteristics and cognitive-behaviour therapy. *British Journal of Disorders of Communication, 22*, 81–92.

Friedl, W., Friedrich, G., and Egger, J. (1990). Personality and coping with stress in patients suffering from functional dysphonia. *Folia Phoniatrica, 42*, 144–149.

Gerritsma, E. J. (1991). An investigation into some personality characteristics of patients with psychogenic aphonia and dysphonia. *Folia Phoniatrica, 43*, 13–20.

House, A. O., and Andrews, H. B. (1987). The psychiatric and social characteristics of patients with functional dysphonia. *Journal of Psychosomatic Research, 3*, 483–490.

Kinzl, J., Biebl, W., and Rauchegger, H. (1988). Functional aphonia: Psychosomatic aspects of diagnosis and therapy. *Folia Phoniatrica, 40*, 131–137.

Milutinovic, Z. (1991). Inflammatory changes as a risk factor in the development of phononeurosis. *Folia Phoniatrica, 43*, 177–180.

Nichol, H., Morrison, M. D., and Rammage, L. A. (1993). Interdisciplinary approach to functional voice disorders: The psychiatrist's role. *Otolaryngology–Head and Neck Surgery, 108*, 643–647.

Pfau, E. M. (1975). Psychologische Untersuchungsergegnisse für Ätiologie der psychogenen Dysphonien. *Folia Phoniatrica, 25,* 298–306.

Rammage, L. A., Nichol, H., and Morrison, M. D. (1987). The psychopathology of voice disorders. *Human Communications Canada, 11,* 21–25.

Roy, N., and Bless, D. M. (2000). Toward a theory of the dispositional bases of functional dysphonia and vocal nodules: Exploring the role of personality and emotional adjustment. In R. D. Kent and M. J. Ball (Eds.), *Voice quality measurement* (pp. 461–480). San Diego, CA: Singular Publishing Group.

Roy, N., Bless, D. M., and Heisey, D. (2000a). Personality and voice disorders: A superfactor trait analysis. *Journal of Speech, Language and Hearing Research, 43,* 749–768.

Roy, N., Bless, D. M., and Heisey, D. (2000b). Personality and voice disorders: A multitrait-multidisorder analysis. *Journal of Voice, 14,* 521–548.

Roy, N., McGrory, J. J., Tasko, S. M., Bless, D. M., Heisey, D., and Ford, C. N. (1997). Psychological correlates of functional dysphonia: An evaluation using the Minnesota Multiphasic Personality Inventory. *Journal of Voice, 11,* 443–451.

Sapir, S. (1995). Psychogenic spasmodic dysphonia: A case study with expert opinions. *Journal of Voice, 9,* 270–281.

Schalen, L., and Andersson, K. (1992). Differential diagnosis and treatment of psychogenic voice disorder. *Clinical Otolaryngology, 17,* 225–230.

White, A., Deary, I. J., and Wilson, J. A. (1997). Psychiatric disturbance and personality traits in dysphonic patients. *European Journal of Disorders of Communication, 32,* 121–128.

Further Readings

Deary, I. J., Scott, S., Wilson, I. M., White, A., MacKenzie, K., and Wilson, J. A. (1998). Personality and psychological distress in dysphonia. *British Journal of Health Psychology, 2,* 333–341.

Friedl, W., Friedrich, G., Egger, J., and Fitzek, I. (1993). Psychogenic aspects of functional dysphonia. *Folia Phoniatrica, 45,* 10–13.

Green, G. (1988). The inter-relationship between vocal and psychological characteristics: A literature review. *Australian Journal of Human Communication Disorders, 16,* 31–43.

Gunther, V., Mayr-Graft, A., Miller, C., and Kinzl, H. (1996). A comparative study of psychological aspects of recurring and non-recurring functional aphonias. *European Archives of Otorhinolaryngology, 253,* 240–244.

House, A. O., and Andrews, H. B. (1988). Life events and difficulties preceding the onset of functional dysphonia. *Journal of Psychosomatic Research, 32,* 311–319.

Koufman, J. A., and Blalock, P. D. (1982). Classification and approach to patients with functional voice disorders. *Annals of Otology, Rhinology, and Laryngology, 91,* 372–377.

Morrison, M. D., and Rammage, L. (1993). Muscle misuse voice disorders: Description and classification. *Acta Otolaryngologica (Stockholm), 113,* 428–434.

Moses, P. J. (1954). *The voice of neurosis.* New York: Grune and Stratton.

Pennebaker, J. W., and Watson, D. (1991). The psychology of somatic symptoms. In L. J. Kirmayer and J. M. Robbins (Eds.), *Current concepts of somatization.* Washington, DC: American Psychiatric Press.

Roy, N., and Bless, D. M. (2000). Personality traits and psychological factors in voice pathology: A foundation for future research. *Journal of Speech, Language, and Hearing Research, 43,* 737–748.

Hypokinetic Laryngeal Movement Disorders

Hypokinetic laryngeal movement disorders are observed most often in individuals diagnosed with the neurological disorder, parkinsonism. Parkinsonism has the following features: bradykinesia, postural instability, rigidity, resting tremor, and freezing (motor blocks) (Fahn, 1986). For the diagnosis to be made, at least two of these five features should be present, and one of the two features should be either tremor or rigidity. Parkinsonism as a syndrome can be classified as idiopathic Parkinson's disease (PD) (i.e., symptoms of unknown cause); secondary (or symptomatic) PD, caused by a known and identifiable cause; or parkinsonism-plus syndromes, in which symptoms of parkinsonism are caused by a known gene defect or have a distinctive pathology. The specific diagnosis depends on findings in the clinical history, the neurological examination, and laboratory tests. No single feature is completely reliable for differentiating among the different causes of parkinsonism.

Idiopathic PD is the most common type of parkinsonism encountered by the neurologist. Pathologically, idiopathic PD affects many structures in the central nervous system (CNS), with preferential involvement of dopaminergic neurons in the substantia nigra pars compacta (SNpc). Lewy bodies, eosinophilic intracytoplasmatic inclusions, can be found in these neurons (Galvin, Lee, and Trojanowski, 2001). Alpha-synuclein is the primary component of Lewy body fibrils (Galvin, Lee, and Trojanowski, 2001). However, only about 75% of patients with the clinical diagnosis of idiopathic PD are found at autopsy to have the pathological CNS changes characteristic of PD (Hughes et al., 1992).

Many patients and their families consider the reduced ability to communicate one of the most difficult aspects of PD. Hypokinetic dysarthria, characterized by a soft voice, monotone, a breathy, hoarse voice quality, and imprecise articulation (Darley, Aronson, and Brown, 1975; Logemann et al., 1978), and reduced facial expression (masked facies) contribute to limitations in communication in the vast majority of individuals with idiopathic PD (Pitcairn et al., 1990). During the course of the disease, approximately 45%–89% of patients will report speech problems (Logemann and Fisher, 1981; Sapir et al., 2002). Repetitive speech phenomena (Benke et al., 2000), voice tremor, and hyperkinetic dysarthria may also be encountered in individuals with idiopathic PD. When hyperkinetic dysarthria is reported in idiopathic PD, it is most frequently seen together with other motor complications (e.g., dyskinesia) of prolonged levodopa therapy (Critchley, 1981).

Logemann et al. (1978) suggested that the clusters of speech symptoms they observed in 200 individuals with PD represented a progression in dysfunction, beginning with disordered phonation in recently diagnosed patients and extending to include disordered articulation and other aspects of speech in more advanced cases. Recent findings by Sapir et al. (2002) are consistent with this suggestion. Sapir et al. (2002) observed voice disorders in individuals with recent onset of PD and low Unified Parkinson Disease Rating Scale (UPDRS) scores; in individuals with longer duration of disease and higher UPDRS scores, they observed a significantly higher incidence of abnormal articulation and fluency, in addition to the disordered voice. Hypokinetic dysarthria of parkinsonism is considered to be a part of basal ganglia damage (Darley, Aronson, and Brown, 1975). However, there are no studies on pathological changes in the hypokinetic dysarthria of idiopathic PD. A significant correlation between neuronal loss and gliosis in SNpc and substantia nigra pars reticulata (SNpr) and severity of hypokinetic dysarthria was found in patients with Parkinson-plus syndromes (Kluin et al., 2001). Speech and voice characteristics may differ between idiopathic PD and Parkinson-plus syndromes (e.g., Shy-Drager syndrome, progressive supranuclear palsy, multisystem atrophy). In addition to the classic hypokinetic symptoms, these patients may have more slurring, a strained, strangled voice, pallilalia, and hypernasality (Countryman, Ramig, and Pawlas, 1994) and their symptoms may progress more rapidly.

Certain aspects of hypokinetic dysarthria in idiopathic PD have been studied extensively. Hypophonia (reduced loudness, monotone, a breathy, hoarse quality) may be observed in as many as 89% of individuals with idiopathic PD (Logemann et al., 1978). Fox and Ramig (1997) reported that sound pressure levels in individuals with idiopathic PD were significantly lower (2–4 dB [30 cm]) across a variety of speech tasks than in an age- and sex-matched control group. Lack of vocal fold closure, including bowing of the vocal cords and anterior and posterior chinks (Hanson, Gerratt, and Ward, 1984; Smith et al., 1995), has been implicated as a cause of this hypophonia. Perez et al. (1996) used videostroboscopic observations to study vocal fold vibration in individuals with idiopathic PD. They reported abnormal phase closure and symmetry and tremor (both at rest and during phonation) in nearly 50% of patients. Whereas reduced loudness and disordered voice quality in idiopathic PD have been associated with glottal incompetence (lack of vocal fold closure—e.g., bowing; Hanson, Gerratt, and Ward, 1984; Smith et al., 1995; Perez et al., 1996), the specific origin of this glottal incompetence has not been clearly defined. Rigidity or fatigue secondary to rigidity, paralysis, reduced thyroarytenoid longitudinal tension secondary to cricothyroid rigidity (Aronson, 1990), and misperception of voice loudness (Ho, Bradshaw, and Iansek 2000; Sapir et al., 2002) are among the explanations. It has been suggested that glottal incompetence (e.g., vocal fold bowing) might be due to loss of muscle or connective tissue volume, either throughout the entire vocal fold or localized near the free margin of the vocal fold. Recent physiological studies of laryngeal function in idiopathic PD have shown a reduced amplitude of electromyographic activity in the thyroarytenoid muscle accompanying glottal incompetence when compared with both aged-matched and younger controls (Baker et al., 1998). These findings and the observation of reduced and variable single motor unit activity in the thyroarytenoid muscle of individuals with idiopathic PD (Luschei et al., 1999) are consistent with a number of hypotheses, the most plausible of which is reduced central drive to laryngeal motor neuron pools.

Although the origin of the hypophonia in PD is currently undefined, Ramig and colleagues (e.g., Fox et al., 2002) have hypothesized that there are at least three features underlying the voice disorder in individuals with PD: (1) an overall neural amplitude scaledown (Penny and Young, 1983) to the laryngeal mechanism (reduced amplitude of neural drive to the muscles of the larynx); (2) problems in sensory perception of effort (Berardelli et al., 1986), which prevents the individual with idiopathic PD from accurately monitoring his or her vocal output; which results in (3) the individual's difficulty in independently generating (through internal cueing or scaling) adequate vocal effort (Hallet and Khoshbin, 1980) to produce normal loudness. Reduced neural drive, problems in sensory perception of effort, and problems scaling adequate vocal output effort may be significant factors underlying the voice problems in individuals with PD.

—Lorraine Olson Ramig, Mitchell F. Brin, Miodrag Velickovic, and Cynthia Fox

References

Aronson, A. E. (1990). *Clinical voice disorders*. New York: Thieme-Stratton.

Baker, K. K., Ramig, L. O., Luschei, E. S., and Smith, M. E. (1998). Thyroarytenoid muscle activity associated with hypophonia in Parkinson disease and aging. *Neurology, 51,* 1592–1598.

Benke, T., Hohenstein, C., Poewe, W., and Butterworth, B. (2000). Repetitive speech phenomena in Parkinson's disease. *Journal of Neurology, Neurosurgery, and Psychiatry, 69,* 319–324.

Berardelli, A., Dick, J. P., Rothwell, J. C., Day, B. L., and Marsden, C. D. (1986). Scaling of the size of the first agonist EMG burst during rapid wrist movements in patients with Parkinson's disease. *Journal of Neurology, Neurosurgery, and Psychiatry, 49,* 1273–1279.

Countryman, S., Ramig, L. O., and Pawlas, A. A. (1994). Speech and voice deficits in Parkinsonian Plus syndromes: Can they be treated? *Journal of Medical Speech-Language Pathology, 2,* 211–225.

Critchley, E. M. (1981). Speech disorders of Parkinsonism: A review. *Journal of Neurology, Neurosurgery, and Psychiatry, 44,* 751–758.

Darley, F. L., Aronson, A. E., and Brown, J. B. (1975). *Motor speech disorders*. Philadelphia: Saunders.

Fahn, S. (1986). Parkinson's disease and other basal ganglion disorders. In A. K. Asbury, G. M. McKhann, and W. I. McDonald (Eds.), *Diseases of the nervous system: Clinical neurobiology*. Philadelphia: Ardmore.

Fox, C., Morrison, C. E., Ramig, L. O., and Sapir, S. (2002). Current perspectives on the Lee Silverman voice treatment (LSVT) for individuals with idiopathic Parkinson's disease. *American Journal of Speech-Language Pathology, 11,* 111–123.

Fox, C., and Ramig, L. (1997). Vocal sound pressure level and self-perception of speech and voice in men and women with idiopathic Parkinson disease. *American Journal of Speech-Language Pathology, 6,* 85–94.

Galvin, J. E., Lee, V. M., and Trojanowski, J. Q. (2001). Synucleinopathies: Clinical and pathological implications. *Archives of Neurology, 58,* 186–190.

Hallet, M., and Khoshbin, S. (1980). A physiological mechanism of bradykinesia. *Brain, 103,* 301–314.

Hanson, D., Gerratt, B., and Ward, P. (1984). Cinegraphic observations of laryngeal function in Parkinson's disease. *Laryngoscope, 94,* 348–353.

Ho, A. K., Bradshaw, J. L., and Iansek, T. (2000). Volume perception in parkinsonian speech. *Movement Disorders, 15,* 1125–1131.

Hughes, A. J., Daniel, S. E., Kilford, L., and Lees, A. J. (1992). Accuracy of clinical diagnosis of idiopathic Parkinson's disease: A clinico-pathological study of 100 cases. *Journal of Neurology, Neurosurgery, and Psychiatry, 55,* 181–184.

Kluin, K. J., Gilman, S., Foster, N. L., Sima, A., D'Amato, C., Bruch, L., et al. (2001). Neuropathological correlates of dysarthria in progressive supranuclear palsy. *Archives of Neurology, 58,* 265–269.

Logemann, J. A., and Fisher, H. B. (1981). Vocal tract control in Parkinson's disease: Phonetic feature analysis of misarticulations. *Journal of Speech and Hearing Disorders, 46,* 348–352.

Logemann, J. A., Fisher, H. B., Boshes, B., and Blonsky, E. (1978). Frequency and concurrence of vocal tract dysfunctions in the speech of a large sample of Parkinson's patients. *Journal of Speech and Hearing Disorders, 43,* 47–57.

Luschei, E. S., Ramig, L. O., Baker, K. L., and Smith, M. E. (1999). Discharge characteristics of laryngeal single motor units during phonation in young and older adults and in persons with Parkinson disease. *Journal of Neurophysiology, 81,* 2131–2139.

Penny, J. B., and Young, A. B. (1983). Speculations on the functional anatomy of basal ganglia disorders. *Annual Review of Neurosciences, 6,* 73–94.

Perez, K., Ramig, L. O., Smith, M., and Dromey, C. (1996). The Parkinson larynx: Tremor and videostroboscopic findings. *Journal of Voice, 10,* 354–361.

Pitcairn, T., Clemie, S., Gray, J., and Pentland, B. (1990). Non-verbal cues in the self-presentation of parkinsonian patients. *British Journal of Clinical Psychology, 29,* 177–184.

Sapir, S., Pawlas, A. A., Ramig, L. O., Countryman, S., et al. (2002). Speech and voice abnormalities in Parkinson disease: Relation to severity of motor impairment, duration of disease, medication, depression, gender, and age. *Journal of Medical Speech-Language Pathology, 9,* 213–226.

Smith, M. E., Ramig, L. O., Dromey, C., et al. (1995). Intensive voice treatment in Parkinson disease: Laryngostroboscopic findings. *Journal of Voice, 9,* 453–459.

Further Readings

Ackerman, H., and Ziegler, W. (1991). Articulatory deficits in Parkinsonian dysarthria. *Journal of Neurology, Neurosurgery, and Psychiatry, 54,* 1093–1098.

Brown, R. G., and Marsden, C. D. (1988). An investigation of the phenomenon of "set" in Parkinson's disease. *Movement Disorders, 3,* 152–161.

Caliguri, M. P. (1989). Short-term fluctuations in orofacial motor control in Parkinson's disease. In K. M. Yorkson and D. R. Beukelman (Eds.), *Recent advances in clinical dysarthria.* Boston: College-Hill Press.

Conner, N. P., Abbs, J. H., Cole, K. J., and Gracco, V. L. (1989). Parkinsonian deficits in serial multiarticulate movements for speech. *Brain, 112,* 997–1009.

Contreras-Vidal, J., and Stelmach, G. (1995). A neural model of basal ganglia-thalamocortical relations in normal and parkinsonian movement. *Biological Cybernetics, 73,* 467–476.

DeLong, M. R. (1990). Primate models of movement disorders of basal ganglia origin. *Trends in Neuroscience, 13,* 281–285.

Forrest, K., Weismer, G., and Turner, G. (1989). Kinematic, acoustic and perceptual analysis of connected speech produced by Parkinsonian and normal geriatric adults. *Journal of the Acoustical Society of America, 85,* 2608–2622.

Jobst, E. E., Melnick, M. E., Byl, N. N., Dowling, G. A., and Aminoff, M. J. (1997). Sensory perception in Parkinson disease. *Archives of Neurology, 54,* 450–454.

Jurgens, U., and von Cramon, D. (1982). On the role of the anterior cingulated cortex in phonation: A case report. *Brain and Language, 15,* 234–248.

Larson, C. (1985). The midbrain periaqueductal fray: A brain-stem structure involved in vocalization. *Journal of Speech and Hearing Research, 28,* 241–249.

Ludlow, C. L., and Bassich, C. J. (1984). Relationships between perceptual ratings and acoustic measures of hypokinetic speech. In M. R. McNeil, J. C. Rosenbek, and A. E. Aronson (Eds.), *Dysarthria of speech: Physiology-acoustics-linguistics-management.* San Diego, CA: College-Hill Press.

Netsell, R., Daniel, B., and Celesia, G. G. (1975). Acceleration and weakness in parkinsonian dysarthria. *Journal of Speech and Hearing Disorders, 40,* 170–178.

Sarno, M. T. (1968). Speech impairment in Parkinson's disease. *Journal of Speech and Hearing Disorders, 49,* 269–275.

Schneider, J. S., Diamond, S. G., and Markham, C. H. (1986). Deficits in orofacial sensorimotor function in Parkinson's disease. *Annals of Neurology, 19,* 275–282.

Solomon, N. P., Hixon, T. J. (1993). Speech breathing in Parkinson's disease. *Journal of Speech and Hearing Research, 36,* 294–310.

Stewart, C., Winfield, L., Hunt, A., et al. (1995). Speech dysfunction in early Parkinson's disease. *Movement Disorders, 10,* 562–565.

Infectious Diseases and Inflammatory Conditions of the Larynx

Infectious and inflammatory conditions of the larynx can affect the voice, swallowing, and breathing to varying extents. Changes can be acute or chronic and can occur in isolation or as part of systemic processes. The conditions described in this article are grouped by etiology.

Infectious Diseases

Viral Laryngotracheitis. Viral laryngotracheitis is the most common infectious laryngeal disease. It is typically associated with upper respiratory infection, for example, by rhinoviruses and adenoviruses. Dysphonia is usually self-limiting but may create major problems for a professional voice user. The larger diameter upper airway in adults makes airway obstruction much less likely than in children.

In a typical clinical scenario, a performer with mild upper respiratory symptoms has to carry on performing but complains of reduced vocal pitch and increased effort on singing high notes. Mild vocal fold edema and erythema may occur but can be normal for this patient group. Thickened, erythematous tracheal mucosa visible between the vocal folds supports the diagnosis.

Hydration and rest may be sufficient treatment. However, if the performer decides to proceed with the show, high-dose steroids can reduce inflammation, and antibiotics may prevent opportunistic bacterial infection. Cough suppressants, expectorants, and steam inhalations may also be useful. Careful vocal warmup should be undertaken before performing, and "rescue" must be balanced against the risk of vocal injury.

Other Viral Infections.   Herpes simplex and herpes zoster infection have been reported in association with vocal fold paralysis (Flowers and Kernodle, 1990; Nishizaki et al., 1997). Laryngeal vesicles, ulceration, or plaques may lead to suspicion of the diagnosis, and antiviral therapy should be instituted early. New laryngeal muscle weakness may also occur in post-polio syndrome (Robinson, Hillel, and Waugh, 1998). Viral infection has also been implicated in the pathogenesis of certain laryngeal tumors. The most established association is between human papillomavirus (HPV) and laryngeal papillomatosis (Levi et al., 1989). HPV, Epstein-Barr virus, and even herpes simplex virus have been implicated in the development of laryngeal malignancy (Ferlito et al., 1997; Garcia-Milian et al., 1998; Pou et al., 2000).

Bacterial Laryngitis.   Bacterial laryngitis is most commonly due to *Hemophilus influenzae, Staphylococcus aureus, Streptococcus pneumoniae,* and beta-hemolytic streptococcus. Pain and fever may be severe, with airway and swallowing difficulties generally overshadowing voice loss. Typically the supraglottis is involved, with the aryepiglottic folds appearing boggy and edematous, often more so than the epiglottis. Unlike in children, laryngoscopy is usually safe in adults and is the best means of diagnosis. Possible underlying causes such as a laryngeal foreign body should be considered. Treatment includes intravenous antibiotics, hydration, humidification, and corticosteroids. Close observation is essential in case airway support is needed. Rarely, infected mucous retention cysts and epiglottic abscesses occur (Stack and Ridley, 1995). Tracheostomy and drainage may be required.

Mycobacterial Infections.   Laryngeal tuberculosis is rare in industrialized countries but must be considered in the differential diagnosis of laryngeal disease, especially in patients with AIDS or other immune deficiencies (Singh et al., 1996). Tuberculosis can infect the larynx primarily, by direct spread from the lungs, or by hematogenous or lymphatic dissemination (Ramandan, Tarayi, and Baroudy, 1993). Most patients have hoarse-

ness and odynophagia, typically out of proportion to the size of the lesion. However, these symptoms are not universally present. The vocal folds are most commonly affected, although all areas of the larynx can be involved. Laryngeal tuberculosis is often difficult to distinguish from carcinoma on laryngoscopy. Chest radiography and the purified protein derivative (PPD) test help establish the diagnosis, although biopsy and histological confirmation may be required. Patients are treated with antituberculous chemotherapy. The laryngeal symptoms usually respond within 2 weeks.

Leprosy is rare in developing countries. Laryngeal infection by *Mycobacterium leprae* can cause nodules, ulceration, and fibrosis. Lesions are often painless but may progress over the years to laryngeal stenosis. Treatment is with antileprosy chemotherapy (Soni, 1992).

Other Bacterial Infections.   Laryngeal actinomycosis can occur in immunocompromised patients and following laryngeal radiotherapy (Nelson and Tybor, 1992). Biopsy may be required to distinguish it from radionecrosis or tumor. Treatment requires prolonged antibiotic therapy.

Scleroma is a chronic granulomatous disease due to *Klebsiella scleromatis.* Primary involvement is in the nose, but the larynx can also be affected. Subglottic stenosis is the main concern (Amoils and Shindo, 1996).

Fungal Laryngitis.   Fungal laryngitis is rare and typically occurs in immunocompromised individuals. Fungi include yeasts and molds. Yeast infections are more frequent in the larynx, with *Candida albicans* most commonly identified (Vrabec, 1993). Predisposing factors in nonimmunocompromised patients include antibiotic and inhaled steroid use, and foreign bodies such as silicone voice prostheses.

The degree of hoarseness in laryngeal candidiasis may not reflect the extent of infection. Pain and associated swallowing difficulty may be present. Typically, thick white exudates are seen, and oropharyngeal involvement can coexist. Biopsy may show epithelial hyperplasia with a pseudocarcinomatous appearance. Potential complications include scarring, airway obstruction, and systemic dissemination.

In mild localized disease, topical nystatin or clotrimazole are usually effective. Discontinuing antibiotics or inhaled steroids should be considered. More severe cases may require oral antifungal azoles such as ketoconazole, fluconazole, or itraconazole. Intravenous amphotericin is efficacious but has potentially severe side effects. It is usually used for invasive or systemic disease.

Less common fungal diseases include blastomycosis, histoplasmosis, and coccidiomycosis. Infection may be confused with laryngeal carcinoma, and special histological stains are usually required for diagnosis. Long-term treatment with amphotericin B may be necessary.

Syphilis.   Syphilis is caused by the spirochete *Treponema pallidum.* Laryngeal involvement is rare but may occur in later stages of the disease. Secondary syphilis may present with laryngeal papules, ulcers and edema that mimic carcinoma, or tuberculous laryngitis. Tertiary syphilis may cause gummas, leading to scarring and stenosis (Lacy, Alderson, and Parker, 1994). Serologic tests are diagnostic. Active disease is treated with penicillin.

Inflammatory Processes

Chronic Laryngitis. Chronic laryngeal inflammation can result from smoking, gastroesophageal reflux (GER), voice abuse, or allergy. Patients often complain of hoarseness, sore throat, a globus sensation, and throat clearing. The vocal folds are usually thickened, dull, and erythematous. Posterior laryngeal involvement usually suggests GER. Besides direct chemical irritation, GER can promote laryngeal muscle misuse, which contributes to wear-and-tear injury (Gill and Morrison, 1998).

Although seasonal allergies may cause vocal fold edema and hoarseness (Jackson-Menaldi, Dzul, and Holland, 1999), it is surprising that allergy-induced chronic laryngitis is not more common. Even patients with significant nasal allergies or asthma have a low incidence of voice problems. The severity of other allergic accompaniments helps the clinician identify patients with dysphonia of allergic cause.

Treatment of chronic laryngitis includes voice rest and elimination of irritants. Dietary modifications and postural measures such as elevating the head of the bed can reduce GER. Proton pump inhibitors can be effective for persistent laryngeal symptoms (Hanson, Kamel, and Kahrilas, 1995).

Traumatic and Iatrogenic Causes. Inflammatory polyps, polypoid degeneration, and contact granuloma can arise from vocal trauma. Smoking contributes to polypoid degeneration, and intubation injury can cause contact granulomas. GER may promote inflammation in all these conditions. Granulomas can also form many years after Teflon injection for glottic insufficiency.

Rheumatoid Arthritis and Systemic Lupus Erythematosus. Laryngeal involvement occurs in almost a third of patients with rheumatoid arthritis (Lofgren and Montgomery, 1962). Patients present with a variety of symptoms. In the acute phase the larynx may be tender and inflamed. In the chronic phase the laryngeal mucosa may appear normal, but cricoarytenoid joint ankylosis may be present. Submucosal rheumatoid nodules or "bamboo nodes" can form in the membranous vocal folds. If the mucosal wave is severely damped, microlaryngeal excision can improve the voice. Corticosteroids can be injected intracordally following excision. Other autoimmune diseases such as systemic lupus erythematosus can cause similar laryngeal pathology (Woo, Mendelsohn, and Humphrey, 1995).

Relapsing Polychondritis. Relapsing polychondritis is an autoimmune disease causing inflammation of cartilaginous structures. The pinna is most commonly affected, although laryngeal involvement occurs in around 50% of cases. Dapsone, corticosteroids, and immunosuppressive drugs have been used to control the disease. Repeated attacks of laryngeal chondritis can cause subglottic scarring, necessitating permanent tracheostomy (Spraggs, Tostevin, and Howard, 1997).

Cicatricial Pemphigoid. This chronic subepithelial bullous disease predominantly involves the mucous membranes. Acute laryngeal lesions are painful, and examination shows mucosal erosion and ulceration. Later, scarring and stenosis may occur, with supraglottic involvement (Hanson, Olsen, and Rogers, 1988). Treatment includes dapsone, systemic or intralesional steroids, and cyclophosphamide. Scarring may require laser excision and sometimes tracheostomy.

Amyloidosis. Amyloidosis is characterized by deposition of acellular proteinaceous material (amyloid) in tissues (Lewis et al., 1992). It can occur primarily or secondary to other diseases such as multiple myeloma or tuberculosis. Deposits may be localized or generalized. Laryngeal involvement is usually due to primary localized disease. Submucosal deposits may affect any part of the larynx but most commonly occur in the ventricular folds. Treatment is by conservative laser excision. Recurrences are frequent.

Sarcoidosis. Sarcoidosis is a multiorgan granulomatous disease of unknown etiology. About 6% of cases involve the larynx, producing dysphonia and airway obstruction. Pale, diffuse swelling of the epiglottis and aryepiglottic folds is characteristic (Benjamin, Dalton, and Croxson, 1995). Systemic or intralesional steroids, antilepromatous therapy, and laser debulking are all possible treatments.

Wegener's Granulomatosis. Wegener's granulomatosis is an idiopathic syndrome characterized by vasculitis and necrotizing granulomas of the respiratory tract and kidneys. The larynx is involved in 8% of cases (Waxman and Bose, 1986). Ulcerative lesions and subglottic stenosis may occur, causing hoarseness and dyspnea. Treatment includes corticosteroids and cyclophosphamide. Laser resection or open surgery is sometimes necessary for airway maintenance.

—*David P. Lau and Murray D. Morrison*

References

Amoils, C., and Shindo, M. (1996). Laryngotracheal manifestations of rhinoscleroma. *Annals of Otology, Rhinology, and Laryngology, 105,* 336–340.

Benjamin, B., Dalton, C., and Croxson, G. (1995). Laryngoscopic diagnosis of laryngeal sarcoid. *Annals of Otology, Rhinology, and Laryngology, 104,* 529–531.

Ferlito, A., Weiss, L., Rinaldo, A., et al. (1997). Clinicopathologic consultation: Lymphoepithelial carcinoma of the larynx, hypopharynx and trachea. *Annals of Otology, Rhinology, and Laryngology, 106,* 437–444.

Flowers, R., and Kernodle, D. (1990). Vagal mononeuritis caused by herpes simplex virus: Association with unilateral vocal cord paralysis. *American Journal of Medicine, 88,* 686–688.

Garcia-Milian, R., Hernandez, H., Panade, L., et al. (1998). Detection and typing of human papillomavirus DNA in benign and malignant tumours of laryngeal epithelium. *Acta Oto-Laryngologica, 118,* 754–758.

Gill, C., and Morrison, M. (1998). Esophagolaryngeal reflux in a porcine animal model. *Journal of Otolaryngology, 27,* 76–80.

Hanson, D., Kamel, P., and Kahrilas, P. (1995). Outcomes of antireflux therapy for the treatment of chronic laryngitis. *Annals of Otology, Rhinology, and Laryngology, 104,* 550–555.

Hanson, R., Olsen, K., and Rogers, R. (1988). Upper aero-digestive tract manifestations of cicatricial pemphigoid. *Annals of Otology, Rhinology, and Laryngology, 97,* 493–499.

Jackson-Menaldi, C., Dzul, A., and Holland, R. (1999). Allergies and vocal fold edema: A preliminary report. *Journal of Voice, 13,* 113–122.

Lacy, P., Alderson, D., and Parker, A. (1994). Late congenital syphilis of the larynx and pharynx presenting at endotracheal intubation. *Journal of Laryngology and Otology, 108,* 688–689.

Levi, J., Delcelo, R., Alberti, V., Torloni, H., and Villa, L. (1989). Human papillomavirus DNA in respiratory papillomatosis detected by in situ hybridization and polymerase chain reaction. *American Journal of Pathology, 135,* 1179–1184.

Lewis, J., Olsen, K., Kurtin, P., and Kyle, R. (1992). Laryngeal amyloidosis: A clinicopathologic and immunohistochemical review. *Otolaryngology–Head and Neck Surgery, 106,* 372–377.

Lofgren, R., and Montgomery, W. (1962). Incidence of laryngeal involvement in rheumatoid arthritis. *New England Journal of Medicine, 267,* 193.

Nelson, E., and Tybor, A. (1992). Actinomycosis of the larynx. *Ear, Nose, and Throat Journal, 71,* 356–358.

Nishizaki, K., Onada, K., Akagi, H., Yuen, K., Ogawa, T., and Masuda, Y. (1997). Laryngeal zoster with unilateral laryngeal paralysis. *ORL: Journal for Oto-rhino-laryngology and Its Related Specialties, 59,* 235–237.

Pou, A., Vrabec, J., Jordan, J., Wilson, D., Wang, S., and Payne, D. (2000). Prevalence of herpes simplex virus in malignant laryngeal lesions. *Laryngoscope, 110,* 194–197.

Ramandan, H., Tarayi, A., and Baroudy, F. (1993). Laryngeal tuberculosis: Presentation of 16 cases and review of the literature. *Journal of Otolaryngology, 22,* 39–41.

Robinson, L., Hillel, A., and Waugh, P. (1998). New laryngeal muscle weakness in post-polio syndrome. *Laryngoscope, 108,* 732–734.

Singh, B., Balwally, A., Nash, M., Har-El, G., and Lucente, F. (1996). Laryngeal tuberculosis in HIV-infected patients: A difficult diagnosis. *Laryngoscope, 106,* 1238–1240.

Soni, N. (1992). Leprosy of the larynx. *Journal of Laryngology and Otology, 106,* 518–520.

Spraggs, P., Tostevin, P., and Howard, D. (1997). Management of laryngotracheobronchial sequelae and complications of relapsing polychondritis. *Laryngoscope, 107,* 936–941.

Stack, B., and Ridley, M. (1995). Epiglottic abscess. *Head and Neck, 17,* 263–265.

Vrabec, D. (1993). Fungal infections of the larynx. *Otolaryngologic Clinics of North America, 26,* 1091–1114.

Waxman, J., and Bose, W. (1986). Laryngeal manifestations of Wegener's granulomatosis: Case reports and review of the literature. *Journal of Rheumatology, 13,* 408–411.

Woo, P., Mendelsohn, J., and Humphrey, D. (1995). Rheumatoid nodules of the larynx. *Otolaryngology–Head and Neck Surgery, 113,* 147–150.

Further Readings

Badaracco, G., Venuti, A., Morello, R., Muller, A., and Marcante, M. (2000). Human papillomavirus in head and neck carcinomas: Prevalence, physical status and relationship with clinical/pathological parameters. *Anticancer Research, 20,* 1305.

Cleary, K., and Batsakis, J. (1995). Mycobacterial disease of the head and neck: Current perspective. *Annals of Otology, Rhinology, and Laryngology, 104,* 830–833.

Herridge, M., Pearson, F., and Downey, G. (1996). Subglottic stenosis complicating Wegener's granulomatosis: Surgical repair as a viable treatment option. *Journal of Thoracic and Cardiovascular Surgery, 111,* 961–966.

Jones, K. (1998). Infections and manifestations of systemic disease in the larynx. In C. W. Cummings, J. M. Fredrickson, L. A. Harker, C. J. Krause, D. E. Schuller, and M. A. Richardson (Eds.), *Otolaryngology—head and neck surgery* (3rd ed., pp. 1979–1988). St Louis: Mosby.

Langford, C., and Van Waes, C. (1997). Upper airway obstruction in the rheumatic diseases. *Rheumatic Diseases Clinics of North America, 23,* 345–363.

Morrison, M., Rammage, L., Nichol, H., Pullan, B., May, P., and Salkeld, L. (2001). *Management of the voice and its disorders* (2nd ed.). San Diego, CA: Singular Publishing Group.

Raymond, A., Sneige, N., and Batsakis, J. (1992). Amyloidosis in the upper aerodigestive tracts. *Annals of Otology, Rhinology, and Laryngology, 101,* 794–796.

Richter, B., Fradis, M., Kohler, G., and Ridder, G. (2001). Epiglottic tuberculosis: Differential diagnosis and treatment. Case report and review of the literature. *Annals of Otology, Rhinology, and Laryngology, 110,* 197–201.

Ridder, G., Strohhacker, H., Lohle, E., Golz, A., and Fradis, M. (2000). Laryngeal sarcoidosis: Treatment with the antileprosy drug clofazimine. *Annals of Otology, Rhinology, and Laryngology, 109,* 1146–1149.

Sataloff, R. (1997). Common infections and inflammations and other conditions. In R. T. Sataloff (Ed.), *Professional voice: The science and art of clinical care* (2nd ed., pp. 429–436). San Diego, CA: Singular Publishing Group.

Tami, T., Ferlito, A., Rinaldo, A., Lee, K., and Singh, B. (1999). Laryngeal pathology in the acquired immunodeficiency syndrome: Diagnostic and therapeutic dilemmas. *Annals of Otology, Rhinology, and Laryngology, 108,* 214–220.

Thompson, L. (2001). Pathology of the larynx, hypopharynx and tarachea. In Y. Fu, B. M. Wenig, E. Abemayor, and B. L. Wenig (Eds.), *Head and neck pathology with clinical correlations* (pp. 369–454). New York: Churchill Livingstone.

Vrabec, J., Molina, C., and West, B. (2000). Herpes simplex viral laryngitis. *Annals of Otology, Rhinology, and Laryngology, 109,* 611–614.

Instrumental Assessment of Children's Voice

Disorders of voice may affect up to 5% of children, and instrumental procedures such as acoustics, aerodynamics, or electroglottography (EGG) may complement auditory-perceptual and imaging procedures by providing objective measures that help in determining the nature and severity of laryngeal pathology. The use of these procedures should take into account the developmental features of the larynx and special problems associated with a pediatric population.

An important starting point is the developmental anatomy and physiology of the larynx. This background is essential in understanding children's vocal function as determined by instrumental assessments. The larynx of the infant and young child differs considerably in its anatomy and physiology from the adult larynx (see ANATOMY OF THE HUMAN LARYNX). The vocal folds in an infant are about 3–5 mm long, and the composition of the folds is uniform. That is, the infant's vocal folds are not only very short compared with those of the adult, but they lack the lamination seen in the adult folds. The lamination has been central to modern theories of phonation, and its absence in infants and marginal development in young children presents interesting challenges to theories of phonation applied to a pediatric population. An early stage of development of the lamina propria begins between 1 and 4 years, with the appearance of the vocal ligament (intermediate and deep layers of the lamina propria). During this same interval, the length of the vocal fold increases (reaching about 7.5 mm by age 5) and the entire laryngeal framework increases in size. The differentiation of the superficial layer of the lamina propria apparently is not complete until at least the age of 12 years.

Studies on the time of first appearance of sexual dimorphism in laryngeal size are conflicting, ranging from 3 years to no sex differences in laryngeal size observable during early childhood. Sexual dimorphism of vocal fold length has been reported to appear at about age 6–7 years. These reported anatomical differences do not appear to contribute to significant differences in vocal fundamental frequency (f_0) between males and females until puberty, at which time laryngeal growth is remarkable, especially in boys. For example, in boys, the anteroposterior dimension of the thyroid cartilage increases threefold, along with increases in vocal fold length.

Acoustic Studies of Children's Voice. Mean f_0 has been one of the most thoroughly studied aspects of the pediatric voice. For infants' nondistress utterances, such as cooing and babbling, mean f_0 falls in the range of 300–600 Hz and appears to be stable until about 9 months, when it begins to decline until adulthood (Kent and Read, 2002). A relatively sharp decline occurs between the ages of 12 months and 3 years, so that by the age of 3 years, the mean f_0 in both males and females is about 250 Hz. Mean f_0 is stable or gradually falling between 6 and 11 years, and the value of 250 Hz may be taken as a reasonable estimate of f_0 in both boys and girls. Some studies report no significant change in f_0 during this developmental period, but Glaze et al. (1988) reported that f_0 decreased with increasing age, height, and weight for boys and girls ages 5–11 years, and Ferrand and Bloom (1996) observed a decrease in the mean, maximum, and range of f_0 in boys, but not in girls, at about 7–8 years of age.

Sex differences in f_0 emerge especially strongly during adolescence. The overall f_0 decline from infancy to adulthood is about one octave for girls and two octaves for boys. There is some question as to when the sex difference emerges. Lee et al. (1999) observed that f_0 differences between male and female children were statistically significant beginning at about age 12 years, but Glaze et al. (1988) observed differences between boys and girls for the age period 5–11 years. Further, Hacki and Heitmuller (1999) reported a lowering of both the habitual pitch and the entire speaking pitch range between the ages of 7 and 8 years for girls and between the ages of 8 and 9 years for boys. Sex differences emerge strongly with the onset of mutation. Hacki and Heitmuller (1999) concluded that the beginning of the mutation occurs at age 10–11 years. Mean f_0 change is pronounced in males between the ages of about 12 and 15 years. For example, Lee et al. (1999) reported a 78% decrease in f_0 for males between these ages. No significant change was observed after the age of 15 years, which indicates that the voice change is effectively complete by that age (Hollien, Green, and Massey, 1994; Kent and Vorperian, 1995).

Other acoustic aspects of children's voices have not been extensively studied. In apparently the only large-scale study of its kind, Campisi et al. (2002) provided normative data for children for the parameters of the Multi-Dimensional Voice Program (MDVP). On the majority of parameters (excluding, of course, f_0), the mean values for children were fairly consistent with those for adults, which simplifies the clinical application of MDVP. However, this conclusion does not apply to the pubescent period, during which variability in amplitude and fundamental frequency increases in both girls and boys, but markedly so in the latter (Boltezar, Burger, and Zargi, 1997). It should also be noted voice training can affect the degree of aperiodicity in children's voices (Dejonckere et al., 1996) (see ACOUSTIC ASSESSMENT OF VOICE).

Aerodynamic Studies of Children's Voice. There are only limited data describing developmental patterns in voice aerodynamics. Table 1 shows normative data for flow, pressure, and laryngeal airway resistance from three sources (Netsell et al., 1994; Keilman and Bader, 1995; Zajac, 1995, 1998). All of the data were collected during the production of /pi/ syllable trains, following the procedure first described by Smitheran and Hixon (1981). Flow appears to increase with age, ranging from 75–79 mL/s in children aged 3–5 years to 127–188 mL/s in adults. Pressure decreases slightly with age, ranging from 8.4 cm H_2O in children ages 3–5 years to 5.3–6.0 cm H_2O in adults. Laryngeal airway pressure decreases with age, ranging from 111–119 cm H_2O/L/s in children aged 3–6 years to 34–43 cm H_2O/L/s in adults. This decrease in laryngeal airway pressure occurs as a function of the rate of flow increase exceeding the rate of pressure decrease across the age range.

Netsell et al. (1994) explained the developmental changes in flow, pressure, and laryngeal airway pressure

Table 1. Aerodynamic normative data from three sources: N (Netsell et al., 1994), K (Keilman & Bader, 1995), and Z (Zajac, 1995, 1998). All data were collected using the methodology described by Smitheran and Hixon (1981). Values shown are means, with standard deviations in parentheses

Reference	Age (yr)	Sex	N	Flow (mL/s)	Pressure (cm H_2O)	LAR (cm H_2O/L/s)
N	3–5	F	10	79 (16)	8.4 (1.3)	111 (26)
N	3–5	M	10	75 (20)	8.4 (1.4)	119 (20)
K	4–7	F&M			7.46 (2.26)	
N	6–9	F	10	86 (19)	7.4 (1.5)	89 (25)
N	6–9	M	9	101 (42)	8.3 (2.0)	97 (39)
Z	7–11	F&M	10	123 (30)	11.4 (2.3)	95.3 (24.4)
K	8–12	F&M			6.81 (2.29)	
N	9–12	F	10	121 (21)	7.1 (1.2)	59 (7)
N	9–12	M	10	115 (42)	7.9 (1.3)	77 (23)
K	13–15	F&M			5.97 (2.07)	
K	4–15	F&M	100	50–150		87.82 (62.95)
N	Adult	F	10	127 (29)	5.3 (1.2)	43 (10)
N	Adult	M	10	188 (51)	6.0 (1.4)	34 (9)

F = female, M = male, N = number of participants, LAR = laryngeal airway resistance.

as secondary to an increasing airway size and decreasing dependence on expiratory muscle forces alone for speech breathing with age. No consistent differences in aerodynamic parameters were observed between female and male children. High standard deviations reflect considerable variation between children of similar ages (see AERODYNAMIC ASSESSMENT OF VOICE).

Electroglottographic Studies of Children's Voice. Although EGG data on children's voice are not abundant, one study provides normative data on a sample of 164 children, 79 girls and 85 boys, ages 3–16 years (Cheyne, Nuss, and Hillman, 1999). Cheyne et al. reported no significant effect of age on the EGG measures of jitter, open quotient, closing quotient, and opening quotient. The means and standard deviations (in parentheses) for these measures were as follows: jitter—0.76% (0.61), open quotient—54.8% (3.3), closing quotient—14.1% (3.8), and opening quotient—31.1% (4.1). These values are reasonably similar to values reported for adults, although caution should be observed because of differences in procedures across studies (Takahashi and Koike, 1975) (see ELECTROGLOTTOGRAPHIC ASSESSMENT OF VOICE).

One of the most striking features of the instrumental studies of children's voice is that, except for f_0 and the aerodynamic measures, the values obtained from instrumental procedures change relatively little from childhood to adulthood. This stability is remarkable in view of the major changes that are observed in laryngeal anatomy and physiology. Apparently, children are able to maintain normal voice quality in the face of considerable alteration in the apparatus of voice production. With the mutation, however, stability is challenged, and the suitability of published normative data is open to question. The maintenance of rather stable values across a substantial period of childhood (from about 5 to 12 years) for many acoustic and EGG parameters holds a distinct advantage for clinical application. It is also clear

that instrumental procedures can be used successfully with children as young as 3 years of age. Therefore, these procedures may play a valuable role in the objective assessment of voice in children.

See also VOICE DISORDERS IN CHILDREN.

—*Ray D. Kent and Nathan V. Welham*

References

Boltezar, I. H., Burger, Z. R., and Zargi, M. (1997). Instability of voice in adolescence: Pathologic condition or normal developmental variation? *Journal of Pediatrics, 130,* 185–190.

Campisi, P., Tewfik, T. L., Manoukian, J. J., Schloss, M. D., Pelland-Blais, E., and Sadeghi, N. (2002). Computer-assisted voice analysis: Establishing a pediatric database. *Archives of Otolaryngology–Head and Neck Surgery, 128,* 156–160.

Cheyne, H. A., Nuss, R. C., and Hillman, R. E. (1999). Electroglottography in the pediatric population. *Archives of Otolaryngology–Head and Neck Surgery, 125,* 1105–1108.

Dejonckere, P. H. (1999). Voice problems in children: Pathogenesis and diagnosis. *International Journal of Pediatric Otorhinolaryngology, 49*(Suppl. 1), S311–S314.

Dejonckere, P. H., Wieneke, G. H., Bloemenkamp, D., and Lebacq, J. (1996). F_0-perturbation and f_0-loudness dynamics in voices of normal children, with and without education in singing. *International Journal of Pediatric Otorhinolaryngology, 35,* 107–115.

Ferrand, C. T., and Bloom, R. L. (1996). Gender differences in children's intonational patterns. *Journal of Voice, 10,* 284–291.

Glaze, L. E., Bless, D. M., Milenkovic, P., and Susser, R. (1988). Acoustic characteristics of children's voice. *Journal of Voice, 2,* 312–319.

Hacki, T., and Heitmuller, S. (1999). Development of the child's voice: Premutation, mutation. *International Journal of Pediatric Otorhinolaryngology, 49*(Suppl. 1), S141–S144.

Hollien, H., Green, R., and Massey, K. (1994). Longitudinal research on adolescent voice change in males. *Journal of the Acoustical Society of America, 96,* 2646–2654.

Keilman, A., and Bader, C. (1995). Development of aerodynamic aspects in children's voice. *International Journal of Pediatric Otorhinolaryngology, 31*, 183–190.

Kent, R. D., and Read, C. (2002). *The acoustic analysis of speech* (2nd ed.). San Diego, CA: Singular/Thompson Learning.

Kent, R. D., and Vorperian, H. K. (1995). Anatomic development of the craniofacial-oral-laryngeal systems: A review. *Journal of Medical Speech-Language Pathology, 3*, 145–190.

Lee, S., Potamianos, A., and Narayanan, S. (1999). Acoustics of children's speech: Developmental changes of temporal and spectral parameters. *Journal of the Acoustical Society of America, 105*, 1455–1468.

Netsell, R., Lotz, W. K., Peters, J. E., and Schulte, L. (1994). Developmental patterns of laryngeal and respiratory function for speech production. *Journal of Voice, 8*, 123–131.

Smitheran, J., and Hixon, T. (1981). A clinical method for estimating laryngeal airway resistance during vowel production. *Journal of Speech and Hearing Disorders, 46*, 138–146.

Takahashi, H., and Koike, Y. (1975). Some perceptual dimensions and acoustical correlates of pathological voices. *Acta Otolaryngolica Supplement (Stockholm), 338*, 1–24.

Zajac, D. J. (1995). Laryngeal airway resistance in children with cleft palate and adequate velopharyngeal function. *Cleft Palate–Craniofacial Journal, 32*, 138–144.

Zajac, D. J. (1998). Effects of a pressure target on laryngeal airway resistance in children. *Journal of Communication Disorders, 31*, 212–213.

Laryngeal Movement Disorders: Treatment with Botulinum Toxin

The laryngeal dystonias include spasmodic dysphonia, tremor, and paradoxical breathing dystonia. All of these conditions are idiopathic and all have distinctive symptoms, which form the basis for diagnosis. In adductor spasmodic dysphonia (ADSD), voice breaks during vowels are associated with involuntary spasmodic muscle bursts in the thyroarytenoid and other adductor laryngeal muscles, although bursts can also occur in the cricothyroid muscle in some persons (Nash and Ludlow, 1996). When voice breaks are absent, however, muscle activation is normal in both adductor and abductor laryngeal muscles (Van Pelt, Ludlow, and Smith, 1994). In the abductor type of spasmodic dysphonia (ABSD), breathy breaks are due to prolonged vocal fold opening during voiceless consonants. The posterior cricoarytenoid muscle is often involved in ABSD, although not in all patients (Cyrus et al., 2001). In the 1980s, "spastic" dysphonia was renamed "spasmodic" dysphonia to denote the intermittent aspect of the voice breaks and was classified as a task-specific focal laryngeal dystonia (Blitzer and Brin, 1991). Abnormalities in laryngeal adductor responses to sensory stimulation are found in both ADSD and ABSD (Deleyiannis et al., 1999), indicating a reduction in the normal central suppression of laryngeal sensorimotor responses in these disorders. ADSD affects 85% of patients with spasmodic dysphonia; the other 15% have ABSD.

Vocal tremor is present in at least one-third of patients with ADSD or ABSD and can also occur in isolation. A 5-Hz tremor can be heard on prolonged vowels, owing to intensity and frequency modulation. Tremor can affect either or both the adductor or abductor muscles, producing voice breaks in vowels or breathy intervals in the abductor type. Voice tremor occurs more often in women, sometimes with an associated head tremor. A variety of muscles may be involved in voice tremor (Koda and Ludlow, 1992).

Intermittent voice breaks are specific to the spasmodic dysphonias, either prolonged glottal stops and intermittent intervals of a strained or strangled voice quality during vowels in ADSD or prolonged voiceless consonants (p, t, k, f, s, h), which are perceived as breathy breaks, in ABSD. Other idiopathic voice disorders, such as muscular tension dysphonia, do not involve intermittent spasmodic changes in the voice. Rather, consistent abnormal hypertense laryngeal postures are maintained during voice production. Such persons may respond to manual laryngeal manipulation (Roy, Ford, and Bless, 1996). Muscular tension dysphonia may be confused with spasmodic dysphonia when ADSD patients develop increased muscle tension in an effort to overcome vocal instability, resulting in symptoms of both disorders. Some patients with voice tremor may also develop muscular tension dysphonia in an effort to overcome vocal instability.

Paradoxical breathing dystonia is rare, with adductory movements of the vocal folds during inspiration that remit during sleep (Marion et al., 1992). It differs from vocal fold dysfunction, which is usually intermittent and often coincides with irritants affecting the upper airway (Christopher et al., 1983; Morrison, Rammage, and Emami, 1999).

Botulinum toxin type A (BTX-A) is effective in treating a myriad of hyperkinetic disorders by partially denervating the muscle. The toxin is injected into muscle, diffuses, and is endocytosed into nerve endings. The toxin cleaves SNAP 25, a vesicle-docking protein essential for acetylcholine release into the neuromuscular junction (Aoki, 2001). When acetylcholine release is blocked, the muscle fibers become temporarily denervated. The effect is reversible: within a few weeks new nerve endings sprout, which may provide synaptic transmission and some reduction in muscle weakness. These nerve endings are later replaced by restitution of the original end-plates (de Paiva et al., 1999). In ADSD, BTX-A injection, either small bilateral injections or a unilateral injection produces a partial chemodenervation of the thyroarytenoid muscle for up to 4 months. Reductions in spasmodic muscle bursts relate to voice improvement (Bielamowicz and Ludlow, 2000). This therapy is effective in least 90% of ADSD patients, as has been demonstrated in a small randomized controlled trial (Truong et al., 1991) and in multiple case series (Ludlow et al., 1988; Blitzer and Brin, 1991; Blitzer, Brin, and Stewart, 1998). BTX-A is less effective in ABSD. When only ABSD patients with cricothyroid muscle spasms are injected in that muscle, significant improvements occur in 60% of cases (Ludlow et al., 1991). Similarly, two-thirds of ABSD patients obtain some degree of benefit from posterior cricoarytenoid injections (Blitzer et al., 1992). When speech symptoms were measured in blinded fashion before and after teatment, BTX-A was less effective in ABSD (Bielamowicz et al., 2001) than in ADSD (Ludlow et al., 1988).

Patients with adductor tremor confined to the vocal folds often receive some benefit from thyroarytenoid muscle BTX-A injections. When objective measures were used (Warrick et al., 2000), BTX-A injection was beneficial in 50% of patients with voice tremors. Either unilateral or bilateral thyroarytenoid injections can be used, although larger doses are sometimes more effective. BTX-A is much less effective, however, for treating tremor than it is in ADSD (Warrick et al., 2000), and it is rarely helpful in patients with abductor tremor.

BTX-A administered as either unilateral or bilateral injections into the thyroarytenoid muscle has been used successfully to treat paradoxical breathing dystonia (Marion et al., 1992; Grillone et al., 1994).

Changes in laryngeal function following BTX-A injection in persons with ADSD are similar, whether the injection was unilateral or bilateral. A few persons report a sense of reduction in laryngeal tension within 8 hours following injection, although voice loudness is not yet reduced. Voice loudness and breaks gradually diminish as BTX-A diffuses through the muscle, causing progressive denervation. Most people report that benefits become apparent the second day, while the side effects of progressive breathiness and swallowing difficulties increase over the 3–5 days after injection. Difficulty swallowing liquids may occur and occasionally results in aspiration. Patients are advised to ingest liquids slowly and in small volumes, by sipping through a straw. The difficulties with swallowing gradually subside between the first and second weeks after an injection (Ludlow, Rhew, and Nash, 1994), possibly as patients learn to compensate. The breathiness resolves somewhat later, reaching normal loudness levels as late as 3–4 weeks after injection, during the period when axonal sprouting may occur (de Paiva et al., 1999). Because improvements in voice volume seem independent of recovery of swallowing, different mechanisms may underlie recovery of these functions.

The benefit is greatest between 1 and 3 months after injection, when the patient's voice is close to normal volume, voice breaks are significantly reduced, and speech is more fluent, with reduced hoarseness (Ludlow et al., 1988). This benefit period differs among the disorders, lasting from 3 to 5 months in ADSD but from 1 to 3 months in other disorders such as ABSD and tremor.

The return of symptoms in ADSD is gradual, usually occurring over a period of about 2 months during endplate reinnervation. To maintain symptom control, most patients return for injection about 3 months before the full return of symptoms. Some individuals, however, maintain benefit for more than a year following injection, returning 2 or more years later for reinjection.

The mechanisms responsible for benefit from BTX-A in laryngeal dystonia likely differ with the different pathophysiologies: although BTX-A is beneficial in many hyperkinetic disorders, it is more effective in some than in others. In all cases BTX-A causes partial denervation, which reduces the force that can be exerted by a muscle following injection. In ADSD, then, the forcefulness of vocal fold hyperadduction is reduced and patients are less able to produce voice breaks even if muscle spasms continue to occur. Central control changes also appear to occur, however, in persons with ADSD following BTX-A injection. When thyroarytenoid muscle injections were unilateral, spasmodic bursts were significantly reduced on both sides of the larynx, and there were also reductions in overall levels of muscle tone (measured in microvolts) and maximum activity levels (Bielamowicz and Ludlow, 2000). Such reductions in muscle activity and spasms may be the result of reductions in muscle spindle and mechanoreceptor feedback, resulting in lower motor neuron pool activity for all the laryngeal muscles. The physiological effects of BTX-A may be greater on the fusimotor system than on muscle fiber innervation (On et al., 1999). Although only one portion of the human thyroarytenoid muscle may contain muscle spindles (Sanders et al., 1998), mucosal mechanoreceptor feedback will also change with reductions in adductory force between the vocal folds following BTX-A injection. Perhaps changes in sensory feedback account for the longer period of benefit in ADSD than in other laryngeal movement disorders, although the duration of side effects is similar in all disorders. Future approaches to altering sensory feedback may also have a role in the treatment of laryngeal dystonia, in addition to efferent denervation by BTX-A.

—*Christy L. Ludlow*

References

Aoki, K. R. (2001). Pharmacology and immunology of botulinum toxin serotypes. *Journal of Neurology, 248*(Suppl. 1), 3–10.

Bielamowicz, S., and Ludlow, C. L. (2000). Effects of botulinum toxin on pathophysiology in spasmodic dysphonia. *Annals of Otology, Rhinology, and Laryngology, 109,* 194–203.

Bielamowicz, S., Squire, S., Bidus, K., and Ludlow, C. L. (2001). Assessment of posterior cricoarytenoid botulinum toxin injections in patients with abductor spasmodic dysphonia. *Annals of Otology, Rhinology, and Laryngology, 110,* 406–412.

Blitzer, A., and Brin, M. F. (1991). Laryngeal dystonia: A series with botulinum toxin therapy. *Annals of Otology, Rhinology, and Laryngology, 100,* 85–89.

Blitzer, A., Brin, M. F., and Stewart, C. F. (1998). Botulinum toxin management of spasmodic dysphonia (laryngeal dystonia): A 12-year experience in more than 900 patients. *Laryngoscope, 108,* 1435–1441.

Blitzer, A., Brin, M., Stewart, C., Aviv, J. E., and Fahn, S. (1992). Abductor laryngeal dystonia: A series treated with botulinum toxin. *Laryngoscope, 102,* 163–167.

Christopher, K. L., Wood, R., Eckert, R. C., Blager, F. B., Raney, R. A., and Souhrada, J. F. (1983). Vocal-cord dysfunction presenting as asthma. *New England Journal of Medicine, 306,* 1566–1570.

Cyrus, C. B., Bielamowicz, S., Evans, F. J., and Ludlow, C. L. (2001). Adductor muscle activity abnormalities in abductor spasmodic dysphonia. *Otolaryngology–Head and Neck Surgery, 124,* 23–30.

de Paiva, A., Meunier, F. A., Molgo, J., Aoki, K. R., and Dolly, J. O. (1999). Functional repair of motor endplates after botulinum neurotoxin type A poisoning: Biphasic switch of synaptic activity between nerve sprouts and their parent terminals. *Proceedings of the National Academy of Sciences of the United States of America, 96,* 3200–3205.

Deleyiannis, F. W., Gillespie, M., Bielamowicz, S., Yamashita, T., and Ludlow, C. L. (1999). Laryngeal long latency response conditioning in abductor spasmodic dysphonia. *Annals of Otology, Rhinology, and Laryngology, 108,* 612–619.

Grillone, G. A., Blitzer, A., Brin, M. F., Annino, D. J., and Saint-Hilaire, M. H. (1994). Treatment of adductor laryngeal breathing dystonia with botulinum toxin type A. *Laryngoscope, 24,* 30.

Koda, J., and Ludlow, C. L. (1992). An evaluation of laryngeal muscle activation in patients with voice tremor. *Otolaryngology–Head and Neck Surgery, 107,* 684–696.

Ludlow, C. L., Naunton, R. F., Sedory, S. E., Schulz, G. M., and Hallett, M. (1988). Effects of botulinum toxin injections on speech in adductor spasmodic dysphonia. *Neurology, 38,* 1220–1225.

Ludlow, C. L., Naunton, R. F., Terada, S., and Anderson, B. J. (1991). Successful treatment of selected cases of abductor spasmodic dysphonia using botulinum toxin injection. *Otolaryngology–Head and Neck Surgery, 104,* 849–855.

Ludlow, C. L., Rhew, K., and Nash, E. A. (1994). Botulinum toxin injection for adductor spasmodic dysphonia. In J. Jankovic and M. Hallett (Eds.), *Therapy with botulinum toxin* (pp. 437–450). New York: Marcel Dekker.

Marion, M. H., Klap, P., Perrin, A., and Cohen, M. (1992). Stridor and focal laryngeal dystonia. *Lancet, 339,* 457–458.

Morrison, M., Rammage, L., and Emami, A. J. (1999). The irritable larynx syndrome. *Journal of Voice, 13,* 447–455.

Nash, E. A., and Ludlow, C. L. (1996). Laryngeal muscle activity during speech breaks in adductor spasmodic dysphonia. *Laryngoscope, 106,* 484–489.

On, A. Y., Kirazli, Y., Kismali, B., and Aksit, R. (1999). Mechanisms of action of phenol block and botulinus toxin type A in relieving spasticity: Electrophysiologic investigation and follow-up. *American Journal of Physical Medicine and Rehabilitation, 78,* 344–349.

Roy, N., Ford, C. N., and Bless, D. M. (1996). Muscle tension dysphonia and spasmodic dysphonia: The role of manual laryngeal tension reduction in diagnosis and management. *Annals of Otology, Rhinology, and Laryngology, 105,* 851–856.

Sanders, I., Han, Y., Wang, J., and Biller, H. (1998). Muscle spindles are concentrated in the superior vocalis subcompartment of the human thyroarytenoid muscle. *Journal of Voice, 12,* 7–16.

Truong, D. D., Rontal, M., Rolnick, M., Aronson, A. E., and Mistura, K. (1991). Double-blind controlled study of botulinum toxin in adductor spasmodic dysphonia. *Laryngoscope, 101,* 630–634.

Van Pelt, F., Ludlow, C. L., and Smith, P. J. (1994). Comparison of muscle activation patterns in adductor and abductor spasmodic dysphonia. *Annals of Otology, Rhinology, and Laryngology, 103,* 192–200.

Warrick, P., Dromey, C., Irish, J. C., Durkin, L., Pakiam, A., and Lang, A. (2000). Botulinum toxin for essential tremor of the voice with multiple anatomical sites of tremor: A crossover design study of unilateral versus bilateral injection. *Laryngoscope, 110,* 1366–1374.

Further Readings

Barkmeier, J. M., Case, J. L., and Ludlow, C. L. (2001). Identification of symptoms for spasmodic dysphonia and vocal tremor: A comparison of expert and nonexpert judges. *Journal of Communication Disorders, 34,* 21–37.

Blitzer, A., Lovelace, R. E., Brin, M. F., Fahn, S., and Fink, M. E. (1985). Electromyographic findings in focal laryngeal dystonia (spastic dysphonia). *Annals of Otology, Rhinology, and Laryngology, 94,* 591–594.

Braun, N., Abd, A., Baer, J., Blitzer, A., Stewart, C., and Brin, M. (1995). Dyspnea in dystonia: A functional evaluation. *Chest, 107,* 1309–1316.

Brin, M. F., Blitzer, A., and Stewart, C. (1998). Laryngeal dystonia (spasmodic dysphonia): Observations of 901 patients and treatment with botulinum toxin. *Advances in Neurology, 78,* 237–252.

Brin, M. F., Stewart, C., Blitzer, A., and Diamond, B. (1994). Laryngeal botulinum toxin injections for disabling stuttering in adults. *Neurology, 44,* 2262–2266.

Cohen, L. G., Ludlow, C. L., Warden, M., Estegui, M. D., Agostino, R., Sedory, S. E., et al. (1989). Blink reflex curves in patients with spasmodic dysphonia. *Neurology, 39,* 572–577.

Davidson, B., and Ludlow, C. L. (1996). Long term effects of botulinum toxin injections in spasmodic dysphonia. *Otolaryngology–Head and Neck Surgery, 105,* 33–42.

Jankovic, J. (1987). Botulinum A toxin for cranial-cervical dystonia: A double-blind, placebo-controlled study. *Neurology, 37,* 616–623.

Jankovic, J. (1988). Cranial-cervical dyskinesias: An overview. *Advances in Neurology, 49,* 1–13.

Jankovic, J., and Linden, C. V. (1988). Dystonia and tremor induced by peripheral trauma: Predisposing factors. *Journal of Neurology, Neurosurgery, and Psychiatry, 51,* 1512–1519.

Lange, D. J., Rubin, M., Greene, P. E., Kang, U. J., Moskowitz, C. B., Brin, M. F., et al. (1991). Distant effects of locally injected botulinum toxin: A double-blind study of single fiber EMG changes. *Muscle and Nerve, 14,* 672–675.

Ludlow, C. L. (1990). Treatment of speech and voice disorders with botulinum toxin. *Journal of the American Medical Association, 264,* 2671–2675.

Ludlow, C. L. (1995). Pathophysiology of the spasmodic dysphonias. In F. Bell-Berti and L. J. Rapheal (Eds.), *Producing speech: Contemporary issues for Katherine Safford Harris* (pp. 291–308). Woodbury, NY: American Institute of Physics.

Ludlow, C. L., VanPelt, F., and Koda, J. (1992). Characteristics of late responses to superior laryngeal nerve stimulation in humans. *Annals of Otology, Rhinology, and Laryngology, 101,* 127–134.

Miller, R. H., Woodson, G. E., and Jankovic, J. (1987). Botulinum toxin injection of the vocal fold for spasmodic dysphonia. *Archives of Otolaryngology–Head and Neck Surgery, 113,* 603–605.

Murry, T., Cannito, M. P., and Woodson, G. E. (1994). Spasmodic dysphonia: Emotional status and botulinum toxin treatment. *Archives of Otolaryngology–Head and Neck Surgery, 120,* 310–316.

Rhew, K., Fiedler, D., and Ludlow, C. L. (1994). Endoscopic technique for injection of botulinum toxin through the flexible nasolaryngoscope. *Otolaryngology–Head and Neck Surgery, 111,* 787–794.

Rosenbaum, F., and Jankovic, J. (1988). Task-specific focal tremor and dystonia: Categorization of occupational movement disorders. *Neurology, 38,* 522–527.

Sapienza, C. M., Walton, S., and Murry, T. (2000). Adductor spasmodic dysphonia and muscular tension dysphonia: Acoustic analysis of sustained phonation and reading. *Journal of Voice, 14,* 502–520.

Sedory-Holzer, S. E., and Ludlow, C. L. (1996). The swallowing side effects of botulinum toxin type A injection in spasmodic dysphonia. *Laryngoscope, 106,* 86–92.

Stager, S. V., and Ludlow, C. L. (1994). Responses of stutterers and vocal tremor patients to treatment with botulinum toxin. In J. Jankovic and M. Hallett (Eds.), *Therapy with botulinum toxin* (pp. 481–490). New York: Marcel Dekker.

Stewart, C. F., Allen, E. L., Tureen, P., Diamond, B. E., Blitzer, A., and Brin, M. F. (1997). Adductor spasmodic dysphonia: Standard evaluation of symptoms and severity. *Journal of Voice, 11,* 95–103.

Witsell, D. L., Weissler, M. C., Donovan, K., Howard, J. F., and Martinkosky, S. J. (1994). Measurement of laryngeal resistance in the evaluation of botulinum toxin injection for treatment of focal laryngeal dystonia. *Laryngoscope, 104,* 8–11.

Zwirner, P., Murry, T., and Woodson, G. E. (1993). A comparison of bilateral and unilateral botulinum toxin treatments for spasmodic dysphonia. *European Archives of Otorhinolaryngology, 250,* 271–276.

Laryngeal Reinnervation Procedures

The human larynx is a neuromuscularly complex organ responsible for three primary and often opposing functions: respiration, swallowing, and speech. The most primitive responsibilities include functioning as a conduit to bring air to the lungs and protecting the respiratory tract during swallowing. These duties are physiologically opposite; the larynx must form a wide caliber during respiration but also be capable of forming a tight sphincter during swallowing. Speech functions are fine-tuned permutations of laryngeal opening and closure against pulmonary airflow. Innervation of this organ is complex, and its design is still being elucidated. Efferent fibers to the larynx from the brainstem motor nuclei travel by way of the vagus nerve to the superior laryngeal nerve (SLN) and the recurrent laryngeal nerves (RLNs). Afferent fibers emanate from intramucosal and intramuscular receptors and travel along pathways that include the SLN (supraglottic larynx) and the RLN (subglottic larynx). Autonomic fibers also innervate the larynx, but these are poorly understood (see also ANATOMY OF THE HUMAN LARYNX).

Reinnervation of the larynx was first reported 1909 by Horsley, who described reanastomosis of a severed RLN. Reports of laryngeal reinnervation spotted the literature over the next several decades, but it was not until the last 30 years that reinnervation techniques were refined and became performed with relative frequency. Surely this is associated with advances in surgical optics as well as microsurgical instrumentation and technique. Indications for laryngeal reinnervation include functional reanimation of the paralyzed larynx, prevention of denervation atrophy, restoration of laryngeal sensation, and modification of pathological innervation (Crumley, 1991; Aviv et al., 1997; Berke et al., 1999).

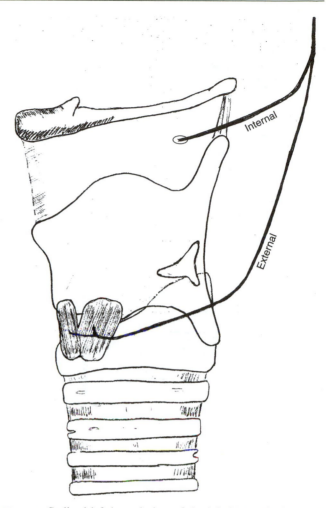

Figure 1. Stylized left lateral view of the left SLN. The internal (sensory) branch pierces the thyrohyoid membrane and terminates in the supraglottic submucosal receptors. The external (motor) branch terminates in the cricothyroid muscle. Branching of the SLN occurs proximally as it exits the carotid sheath.

Anatomy and Technique of Reinnervation. The technique of reinnervation is similar for both sensory and motor systems. The nerve in question is identified through a transcervical approach. Usually a horizontal skin incision is placed into a neck skin crease at about the level of the cricoid cartilage. Subplatysmal flaps are elevated and retracted. The larynx is further exposed after splitting the strap muscles in the midline. Sensation to the supraglottic mucosal is supplied via the internal branch of the SLN. This structure is easily identified as it pierces the thyrohyoid membrane on either side (Fig. 1). The motor innervation of the larynx is somewhat more complicated. All of the intralaryngeal muscles are innervated by the RLN. This nerve approaches the larynx from below in the tracheoesophageal groove. The nerve enters the larynx from deep to the cricothyroid joint and immediately splits into an anterior and a posterior division (Fig. 2). The anterior division supplies all of the laryngeal adductors except the cricothyroid muscle; the posterior division supplies the only abductor of the

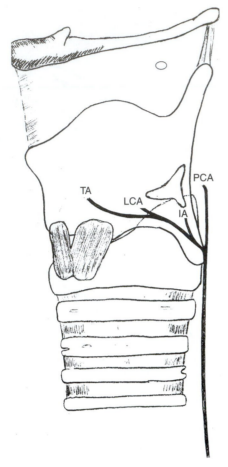

Figure 2. Stylized left lateral view of the left RLN. The branching pattern is quite consistent from patient to patient. The RLN divides into an anterior and a posterior division just deep to the cricothyroid joint. The posterior division travels to the posterior cricoarytenoid (PCA) muscle. The anterior division gives off branches at the interarytenoid (IA) and lateral cricoarytenoid (LCA) muscles and then terminates in the midportion of the thyroarytenoid (TA) muscle. The branches to the TA and LCA are easily seen through a large inferiorly based cartilage window reminiscent of those done for thyroplasty. If preserved during an anterior approach, the inferior cornu of the thyroid cartilage protects the RLN's posterior division and the IA branch during further dissection.

larynx, the posterior cricoarytenoid muscle. The anterior division further arborizes to innervate each of the intrinsic adductors in a well-defined order: the interarytenoid followed by the lateral cricoarytenoid, and lastly the thyroarytenoid muscles. The interarytenoid muscle is thought to receive bilateral innervation, while the other muscles all receive unilateral innervation. The external branch of the SLN innervates the only external adductor of the larynx—the cricothyroid muscle. Although the SLN and the main trunk of the RLN can be approached without opening the larynx, the adductor branches of the RLN can only be successfully approached after opening

the thyroid cartilage. A large inferiorly based window is made in the thyroid lamina and centered over the inferior tubercle. Once the cartilage is opened the anterior branch can be seen coursing obliquely toward the terminus in the midportion of the thyroarytenoid muscle. The posterior division is approached by rotation of the larynx, similar to an external approach to the arytenoid. Identification and dissection of the fine distal nerve branches is usually carried out under louposcopic or microscopic magnification using precision instruments.

Once the damaged nerve is identified, it is severed sharply with a single cut of a sharp instrument. This is important to avoid crushing trauma to the nerve stump. The new motor or sensory nerve is brought into the field under zero tension and then anastomosed with several epineural sutures of fine microsurgical material (9-0 or 10-0 nylon or silk). The anastomosis must be tension-free. The donor nerve is still connected to its proximal (motor) or distal (sensory) cell bodies. Selection of the appropriate donor nerve is discussed subsequently.

Over the next 3–9 months healing occurs, with neurontization of the motor end-plates or the sensory receptors. Although physiological reinnervation is the goal, relatively few reports have demonstrated true volitional movement. Typically, one can hope to prevent muscle atrophy and help restore muscle bulk. Sensory reinnervation is less clear.

Prior to the microsurgical age, most reinnervation procedures of the larynx were carried out with nerve-muscle pedicle implantation into the affected muscle. With modern techniques, end-to-end nerve-nerve anastomosis with epineural suture fixation is a superior and far more reliable technique of reinnervation.

Reinnervation for Laryngeal Paralysis. Paralysis of the larynx is described as unilateral or bilateral. The diagnosis is made on the basis of history and physical examination including laryngoscopic findings, and sometimes on the basis of laryngeal electromyography or radiographic imaging. The unilaterally paralyzed larynx is more common and is characterized by a lateralized vocal cord that prevents complete glottic closure during laryngeal tasks. The patient seeks care for dysphonia and aspiration or cough during swallowing. The etiology is commonly idiopathic, but the condition may be due to inflammatory neuropathy, iatrogenic trauma, or neoplastic invasion of the recurrent nerve. Although many patients are successfully treated with various static procedures, one can argue that, theoretically, the best results would restore the organ to its preexisting physiological state. Over the past 20 years there has been increased interest in physiological restoration, a concept championed by Crumley (Crumley, 1983, 1984, 1991; Crumley, Izdebski, and McMicken, 1988). A series of patients with unilateral vocal cord paralysis were treated with anastomosis of the distal RLN trunk to the ansa cervicalis. The ansa cervicalis is a good example of an acceptable motor donor nerve (Crumley, 1991; Berke et al., 1999). This nerve normally supplies motor neurons to the strap muscles (extrinsic accessory muscles of the larynx), whose function is to elevate and lower the larynx during swallowing. Fortunately, when the ansa cervicalis is sacrificed, the patient does not have noticeable disability. The size match to the RLN is excellent when using either the whole nerve bundle for main trunk anastomosis or an easily identifiable fascicle for connection to the anterior branch.

Hemilaryngeal reinnervation with the ansa cervicalis has been shown to improve voicing in those patients undergoing the procedure (Crumley and Izdebski, 1986; Chhetri et al., 1999). Evaluation of these patients, however, does not demonstrate restoration of normal muscular physiology. The affected vocal cord has good bulk, but volitional movement typically is not restored. Proponents of other techniques have argued that the ansa cervicalis may not have enough axons to properly regenerate the RLN, or that synkinesis has occurred (Paniello, Lee, and Dahm, 1999). Synkinesis refers to mass firing of a motor nerve that can occur after reinnervation. In the facial nerve, for example, one may see mass movement of the face with volitional movement because all the braches are essentially acting as one. The RLN contains both abductor and adductor (as well as a small amount of sensory and autonomic) fibers. With reinnervation, one may hypothesize that mass firing of all fibers cancels the firings of individual fibers out and thus produces a static vocal cord. With this concept in mind, some have recommended combining reinnervation with another static procedure to augment results (combination with arytenoid adduction) or to avoid the potential for synkinesis by performing the anastomosis of the donor nerve to the anterior branch of the recurrent nerve (Green et al., 1992; Nasri et al., 1994; Chhetri et al., 1999).

Paniello has proposed that the ansa cervicalis is not the best donor nerve to the larynx (Paniello, Lee, and Dahm, 1999). He suggests that the hypoglossal nerve would be more appropriate because of increased axon bulk and little donor morbidity. Animal experiments with this technique have demonstrated volitional and reflexive movement of the reinnervated vocal cord.

Neurological bilateral vocal cord paralysis is often post-traumatic or iatrogenic. These patients are troubled by a fixed small airway and often find themselves tracheotomy dependent. Therapy is directed at restoring airway caliber while avoiding aspiration. Voicing issues are usually considered secondary to the airway concerns. Although most practitioners currently treat with static techniques, physiological restoration would be preferred. In the 1970s, Tucker advocated reinnervation of the posterior cricoarytenoid with a nerve muscle pedicle of the sternohyoid muscle and ansa cervicalis (Tucker, 1978). Although his results were supportive of his hypothesis, many have had trouble repeating them. More recently, European groups have studied phrenic nerve to posterior branch of the RLN transfers (van Lith-Bijl et al., 1997, 1998). The phrenic nerve innervates the diaphragm and normally fires with inspiration; it has been shown that one of its nerve roots can be sacrificed without paralysis of the diaphragm. Others have suggested use of the SLN as a motor source for the posterior cricoarytenoid muscle (Maniglia et al., 1989). Most techniques of reinnervation for bilateral vocal cord paralysis still have not enjoyed the success of unilateral reinnervation and are only performed by a few practitioners. The majority of patients with bilateral vocal cord paralysis undergo a static procedure such as cordotomy, arytenoidectomy, or tracheotomy to improve their airway.

Sensory Palsy. Recent work has highlighted the importance of laryngeal sensation. After development of an air-pulse quantification system to measure sensation, it was shown that patients with stroke and dysphagia have a high incidence of laryngosensory deficit. Studies performed in the laboratory demonstrated that reanastomosis of the internal branch of the SLN restored protective laryngeal reflexes (Blumin, Berke, and Blackwell, 1999). Clinically, anastomosis of the greater auricular nerve to the internal branch of the SLN has been successfully used to restore sensation to the larynx (Aviv et al., 1997).

Modification of Dystonia. Spasmodic dysphonia is an idiopathic focal dystonia of the larynx. The majority of patients have the adductor variety, characterized by intermittent and paroxysmal spasms of the vocal cords during connected speech. The mainstay of treatment for this disorder is botulinum toxin (Botox) injections into the affected laryngeal adductor muscles. Unfortunately, the effect of Botox is temporary, and repeated injections are needed indefinitely. A laryngeal denervation and reinnervation procedure has been designed to provide a permanent alternative to Botox treatment (Berke et al., 1999). In this procedure, the distalmost branches of the laryngeal adductors are severed from their muscle insertion. These "bad" nerve stumps are then sutured outside the larynx to avoid spontaneous reinnervation. A fascicle of the ansa cervicalis is then suture-anastomosed to the distal thyroarytenoid branch for reinnervation. Reinnervation maintains tone of the thyroarytenoid, thus preventing atrophy and theoretically protecting that muscle by occupying the motor end-plates with neurons unaffected by the dystonia. This approach has had great success, with about 95% of patients achieving freedom from further therapy.

Laryngeal Transplantation. Transplantation of a physiologically functional larynx is the sought-after grail of reinnervation. For a fully functional larynx, eight nerves would be anastomosed—bilateral anterior and posterior branches of the RLN and bilateral external and internal branches of the SLN. To date, success has been reliably achieved in the canine model (Berke et al., 1993) and partially achieved in one human (Strome et al., 2001). Current research has been aimed at preventing transplant rejection. The technique of microneural, microvascular, and mucosal anastomosis has been well worked out in the animal model.

—Joel H. Blumin and Gerald S. Berke

References

Aviv, J. E., Mohr, J. P., Blitzer, A., Thomson, J. E., and Close, L. G. (1997). Restoration of laryngopharyngeal sensation by neural anastomosis. *Archives of Otolaryngology–Head and Neck Surgery, 123,* 154–160.

Berke, G. S., Blackwell, K. E., Gerratt, B. R., Verneil, A., Jackson, K. S., and Sercarz, J. A. (1999). Selective laryngeal adductor denervation-reinnervation: A new surgical treatment for adductor spasmodic dysphonia. *Annals of Otology, Rhinology, and Laryngology, 108,* 227–231.

Berke, G. S., Ye, M., Block, R. M., Sloan, S., and Sercarz, J. (1993). Orthotopic laryngeal transplantation: Is it time? *Laryngoscope, 103,* 857–864.

Blumin, J. H., Ye, M., Berke, G. S., and Blackwell, K. E. (1999). Recovery of laryngeal sensation after superior laryngeal nerve anastomosis. *Laryngoscope, 109,* 1637–1641.

Chhetri, D. K., Gerratt, B. R., Kreiman, J., and Berke, G. S. (1999). Combined arytenoid adduction and laryngeal reinnervation in the treatment of vocal fold paralysis. *Laryngoscope, 109,* 1928–1936.

Crumley, R. L. (1983). Phrenic nerve graft for bilateral vocal cord paralysis. *Laryngoscope, 93,* 425–428.

Crumley, R. L. (1984). Selective reinnervation of vocal cord adductors in unilateral vocal cord paralysis. *Annals of Otology, Rhinology, and Laryngology, 93,* 351–356.

Crumley, R. L. (1991). Update: Ansa cervicalis to recurrent laryngeal nerve anastomosis for unilateral laryngeal paralysis. *Laryngoscope, 101,* 384–387.

Crumley, R. L., Izdebski, K. (1986). Voice quality following laryngeal reinnervation by ansa hypoglossi transfer. *Laryngoscope, 96,* 611–616.

Crumley, R. L., Izdebski, K., and McMicken, B. (1988). Nerve transfer versus Teflon injection for vocal cord paralysis: A comparison. *Laryngoscope, 98,* 1200–1204.

Green, D. C., Berke, G. S., Graves, M. C., Natividad, M. (1992). Physiologic motion after vocal cord reinnervation: A preliminary study. *Laryngoscope, 102,* 14–22.

Horsley, J. S. (1909). Suture of the recurrent laryngeal nerve with report of a case. *Transactions of the Southern Surgical Gynecology Association, 22,* 161–167.

Maniglia, A. J., Dodds, B., Sorensen, K., Katirji, M. B., and Rosenbaum, M. L. (1989). Newer technique of laryngeal reinnervation: Superior laryngeal nerve (motor branch) as a driver of the posterior cricoarytenoid muscle. *Annals of Otology, Rhinology, and Laryngology, 98,* 907–909.

Nasri, S., Sercarz, J. A., Ye, M., Kreiman, J., Gerratt, B. R., and Berke, G. S. (1994). Effects of arytenoid adduction on laryngeal function following ansa cervicalis nerve transfer for vocal fold paralysis in an *in vivo* canine model. *Laryngoscope, 104,* 1187–1193.

Paniello, R. C., Lee, P., and Dahm, J. D. (1999). Hypoglossal nerve transfer for laryngeal reinnervation: A preliminary study. *Annals of Otology, Rhinology, and Laryngology, 108,* 239–244.

Strome, M., Stein, J., Esclamado, R., Hicks, D., Lorenz, R. R., Braun, W., et al. (2001). Laryngeal transplantation and 40-month follow-up. *New England Journal of Medicine, 3443,* 1676–1679.

Tucker, H. M. (1978). Human laryngeal reinnervation: Long term experience with the nerve muscle pedicle technique. *Laryngoscope, 88,* 598–604.

van Lith-Bijl, J. T., Stolk, R. J., Tonnaer, J. A. D. M., Groenhout, C., Konings, P. N. M., and Mahieu, H. F. (1997). Selective laryngeal reinnervation with separate phrenic and ansa cervicalis nerve transfers. *Archives of Otolaryngology–Head and Neck Surgery, 123,* 406–411.

van Lith-Bijl, J. T., Stolk, R. J., Tonnaer, J. A. D. M., Groenhout, C., Konings, P. N. M., and Mahieu, H. F. (1998). Laryngeal abductor reinnervation with a phrenic nerve transfer after a 9-month delay. *Archives of Otolaryngology–Head and Neck Surgery, 124,* 393–398.

Further Readings

Benninger, M. S., Crumley, R. L., Ford, C. N., Gould, W. J., Hanson, D. G., Ossoff, R. H., et al. (1994). Evaluation and treatment of the unilateral paralyzed vocal fold. *Otolaryngology–Head and Neck Surgery, 111,* 497–508.

Crumley, R. L. (1989). Laryngeal synkinesis: Its significance to the laryngologist. *Annals of Otology, Rhinology, and Laryngology, 98,* 87–92.

Crumley, R. L. (1991). Muscle transfer for laryngeal paralysis: Restoration of inspiratory vocal cord abduction by phrenicomohyoid transfer. *Archives of Otolaryngology–Head and Neck Surgery, 117,* 1113–1117.

Crumley, R. L. (2000). Laryngeal synkinesis revisited. *Annals of Otology, Rhinology, and Laryngology, 109,* 365–371.

Flint, P. W., Downs, D. H., and Coltrera, M. D. (1991). Laryngeal synkinesis following reinnervation in the rat: Neuroanatomic and physiologic study using retrograde fluorescent tracers and electromyography. *Annals of Otology, Rhinology, and Laryngology, 100,* 797–806.

Jacobs, I. N., Sanders, I., Wu, B. L., and Biller, H. F. (1990). Reinnervation of the canine posterior cricoarytenoid muscle with sympathetic preganglionic neurons. *Annals of Otology, Rhinology, and Laryngology, 99,* 167–174.

Kreyer, R., and Pomaroli, A. (2000). Anastomosis between the external branch of the superior laryngeal nerve and the recurrent laryngeal nerve. *Clinical Anatomy, 13,* 79–82.

Marie, J. P., Lerosey, Y., Dehesdin, D., Tadie, M., and Andrieu-Guitrancourt, J. (1999). Cervical anatomy of phrenic nerve roots in the rabbit. *Annals of Otology, Rhinology, and Laryngology, 108,* 516–521.

Paniello, R. C., West, S. E., and Lee, P. (2001). Laryngeal reinnervation with the hypoglossal nerve: I. Physiology, histochemistry, electromyography, and retrograde labeling in a canine model. *Annals of Otology, Rhinology, and Laryngology, 110,* 532–542.

Peterson, K. L., Andrews, R., Manek, A., Ye, M., and Sercarz, J. A. (1998). Objective measures of laryngeal function after reinnervation of the anterior and posterior recurrent laryngeal nerve branches. *Laryngoscope, 108,* 889–898.

Sercarz, J. A., Nguyen, L., Nasri, S., Graves, M. C., Wenokur, R., and Berke, G. S. (1997). Physiologic motion after laryngeal nerve reinnervation: A new method. *Otolaryngology–Head and Neck Surgery, 116,* 466–474.

Tucker, H. M. (1999). Long-term preservation of voice improvement following surgical medialization and reinnervation for unilateral vocal fold paralysis. *Journal of Voice, 13,* 251–256.

van Lith-Bijl, J. T., and Mahieu, H. F. (1998). Reinnervation aspects of laryngeal transplantation. *European Archives of Otorhinolaryngology, 255,* 515–520.

Weed, D. T., Chongkolwatana, C., Kawamura, Y., Burkey, B. B., Netterville, J. L., Ossoff, R. H., et al. (1995). Reinnervation of the allograft larynx in the rat laryngeal transplant model. *Otolaryngology–Head and Neck Surgery, 113,* 517–529.

Zheng, H., Li, Z., Zhou, S., Cuan, Y., and Wen, W. (1996). Update: laryngeal reinnervation for unilateral vocal cord paralysis with the ansa cervicalis. *Laryngoscope, 106,* 1522–1527.

Zheng, H., Zhou, S., Chen, S., Li, Z., and Cuan, Y. (1998). An experimental comparison of different kinds of laryngeal muscle reinnervation. *Otolaryngology–Head and Neck Surgery, 119,* 540–547.

Laryngeal Trauma and Peripheral Structural Ablations

Alterations of the vibratory, articulatory, or resonance system consequent to traumatic injury or the treatment of disease can significantly alter the functions of both voice and speech, and potentially deglutition and swallowing. In some instances, subsequent changes to the larynx and oral peripheral system may be relatively minor and without substantial consequence to the individual. In other instances these changes may result in dramatic alteration of one or more anatomical structures necessary for normal voice and speech production, in addition to other oral functions. Traumatic injury and surgical treatment for disease also may affect isolated structures of the peripheral speech mechanism, or may have more widespread influences on entire speech subsystems (e.g., articulatory, velopharyngeal) and the related structures necessary for competent and effective verbal communication.

Laryngeal Trauma

Trauma to the larynx is a relatively rare clinical entity. Estimates in the literature indicate that acute laryngeal trauma accounts for 1 in 15,000 to 1 in 42,000 emergency room visits. A large number of such traumatic injuries are the result of accidental blunt trauma to the neck; causes include motor vehicle collisions, falls, athletic injuries, and the like. Another portion of these injuries are the result of violence, such as shooting or stabbing, which may result in penetrating injuries not only of the larynx but also of other critical structures in the neck. Blunt laryngeal trauma is most commonly reported in persons less than 30 years old.

In cases of blunt trauma to the larynx, the primary presenting symptoms are hoarseness, pain, dyspnea (shortness of breath), dysphagia, and swelling of the tissues of the neck (cervical emphysema). Injuries may involve fractures of laryngeal cartilages, partial or complete dislocations, lacerations of soft tissues, or combined types of injury. Because laryngeal trauma, no matter how minor, holds real potential to affect breathing, medical intervention is first directed at determining airway patency and, when necessary, maintaining an adequate airway through emergency airway management (Schaefer, 1992). When airway compromise is observed, emergency tracheotomy is common. Laryngeal trauma is truly an emergency medical condition. When injuries are severe, additional surgical treatment may be warranted. Thus, whereas vocal disturbances are possible, the airway is of primary concern; changes to the voice are of secondary importance.

Injuries to the intrinsic structures of the oral cavity are also rare, although when they do occur, changes in speech, deglutition, and swallowing may exist. Although the clinical literature is meager in relation to injuries of the lip, alveolus, floor of the mouth, tongue, hard palate, and velum, such injuries or their medical treatment may have a significant impact on speech. Trauma to the mandible also can directly impact verbal communication. Unfortunately, the literature in this area is sparse, and information on speech outcomes following injuries of this type is frequently anecdotal. However, in addressing any type of traumatic injury to the peripheral structures of the speech mechanism, assessment methods typically employed with the dysarthrias may be most appropriate (e.g., Dworkin, 1991). In this regard, the point-place system may provide essential information on the extent and degree of impairment of speech subsystems (Netsell and Daniel, 1979).

Speech Considerations. Speech management initially focuses on identifying which subsystems are impaired, the severity of impairment, and the consequent reduction in speech intelligibility and communicative proficiency. A comprehensive evaluation that involves aerodynamic, acoustic, and auditory-perceptual components is essential. Information from each of these areas is valuable in identifying the problem, developing management strategies, and monitoring patient progress. Because of variability in the extent of traumatic injuries, the literature on the dysarthrias often provides a useful framework for establishing clinical goals and evaluating treatment effectiveness.

Peripheral Structural Changes Resulting from Surgical Ablation

In contrast to peripheral structural changes due to traumatic injury, structural changes due to surgical ablation for oral cancer also result in alterations in functions necessary for speech or swallowing. The treatment itself has clear potential to affect speech production, but changes in speech may be variable and ultimately depend on the structures treated.

Malignant Conditions Affecting Peripheral Structures of the Speech System. Head and neck squamous cell carcinoma may occur in the epithelial tissue of the mouth, nasal cavity, pharynx, or larynx. Tumors of the head and neck account for approximately 5% of all malignancies in men and 2% of all malignancies in women (Franceschi et al., 2000). The majority of head and neck cancers involve squamous epithelial tissue. These tumors have the potential to be invasive; therefore, the potential for spread of disease is substantial, and radical dissection of regional lymphatics is often required. Because of the possibility of disease spread, radiation therapy is commonly used to eliminate occult disease, and this treatment may have negative consequences on vocal and speech functions.

As tumors increase in size, they may invade adjacent tissue, which frequently requires more extensive treatment because of the threat of distant spread of disease. Some individuals are asymptomatic at the time of diagnosis; others report pain, difficulty swallowing (dysphagia), or difficulty breathing. The destructive nature of a malignant tumor may cause adjacent muscular structures of the tongue or floor of mouth to become fixed. In other situations, the tumor may encroach on the nerve supply, which is likely to result in loss of sensation (paresthesia), paralysis, or pain. In both circumstances, the potential for metastatic spread of disease is substantial.

Current treatment protocols for tumors involving structures of the peripheral speech mechanism include surgery, radiotherapy, or chemotherapy, alone or in combination. The choice of modality usually depends on tumor location, disease stage, cell type, and other factors. Each treatment modality is associated with some additional morbidity that can significantly affect structure, function, cosmesis, and quality of life. Surgery carries a clear potential for anatomical and physiological changes that may directly alter speech and swallowing, while at the same time creating significant cosmetic deformities. Similarly, radiotherapy is commonly associated with a range of side effects. Radiation delivered to the head and neck affects both abnormal and normal tissues. Salivary glands may be damaged, with a resulting decrease in salivary flow leading to a dry mouth (xerostomia). This decrease in saliva may then challenge normal oral hygiene and health, which may result in dental caries following radiation treatment. Osteoradionecrosis may result in the exposure of bone, tissue changes, or infection, which usually cause significant discomfort to the individual. Osteoradionecrosis may be decreased if the radiation exposure is limited to less than 60 cGy (Thorn et al., 2000). In some cases, surgery may be necessary to debride infected tissue or to remove damaged bone, with a subsequent need for grafting. Hyperbaric oxygen therapy is sometimes used to reduce the degree of osteoradionecrosis (Marx, Johnson, and Kline, 1985). This therapy facilitates oxygen uptake in blood and related tissues, which in turn improves vascularity, thus reducing tissue damage and related osteoradionecrotic changes following extractions (Marx, 1983a, 1983b).

Once primary medical treatment (surgery, radiotherapy) has been completed, the goals of rehabilitation are to maintain or restore anatomical structure and physiological function. However, if the lesion is extensive and destructive, with distant spread, and subsequent treatment is contraindicated, palliative care may be initiated instead. Palliative care focuses on pain control and maintaining some level of nutrition, respiration, and human dignity.

Defects of the Maxilla and Velum.   Surgery is the preferred method for treating cancer of the maxilla. Such procedures vary in the extent of resection and may be performed transorally or transfacially. Because surgical extirpation of maxillary tumors may involve extensive resection, a significant reduction in the essential structures for speech may exist post-treatment. Surgical reduction of the gum ridge (alveolus) as well as the hard and soft palates may occur. Although defects of the alveolus may be augmented quite well prosthetically, more significant surgical resections of the hard and soft palate frequently have a dramatic influence on speech production. The primary deficit observed is velopharyngeal incompetence due to structural defects that eliminate the ability to effectively seal the oral cavity from the nasal cavity (Brown et al., 2000).

When considerable portions of both the hard and the soft palate are removed, the integrity of the oral valve for articulatory shaping and the subsequent demands of the resonance system are substantially affected, often with profound influences on oral communication. The goals of rehabilitation include reducing the surgical defect through prosthetic management so that the individual can eat, drink, and attain some level of functional speech. Rehabilitation involves a multidisciplinary team and occurs over several months, during which the postsurgical anatomy changes and the prosthesis is changed in tandem. Healing and other effects of treatment also need to be addressed during this period.

Defects of the Tongue, Floor of Mouth, Alveolus, Lip, and Mandible.   Surgery for traumatic injury or tumors that invade the mandible, tongue, and floor of the mouth is frequently more radical than surgery for injuries or tumors of the maxilla. The mandible and tongue are movable structures that are intricately involved in swallowing and speech production. Focal excisions may not result in any significant level of noticeable change in deglutition, swallowing, or speech. However, when larger resections are performed on the tongue (partial or total glossectomy) or floor of the mouth, reconstruction with one of a variety of flap procedures is necessary. Large resections and reconstructions also increase the potential for speech disruption because of limited mobility of the reconstructed areas (e.g., portions of the tongue). Defects in the alveolar ridge or lip may have variable effects on speech and general oral function. The literature in this area is scant to nonexistent; however, changes to the lip and alveolus may certainly limit the production of specific speech sounds. For example, anterior sounds in which the lip is an active articulator (e.g., labiodental sounds), sounds that rely on pressure build-up (e.g., stop-plosive sounds), or sounds that require a fixed position for continuous generation or oral airway turbulence (e.g., lingual-alveolar sounds), among others, may be altered by surgical ablation of these structures. In many instances, these types of problems can be addressed using methods commonly employed for articulation therapy. Slowing the speech rate may help to augment articulatory precision in the presence of such defects following surgical treatment.

Isolated mandibular tumors are rare, but regional spread of cancer to the mandible from other oral structures is not uncommon. Extended lesions involving the mandible often require surgical resection. Because cancer has invaded bone, resections are often substantial, subsequently requiring reconstruction with donor bone or plate reconstruction methods. However, changes in the mobility of the mandible pose a risk for changes in the overall acoustic structure of speech due to changes in oral resonance. Prosthetic rehabilitation for jaw defects resulting from injury or malignancy is essential (Adisman, 1990). However, mandibular reconstructions may permit the individual to manipulate the mandible with relative efficiency for speech and swallowing movements. Again, this area is not well documented in the clinical literature.

Oral Articulatory Evaluation. Total or partial removal of the tongue (glossectomy) or resection of the anterior maxilla or mandible results in significant speech impairment. The results of peripheral structural ablations of the oral speech system are best addressed using the methods recommended for treatment of the dysarthrias (e.g., Kent et al., 1989). Acoustic analysis, including evaluation of formant frequency, amplitude, and spectral moments, is of clinical value (Gillis and Leonard, 1982; Leonard and Gillis, 1982; Tobey and Lincks, 1989). Acoustic considerations relative to speech intelligibility should also be addressed in this population using tools developed for the dysarthrias (Kent et al., 1989).

Prosthetic Management. To optimize the care of each patient, the expertise of multiple professionals, including a dentist, prosthodontist, head and neck surgeon, prosthetist, speech-language pathologist, and radiologist, is necessary. Surgical treatment of maxillary tumors can result in a variety of problems postsurgically. For example, leakage of food or drink into the nasal cavity significantly disrupts eating and drinking. This may be compounded by difficulties in chewing food or by dysphagia, so that nutritional problems must always be considered. Additionally, such surgical defects reduce articulatory precision and change the acoustic structure of speech because of changes in the volume of the vocal tract as well as resultant hypernasality and nasal emission (abnormal and perhaps excessive flow of air through the nasal cavity). Together, these types of changes to the peripheral oral structures will almost certainly result in decreased speech intelligibility and communication. In order for speech improvement to occur, the surgical defect must be augmented with a prosthesis. This is typically a multistage process, with the first obturator being placed in situ at the time of surgery. The initial obturator is maintained for 1–2 weeks, at which time an interim device is fabricated. Most individuals use the interim device until complete healing has occurred and related treatments are completed, usually anywhere from 3 to 6 months after surgery. At this time a final or definitive obturator is fabricated. Although some minor adjustments to the definitive prosthesis are not uncommon, this obturator will be maintained permanently (Desjardins, 1977, 1978; Anderson et al., 1992).

Prosthetic Management of Surgical Defects. Early oral rehabilitation is essential, for reasons that go beyond speech concerns. The surgical obturator allows careful packing of the wound site, keeps food and other debris from entering the wound, permits eating, drinking, and swallowing without a nasogastric tube, and allows immediate oral communication (Doyle, 1999; Leeper and Gratton, 1999). However, certain factors may alter the course of rehabilitation. Fabrication of a prosthesis is more difficult when teeth are absent, as this creates problems in fitting and retention of the prosthesis, which may result in secondary problems. When the jaw is disrupted, changes in symmetry may emerge that may influence chewing and swallowing. For soft palate defects, early prostheses can be modified throughout the course of treatment to facilitate swallowing and speech. Because respiration is paramount, the devices must be created so that they do not impede normal breathing.

In general, intraoral prostheses for those with surgical defects of peripheral oral structures seek to maintain the oral and nasal cavities as separate entities and to reduce velopharyngeal orifice area. Reduction of surgically induced velopharyngeal incompetence is essential to enhancing residual speech capabilities, particularly following larger resections of the maxilla. In addition to the obvious defects in the structural integrity of the peripheral oral mechanism, treatment may disrupt neural processes, including both afferent and efferent components of the system. As such, speech assessment must evaluate the motor capacity as well as the capacity of the sensory system.

When reductions in the ability of the tongue to approximate superior structures of the oral cavity exist after treatment, attempts to facilitate this ability may be achieved by constructing a "palatal drop" prosthesis, which supplements lingual inability by bringing the new hard palate inferior in the oral cavity. The individual may then have greater ability to make the necessary oral contacts to improve articulatory precision and speech intelligibility (e.g., Aramany et al., 1982; Gillis and Leonard, 1983). Such a prosthesis is useful in patients who have healed after undergoing a maxillectomy or maxillary-mandibular resection. Prosthetic adaptations of this type may also benefit eating and swallowing. These devices serve both speech and swallowing by helping to reduce velopharyngeal defects.

Speech Assessment

Systematic assessment of the peripheral speech mechanism includes formal evaluation of all subsystems—respiratory, laryngeal, velopharyngeal, and articulatory. As each component of the system is assessed, its relative contributions to the overall speech deficits observed can be better defined for purposes of treatment monitoring. Subsystem evaluation may entail instrumentally based assessments (speech aerodynamics and acoustics), which elicit information on the aeromechanical relationship to oral port size and tongue–hard palate valving (Warren and DuBois, 1964), auditory-perceptual evaluations of speech or voice parameters, and measures of speech intelligibility (Leeper, Sills, and Charles, 1993; Leeper and

Gratton, 1999). Use of Netsell and Daniel's (1979) physiological model allows the clinician to identify the relative contribution of each speech subsystem and to target appropriate therapy techniques in an effort to optimize the system. The physiologic approach also permits continuous evaluation of each component in a comparative manner for prosthesis-in and prosthesis-out conditions. Such evaluations aid in fine-tuning prosthetic management.

Once obturation occurs, direct speech treatment goals may include improving the control of the respiratory support system for speech, determining and maintaining the optimal speech rate, increasing the accuracy of specific sound production (or potentially the directed compensation of sound substitutions), improving intelligibility through overarticulation, modulating vocal intensity to improve oral resonance, and related tasks that seek to improve intelligibility. Treatment goals may best be achieved by using the methods previously described for the dysarthrias (Dworkin, 1991).

—Philip C. Doyle

References

Adisman, I. (1990). Prosthesis serviceability for acquired jaw defects. *Dental Clinics of North America, 34,* 265–284.

Anderson, J. D., Awde, J. D., Leeper, H. A., and Sills, P. S. (1992). Prosthetic management of the head and neck cancer patient. *Canadian Journal of Oncology, 2,* 110–118.

Aramany, M. A., Downs, J. A., Beery, Q. C., and Ayslan, F. (1982). Prosthodontic rehabilitation for glossectomy patients. *Journal of Prosthetic Dentistry, 48,* 78–81.

Brown, J. S., Rogers, S. N., McNally, D. N., and Boyle, M. (2000). A modified classification for the maxillectomy defect. *Head and Neck, 22,* 17–26.

Desjardins, R. P. (1977). Early rehabilitative management of the maxillectomy patient. *Journal of Prosthetic Dentistry, 38,* 311–318.

Desjardins, R. P. (1978). Obturator design for acquired maxillary defects. *Journal of Prosthetic Dentistry, 39,* 424–435.

Doyle, P. C. (1999). Postlaryngectomy speech rehabilitation: Contemporary concerns in clinical care. *Journal of Speech-Language Pathology and Audiology, 23,* 109–116.

Dworkin, J. P. (1991). *Motor speech disorders: A treatment guide.* St. Louis: Mosby.

Franceschi, S., Bidoli, E., Herrero, R., and Munoz, N. (2000). Comparison of cancers of the oral cavity and pharynx worldwide: Etiological clues. *Oral Oncology, 36,* 106–115.

Gillis, R. E., and Leonard, R. J. (1983). Prosthetic treatment for speech and swallowing in patients with total glossectomy. *Journal of Prosthetic Dentistry, 50,* 808–814.

Kent, R. D., Weismer, G., Kent, J. F., and Rosenbek, J. C. (1989). Toward phonetic intelligibility testing in dysarthria. *Journal of Speech and Hearing Disorders, 54,* 482–499.

Leeper, H. A., and Gratton, D. G. (1999). Oral prosthetic rehabilitation of individuals with head and neck cancer: A review of current practice. *Journal of Speech-Language Pathology and Audiology, 23,* 117–133.

Leeper, H. A., Sills, P. S., and Charles, D. (1993). Prosthodontic management of maxillofacial and palatal defects. In K. T. Moller and C. D. Starr (Eds.), *Cleft palate: Interdisciplinary issues and treatment* (p. 145). Austin, TX: Pro-Ed.

Leonard, R. J., and Gillis, R. E. (1982). Effects of a prosthetic tongue on vowel intelligibility and food management in a patient with total glossectomy. *Journal of Speech and Hearing Disorders, 47,* 25–29.

Marx, R. E. (1983a). Osteoradionecrosis: A new concept of its pathophysiology. *Journal of Oral and Maxillofacial Surgery, 41,* 283–288.

Marx, R. E. (1983b). A new concept in the treatment of osteoradionecrosis. *Journal of Oral and Maxillofacial Surgery, 41,* 351–357.

Marx, R. E., Johnson, R. P., and Kline, S. N. (1985). Prevention of osteoradionecrosis: A randomized prospective clinical trial of hyperbaric oxygen vs. penicillin. *Journal of the American Dental Association, 111,* 49–54.

Netsell, R., and Daniel, B. (1979). Dysarthria in adults: Physiologic approach to rehabilitation. *Archives of Physical Medicine and Rehabilitation, 60,* 502–508.

Schaefer, S. D. (1992). The acute management of external laryngeal trauma. *Archives of Otolaryngology–Head and Neck Surgery, 118,* 598–604.

Thorn, J. J., Hansen, H. S., Specht, L., and Bastholt, L. (2000). Osteoradionecrosis of the jaws: Clinical characteristics and relation to the field of irradiation. *Journal of Oral and Maxillofacial Surgery, 58,* 1088–1093.

Tobey, E. A., and Lincks, J. (1989). Acoustic analyses of speech changes after maxillectomy and prosthodontic management. *Journal of Prosthetic Dentistry, 62,* 449–455.

Warren, D. W., and DuBois, A. B. (1964). A pressure-flow technique for measuring velopharyngeal orifice area during spontaneous speech. *Cleft Palate Journal, 1,* 52–71.

Further Readings

Balogh, J., and Sutherland, S. (1983). Osteoradionecrosis of the mandible: A review. *American Journal of Otolaryngology, 13,* 82.

Batsakis, J. G. (1979). Squamous cell carcinomas of the oral cavity and the oropharynx. In J. G. Batsakis (Ed.), *Tumours of the head and neck: Clinical and pathological considerations* (2nd ed.). Baltimore: Williams and Wilkins.

Beumer, J., Curtis, T., and Marunick, M. (1996). *Maxillofacial rehabilitation: Prosthodontic and surgical considerations.* St. Louis: Ishiyaki EuroAmerica.

Cherian, T. A., and Raman, V. R. R. (1993). External laryngeal trauma: Analysis of 30 cases. *Journal of Laryngology and Otology, 107,* 920–923.

Doyle, P. C. (1994). *Foundations of voice and speech rehabilitation following laryngeal cancer* (pp. 97–122). San Diego, CA: Singular Publishing Group.

Gussack, G. S., Jurkovich, G. J., and Luterman, A. (1986). Laryngotracheal trauma. *Laryngoscope, 96,* 660–665.

Goldenberg, D., Golz, A., Flax-Goldenberg, R., and Joachims, H. Z. (1997). Severe laryngeal injury cased by blunt trauma to the neck: A case report. *Journal of Laryngology and Otology, 111,* 1174–1176.

Haribhakti, V., Kavarana, N., and Tibrewala, A. (1993). Oral cavity reconstruction: An objective assessment of function. *Head and Neck, 15,* 119–124.

Hassan, S. J., and Weymuller, E. A. (1993). Assessment of quality of life in head and neck cancer patients. *Head and Neck, 15,* 485–496.

Jewett, B. S., Shockley, W. W., and Rutledge, R. (1999). External laryngeal trauma analysis of 392 patients. *Archives of Otolaryngology–Head and Neck Surgery, 125,* 877–880.

Kornblith, A. B., Zlotolow, I. M., Gooen, J., Huryn, J. M., Lerner, T., Strong, E. W., Shah, J. P., Spiro, R. H., and

Holland, J. C. (1996). Quality of life of maxillectomy patients using an obturator prosthesis. *Head and Neck, 18,* 323–334.

Lapointe, H. J., Lampe, H. B., and Taylor, S. M. (1996). Comparison of maxillectomy patients with immediate versus delayed obturator prosthesis placement. *Journal of Otolaryngology, 25,* 308–312.

Light, J. (1997). Functional assessment testing for maxillofacial prosthetics. *Journal of Prosthetic Dentistry, 77,* 388–393.

List, M. A., Ritter-Sterr, C. A., Baker, T. M., Colangelo, L. A., Matz, G., Pauloksi, B. R., and Logemann, J. A. (1996). Longitudinal assessments of quality of life in laryngeal cancer patients. *Head and Neck, 18,* 1–10.

Logemann, J. A., Kahrilas, P. J., Hurst, P., Davis, J., and Krugler, C. (1989). Effects of intraoral prosthetics on swallowing in patients with oral cancer. *Dysphagia, 4,* 118–120.

Mahanna, G. K., Beukelman, D. R., Marshall, J. A., Gaebler, C. A., and Sullivan, M. (1998). Obturator prostheses after cancer surgery: An approach to speech outcome assessment. *Journal of Prosthetic Dentistry, 79,* 310–316.

Myers, E. M., and Iko, B. O. (1987). The management of acute laryngeal trauma. *Journal of Trauma, 4,* 448–452.

Pauloski, B., Logemann, J., Rademaker, A., McConnel, F., Heiser, M., Cardinale, S., et al. (1993). Speech and swallowing function after anterior tongue and floor of mouth resection with distal flap reconstruction. *Journal of Speech and Hearing Research, 36,* 267–276.

Robbins, K., Bowman, J., and Jacob, R. (1987). Postglossectomy deglutitory and articulatory rehabilitation with palatal augmentation prosthesis. *Archives of Otolaryngology–Head and Neck Surgery, 113,* 1214–1218.

Sandor, G. K. B., Leeper, H. A., and Carmichael, R. P. (1997). Speech and velopharyngeal function. *Oral and Maxillofacial Surgery Clinics of North America, 9,* 147–165.

Schaefer, S. D., and Close, L. C. (1989). Acute management of laryngeal trauma. *Annals of Otology, Rhinology, and Laryngology, 98,* 98–104.

Warren, D. W. (1979). PERCI: A method for rating palatal efficiency. *Cleft Palate Journal, 16,* 279–285.

Wedel, A., Yontchev, E., Carlsson, G., and Ow, R. (1994). Masticatory function in patients with congenital and acquired maxillofacial defects. *Journal of Prosthetic Dentistry, 72,* 303–308.

Psychogenic Voice Disorders: Direct Therapy

Psychogenic voice disorder refers to a voice disorder that is a manifestation of some *confirmed* psychological disequilibrium (Aronson, 1990). In its purest form, the psychogenic voice disorder is not associated with structural laryngeal changes or frank central or peripheral nervous system pathology. It is asserted that the larynx, by virtue of its neural connections to emotional centers within the brain, is vulnerable to excess or poorly regulated musculoskeletal tension arising from stress, conflict, fear, and emotional inhibition (Case, 1996). Such dysregulated laryngeal muscle tension can interfere with normal voice and give rise to complete aphonia (i.e., whispered speech) or partial voice loss (dysphonia). Although numerous theories have been offered to explain psychogenic voice loss, the precise mechanisms underlying such psychologically based disorders have not been fully elucidated (see FUNCTIONAL VOICE DISORDERS for a review). Despite considerable controversy surrounding causal mechanisms, the clinical voice literature is replete with evidence that symptomatic voice therapy for psychogenic disorders can often result in rapid and dramatic voice improvement (Koufman and Blalock, 1982; Aronson, 1990; Milutinovic, 1990; Carding and Horsley, 1992; Roy and Leeper, 1993; Gunther et al., 1996; Roy et al., 1997; Andersson and Schalen, 1998; Carding, Horsley, and Docherty, 1999; Stemple, 2000). The following discussion considers voice therapy techniques aimed at directly alleviating vocal symptoms without specific attention to the putative psychological dysfunction underlying the disorder.

Before symptomatic therapy is begun, the laryngological findings are reviewed with the patient, and he or she is reassured regarding the absence of any structural laryngeal pathology. An explanation of the problem is then provided by the clinician. While the specific approach and emphasis vary among clinicians, the discussion typically includes some explanation of the untoward effects of excess or dysregulated muscle tension on voice production and its probable link to stress, situational conflicts, or other psychological precursors that were identified during the interview. The confident clinician provides brief information regarding the therapy plan and the likelihood of a positive outcome.

Because excess or dysregulated laryngeal muscle tension is frequently offered as the proximal cause of the psychogenic voice disorder, many voice therapies including yawn-sigh resonant voice therapy, visual and electromyographic biofeedback, chewing therapy, progressive relaxation, and circumlaryngeal massage aimed at reducing or rebalancing such tension (Boone and McFarlane, 2000). Prolonged hypercontraction of laryngeal muscles is often associated with elevation of the larynx and hyoid bone, with associated pain and discomfort when the circumlaryngeal region is palpated. Aronson (1990) and Roy and Bless (1998) have described manual techniques to determine the presence and degree of laryngeal musculoskeletal tension, as well as methods to relieve such tension during the diagnostic assessment and management session. Circumlaryngeal massage is one such treatment approach. Skillfully applied, systematic kneading of the extralaryngeal region is believed to stretch muscle tissue and fascia, promote local circulation with removal of metabolic wastes, relax tense muscles, and relieve pain and discomfort associated with muscle spasms. The hypothesized physical effect of such massage is reduced laryngeal height and stiffness and increased mobility. Once the larynx is "released" and range of motion is normalized, proportional improvement in voice is said to follow. Improvement in voice and reductions in pain and laryngeal height suggest a relief of tension (Roy and Ferguson, 2001). In a similar vein, Roy and Bless (1998) also recently described a number of manual laryngeal reposturing techniques that can stimulate improved voice and briefly interrupt patterns of muscle misuse. These brief moments of voice improvement associated with laryngeal reposturing maneuvers are immediately identified for the patient and reinforced. Digital cues can then be faded and the patient taught to rely on sensory feedback (auditory, kinesthetic, and proprioceptive) to maintain improved laryngeal positioning and muscle balance. Any partial relapses or return of abnormal voice during the therapy process can be dealt with by reassurance, verbal reinstruction, or manual cueing. Once the larynx is correctly positioned, recovery of normal voice can occur rapidly.

Certain patients with psychogenic dysphonia and aphonia appear to have lost kinesthetic awareness and volitional control over voice production for speech and communication purposes, yet display normal voicing for vegetative or nonspeech acts. For instance, some aphonic and severely dysphonic patients may be able to clear the throat, grunt, cough, sigh, gargle, laugh, hum, or produce a high-pitched squeak with normal or near-normal voice quality. Such preserved voicing for non-speech purposes represents a clue to the capacity for normal phonation. In symptomatic therapy, then, the patient is asked to produce such vocal behaviors. The goal of these voice maneuvers is to elicit even a brief trace of clearer voice so that it may be shaped toward normal quality or extended to longer utterances. These efforts follow a trial-and-error pattern and require the seasoned clinician to be constantly vigilant, listening for any brief moments of clearer voice. When improved voice is elicited, it is instantly reinforced, and the clinician provides immediate feedback regarding the positive change. During this process, the patient needs to be an active participant and is encouraged to continually self-monitor the type and manner of voice produced. Once this brief but relatively normal voice is reliably achieved, it is shaped and extended into sustained vowels, words, simple phrases, and oral reading. When this phase of intervention is successful, the patient is then engaged in casual conversation that begins with basic biographical information and proceeds to brief narratives, and then conversation about any topic and with anyone in the clinical setting. If established, the restored voice is usually maintained without compensatory effort and may improve further during conversation. Finally, the clinician should debrief the patient regarding the cause of the voice improvement, discuss the patient's feelings about the improved voice, and review possible causes of the problem and the prognosis for maintaining normal voice.

Certainly, direct symptomatic therapy for psychogenic voice disorders can produce rapid changes; however, in some cases voice therapy can be a frustrating and protracted experience for both clinician and patient (Bridger and Epstein, 1983; Fex et al., 1994). The rate of improvement during therapy for psychogenic voice disorders varies. Patients may progress gradually through various stages of dysphonia on their way to normal voice recovery. Other patients will appear to experience sudden return of voice without necessarily transitioning through phases of decreasing severity (Aronson, 1990).

Because there are few studies directly comparing the effectiveness of specific therapy techniques, not much is known about whether one therapy approach for psychogenic voice disorder is superior to another. Although signs of improvement should typically be observed within the first session, some patients may need an extended, intensive treatment session or several sessions, depending on several variables, including the therapy techniques selected, clinician experience and confidence in administering the approach, and patient motivation and tolerance, to mention only a few.

The anecdotal clinical literature suggests that the prognosis for sustained removal of abnormal symptoms in psychogenic aphonia or dysphonia may depend on several factors. First, the time between the onset of voice problem and the initiation of therapy may be important. The sooner voice therapy is initiated following the onset of the voice problem, the better the prognosis. If months or years have elapsed, it may be more difficult to eliminate the abnormal symptoms. Second, the more extreme the voice symptoms, the better the prognosis for improvement. Aphonia and extreme tension, according to some authorities, may be easier to modify than intermittent or mild dysphonia. Third, if significant secondary gain is present, this may interfere with progress and contribute to a poorer treatment outcome. Finally, if the underlying psychological triggers are no longer active, then normal voice should be established quickly and improvement should be sustained (Aronson, 1990; Duffy, 1995; Case, 1996; Colton and Casper, 1996). As a caveat, however, the foregoing observations have rarely been studied in any objective manner; therefore they are best regarded as clinical impressions rather than factual statements.

The long-term effectiveness of direct voice therapy for psychogenic voice disorders also has not been rigorously evaluated (Pannbacker, 1998; Ramig and Verdolini, 1998). Most clinicians report that relapse is infrequent and isolated, yet others report more frequent post-treatment recurrences. Of the few investigations that exist, the results regarding the durability of voice improvement following direct therapy are mixed (Gunther et al., 1996; Roy et al., 1997; Andersson and Schalen, 1998; Carding, Horsley, and Docherty, 1999). It should be acknowledged that following direct voice therapy, only the symptom of psychological disturbance has been removed, not the disturbance itself (Brodnitz, 1962; Kinzl, Biebl, and Rauchegger, 1988). Therefore, the nature of psychological dysfunction needs to be better understood. If the situational, emotional, or personality features that contributed to the development of the psychogenic voice disorder remain unchanged following behavioral treatment, it would be logical to expect that such persistent factors would increase the probability of future recurrences (Nichol, Morrison, and Rammage, 1993; Andersson and Schalen, 1998). Therefore, in some cases, post-treatment referral to a psychiatrist or psychologist may be necessary to achieve more enduring improvements in the patient's emotional adjustment and voice function (Butcher, Elias, and Raven, 1993; Roy et al., 1997).

In summary, psychogenic voice disorders are powerful examples of the intimate connection between mind and body. These voice disorders, which occur in the absence of structural laryngeal pathology, often represent some of the most severely disturbed voices encountered by voice pathologists. In an experienced clinician's hands, direct symptomatic therapy for psychogenic voice disorders can produce rapid and remarkable restoration of normal voice. Much remains to be learned regarding the underlying bases of these disorders and the long-term effect of direct therapeutic interventions.

See also FUNCTIONAL VOICE DISORDERS.

—*Nelson Roy*

References

Andersson, K., and Schalen, L. (1998). Etiology and treatment of psychogenic voice disorder: Results of a follow-up study of thirty patients. *Journal of Voice, 12,* 96–106.

Aronson, A. E. (1990). *Clinical voice disorders: An interdisciplinary approach* (3rd ed.). New York: Thieme.

Boone, D. R., and McFarlane, S. C. (2000). *The voice and voice therapy* (6th ed.). Boston: Allyn and Bacon.

Bridger, M. M., and Epstein, R. (1983). Functional voice disorders: A review of 109 patients. *Journal of Laryngology and Otology, 97,* 1145–1148.

Brodnitz, F. S. (1962). Functional disorders of the voice. In N. M. Levin (Ed.), *Voice and speech disorders: Medical aspects* (pp. 453–481). Springfield, IL: Charles C Thomas.

Butcher, P., Elias, A., and Raven, R. (1993). *Psychogenic voice disorders and cognitive behaviour therapy.* San Diego, CA: Singular Publishing Group.

Butcher, P., Elias, A., Raven, R., Yeatman, J., and Littlejohns, D. (1987). Psychogenic voice disorder unresponsive to speech therapy: Psychological characteristics and cognitive-behaviour therapy. *British Journal of Disorders of Communication, 22,* 81–92.

Carding, P., and Horsley, I. (1992). An evaluation study of voice therapy in non-organic dysphonia. *European Journal of Disorders of Communication, 27,* 137–158.

Carding, P., Horsley, I., and Docherty, G. (1999). A study of the effectiveness of voice therapy in the treatment of 45 patients with nonorganic dysphonia. *Journal of Voice, 13,* 72–104.

Case, J. L. (1996). *Clinical management of voice disorders* (3rd ed.). Austin, TX: Pro-Ed.

Colton, R., and Casper, J. K. (1996). *Understanding voice problems: A physiological perspective for diagnosis and treatment.* Baltimore: Williams and Wilkins.

Duffy, J. R. (1995). *Motor speech disorders: Substrates, differential diagnosis, and management.* St. Louis: Mosby.

Fex, F., Fex, S., Shiromoto, O., and Hirano, M. (1994). Acoustic analysis of functional dysphonia: Before and after voice therapy (Accent Method). *Journal of Voice, 8,* 163–167.

Gunther, V., Mayr-Graft, A., Miller, C., and Kinzl, H. (1996). A comparative study of psychological aspects of recurring and non-recurring functional aphonias. *European Archives of Otorhinolaryngology, 253,* 240–244.

Kinzl, J., Biebl, W., and Rauchegger, H. (1988). Functional aphonia: Psychosomatic aspects of diagnosis and therapy. *Folia Phoniatrica, 40,* 131–137.

Koufman, J. A., and Blalock, P. D. (1982). Classification and approach to patients with functional voice disorders. *Annals of Otology, Rhinology, and Laryngology, 91,* 372–377.

Milutinovic, Z. (1990). Results of vocal therapy for phono-neurosis: Behavior approach. *Folia Phoniatrica, 42,* 173–177.

Nichol, H., Morrison, M. D., and Rammage, L. A. (1993). Interdisciplinary approach to functional voice disorders: The psychiatrist's role. *Otolaryngology–Head and Neck Surgery, 108,* 643–647.

Pannbacker, M. (1998). Voice treatment techniques: A review and recommendations for outcome studies. *American Journal of Speech-Language Pathology, 7,* 49–64.

Ramig, L. O., and Verdolini, K. (1998). Treatment efficacy: Voice disorders. *Journal of Speech, Language, and Hearing Research, 41*(Suppl.), S101–S116.

Roy, N., and Bless, D. M. (1998). Manual circumlaryngeal techniques in the assessment and treatment of voice disorders. *Current Opinion in Otolaryngology and Head and Neck Surgery, 6,* 151–155.

Roy, N., Bless, D. M., Heisey, D., and Ford, C. F. (1997). Manual circumlaryngeal therapy for functional dysphonia: An evaluation of short- and long-term treatment outcomes. *Journal of Voice, 11,* 321–331.

Roy, N., and Ferguson, N. A. (2001). Formant frequency changes following manual circumlaryngeal therapy for functional dysphonia: Evidence of laryngeal lowering? *Journal of Medical Speech-Language Pathology, 9,* 169–175.

Roy, N., and Leeper, H. A. (1993). Effects of the manual laryngeal musculoskeletal tension reduction technique as a treatment for functional voice disorders: Perceptual and acoustic measures. *Journal of Voice, 7,* 242–249.

Roy, N., McGrory, J. J., Tasko, S. M., Bless, D. M., Heisey, D., and Ford, C. N. (1997). Psychological correlates of functional dysphonia: An evaluation using the Minnesota Multiphasic Personality Inventory. *Journal of Voice, 11,* 443–451.

Schalen, L., and Andersson, K. (1992). Differential diagnosis and treatment of psychogenic voice disorder. *Clinical Otolaryngology, 17,* 225–230.

Stemple, J. (2000). *Voice therapy: Clinical studies* (2nd ed.). San Diego, CA: Singular Publishing Group.

The Singing Voice

The functioning of the voice organ in singing is similar to that in speech. Thus, the origin of the sound is the *voice source*—the pulsating airflow through the glottis. The voice source is mainly controlled by three physiological factors, subglottal pressure, length and stiffness of the vocal folds, and the degree of glottal adduction. These control parameters determine vocal loudness, F0, and mode of phonation, respectively. The voice source is a complex tone composed of a series of harmonic partials of amplitudes decreasing by about 12 dB per octave as measured in flow units. It propagates through the vocal tract and is thereby filtered in a manner determined by its resonance or *formant frequencies*. These frequencies are determined by the vocal tract shape. For most vowel sounds, the two lowest formant frequencies determine vowel quality, while the higher formant frequencies belong to the personal voice characteristics.

Breathing.   Subglottal pressure determines vocal loudness and is therefore used for expressive purposes in singing. It is also varied with F0, such that higher pitches are sung with higher subglottal pressures than lower pitches. As a consequence, singers need to vary subglottal pressure constantly, adapting it to both loudness and pitch. This is in sharp contrast to speech, where subglottal pressure is much more constant. Singers therefore need to develop a virtuosic control of the breathing apparatus. In addition, subglottal pressures in singing are varied over a larger range than in speech. Thus, while in loud speech subglottal pressure may be raised to 1.5 or 2 kPa, singers may use pressures as high as 4 or 6 kPa for loud tones sung at high pitches.

Subglottal pressure is determined by active forces produced by the breathing muscles and passive forces produced by gravity and the elasticity of the breathing apparatus. Elasticity, generated by the lungs and the rib cage, varies with lung volume. At high lung volumes, elasticity produces an exhalatory force that may amount to 3 kPa or more. At low lung volumes, elasticity contributes an inhalatory force. Whereas in conversational speech, no more than about 15%–20% of the total lung capacity is used, classically trained singers use an average lung volume range that is more than twice as large and occasionally may vary from 100% to 0% of the total vital capacity in long phrases.

As the elasticity forces change from exhalatory at high lung volumes to inhalatory at low lung volumes, they reach an equilibrium at a certain lung volume. This lung volume is called the functional residual capacity (FRC). In tidal breathing, inhalations are started from FRC. In both speech and singing, lung volumes above FRC are preferred. Because much higher lung volumes are used in singing than in speech, singers need to deal with much greater exhalatory elasticity forces.

Voice Source. The airflow waveform of the voice source is characterized by quasi-triangular pulses, produced when the vocal folds open the glottis, and followed by horizontal portions near or at zero airflow, produced when the folds close the glottis more or less completely (Fig. 1).

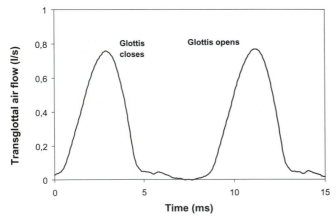

Figure 1. Typical flow glottogram showing transglottal airflow versus time.

The acoustic significance of the waveform is straightforward. The slope of the source spectrum is determined mainly by the negative peak of the differentiated flow waveform, frequently referred to as the maximum flow declination rate. It represents the main excitation of the vocal tract. This steepness is linearly related to the subglottal pressure in such a way that a doubling of subglottal pressure causes an SPL increase of about 10 dB. The amplitude gain of higher partials is greater than that of lower partials. Thus, if the sound level of a vowel sound is increased by 10 dB, the partials near 3 kHz typically increase by about 17 dB.

The air volume contained in a flow pulse is decisive to the amplitude of the source spectrum fundamental and is strongly influenced by the overall glottal adduction force. Thus, for a given subglottal pressure, a firmer adduction produces a smaller air volume in a pulse, which reduces the amplitude of the fundamental. An exaggerated glottal adduction thus attenuates the fundamental. This phonation mode is generally referred to as hyperfunctional or pressed. The opposite extreme—that is, the habitual use of too faint adduction—is called hypofunctional and prevents the vocal folds from closing the glottis also during the vibratory cycle. As a result, airflow escapes the glottis during the quasi-closed phase. This generates noise and produces a strong fundamental. This phonation mode is often referred to as breathy.

In classical singing, pressed phonation is typically avoided. Instead, singers seem to strive to reduce glottal adduction to the minimum that will still result in glottal closure during the closed phase. This generates a source spectrum with strong high partials and a strong fundamental. This type of phonation has been called flow phonation or resonant voice. In nonclassical singing, on the other hand, pressed phonation is occasionally used for high, loud tones, apparently for expressive purposes.

A main characteristic of classical singing is the vibrato. It corresponds to a quasi-periodic modulation of F0 (Fig. 2). The pitch perceived from a vibrato tone corresponds to its average F0. The modulation frequency, mostly between 5 and 7 Hz, is generally referred to as the vibrato rate and is rather constant for a singer. Curiously enough, however, it tends to increase somewhat toward the end of tones. The peak-to-peak modulation range is varied between nil and less than two semitones, or $F0 \cdot 2^{1/6}$. With increasing age, singers' vibrato rates tend to decrease by about one-half hertz per decade of years, and vibrato extent tends to increase by about 15 cent per decade.

The vibrato is generated by a rhythmical pulsation of the cricothyroid muscles. When contracting, these muscles cause a stretching of the vocal folds, and so raise F0. The neural origin of this pulsation is not understood. One possibility is that it emanates from a cocontraction of the cricothyroid and vocalis muscles.

In speech, pitch is perceived in a continuous fashion, such that a continuous variation in F0 is heard as a continuous variation of pitch. In music, on the other hand, pitch is perceived categorically, where the categories are scale tones or the intervals between them. Thus,

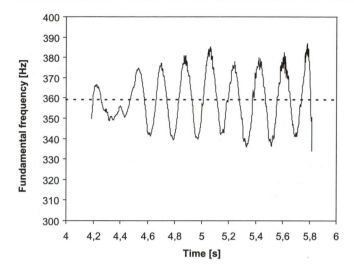

Figure 2. Example of vibrato.

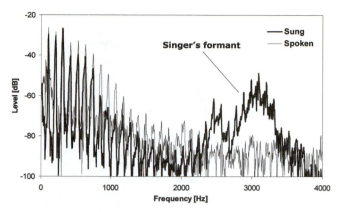

Figure 3. Spectra of the vowel [u] as spoken and sung by a classically trained baritone singer.

the F0 continuum is divided logarithmically into a series of bins, each of which corresponds to a scale tone. The width of each scale tone is approximately 6% wide, and the center frequency of a scale tone is $2^{1/12}$ higher than its lower neighbor.

The demands for pitch accuracy are quite high in singing. Experts generally find that a tone is out of tune when it deviates from the target F0 by more than about 7 cent, or 0.07 of a semitone interval. This corresponds to less than one-tenth of a typical vibrato extent. The target F0 generally agrees with equal-tempered tuning, where the interval between adjacent scale tones corresponds to the F0 ratio of $1:2^{1/12}$. However, apparently depending on the musical context, the target F0 for a scale tone may deviate from its value in equal-tempered tuning by about a tenth of a semitone interval.

Resonance. The formant frequencies in classical singing differ between voice classifications. Thus, basses have lower formant frequencies than baritones, who have lower formant frequencies than tenors. These differences probably reflect differences in vocal tract length. The formant frequencies also deviate from those typically found in speech. For example, the second formant of the vowel [i] is generally considerably lower in classical singing than in speech, such that the vowel quality approaches that of the vowel [y].

These formant frequency deviations are related to the *singer's formant*, a marked spectrum envelope peak between approximately 2.5 and 3 kHz, that appears in all voiced sounds produced by classically trained male singers and altos (Fig. 3). It is produced by a clustering of F3, F4, and F5. This clustering seems to be achieved by combining a narrow opening of the larynx tube with a wide pharynx. If the area ratio between the larynx tube opening and the pharynx approximates 1:6 or less, the larynx tube acts as a separate resonator in the sense that its resonance frequency is rather insensitive to the cross-sectional area in the remaining parts of the vocal tract.

Its resonance frequency can be somewhere between 2.5 and 3 kHz. If this resonance is appropriately tuned, it will provide a formant cluster.

A common method to achieve a wide pharynx seems to be to lower the larynx, which is typically observed in classically trained singers. Lowering the larynx lengthens the pharynx cavity. As F2 of the vowel [i] is mainly dependent on the pharynx length, it will be lowered by a lowering of the larynx. In nonclassical singing, more speechlike formant frequencies are used, and no singer's formant is produced.

The center frequency of the singer's formant varies between voice classifications. On average, it tends to be about 2.4, 2.6, and 2.8 kHz for basses, baritones, and tenors, respectively. These differences, which contribute significantly to the characteristic voice qualities of these classifications, probably reflect differences in vocal tract length.

The singer's formant spectrum peak is particularly prominent in bass and baritone singers. In tenors and altos it is less prominent and in sopranos it is generally not observable. Thus, sopranos do not seem to produce a singer's formant.

The singer's formant seems to serve the purpose of enhancing the voice when accompanied by a loud orchestra. The long-term-average spectrum of a symphonic orchestra typically shows a peak near 0.5 kHz followed by a descent of about 9 dB per octave toward higher frequencies (Fig. 4). Therefore, the sound level of an orchestra is comparatively low in the frequency region of the singer's formant, so that the singer's formant makes the singer's voice easier to perceive. As the singer's formant is produced mainly by vocal tract resonance, it can be regarded as a manifestation of vocal economy. It does not appear in nonclassical singing, where the soloist is provided with a sound amplification system that takes care of audibility problems. Also, it is absent or much less prominent among choral singers, whose voices are supposed to blend, such that individual singers' voices are difficult to discern.

The approximate pitch range of a singer is about two octaves. Typical ranges for basses, baritones, tenors,

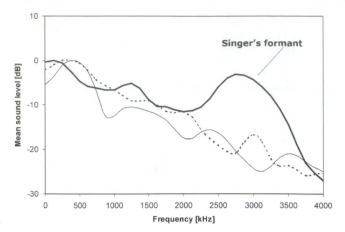

Figure 4. Long-term-average spectrum of an orchestra with and without a tenor soloist (heavy solid and dashed curves). The thin solid curve shows a rough approximation of a corresponding analysis of neutral speech at conversational loudness.

altos, and sopranos are E2–E4 (82–330 Hz), G2–G4 (98–392 Hz), C3–C5 (131–523 Hz), F3–F5 (175–698 Hz), and C4–C6 (262–1047 Hz), respectively. This implies that F0 is often higher than the typical value of F1 in some vowels. Singers, however, seem to avoid the situation in which F0 is higher than F1. Instead, they increase F1 so that it is always higher than F0. For the vowel [a], this is achieved by widening the jaw opening; the higher the pitch, the wider the jaw opening. For other vowels, singers seem first to reduce the tongue constriction of the vocal tract, and resort to a widening of the jaw opening when the effect of this neutralization of the articulation fails to produce further increase of F1.

Because F1 and F2 are decisive to the perception of vowels, the substantial departures from the typical formant frequency values in speech affect vowel identification. Yet vowel identification is surprisingly successful also at high F0. Most isolated vowel sounds can be correctly identified up to an F0 of about 500 Hz. Above this frequency, identification deteriorates quickly and remains low for most vowels at F0 higher than 700 Hz. In reality, however, text intelligibility can be greatly improved by consonants.

Health Risks. Because singers are extremely dependent on the perfect functioning of their voices, they often need medical attention. A frequent origin of their voice disorders is a cold, which typically causes dryness of the glottal mucosa. This disturbs the normal function of the vocal folds. Also relevant would be their use of high subglottal pressures. An inappropriate vocal technique, sometimes associated with a habitually exaggerated glottal adduction or with singing in a too high pitch range, also tends to cause voice disorders, which in some cases may lead to developing vocal nodules. Such nodules generally disappear after voice rest, and surgical treatment is mostly considered inappropriate.

See also VOICE ACOUSTICS.

—*Johan Sundberg*

References

Sundberg, J. (1987). *The science of the singing voice.* DeKalb, IL: Northern Illinois University Press.
Titze, I. (1994). *Principles of voice production.* Englewood Cliffs, NJ: Prentice Hall.

Vocal Hygiene

Vocal hygiene has been part of the voice treatment literature continuously since the publication of Mackenzie's *The Hygiene of Vocal Organs*, in 1886. In it the author, a noted otolaryngologist, described many magical prescriptions used by famous singers to care for their voices. In 1911, a German work by Barth included a chapter with detailed discussion of vocal hygiene. The ideas about vocal hygiene expressed in this book were similar to those expressed in the current literature. Concern was raised about the effects of tobacco, alcohol, loud and excessive talking, hormones, faulty habits, and diet on the voice. Another classic text was *Diseases and Injuries of the Larynx*, published in 1942. The authors, Jackson and Jackson, implicated various vocal abuses as the primary causes of voice disorders, and cited rest and refraint from the behavior as the appropriate treatment. Luchsinger and Arnold (1965) stressed the need for attention to the physiological norm as the primary postulate of vocal hygiene and preventive laryngeal medicine. Remarkably, these authors discussed the importance of this type of attention not only for teachers and voice professionals, but also for children in the classroom. Subsequently, virtually all voice texts have addressed the issue of vocal hygiene.

Both the general public and professionals in numerous disciplines commonly use the term *hygiene*. The 29th edition of *Dorland's Medical Dictionary* defines it as "the science of health and its preservation." Thus, we can take vocal hygiene to mean the science of vocal health and the proper care of the vocal mechanism. Despite long-held beliefs about the value of certain activities most frequently discussed as constituting vocal hygiene, the science on which these ideas are based was, until quite recently, more implied and deduced than specific.

Patient education and vocal hygiene are both integral to voice therapy. Persons who are educated about the structure and function of the phonatory mechanism are better able to grasp the need for care to restore it to health and to maintain its health. Thus, the goal of patient education is understanding. Vocal hygiene, on the other hand, focuses on changing an individual's vocal behavior. In some instances, a therapy program may be based completely on vocal hygiene. More frequently, however, vocal hygiene is but one spoke in a total therapy program that also includes directed instruction in voice production techniques.

Although there are commonalities among vocal hygiene programs regardless of the pathophysiology of the voice disorder, that pathophysiology should dictate some specific differences in the vocal hygiene approach. In addition to the nature of the voice disorder, factors such as timing of the program relative to surgery (i.e., pre or post), and whether the vocal hygiene training stands alone or is but one aspect of a more extensive therapy process, must also inform specific aspects of the vocal hygiene program.

Hydration and environmental humidification are particularly important to the health of the voice, and, as such, should be a focus of all vocal hygiene programs. A number of authors have studied the effects of hydration and dehydration of vocal fold mucosa and viscosity of the folds on phonation threshold pressure (PTP). (PTP is the minimum subglottal pressure required to initiate and maintain vocal fold vibration.) For example, Verdolini et al. (1990, 1994) studied PTP in normal speakers subjected to hydrating and dehydrating conditions. Both PTP and self-perceived vocal effort were lower after hydration. Jiang, Ng, and Hanson (1999) showed that vocal fold oscillations cease in a matter of minutes in fresh excised canine larynges deprived of humidified air. Rehydration by dripping saline onto the folds restored the oscillations, demonstrating the need for hydration and surface moisture for lower PTP.

In one light, viscosity is a measure of the resistance to deformation of the vocal fold tissue. Viscosity is increased by hydration and decreased by drying—hence the importance of vocal fold hydration to ease of phonation. Moreover, it appears that the body has robust cellular and neurophysiological mechanims to conserve the necessary hydration of airway tissues. In a study of patients undergoing dialysis, rapid removal of significant amounts of body water increased PTP and was associated with symptoms of mild vocal dysfunction in some patients. Restoration of the body fluid reversed this trend (Fisher et al., 2001). Jiang, Lin, and Hanson (2000) noted the presence of mucous glands in the tissue of the vestibular folds and observed that these glands distribute a very important layer of lubricating mucus to the surface of the vocal folds. Environmental hydration facilitates the vocal fold vibratory behavior, mainly because of the increased water content in this mucous layer and in the superficial epithelium. The viscosity of secretions is thickened with ingestion of foods or medications with a drying or diuretic effect, radiation therapy, inadequate fluid intake, and the reduction in mucus production in aging.

Thus, there appear to be a number of mechanisms, not yet fully understood, by which the hydration of vocal fold mucosa and the viscosity of the vocal folds are directly involved in the effort required to initiate and maintain phonation. Both environmental humidity and surface hydration are important physiological factors in determining the energy needed to sustain phonation. External or superficial hydration may occur as a by-product of drinking large amounts of water, which increases the secretions in and around the larynx and lowers the viscosity of those secretions. Steam inhalation and environmental humidification further hydrate the surface of the vocal folds, and mucolytic agents may decrease the viscosity of the vocal folds. Clearly, the lower the phonation threshold pressure, the less air pressure is required and the greater is the ease of pho-

nating. Many questions remain in this area, such as the most effective method of hydration.

Other major components of vocal hygiene programs are reducing vocal intensity by eliminating shouting or speaking above high ambient noise levels, avoiding frequent throat clearing and other phonotraumatic behaviors. The force of collision (or impact) of the vocal folds has been described by Titze (1994) as proportional to vibrational amplitude and vibrational frequency. This was explored further in phonation by Jiang and Titze (1994), who showed that intraglottal contact increases with increased vocal fold adduction. Titze (1994) theorized that if a vibrational dose reaches and exceeds a threshold level in a predisposed individual, tissue injury will probably ensue. This lends support to the widespread belief that loud and excessive voice use, and indeed other forms of harsh vocal productions, can cause vocal fold pathology. It also supports the view that teachers and others in vocally demanding professions are prone to vibration overdose, with inadequate recovery time. Thus, the stage is set for cyclic tissue injury, repair, and eventual voice or tissue change.

The complexity of vocal physiology suggests a direct connection between viscosity and hydration, phonation threshold pressure, and the effects of collision and shearing forces. The greater the viscosity of vocal fold tissue, the higher the PTP that is required and the greater is the internal friction or shearing force in the vocal fold. These effects may explain vocal fold injuries, particularly with long-term vocal use that involves increased impact stress on the tissues during collision and shearing stresses (Jiang and Titze, 1994). Thus, issues of collision and the impact forces associated with increased loudness and phonotraumatic vocalization are appropriately addressed in vocal hygiene programs and in directed therapy approaches.

Reflux, both gastroesophageal and laryngopharyngeal, affects the health of the larynx and pharynx. Gastric acid and gastric pepsin, the latter implicated in the delayed healing of submucosal laryngeal injury (Koufman, 1991), have been found in refluxed material. Laryngopharyngeal reflux has been implicated in a long list of laryngeal conditions, including chronic or intermittent dysphonia, vocal fatigue, chronic throat clearing, reflux laryngitis, vocal nodules, and malignant tissue changes. Treatment may include dietary changes, lifestyle modifications, and medication. Surgery is usually a treatment of last resort. Caffeine, tobacco, alcohol, fried foods, and excessive food intake have all been implicated in exacerbating the symptoms of laryngopharyngeal reflux. Thus, vocal hygiene programs that address healthy diet and lifestyle and that include reflux precautions appear to be well-founded. It is now common practice for patients scheduled for any laryngeal surgery to be placed on a preoperative course of antireflux medication that will be continued through the postoperative healing stage. Although this is clearly a medical treatment, the speech-language pathologist should provide information and supportive guidance through vocal hygiene instruction to ensure that patients follow the prescribed protocol.

An unanswered question is whether a vocal hygiene therapy program alone is adequate treatment for vocal problems. Roy et al. (2001) found no significant improvement in a group of teachers with voice disorders after a course of didactic training in vocal hygiene. Teachers who received a directed voice therapy program (Vocal Function Exercises), however, experienced significant improvement. It should be noted that the vocal hygiene program used in this study, being purely didactic and requiring no activity on the part of the participants, might more appropriately be described as a patient education program. Chan (1994) reported that a group of non-voice-disordered kindergarten teachers did show positive behavioral changes following a program of vocal education and hygiene. In another study, Roy et al. (2002) examined the outcome of voice amplification versus vocal hygiene instruction in a group of voice-disordered teachers. Most pairwise contrasts directly comparing the effects of the two approaches failed to reach significance. Although the vocal hygiene group showed changes in the desired direction on all dependent measures, the study results suggest that the benefits of amplification may have exceeded those of vocal hygiene instruction. Of note, the amplification group reported higher levels of extraclinical compliance with the program than the vocal hygiene group. This bears out the received wisdom that it is easier to take a pill—or wear an amplification device—than to change habits.

Although study results are mixed, there is insufficient evidence to suggest that vocal hygiene instruction be abandoned. The underlying rationale for vocal hygiene is sufficiently compelling that a vocal hygiene program should continue to be a component of a broad-based voice therapy intervention.

—*Janina K. Casper*

References

Barth, E. (1911). *Einfuhrung in die Physiologie, Pathologie und Hygiene der Menschlichen Stimme und Sprache*. Leipzig: Thieme.

Chan, R. W. (1994). Does the voice improve with vocal hygiene education? A study of some instrumental voice measures in a group of kindergarten teachers. *Journal of Voice, 8*, 279–291.

Fisher, K. V., Ligon, J., Sobecks, J. L., and Rose, D. M. (2001). Phonatory effects of body fluid removal. *Journal of Speech, Language, and Hearing Research, 44*, 354–367.

Jackson, C., and Jackson, C. L. (1942). *Diseases and injuries of the larynx*. New York: Macmillan.

Jiang, J., Lin, E., and Hanson, D. (2000). Vocal fold physiology. *Otolaryngologic Clinics of North America, 1*, 699–718.

Jiang, J., Ng, J., and Hanson, D. (1999). The effects of rehydration on phonation in excised canine larynges. *Journal of Voice, 13*, 51–59.

Jiang, J., and Titze, I. R. (1994). Measurement of vocal fold intraglottal pressure and impact stress. *Journal of Voice, 8*, 132–144.

Koufman, J. A. (1991). The otolaryngologic manifestations of gastroesophageal reflux disease: A clinical investigation of 225 patients using ambulatory 24 hr pH monitoring and an experimental investigation of the role of acid and pepsin in the development of laryngeal injury. *Laryngoscope, 101*(Suppl. 53), 1–78.

Luchsinger, R., and Arnold, G. E. (1965). *Voice-speech-language*. Belmont, CA: Wadsworth.

Mackenzie, M. (1886). *The hygiene of vocal organs*. London: Macmillan.

Roy, N., Gray, S. D., Simon, M., Dove, H., Corbin-Lewis, K., and Stemple, J. C. (2001). An evaluation of the effects of two treatment approaches for teachers with voice disorders: A prospective randomized clinical trial. *Journal of Speech, Language, and Hearing Research, 44*, 286–296.

Roy, N., Weinrich, V., Gray, S. D., Tanner, K., Toledo, S. W., Dove, H., et al. (2001). Voice amplification versus vocal hygiene instruction for teachers with voice disorders: A treatment outcome study. *Journal of Speech, Language, and Hearing Research, 44*, 286–296.

Titze, I. R. (1994). *Principles of voice production*. Englewood Cliffs, NJ: Prentice Hall.

Verdolini, K., Titze, I. R., and Fennell, A. (1994). Dependence of phonatory effort on hydration level. *Journal of Speech, Language, and Hearing Research, 37*, 1001–1007.

Verdolini-Marsten, K., Titze, I., and Druker, D. (1990). Changes in phonation threshold pressure with induced conditions of hydration. *Journal of Voice, 4*, 142–151.

Vocal Production System: Evolution

The human vocal production system is similar in broad outline to that of other terrestrial vertebrates. All tetrapods (nonfish vertebrates: amphibians, reptiles, birds, and mammals) inherit from a common ancestor three key components: (1) a respiratory system with lungs; (2) a larynx that acts primarily as a quick-closing gate to protect the lungs, and often secondarily to produce sound; and (3) a supralaryngeal vocal tract which filters this sound before emitting it into the environment. Despite this shared plan, a wide variety of interesting modifications of the vocal production system are known. The functioning of the basic tetrapod vocal production system can be understood within the theoretical framework of the myoelastic-aerodynamic and source/filter theories familiar to speech scientists.

The lungs and attendant respiratory musculature provide the air stream powering phonation. In primitive air-breathing vertebrates, the lungs were inflated by rhythmic compression of the oral cavity, or "buccal pumping," and this system is still used by lungfish and amphibians (Brainerd and Ditelberg, 1993). Inspiration by active expansion of the thorax evolved later, in the ancestor of reptiles, birds, and mammals. This was powered originally by the intercostal muscles (as in lizards or crocodilians) and later (in mammals only) by a muscular diaphragm (Liem, 1985). Phonation is typically powered by passive deflation of the elastic lungs, or in some cases by active compression of the hypaxial musculature. In many frogs, air expired from the lungs during phonation is captured in an elastic air sac, which then deflates, returning the air to the lungs. This allows frogs to produce multiple calls from the same volume of air. The inflated sac also increases the efficiency with which sound is radiated into the environment (Gans, 1973).

The lungs are protected by a larynx in all tetrapods. This structure primitively includes a pair of barlike cartilages that can be separated (for breathing) or pushed together (to seal the airway) (Negus, 1949). Expiration through the partially closed larynx creates a turbulent hiss—perhaps the most primitive vocalization, which virtually all tetrapods can produce. However, more sophisticated vocalizations became possible after the innovation of elastic membranes within the larynx, the vocal cords, which are found in most frogs, vocal reptiles (geckos, crocodilians), and mammals. Although the larynx in these species can support a wide variety of vocalizations, its primary function as a protective gateway appears to have constrained laryngeal anatomy. In birds, a novel phonatory structure called the syrinx evolved at the base of the trachea. Dedicated to vocal production, and freed from the necessity of tracheal protection, the avian syrinx is a remarkably diverse structure underlying the great variety of bird sounds (King, 1989).

Although our knowledge of animal phonation is still limited, phonation in nonhumans appears to follow the principles of the myoelastic-aerodynamic theory of human phonation. The airflow from the lungs sets the vocal folds (or syringeal membranes) into vibration, and the rate of vibration is passively determined by the size and tension of these tissues. Vibration at a particular frequency does not typically require neural activity at that frequency. Thus, relatively normal phonation can be obtained by blowing moist air through an excised larynx, and rodents and bats can produce ultrasonic vocalizations at 40 kHz and higher (Suthers and Fattu, 1973). However, cat purring relies on an active tensing of the vocal fold musculature at the 20–30 Hz fundamental frequency of the purr (Frazer Sissom, Rice, and Peters, 1991). During phonation, the movements of the vocal folds can be periodic and stable (leading to tonal sounds) or highly aperiodic or even chaotic (e.g., in screams); while such aperiodic vocalizations are rare in nonpathological human voices, they can be important in animal vocal repertoires (Fitch, Neubauer, and Herzel, 2002).

Because the length of the vocal folds determines the lowest frequency at which they could vibrate (Titze, 1994), with long folds producing lower frequencies, one might expect that a low fundamental would provide a reliable indication of large body size. However, the size of the larynx is not tightly constrained by body size. Thus, a huge larynx has independently evolved in many mammal species, probably in response to selection for low-pitched voices (Fig. 1*A*, *B*). For example, in howler monkeys (genus *Alouatta*) the larynx and hyoid have grown to fill the space between mandible and sternum, giving these small monkeys remarkably impressive and low-pitched voices (Kelemen and Sade, 1960). The most extreme example of laryngeal hypertrophy is seen in the hammerhead bat *Hypsignathus monstrosus*, in which the larynx of males expands to fill the entire thoracic cavity, pushing the heart, lungs, and trachea down into the abdomen (Schneider, Kuhn, and Keleman, 1967). A similar though less impressive increase in larynx dimensions is observed in human males and is partially responsible for the voice change at puberty (Titze, 1989).

Sounds created by the larynx must pass through the air contained in the pharyngeal, oral, and nasal cavities, collectively termed the supralaryngeal vocal tract or simply vocal tract. Like any column of air, this air has mass and elasticity and vibrates preferentially at certain resonant frequencies. Vocal tract resonances are termed formants (from the Latin *formare*, to shape): they act as filters to shape the spectrum of the vocal output. Because all tetrapods have a vocal tract, all have formants. Formant frequencies are determined by the length and shape of the vocal tract. Because the vocal tract in mammals rests within the confines of the head, and skull size and body size are tightly linked (Fitch, 2000b), formant frequencies provide a possible indicator of body size not as easily "faked" as the laryngeal cue of fundamental frequency. Large animals have long vocal tracts and low formants. Together with demonstrations of formant perception by nonhuman animals (Sommers et al., 1992; Fitch and Kelley, 2000), this suggests that formants may have provided a cue to size in primitive vertebrates (Fitch, 1997). However, it is possible to break the anatomical link between vocal tract length and body size, and some intriguing morphological adaptations have arisen to elongate the vocal tract (presumably resulting from selection to sound larger; Fig. 1*C–E*). Elongations of the nasal vocal tract are seen in the long nose of male proboscis monkeys or the impressive nasal crests of hadrosaur dinosaurs (Weishampel, 1981). Vocal tract elongation can also be achieved by lowering the larynx; this is seen in extreme form in the red deer *Cervus elaphus*, which retract the larynx to the sternum during territorial roaring (Fitch and Reby, 2001). Again, a similar change occurs in human males at puberty: the larynx descends slightly to give men a longer vocal tract and lower formants than same-sized women (Fitch and Giedd, 1999).

Human speech is thus produced by the same conservative vocal production system of lungs, larynx, and vocal tract shared by all tetrapods. However, the evolution of the human speech apparatus involved several important changes. One was the loss of laryngeal air sacs. All great apes posses large balloon-like sacs that open into the larynx directly above the glottis (Negus, 1949; Schön Ybarra, 1995). Parsimony suggests that the common ancestor of apes and humans also had such air sacs, which were subsequently lost in human evolution. However, air sacs are occasionally observed in humans in pathological situations, a laryngocele is a congenital or acquired air sac that is attached to the larynx through the laryngeal ventricle at precisely the same location as in the great apes (Stell and Maran, 1975). Because the function of air sacs in ape vocalizations is not understood, the significance of their loss in human evolution is unknown.

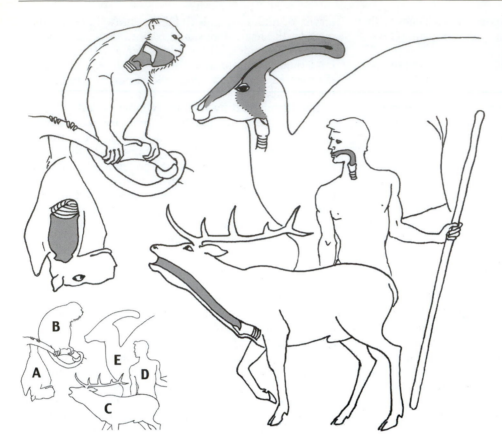

Figure 1. Examples of unusual vocal adaptations among vertebrates (not to scale). **A**, Hammerheaded bat, *Hypsignathus monstrosus*, has a huge larynx (gray) enlarged to fill the thoracic cavity. **B**, Howler monkeys *Alouatta* spp. have the largest relative larynx size among primates, which together with the enlarged hyoid fills the space beneath the mandible (larynx and hyoid shown in gray). **C**, Male red deer *Cervus elaphus* have a permanently descended larynx, which they lower to the sternum when roaring, resulting in an extremely elongated vocal tract (shown in gray). **D**, Humans—*Homo sapiens*—have a descended larynx, resulting in an elongated "two-tube" vocal tract (shown in gray). **E**, The now extinct duck-billed dinosaur *Parasaurolophus* had a hugely elongated nasal cavity (shown in gray) that filled the bony crest adorning the skull.

A second change in the vocal production system during human evolution was the descent of the larynx from its normal mammalian position high in the throat to a lower position in the neck (Negus, 1949). In the 1960s, speech scientists realized that this "descended larynx" allows humans to produce a wider variety of formant patterns than would be possible with a high larynx (Lieberman, Klatt, and Wilson, 1969). In particular, the "point vowels" /i, a, u/ seem to be impossible to attain unless the tongue body is bent and able to move freely within the oropharyngeal cavity. Given the existence of these vowels in virtually all languages (Maddieson, 1984), speech typical of modern humans appears to require a descended larynx. Of course, all mammals can produce a diversity of sounds, which could have served a simpler speech system. Also, most mammals appear to lower the larynx during vocalization (Fitch, 2000a), lessening the gap between humans and other animals. Despite these caveats, the descended larynx is clearly an important component of human spoken language (Lieberman, 1984). The existence of nonhuman mammals with a descended larynx raises the possibility that this trait initially arose to exaggerate size in early hominids and was later coopted for use in speech (Fitch and Reby, 2001). Finally, recent fossils suggest that an expansion of the thoracic intervertebral canal occurred during the evolution of *Homo* some time after the earliest *Homo erectus* (MacLarnon and Hewitt, 1999). This change

may be associated with an increase in breathing control necessary for singing and speech in our own species.

See also VOCALIZATION, NEURAL MECHANISMS OF.

—*W. Tecumseh Fitch*

References

Brainerd, E. L., and Ditelberg, J. S. (1993). Lung ventilation in salamanders and the evolution of vertebrate air-breathing mechanisms. *Biological Journal of the Linnean Society, 49,* 163–183.

Fitch, W. T. (1997). Vocal tract length and formant frequency dispersion correlate with body size in rhesus macaques. *Journal of the Acoustical Society of America, 102,* 1213–1222.

Fitch, W. T. (2000a). The phonetic potential of nonhuman vocal tracts: Comparative cineradiographic observations of vocalizing animals. *Phonetica, 57,* 205–218.

Fitch, W. T. (2000b). Skull dimensions in relation to body size in nonhuman mammals: The causal bases for acoustic allometry. *Zoology, 103,* 40–58.

Fitch, W. T., and Giedd, J. (1999). Morphology and development of the human vocal tract: A study using magnetic resonance imaging. *Journal of the Acoustical Society of America, 106,* 1511–1522.

Fitch, W. T., and Kelley, J. P. (2000). Perception of vocal tract resonances by whooping cranes, *Grus americana. Ethology, 106,* 559–574.

Fitch, W. T., Neubauer, J., and Herzel, H. (2002). Calls out of chaos: The adaptive significance of nonlinear phenomena in mammalian vocal production. *Animal Behaviour*, *63*, 407–418.

Fitch, W. T., and Reby, D. (2001). The descended larynx is not uniquely human. *Proceedings of the Royal Society, Biological Sciences*, *268*, 1669–1675.

Frazer Sissom, D. E., Rice, D. A., and Peters, G. (1991). How cats purr. *Journal of Zoology (London)*, *223*, 67–78.

Gans, C. (1973). Sound production in the Salientia: Mechanism and evolution of the emitter. *American Zoologist*, *13*, 1179–1194.

Kelemen, G., and Sade, J. (1960). The vocal organ of the howling monkey (*Alouatta palliata*). *Journal of Morphology*, *107*, 123–140.

King, A. S. (1989). Functional anatomy of the syrinx. In A. S. King and J. McLelland (Eds.), *Form and function in birds* (pp. 105–192). New York: Academic Press.

Lieberman, P. (1984). *The biology and evolution of language*. Cambridge, MA: Harvard University Press.

Lieberman, P. H., Klatt, D. H., and Wilson, W. H. (1969). Vocal tract limitations on the vowel repertoires of rhesus monkey and other nonhuman primates. *Science*, *164*, 1185–1187.

Liem, K. F. (1985). Ventilation. In M. Hildebrand (Ed.), *Functional vertebrate morphology* (pp. 185–209). Cambridge, MA: Belknap Press/Harvard University Press.

MacLarnon, A., and Hewitt, G. (1999). The evolution of human speech: The role of enhanced breathing control. *American Journal of Physical Anthropology*, *109*, 341–363.

Maddieson, I. (1984). *Patterns of sounds*. Cambridge, UK: Cambridge University Press.

Negus, V. E. (1949). *The Comparative anatomy and physiology of the larynx*. New York: Hafner.

Schneider, R., Kuhn, H.-J., and Kelemen, G. (1967). Der Larynx des männlichen *Hypsignathus monstrosus* Allen, 1861 (Pteropodidae, Megachiroptera, Mammalia). *Zeitschrift für wissenschaftliche Zoologie*, *175*, 1–53.

Schön Ybarra, M. (1995). A comparative approach to the nonhuman primate vocal tract: Implications for sound production. In E. Zimmerman and J. D. Newman (Eds.), *Current topics in primate vocal communication* (pp. 185–198). New York: Plenum Press.

Sommers, M. S., Moody, D. B., Prosen, C. A., and Stebbins, W. C. (1992). Formant frequency discrimination by Japanese macaques (*Macaca fuscata*). *Journal of the Acoustical Society of America*, *91*, 3499–3510.

Stell, P. M., and Maran, A. G. D. (1975). Laryngocoele. *Journal of Laryngology and Otology*, *89*, 915–924.

Suthers, R. A., and Fattu, J. M. (1973). Mechanisms of sound production in echolocating bats. *American Zoologist*, *13*, 1215–1226.

Titze, I. R. (1989). Physiologic and acoustic differences between male and female voices. *Journal of the Acoustical Society of America*, *85*, 1699–1707.

Titze, I. R. (1994). *Principles of voice production*. Englewood Cliffs, NJ: Prentice Hall.

Weishampel, D. B. (1981). Acoustic analysis of potential vocalization in lambeosaurine dinosaurs (Reptilia: Ornithischia). *Paleobiology*, *7*, 252–261.

Vocalization, Neural Mechanisms of

The capacity for speech and language separates humans from other animals and is the cornerstone of our intellectual and creative abilities. This capacity evolved from rudimentary forms of communication in the ancestors of humans. By studying these mechanisms in animals that represent stages of phylogenetic development, we can gain insight into the neural control of human speech that is necessary for understanding many disorders of human communication.

Vocalization is an integral part of speech and is widespread in mammalian aural communication systems. The limbic system, a group of neural structures controlling motivation and emotion, also controls most mammalian vocalizations. Although there are little supporting empirical data, many human emotional vocalizations probably involve the limbic system. This discussion considers the limbic system and those neural mechanisms thought to be necessary for normal speech and language to occur.

The anterior cingulate gyrus (ACG), which lies on the mesial surface of the frontal cortex just above and anterior to the genu of the corpus callosum, is considered part of the limbic system (Fig. 1). Electrical stimulation of the ACG in monkeys elicits vocalization and autonomic responses (Jürgens, 1994). Monkeys become mute when the ACG is lesioned, and single neurons in the ACG become active with vocalization or in response to vocalizations from conspecifics (Sutton, Larson, and Lindeman, 1974; Müller-Preuss, 1988; West and Larson, 1995). Electrical stimulation of the ACG in humans may also result in oral movements or postural distortions representative of an "archaic" level of behavior (Brown, 1988). Damage to the ACG in humans results in akinetic mutism that is accompanied by open eyes, a fixed gaze, lack of limb movement, lack of apparent affect, and nonreactance to painful stimuli (Jürgens and von Cramon, 1982). These symptoms reflect a lack of drive to initiate vocalization and many other behaviors (Brown, 1988). During recovery, a patient's ability to communicate gradually returns, first as a whisper, then with vocalization. However, the vocalizations lack prosodic features and are characterized as expressionless (Jürgens and von Cramon, 1982). These observations support the view that the ACG controls motivation for primitive forms of behavior, including prelinguistic vocalization.

The ACG has reciprocal connections with several cortical and subcortical sites, including a premotor area homologous with Broca's area, the superior temporal gyrus, the posterior cingulate gyrus, and the supplementary motor area (SMA) (Müller-Preuss, Newman, and Jürgens, 1980). Electrical stimulation of the SMA elicits vocalization, speech arrests, hesitation, distortions, and palilalic iterations (Brown, 1988). Damage to the SMA may result in mutism, poor initiation of speech, or repetitive utterances, and during recovery, patients often go through a period in which the production of

The Human Brain

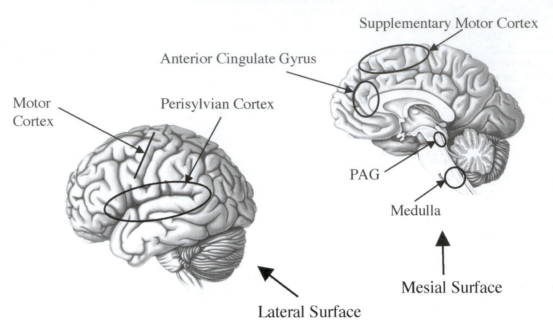

Figure 1. The lateral and mesial surface of the human brain.

propositional speech remains severely impaired but nonpropositional speech (e.g., counting) remains relatively unaffected (Brown, 1988). Studies of other motor systems in primates suggest that the SMA is involved in selection and initiation of a remembered motor act or the correct sequencing of motor acts (Picard and Strick, 1997). Speech and vocalization fall into these categories, as both are remembered and require proper sequencing. Output from the SMA to other vocalization motor areas is a subsequent stage in the execution of vocalization.

The ACG is also connected with the perisylvian cortex of the left hemisphere (Müller-Preuss, Newman, and Jürgens, 1980), an area important for speech and language. Damage to Broca's area may cause total or partial mutism, along with expressive aphasia or apraxia (Duffy, 1995). However, vocalization is less frequently affected than speech articulation or language (Duffy, 1995), and the effect is usually temporary. In some cases, aphonia may arise from widespread damage, and recovery following therapy may suggest a diffuse, motivational, or psychogenic etiology (Sapir and Aronson, 1987). Mutism seems to occur more frequently when the opercular region of the pre- and postcentral gyri is damaged bilaterally or when the damage extends deep into the cortex, affecting the insula and possibly the basal ganglia (Jürgens, Kirzinger, and von Cramon, 1982; Starkstein, Berthier, and Leiguarda, 1988; Duffy, 1995). Additional evidence linking the insula to vocalization comes from recent studies of apraxia in humans (Dronkers, 1996) and findings of increased blood flow in the insula during singing (Perry et al., 1999). Further research is necessary to determine whether the opercular cortex alone or deeper structures (e.g., insula) are im-

portant for vocalization. In specific cases, it is necessary to know whether mutism results from psychogenic or physiological mechanisms.

The perisylvian cortex may control vocalization by one or more pathways to the medulla. The perisylvian cortex is reciprocally connected to the ACG, which projects to midbrain mechanisms involved in vocalization. The perisylvian cortex also projects directly to the medulla, where motor neurons controlling laryngeal muscles are located (Kuypers, 1958). These neuroanatomical projections are supported by observations of a short time delay (13 ms) between stimulation of the cortex and excitation of laryngeal muscles (Ludlow and Lou, 1996). The perisylvian cortex also includes the right superior temporal gyrus and Heschl's gyrus, which are preferentially active for perception of complex tones, singing, perception of one's own voice, and perhaps control of the voice by self-monitoring auditory feedback (Perry et al., 1999; Belin et al., 2000).

The other widely studied limbic system structure known for its role in vocalization, is the midbrain periaqueductal gray (PAG) (Jürgens, 1994). Lesions of the PAG in humans and animals lead to mutism (Jürgens, 1994). Electrical and chemical stimulation of the PAG in many animal species elicits species-specific vocalizations (Jürgens, 1994). A variety of techniques have shown that PAG neurons, utilizing excitatory amino acid transmitters (glutamate), activate or suppress coordinated groups of oral, facial, respiratory, and laryngeal muscles for species-specific vocalization (Larson, 1991; Jürgens, 1994). The specific pattern of activation or suppression is determined by descending inputs from the ACG and limbic system, along with sensory feedback from the auditory, laryngeal and respiratory systems (Davis, Zhang, and Bandler, 1993; Ambalavanar et al., 1999). The resultant vocalizations convey the affective state of the organism. Although this system probably is responsible for emotional vocalizations in humans, it is unknown whether this pathway is involved in normal, nonemotive speech and language.

Neurons of the PAG project to several sites in the pons and medulla, one of which is the nucleus retroambiguus (NRA) (Holstege, 1989). The NRA in turn projects to the nucleus ambiguus (NA) and spinal cord motor neurons of the respiratory muscles. Lesions of the NRA eliminate vocalizations evoked by PAG stimulation (Shiba et al., 1997), and stimulation of the NRA elicits vocalization (Zhang, Bandler, and Davis, 1995). Thus, the NRA lies functionally between the PAG and motor neurons of laryngeal and respiratory muscles controlling vocalization and may play a role in coordinating these neuronal groups (Shiba et al., 1997; Luthe, Hausler, and Jürgens, 2000).

The PAG also projects to the parvocellular reticular formation, where neurons modulate their activity with temporal and acoustical variations in monkey calls, and lesions alter the acoustical structure of vocalizations (Luthe, Hausler, and Jürgens, 2000). These data suggest that the parvocellular reticular formation is important for the regulation of vocal quality and pitch.

Finally, the NA contains laryngeal motor neurons and is crucial to vocalization. Motor neurons in the NA control laryngeal muscles during vocalization, swallowing, and respiration (Yajima and Larson, 1993), and lesions of the NA abolish vocalizations elicited by PAG stimulation (Jürgens and Pratt, 1979). The NA receives projections either indirectly from the PAG, by way of

the NRA (Holstege, 1989), or directly from the cerebral cortex (Kuypers, 1958). Sensory feedback for the reflexive control of laryngeal muscles flows through the superior and recurrent laryngeal nerves to the nucleus of the solitary tract and spinal nucleus of the trigeminal nerve (Tan and Lim, 1992).

In summary, vocalization is controlled by two pathways, one that is primitive and found in most animals, and one that is found only in humans and perhaps anthropoid apes (Fig. 2). The pathway found in all mammals extends from the ACG through the limbic system and midbrain PAG to medullary and spinal motor neurons, and seems to control most emotional vocalizations. Voluntary vocal control, found primarily in humans, aided by sensory feedback, may be exerted through a direct pathway from the motor cortex to the medulla. The tendency for vocalization and human speech to be strongly affected by emotions may suggest that all vocalizations rely at least in part on the ACG-PAG pathway. Details of how these two parallel pathways are integrated are unknown.

See also VOCAL PRODUCTION SYSTEM: EVOLUTION.

—*Charles R. Larson*

References

Ambalavanar, R., Tanaka, Y., Damirjian, M., and Ludlow, C. L. (1999). Laryngeal afferent stimulation enhances fos immunoreactivity in the periaqueductal gray in the cat. *Journal of Comparative Neurology*, *409*, 411–423.

Belin, P., Zatorre, R. J., Ladaille, P., Ahad, P., and Pike, B. (2000). Voice-selective areas in human auditory cortex. *Nature*, *403*, 309–312.

Brown, J. (1988). Cingulate gyrus and supplementary motor correlates of vocalization in man. In J. D. Newman (Ed.), *The physiological control of mammalian vocalization* (pp. 227–243). New York: Plenum Press.

Davis, P. J., Zhang, S. P., and Bandler, R. (1993). Pulmonary and upper airway afferent influences on the motor pattern of vocalization evoked by excitation of the midbrain periaqueductal gray of the cat. *Brain Research*, *607*, 61–80.

Dronkers, N. F. (1996). A new brain region for coordinating speech articulation. *Nature*, *384*, 159–161.

Duffy, J. R. (1995). *Motor speech disorders*. St. Louis: Mosby.

Holstege, G. (1989). An anatomical study on the final common pathway for vocalization in the cat. *Journal of Comparative Neurology*, *284*, 242–252.

Jürgens, U. (1994). The role of the periaqueductal grey in vocal behaviour. *Behavioural Brain Research*, *62*, 107–117.

Jürgens, U., Kirzinger, A., and von Cramon, D. (1982). The effects of deep-reaching lesions in the cortical face area on phonation: A combined case report and experimental monkey study. *Cortex*, *18*, 125–140.

Jürgens, U., and Pratt, R. (1979). Role of the periaqueductal grey in vocal expression of emotion. *Brain Research*, *167*, 367–378.

Jürgens, U., and von Cramon, D. (1982). On the role of the anterior cingulate cortex in phonation: A case report. *Brain and Language*, *15*, 234–248.

Kuypers, H. G. H. M. (1958). Corticobulbar connexions to the pons and lower brain-stem in man. *Brain*, *81*, 364–388.

Larson, C. R. (1991). On the relation of PAG neurons to laryngeal and respiratory muscles during vocalization in the monkey. *Brain Research*, *552*, 77–86.

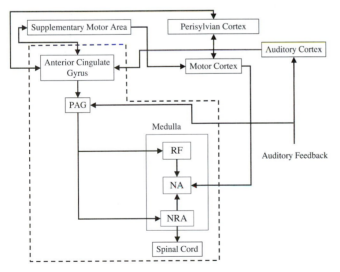

Figure 2. Block diagram and arrows indicating known connections between principal structures involved in vocalization. Structures inside the dashed box are involved in vocalization in other mammals as well as in humans. Structures outside the dashed box may be found only in humans and perhaps anthropoid apes. NA, nucleus ambiguous; NRA, nucleus retroambiguus; PAG, periaqueductal gray; RF, reticular formation.

Ludlow, C. L., and Lou, G. (1996). Observations on human laryngeal muscle control. In P. J. Davis and N. H. Fletcher (Eds.), *Vocal fold physiology: Controlling complexity and chaos* (pp. 201–218). San Diego: Singular Publishing Group.

Luthe, L., Hausler, U., and Jürgens, U. (2000). Neuronal activity in the medulla oblongata during vocalization: A single-unit recording study in the squirrel monkey. *Behavioural Brain Research, 116,* 197–210.

Müller-Preuss, P. (1988). Neural correlates of audio-vocal behavior: Properties of anterior limbic cortex and related areas. In J. D. Newman (Ed.), *The physiological control of mammalian vocalization* (pp. 245–262). New York: Plenum Press.

Müller-Preuss, P., Newman, J. D., and Jürgens, U. (1980). Anatomical and physiological evidence for a relationship between the "cingular" vocalization area and the auditory cortex in the squirrel monkey. *Brain Research, 202,* 307–315.

Perry, D. W., Zatorre, R. J., Petrides, M., Alivisatos, B., Meyer, E., and Evans, A. C. (1999). Localization of cerebral activity during simple singing. *NeuroReport, 10,* 3453–3458.

Picard, N., and Strick, P. L. (1997). Activation on the medial wall during remembered sequences of reaching movements in monkeys. *Journal of Neurophysiology, 77,* 2197–2201.

Sapir, S., and Aronson, A. E. (1987). Coexisting psychogenic and neurogenic dysphonia: A source of diagnostic confusion. *British Journal of Disorders of Communication, 22,* 73–80.

Shiba, K., Umezaki, T., Zheng, Y., and Miller, A. D. (1997). The nucleus retroambigualis controls laryngeal muscle activity during vocalization in the cat. *Experimental Brain Research, 115,* 513–519.

Starkstein, S. E., Berthier, M., and Leiguarda, R. (1988). Bilateral opercular syndrome and crossed aphemia due to a right insular lesion: A clinicopathological study. *Brain and Language, 34,* 253–261.

Sutton, D., Larson, C., and Lindeman, R. C. (1974). Neocortical and limbic lesion effects on primate phonation. *Brain Research, 71,* 61–75.

Tan, C. K., and Lim, H. H. (1992). Central projection of the sensory fibres of the recurrent laryngeal nerve of the cat. *Acta Anatomica, 143,* 306–308.

West, R. A., and Larson, C. R. (1995). Neurons of the anterior mesial cortex related to faciovocal behavior in the awake monkey. *Journal of Neurophysiology, 74,* 1156–1169.

Yajima, Y., and Larson, C. R. (1993). Multifunctional properties of ambiguous neurons identified electrophysiologically during vocalization in the awake monkey. *Journal of Neurophysiology, 70,* 529–540.

Zhang, S. P., Bandler, R., and Davis, P. J. (1995). Brain stem integration of vocalization: Role of the nucleus retroambigualis. *Journal of Neurophysiology, 74,* 2500–2512.

Further Readings

Adametz, J., and O'Leary, J. L. (1959). Experimental mutism resulting from periaqueductal lesions in cats. *Neurology, 9,* 636–642.

Aronson, A. E. (1985). *Clinical voice disorders.* New York: Thieme-Stratton.

Barris, R. W., and Schuman, H. R. (1953). Bilateral anterior cingulate gyrus lesions. *Neurology, 3,* 44–52.

Botez, M. I., and Barbeau, A. (1971). Role of subcortical structures, and particularly of the thalamus, in the mechanisms of speech and language. *International Journal of Neurology, 8,* 300–320.

Brown, J. W., and Perecman, E. (1985). Neurological basis of language processing. In J. K. Darby (Ed.), *Speech and language evaluation in neurology: Adult disorders* (pp. 45–81). New York: Grune and Stratton.

Davis, P. J., and Nail, B. S. (1984). On the location and size of laryngeal motoneurons in the cat and rabbit. *Journal of Comparative Neurology, 230,* 13–32.

Gemba, H., Miki, N., and Sasaki, K. (1995). Cortical field potentials preceding vocalization and influences of cerebellar hemispherectomy upon them in monkeys. *Brain Research, 69,* 143–151.

Jonas, S. (1987). The supplementary motor region and speech. In E. Perecman (Ed.), *The frontal lobes revisited.* New York: IRBN Press.

Jürgens, U. (1982). Amygdalar vocalization pathways in the squirrel monkey. *Brain Research, 241,* 189–196.

Jürgens, U. (2000). Localization of a pontine vocalization-controlling area. *Journal of the Acoustical Society of America, 108,* 1393–1396.

Jürgens, U., and Zwirner, P. (2000). Individual hemispheric asymmetry in vocal fold control of the squirrel monkey. *Behavioural Brain Research, 109,* 213–217.

Kalia, M., and Mesulam, M. (1980). Brainstem projections of sensory and motor components of the vagus complex in the cat: II. Laryngeal, tracheobronchial, pulmonary, cardiac, and gastrointestinal branches. *Journal of Comparative Neurology, 193,* 467–508.

Kirzinger, A., and Jürgens, U. (1982). Cortical lesion effects and vocalization in the squirrel monkey. *Brain Research, 233,* 299–315.

Kirzinger, A., and Jürgens, U. (1991). Vocalization-correlated single-unit activity in the brain stem of the squirrel monkey. *Experimental Brain Research, 84,* 545–560.

Lamandella, J. T. (1977). The limbic system in human communication. In J. Whitaker and H. A. Whitaker (Eds.), *Studies in neurolinguistics* (vol. 3, pp. 157–222). New York: Academic Press.

Larson, C. R. (1975). *Effects of cerebellar lesions on conditioned monkey phonation.* Unpublished doctoral dissertation, University of Washington, Seattle.

Larson, C. R., Wilson, K. E., and Luschei, E. S. (1983). Preliminary observations on cortical and brainstem mechanisms of laryngeal control. In D. M. Bless and J. H. Abbs (Eds.), *Vocal fold physiology: Contemporary research and clinical issues.* San Diego, CA: College-Hill Press.

Ludlow, C. L., Schulz, G. M., Yamashita, T., and Deleyiannis, F. W.-B. (1995). Abnormalities in long latency responses to superior laryngeal nerve stimulation in adductor spasmodic dysphonia. *Annals of Otology, Rhinology, and Laryngology, 104,* 928–935.

Marshall, R. C., Gandour, J., and Windsor, J. (1988). Selective impairment of phonation: A case study. *Brain and Language, 35,* 313–339.

Müller-Preuss, P., and Jürgens, U. (1976). Projections from the "cingular" vocalization area in the squirrel monkey. *Brain Research, 103,* 29–43.

Ortega, J. D., DeRosier, E., Park, S., and Larson, C. R. (1988). Brainstem mechanisms of laryngeal control as revealed by microstimulation studies. In O. Fujimura (Ed.), *Vocal physiology: Voice production, mechanisms and functions* (vol. 2, pp. 19–28). New York: Raven Press.

Paus, T., Petrides, M., Evans, A. C., and Meyer, E. (1993). Role of the human anterior cingulate cortex in the control of oculomotor, manual and speech responses: A positron emission tomography study. *Journal of Neurophysiology, 70,* 453–469.

Penfield, W., and Welch, K. (1951). The supplementary motor area of the cerebral cortex. *Archives of Neurology and Psychiatry, 66*, 289–317.

von Cramon, D., and Jürgens, U. (1983). The anterior cingulate cortex and the phonatory control in monkey and man. *Neurosciences and Biobehavior Review, 7*, 423–425.

Ward, A. A. (1948). The cingular gyrus: Area 24. *Journal of Neurophysiology, 11*, 13–23.

Zatorre, R. J., and Samson, S. (1991). Role of the right temporal neocortex in retention of pitch in auditory short-term memory. *Brain, 114*, 2403–2417.

Voice Acoustics

The basic acoustic source during normal phonation is a waveform consisting of a quasi-periodic sequence of pulses of volume velocity $U_s(t)$ that pass between the vibrating vocal folds (Fig. 1*A*). For modal vocal fold vibration, the volume velocity is zero in the time interval between the pulses, and there is a relatively abrupt discontinuity in slope at the time the volume velocity decreases to zero. The periodic nature of this waveform is reflected in the harmonic structure of the spectrum (Fig. 1*B*). The amplitudes of the harmonics at high frequencies decrease as $1/f^2$, where f = frequency, i.e., at about -12 dB per octave. The frequency of this source waveform varies from one individual to another and within an utterance. In the time domain (Fig. 1*A*), a change in frequency is represented in the number of pulses per second; in the frequency domain (Fig. 1*B*), the frequency is represented by the spacing between the harmonics. The shape of the individual pulses can also vary with the speaker, and during an utterance the shape can be modified depending on the position within the utterance and the prominence of the syllable.

When the position and tension of the vocal folds are properly adjusted, a positive pressure below the glottis will cause the vocal folds to vibrate. As the cross-sectional area of the glottis changes during a cycle of vibration, the airflow is modulated. During the open phase of the cycle, the impedance of the glottal opening is usually large compared with the impedance looking into the vocal tract from the glottis. Thus, in most cases it is reasonable to represent the glottal source as a volume-velocity source that produces similar glottal pulses for different vocal tract configurations.

This source $U_s(t)$ is filtered by the vocal tract, as depicted in Figure 2. The volume velocity at the lips is $U_m(t)$, and the output sound pressure at a distance r from the lips is $p_r(t)$. The magnitudes of the spectral components of $U_s(f)$ and $p_r(f)$ are shown below the corresponding waveforms in Figure 2. When a non-nasal vowel is produced, the vocal tract transfer function $T(f)$, defined as the ratio $U_m(f)/U_s(f)$, is an all-pole transfer function. The sound pressure p_r is related to U_m by a radiation characteristic $R(f)$. The magnitude of this radiation characteristic is approximately

$$|R(f)| = \frac{\rho \cdot 2\pi f}{4\pi r}, \tag{1}$$

where ρ = density of air. Thus we have

$$p_r(f) = U_s(f) \cdot T(f) \cdot R(f). \tag{2}$$

The magnitude of $p_r(f)$ can be written as

$$|p_r(f)| = |U_s(f) \cdot 2\pi f| \, |T(f)| \cdot \frac{\rho}{4\pi r}. \tag{3}$$

The expression $|U_s(f) \cdot 2\pi f|$ is the magnitude of the Fourier transform of the derivative $U_s'(t)$. Thus the output sound pressure can be considered to be the result of filtering $U_s'(t)$ by the vocal tract transfer function $T(f)$, multiplied by a constant. That is, the derivative $U_s'(t)$ can be viewed as the effective excitation of the vocal tract.

For the ideal or modal volume-velocity waveform (Fig. 1), this derivative has the form shown in Figure 3*A* (Fant, Liljencrants, and Lin, 1985). Each pulse has a sequence of two components: (1) an initial smooth portion where the waveform is first positive, then passes through zero (corresponding to the peak of the pulse in Fig. 1), and then reaches a maximum negative value; and (2) a second portion where the waveform returns abruptly to zero, corresponding to the discontinuity in

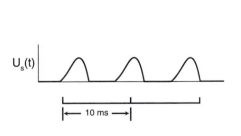

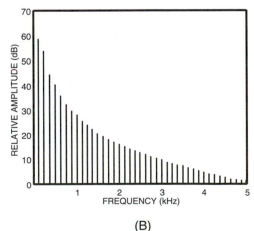

Figure 1. A, Idealized waveform of glottal volume velocity $U_s(t)$ for modal vocal fold vibration for an adult male speaker. **B**, Spectrum of waveform in **A**.

(A)   (B)

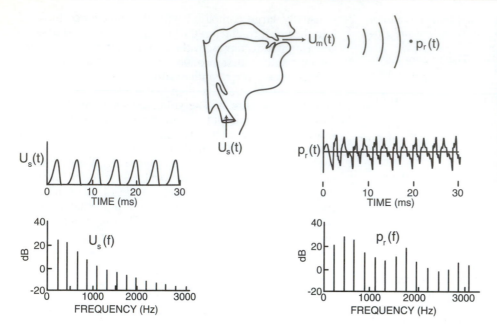

Figure 2. Schema showing how the acoustic source at the glottis is filtered by the vocal tract to yield a volume velocity $U_m(t)$ at the lips, which is radiated to obtain the sound pressure $p_r(t)$ at some distance from the lips. At the left of the figure both the source waveform $U_s(t)$ and its spectrum $U_s(f)$ are shown. At the right is the waveform $p_r(t)$ and spectrum $p_r(f)$ of the sound pressure. (Adapted with permission from Stevens, 1994.)

slope of the original waveform $U_s(t)$ at the time the vocal folds come together. The principal acoustic excitation of the vocal tract occurs at the time of this discontinuity. For this ideal or modal derivative waveform, the spectrum (Fig. 3B) at high frequencies decreases as $1/f$, i.e., at −6 dB/octave, reflecting the discontinuity at closure.

For normal speech production, there are several ways in which the glottal waveform can differ from the modal waveform (or its derivative). One obvious attribute is the frequency f_0 of the glottal pulses, which is controlled primarily by changing the tension of the vocal folds, although the subglottal pressure also influences the frequency, particularly when the folds are relatively slack (Titze, 1989). Increasing or decreasing the subglottal pressure P_s causes increases or decreases in the amplitude of the glottal pulses, or, more specifically, in the magnitude of the discontinuity in slope at the time of glottal closure. The magnitude of the glottal excitation

increases roughly as $P_s^{3/2}$ (Ladefoged and McKinney, 1963; Isshiki, 1964; Tanaka and Gould, 1983).

Changes in the configuration of the membranous and cartilaginous portions of the vocal folds relative to the modal configuration can lead to changes in the waveform and spectrum of the glottal source. For some speakers and for some styles of speaking, the vocal folds and arytenoid cartilages are configured such that the glottis is never completely closed during a cycle of vibration, introducing several acoustic consequences. First, the speed with which the vocal folds approach the midline is reduced; the effect on the derivative waveform $U_s'(t)$ is that the maximum negative value is reduced (that is, it is less negative). Thus, the excitation of the vocal tract and the overall amplitude of the output are decreased. Second, there is continuing airflow throughout the cycle. The inertia of the air in the glottis and supraglottal airways prevents the occurrence of the

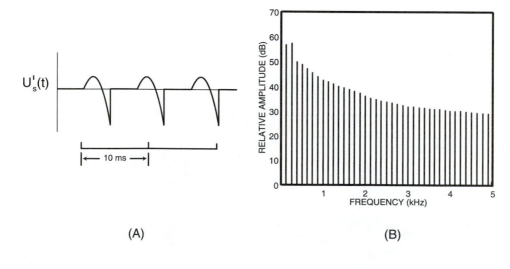

(A)   (B)

Figure 3. A, Derivative $U_s'(t)$ of the modal volume-velocity waveform in Figure 1. **B,** Spectrum of waveform in **A.**

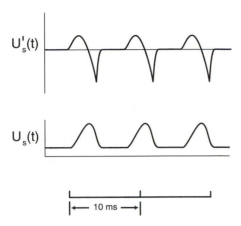

Figure 4. Schematized representation of volume velocity waveform $U_s(t)$ and its derivative $U_s'(t)$ when the glottis is never completely closed within a cycle of vibration.

abrupt discontinuity in $U_s'(t)$ that occurs at the time of vocal fold closure in modal phonation (Rothenberg, 1981). Rather, there is a non-zero *return phase* following the maximum negative peak, during which $U_s'(t)$ gradually returns to zero (Fant, Liljencrants, and Lin, 1985). The derivative waveform $U_s'(t)$ then has a shape that is schematized in Figure 4. The corresponding waveform $U_s(t)$ is shown below the waveform $U_s'(t)$. The spectral consequence of this non-zero return phase is a reduction in the high-frequency spectrum amplitude of $U_s'(t)$ relative to the low-frequency spectrum amplitude. A third consequence of a somewhat abducted glottal configuration is an increased loss of acoustic energy from the vocal tract through the partially open glottis and into the subglottal airways. This energy loss affects the vocal tract filter rather than the source waveform. It is most apparent in the first formant range and results in an increased bandwidth of F1, causing a reduction in A1, the amplitude of the first-formant prominence in the

spectrum (Hanson, 1997). The three consequences just described lead to a vowel for which the spectrum amplitude A1 in the F1 range is reduced and the amplitudes of the spectral prominences due to higher formants are reduced relative to A1.

Still another consequence of glottal vibration with a partially open glottis is that there is increased average airflow through the glottis, as shown in the $U_s(t)$ waveform in Figure 4. This increased flow causes an increased amplitude of noise generated by turbulence in the vicinity of the glottis. Thus, in addition to the quasi-periodic source, there is an *aspiration* noise source with a continuous spectrum (Klatt and Klatt, 1990). Since the flow is modulated by the periodic fluctuation in glottal area, the noise source is also modulated. This type of phonation has been called "breathy-voiced."

The aspiration noise source can be represented as an equivalent acoustic volume-velocity source that is added to the periodic source. In contrast to the periodic source, the noise source has a spectrum that tilts upward with increasing frequency. It appears to have a broad peak at high frequencies, around 2–4 kHz (Stevens, 1998). Figure 5A shows estimated spectra of the periodic and noise components that would occur during modal phonation. The noise component is relatively weak, and is generated only during the open phase of glottal vibration. Phonation with a more abducted glottis of the type represented in Figure 4 leads to greater noise energy and reduced high-frequency amplitude of the periodic component, and the noise component may dominate the periodic component at high frequencies (Fig. 5B). With breathy-voiced phonation, the individual harmonics corresponding to the periodic component may be obscured by the noise component at high frequencies. At low frequencies, however, the harmonics are well defined, since the noise component is weak in this frequency region.

Figure 6 shows spectra of a vowel produced by a speaker with modal glottal vibration (*A*) and the same vowel produced by a speaker with a somewhat abducted

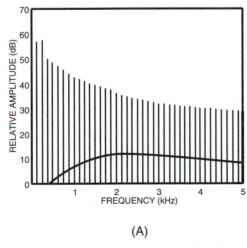

(A)

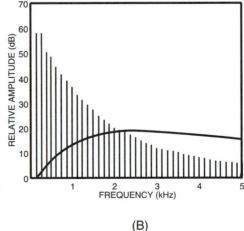

(B)

Figure 5. Schematized representation of spectra of the effective periodic and noise components of the glottal source for modal vibration (**A**) and breathy voicing (**B**). The spectrum of the periodic component is represented by the amplitudes of the harmonics. The spectrum of the noise is calculated with a bandwidth of about 300 Hz.

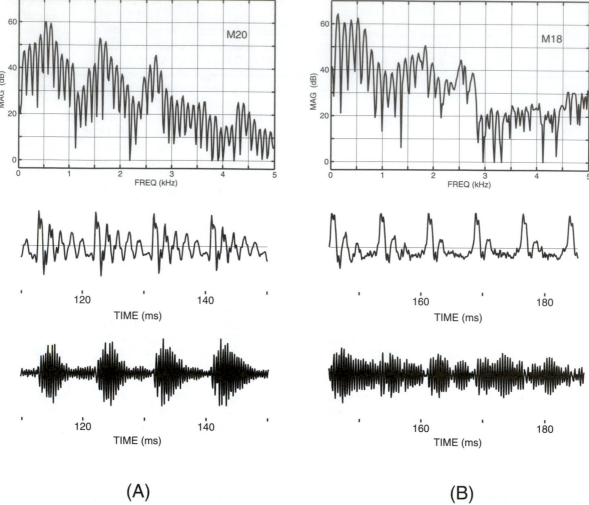

(A)   (B)

Figure 6. A, Spectrum of the vowel /ɛ/ produced by a male speaker with approximately modal phonation. Below the spectrum are waveforms of this vowel before and after being filtered with a bandpass filter centered on F3, with a bandwidth of 600 Hz. The individual glottal pulses as filtered by F3 of the vowel are evident. **B,** Spectrum of the vowel /ɛ/ produced by a male speaker who apparently phonated with a glottal chink. The waveforms below are as described in A. The noise in the waveform in the F3 region (and above) obscures the individual glottal pulses. The spectra are from Hanson and Chuang (1999). See text.

glottis (*B*). Below the spectra are waveforms of the vowel before and after being filtered by a broad bandpass filter (bandwidth of 600 Hz) centered on the third-formant frequency F3. Filtered waveforms of this type have been used to highlight the presence of noise at high frequencies during phonation by a speaker with a breathy voice (Klatt and Klatt, 1990). The noise is also evident in the spectrum at high frequencies for the speaker of Figure 6B. Comparison of the two spectra in Figure 6 also shows the greater spectrum tilt and the reduced prominence of the first formant peak associated with an abducted glottis, as already noted.

As the average glottal area increases, the transglottal pressure required to maintain vibration (phonation threshold pressure) increases. Therefore, for a given subglottal pressure an increase in the glottal area can lead to cessation of vocalfold vibration.

Adduction of the vocal folds relative to their modal configuration can also lead to changes in the source waveform. As the vocal folds are adducted, pressed voicing occurs, in which the glottal pulses are narrower and of lower amplitude than in modal phonation, and may occur aperiodically (glottalization). In addition, phonation-threshold pressure increases, eventually reaching a point where the folds no longer vibrate.

The above description of the glottal vibration pattern for various degrees of glottal abduction and adduction suggests that there is an optimum glottal width that gives rise to a maximum in sound energy (Hanson and Stevens, 2002). This optimum configuration has been examined experimentally by Verdolini et al. (1998).

There are substantial individual and sex differences in the degree to which the folds are abducted or adducted during phonation. These differences lead to significant

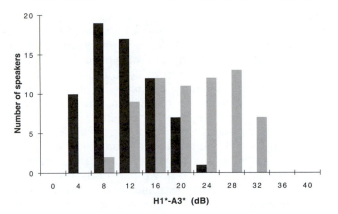

Figure 7. Distributions of H1*-A3*, a measure that reflects the reduction of the high-frequency spectrum relative to the low-frequency spectrum, for male (black bars) and female (gray bars) speakers. H1 is the amplitude of the first harmonic and A3 is the amplitude of the strongest harmonic in the F3 peak. The asterisks indicate that corrections have been applied to H1 and A3, as described in the text. (Adapted with permission from Hanson and Chuang, 1999.)

differences in the waveform and spectrum of the glottal source, and consequently in the spectral characteristics of vowels generated by these sources (Hanson, 1997; Hanson and Chuang, 1999). Similar observations have also been made by Holmberg, Hillman, and Perkell (1988) using different measurement techniques. One acoustic measure that reflects the reduction of the high-frequency spectrum amplitude relative to the low-frequency spectrum amplitude is the difference H1*-A3* (in dB) between the amplitude of the first harmonic and the amplitude of the third-formant spectrum prominence. (The asterisks indicate that corrections are made in H1 due to the possible influence of the first formant, and in A3 due to the influence of the frequencies of the first and second formants.) Distributions of values of H1*-A3* are given in Figure 7 for a population of 22 female and 21 male speakers. The female speakers appear to have a greater spectrum tilt on average, suggesting a somewhat less abrupt glottal closure during a cycle and a greater tendency for lack of complete closure throughout the cycle. Note the substantial ranges of 20 dB or more within each sex.

—*Kenneth N. Stevens and Helen M. Hanson*

References

Fant, G., Liljencrants, J., and Lin, Q. G. (1985). A four-parameter model of glottal flow. *Speech Transmission Laboratory Quarterly Progress and Status Report, 4,* 1–13. Stockholm: Royal Institute of Technology.

Hanson, H. M. (1997). Glottal characteristics of female speakers: Acoustic correlates. *Journal of the Acoustical Society of America, 101,* 466–481.

Hanson, H. M., and Chuang, E. S. (1999). Glottal characteristics of male speakers: Acoustic correlates and comparison with female data. *Journal of the Acoustical Society of America, 106,* 1094–1077.

Hanson, H. M., and Stevens, K. N. (2002). A quasiarticulatory approach to controlling acoustic source parameters in a Klatt-type formant synthesizer using HLsyn. *Journal of the Acoustical Society of America, 112,* 1158–1182.

Holmberg, E. B., Hillman, R. E., and Perkell, J. S. (1988). Glottal airflow and transglottal air pressure measurements for male and female speakers in soft, normal, and loud voice. *Journal of the Acoustical Society of America, 84,* 511–529.

Isshiki, N. (1964). Regulatory mechanism of voice intensity variation. *Journal of Speech and Hearing Research, 7,* 17–29.

Klatt, D. H., and Klatt, L. C. (1990). Analysis, synthesis, and perception of voice quality variations among female and male talkers. *Journal of the Acoustical Society of America, 87,* 820–857.

Ladefoged, P., and McKinney, N. P. (1963). Loudness, sound pressure, and subglottal pressure in speech. *Journal of the Acoustical Society of America, 35,* 454–460.

Rothenberg, M. (1981). Acoustic interaction between the glottal source and the vocal tract. In K. N. Stevens and M. Hirano (Eds.), *Vocal fold physiology* (pp. 305–323). Tokyo: University of Tokyo Press.

Stevens, K. N. (1994). Scientific substrates of speech production. In F. D. Minifie (Ed.), *Introduction to communication sciences and disorders* (pp. 399–437). San Diego, CA: Singular Publishing Group.

Stevens, K. N. (1998). *Acoustic phonetics.* Cambridge, MA: MIT Press.

Tanaka, S., and Gould, W. J. (1983). Relationships between vocal intensity and noninvasively obtained aerodynamic parameters in normal subjects. *Journal of the Acoustical Society of America, 73,* 1316–1321.

Titze, I. R. (1989). On the relation between subglottal pressure and fundamental frequency in phonation. *Journal of the Acoustical Society of America, 85,* 901–912.

Verdolini, K., Drucker, D. G., Palmer, P. M., and Samawi, H. (1998). Laryngeal adduction in resonant voice. *Journal of Voice, 12,* 315–327.

Voice Disorders in Children

Investigations of voice using aerodynamic techniques have been reported for more than 30 years. Investigators realized early on that voice production is an aeromechanical event and that vocal tract aerodynamics reflect the interactions between laryngeal anatomy and complex physiological events. Aerodynamic events do not always have a one-to-one correspondence with vocal tract physiology in a dynamic biological system, but careful control of stimuli and a good knowledge of laryngeal physiology make airflow and air pressure measurements invaluable tools.

Airflow (rate of air movement or velocity) and air pressure (force per unit area of air molecules) in the vocal tract are good reflectors of vocal physiology. For example, at a simple level, airflow through the glottis (Vg) is an excellent indicator of whether the vocal folds are open or closed. When the vocal folds are open, there is airflow through the glottis, and when the vocal folds are completely closed, there is zero airflow. With other physiological events held constant, the amount of airflow can be an excellent indicator of the degree of opening between the vocal folds.

Subglottal air pressure directly reflects changes in the size of the subglottal air cavity. A simplified version of Boyle's law predicts the relationship in that a particular pressure (P) in a closed volume (V) of air must equal a constant (K), that is, $K = PV$. Subglottal air pressure will increase when the size of the lungs is decreased; conversely, subglottal pressure will decrease when the size of the lungs is made larger. Changes in subglottal air pressure are mainly regulated through muscular forces controlling the size of the rib cage, with glottal resistance or glottal flow used to help increase or decrease the pressures (the glottis can be viewed as a valve that helps regulate pulmonary flows and pressures).

A small number of classic studies used average airflow and intraoral air pressure to investigate voice production in children (Subtelny, Worth, and Sakuda, 1966; Arkebauer, Hixon, and Hardy, 1967; Van Hattum and Worth, 1967; Beckett, Theolke and Cowan, 1971; Diggs, 1972; Bernthal and Beukelman, 1978; Stathopoulos and Weismer, 1986). Measures of flow and pressure were used to reflect laryngeal and respiratory function. During voice production, children produce lower average airflow than adults, and boys tend to produce higher average airflow than girls of the same age. Supraglottal and glottal airway opening most likely account for the different average airflow values as a function of age and sex. Assuming that pressure is the same across all speakers, a smaller supraglottal or glottal opening yields a higher resistance at the constriction and therefore a restricted or lower flow of air. The findings related to intraoral air pressure have indicated that children produce higher intraoral air pressures than adults, especially because they tend to speak at higher sound pressure levels (SPLs). The higher pressures produced by children versus adults reflect two physiological events. First, children tend to speak at a higher SPL than adults, and second, children's airways are smaller and less compliant than adults' (Stathopoulos and Weismer, 1986). Intuitively, it would appear that the greater peak intraoral air pressure in children should lead to a greater magnitude of oral airflow. It is likely that children's smaller glottal and supraglottal areas substantially counteract the potentially large flows resulting from their high intraoral air pressures.

Children were found to be capable of maintaining the same linguistic contrasts as adults through manipulation of physiological events such as lung cavity size and driving pressure, and laryngeal and articulatory configuration. Other intraoral air pressure distinctions in children are similar to the overall trends described for adult pressures. Like adults, children produce higher pressures during (1) voiceless compared to voiced consonants, (2) prevocalic compared to postvocalic consonants, (3) stressed compared to unstressed syllables, and (4) stops compared to fricatives.

In the 1970s and 1980s, two important aerodynamic techniques relative to voice production were developed that stimulated new ways of analyzing children's aero-

dynamic vocal function. The first technique was inverse filtering of the easily accessible oral airflow signal (Rothenberg, 1977). Rothenberg's procedure allowed derivation of the glottal airflow waveform. The derived volume velocity waveform provides airflow values, permitting detailed, quantifiable analysis of vocal fold physiology. The measures made from the derived volume velocity waveform can be related to the speed of opening and closing of the vocal folds, the closed time of the vocal folds, the amplitude of vibration, the overall shape of the vibratory waveform, and the degree of glottal opening during the closed part of the cycle.

The second aerodynamic technique developed was for the estimation of subglottal pressure and laryngeal airway resistance (Rlaw) through noninvasive procedures (Lofqvist, Carlborg, and Kitzing, 1982; Smitheran and Hixon, 1981). Subglottal air pressure is of primary importance, because it is responsible for generating the pressure differential causing vocal fold vibration (the pressure that drives the vocal folds). Subglottal pressure is also important for controlling sound pressure level and for contributing to changes in fundamental frequency—all factors essential for normal voice production. The estimation of Rlaw offers a more general interpretation of laryngeal dynamics and can be used as a screening measure to quantify values outside normal ranges of vocal function.

Measures made using the Smitheran and Hixon (1981) technique include the following:

1. *Average oral air flow:* Measured during the open vowel /ɑ/ at midpoint to obtain an estimate of laryngeal airflow.
2. *Intraoral air pressure:* Measured peak pressure during the voiceless [p] to obtain an estimate of subglottal pressure.
3. *Estimated laryngeal airway resistance:* Calculated by dividing the estimated subglottal pressure by estimated laryngeal airflow. This calculation is based on analogy with Olm's law, $R = V/I$, where R = resistance, V = voltage, and I = current. In the speech system, R = laryngeal airway resistance, V = subglottal pressure (P), and I = laryngeal airflow (V). Thus, $R = P/V$.

Measures made using the derived glottal airflow waveform important to vocal fold physiology include the following (Holmberg, Hillman, and Perkell, 1988):

1. *Airflow open quotient:* This measure is comparable to the original open quotient defined by Timcke, von Leden, and Moore (1958). The open time of the vocal folds (defined as the interval of time between the instant of opening and the instant of closing of the vocal cords) is divided by the period of the glottal cycle. Opening and closing instants on the airflow waveform are taken at a point equal to 20% of alternating airflow (OQ-20%).
2. *Speed quotient:* The speed quotient is determined as the time it takes for the vocal folds to open divided by the time it takes for the vocal folds to close. Opening

and closing instants on the waveform are taken at a point equal to 20% of alternating air flow. The measure reflects how fast the vocal folds are opening and closing and the asymmetry of the opening and closing phases.

3. *Maximum flow declination rate:* The measure is obtained during the closing portion of the vocal fold cycle and reflects the fastest rate of airflow shut-off. Differentiating the airflow waveform and then identifying the greatest negative peak on differentiated waveform locates the fastest declination. The flow measure corresponds to how fast the vocal folds are closing.

4. *Alternating glottal airflow:* This measure is calculated by taking the glottal airflow maximum minus minimum. This measure reflects the amplitude of vibration and can reflect the glottal area during vibratory cycle.

5. *Minimum flow:* This measure is calculated by subtracting minimum flow from zero. It is indicative of airflow leak due to glottal opening during the closed part of the cycle.

Additional measures important to vocal fold physiology include the following:

6. *Fundamental frequency:* This measure is obtained from the inverse-filtered waveform by means of a peak-picking program. It is the lowest vibrating frequency of the vocal folds and corresponds perceptually to pitch.

7. *Sound pressure level:* This measure is obtained at the midpoint of the vowel from a microphone signal and corresponds physically to vocal intensity and perceptually to loudness.

Voice production arises from a multidimensional system of anatomical, physiological, and neurological components and from the complex coordination of these biological systems. Many of the measures listed above have been used to derive vocal physiology. Stathopoulos and Sapienza (1997) empirically explored applying objective voice measures to children's productions and discussed the data relative to developmental anatomical data (Stathopoulos, 2000). From these cross-sectional data as a function of children's ages, a clearer picture of child vocal physiology has emerged. Because the anatomical structure in children is constantly growing and changing, children continually alter their movements to make their voices sound "normal." Figures 1 through 7 show cross-sectional vocal aerodynamic data obtained in children ages 4–14 years. One of the striking features that emerge from the aerodynamic data is the change in function at 14 years of age for boys. After that age, boys and men functionally group together, while women and children seem to have more in common aerodynamically and physiologically. The data are discussed in relation to their physiological implications.

Estimated subglottal pressure: Children produce higher subglottal pressures than adults, and all speakers produce higher pressures when they produce higher

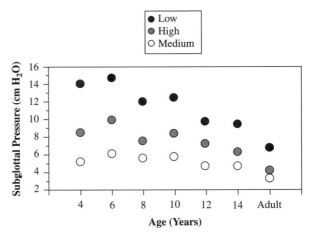

Figure 1. Estimated subglottal pressure as a function of age and sound pressure level.

SPLs (Fig. 1). Anatomical differences in the upper and lower airway will affect the aerodynamic output of the vocal tract. The increased airway resistance in children could substantially increase tracheal pressures (Muller and Brown, 1980).

Airflow open quotient (OQ-20%): Open quotient has traditionally been very closely correlated with SPL. In adults, it is widely believed that as SPL increases, the open quotient decreases. That is, the vocal folds remain closed for a longer proportion of the vibratory cycle as vocal intensity increases. As seen in Figures 2*A* and 2*B*, which show data from a wide age span and both sexes, only adults and older teenagers produce lower open quotients for higher SPLs. It is notable that the younger children and women produce higher OQ-20%, indicating that the vocal folds are open for a longer proportion of the cycle than in men and older boys, regardless of vocal intensity.

Maximum flow declination rate (MFDR): Children and adults regulate their airflow shut-off through a combination of laryngeal and respiratory strategies. Their MFDRs range from about 250 cc/s/s for comfortable levels of SPL to about 1200 cc/s/s for quite high SPLs. In children and adults, MFDR increases as SPL increases (Fig. 3). Increasing MFDR as SPL increases affects the acoustic waveform by emphasizing the high-frequency components of the acoustic source spectra (Titze, 1988).

Alternating glottal airflow: Fourteen-year-old boys and men produce higher alternating glottal airflows than younger children and women during vowel production for the high SPLs (Fig. 4). We can interpret the flow data to indicate that older boys and men produce higher alternating glottal airflows because of their larger laryngeal structures and greater glottal areas. Additionally, men and boys increase their amplitude of vibration during the high SPLs more than women and children do. Greater SPLs result in greater lateral excursion of the vibrating vocal folds; hence the higher alternating glottal airflows for adults. Younger children also increase their

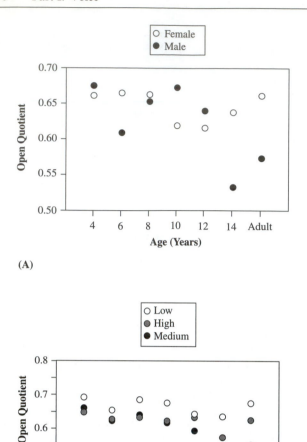

(A)

(B)

Figure 2. A, Airflow open quotient as a function of age and sex. **B,** Airflow open quotient as a function of age and sound pressure level.

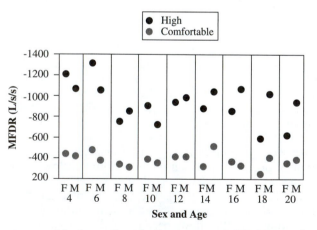

Figure 3. Maximum flow declination rate (MFDR) as a function of age, sex, and sound pressure level.

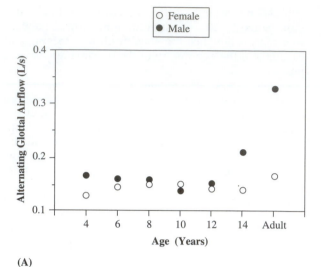

(A)

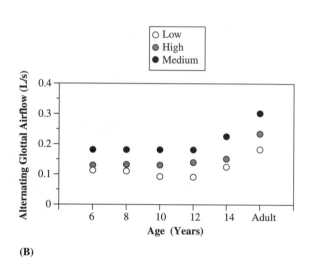

(B)

Figure 4. A, Alternating glottal airflow as a function of age and sex. **B,** Alternating glottal airflow as a function of age and sound pressure level.

amplitude of vibration when they increase their SPL, and we would assume an increase in the alternating flow values. The interpretation is somewhat complicated by the fact that younger children and women have a shorter vocal fold length and smaller area (Flanagan, 1958), thereby limiting airflow through the glottis.

Fundamental frequency: As expected, older boys and men produce lower fundamental frequencies than women and younger children. An interesting result predicted by Titze's (1988) modeling data is that the 4- and 6-year-olds produce unusually high f_0 values when they increase their SPL to high levels (Fig. 5). Changes in fundamental frequency are more easily effected by increasing tracheal pressure when the vocal fold is characterized by a smaller effective vibrating mass, as in young children ages 4–6 years.

Laryngeal airway resistance: Children produce voice with higher Rlaw than 14-year-olds and adults, and all speakers increase their Rlaw when increasing their SPL (Fig. 6). Since Rlaw is calculated by dividing subglottal

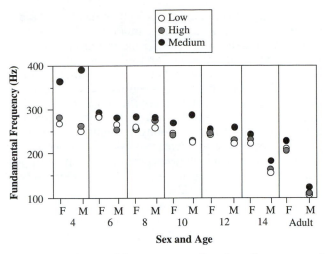

Figure 5. Fundamental frequency as a function of age, sex, and sound pressure level.

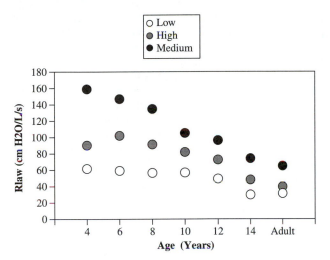

Figure 6. Laryngeal airway resistance as a function of age and sound pressure level.

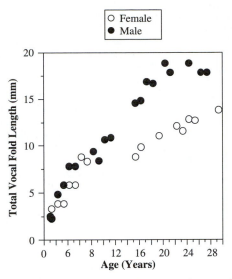

Figure 7. Length of vocal fold as a function of age and sex.

pressure by laryngeal airflow, the high Rlaw for high SPL is largely due to higher values of subglottal pressure, since the average glottal airflow is the same across age groups. A basic assumption needs to be discussed here, and that is, that glottal airflow will increase when subglottal air pressure increases if laryngeal configuration/resistance is held constant. The fact that subglottal pressure increases for high SPLs but flow does not increase clearly indicates that Rlaw must be increasing. Physiologically, the shape and configuration of the laryngeal airway must be decreasing in size to maintain the constant airflow in the setting of increasing subglottal pressures. In sum, children and adults alike continually modify their glottal airway to control the important variables of subglottal pressure and SPL.

The cross-sectional aerodynamic data, and in particular the flow data, make a compelling argument that the primary factor affecting children's vocal physiology is the size of their laryngeal structure. A general scan of the cross-sectional data discussed here shows a change in

vocal function at age 14 in boys. It is not merely coincidental that at 14 years, male larynges continue to increase in size to approximate the size of adult male larynges, whereas larynges in teenage girls plateau and approximate the size of adult female larynges (Fig. 7). Regardless of whether it is size or other anatomical factors affecting vocal function, it is clear that use of an adult male model for depicting normal vocal function is inappropriate for children. Age- and sex-appropriate aerodynamic, acoustic, and physiological models of normal voice need to be referred to for the diagnosis and remediation of voice disorders.

See also INSTRUMENTAL ASSESSMENT OF CHILDREN'S VOICE.

—Elaine T. Stathopoulos

References

Arkebauer, H. J., Hixon, T. J., and Hardy, J. C. (1967). Peak intraoral air pressure during speech. *Journal of Speech and Hearing Research, 10,* 196–208.

Beckett, R. L., Theolke, W. M., and Cowan, L. A. (1971). Normative study of airflow in children. *British Journal of Disorders in Communication, 6,* 13–17.

Bernthal, J. E., and Beukelman, D. R. (1978). Intraoral air pressure during the production of /p/ and /b/ by children, youths, and adults. *Journal of Speech and Hearing Research, 21,* 361–371.

Diggs, C. C. (1972). *Intraoral air pressure for selected English consonants: A normative study of children.* Unpublished master's thesis, Purdue University, Lafayette, Indiana.

Flanagan, J. L. (1958). Some properties of the glottal sound source. *Journal of Speech and Hearing Disorders, 1,* 99–116.

Holmberg, E. B., Hillman, R. B., and Perkell, J. (1988). Glottal airflow and transglottal air pressure measurements for male and female speakers in soft, normal, and loud voice. *Journal of the Acoustical Society of America, 84,* 511–529.

Lofqvist, A., Carlborg, B., and Kitzing, P. (1982). Initial validation of an indirect measure of subglottal pressure during vowels. *Journal of Acoustical Society of America, 72,* 633–635.

Muller, E. M., and Brown, W. S. (1980). Variations in the supraglottal air pressure waveform and their articulatory interpretation. *Speech and Language Advance in Basic Research and Practice, 4,* 318–389.

Rothenberg, M. (1977). Measurement of airflow in speech. *Journal of Speech and Hearing Research, 20,* 155–176.

Smitheran, J. R., and Hixon, T. J. (1981). A clinical method for estimating laryngeal airway resistance during vowel production. *Journal of Speech, Language, and Hearing Research, 46,* 138–146.

Stathopoulos, E. T. (2000). A review of the development of the child voice: An anatomical and functional perspective. In P. White (Ed.), *Child voice.* International Symposium. Stockholm, Sweden: KTH Voice Research Centre.

Stathopoulos, E. T., and Sapienza, C. M. (1997). Developmental changes in laryngeal and respiratory function with variations in sound pressure level. *Journal of Speech, Language, and Hearing Research, 40,* 595–614.

Stathopoulos, E. T., and Weismer, G. (1986). Oral airflow and air pressure during speech production: A comparative study of children, youths, and adults. *Folia Phoniatrica, 37,* 152–159.

Subtelny, J. D., Worth, J. H., and Sakuda, M. (1966). Intraoral air pressure and rate of flow during speech. *Journal of Speech and Hearing Research, 9,* 498–515.

Timcke, R., von Leden, H., and Moore, P. (1958). Laryngeal vibrations: Measurements of the glottic wave. *AMA Archives of Otolaryngology, 68,* 1–19.

Titze, I. R. (1988). Regulation of vocal power and efficiency by subglottal pressure and glottal width. In O. Fujimura (Ed.), *Vocal fold physiology: Voice production, mechanisms, and functions* (pp. 227–238). New York: Raven Press.

Van Hattum, R. J., and Worth, J. H. (1967). Airflow rates in normal speakers. *Cleft Palate Journal, 4,* 137–147.

Voice Disorders of Aging

Voice disorders afflict up to 12% of the elderly population (Shindo and Hanson, 1990). Voice disorders in elderly persons can result from normal age-related changes in the voice production mechanism or from pathological conditions separate from normal aging (Linville, 2001). However, distinguishing between pathology and normal age-related changes can be difficult. Indeed, a number of investigators have concluded that the vast majority of elderly patients with voice disorders suffer from a disease process associated with aging rather than from a disorder involving physiological aging alone (Morrison and Gore-Hickman, 1986; Woo, Casper, Colton, and Brewer, 1992). Therefore, a thorough medical examination and history are required to rule out pathological processes affecting voice in elderly patients (Hagen, Lyons, and Nuss, 1996). In addition, stroboscopic examination of the vocal folds is recommended to detect abnormalities of mucosal wave and amplitude of vocal fold vibration that affect voice production (Woo et al., 1992).

A number of pathological conditions that affect voice are prevalent in the elderly population simply because of

advanced age. Such conditions include neurological disorders, benign lesions, trauma, inflammatory processes, and endocrine disorders (Morrison and Gore-Hickman, 1986; Woo et al., 1992). Carcinoma of the head and neck occasionally occurs late in life, although more commonly it is diagnosed between the ages of 50 and 70 (Leon et al., 1998). Interestingly, multiple etiologic factors related to a voice disorder are more common in elderly patients than in younger adults. In addition, elderly persons are at increased risk for laryngeal side effects from pharmacological agents, since prescription and nonprescription drugs are used disproportionately by the elderly (Linville, 2001).

Elderly patients often exhibit neurological voice disorders, particularly in later stages of old age. Estimates of the incidence of peripheral laryngeal nerve damage in elderly dysphonic patients range from 7% to 21%. Generally, peripheral paralysis in the elderly tends to be associated with disease processes associated with aging (such as lung neoplasm), as opposed to idiopathic peripheral paralysis, which occurs infrequently (Morrison and Gore-Hickman, 1986; Woo et al., 1992). Symptoms of peripheral paralysis include glottic insufficiency, reduced loudness, breathiness, and diplophonia. Voice therapy for peripheral paralysis frequently involves increasing vocal fold adductory force to facilitate closure of the glottis and improving breath support to minimize fatigue and improve speech phrasing. After age 60, central neurological disorders such as stroke, focal dystonia, Parkinson's disease, Alzheimer's disease, and essential tremor also occur frequently. Treatment for central disorders involves attention to specific deficits in vocal fold function such as positioning deficits, instability of vibration, and incoordination of movements. Functioning of the velopharynx, tongue, jaw, lips, diaphragm, abdomen, and rib cage may also be compromised and may require treatment. Treatment may focus on vocal fold movement patterns, postural changes, coordination of respiratory and phonatory systems, respiratory support, speech prosody, velopharyngeal closure, or speech intelligibility. In some cases, augmentative communication strategies might be used, or medical treatment may be combined with speech or voice therapy to improve outcomes (Ramig and Scherer, 1992).

A variety of benign vocal lesions are particularly prevalent in the elderly, including Reineke's edema, polypoid degeneration, unilateral sessile polyp, and benign epithelial lesions with variable dysplastic changes (Morrison and Gore-Hickman, 1986; Woo et al., 1992). Reineke's edema and polypoid degeneration occur more commonly in women and are characterized by chronic, diffuse edema extending along the entire length of the vocal fold. The specific site of the edema is the superficial layer of the lamina propria. Although the etiology of Reineke's edema and polypoid degeneration is uncertain, reflux, cigarette smoking, and vocal abuse/misuse have been mentioned as possible causal factors (Koufman, 1995; Zeitels et al., 1997). Some degree of edema and epithelial thickening is a normal accompaniment of aging in some individuals. The reason why women are at greater risk than men for developing pathological epithelial changes as they age is unknown, although differences in vocal use patterns could be a factor. That is, elderly women may be more likely to develop hypertensive phonatory patterns in an effort to compensate for the age-related pitch lowering that accompanies vocal fold thickening and edema (Linville, 2001).

The incidence of functional hypertensive dysphonia among elderly speakers is disputed. Some investigators report significant evidence of phonatory behaviors consistent with hypertension, such as hyperactivity of the ventricular vocal folds in the elderly population (Hagen, Lyons, and Nuss, 1996; Morrison and Gore-Hickman, 1986). Others report a low incidence of vocal fold lesions commonly associated with hyperfunction (vocal nodules, pedunculated polyps), as well as relatively few cases of functional dysphonia without tissue changes (Woo et al., 1992). Clinicians are in agreement, however, that elderly patients need to be evaluated for evidence of hypertensive phonation and provided with therapy to promote more relaxed phonatory adjustments when evidence of hypertension is found, such as visible tension in the cervical muscles, a report of increased phonatory effort, a pattern of glottal attack, high laryngeal position, and/or anteroposterior laryngeal compression.

Inflammatory conditions such as pachydermia, laryngitis sicca, and nonspecific laryngitis also are diagnosed with some regularity in the elderly (see INFECTIOUS DISEASES AND INFLAMMATORY CONDITIONS OF THE LARYNX). These conditions might arise as a consequence of smoking, reflux, medications, or poor hydration and often coexist with vocal fold lesions that may be either benign or malignant. Age-related laryngeal changes such as mucous gland degeneration might be a factor in development of laryngitis sicca (Morrison and Gore-Hickman, 1986; Woo et al., 1992). Gastroesophageal reflux disease (GERD) is another inflammatory condition that is reported to occur with greater frequency in the elderly (Richter, 2000). Since GERD has been present for a longer time in the elderly in comparison with younger adults, it is a more complicated disease in this group. Often elderly patients report less severe heartburn but have more severe erosive damage to the esophagus (Katz, 1998; Richter, 2000).

Because of advanced age, elderly patients may be at increased risk for traumatic injury to the vocal folds. Trauma might manifest as granuloma or scar tissue from previous surgical procedures requiring general anesthesia, or from other traumatic vocal fold injuries. Vocal fold scarring may be present as a consequence of previous vocal fold surgery, burns, intubation, inflammatory processes, or radiation therapy for glottic carcinoma (Morrison and Gore-Hickman, 1986; Kahane and Beckford, 1991).

Age-related changes in the endocrine system also affect the voice. Secretion disorders of the thyroid (both hyperthyroidism and hypothyroidism) occur commonly in the elderly and often produce voice symptoms, either as a consequence of altered hormone levels or as a result of increased pressure on the recurrent laryngeal nerve. In addition, voice changes are possible with thyroidectomy, even if the procedure is uncomplicated (e.g.,

Debruyne et al., 1997; Francis and Wartofsky, 1992; Sataloff, Emerich, and Hoover, 1997). Elderly persons also may experience vocal symptoms as a consequence of hypoparathyroidism or hyperparathyroidism, or from neuropathic disturbances resulting from diabetes (Maceri, 1986).

Lifestyle factors and variability among elderly speakers often blur the distinction between normal and disordered voice. Elderly persons differ in the rate and extent to which they exhibit normal age-related anatomical, physiological, and neurological changes. They also differ in lifestyle. These factors result in considerable variation in phonatory characteristics, articulatory precision habits, and respiratory function capabilities among elderly speakers (Linville, 2001).

Lifestyle factors can either postpone or exacerbate the effects of aging on the voice. Although a potentially limitless combination of environmental factors combine to affect aging, perhaps the most controllable and potentially significant lifestyle factors are physical fitness and cigarette smoking. The elderly population is extremely variable in fitness levels. The rate and extent of decline in motor and sensory performance with aging varies both within and across elderly individuals (Finch and Schneider, 1985). Declines in motor performance are directly related to muscle use and can be minimized by a lifestyle that includes exercise. The benefits of daily exercise include facilitated muscle contraction, enhanced nerve conduction velocity, and increased blood flow (Spirduso, 1982; Finch and Schneider, 1985; De Vito et al., 1997). A healthy lifestyle that includes regular exercise may also positively influence laryngeal performance, although a direct link has yet to be established (Ringel and Chodzko-Zajko, 1987). However, there is evidence that variability on measures of phonatory function in elderly speakers is reduced by controlling for a speaker's physiological condition (Ramig and Ringel, 1983). Physical conditioning programs that include aerobic exercise often are recommended for aging professional singers to improve respiratory and abdominal conditioning and to avoid tremolo, as well as to improve endurance, accuracy, and agility. Physical conditioning is also important in nonsingers to prevent dysphonia in later life (Sataloff, Spiegel, and Rosen, 1997; Linville, 2001).

The effects of smoking coexist with changes related to normal aging in elderly smokers. Smoking amplifies the impact of normal age-related changes in both the pulmonary and laryngeal systems. Elderly smokers demonstrate accelerated declines in pulmonary function, even if no pulmonary disease is detected (Hill and Fisher, 1993; Lee et al., 1999). Smoking also has a definite effect on the larynx and alters laryngeal function. Clinicians must consider smoking history in assessing an elderly speaker's voice (Linville, 2001).

Clinicians also must be mindful of the overall health status of older patients presenting with voice disorders. Elderly dysphonic patients often are in poor general health and have a high incidence of systemic illness. Pulmonary disease and hypertensive cardiac disease have been cited as particularly prevalent in elderly voice patients (Woo et al., 1992). If multiple health problems are present, elderly dysphonic patients may be less compliant in following therapeutic regimens, or treatment for voice problems may need to be postponed. In general, the diagnosis and treatment of voice disorders are more complicated if multiple medical conditions are present (Linville, 2001).

—*Sue Ellen Linville*

References

Debruyne, F., Ostyn, F., Delaere, P., Wellens, W., and Decoster, W. (1997). Temporary voice changes after uncomplicated thyroidectomy. *Acta Oto-Rhino-Laryngologica (Belgium), 51,* 137–140.

De Vito, G., Hernandez, R., Gonzalez, V., Felici, F., and Figura, F. (1997). Low intensity physical training in older subjects. *Journal of Sports Medicine and Physical Fitness, 37,* 72–77.

Finch, C., and Schneider, E. (1985). *Handbook of the biology of aging.* New York: Van Nostrand Reinhold.

Francis, T., and Wartofsky, L. (1992). Common thyroid disorders in the elderly. *Postgraduate Medicine, 92,* 225.

Hagen, P., Lyons, F., and Nuss, D. (1996). Dysphonia in the elderly: Diagnosis and management of age-related voice changes. *Southern Medical Journal, 89,* 204–207.

Hill, R., and Fisher, E. (1993). Smoking cessation in the older chronic smoker: A review. In D. Mahler (Ed.), *Lung biology in health and disease* (vol. 63, pp. 189–218). New York: Marcel Dekker.

Kahane, J., and Beckford, N. (1991). The aging larynx and voice. In D. Ripich (Ed.), *Handbook of geriatric communication disorders.* Austin, TX: Pro-Ed.

Katz, P. (1998). Gastroesophageal reflux disease. *Journal of the American Geriatrics Society, 46,* 1558–1565.

Koufman, J. (1995). Gastroesophageal reflux and voice disorders. In C. Korovin and W. Gould (Eds.), *Diagnosis and treatment of voice disorders* (pp. 161–175). New York: Igaku-Shoin.

Lee, H., Lim, M., Lu, C., Liu, V., Fahn, H., Zhang, C., et al. (1999). Concurrent increase of oxidative DNA damage and lipid peroxidation together with mitochondrial DNA mutation in human lung tissues during aging: Smoking enhances oxidative stress on the aged tissues. *Archives of Biochemistry and Biophysics, 362,* 309–316.

Leon, X., Quer, M., Agudelo, D., Lopez-Pousa, A., De Juan, M., Diez, S., and Burgues, J. (1998). Influence of age on laryngeal carcinoma. *Annals of Otology, Rhinology, and Laryngology, 107,* 164–169.

Linville, S. E. (2001). *Vocal aging.* San Diego, CA: Singular Publishing Group.

Maceri, D. (1986). Head and neck manifestations of endocrine disease. *Otolaryngologic Clinics of North America, 19,* 171–180.

Morrison, M., and Gore-Hickman, P. (1986). Voice disorders in the elderly. *Journal of Otolaryngology, 15,* 231–234.

Ramig, L., and Ringel, R. (1983). Effects of physiological aging on selected acoustic characteristics of voice. *Journal of Speech and Hearing Research, 26,* 22–30.

Ramig, L., and Scherer, R. (1992). Speech therapy for neurologic disorders of the larynx. In A. Blitzer, M. Brin, C. Sasaki, S. Fahn, and K. Harris (Eds.), *Neurologic disorders of the larynx* (pp. 163–181). New York: Thieme Medical Publishers.

Richter, J. (2000). Gastroesophageal disease in the older patient: Presentation, treatment, and complications. *American Journal of Gastroenterology, 95,* 368–373.

Ringel, R., and Chodzko-Zajko, W. (1987). Vocal indices of biological age. *Journal of Voice, 1,* 31–37.

Sataloff, R., Emerich, K., and Hoover, C. (1997). Endocrine dysfunction. In R. Sataloff (Ed.), *Professional voice: The science and art of clinical care* (pp. 291–297). San Diego, CA: Singular Publishing Group.

Sataloff, R., Spiegel, J., and Rosen, D. (1997). The effects of age on the voice. In R. Sataloff (Ed.), *Professional voice: The science and art of clinical care* (pp. 259–267). San Diego, CA: Singular Publishing Group.

Shindo, M., and Hanson, S. (1990). Geriatric voice and laryngeal dysfunction. *Otolaryngologic Clinics of North America, 23,* 1035–1044.

Spirduso, W. (1982). Physical fitness in relation to motor aging. In J. Mortimer, F. Pirozzolo, and G. Maletta (Eds.), *The aging motor system* (pp. 120–151). New York: Praeger.

Woo, P., Casper, J., Colton, R., and Brewer, D. (1992). Dysphonia in the aging: Physiology versus disease. *Laryngoscope, 102,* 139–144.

Zeitels, S., Hillman, R., Bunting, G., and Vaughn, T. (1997). Reineke's edema: Phonatory mechanisms and management strategies. *Annals of Otology, Rhinology, and Laryngology, 106,* 533–543.

Further Readings

Abitbol, J., Abitbol, P., and Abitbol, B. (1999). Sex hormones and the female voice. *Journal of Voice, 13,* 424–446.

Benjamin, B. (1997). Speech production of normally aging adults. *Seminars in Speech and Language, 18,* 135–141.

Benninger, M., Alessi, D., Archer, S., Bastian, R., Ford, C., Koufman, J., et al. (1996). Vocal fold scarring: Current concepts and management. *Otolaryngology–Head and Neck Surgery, 115,* 474–482.

Finucane, P., and Anderson, C. (1995). Thyroid disease in older patients: Diagnosis and treatment. *Drugs and Aging, 6,* 268–277.

Hirano, M., Kurita, S., and Sakaguchi, S. (1989). Ageing of the vibratory tissue of human vocal folds. *Acta Otolaryngologica, 107,* 428–433.

Hoit, J., and Hixon, T. (1987). Age and speech breathing. *Journal of Speech and Hearing Research, 30,* 351–366.

Hoit, J., Hixon, T., Altman, M., and Morgan, W. (1989). Speech breathing in women. *Journal of Speech and Hearing Research, 32,* 353–365.

Kahane, J. (1990). Age-related changes in the peripheral speech mechanism: Structural and physiological changes. In *Proceedings of the Research Symposium on Communicative Sciences and Disorders and Aging* (ASHA Reports No. 19). Rockville, MD: American Speech-Language-Hearing Association, pp. 75–87.

Koch, W., Patel, H., Brennan, J., Boyle, J., and Sidransky, D. (1995). Squamous cell carcinoma of the head and neck in the elderly. *Archives of Otolaryngology–Head and Neck Surgery, 121,* 262–265.

Linville, S. E. (1992). Glottal gap configurations in two age groups of women. *Journal of Speech and Hearing Research, 35,* 1209–1215.

Linville, S. E. (2000). The aging voice. In R. D. Kent and M. J. Ball (Eds.), *Voice quality measurement* (pp. 359–376). San Diego, CA: Singular Publishing Group.

Liss, J., Weismer, G., and Rosenbek, J. (1990). Selected acoustic characteristics of speech production in very old males. *Journal of Gerontology Psychological Sciences, 45,* P35–P45.

Lu, F., Casiano, R., Lundy, D., and Xue, J. (1998). Vocal evaluation of thyroplasty type I in the treatment of non-paralytic glottic incompetence. *Annals of Otology, Rhinology, and Laryngology, 103,* 547–553.

Luborsky, M., and McMullen, D. (1999). Culture and aging. In J. Cavanaugh and S. Whitbourne (Eds.), *Gerontology: An interdisciplinary perspective* (pp. 65–90). New York: Oxford University Press.

Lundy, D., Silva, C., Casiano, R., Lu, F. L., and Xue, J. (1998). Cause of hoarseness in elderly patients. *Otolaryngology–Head and Neck Surgery, 118,* 481–485.

Morrison, M., Rammage, L., and Nichol, H. (1989). Evaluation and management of voice disorders in the elderly. In J. Goldstein, H. Kashima, and C. Koopermann (Eds.), *Geriatric otorhinolaryngology.* Philadelphia: B.C. Decker.

Murry, T., Xu, J., and Woodson, G. (1998). Glottal configuration associated with fundamental frequency and vocal register. *Journal of Voice, 12,* 44–49.

Omori, K., Slavit, D., Kacker, A., and Blaugrund, S. (1998). Influence of size and etiology of glottal gap in glottic incompetence dysphonia. *Laryngoscope, 108,* 514–518.

Omori, K., Slavit, D., Matos, C., Kojima, H., Kacker, A., and Blaugrund, S. (1997). Vocal fold atrophy: Quantitative glottic measurement and vocal function. *Annals of Otology, Rhinology, and Laryngology, 106,* 544–551.

Owens, N., Fretwell, M. D., Willey, C., and Murphy, S. S. (1994). Distinguishing between the fit and frail elderly, and optimizing pharmacotherapy. *Drugs and Aging, 4,* 47–55.

Ramig, L., Gray, S., Baker, K., Corbin-Lewis, K., Buder, E., Luschei, E., et al. (2001). The aging voice: A review, treatment data and familial and genetic perspectives. *Folia Phoniatrica et Logopedica, 53,* 252–265.

Sinard, R., and Hall, D. (1998). The aging voice: How to differentiate disease from normal changes. *Geriatrics, 53,* 76–79.

Slavit, D. (1999). Phonosurgery in the elderly: A review. *Ear, Nose, and Throat Journal, 78,* 505–512.

Tanaka, S., Hirano, M., and Chijiwa, K. (1994). Some aspects of vocal fold bowing. *Annals of Otology, Rhinology, and Laryngology, 103,* 357–362.

Tolep, K., Higgins, N., Muza, S., Criner, G., and Kelsen, S. (1995). Comparison of diaphragm strength between healthy adult elderly and young men. *American Journal of Respiratory and Critical Care Medicine, 152,* 677–682.

Weismer, G., and Liss, J. (1991). Speech motor control and aging. In D. Ripich (Ed.), *Handbook of geriatric communication disorders.* Austin, TX: Pro-Ed.

Voice Production: Physics and Physiology

When the vocal folds are near each other, a sufficient transglottal pressure will set them into oscillation. This oscillation produces cycles of airflow that create the acoustic signal known as phonation, the voicing sound source, the voice signal, or more generally, voice. This article discusses some of the mechanistic aspects of phonation.

The most general expression of forces in the larynx dealing with motion of the vocal folds during phonation is

$$F(x) = mx'' + bx' + kx, \tag{1}$$

where $F(x)$ is the air pressure forces on the vocal fold tissues, m is the mass of the tissue in motion, b is a viscous coefficient, k is a spring constant coefficient, x is the position of the tissue from rest, x' is the velocity of the tissue, and x'' is the acceleration of the tissue. In multi-mass models of phonation (e.g., Ishizaka and Flanagan, 1972), this equation is used for each mass proposed. Each term on the right-hand side characterizes forces in the tissue, and the left-hand side represents the external forces. This equation emphasizes the understanding that mass, viscosity, and stiffness each play a role in the motion (normal or abnormal) of the vocal folds, that these are associated with the acceleration, velocity, and displacement of the tissue, respectively, and they are balanced by the external air pressure forces acting on the vocal folds.

Glottal adduction has three parts. (1) How close the vocal processes are to each other determines the posterior prephonatory closeness of the membranous vocal folds. (2) The space created by the intercartilaginous glottis determines the "constant" opening there through which some or all of the DC (baseline) air will flow. (3) The closeness of the membranous vocal folds partly determines whether vocal fold oscillation can take place. To permit oscillation, the vocal folds must be within the *phonatory adductory range* (not too far apart, and yet not too overly compressed; Scherer, 1995), and the transglottal pressure must be at or greater than the *phonatory threshold pressure* (Titze, 1992) for the prevailing conditions of the vocal fold tissues and adduction.

The fundamental frequency F0, related to the pitch of the voice, will tend to rise if the tension of the tissue in motion increases, and will tend to fall if the length, mass, or density increases. The most general expression to date for pitch control has been offered by Titze (1994), viz.,

$$F0 = (0.5/L)\sqrt{(s_p/\rho)} * (1 + (d_a/d) * (s_{am}/s_p) * a_{TA})^{0.5}, \tag{2}$$

where L is the vibrating length of the vocal folds, s_p is the passive tension of the tissue in motion, d_a/d is the ratio of the depth of the thyroarytenoid (TA) muscle in vibration to the total depth in vibration (the other tissue in motion is the more medial mucosal tissue), s_{am} is the maximum active stress that the TA muscle can produce, a_{TA} is the activity level of the TA muscle, and ρ is the density of the tissue in motion. When the vocal folds are lengthened by rotation of the thyroid and cricoid cartilages through the contraction of the cricothyroid (CT) muscles, the passive stretching of the vocal folds increases their passive tension, and thus L and s_p tend to counter each other, with s_p being more dominant (F0 generally rises with vocal fold elongation). Increasing subglottal pressure increases the lateral amplitude of motion of the vocal folds, thus increasing s_p (via greater passive stretch; Titze, 1994) and d_a, thereby increasing

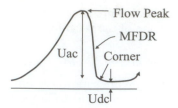

Figure 1. One cycle of glottal airflow. Uac is the varying portion of the waveform, and Udc is the offset or bias flow. The flow peak is the maximum flow in the cycle, MFDR is the maximum flow declination rate (derivative of the flow), typically located on the right-hand side of the flow pulse, and the corner curvature at the end of the flow pulse describes how sharp the corner "shut-off" is. The flow peak, MFDR, and corner sharpness are all important for the spectral aspects of the flow pulse (see text).

F0. Increasing the contraction of the TA muscle (a_{TA}) would tend to stiffen the muscle and shorten the vocal fold length (L), both of which would raise F0 but at the same time decrease the passive tension (s_p) and the depth of vibration (d_a), which would decrease F0. Typically, large changes in F0 are associated with increased contraction of both the CT and TA muscles (Hirano, Ohala, and Vennard, 1969; Titze, 1994). Thus, the primary control for F0 is through the coordinative contraction of the TA and CT muscles, and subglottal pressure. F0 control, including the differentiated contraction of the complex TA muscle, anterior pull by the hyoid bone (Honda, 1983), cricoid tilt via tracheal pull (Sundberg, Leanderson, and von Euler, 1989), and the associations with adduction and vocal quality all need much study.

The intensity of voiced sounds, related to the loudness of the voice, is a combination and coordination of respiratory, laryngeal, and vocal tract aspects. Intensity increases with an increase in subglottal pressure, which itself depends on both lung volume reduction (an increase in air pressure in the lungs) and adduction of the vocal folds (which offers resistance to the flow of air from the lungs). An increase in the subglottal pressure during phonation can affect the cyclic glottal flow waveform (Fig. 1) by increasing its flow peak, increasing the maximum flow declination rate (MFDR, the maximum rate that the flow shuts off as the glottis is closing), and the sharpness of the baseline corner when the flow is near zero (or near its minimum value in the cycle). Greater peak flow, MFDR, and corner sharpness respectively increase the intensity of F0, the intensity of the first formant region (at least), and the intensity of the higher partials (Fant, Liljencrants, and Lin, 1985; Gauffin and Sundberg, 1989). Glottal adduction level greatly affects the source spectrum or quality of the voice, increasing the negative slope of the spectrum as one changes voice production from highly compressed voice (a relatively flat spectrum) to normal adduction to highly breathy voice (a relatively steep spectrum) (Scherer, 1995). The vocal tract filter function will augment the spectral intensity values of the glottal flow source in the region of the formants (resonances), and will decrease their intensity values in the valleys of the resonant structure (Titze, 1994). The radiation away from the lips will increase the spectrum slope (by about 6 dB per octave).

Maintenance of vocal fold oscillation during phonation depends on the tissue characteristics mentioned above, as well as the changing shape of the glottis and the changing intraglottal air pressures during each cycle. During glottal opening, the shape of the glottis corresponding to the vibrating vocal folds is convergent (wider in the lower glottis, narrower in the upper glottis), and the pressures on the walls of the glottis are positive due to this shape and to the (always) positive subglottal pressure (for normal egressive phonation) (Fig. 2). This positive pressure separates the folds during glottal opening. During glottal closing, the shape of the glottis is divergent (narrower in the lower glottis, wider in the upper glottis), and the pressures on the walls of the lower glottis are negative because of this shape (Fig. 2), and negative throughout the glottis when there also is rarefaction (negative pressure) of the supraglottal region. This alternation in glottal shape and intraglottal pressures, along with the alternation of the internal forces of the vocal folds, maintains the oscillation of the vocal folds. The exact glottal shape and intraglottal pressure changes, however, need to be established in the human larynx for the wide range of possible phonatory and vocal tract acoustic conditions.

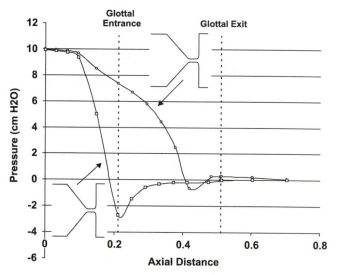

Figure 2. Pressure profiles within the glottis. The upper trace corresponds to the data for a glottis with a 10° convergence and the lower trace to data for a glottis with a 10° divergence, both having a minimal glottal diameter of 0.04 cm (using a Plexiglas model of the larynx; Scherer and Shinwari, 2000). The transglottal pressure was 10 cm H_2O in this illustration. Glottal entrance is at the minimum diameter position for the divergent glottis. The length of the glottal duct was 0.3 cm. Supraglottal pressure was taken to be atmospheric (zero). The convergent glottis shows positive pressures and the divergent glottis shows negative pressures throughout most of the glottis. The curvature at the glottal exit of the convergent glottis prevents the pressures from being positive throughout (Scherer, DeWitt, and Kucinschi, 2001).

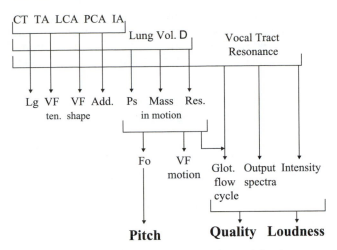

Figure 3. Factors leading to pitch, quality, and loudness production. See text.

When the two medial vocal fold surfaces are not mirror images of each other across the midline, the geometric asymmetry creates different pressures on the two sides (i.e., pressure asymmetries; Scherer et al., 2001, 2002) and therefore different driving forces on the two sides. Also, if there is tissue asymmetry, that is, if the two vocal folds themselves do not have equal values of tension (stiffness) and mass, one vocal fold may not vibrate like the other one, creating roughness, subharmonics, and cyclic groupings (Isshiki and Ishizaka, 1976; Gerratt et al., 1988; Wong et al., 1991; Titze, Baken, and Herzel, 1993; Steinecke and Herzel, 1995).

Figure 3 summarizes some basic aspects of phonation. The upper left suggests muscle contraction effects of vocal fold length (via CT and TA action), adduction (via TA, lateral cricoarytenoid, posterior cricoarytenoid, and interarytenoid muscle contraction), tension (via CT, TA, and adduction), and glottal shape (via vocal fold length, adduction, and TA rounding effect). When lung volume reduction is then employed, glottal airflow and subglottal pressure are created, resulting in motion of the vocal folds (if the adduction and pressure are sufficient), glottal flow resistance (transglottal pressure divided by the airflow), and the fundamental frequency (and pitch) of the voice. With the vocal tract included, the glottal flow is affected by the resonances of the vocal tract (pressures acting at the glottis level) and the inertance of the air of the vocal tract (to skew the glottal flow waveform to the right; Rothenberg, 1983), and the output spectra (quality) and intensity (loudness) result from the combination of the glottal flow, resonance, and radiation from the lips.

Many basic issues of glottal aerodynamics, aeroacoustics, and modeling remain unclear for both normal and abnormal phonation. The glottal flow (the volume velocity flow) is considered a primary sound source, and the presence of the false vocal folds may interfere with the glottal jet and create a secondary sound source

(Zhang et al., 2001). The turbulence and vorticities of the glottal flow may also contribute sound sources (Zhang et al., 2001). The false vocal folds themselves may contribute significant control of the flow resistance through the larynx, from more resistance (decreasing the flow if the false folds are quite close) to less resistance (increasing the glottal flow when the false folds are in an intermediate position) (Agarwal and Scherer, in press). Computer modeling needs to be practical, as in two-mass modeling (Ishizaka and Flanagan, 1972), but also closer to physiological reality, as in finite element modeling (Alipour, Berry, and Titze, 2000; Alipour and Scherer, 2000). The most complete approach so far is to combine finite element modeling of the tissue with computational fluid dynamics of the flow (to solve the Navier-Stokes equations; Alipour and Titze, 1996). However, we still need models of phonation that are helpful in describing and predicting subtle aspects of laryngeal function necessary for differentiating vocal pathologies, phonation styles and types, and approaches for phonosurgery, as well as for providing rehabilitation and training feedback for clients.

See also VOICE ACOUSTICS.

—*Ron Scherer*

References

Agarwal, M., Scherer, R. C., and Hollien, H. (in press). The false vocal folds: Shape and size in coronal view during phonation. *Journal of Voice*.

Alipour, F., Berry, D. A., and Titze, I. R. (2000). A finite-element model of vocal-fold vibration. *Journal of the Acoustical Society of America, 108*, 3003–3012.

Alipour, F., and Scherer, R. C. (2000). Vocal fold bulging: Effects on phonation using a biophysical computer model. *Journal of Voice, 14*, 470–483.

Alipour, F., and Titze, I. R. (1996). Combined simulation of airflow and vocal fold vibrations. In P. Davis and N. Fletcher (Eds.), *Vocal fold physiology: Controlling complexity and chaos* (pp. 17–29). San Diego, CA: Singular Publishing Group.

Fant, G., Liljencrants, J., and Lin, Q. (1985). A four-parameter model of glottal flow. *Speech Transmission Laboratory Quarterly Progress and Status Report, 4*, 1–13. Stockholm: Royal Institute of Technology.

Gauffin, J., and Sundberg, J. (1989). Spectral correlates of glottal voice source waveform characteristics. *Journal of Speech and Hearing Research, 32*, 556–565.

Gerratt, B. R., Precoda, K., Hanson, D., and Berke, G. S. (1988). Source characteristics of diplophonia. *Journal of the Acoustical Society of America, 83*, S66.

Hirano, M., Ohala, J., and Vennard, W. (1969). The function of the laryngeal muscles in regulating fundamental frequency and intensity of phonation. *Journal of Speech and Hearing Research, 12*, 616–628.

Honda, K. (1983). Relationship between pitch control and vowel articulation. In D. M. Bless and J. H. Abbs (Eds.), *Vocal fold physiology: Contemporary research and clinical issues*. San Diego, CA: College-Hill Press.

Ishizaka, K., and Flanagan, J. L. (1972). Synthesis of voiced sounds from a two-mass model of the vocal cords. *Bell System Technology Journal, 51*, 1233–1268.

Isshiki, N., and Ishizaka, K. (1976). Computer simulation of pathological vocal cord vibration. *Journal of the Acoustical Society of America, 60,* 1193–1198.

Rothenberg, M. (1983). An interactive model for the voice source. In D. M. Bless and J. H. Abbs (Eds.), *Vocal fold physiology: Contemporary research and clinical issues* (pp. 155–165). San Diego, CA: College-Hill Press.

Scherer, R. C. (1995). Laryngeal function during phonation. In J. S. Rubin, R. T. Sataloff, G. S. Korovin, and W. J. Gould (Eds.), *Diagnosis and treatment of voice disorders* (pp. 86–104). New York: Igaku-Shoin.

Scherer, R. C., DeWitt, K., and Kucinschi, B. R. (2001). The effect of exit radii on intraglottal pressure distributions in the convergent glottis. *Journal of the Acoustical Society of America, 110,* 2267–2269.

Scherer, R. C., and Shinwari, D. (2000). Glottal pressure profiles for a diameter of 0.04 cm. *Journal of the Acoustical Society of America, 107,* 2905 (A).

Scherer, R. C., Shinwari, D., DeWitt, K., Zhang, C., Kucinschi, B., and Afjeh, A. (2001). Intraglottal pressure profiles for a symmetric and oblique glottis with a divergence angle of 10 degrees. *Journal of the Acoustical Society of America, 109,* 1616–1630.

Scherer, R. C., Shinwari, D., De Witt, K. J., Zhang, C., Kucinschi, B. R., and Afjeh, A. A. (2002). Intraglottal pressure profiles for a symmetric and oblique glottis with a uniform duct. *Journal of the Acoustical Society of America, 112*(4), 1253–1256.

Steinecke, I., and Herzel, H. (1995). Bifurcations in an asymmetric vocal-fold model. *Journal of the Acoustical Society of America, 97,* 1874–1884.

Sundberg, J., Leanderson, R., and von Euler, C. (1989). Activity relationship between diaphragm and cricothyroid muscles. *Journal of Voice, 3,* 225–232.

Titze, I. R. (1992). Phonation threshold pressure: A missing link in glottal aerodynamics. *Journal of the Acoustical Society of America, 91,* 2926–2935.

Titze, I. R. (1994). *Principles of voice production.* Englewood Cliffs, NJ: Prentice Hall.

Titze, I. R., Baken, R. J., and Herzel, H. (1993). Evidence of chaos in vocal fold vibration. In I. R. Titze (Ed.), *Vocal fold physiology: Frontiers in basic science* (pp. 143–188). San Diego, CA: Singular Publishing Group.

Wong, D., Ito, M. R., Cox, N. B., and Titze, I. R. (1991). Observation of perturbations in a lumped-element model of the vocal folds with application to some pathological cases. *Journal of the Acoustical Society of America, 89,* 383–394.

Zhang, C., Zhao, W., Frankel, S. H., and Mongeau, L. (2001). Computational aeroacoustics of phonation: Effect of subglottal pressure, glottal oscillation frequency, and ventricular folds. *Journal of the Acoustical Society, 109,* 2412 (A).

Voice Quality, Perceptual Evaluation of

Voice quality is the auditory perception of acoustic elements of phonation that characterize an individual speaker. Thus, it is an interaction between the acoustic speech signal and a listener's perception of that signal. Voice quality has been of interest to scholars for as long as people have studied speech. The ancient Greeks associated certain kinds of voices with specific character traits; for example, a nasal voice indicated a spiteful and immoral character. Ancient writers on oratory emphasized voice quality as an essential component of polished speech and described methods for conveying a range of emotions appropriately, for cultivating power, brilliance, and sweetness, and for avoiding undesirable characteristics like roughness, brassiness, or shrillness (see Laver, 1981, for review).

Evaluation of vocal quality is an important part of the diagnosis and treatment of voice disorders. Patients usually seek clinical care because of their own perception of a voice quality deviation, and most often they judge the success of treatment for the voice problem by improvement in their voice quality. A clinician may also judge success by documenting changes in laryngeal anatomy or physiology, but in general, patients are more concerned with how their voices sound after treatment. Researchers from other disciplines are also interested in measuring vocal quality. For example, linguists are interested in how changes in voice quality can signal changes in meaning; psychologists are concerned with the perception of emotion and other personal information encoded in voice; engineers seek to develop algorithms for signal compression and transmission that preserve voice quality; and law enforcement officials need to assess the accuracy of speaker identifications.

Despite this long intellectual history and the substantial cross-disciplinary importance of voice quality, measurement of voice quality is problematic, both clinically and experimentally. Most techniques for assessing voice quality fall into one of two general categories: perceptual assessment protocols, or protocols employing an acoustic or physiologic measurement as an index of quality. In perceptual assessments, a listener (or listeners) rates a voice on a numerical scale or a set of scales representing the extent to which the voice is characterized by critical aspects of voice quality. For example, Fairbanks (1960) recommended that voices be assessed on 5-point scales for the qualities harshness, hoarseness, and breathiness. In the GRBAS protocol (Hirano, 1981), listeners evaluate voices on the scales Grade (or extent of pathology), Roughness, Breathiness, Asthenicity (weakness or lack of power in the voice), and Strain, with each scale ranging from 0 (normal) to 4 (severely disordered). A recent revision to this protocol (Dejonckere et al., 1998) has expanded it to GIRBAS by adding a scale for Instability. Many other similar protocols have been proposed. For example, the Wilson Voice Profile System (Wilson, 1977) includes 7-point scales for laryngeal tone, laryngeal tension, vocal abuse, loudness, pitch, vocal inflections, pitch breaks, diplophonia (perception of two pitches in the voice), resonance, nasal emission, rate, and overall vocal efficiency. A 13-scale protocol proposed by Hammarberg and Gauffin (1995) includes scales for assessing aphonia (lack of voice), breathiness, tension, laxness, creakiness, roughness, gratings, pitch instability, voice breaks, diplophonia, falsetto, pitch, and loudness. Even more elaborate protocols have been proposed by Gelfer (1988; 17 parameters) and Laver (approximately

50 parameters; e.g., Greene and Mathieson, 1989). Methods like visual-analog scaling (making a mark on an undifferentiated line to indicate the amount of a quality present) or direct magnitude estimation (assigning any number—as opposed to one of a finite number of scale values—to indicate the amount of a quality present) have also been applied in efforts to quantify voice quality. Ratings may be made with reference to "anchor" stimuli that exemplify the different scale values, or with reference to a listener's own internal standards for the different levels of a quality.

The usefulness of such protocols for perceptual assessment is limited by difficulties in establishing the correct and adequate set of scales needed to document the sound of a voice. Researchers have never agreed on a standardized set of scales for assessing voice quality, and some evidence suggests that differences between listeners in perceptual strategies are so large that standardization efforts are doomed to failure (Kreiman and Gerratt, 1996). In addition, listeners are apparently unable to agree in their ratings of voices. Evidence suggests that on average, more than 60% of the variance in ratings of voice quality is due to factors other than differences between voices in the quality being rated. For example, scale ratings may vary depending on variable listener attention, difficulty isolating single perceptual dimensions within a complex acoustic stimulus, and differences in listeners' previous experience with a class of voices (Kreiman and Gerratt, 1998). Evidence suggests that traditional perceptual scaling methods are effectively matching tasks, where external stimuli (the voices) are compared to stored mental representations that serve as internal standards for the various rating scales. These idiosyncratic, internal standards appear to vary with listeners' previous experience with voices (Verdonck de Leeuw, 1998) and with the context in which a judgment is made, and may vary substantially across listeners as well as within a given listener. In addition, severity of vocal deviation, difficulty isolating individual dimensions in complex perceptual contexts, and factors like lapses in attention can also influence perceptual measures of voice (de Krom, 1994). These factors (and possibly others) presumably all add uncontrolled variability to scalar ratings of vocal quality, and contribute to listener disagreement (see Gerratt and Kreiman, 2001, for review).

In response to these substantial difficulties, some researchers suggest substituting objective measures of physiologic function, airflow, or the acoustic signal for these flawed perceptual measures, for example, using a measure of acoustic frequency perturbation as a de facto measure of perceived roughness (see ACOUSTIC ASSESSMENT OF VOICE). This approach reflects the prevailing view that listeners are inherently unable to agree in their perception of such complex auditory stimuli. Theoretical and practical difficulties also beset this approach. Theoretically, we cannot know the perceptual importance of particular aspects of the acoustic signal without valid measures of that perceptual response, because voice quality is by definition the perceptual response to a particular acoustic stimulus. Thus, acoustic measures that purport to quantify vocal quality can only derive their validity as measures of voice quality from their causal association with auditory perception. Practically, consistent correlations have never been found between perceptual and instrumental measures of voice, suggesting that such instrumental measures are not stable indices of perceived quality. Finally, correlation does not imply causality: simply knowing the relationship of an acoustic variable to a perceptual one does not necessarily illuminate its contribution to perceived quality. Even if an acoustic variable were important to a listener's judgment of vocal quality, the nature of that contribution would not be revealed by a correlation coefficient. Further, given the great variability in perceptual strategies and habits that individual listeners demonstrate in their use of traditional rating scales, the overall correlation between acoustic and perceptual variables, averaged across samples of listeners and voices, fails to provide useful insight into the perceptual process. (See Kreiman and Gerratt, 2000, for an extended review of these issues.)

Gerratt and Kreiman (2001) proposed an alternative solution to this dilemma. They measured vocal quality by asking listeners to copy natural voice samples with a speech synthesizer. In this method, listeners vary speech synthesis parameters to create an acceptable auditory match to a natural voice stimulus. When a listener chooses the best match to a test stimulus, the synthesis settings parametrically represent the listener's perception of voice quality. Because listeners directly compare each synthetic token they create with the target natural voice, they need not refer to internal standards for particular voice qualities. Further, listeners can manipulate acoustic parameters and hear the result of their manipulations immediately. This process helps listeners focus attention on individual acoustic dimensions, reducing the perceptual complexity of the assessment task and the associated response variability. Preliminary evaluation of this method demonstrated near-perfect agreement among listeners in their assessments of voice quality, presumably because this analysis-synthesis method controls the major sources of variance in quality judgments while avoiding the use of dubiously valid scales for quality. These results indicate that listeners do in fact agree in their perceptual assessments of pathological voice quality, and that tools can be devised to measure perception reliably. However, how such protocols will function in clinical (rather than research) applications remains to be demonstrated. Much more research is certainly needed to determine a meaningful, parsimonious set of acoustic parameters that successfully characterizes all possible normal and pathological voice qualities. Such a set could obviate the need for voice quality labels, allowing researchers and clinicians to replace quality labels with acoustic parameters that are causally linked to auditory perception, and whose levels objectively, completely, and validly specify the voice quality of interest.

—Bruce Gerratt and Jody Kreiman

References

de Krom, G. (1994). Consistency and reliability of voice quality ratings for different types of speech fragments. *Journal of Speech and Hearing Research, 37*, 985–1000.

Dejonckere, P. H., Remacle, M., Fresnel-Elbaz, E., Woisard, V., Crevier, L., and Millet, B. (1998). Reliability and clinical relevance of perceptual evaluation of pathological voices. *Revue de Laryngologie Otologie Rhinologie, 119*, 247–248.

Fairbanks, G. (1960). *Voice and articulation drillbook.* New York: Harper.

Gelfer, M. P. (1988). Perceptual attributes of voice: Development and use of rating scales. *Journal of Voice, 2*, 320–326.

Gerratt, B. R., and Kreiman, J. (2001). Measuring vocal quality with speech synthesis. *Journal of the Acoustical Society of America, 110*, 2560–2566.

Greene, M. C. L., and Mathieson, L. (1989). *The voice and its disorders.* London: Whurr.

Hammarberg, B., and Gauffin, J. (1995). Perceptual and acoustic characteristics of quality differences in pathological voices as related to physiological aspects. In O. Fujimura and M. Hirano (Eds.), *Vocal fold physiology: Voice quality control* (pp. 283–303). San Diego, CA: Singular Publishing Group.

Hirano, M. (1981). *Clinical examination of voice.* New York: Springer-Verlag.

Kreiman, J., and Gerratt, B. R. (1996). The perceptual structure of pathologic voice quality. *Journal of the Acoustical Society of America, 100*, 1787–1795.

Kreiman, J., and Gerratt, B. R. (1998). Validity of rating scale measures of voice quality. *Journal of the Acoustical Society of America, 104*, 1598–1608.

Kreiman, J., and Gerratt, B. R. (2000). Measuring vocal quality. In R. D. Kent and M. J. Ball (Eds.), *Voice quality measurement* (pp. 73–102). San Diego, CA: Singular Publishing Group.

Laver, J. (1981). The analysis of vocal quality: From the classical period to the 20th century. In R. Asher and E. Henderson (Eds.), *Toward a history of phonetics* (pp. 79–99). Edinburgh: Edinburgh University Press.

Verdonck de Leeuw, I. M. (1998). Perceptual analysis of voice quality: Trained and naive raters, and self-ratings. In G. de Krom (Ed.), *Proceedings of Voicedata98 Symposium on Databases in Voice Quality Research and Education* (pp. 12–15). Utrecht, the Netherlands: Utrecht Institute of Linguistics.

Wilson, F. B. (1977). *Voice disorders.* Austin; TX: Learning Concepts.

Further Readings

Gerratt, B. R., and Kreiman, J. (2001). Measuring vocal quality with speech synthesis. *Journal of the Acoustical Society of America, 110*, 2560–2566.

Kent, R. D., and Ball, M. J. (2000). *Voice quality measurement.* San Diego, CA: Singular Publishing Group.

Kreiman, J., and Gerratt, B. R. (2000). Sources of listener disagreement in voice quality assessment. *Journal of the Acoustical Society of America, 108*, 1867–1879.

Kreiman, J., Gerratt, B. R., Kempster, G., Erman, A., and Berke, G. S. (1993). Perceptual evaluation of voice quality: Review, tutorial, and a framework for future research. *Journal of Speech and Hearing Research, 36*, 21–40.

Voice Rehabilitation After Conservation Laryngectomy

Partial or conservation laryngectomy procedures are performed not only to surgically remove a malignant lesion from the larynx, but also to preserve some functional valving capacity of the laryngeal mechanism. Retention of adequate valvular function allows conservation of some degree of vocal function and safe swallowing. As such, the primary goal of conservation laryngectomy procedures is cancer control and oncologic safety, with a secondary goal of maintaining upper airway sphincteric function and phonatory capacity postsurgery. However, conservation laryngectomy will always necessitate tissue ablation, with disruption of the vibratory integrity of at least one vocal fold (Bailey, 1981). From the standpoint of voice production, any degree of laryngeal tissue ablation has direct and potentially highly negative implications for the functional capacity of the postoperative larynx. Changes in laryngeal structure result in aerodynamic, vibratory, and ultimately acoustic changes in the voice signal (Berke, Gerratt, and Hanson, 1983; Rizer, Schecter, and Coleman, 1984; Doyle, 1994).

Vocal characteristics following conservation laryngectomy are a consequence of anatomical influences and the resultant physiological function of the postsurgical laryngeal sphincter, as well as secondary physiological compensation. In some instances, this level of compensation may facilitate the communicative process, but in other instances such compensations may be detrimental to the speaker's communicative effectiveness (Doyle, 1997). Perceptual observations following a variety of conservation laryngectomy procedures have been diverse, but data clearly indicate perceived changes in voice quality, the degree of air leakage through the reconstructed laryngeal sphincter, the appearance of compensatory hypervalving, and other features (Blaugrund et al., 1984; Leeper, Heeneman, and Reynolds, 1990; Hoasjoe et al., 1992; Doyle et al., 1995; Keith, Leeper, and Doyle, 1996). Two factors in particular, glottic insufficiency and the relative degree of compliance and resistance to airflow offered by the reconstructed valve, appear to play a significant role in compensatory behaviors influencing auditory-perceptual assessments of voice quality (Doyle, 1997). Excessive closure of the laryngeal mechanism at either glottic or supraglottic (or both) levels might decrease air escape, but may also create abnormalities in voice quality due to active (volitional) hyperclosure (Leeper, Heeneman, and Reynolds, 1990; Doyle et al., 1995; Keith, Leeper, and Doyle, 1996; Doyle, 1997). Similarly, volitional, compensatory adjustments in respiratory volume in an effort to drive a noncompliant voicing source characterized by postsurgical increases in its resistance to airflow may negatively influence auditory-perceptual judgments of the voice by listeners. This may then call attention to the voice, with varied degrees of social penalty. In this regard, the ultimate postsurgical effects of conservation laryngectomy on voice quality may result in unique limitations for men and women, and as such require clinical consideration.

The clinical evaluation of individuals who have undergone conservation laryngectomy initially focuses on identifying behaviors that hold the greatest potential to negatively alter voice quality. Excessive vocal effort and a harsh, strained voice quality are commonly observed (Doyle et al., 1995). Standard evaluation may include videoendoscopy (via both rigid and flexible endoscopy) and acoustic, aerodynamic, and auditory-perceptual assessment. Until recently, only limited comprehensive data on vocal characteristics of those undergoing conservation laryngectomy have been available. Careful, systematic perceptual assessment has direct clinical implications in that information from such an assessment will lead to the definition of treatment goals and methods of monitoring potential progress. A comprehensive framework for the evaluation and treatment of voice alterations in those who have undergone conservation laryngectomy is available (Doyle, 1977).

Depending on the auditory-perceptual character of the voice, the clinician should be able to discern functional (physiological) changes to the sphincter that may have a direct influence on voice quality. Those auditory-perceptual features that most negatively affect overall voice quality should form the initial targets for therapeutic intervention. For example, the speaker's attempt to increase vocal loudness may create a level of hyperclosure that is detrimental to judgments of voice quality. Although the rationale for such "abnormal" behavior is easily understood, the speaker must understand the relative levels of penalty it creates in a communicative context. Further treatment goals should focus on (1) enhancing residual vocal functions and capacities, and (2) efforts to reduce or eliminate compensatory behaviors that negatively alter the voice signal (Doyle, 1997). Thus, primary treatment targets will frequently address changes in voice quality and/or vocal effort. Increased effort may be compensatory in an attempt to alter pitch or loudness, or simply to initiate the generation of voice. Clinical assessment should determine whether voice change is due to under- or overcompensation for the disrupted sphincter. Therefore, strategies for voice therapy must address changes in anatomical and physiological function, the contributions of volitional compensation, and whether changes in voice quality may be the result of multiple factors.

Voice therapy strategies for those who have undergone conservation laryngectomy have evolved from strategies used in traditional voice therapy (e.g., Colton and Casper, 1990; Boone and McFarland, 1994). Doyle (1997) has suggested that therapy following conservation laryngectomy should focus on "(1) smooth and easy phonation; (2) a slow, productive transition to voice generation at the initiation of voice and speech production, (3) increasing the length of utterance in conjunction with consistently easy phonation, and (4) control of speech rate via phrasing." The intent is to improve vocal efficiency and generate the best voice quality without excessive physical effort. Clinical goals that focus on "easy" voice production without excessive speech rate are appropriate targets. Common facilitation methods may involve the use of visual or auditory feedback, ear training, and respiration training (Boone, 1977; Boone and McFarland, 1994; Doyle, 1997).

Maladaptive compensations following conservation laryngectomy often tend to be hyperfunctional behaviors. However, a subgroup of individuals may present with weak and inaudible voices because of pain or discomfort in the early postsurgical period. Such compensations may remain when the discomfort has resolved, and may result in perceptible limitations in verbal communication. In such cases of hypofunctional behavior, voice therapy is usually directed toward facilitating increased approximation of the laryngeal valve by means of traditional voice therapy methods (Boone, 1977; Colton and Casper, 1990). A weak voice requires the clinician to orient therapy tasks toward systematically increasing glottal resistance. Although a "rough" or "effortful" voice may be judged as abnormal, it may be preferable for some speakers when compared to a breathy voice quality. This is of particular importance when evaluating goals and potential voice outcomes relative to the speaker's sex.

The physical and psychological demands placed on the patient during initial attempts at voicing might increase levels of tension that ultimately may reduce the individual's phonatory capability. Those individuals who exhibit increased fundamental frequency, excessively aperiodic voices, or intermittent voice stoppages may be experiencing problems that result from postoperative physiological overcompensation because they are struggling to produce voice. Many individuals who have undergone conservative laryngectomy may demonstrate considerable effort during attempts at postsurgical voice production, particularly early during treatment. Because active glottic hypofunction is infrequently noted in those who have undergone conservative laryngectomy, clinical tasks that focus on reducing overcompensation (i.e., hyperfunctional closure) are more commonly used.

See also LARYNGECTOMY.

—*Philip C. Doyle*

References

Bailey, B. J. (1981). Partial laryngectomy and laryngoplasty. *Laryngoscope, 81,* 1742–1771.

Berke, G. S., Gerratt, B. R., and Hanson, D. G. (1983). An acoustic analysis of the effects of surgical therapy on voice quality. *Otolaryngology–Head and Neck Surgery, 91,* 502–508.

Blaugrund, S. M., Gould, W. J., Haji, T., Metzler, J., Bloch, C., and Baer, T. (1984). Voice analysis of the partially ablated larynx: A preliminary report. *Annals of Otology, Rhinology, and Laryngology, 93,* 311–317.

Boone, D. R. (1977). *The voice and voice therapy* (2nd ed.). Englewood Cliffs, NJ: Prentice Hall.

Boone, D. R., and McFarlane, S. C. (1994). *The voice and voice therapy* (5th ed.). Englewood Cliffs, NJ: Prentice Hall.

Colton, R. H., and Casper, J. K. (1990). *Understanding voice problems: A physiological perspective for diagnosis and treatment.* Baltimore: Williams and Wilkins.

Doyle, P. C. (1994). *Foundations of voice and speech rehabilitation following laryngeal cancer.* San Diego, CA: Singular Publishing Group.

Doyle, P. C. (1997). Voice refinement following conservation surgery for cancer of the larynx: A conceptual model for therapeutic intervention. *American Journal of Speech-Language Pathology, 6,* 27–35.

Doyle, P. C., Leeper, H. A., Houghton-Jones, C., Heeneman, H., and Martin, G. F. (1995). Perceptual characteristics of hemilaryngectomized and near-total laryngectomized male speakers. *Journal of Medical Speech-Language Pathology, 3,* 131–143.

Hoasjoe, D. R., Martin, G. F., Doyle, P. C., and Wong, F. S. (1992). A comparative acoustic analysis of voice production by near-total laryngectomy and normal laryngeal speakers. *Journal of Otolaryngology, 21,* 39–43.

Keith, R. L., Leeper, H. A., and Doyle, P. C. (1996). Microacoustical measures of voice following near-total laryngectomy. *Otolaryngology–Head and Neck Surgery, 113,* 698–694.

Leeper, H. A., Heeneman, H., and Reynolds, C. (1990). Vocal function following vertical hemilaryngectomy: A preliminary investigation. *Journal of Otolaryngology, 19,* 62–67.

Rizer, F. M., Schecter, G. L., and Coleman, R. F. (1984). Voice quality and intelligibility characteristics of the reconstructed larynx and pseudolarynx. *Otolaryngology–Head and Neck Surgery, 92,* 635–638.

Further Readings

Biacabe, B., Crevier-Buchman, L., Hans, S., Laccourreye, O., and Brasnu, D. (1999). Vocal function after vertical partial laryngectomy with glottic reconstruction by false vocal fold flap: Durational and frequency measures. *Laryngoscope, 109,* 698–704.

Crevier-Buchman, L., Laccourreye, O., Wuyts, F. L., Monfrais-Pfauwadel, M., Pillot, C., and Brasnu, D. (1998). Comparison and evolution of perceptual and acoustic characteristics of voice after supracricoid partial laryngectomy with cricohyoidoepiglottopexy. *Acta Otolaryngologica, 118,* 594–599.

DeSanto, L. W., Pearson, B. W., and Olsen, K. D. (1989). Utility of near-total laryngectomy for supraglottic, pharyngeal, base-of-tongue, and other cancers. *Annals of Otology, Rhinology, and Laryngology, 98,* 2–7.

De Vincentiis, M., Minni, A., Gallo, A., and DiNardo, A. (1998). Supracricoid partial laryngectomies: Oncologic and functional results. *Head and Neck, 20,* 504–509.

Fung, K., Yoo, J., Leeper, H. A., Hawkins, S., Heeneman, H., Doyle, P. C., et al. (2001). Vocal function following radiation for non-laryngeal versus laryngeal tumors of the head and neck. *Laryngoscope, 111,* 1920–1924.

Gavilan, J., Herranz, J., Prim, P., and Rabanal, I. (1996). Speech results and complications of near-total laryngectomy. *Annals of Otology, Rhinology, and Laryngology, 105,* 729–733.

Hanamitsu, M., Kataoka, H., Takeuchi, E., and Kitajima, K. (1999). Comparative study of vocal function after near-total laryngectomy. *Laryngoscope, 109,* 1320–1323.

Kirchner, J. A. (1975). Growth and spread of laryngeal cancer as related to partial laryngectomy. *Laryngoscope, 85,* 1516–1521.

Kirchner, J. A. (1984). Pathways and pitfalls in partial laryngectomy. *Annals of Otology, Rhinology, and Laryngology, 93,* 301–305.

Kirchner, J. A. (1989). What have whole organ sections contributed to the treatment of laryngeal cancer? *Annals of Otology, Rhinology, and Laryngology, 98,* 661–667.

Lefebvre, J. (1998). Larynx preservation: The discussion is not closed. *Otolaryngology–Head and Neck Surgery, 118,* 389–393.

Pressman, J. J. (1956). Submucosal compartmentalization of the larynx. *Annals of Otology, Rhinology, and Laryngology, 65,* 766–773.

Robbins, K. T., and Michaels, L. (1985). Feasibility of subtotal laryngectomy based on whole-organ examination. *Archives of Otolaryngology, 111,* 356–360.

Tucker, G. (1964). Some clinical inferences from the study of serial laryngeal sections. *Laryngoscope, 73,* 728–748.

Tucker, G. F., and Smith, H. R. (1982). A histological demonstration of the development of laryngeal connective tissue compartments. *Transactions of the American Academy of Ophthalmology and Otolaryngology, 66,* 308–318.

Voice Therapy: Breathing Exercises

Breathing—the mechanical process of moving air in and out of the lungs—plays an important role in both speech and voice production; however, the emphasis placed on breathing exercises relative to voice disorders in the published literature is mixed. A review of voice therapy techniques by Casper and Murray (2000) did not suggest any breathing exercises for voice disorders. Some books on voice and voice disorders have no discussion of changing breathing behavior relative to voice disorders (Case, 1984; Colton and Casper, 1996), others do (e.g., Aronson, 1980; Boone and McFarlane, 2000; Cooper, 1973; Stemple, Glaze, and Gerdeman, 1995). Although breathing exercises are advocated by some, little is known about the role played by breathing, either directly or indirectly, in disorders of the voice. Reed (1980) noted the lack of empirical evidence that breathing exercises were useful in ameliorating voice disorders.

At present, then, there is a paucity of data on the relationship of breathing to voice disorders. The data that do exist generally describe the breathing patterns that accompany voice disorders, but there are no data on what kind of breathing behavior might contribute to voice disorders. For example, Sapienza, Stathopoulos, and Brown (1997) studied breathing kinematics during reading in ten women with vocal fold nodules. They found that the women used more air per syllable, more lung volume per phrase, and initiated breath groups at higher lung volumes than women without vocal nodules. However, as the authors point out, the breathing behavior observed in the women with nodules was most likely in response to inefficient valving at the larynx and did not cause the nodules.

Normal Breathing

When assessing and planning therapy for disorders of the voice, it is important to know what normal function is. Hixon (1975) provides a useful parameterization of breathing for speech that includes volume, pressure, flow, and body configuration or shape. For conversational speech in the upright body position, the following apply. Lung volume is the amount of air available for speaking or vocalizing. The volumes used for speech are usually within the midvolume range of vital capacity (VC), beginning at 60% VC and ending at around 40% VC (Hixon, 1973; Hixon, Mead, and Goldman, 1976; Hoit et al., 1989). This volume range is efficient and economical, in that extra effort is not required to overcome recoil forces (Hixon, Mead, and Goldman, 1976). Most lung volume exchange for speech is brought about by rib cage displacement and not by displacement of the abdomen (Hixon, 1973). The rib cage is efficient in displacing lung volume because it covers a greater surface area of the lungs, it consists of muscle fiber types that are able to generate fast and accurate pressure changes, and it is well endowed with spindle organs for purposes of sensory feedback. Pressure (translaryngeal pressure) is related to the intensity of the voice (Bouhuys, Proctor, and Mead, 1966). Pressure for conversational speech is typically around 4–7 cm H_2O, or 0.4–0.7 kPa (Isshiki, 1964; Stathopoulos and Sapienza, 1993). Pressure is generated by both muscular and inherent recoil forces, and the interworking of these forces depends on the level of lung volume (Hixon, Mead, and Goldman, 1976). Reference to flow is in the macro sense and denotes shorter inspiratory durations relative to longer expiratory durations. This difference in timing reflects the speaker's desire to maintain the flow of speech in his or her favor. In the upright body position, body configuration refers to the size of the abdomen relative to the size of rib cage. For speech production in the upright body position, the abdomen is smaller and the rib cage is larger relative to relaxation (Hixon, Goldman, and Mead, 1973).

The upright body configuration provides an economical and efficient mechanical advantage to the breathing apparatus. The abdomen not only produces lung volume change in the expiratory direction, it also optimizes the function of the diaphragm and rib cage. It does so in two ways. First, inward abdominal placement lifts the diaphragm and the rib cage (Goldman, 1974). This action positions the expiratory muscle fibers of the rib cage and muscle fibers of the diaphragm on a more favorable portion of their length-tension curve. This allows quicker and more forceful contractions for both inspiration and expiration while using less neural energy. Second, this inward abdominal position as it is maintained provides a platform against which the diaphragm and rib cage can push in order to produce the necessary pressures and flows for speech. If the abdomen did not offer resistance to the rib cage during the expiratory phase of speech breathing, it would be forced outward and would move in a paradoxical manner during expiration. Paradoxical motion results in reduced economy of movement, or wasted motion. Thus, the pressure generated by the rib cage would alter the shape of the breathing apparatus and would not assist in developing as rapid and as large an alveolar pressure change (Hixon and Weismer, 1995).

Effects of Posture

Although much is known about speech breathing, little of this information has found its way into the clinical literature and been applied to voice therapy. As a result, only one breathing technique to improve voice production is usually described: The client is placed supine and increased outward movement of the abdomen is observed as the client breathes at rest.

The changes that occur in speech breathing with a switch from the upright position are numerous and reflect the different effects of gravity (see Hoit, 1995, for a comprehensive tutorial). In supine speech breathing involves approximately 20% less of VC. The change of body configuration from the upright position to the supine position means that rib cage volume decreases and abdominal volume increases. This modification changes the mechanics of the breathing muscles and requires a different motor control strategy for speech production. For example, in the supine position there is little or no muscular activity of the abdomen during speaking, whereas in the upright body position the abdominal muscles are quite active (Hixon, Mead, and Goldman, 1976; Hoit et al., 1988). In light of the mechanical and neural control issues discussed earlier, it seems unwarranted to position an individual supine to teach "natural" breathing for speech and voice. With regard to breathing at rest, it should be noted that this task is not specific to speech. Kelso, Saltzman, and Tuller (1986) hypothesize that the control of speech is task-specific. Hixon (1982) showed kinematic data from a patient with Friedreich's ataxia whose abdominal wall was assumed to be paralyzed because it showed no inward displacement and no movement during speech. However, when this patient laughed, his abdominal wall was displaced inward and displayed a great amount of movement. As Hoit (1995) points out, it seems unlikely that techniques for changing breathing behavior learned in a resting, supine position would generalize to an upright body position. It seems curious why this technique is advocated. It may be that this technique does not change breathing behavior but is effective in relaxing individuals with voice disorders. Relaxation techniques have been advocated to reduce systemic muscular tension in individuals with voice disorders (Boone and McFarlane, 2000; Greene and Mathieson, 1989), and breathing exercises are known to be beneficial in reducing heart rate and blood pressure (Grossman et al., 2001; Han, Stegen, Valck, Clement, and Woestijne, 1996).

Other Approaches

If learning breathing techniques in the supine position is not useful, what else might be done with the breathing apparatus to ameliorate voice disorders? Perhaps modifying lung volume would be useful. Hixon and Putnam (1983) described breathing behavior in a 30-year-old woman (a local television broadcaster) with a functional voice problem. Although she had a normal voice and no positive laryngeal signs, audible inspiratory turbulence was evident during her broadcasts. Using breathing kinematic measurement techniques, Hixon and Putnam found that this person spoke in the lower range of her VC, between 45% and 10%. They believed the noisy inspirations were due to the turbulence created by increased resistance in the lower airways that occurs at low lung volume. Therefore, it is possible the telecaster's noisy inspirations could have been eliminated or reduced if she were to produce speech at higher (more normal) lung volumes. However, the authors did not report any attempts to modify lung volume. Of note, the woman said that when she spoke at lower lung volumes, her voice sounded more authoritative, and that her voice seemed to be much lighter when she spoke at higher lung volumes.

When a person inspires to higher lung volumes, the downward movement of the diaphragm pulls on the trachea, and this pulling is believed to generate passive adductory forces on the vocal folds (Zenker and Zenker, 1960). Solomon, Garlitz, and Milbrath (2000) found that in men, there was a tendency for laryngeal airway resistance to be reduced during syllable production at high lung volumes compared with low lung volumes. Milstein (1999), using video-endoscopic and breathing kinematic analysis, found that at high lung volumes, the laryngeal area appeared more dilated and the larynx was in a lower vertical position in the neck than during phonation at lower lung volumes. Plassman and Lansing (1990) showed that with training, individuals can produce consistently higher lung volumes during inspiration.

Even after the call by Reed (1980) more than 20 years ago for more empirical data on breathing exercises to treat voice disorders, little has been done. More research in this area is decisively needed. Research efforts should focus first on how and whether abnormal breathing behavior contributes to voice disorders. Then researchers should examine what techniques are viable for changing this abnormal breathing behavior—if it exists. Efficacy research is of great importance because of the reluctance of third-party insurers to cover voice disorders.

—*Peter Watson*

References

Aronson, A. (1980). *Clinical voice disorders: An interdisciplinary approach.* New York: B.C. Decker.

Boone, D., and McFarlane, S. (2000). *The voice and voice therapy* (6th ed.). Boston: Allyn and Bacon.

Bouhuys, A., Proctor, D. F., and Mead, J. (1966). Kinetic aspects of singing. *Journal of Applied Physiology, 21,* 483–496.

Case, J. (1984). *Clinical management of voice disorders.* Rockville, MD: Aspen.

Casper, J., and Murray, T. (2000). Voice therapy methods in dysphonia. *Otolaryngologic Clinics of North America, 33,* 983–1002.

Colton, R., and Casper, J. (1996). *Understanding voice problems* (2nd ed.). Baltimore: Williams and Wilkins.

Cooper, M. (1973). *Modern techniques of vocal rehabilitation.* Springfield: Charles C. Thomas.

Goldman, M. (1974). Mechanical coupling of the diaphragm and rib cage. In L. Pengally, A. Rebuk, and C. Reed (Eds.), *Loaded breathing* (pp. 50–63). London: Churchill Livingstone.

Greene, M., and Mathieson, L. (1989). *The voice and its disorders* (5th ed.). London: Whurr.

Grossman, E., Grossman, A., Schein, M., Zimlichman, R., and Gavish, B. (2001). Breathing-control lowers blood pressure. *Journal of Human Hypertension, 14,* 263–269.

Han, J., Stegen, K., Valck, C. D., Clement, J., and van de Woestijne, K. (1996). Influence of breathing therapy on complaints, anxiety and breathing pattern in patients with hyperventilation syndrome and anxiety disorders. *Journal of Psychosomatic Research, 41,* 481–493.

Hixon, T. (1975). *Respiratory-laryngeal evaluation.* Paper presented at the Veterans Administration Workshop on Motor Speech Disorders, Madison, WI.

Hixon, T., and Putnam, A. (1983). Voice abnormalities in relation to respiratory kinematics. *Seminars in Speech and Language, 5,* 217–231.

Hixon, T., and Weismer, G. (1995). Perspectives on the Edinburgh study of speech breathing. *Journal of Speech and Hearing Research, 38,* 42–60.

Hixon, T. J. (1973). Respiratory function in speech. In F. D. Minifie, T. J. Hixon, and F. Williams (Eds.), *Normal aspects of speech, hearing, and language.* Englewood Cliffs, NJ: Prentice-Hall.

Hixon, T. J. (1982). Speech breathing kinematics and mechanism inferences therefrom. In S. Grillner, B. Lindblom, J. Lubker, and A. Persson (Eds.), *Speech motor control* (pp. 75–93). Oxford, UK: Pergamon Press.

Hixon, T. J., Goldman, M. D., and Mead, J. (1973). Kinematics of the chest wall during speech production: Volume displacements of the rib cage, abdomen, and lung. *Journal of Speech and Hearing Research, 16,* 78–115.

Hixon, T. J., Mead, J., and Goldman, M. D. (1976). Dynamics of the chest wall during speech production: Function of the thorax, rib cage, diaphragm, and abdomen. *Journal of Speech and Hearing Research, 19,* 297–356.

Hoit, J. (1995). Influence of body position on breathing and its implications for the evaluation and treatment of voice disorders. *Journal of Voice, 9,* 341–347.

Hoit, J. D., Hixon, T. J., Altman, M. E., and Morgan, W. J. (1989). Speech breathing in women. *Journal of Speech and Hearing Research, 32,* 353–365.

Hoit, J. D., Plassman, B. L., Lansing, R. W., and Hixon, T. J. (1988). Abdominal muscle activity during speech production. *Journal of Applied Physiology, 65,* 2656–2664.

Isshiki, N. (1964). Regulatory mechanisms of voice intensity variation. *Journal of Speech and Hearing Research, 7,* 17–29.

Kelso, J. A. S., Saltzman, E. L., and Tuller, B. (1986). The dynamic perspective on speech production: Data and theory. *Journal of Phonetics, 14,* 29–59.

Milstein, C. (1999). *Laryngeal function associated with changes in lung volume during voice and speech production in normal speaking women.* Unpublished dissertation, University of Arizona, Tucson.

Plassman, B., and Lansing, R. (1990). Perceptual cues used to reproduce an inspired lung volume. *Journal of Applied Physiology, 69,* 1123–1130.

Reed, C. (1980). Voice therapy: A need for research. *Journal of Speech and Hearing Disorders, 45,* 157–169.

Sapienza, C. M., Stathopoulos, E. T., and W. S. Brown, J. (1997). Speech breathing during reading in women with vocal nodules. *Journal of Voice, 11,* 195–201.

Solomon, N., Garlitz, S., and Milbrath, R. (2000). Respiratory and laryngeal contributions to maximum phonation duration. *Journal of Voice, 14,* 331–340.

Stathopoulos, E. T., and Sapienza, C. (1993). Respiratory and laryngeal function of women and men during vocal intensity variation. *Journal of Speech and Hearing Research*, *36*, 64–75.

Stemple, J., Glaze, L., and Gerdeman, B. (1995). *Clinical voice pathology: Theory and management* (2nd ed.). San Diego, CA: Singular Publishing Group.

Zenker, W., and Zenker, A. (1960). Über die Regelung der Stimmlippenspannung durch von aussen eingreifende Mechansimen. *Folia Phoniatricia*, *12*, 1–36.

Further Readings

Agostoni, E., and Mead, J. (1986). Statics of the respiratory system. In P. T. Macklem and J. Mead (Eds.), *The respiratory system* (3rd ed., vol. 3, pp. 387–409). Bethesda, MD: American Physiological Society.

Druz, W. S., and Sharp, J. T. (1981). Activity of respiratory muscles in upright and recumbent humans. *Journal of Applied Physiolgy, Respiration, and Environment*, *51*, 1552–1561.

Goldman-Eisler. (1968). The significance of breathing in speech. In *Psycholinguistics: Experiments in spontaneous speech* (pp. 100–106). New York: Academic Press.

Konno, K., and Mead, J. (1967). Measurement of the separate volume changes of rib cage and abdomen during breathing. *Journal of Applied Physiology*, *22*, 407–422.

Lansing, R. W., and Banzett, R. B. (1996). Psychophysical methods in the study of respiratory sensation. In L. Adams and A. Guz (Eds.), *Respiratory sensation*. New York: Marcel Dekker.

Loring, S. H., and Bruce, E. N. (1986). Methods for study of the chest wall. In P. T. Macklem and J. Mead (Eds.), *Handbook of physiology* (vol. 3, pp. 415–428). Betheseda, MD: American Physiological Society.

Loring, S., Mead, J., and Griscom, N. T. (1985). Dependence of diaphragmatic length on lung volume and thoracoabdominal configuration. *Journal of Applied Physiology*, *59*, 1961–1970.

McFarland, D. H., and Smith, A. (1989). Surface recordings of respiratory muscle activity during speech: Some preliminary findings. *Journal of Speech and Hearing Research*, *32*, 657–667.

Mead, J., and Agostoni, E. (1986). Dynamics of breathing. In P. T. Macklem and J. Mead (Eds.), *The respiratory system* (3rd ed., vol. 3, pp. 411–427). Bethesda, MD: American Physiological Society.

Mitchell, H., Hoit, J., and Watson, P. (1996). Cognitive-linguistic demands and speech breathing. *Journal of Speech and Hearing Research*, *39*, 93–104.

Porter, R. J., Hogue, D. M., and Tobey, E. A. (1994). Dynamic analysis of speech and non-speech respiration. In F. Bell-Berti and L. J. Raphael (Eds.), *Studies in speech production: A Festschrift for Katherine Safford Harris* (pp. 1–25). Washington, DC: American Institute of Physics.

Smith, J. C., and Loring, S. H. (1986). Passive mechanical properties of the chest wall. In P. T. Macklem and J. Mead (Eds.), *Handbook of physiology* (vol. 3, pp. 429–442). Betheseda, MD: American Physiological Society.

Watson, P. J., and Hixon, T. J. (1985). Respiratory kinematics in classical (opera) singers. *Journal of Speech and Hearing Research*, *28*, 104–122.

Watson, P., Hixon, T., and Maher, M. (1987). To breathe or not to breathe—that is the question: An investigation of speech breathing kinematics in world-class Shakespearean actors. *Journal of Voice*, *1*, 269–272.

Watson, P. J., Hixon, T. J., Stathopoulos, E. T., and Sullivan, D. R. (1990). Respiratory kinematics in female classical singers. *Journal of Voice*, *4*, 120–128.

Watson, P. J., Hoit, J. D., Lansing, R. W., and Hixon, T. J. (1989). Abdominal muscle activity during classical singing. *Journal of Voice*, *3*, 24–31.

Webb, R., Williams, F., and Minifie, F. (1967). Effects of verbal decision behavior upon respiration during speech production. *Journal of Speech and Hearing Research*, *10*, 49–56.

Winkworth, A. L., and Davis, P. J. (1997). Speech breathing and the lombard effect. *Journal of Speech, Language, and Hearing Research*, *40*, 159–169.

Winkworth, A. L., Davis, P. J., Ellis, E., and Adams, R. D. (1994). Variability and consistency in speech breathing during reading: Lung volumes, speech intensity, and linguistic factors. *Journal of Speech and Hearing Research*, *37*, 535–556.

Voice Therapy: Holistic Techniques

Whenever a voice disorder is present, a change in the normal functioning of the physiology responsible for voice production may be assumed. These physiological events are measurable and may be modified by voice therapy. Normal voice production depends on a relative balance among airflow, supplied by the respiratory system; laryngeal muscle strength, balance, coordination, and stamina; and coordination among these and the supraglottic resonators (pharynx, oral cavity, nasal cavity). Any disturbance in the relative physiological balance of these vocal subsystems may lead to or be perceived as a voice disorder. Disturbances may occur in respiratory volume, power, pressure, and flow, and may manifest in vocal fold tone, mass, stiffness, flexibility, and approximation. Finally, the coupling of the supraglottic resonators and the placement of the laryngeal tone may cause or be implicated in a voice disorder (Titze, 1994).

The overall causes of vocal disturbances may be mechanical, neurological, or psychological. Whatever the cause, one management approach is direct modification of the inappropriate physiological activity through direct exercise and manipulation. When all three subsystems of voice are addressed in one exercise, this is considered holistic voice therapy. Examples of holistic voice therapy include Vocal Function Exercises (Stemple, Glaze, and Klaben, 2000), Resonant Voice Therapy (Verdolini, 2000), the Accent Method of voice therapy (Kotby, 1995; Harris, 2000), and the Lee Silverman Voice Treatment (Ramig, 2000). The following discussion considers the use of Vocal Function Exercises to strengthen and balance the vocal mechanism.

The Vocal Function Exercise program is based on an assumption that has not been proved empirically. Nonetheless, this assumption and the clinical logic that follows have been supported through many years of clinical experience and observation, as well as several efficacy studies (Stemple, 1994; Sabol, Lee, and Stemple, 1995; Roy et al., 2001). In a double-blind, placebo-controlled study, Stemple et al. (1994) demonstrated that Vocal Function Exercises were effective in enhancing voice production in young women without vocal pathology. The primary physiological effects were reflected in increased phonation volumes at all pitch levels, decreased airflow rates, and a subsequent increase in maximum phonation times. Frequency ranges were extended significantly in the downward direction.

Sabol, Lee, and Stemple (1995), experimenting with the value of Vocal Function Exercises in the practice regimen of singers, used graduate students of opera as subjects. Significant improvements in the physiologic measurements of voice production were achieved, including increased airflow volume, decreased airflow rates, and increased maximum phonation time, even in this group of superior voice users.

Roy et al. (2001) studied the efficacy of Vocal Function Exercises in a population with voice pathology. Teachers who reported experiencing voice disorders were randomly assigned to three groups: Vocal Function Exercises, vocal hygiene, and control groups. For 6 weeks the experimental groups followed their respective therapy programs and were monitored by speech-language pathologists trained by the experimenters in the two approaches. Pre- and post-testing of all three groups using the Voice Handicap Index (VHI; Jacobson et al., 1997) revealed significant improvement in the Vocal Function Exercise group, and no improvement in the vocal hygiene group. Subjects in the control group rated themselves worse.

The laryngeal mechanism is similar to other muscle systems and may become strained and imbalanced for a variety of reasons (Saxon and Schneider, 1995). Indeed, the analogy that we often draw with patients is a comparison of knee rehabilitation with rehabilitation of the voice. Both the knee and the larynx consist of muscle, cartilage, and connective tissue. When the knee is injured, rehabilitation includes a short period of immobilization to reduce the effects of the acute injury. The immobilization is followed by assisted ambulation, and then the primary rehabilitation begins, in the form of systematic exercise. This exercise is designed to strengthen and balance all of the supportive knee muscles for the purpose of returning the knee as close to its normal functioning as possible.

Rehabilitation of the voice may also involve a short period of voice rest after acute injury or surgery to permit healing of the mucosa to occur. The patient may then begin conservative voice use and follow through with all of the management approaches that seem necessary. Full voice use is then resumed quickly, and the therapy program often is successful in returning the patient to normal voice production. Often, however, patients are not fully rehabilitated because an important step was neglected—the systematic exercise program to regain the balance among airflow, laryngeal muscle activity, and supraglottic placement of the tone.

A series of laryngeal muscle exercises was first described by Bertram Briess (1957, 1959). Briess suggested that for the voice to be most effective, the intrinsic muscles of the larynx must be in equilibrium. Briess's exercises concentrated on restoring the balance in the laryngeal musculature and decreasing tension of the hyperfunctioning muscles. Unfortunately, many assumptions Briess made regarding laryngeal muscle function were incorrect, and his therapy methods were not widely followed. The concept of direct exercise to strengthen voice production persisted. Barnes (1977) described a modification of Briess's work that she termed Briess Exercises. These exercises were modified and expanded by Stemple (1984) into Vocal Function Exercises. The exercise program strives to balance and strengthen the subsystems of voice production, whether the disorder is one of vocal hyperfunction or hypofunction.

The exercises are simple to teach and, when presented appropriately, seem reasonable to patients. Indeed, many patients are enthusiastic to have a concrete program, similar in concept to physical therapy, during which they may plot the progress of their return to vocal efficiency. The program begins by describing the problem to the patient, using illustrations as needed or the patient's own stroboscopic evaluation video. The patient is then taught a series of four exercises to be practiced at home, two times each, twice a day, preferably morning and evening. These exercises include the following:

1. Sustain the /i/ vowel for as long as possible on a musical note: F above middle C for females and boys, F below middle C for males. (Pitches may be modified up or down to fit the needs of the patient. Seldom are they modified by more than two scale steps in either direction.)

The goal of the exercise is based on airflow volume. In our clinic, the goal is based on reaching 80–100 mL/s of airflow. So, if the flow volume is 4000 mL, the goal is 40–45 s. When airflow measurements are not available, the goal is equal to the longest /s/ that the patient is able to sustain. Placement of the tone should be in an extreme forward focus, almost but not quite nasal. All exercises are produced as softly as possible, but not breathy. The voice must be engaged. This is considered a warm-up exercise.

2. Glide from your lowest note to your highest note on the word *knoll*.

The goal is to achieve no voice breaks. The glide requires the use of all laryngeal muscles. It stretches the vocal folds and encourages a systematic, slow engagement of the cricothyroid muscles. The word *knoll* encourages a forward placement of the tone as well as an expanded open pharynx. The patient's lips are to be rounded, and a sympathetic vibration should be felt on the lips. (A lip trill, tongue trill, or the word *whoop* may also be used.) Voice breaks will typically occur in the transitions between low and high registers. When breaks occur, the patient is encouraged to continue the glide without hesitation. When the voice breaks at the top of the current range and the patient typically has more range, the glide may be continued without voice as the folds will continue to stretch. Glides improve muscular control and flexibility. This is considered a stretching exercise.

3. Glide from your highest note to your lowest note on the word *knoll*.

The goal is to achieve no voice breaks. The patient is instructed to feel a half-yawn in the throat throughout this exercise. By keeping the pharynx open and focusing the sympathetic vibration at the lips, the downward glide encourages a slow, systematic engagement of the thyroarytenoid muscles without the presence of a back-focused growl. In fact, no growl is permitted. (A lip trill, tongue trill, or the word *boom* may also be used.) This is considered a contracting exercise.

4. Sustain the musical notes C-D-E-F-G for as long as possible on the word *knoll* minus the *kn*. The range should be around middle C for females and boys, an octave below middle C for men.

The goal is the same as for exercise 1. The *-oll* is produced with an open pharynx and constricted, sympathetically vibrating lips. The shape of the pharynx in respect to the lips is like an inverted megaphone. This exercise may be tailored to the patient's present vocal ability. Although the basic range of middle C (an octave lower for men) is appropriate for most voices, the exercises may be customized up or down to fit the current vocal condition or a particular voice type. Seldom, however, is the exercise shifted more than two scale steps in either direction. This is considered a low-impact adductory power exercise.

The quality of the tone is also monitored for voice breaks, wavering, and breathiness. Tone quality improves as times increase and pathologic conditions begin to resolve. All exercises are done as softly as possible. It is much more difficult to produce soft tones; therefore, the vocal subsystems will receive a better workout than if louder tones are produced. Extreme care is taken to teach the production of a forward tone that lacks tension. In addition, attention is paid to the glottal onset of the tone. The patient is asked to breathe in deeply, with attention paid to training abdominal breathing, posturing the vowel momentarily, and then initiating the exercise gesture without a forceful glottal attack or an aspirated breathy attack. It is explained to the patient that maximum phonation times increase as the efficiency of the vocal fold vibration improves. Times do not increase with improved lung capacity. (Even aerobic exercise does not improve lung capacity, but rather the efficiency of oxygen exchange with the circulatory system, thus giving the sense of more air.)

The musical notes are matched to the notes produced by an inexpensive pitch pipe that the patient purchases for use at home, or a tape recording of live voice doing the exercises may be given to the patient for home use. Many patients find the tape-recorded voice easier to match than the pitch pipe. We have found that patients who think they are "tone deaf" can often be taught to

approximate the correct notes well with practice and guidance from the voice pathologist.

Finally, patients are given a chart on which to mark their sustained times, which is a means of plotting progress. Progress is monitored over time and, because of normal daily variability, patients are encouraged not to compare today with tomorrow, and so on. Rather, weekly comparisons are encouraged. The estimated time of completion for the program is 6–8 weeks. Some patients experience minor laryngeal aching for the first day or two of the program, similar to the muscle aching that might occur with any new muscular exercise. As this discomfort will soon subside, they are encouraged to continue the program through the discomfort should it occur.

When the patient has reached the predetermined therapy goal, and the voice quality and other vocal symptoms have improved, then a tapering maintenance program is recommended. Although some professional voice users choose to remain in peak vocal condition, many of our patients desire to taper the exercise program. The following systematic taper is recommended:

· Full program, 2 times each, 2 times per day
· Full program, 2 times each, 1 time per day (morning)
· Full program, 1 time each, 1 time per day (morning)
· Exercise 4, 2 times each, 1 time per day (morning)
· Exercise 4, 1 time each, 1 time per day (morning)
· Exercise 4, 1 time each, 3 times per week (morning)
· Exercise 4, 1 time each, 1 time per week (morning)

Each taper should last 1 week. Patients should maintain 85% of their peak time; otherwise they should move up one step in the taper until the 85% criterion is met.

Vocal Function Exercises provide a holistic voice treatment program that attends to the three major subsystems of voice production. The program appears to benefit patients with a wide range of voice disorders because it is reasonable in regard to time and effort. It is similar to other recognizable exercise programs: the concept of physical therapy for the vocal folds is understandable; progress may be easily plotted, which is inherently motivating; and it appears to balance and strengthen the relationships among airflow, laryngeal muscle activity, and supraglottic placement.

—*Joseph Stemple*

References

Barnes, J. (1977, October). *Briess exercises.* Workshop presented at the Southwestern Ohio Speech and Hearing Association, Cincinnati, OH.

Behrman, A., and Orlikoff, R. (1997). Instrumentation in voice assessment and treatment: What's the use? *American Journal of Speech-Language Pathology, 6*(4), 9–16.

Bless, D. (1991). Assessment of laryngeal function. In C. Ford and D. Bless (Eds.), *Phonosurgery* (pp. 91–122). New York: Raven Press.

Briess, B. (1957). Voice therapy: Part 1. Identification of specific laryngeal muscle dysfunction by voice testing. *Archives of Otolaryngology, 66,* 61–69.

Briess, B. (1959). Voice therapy: Part II. Essential treatment phases of laryngeal muscle dysfunction. *Archives of Otolaryngology, 69*, 61–69.

Harris, S. (2000). The accent method of voice therapy. In J. Stemple (Ed.), *Voice therapy: Clinical studies* (2nd ed., pp. 62–75). San Diego, CA: Singular Publishing Group.

Hicks, D. (1991). Functional voice assessment: What to measure and why. In *Assessment of speech and voice production: Research and clinical applications* (pp. 204–209). Bethesda, MD: National Institute of Deafness and Other Communicative Disorders.

Jacobson, B., Johnson, A., Grywalski, C., Silbergleit, A., Jacobson, G., Benninger, M., and Newman, C. (1997). The Voice Handicap Index (VHI): Development and validation. *American Journal of Speech-Language Pathology, 6*(3), 66–70.

Kotby, N. (1995). *The accent method of voice therapy.* San Diego, CA: Singular Publishing Group.

Ramig, L. (2000). Lee Silverman voice treatment for individuals with neurological disorders: Parkinson disease. In J. Stemple (Ed.), *Voice therapy: Clinical studies* (2nd ed., pp. 76–81). San Diego, CA: Singular Publishing Group.

Roy, N., Gray, S., Simon, M., Dove, H., Corbin-Lewis, K., and Stemple, J. (2001). An evaluation of the effects of two treatment approaches for teachers with voice disorders: A prospective randomized clinical trial. *Journal of Speech and Hearing Research, 44*, 286–296.

Sabol, J., Lee, L., and Stemple, J. (1995). The value of vocal function exercises in the practice regimen of singers. *Journal of Voice, 9*, 27–36.

Saxon, K., and Schneider, C. (1995). *Vocal exercise physiology.* San Diego, CA: Singular Publishing Group.

Stemple, J. (1984). *Clinical voice pathology: Theory and management* (1st ed.). Columbus, OH: Merrill.

Stemple, J. (2000). Vocal function exercises. In J. Stemple (Ed.), *Voice therapy: Clinical studies* (2nd ed., pp. 34–46). San Diego, CA: Singular Publishing Group.

Stemple, J., Glaze, L., and Klaben, B. (2000). *Clinical voice pathology: Theory and management* (3rd ed.). San Diego, CA: Singular Publishing Group.

Stemple, J., Lee, L., D'Amico, B., and Pickup, B. (1994). Efficacy of vocal function exercises as a method of improving voice production. *Journal of Voice, 8*, 271–278.

Titze, I. (1991). Measurements for assessment of voice disorders. In *Assessment of speech and voice production: Research and clinical applications* (pp. 42–49). Bethesda, MD: National Institute of Deafness and Other Communicative Disorders.

Titze, I. (1994). *Principles of voice production.* Englewood Cliffs, NJ: Prentice-Hall.

Verdolini, K. (2000). Resonant voice therapy. In J. Stemple (Ed.), *Voice therapy: Clinical studies* (2nd ed., pp. 46–62). San Diego, CA: Singular Publishing Group.

Voice Therapy for Adults

Voice therapy for adults may be motivated by functional, health-related, or diagnostic considerations. Functional issues are the usual indication. Adults with voice problems often experience significant functional disruptions in occupational, social, communicative, physical, or emotional domains, and in selected populations, voice therapy is effective in reducing such disruptions. Health-related concerns are less common precipitants of voice therapy in adults. However, physical disease such as cancerous, precancerous, inflammatory, or neurogenic disease may exist and may be exacerbated by behavioral factors such as smoking, diet, hydration, or phonotrauma. Voice therapy may be a useful adjunct to medical or surgical treatment in these cases. Finally, voice therapy may be indicated in cases of diagnostic uncertainty. A classic situation is the need to distinguish between functional and neurogenic conditions. The restoration of a normal or near-normal voice with therapy may suggest a functional origin of the problem. Lack of voice restoration suggests the need for further clinical studies to rule out neurological causes.

Voice therapy can be characterized with reference to several different classification schemes, which results in a certain amount of nosological confusion. Many of the conditions listed in the various classifications map to several different voice therapy options, and by the same token, each therapy option maps to multiple classifications. Here we review voice therapy in relation to (1) vocal biomechanics and (2) a specific therapy approach—roughly the "what" and "how" of voice therapy.

Vocal Biomechanics. The preponderance of voice problems that are amenable to voice therapy involve some form of abnormality in vocal fold adduction. Phonotraumatic lesions such as nodules, polyps, and nonspecific inflammation consequent on voice use are traceable to hyperadduction resulting from vocal fold impact stress. Adduction causes monotonic increases in impact stress (Jiang and Titze, 1994). In turn, impact stress appears to be a primary cause of phonotrauma (Titze, 1994). Thus, therapy targeting a reduction in adduction is indicated in cases of hyperadduction. Another large group of diagnostic conditions involves hypoadduction of the vocal folds. Examples include vocal fold paralysis, paresis, atrophy, bowing, and nonadducted hyperfunction (muscle tension dysphonia; for a discussion, see Hillman et al., 1989). Treatment that increases vocal fold closure is indicated in such cases.

Voice therapy addresses adductory deviations using a variety of biomechanical solutions. The traditional approach to hyperadduction and its sequelae has targeted the use of widely separated vocal folds and small-amplitude oscillations during voice production; examples are use of a "quiet, breathy voice" (Casper et al., 1989; Casper, 1993) or quiet "yawn-sigh" phonation (Boone and McFarlane, 1993). This general approach is sensible for the reduction of hyperadduction and thus phonotraumatic changes, in that vocal fold impact stress, and phonotrauma, should be reduced by it. There is evidence that the quiet, breathy voice approach is effective in reducing signs and symptoms of phonotraumatic lesions for individuals who use it outside the clinic (Verdolini-Marston et al., 1995). However, individuals may also restrict their use of a quiet, breathy voice extraclinically because it is functionally limiting (Verdolini-Marston et al., 1995).

The traditional approach to hypoadduction has involved "pushing" and "pulling" exercises, which should reduce the glottal gap (e.g., Boone and McFarlane, 1994). Indeed, some data corroborate clinicians' impressions that this approach can increase voice intensity in individuals with glottal incompetence (Yamaguchi et al., 1993).

A more recent approach to treating adductory abnormalities has focused on the use of a single "ideal" vocal fold configuration as the target for both hyperadduction and hypoadduction. The configuration involves barely separated vocal folds, which is "ideal" because it optimizes the trade-off between voice output strength (relatively strong) and vocal fold impact stress, and thus reduces the potential for phonotraumatic injury (Berry et al., 2001). Voice produced with this intermediate laryngeal configuration has been called "resonant voice," perceptually corresponding to anterior oral vibratory sensations during "easy" voicing (Verdolini et al., 1998). Programmatic approaches to resonant voice training have shown reductions in phonatory effort, voice quality, and laryngeal appearance (Verdolini-Marston et al., 1995), as well as reductions in functional disruptions due to voice problems in individuals with conditions known or presumed to be related to hyperadduction, such as nodules. Moreover, there is evidence that individuals use this type of voicing outside the clinic more than the traditional "quiet, breathy voice" because it is functionally tractable (Verdolini-Marston et al., 1995). Resonant voice training may also be useful in improving vocal and functional status in individuals with hypoadducted dysphonia. Recent theoretical modeling has indicated that nonlinear source (vocal fold)–filter (vocal tract) interactions are critical in maximizing voice output germane to resonant voice and other voice types (Titze, 2002).

A relatively small number of clinical cases involve vocal fold elongation abnormalities as the salient feature of the vocal condition. Often, the medical condition involves cricothyroid paresis, although thyroarytenoid paresis may also be implicated. Voice therapy has been less successful in treating such conditions. Other elongation abnormalities are functional, as in mutational falsetto. The clinical consensus is that voice therapy generally is useful in treating mutational falsetto.

Finally, in addition to addressing laryngeal kinematics, voice therapy usually also addresses nonphonatory aspects of biomechanics that influence the vocal fold mucosa. Such issues are addressed in voice hygiene programs (see VOICE HYGIENE). Mucosal performance and mucosal vulnerability to trauma are the key concerns. The primary issues targeted are hydration and behavioral control of laryngopharyngeal reflux. Dehydration increases the pulmonary effort required for phonation, whereas hydration decreases it and also decreases laryngeal phonotrauma (e.g., Titze, 1988; Verdolini, Titze, and Fennell, 1994; Solomon and DiMattia, 2000). Thus, hydration regimens are appropriate for individuals with voice problems and dehydration (Verdolini-Marston, Sandage, and Titze, 1994). There is increasing support for the view that laryngopharyngeal reflux plays a role in a wide range of laryngeal diseases, including inflammatory and even neurogenic and malignant disease. Voice therapy can play a supportive role to the medical or surgical treatment of laryngopharyngeal reflux by educating patients regarding behavioral issues such as diet and sleeping position. Some data are consistent with the view that control of laryngopharyngeal reflux can improve both laryngeal appearance and voice symptoms in individuals with a diagnosis of laryngopharyngeal reflux (Shaw et al., 1996; Hamdan et al., 2001). However, vocal hygiene programs alone in voice therapy apparently produce little benefit if they are not coupled with voice production work.

Specific Therapy Approach. Recently, interest has emerged in cognitive mechanisms involved in skill acquisition and factors affecting patient compliance as related to voice training and therapy models. Speech-language pathologists may train individuals to acquire the basic biomechanical changes described in preceding paragraphs, and others. The traditional approach is eclectic and entails implementing a series of facilitating techniques such as the "yawn-sigh" and "push-pull" techniques, as well as other maneuvers, such as altering the tongue position, changing the loudness of the voice, using chant talk, and using digital manipulation. Facilitating techniques are used by many clinicians and are generally considered effective. However, formal efficacy data are lacking for most of the techniques. An exception is digital manipulation, specifically manual circumlaryngeal therapy (laryngeal massage), used for idiopathic, presumably hyperfunctional dysphonia. Brief courses of aggressive laryngeal massage by skilled practitioners have dramatically improved voice in individuals with this condition (Roy et al., 1997). Also, variants of "yawn-sigh" phonation, such as falsetto and breathy voicing, may temporarily improve symptoms of adductory spasmodic dysphonia and increase the duration of the effectiveness of botulinum toxin injections (Murry and Woodson, 1995).

Several programmatic approaches to voice therapy have been developed, some of which have been submitted to formal clinical studies. An example is the Lee Silverman Voice Treatment (LSVT). This treatment uses "loud" voice to treat not only hypoadduction and hypophonia, but also prosodic and articulatory deficiencies in individuals with Parkinson's disease. LSVT utilizes a predetermined hierarchy of speech tasks in 16 therapy sessions delivered over 4 weeks. In comparison with control and alternative treatment groups, LSVT has increased vocal loudness and voice inflection for as long as 2 years following therapy termination (Ramig, Sapir, Fox et al., 2001; Ramig, Sapir, Countryman et al., 2001). Critical aspects of LSVT that may contribute to its success include a large number of repetitions of the target "loud voice" in a variety of physical contexts.

Another programmatic approach to voice therapy, the Lessac-Madsen Resonant Voice Therapy (LMRVT), was developed for individuals with either hyper- or hypoadducted voice problems associated with nodules, polyps, nonspecific phonotraumatic changes, paralysis, paresis, atrophy, bowing, and sulcus vocalis. LMRVT targets the use of barely touching or barely separated vocal folds for phonation, a configuration considered to be ideal because it maximizes the ratio of voice output intensity to vocal fold impact intensity (Berry et al., 2001). In LMRVT, eight structured therapy sessions typically are delivered over 8 weeks. Training emphasizes sensory processing and the extension of "resonant voice" to a variety of communicative and emotional environments. Data on preliminary versions of LMRVT indicate that it is as useful as quiet, breathy voice training for sorority women with phonotrauma or the use of amplification for teachers with voice problems in reducing various combinations of phonatory effort, voice quality, laryngeal appearance, and functional status (Verdolini-Marston et al., 1995).

Another programmatic approach to voice therapy for both hyper- and hypoadducted conditions is called Vocal Function Exercises (VFE; Stemple et al., 1994). This approach targets similar vocal fold biomechanics as LMRVT, that is, vocal folds that are barely touching or barely separated, for phonation. Training consists of repeating maximally sustained vowels and pitch glides twice daily over a period of 4–6 weeks. Carryover exercises to conversational speech may also be used. A 6-week program of VFE in teachers with voice problems resulted in greater self-perceived voice improvement, greater phonatory ease, and better voice clarity than that achieved with vocal hygiene treatment alone (Roy et al., 2001).

Another program, Accent Therapy, addresses the ideal laryngeal configuration—barely touching or barely separated vocal folds—in individuals with hyper- and hypoadducted conditions (Smith and Thyme, 1976). Training entails the use of specified rhythmic, prosodically stressed vocal repetitions, beginning with sustained consonants and progressing to phrases and extended speech. The Accent Method is more widely used in Europe and Asia than in the United States.

Electromyographic biofeedback has been reported to be effective in reducing laryngeal hyperfunction and laryngeal appearance in individuals with voice problems linked to hyperadduction (nodules). Also, visual feedback using videoendoscopy may be useful in treating numerous voice conditions; specific clinical observations have been reported relative to ventricular phonation (Bastian, 1987).

Finally, some clinicians have found that sensory differentiation exercises may help in the treatment of repetitive strain injury—one of the fastest growing occupational injuries. Repetitive strain injury involves decreased use of manual digits or voice and pain subsequent to overuse. Attention to sensory differentiation in the treatment of repetitive strain injury is motivated by reports of fused representation for groups of movements in sensory cortex following extensive digit use (e.g., Byl, Merzenich, and Jenkins, 1996).

—*Katherine Verdolini*

References

Bastian, R. W. (1987). Laryngeal image biofeedback for voice disorder patients. *Journal of Voice, 1*, 279–282.

Berry, D. A., Verdolini, K., Montequin, D. W., Hess, M. M., Chan, R. W., and Titze, I. R. (2001). A quantitative output-cost ratio in voice production. *Journal of Speech-Language-Hearing Research, 44*, 29–37.

Boone, D. R., and McFarlane, S. C. (1993). A critical view of the yawn-sigh as a voice therapy technique. *Journal of Voice, 7*, 75–80.

Boone, D. R., and McFarlane, S. C. (1994). *The voice and voice therapy* (5th ed.). Englewood Cliffs, NJ: Prentice Hall.

Byl, N. N., Merzenich, M. M., and Jenkins, W. M. (1996). A primate genesis model of focal dystonia and repetitive strain injury: I. Learning-induced dedifferentiation of the representation of the hand in the primary somatosensory cortex in adult monkeys. *Neurology, 47*, 508–520.

Casper, J. K. (1993). Objective methods for the evaluation of vocal function. In J. Stemple (Ed.), *Voice therapy: Clinical methods* (pp. 39–45). St. Louis: Mosby–Year Book.

Casper, J. K., Colton, R. H., Brewer, D. W., and Woo, P. (1989). *Investigation of selected voice therapy techniques.* Paper presented at the 18th Symposium of the Voice Foundation, Care of the Professional Voice, New York.

Hamdan, A. L., Sharara, A. I., Younes, A., and Fuleihan, N. (2001). Effect of aggressive therapy on laryngeal symptoms and voice characteristics in patients with gastroesophageal reflux. *Acta Otolaryngologica, 121*, 868–872.

Hillman, R. E., Holmberg, E. B., Perkell, J. S., Walsh, M., and Vaughan, C. (1989). Objective assessment of vocal hyperfunction: An experimental framework and initial results. *Journal of Speech and Hearing Research, 32*, 373–392.

Jiang, J. J., and Titze, I. R. (1994). Measurement of vocal fold intraglottal stress and impact stress. *Journal of Voice, 8*, 132–144.

Koufman, J. A., Amin, M. R., and Panetti, M. (2000). Relevance of reflux in 113 consecutive patients with laryngeal and voice disorders. *Otolaryngology–Head and Neck Surgery, 123*, 385–388.

Murry, T., and Woodson, G. (1995). Combined-modality treatment of adductor spasmodic dysphonia with botulinum toxin and voice therapy. *Journal of Voice, 6*, 271–276.

Ramig, L. O., Sapir, S., Countryman, S., Pawlas, A. A., O'Brien, C., Hoehn, M., et al. (2001). Intensive voice treatment (LSVT) for patients with Parkinson's disease: A 2 year follow up. *Journal of Neurology, Neurosurgery, and Psychiatry, 71*, 493–498.

Ramig, L. O., Sapir, S., Fox, C., and Countryman, S. (2001). Changes in vocal loudness following intensive voice treatment (LSVT) in individuals with Parkinson's disease: A comparison with untreated patients and normal age-matched controls. *Movement Disorders, 16*, 79–83.

Roy, N., Gray, S. D., Simon, M., Dove, H., Corbin-Lewis, K., and Stemple, J. C. (2001). An evaluation of the effects of two treatment approaches for teachers with voice disorders: A prospective randomized clinical trial. *Journal of Speech-Language-Hearing Research, 44*, 286–296.

Shaw, G. Y., Searl, J. P., Young, J. L., and Miner, P. B. (1996). Subjective, laryngoscopic, and acoustic measurements of laryngeal reflux before and after treatment with omeprazole. *Journal of Voice, 10*, 410–418.

Smith, S., and Thyme, K. (1976). Statistic research on changes in speech due to pedagogic treatment (the accent method). *Folia Phoniatrica, 28*, 98–103.

Solomon, N. P., and Di Mattia, M. S. (2000). Effects of a vocally fatiguing task and systemic hydration on phonation threshold pressure. *Journal of Voice, 14*, 341–362.

Stemple, J. C., Lee, L., D'Amico, and Pickup, B. (1994). Efficacy of vocal function exercises as a method of improving voice production. *Journal of Voice, 8*, 271–278.

Titze, I. R. (1994). Mechanical stress in phonation. *Journal of Voice, 8*, 99–105.

Titze, I. R. (2002). Regulating glottal airflow in phonation: Application of the maximum power transfer theorem to a low dimensional phonation model. *Journal of the Acoustical Society of America, 111*, 367–376.

Verdolini, K. (2000). Case study: Resonant voice therapy. In J. Stemple (Ed.), *Voice therapy: Clinical studies* (2nd ed., pp. 46–62). San Diego, CA: Singular Publishing Group.

Verdolini, K., Druker, D. G., Palmer, P. M., and Samawi, H. (1998). Laryngeal adduction in resonant voice. *Journal of Voice, 12*, 315–327.

Verdolini, K., Titze, I. R., and Fennell, A. (1994). Dependence of phonatory effort on hydration level. *Journal of Speech and Hearing Research, 37*, 1001–1007.

Verdolini-Marston, K., Burke, M. K., Lessac, A., Glaze, L., and Caldwell, E. (1995). Preliminary study of two methods of treatment for laryngeal nodules. *Journal of Voice, 9*, 74–85.

Verdolini-Marston, K., Sandage, M., and Titze, I. R. (1994). Effect of hydration treatments on laryngeal nodules and polyps and related voice measures. *Journal of Voice, 8*, 30–47.

Yamaguchi, H., Yotsukura, Y., Hirosaku, S., Watanabe, Y., Hirose, H., Kobayashi, N., and Bless, D. (1993). Pushing exercise program to correct glottal incompetence. *Journal of Voice, 7*, 250–256.

Further Readings

Boone, D. R., McFarlane, S. C. (1994). *The voice and voice therapy* (5th ed.). Englewood Cliffs, NJ: Prentice Hall.

Colton, R., and Casper, J. K. (1996). *Understand voice problems: A physiological perspective for diagnosis and treatment* (2nd ed.). Baltimore: Williams and Wilkins.

Kotby, M. N. (1995). *The Accent Method of voice therapy*. San Diego, CA: Singular Publishing Group.

Stemple, J. C. (2000). *Voice therapy: Clinical studies* (2nd ed.). San Diego, CA: Singular/Thompson Learning.

Stemple, J. C., Glaze, L. E., and Gerdeman, R. K. (1995). *Clinical voice pathology: Theory and management* (2nd ed.). San Diego, CA: Singular Publishing Group.

Titze, I. R. (1994). *Principles of voice production*. Englewood Cliffs, NJ: Prentice Hall.

Verdolini, K., and Krebs, D. (1999). Some considerations on the science of special challenges in voice training. In G. Nair, *Voice tradition and technology: A state-of-the-art studio* (pp. 227–239). San Diego, CA: Singular Publishing Group.

Verdolini, K., Ostrem, J., DeVore, K., and McCoy, S. (1998). *National Center for Voice and Speech's guide to vocology*. Iowa City, IA: National Center for Voice and Speech.

Verdolini, K., and Ramig, L. (2001). Review: Occupational risks for voice problems. *Journal of Logopedics, Phoniatrics, and Vocology, 26*, 37–46.

Voice Therapy for Neurological Aging-Related Voice Disorders

Introduction

The neurobiological changes that a person undergoes with advancing age produce structural and functional changes in all of the organs and organ systems in the body. The upper respiratory system, the larynx, vocal tract, and oral cavity all reflect both normal and abnormal changes that result from aging. In 1983, Ramig and Ringel suggested that age-related changes of the voice must be viewed as part of the normal process of physiological aging of the entire body (Ramig and Ringel, 1983). Neurological, musculoskeletal, and circulatory remodeling account for changes in laryngeal function and vocal output in older adults. These changes, however, do not necessarily result in abnormal voice quality. A thorough laryngological examination coupled with a complete voice assessment will likely reveal obvious voice disorders associated with aging. It still remains for the clinicians along with the help of the patient to identify and distinguish normal age-related voice changes from voice disorders. This entry describes neurological aging-related voice disorders and their treatment options. Traumatic or idiopathic vocal fold paralysis is described in another entry, as is Parkinson's disease. This article focuses on neurologically based voice disorders associated with general aging.

Voice production in the elderly is associated with other bodily changes that occur with advancing age (Chodzko-Zajko and Ringel, 1987), although changes in specific organs may derive from various causes and mechanisms. The effects of normal aging are somewhat similar across organ systems. Aging of the vocal organs, like other organ systems, is associated with decreased strength, accuracy, endurance, speed, coordination, organ system interaction (i.e., larynx and respiratory systems), nerve conduction velocity, circulatory function, and chemical degradation at synaptic junctions.

Anatomical (Hirano, Kurita, and Yukizane, 1989; Kahane, 1987) and histological studies (Luchsinger and Arnold, 1965) clearly demonstrate that differences in structure and function do exist as a result of aging. The vocal fold epithelium, the layers of the lamina propria, and the muscles of the larynx change with aging. The vocal folds lose collaginous fibers, leading to increased stiffness.

The neurological impact to the aging larynx includes central and peripheral motor nervous system changes. Central nervous system changes include nerve cell losses in the cortex of the frontal, parietal, and temporal lobes of the brain. This results in the slowing of motor movements (Scheibel and Scheibel, 1975). Nerve conduction velocity also contributes to speed of voluntary movements such as pitch changes, increased loudness, and speed of articulation (Leonard et al., 1997). Nervous system changes are also associated with tremor, a

Table 1. Diagnoses of Subjects Age 65 and Older Seen at the University of Pittsburgh Voice Center

Diagnosis	N	%
Vocal fold atrophy	46	23
Vocal fold paralysis	39	19
Laryngopharyngeal reflux	32	16
Parkinson's disease	26	13
Essential tremor	8	4
Other neurological disorders	16	8
Muscular tension dysphonia—primary	15	7
Muscular tension dysphonia—secondary	38	19
Edema	14	6
Spasmodic dysphonia	7	3

N = 205. The total number of diagnoses is larger since some patients had more than one diagnosis.

condition seen more in the elderly than in young individuals. Finally, dopaminergic changes which decline with aging may also affect the speed of motor processing (Morgan and Finch, 1988).

The peripheral changes that occur in the elderly are thought to be broadly related to environmental effects of trauma (Woo et al., 1992), selective denervation of type II fast twitch muscle fibers (Lexell, 1997) and decrease in distal and motor neurons, resulting in decreased contractile strength and an increase in muscle fatigue (Doherty and Brown, 1993).

Voice Changes Related to Neurological Aging

The central and peripheral degeneration and concomitant regenerative neural changes that occur with neurological aging may result in a number of voice disorders. Excluding vocal fold paralysis, these neurological changes account for disorders of voice quality and overall vocal output. Murry and Rosen reported on 205 patients 65 years of age and older. Table 1 shows the diagnosis of this group (Murry and Rosen, 1999).

The most common symptoms reported by this group of patients are shown in Table 2.

Neurological changes to the voice accompanying aging are related to decreased neurological structure and

Table 2. The Most Common Voice Symptoms Reported by Patients 65 Years of Age and Older

Symptom	% of Patients
Loss of volume	28
Raspy or hoarse voice	24
Vocal fatigue	22
Difficulty breathing during speech	18
Talking in noisy environments	15
Loss of clarity	16
Tremor	7
Intermittent voice loss	6
Articulation-related problems	5

Total exceeds 100% as some individuals reported more than one complaint.

function which result in patient perceived and listener perceived vocal dysfunction. Indeed, if the neuromotor systems are intact and the elderly patient is healthy, the speaking and singing voice is not likely to be perceived as "old" nor function as "old" (McGlone and Hollien, 1963). Conversely, the voice may be perceived as "old" not solely due to neurological changes in the larynx and upper airway, but due to muscular weakness of the upper body (Ramig and Ringel, 1983), cardiovascular changes (Orlikoff, 1990), or decreased hearing acuity resulting in excessive vocal force (Chodzko-Zajko and Ringel, 1987).

There are, however, certain aspects of voice production that are characteristically associated with age-related neuropathy. The clinical examination of elderly individuals who complain of voice disorders should specifically address and test for loss of vocal range and volume, vocal fatigue, increased breathy quality during extended conversations, presence of tremor, and pitch breaks (especially breaks into falsetto and hoarse voice quality). Elderly singers should be evaluated for pitch inaccuracies, increased breathiness, and changes in vibrato (Tanaka, Hirano, and Chijina, 1994).

A careful examination of the elderly patient with a complaint about his or her voice consists of an extensive history including medications, previous surgeries, and current and previously diagnosed diseases. Acoustic, perceptual, and physiological assessment of vocal function may reveal evidence of tremor, vocal volume deficiencies, and/or vocal fatigue. Examination of the larynx and vocal folds via flexible endoscopy as well as strobo-videolaryngoscopy is essential to reveal vocal use patterns, asymmetrical vibration, scarring, tremor (of the larynx or other structures), atrophy, or lesions. In the absence of suspected malignancies or frank aspiration due to lack of glottic closure, voice therapy is the treatment of choice for most elderly patients with neurological aging-related dysphonias.

Treatments for Neurological Aging-Related Voice Disorders

Treatments for elderly patients with mobile vocal folds presenting with dysphonia include behavioral, pharmacological, and surgical approaches. A review of surgical treatments can be found in Ford (1986), Koufman (2000), Postma (1998), and Durson (1996). The use of medications and their relationship to vocal production and vocal aging can be found in the work of Sataloff and colleagues (1997) and Vogel (1995).

Voice therapy for neurological aging-related voice disorders varies, depending on the patient's complaints, diagnosis, and vocal use requirements. The most common needs of patients with neurological age-related voice disorders are to increase loudness and endurance, to reduce hoarseness or breathy voice qualities, and to maintain a broad pitch range for singing. These needs are met with vocal education including awareness of vocal hygiene; direct vocal exercises; and management of the vocal environment. Prior to voice therapy, and as part of the diagnostic process, a thorough audiological assessment of the patient should be done. If the patient wears a hearing aid or aids, he or she should wear them for the therapy sessions.

Vocal Education

Vocal education coupled with vocal hygiene provides the patient with an understanding of the aging process as it relates to voice use. An understanding of how all body organ systems are affected by normal aging helps to explain why the voice may not have the same quality, pitch range, endurance, or loudness that was present in earlier years. Since the voice is the product of respiratory and vocal tract functions, all of the systems that contribute to the aging of these organs are responsible for the final vocal output. Recently, Murry and Rosen published a vocal education and hygiene program for patients (Murry and Rosen, 2000). This program is an excellent guide for all aging patients with neurological voice disorders. Nursing homes, senior citizen residences, and geriatric specialists should consider offering this outline as the first step in patient education when patients complain of voice disorders.

Direct Voice Therapy

Voice therapy is one treatment modality for almost all types of neurological aging-related voice disorders. The recent explosion of knowledge about the larynx is matched by an equal growth of interest in its physiology, its disorders, and their treatment. Increased use of laryngeal imaging and knowledge of laryngeal physiology have provided a base for behavioral therapy that is increasingly focused on the specific nature of the observed pathophysiology. While treatment is designed to restore maximum vocal function, the aging process of weakness, muscle wasting, and system endurance may not restore the voice to its youthful characteristics. Rather, the desired goals should be effective vocal communication and forestalling continued vocal deterioration (Sataloff et al., 1997).

Specific techniques for the aging voice have evolved from our understanding of the aging neuromuscular process. Confidential voice is the voice that one might typically use to describe or discuss confidential matters. Theoretically, it is produced with minimal vocal fold contact. The confidential voice technique is used to (1) eliminate hyperfunctional and traumatic behaviors; (2) allow lesions such as vocal nodules to heal in the absence of continued pounding; (3) eliminate excessive muscular tension and vocal fatigue; (4) reset the internal volume meter; and (5) force a heightened awareness of voice use and the vocal environment. The goal is to create healthier vocal folds and a neutral state from which healthy voice use can be taught and developed through a variety of other techniques (Verdolini-Marston, Burke, and Lessass, 1995; Leddy, Samlan, and Poburka, 1997).

The confidential voice technique is appropriately used to treat benign lesions, muscle tension dysphonia, hyperfunctional dysphonia, and vocal fatigue in the early postoperative period. It is not appropriate for treatment of vocal fold paralysis, conditions with incomplete glottal closure, or a scarred vocal fold.

Resonant voice, or voice with forward focus, usually refers to an easy voice associated with vibratory sensations in facial bones (Verdolini-Marston, Burke, and Lessass, 1995). Therapy focuses on the production of this voice primarily through feeling and hearing. Exercises to place the vocal mechanism in a specific manner coupled with humming help the patient identify to optimum pitch/placement for maximum voice quality. Resonant voice therapy is described as being useful in the treatment of vocal fold lesions, functional voice problems, mild vocal atrophy, and paralysis.

Manual circumlaryngeal massage (manual laryngeal musculoskeletal tension reduction) is a direct, hands-on approach in which the clinician massages and manipulates the laryngeal area in a particular manner while observing changes in voice quality as the patient phonates. The technique was first proposed by Aronson (1990) and later elaborated by Morrison and Rammage (1993). Roy and colleagues reported on their use of the massage technique in controlled studies (Roy, Bless, and Heisey, 1997). They reported almost normal voice following a single session in 93% of 17 subjects with hyperfunctional dysphonia.

General body massage in which muscles are kneaded and manipulated is known to reduce muscle tensions. This concept is adapted to massage the muscles in the laryngeal area. One focus of the circumlaryngeal massage is to relieve the contraction of those muscles and allow the larynx to lower. This technique is most often used with patients who report neck or upper body tension or stiffness, tenderness in the neck muscles, odynophonia, or those who demonstrate rigid postures. Vocal function exercises are designed to pinpoint and exercise specific laryngeal muscles. The four steps address warm-up of the muscles, stretching and contracting of muscles, and building muscle power. The softness of the productions is said to increase muscular and respiratory effort and control. The exercises are hypothesized to restrengthen and balance laryngeal musculature, to improve vocal fold flexibility and movement, and to rebalance airflow (Stemple, Glaze, and Gerdeman, 1995).

Ramig and colleagues developed a structured intensive therapy program, the Lee Silverman voice treatment program, of four sessions per week for 4 weeks specifically for patients with idiopathic Parkinson's disease (Ramig, Bonitati, and Lemke, 1994). Since then, the efficacy of the treatment for this population has been extended to include aging patients and patients with other forms of progressive neurological disease. This treatment method of voice therapy may be the most promising of all for neurological aging-related voice disorders.

The Lee Silverman voice treatment program is based on the principle that, to counteract the physical effects of reduced amplitude of motor acts including voice and speech production, rigidity, bradykinesia, and reduction in respiratory effort, it is necessary to push the entire phonatory mechanism to exert greater effort by focusing on loudness. To increase loudness, the respiratory system must provide more driving power, and the vocal folds must adduct more completely. Indeed, it seems that the respiratory, the laryngeal, and the articulatory mechanisms all benefit from the effort to increase loudness.

The program is highly structured and involves five essential concepts: (1) voice is the focus; (2) a high degree of effort is required; (3) treatment is intensive; (4) the patient's self-perception must be calibrated; and (5) productions and outcomes are quantified. The scope of this article does not permit inclusion of the extensive literature available on this method or an extensive description of the therapy protocol, which is available in published form.

The accent method, originally developed by Smith, has been used to treat all types of dysphonias (Smith and Thyme, 1976). It has been adopted more widely abroad than in the United States and focuses on breathing as the underlying control mechanism of vocal output and uses accentuated and rhythmic movements of the body and then of voicing. Easy voice production with an open-throat feeling is stressed, and attention is paid primarily to an abdominal/diaphragmatic breathing pattern. This method is useful for treating those individuals with vocal fatigue, endurance problems, or overall volume weakness.

All voice therapy is a directed way of changing a particular behavior or set of behaviors. Regardless of the methods used, voice therapy demands the cooperation of the patient in ways that may be novel and unusual. Voice therapy differs from the medical approach, which requires only that a pill be taken or an injection received. It differs from the surgical approach, wherein the surgeon does the work. It differs from the work of voice and acting coaches, who work to enhance and strengthen a normal voice. Voice clinicians work with individuals who never thought about the voice until they acquired a voice disorder. They are primarily interested in rapid restoration of normal voice, a task that cannot always be accomplished.

Vocal Tremor

One neurological aging-related disorder that often resists change is vocal tremor. Tremor often accompanies many voice disorders having a neurological component. Vocal tremor has been treated in the past with medications, and in some cases with laryngeal framework surgery, when vocal fold atrophy is also diagnosed. The specific therapeutic techniques presented in this article may also be helpful in reducing the perception of tremor especially those that focus on increasing vocal fold closure (i.e., Lee Silverman voice treatment and the Accent Method).

Finally, the treatment of aging-related dysphonias should include techniques used in training singers and actors (Sataloff et al., 1997). General physical conditioning, warmup, increased respiratory function exercises, and the ability to monitor voice change help to maintain voice or retard vocal weakness, fatigue, and loss of clear voice quality.

The vocal environment should not be ignored as a factor in communication for patients with neurological aging-related voice disorders. Voice use is maximized in environments where background noise is minimal, sound absorption materials such as rugs and cushions are used in large meeting rooms, and proper lighting is available to help with visual components of communication.

Summary

Progressive neurological aging-related disorders offer a challenge to the speech-language pathologist. In the absence of surgery for vocal fold paralysis, the patient with mobile vocal folds and a neurological disorder may benefit from specific exercises to maintain vocal communication. Diagnosis, which identifies the vocal use habits of the patient is critical to identify strategies and the specific exercises needed to maintain and/or improve voice production.

See also VOICE DISORDERS OF AGING.

—*Thomas Murry*

References

Aronson, A. E. (1990). *Clinical voice disorders*. New York: Thieme-Stratton.

Brody, H. (1992). The aging brain. *Acta Neurologica Scandanavica (Supplement)*, *137*, 40–44.

Chodzko-Zajko, W. J., and Ringel, R. L. (1987). Physiological aspects of aging. *Journal of Voice*, 18–26.

Doherty, T., and Brown, W. (1993). The estimated numbers and relative sizes of the nar motor units as selected by multiple point stimulation in young and older adults. *Muscle and Nerve, 16*, 355–366.

Durson, G., Sataloff, R. T., and Speigel, J. R. (1996). Superior laryngeal nerve paresis and paralysis. *Journal of Voice, 10*, 206–211.

Ford, C. N. (1986). Histologic studies on the fate of soluble collagen injected into canine vocal folds. *Laryngoscope, 96*, 1248–1257.

Hirano, M., Kurita, S., and Yukizane, K. (1989). Asymmetry of the laryngeal framework: A morphologic study of cadaver larynges. *Annals of Otology, Rhinology, and Laryngology, 98*, 135–140.

Hollien, H., and Shipp, T. (1972). Speaking fundamental frequency and chronological age in males. *Journal of Speech and Hearing Research, 15*, 155–159.

Kahane, J. C. (1987). Connective tissue changes in the larynx and their effects on voice. *Journal of Voice, 1*, 27–30.

Koufman, J. A., Postma, G. N., Cummins, M. M., and Blalock, P. D. (2000). Vocal fold paresis. *Otolaryngology–Head and Neck Surgery, 122*, 537–541.

Leddy, M., Samlan, R., and Poburka, B. (1997). Effective treatments for hyperfunctional voice disorders. *Advances for Speech-Language Pathologists and Audiologists, 14*, 18.

Leonard, C., Matsumoto, T., Diedrich, P., and McMillan, J. (1997). Changes in neural modulation and motor control during voluntary movements of older individuals. *Journal of Gerontology, Medical Sciences, 52A*, M320–M325.

Lexell, J. (1997). Evidence for nervous system degeneration with advancing age. *Journal of Nutrition, 127*, 1011S–1013S.

Luchsinger, R., and Arnold, G. E. (1965). *Voice, speech, language: Clinical communicology—Its physiology and pathology*. Belmont, CA: Wadsworth.

McGlone, R., and Hollien, H. (1963). Vocal pitch characteristics of aged women. *Journal of Speech and Hearing Research, 6*, 164–170.

Morgan, D., and Finch, C. (1988). Dopaminergic changes in the basal ganglia: A generalized phenomenon of aging in mammals. *Annuals of the New York Academy of Sciences, Part III. Central Neuronal Alterations Related to Motor Behavior Control in Normal Aging: Basil Ganglia*, 145–159.

Morrison, M. D., and Ramage, L. A. (1993). Muscle misuse voice disorders: Description and classification. *Acta Otolaryngologica, 113*, 428–434.

Murry, T., Rosen, C. A. (1999). Vocal aging: Treatment options (abstr.). In *Proceedings of 2nd World Voice Congress*. São Paulo, Brazil.

Murry, T., and Rosen, C. A. (2000). Vocal education for the professional voice user and singer. In C. A. Rosen and T. Murry (Eds.), *Otolaryngologic Clinics of North America, 33*, 967–982.

Orlikoff, R. F. (1990). The relationship of age and cardiovascular health to certain acoustic characteristics of male voices. *Journal of Speech and Hearing Research, 33*, 450–457.

Postma, G. N., Blalock, P. D., and Koufman, J. A. (1998). Bilateral medialization laryngoplasty. *Laryngoscope, 108*, 1429–1434.

Ramig, L., and Ringel, R. L. (1983). Effects of physiological aging on selected acoustic characteristics of voice. *Journal of Speech and Hearing Research, 26*, 22–30.

Ramig, L. O., Bonitati, C. M., and Lemke, J. H. (1994). Voice treatment for patients with Parkinson's disease: Development of an approach and preliminary efficacy data. *Journal of Medical Speech-Language Pathology, 2*, 191–209.

Rosenburg, S., Malmgren, L. T., and Woo, P. (1989). Age-related change in the internal branch of the rat superior laryngeal nerve. *Archives of Otolaryngology–Head and Neck Surgery, 115*, 78–86.

Roy, N., Bless, D. M., and Heisey, D. (1997). Manual circumlaryngeal therapy for functional dysphonia: An evaluation of short- and long-term treatment outcomes. *Journal of Voice, 11*, 321–331.

Sataloff, R. T., Emerich, K. A., and Hoover, C. A. (1997). Endocrine dysfunction. In R. T. Sataloff (Ed.), *Professional voice* (pp. 291–299). San Diego, CA: Singular Publishing Group.

Sataloff, R. T., Rosen, D. C., Hawkshaw, M., and Spiegel, J. R. (1997). The aging adult voice. *Journal of Voice, 11*, 156–160.

Scheibel, M., and Scheibel, A. (1975). Structural changes in the aging brain. In H. Brody (Ed.), *Clinical morphological and neuromechanical aspects of the aging nervous system*. New York: Raven Press.

Smith, S., and Thyme, K. (1976). Statistic research on changes in speech due to pedagogic treatment (the accent method). *Folia Phoniatrica, 28*, 98–103.

Stemple, J. C., Glaze, L. E., and Gerdeman, B. K. (1995). *Clinical voice pathology* (2nd ed.). San Diego, CA: Singular Publishing Group.

Tanaka, S., Hirano, M., and Chijina, K. (1994). Some aspects of vocal fold bowing. *Annals of Otology, Rhinology, and Laryngology, 103*, 357–362.

Verdolini-Marston, K., Burke, M. K., and Lessas, A. (1995). A preliminary study on two methods of treatment for laryngeal nodules. *Journal of Voice, 9*, 74–85.

Vogel, D., and Carter, J. (1995). *The effects of drugs on communication disorders*. San Diego, CA: Singular Publishing Group.

Woo, P., Casper, J., Colton, R., and Brewer, D. (1992). Dsyphonia in the aging: Physiology versus disease. *Laryngoscope, 102*, 139–144.

Voice Therapy for Professional Voice Users

A professional voice user is a person whose job function critically depends on use of the voice. Not only singers and actors but teachers, lawyers, clergy, counselors, air traffic controllers, telemarketers, firefighters, police, and auctioneers are among those who use their voices significantly in their line of work.

Probably the preponderance of professional voice users who seek treatment for voice problems have voice-induced conditions. Typically, such conditions involve either phonotrauma or functional problems. The full range of non-use-related vocal pathologies may occur in professional voice users as well, at about the same rate as in the population at large. However, special considerations may be required in therapy for professional voice users because of their job demands.

The teaching profession is at highest risk for voice problems. In 1999, teachers made up between 5% and 6% of the employed population in the United States. At any given time, between one-fifth and one-half of teachers in the United States and elsewhere are experiencing a voice problem (Sapir et al., 1993; Russell, Oates, and Greenwood, 1998; E. Smith et al., 1998). Voice problems appear to occur at about the same rates among singers. Other occupations at risk for voice problems are lawyers, clergy, telemarketers, and possibly even counselors and social workers. Increasingly, phonotrauma is considered an occupational hazard in these populations (Villkman, 2000).

A new occupational hazard for voice problems has recently surfaced in the form of repetitive strain injury. This condition, one of the fastest growing occupational injuries in the United States in general, involves weakness and pain from somatic overuse. Symptoms of repetitive strain injury typically begin in the fingers after keyboard use. However, laryngeal symptoms may develop if the individual replaces the keyboard with voice recognition software.

The consequences of voice problems for professionals are not trivial and may include temporary or permanent loss of work. Conservative estimates of costs associated with voice problems in teachers alone are on the order of $2 billion annually in the United States (Verdolini and Ramig, 2001). Thus, voice problems can be devastating both occupationally and personally to many professional voice users.

The goal of treatment for professional voice users is to restore the best possible voice use—and, where relevant, anatomy and physical function—relative to the job in question. Vocal hygiene, including hydration and reflux control, plays a role in most treatment programs for professional voice users (see VOCAL HYGIENE). Surgical management may be appropriate in selected cases. However, for most professional voice users, the mainstay of intervention for voice problems is behavioral work on voice production, or voice therapy.

Traditional therapy for phonotrauma in professional groups that use the voice quantitatively (e.g., teachers, clergy, attorneys), that is, over an extended period of time or at sustained loudness, has emphasized voice conservation. In this approach, however, individuals are limited at least as much by the treatment as by the disease. The current emphasis is on training individuals to meet their voice needs while they recover from existing problems, and to prevent new ones. An intermediate vocal fold configuration, involving slight separation of the vocal processes during phonation, appears relevant to this goal (Berry et al., 2001). A variety of training methods are available for this approach to vocalization, including Lessac-Madsen resonant voice therapy (Verdolini, 2000), Vocal Function Exercises (Stemple et al., 1994), the Accent Method (S. Smith and Thyme, 1976), and flow mode therapy (see, e.g., Gauffin and Sundberg, 1989). Training in this general laryngeal configuration appears to be more effective than vocal hygiene intervention alone and more effective than intensive respiratory training in reducing self-reported functional problems due to voice in at least one class of professional voice users, teachers (Roy et al., 2001).

Therapy for individuals with qualitative both qualitative voice needs recognizes that a special sound of the voice is required occupationally. Therapy for performers—singers and actors—with voice problems is conceptually challenging, for many reasons. Vocal performers have exacting voice needs, which may be complicated by pathology; the voice training of singers and actors is not standardized; few scientific studies on training efficacy exist; and performers are subject to a suite of special personality, career, and lifestyle issues. All of these factors make many speech-language practitioners feel that a specialty focus on vocology is important in working with performing artists.

Voice therapy for performers often replicates voice pedagogy methods. The primary differences are an emphasis on injury reduction and a shorter-term intervention, with specific, measurable goals, in voice therapy. The most comprehensive technical framework for professional voice training in general has been proposed by Estill (2000). The system identifies 11 or 12 physical "degrees of freedom," such as voice onset type, false vocal fold position, laryngeal height, palatal position, and aryepiglottic space, that are independently varied to create "recipes" for a variety of sung and spoken voice qualities. Research conducted thus far has corroborated some aspects of the approach (e.g., Titze, 2002). The system recently has gained currency in voice therapy as well as vocal pedagogy. Voice training for acting tends to be less technically oriented and more "meaning driven" than singing training (e.g. Linklater, 1997).

However, exceptions exist. Also, theatre and increasingly singing training and voice therapy incorporate general body work (alignment, movement) as a central part of training.

In respect to training modalities, traditional speech-language pathology models tend to be more analytical and less experiential than typical performing arts models of training. The motor learning literature indicates that the performers may be right. The literature describes a critical dependence of motor learning on sensory processing and deemphasizes mechanical instruction (Verdolini, 1997; see also Wulf, Höß, and Prinz, 1998). The motor learning literature also clearly indicates the need for special attention to transfer in training. Skills acquired in a clinic or studio may transfer poorly to untrained stimuli in untrained environments if less specific transfer exercises are used. Biofeedback may be a useful adjunct to voice therapy and training; however, cautions exist. Terminal biofeedback, provided after the completion of performance, contributes to greater learning than on-line feedback, which occurs during ongoing performance (Armstrong, 1970, cited in Schmidt and Lee, 1999, pp. 316–317). Also, systematic fading of biofeedback support appears critical for transfer.

The voice therapist may need to address special challenges in the physical and political environments of performers. Stage environments can be frankly toxic, and compromising to vocal and overall physical health. Specific noxious substances that have been measured on stages include aromatic diisocyanates, *Penicillium frequentans* and formaldehyde in cork granulate, cobalt and aluminum (pigment components), and alveolar-size quartz sand (Richter et al., 2002). Open-air performing environments can present particular vocal challenges to performers, especially if these are unmiked. Heavy costumes weighing 80–90 lb or more and unusual, contorted postures required during vocal performance may add further challenges and may even contribute to injury.

Politically, performers may find themselves contractually linked to heavy performance schedules without the possibility of rest if they are ill or vocally indisposed. Performers are threatened with loss of income, loss of health care benefits, and loss of professional reputation if they refuse to perform when they should not. Another political issue has to do with directors' drive toward meeting commercial goals. Such goals may dictate vocal practices that are at odds with performers' best interest. Directors and producers may sometimes show little concern for performers' vocal health, because numerous vocalists are available to replace injured ones who are unwilling or unable to perform.

It is probably safe to say that individuals who are drawn to vocal performance are more extroverted, and more emotionally variable, on average, than many individuals in the population at large. The vocal practitioner should be comfortable dealing with performers' individual personal styles. Moreover, mental attitude toward performance plays a central role in the performing domain. The principles of sports psychology fully apply to the performing arts. A robust finding is that intermediate anxiety levels, as opposed to low or high anxiety, tend to maximize physical performance. Performers need to find ways to establish intermediate arousal states and stay there even in high-stress situations. Also, the direction of attention appears key for distinguishing "chokers" (people who tend to perform poorly under pressure) from persons who perform well under high stress. According to some reports, chokers tend to show a predominance of left hemisphere activation when under the gun, implying verbal analytic thinking and evaluative self-awareness. High-level performers tend to show more distributed brain activation, including right-hemisphere activity consistent with imagery and target awareness (Crews, 2001). Many other findings from the sports psychology literature are applicable to attitude issues in vocal performance.

Vocal performers may have erratic lifestyles that are linked to their jobs. Touring groups literally may live on buses. Exercise and fresh air may be restricted. Daily routines may be nonexistent. Pay may be poor and sporadic. Benefits often are not provided unless the performers belong to a union. Vocal performers with voice problems often cannot pay for treatment because their voice problems lead to lack of employment and thus lack of income and benefits. Clinics wishing to work with professional voice users should be equipped to provide some form of fiscal support for treatment.

Practitioners working with vocal performers agree that no single individual can fully assist a vocalist with voice problems. Rather, convergent efforts are required across specialities, to minimally include an otolaryngologist, speech-language pathologist, voice teacher or coach, and, patient. Different individuals take the lead, depending on the issues at hand. The physician is responsible for medical issues. The speech-language pathologist and voice teacher generally work together on technical issues. The voice teacher is the most appropriate person to address career issues with the performer, particularly issues that bear on a potential mismatch between the individual's aspirations and capabilities. The importance of communication across individuals within the team cannot be overemphasized.

—*Katherine Verdolini*

References

Berry, D. A., Verdolini, K., Montequin, D. W., Hess, M. M., Chan, R. W., and Titze, I. R. (2001). A quantitative output-cost ratio in voice production. *Journal of Speech-Language-Hearing Research, 44,* 29–37.

Crews, D. (2001). First prize: Putting under stress. *Golf, 43,* 94–96.

Estill, J. (2000). *Level one primer of basic figures.* Santa Rosa, CA: Estill Voice Training Systems.

Gauffin, J., and Sundberg, J. (1989). Spectral correlates of glottal voice source waveform characteristics. *Journal of Speech and Hearing Research, 32,* 556–565.

Lessac, A. (1997). *The use and training of the human voice: Bio-dynamic approach to vocal life.* Mountain View, CA: Mayfield.

Linklater, K. (1997). Thoughts on theatre, therapy and the art of voice. In M. Hampton and B. Acker (Eds.), *The vocal vision* (pp. 3–12). New York: Applause.

Richter, B., Löhle, E., Knapp, B., Weikert, M., Schlömicher-Their, J., and Verdolini, K. (2002). Harmful substances on the opera stage: Possible negative effects on singers' respiratory tract. *Journal of Voice, 16,* 72–80.

Roy, N., Gray, S. D., Simon, M., Dove, H., Corbin-Lewis, K., and Stemple, J. C. (2001). An evaluation of the effects of two treatment approaches for teachers with voice disorders: A prospective randomized clinical trial. *Journal of Speech-Language-Hearing Research, 44,* 286–296.

Russell, A., Oates, J., and Greenwood, K. M. (1998). Prevalence of voice problems in teachers. *Journal of Voice, 12,* 467–479.

Sapir, S., Keidar, A., and Marthers-Schmidt, B. (1993). Vocal attrition in teachers: Survey findings. *European Journal of Disorders of Communication, 27,* 129–135.

Schmidt, R. A., and Lee, T. D. (1999). *Motor control and learning: A behavioral emphasis* (3rd ed.). Champaign, IL: Human Kinetics.

Smith, E., Lemke, J., Taylor, M., Kirchner, H. L., and Hoffman, H. (1998). Frequency of voice problems among teachers and other occupations. *Journal of Voice, 12,* 480–499.

Smith, S., and Thyme, K. (1976). Statistic research on changes in speech due to pedagogic treatment (the accent method). *Folia Phoniatrica, 28,* 98–103.

Stemple, J. C., Lee, L., D'Amico, B., and Pickup, B. (1994). Efficacy of vocal function exercises as a method of improving voice production. *Journal of Voice, 83,* 271–278.

Titze, I. R. (2002). Regulating glottal airflow in phonation: Application of the maximum power transfer theorem to a low dimensional phonation model. *Journal of the Acoustical Society of America, 111*(1 Pt 1), 367–376.

Verdolini, K. (1997). Principles of skill acquisition: Implications for voice training. In M. Hampton and B. Acker (Eds.), *The vocal vision: Views on voice* (pp. 65–80). New York: Applause.

Verdolini, K. (2000). Case study: Resonant voice therapy. In J. Stemple (Ed.), *Voice therapy: Clinical studies* (2nd ed., pp. 46–62). San Diego, CA: Singular Publishing Group.

Verdolini, K., and Ramig, L. O. (2001). Review: Occupational risks for voice problems. *Logopedics, Phoniatrics, Vocology, 26,* 37–46.

Villkman, E. (2000). Voice problems at work: A challenge for occupational safety and health arrangement. *Folia Phoniatrica et Logopaedica, 52,* 120–125.

Wulf, G., Höß, M., and Prinz, W. (1998). Instructions for motor learning: Differential effects of internal versus external focus of attention. *Journal of Motor Behavior, 30,* 169–179.

Further Readings

DeVore, K., Verdolini, K. (1998). Professional speaking voice training and applications to speech-language pathology. *Current Opinion in Otolaryngology–Head and Neck Surgery, 6,* 145–150.

Hampton, M., and Acker, B. (Eds.), *The vocal vision: Views on voice.* New York: Applause.

Lessac, A. (1996). *The use and training of the human voice: A practical approach to speech and voice dynamics* (3rd ed.). Mountain View, CA: Mayfield.

Linklater, K. (1976). *Freeing the natural voice.* New York: Drama Book Specialists.

Machlin, E. (1992). *Speech for the stage* (rev. ed.). New York: Theatre Arts Books.

Maisel, E. (1974). *The Alexander technique: The essential writings of F. Matthias Alexander*. London: Thames and Hudson.

Miller, R. (1977). *English, French, German and Italian techniques of singing: A study in national tonal preferences and how they relate to functional efficiency*. Metuchen, NJ: Scarecrow Press.

Nair, G. (1999). *Voice tradition and technology: A state-of-the-art studio*. San Diego, CA: Singular Publishing Group.

Orlick, T. (2000). *In pursuit of excellence*. Champaign, IL: Human Kinetics.

Raphael, B. N. (1997). Special considerations relating to members of the acting profession. In R. T. Sataloff (Ed.), *Professional voice: The science and art of clinical care* (2nd ed., pp. 203–205). San Diego, CA: Singular Publishing Group.

Rodenburg, P. (1997). *The actor speaks*. London: Methuen Drama.

Schmidt, R. A., and Lee, T. D. (1999). *Motor control and learning: A behavioral emphasis* (3rd ed.). Champaign, IL: Human Kinetics.

Sataloff, R. T. (1997). *Professional voice: The science and art of clinical care* (2nd ed.). San Diego, CA: Singular Publishing Group.

Skinner, E., Monich, T., and Mansell, L. (1990). *Speak with distinction* (rev. ed.). New York: Applause.

Sundberg, J. (1977, March). The acoustics of the singing voice. *Scientific American, 236*, 82–91.

Sundberg, J. (1987). *The science of the singing voice*. DeKalb, IL: Northern Illinois University Press.

Thurman, L., and Welch, G. (1997). *Body mind and voice: Foundations of voice education*. Collegeville, MN: Voice-Care Network.

Verdolini, K., Ostrem, J., DeVore, K., and McCoy, S. (1998). *National Center for Voice and Speech's guide to vocology*. Iowa City, IA: National Center for Voice and Speech.

Verdolini, K., and Ramig, L. O. (2001). Review: Occupational risks for voice problems. *Logopedics, Phoniatrics, Vocology, 26*, 37–46.

Part II: Speech

Apraxia of Speech: Nature and Phenomenology

Apraxia of speech is

a phonetic-motoric disorder of speech production caused by inefficiencies in the translation of a well-formed and filled phonologic frame to previously learned kinematic parameters assembled for carrying out the intended movement, resulting in intra- and inter-articulator temporal and spatial segmental and prosodic distortions. It is characterized by distortions of segments, intersegment transitionalization resulting in extended durations of consonants, vowels and time between sounds, syllables and words. These distortions are often perceived as sound substitutions and the misassignment of stress and other phrasal and sentence-level prosodic abnormalities. Errors are relatively consistent in location within the utterance and invariable in type. It is not attributable to deficits of muscle tone or reflexes, nor to deficits in the processing of auditory, tactile, kinesthetic, proprioceptive, or language information. (McNeil, Robin, and Schmidt, 1997, p. 329)

The kernel perceptual behaviors that differentiate apraxia of speech (AOS) from other motor speech disorders and from phonological paraphasia are (1) lengthened segment (slow movements) and intersegment (segment segregation) durations (overall slowed speech), resulting in (2) abnormal prosody across multisyllable words and phrases, with a tendency to make errors on more stressed than unstressed syllables; (3) relatively consistent trial-to-trial location of errors and relatively nonvariable error types; and (4) impaired measures of coarticulation. Although apraxic speakers may produce a preponderance of sound substitutions, these substitutions do not serve as evidence of either AOS or phonemic paraphasia. Sound distortions serve as evidence of a motor-level mechanism or influence in the absence of an anatomical explanation; however, they are not localizable to one part of the motor control architecture and, taken alone, do not differentiate AOS from the dysarthrias. Acoustically well-produced (nondistorted) sound-level serial order (e.g., perseverative, anticipatory, and exchange) errors that cross word boundaries are not compatible with motor planning- or programming-generated mechanisms and are attributable to the phonological encoding mechanism.

Although this motor speech disorder has a languorous and tortuous theoretical and clinical history and is frequently confused with other motor speech disorders and with phonemic paraphasia, a first-pass estimate of some of its epidemiological characteristics has been presented by McNeil, Doyle, and Wambaugh (2000).

Based on retrospective analysis of the records of 3417 individuals evaluated at the Mayo Clinic for acquired neurogenic communication disorders, including dysarthria, AOS, aphasia, and other neurogenic speech, language, and cognitive disorders, Duffy (1995) reported a 4.6% prevalence of AOS. Based on this same retrospective analysis of 107 patient records indicating a diagnosis of AOS, Duffy reported that 58% had a vascular etiology and 6% presented with a neoplasm. One per-

cent presented with a seizure disorder and 16% had a diagnosis of degenerative disease, including Creutzfeldt-Jakob disease and leukoencephalopathy (of the remaining, 9% were unspecified, 4% were associated with dementia, and 3% were associated with primary progressive aphasia). In 15% of cases the AOS was traumatically induced (12% neurosurgically and 3% concomitant with closed head injury), and in the remaining cases the cause was undetermined or was of mixed etiology. Without doubt, these proportions are influenced by the type of patients typically seen at the Mayo Clinic, and may not be representative of other patient care sites.

Among all of the acquired speech and language pathologies of neurological origin, AOS may be the most infrequent. Its occurrence unaccompanied by dysarthria, aphasia, limb apraxia, or oral-nonspeech apraxia is extremely rare. Comorbidity estimates averaged across studies and summarized by McNeil, Doyle, and Wambaugh (2000) indicated an AOS/oral-nonspeech apraxia comorbidity of 68%, an AOS/limb apraxia comorbidity of 67%, an AOS/limb apraxia and oral-nonspeech apraxia comorbidity of 83%, an AOS/aphasia comorbidity of 81%, and an AOS/dysarthria comorbidity of 31%. Its frequent co-occurrence with other disorders and its frequent diagnostic confusion with those disorders that share surface features with it suggest that the occurrence of AOS in isolation (pure AOS) is extremely rare.

The lesion responsible for AOS has been studied since Darley (1968) and Darley, Aronson, and Brown (1975) proposed it as a neurogenic speech pathology that is theoretically and clinically different from aphasia and the dysarthrias. Because Darley defined AOS as a disorder of motor programming, the responsible lesion has been sought in the motor circuitry, especially in Broca's area. Luria (1966) proposed that the frontal lobe mechanisms for storing and accessing motor plans or programs for limb gestures or for speech segments were represented in Broca's area. He also proposed the facial region of the postcentral gyrus in the parietal lobe as a critical area governing coordinated movement between gestures (speech or nonspeech). AOS-producing lesions subtending Broca's area (Mohr et al., 1978) as well as those in the postcentral gyrus (Square, Darley, and Sommers, 1982; Marquardt and Sussman, 1984; McNeil et al., 1990) have received support. Retrospective studies of admittedly poorly defined and poorly described persons purported to have AOS (e.g., Kertesz, 1984) do not show a single site or common cluster of lesion sites responsible for the disorder. Prospective studies of the AOS-producing lesion have been undertaken by a number of investigators. Deutsch (1984) was perhaps the first to conduct a prospective search, with a result that set the stage for most of the rest of the results to follow. He found that 50% of his AOS subjects (N = 18) had a lesion in the frontal lobe and 50% had posterior lesions. Marquardt and Sussman's (1984) prospective study of 12 subjects with AOS also failed to reveal a consistent relationship among lesion location (cortical versus subcortical, anterior versus posterior), lesion volume, and the presence or absence of AOS. Dronkers (1997) reported that 100% of 25 individuals with AOS had a discrete left hemispheric cortical lesion in the precentral gyrus of the insula. One hundred percent of a control group of 19 individuals with left hemispheric lesions in the same arterial distribution as the AOS subjects but without the presence of AOS were reported to have had a complete sparing of this specific region of the insula. McNeil et al. (1990) reported computed tomographic lesion data from four individuals with AOS unaccompanied by other neurogenic speech or language pathologies. The only common lesion site for these "pure" apraxic speakers was in the facial region of the left postcentral gyrus. Two of the four AOS subjects had involvement of the insula, while two of three subjects with phonemic paraphasia (diagnosed with conduction aphasia) had a lesion in the insula. Two of the four subjects with AOS and one of the three subjects with conduction aphasia evinced involvement of Broca's area. The unambiguous results of the Dronkers study notwithstanding, the lesions responsible for AOS remain open to study. It is clear, however, that the major anterior/posterior divisions common to aphasiology and traditional neurology as sites responsible for nonfluent/fluent (respectively) disorders of speech production are challenged by the AOS/lesion data that are available to date.

Theoretical Accounts

The study of and clinical approach to AOS operate under a scientific paradigm generally consistent with the mechanisms ascribed to apraxia. That is, the majority of practitioners view AOS as a disorder of previously learned movements that is different from other speech movement disorders (i.e., the dysarthrias). The diagnosis can be confidently applied when assurance can be obtained that the person has the cognitive or linguistic knowledge underlying the intended movement and the fundamental structural and sensorimotor abilities to carry out the movement. Additionally, most definitions of apraxia suggest an impairment of movements carried out volitionally but executed successfully when performed automatically. The diagnosis requires that patients display the ability to process the language underlying the movement. These criteria are generally consistent with those used for the identification of other apraxias, including oral nonspeech (buccofacial), writing (agraphic), and limb apraxia.

Although AOS is predominantly viewed as a disorder of motor programming (Wertz, LaPointe, and Rosenbek, 1984), derived from its historical roots based in other apraxias (particularly limb-kinetic apraxia; McNeil, Doyle, and Wambaugh, 2000), there are competing theories. Whiteside and Varley (1998) proposed a deficit of the direct phonetic encoding route to account for AOS. In this theory, normal speech production involves the retrieval from storage of verbal motor patterns for frequently used syllables (the direct route), or the patterns are calculated anew (presumably from smaller verbal motor patterns) by an indirect route. Speech produced by normal speakers for infrequently occurring syllables, using the indirect route, are said to share many of the core features of apraxic speakers, such as (1) articulatory prolongation, (2) syllable segregation, (3) inability to increase the speech rate and maintain articulatory integrity, and (4) reduced coarticulation. AOS is therefore proposed to be a deficit of the direct encoding route, with a reliance on the indirect encoding route.

Based on experimental evidence that the phonological similarity effect should not be present in persons with AOS, Rogers and Storkel (1998, 1999) hypothesized a reduced buffer capacity as the mechanism responsible for AOS. In this account, the apraxic speaker with a reduced buffer capacity is required to reload or reprogram the appropriate (unspecified) buffer in a feature-by-feature, sound-by-sound, syllable-by-syllable, or motor-control-variable-by-motor-control-variable fashion. This requirement would give rise to essentially the same observable features of AOS as those commonly used to define the entity and consistent with the observable features discussed earlier.

Van der Merwe (1997) proposed a model of sensorimotor speech disorders in which AOS is defined as a disorder of motor planning. Critical to this view is the separation of motor plans from motor programs. In this model, motor plans carry information (e.g., lip rounding, jaw depression, glottal closure, raising or lowering of the tongue tip, interarticulator phasing/coarticulation) that is articulator-specific, not muscle-specific. Motor plans are derived from specific speech sounds and specify the spatial and temporal goals of the planned unit. Motor programs, on the other hand, specify the movement parameters (e.g., muscle tone, direction, force, range, and rate of movement) of specific muscles or muscle groups. For Van der Merwe, disorders of motor programs result in the dysarthrias and cannot account for the different set of physiological and behavioral signs of AOS. The attributes ascribed to motor plans in this model are consistent with the array of cardinal behavioral features of AOS.

Though their view is expanded from the traditional view of AOS as simply a disorder of motor programming, McNeil, Doyle, and Wambaugh (2000) argue that a combined motor planning and motor programming impairment as specified by Van der Merwe (1997) is required to account for the array of well-established perceptual, acoustic, and physiological features.

Other theoretical accounts of AOS include the overspecification of phonological representations theory of Dogil, Mayer, and Vollmer (1994) and the coalitional/dynamical systems breakdown theory of Kelso and Tuller (1981). These accounts have received considerably less examination in the literature and will not be described here.

AOS is an infrequently occurring pathology that is clinically recognized by most professionals dedicated to the management of speech production disorders. It is classified as a motor speech disorder in the scientific literature. When it occurs, it is frequently accompanied by other speech, language, and apraxic disorders. Its defining features are not widely agreed upon; however, evidence from perceptual, acoustic, kinematic, aerodynamic, and electromyographic studies, informed by recent models of speech motor control and phonological encoding, have led to clearer criteria for subject/patient selection and a resurgence of interest in its proposed mechanisms. The lesions responsible for acquired AOS remain a matter for future study.

See also APRAXIA OF SPEECH: TREATMENT; DEVELOPMENTAL APRAXIA OF SPEECH.

—*Malcolm R. McNeil and Patrick J. Doyle*

References

Darley, F. L. (1968). *Apraxia of speech: 107 years of terminological confusion*. Paper presented at the American Speech and Hearing Association Convention, Denver.

Darley, F. L., Aronson, A. E., and Brown, J. (1975). *Motor speech disorders*. Philadelphia: Saunders.

Deutsch, S. (1984). Prediction of site of lesion from speech apraxic error patterns. In J. C. Rosenbek, M. R. McNeil, and A. E. Aronson (Eds.), *Apraxia of speech: Physiology, acoustics, linguistics, management* (pp. 113–134). San Diego, CA: College-Hill Press.

Dogil, G., Mayer, J., and Vollmer, K. (1994). *A representational account for apraxia of speech*. Paper presented at the Fourth Symposium of the International Clinical Phonetics and Linguistics Association, New Orleans, LA.

Dronkers, N. F. (1997). A new brain region for coordinating speech coordination. *Nature, 384*, 159–161.

Duffy, J. R. (1995). *Motor speech disorders: Substrates, differential diagnosis and management*. St. Louis: Mosby.

Kelso, J. A. S., and Tuller, B. (1981). Toward a theory of apractic syndromes. *Brain and Language, 12*, 224–245.

Kertesz, A. (1984). Subcortical lesions and verbal apraxia. In J. C. Rosenbek, M. R. McNeil, and A. E. Aronson (Eds.), *Apraxia of speech: Physiology, acoustics, linguistics, management* (pp. 73–90). San Diego, CA: College-Hill Press.

Luria, A. R. (1966). *Human brain and psychological processes*. New York: Harper.

Marquardt, T., and Sussman, H. (1984). The elusive lesion-apraxia of speech link in Broca's aphasia. In J. C. Rosenbek, M. R. McNeil, and A. E. Aronson (Eds.), *Apraxia of speech: Physiology, acoustics, linguistics, management* (pp. 91–112). San Diego, CA: College-Hill Press.

McNeil, M. R., Doyle, P. J., and Wambaugh, J. (2000). Apraxia of speech: A treatable disorder of motor planning and programming. In S. E. Nadeau, L. J. Gonzalez Rothi, and B. Crosson (Eds.), *Aphasia and language: Theory to practice* (pp. 221–266). New York: Guilford Press.

McNeil, M. R., Robin, D. A., and Schmidt, R. A. (1997). Apraxia of speech: Definition, differentiation, and treatment. In M. R. McNeil (Ed.), *Clinical management of sensorimotor speech disorders* (pp. 311–344). New York: Thieme.

McNeil, M. R., Weismer, G., Adams, S., and Mulligan, M. (1990). Oral structure nonspeech motor control in normal dysarthric aphasic and apraxic speakers: Isometric force and static position control. *Journal of Speech and Hearing Research, 33*, 255–268.

Mohr, J. P., Pessin, M. S., Finkelstein, S., Funkenstein, H., Duncan, G. W., and Davis, K. R. (1978). Broca aphasia: Pathological and clinical. *Neurology, 28*, 311–324.

Rogers, M. A., and Storkel, H. (1998). Reprogramming phonologically similar utterances: The role of phonetic features in pre-motor encoding. *Journal of Speech and Hearing Research, 41*, 258–274.

Rogers, M. A., and Storkel, H. L. (1999). Planning speech one syllable at a time: The reduced buffer capacity hypothesis in apraxia of speech. *Aphasiology, 13*, 793–805.

Square, P. A., Darley, F. L., and Sommers, R. I. (1982). An analysis of the productive errors made by pure apractic speakers with differing loci of lesions. *Clinical Aphasiology, 10*, 245–250.

Van der Merwe, A. (1997). A theoretical framework for the characterization of pathological speech sensorimotor control. In M. R. McNeil (Ed.), *Clinical management of sensorimotor speech disorders* (pp. 1–25). New York: Thieme.

Wertz, R. T., LaPointe, L. L., and Rosenbek, J. C. (1984). *Apraxia of speech in adults: The disorder and its management*. Orlando, FL: Grune and Stratton.

Whiteside, S. P., and Varley, R. A. (1998). A reconceptualisation of apraxia of speech: A synthesis of evidence. *Cortex, 34*, 221–231.

Further Readings

Ballard, K. J., Granier, J. P., and Robin, D. A. (2000). Understanding the nature of apraxia of speech: Theory, analysis and treatment. *Aphasiology, 14*, 969–995.

Code, C. (1998). Models, theories and heuristics in apraxia of speech. *Clinical Linguistics and Phonetics, 12*, 47–65.

Croot, K. (2001). Integrating the investigation of apraxic, aphasic and articulatory disorders in speech production: A move towards sound theory. *Aphasiology, 15*, 58–62.

Dogil, G., and Mayer, J. (1998). Selective phonological impairment: A case of apraxia of speech. *Phonology, 15*, 143–188.

Geshwind, N. (1975). The apraxias: Neural mechanisms of disorders of learned movement. *American Scientist, 63*, 188–195.

Goodglass, H. (1992). Diagnosis of conduction aphasia. In S. E. Kohn (Ed.), *Conduction aphasia* (pp. 3–50). Hillsdale, NJ: Erlbaum.

Keele, S. W., Cohen, A., and Ivry, R. (1990). Motor programs: Concepts and issues. In M. Jeannerod (Ed.), *Attention and performance: XIII. Motor representation and control* (pp. 77–110). Hillsdale, NJ: Erlbaum.

Kent, R. D., and McNeil, M. R. (1987). Relative timing of sentence repetition in apraxia of speech and conduction aphasia. In J. H. Ryalls (Ed.), *Phonetic approaches to speech production in aphasia and related disorders* (pp. 181–220). Boston: College-Hill Press.

Kent, R. D., and Rosenbek, J. C. (1983). Acoustic patterns of apraxia of speech. *Journal of Speech and Hearing Research, 26*, 231–249.

Lebrun, Y. (1990). Apraxia of speech: A critical review. *Neurolinguistics, 5*, 379–406.

Martin, A. D. (1974). Some objections to the term apraxia of speech. *Journal of Speech and Hearing Disorders, 39*, 53–64.

McNeil, M. R., and Kent, R. D. (1990). Motoric characteristics of adult aphasic and apraxic speakers. In G. E. Hammond (Ed.), *Cerebral control of speech and limb movements* (pp. 349–386). Amsterdam: North-Holland.

Mlcoch, A. G., and Noll, J. D. (1980). Speech production models as related to the concept of apraxia of speech. In N. J. Lass (Ed.), *Speech and language: Advances in basic research and practice* (vol. 4, pp. 201–238). New York: Academic Press.

Miller, N. (1986). *Dyspraxia and its management.* Rockville, MD: Aspen.

Miller, N. (2001). Dual or duel route? *Aphasiology, 15,* 62–68.

Rogers, M. A., and Spencer, K. A. (2001). Spoken word production without assembly: Is it possible? *Aphasiology, 15,* 68–74.

Rosenbek, J. C. (2001). Darley and apraxia of speech in adults. *Aphasiology, 15,* 261–273.

Rosenbek, J. C., Kent, R. D., and LaPointe, L. L. (1984). Apraxia of speech: An overview and some perspectives. In J. C. Rosenbek, M. R. McNeil, and A. E. Aronson (Eds.), *Apraxia of speech: Physiology, acoustics, linguistics, management* (pp. 1–72). San Diego, CA: College-Hill Press.

Rothi, L. J. G., and Heilman, K. M. (Eds.). (1997). *Apraxia: The neuropsychology of action.* East Sussex, UK: Psychology Press.

Roy, E. A. (Ed.). (1985). *Neuropsychological studies of apraxia and related disorders.* Amsterdam: North-Holland.

Square-Storer, P. A. (Ed.). (1989). *Acquired apraxia of speech in aphasic adults.* London: Taylor and Francis.

Varley, R., and Whiteside, S. P. (2001). What is the underlying impairment in acquired apraxia of speech? *Aphasiology, 15,* 39–84.

Ziegler, W. (2001). Apraxia of speech is not a lexical disorder. *Aphasiology, 15,* 74–77.

Ziegler, W., and von Cramon, D. (1985). Anticipatory coarticulation in a patient with apraxia of speech. *Brain and Language, 26,* 117–130.

Ziegler, W., and von Cramon, D. (1986). Disturbed coarticulation in apraxia of speech: Acoustic evidence. *Brain and Language, 29,* 3–47.

Apraxia of Speech: Treatment

In the years since Darley (1968) first described apraxia of speech (AOS) as an articulatory programming disorder that could not be accounted for by disrupted linguistic or fundamental motor processes, considerable work has been done to elucidate the perceptual, acoustic, kinematic, aerodynamic, and electromyographic features that characterize AOS (cf. McNeil, Robin, and Schmidt, 1997; McNeil, Doyle, and Wambaugh, 2000). Explanatory models consistent with these observations have been proposed (Van der Merwe, 1997).

Overwhelmingly, the evidence supports a conceptualization of AOS as a

neurogenic speech disorder caused by inefficiencies in the specification of intended articulatory movement parameters or motor programs which result in intra- and interarticulator temporal and spatial segmental and prosodic distortions. Such movement distortions are realized as extended segmental, intersegmental transitionalization, syllable and word durations, and are frequently perceived as sound substitutions, the misassignment of stress, and other phrasal and sentence-level prosodic abnormalities. (McNeil, Robin, and Schmidt, 1997, p. 329)

Traditional and contemporary conceptualizations of the disorder have resulted in specific assumptions regarding appropriate tactics and targets of intervention, and a number of treatment approaches have been proposed that seek to enhance (1) postural shaping and phasing of the articulators at the segmental and syllable levels, and (2) segmental sequencing of longer speech units (Square-Storer and Hayden, 1989).

More recently, arguments supporting the application of motor learning principles (Schmidt, 1988) for the purposes of specifying the structure of AOS treatment sessions have been proposed, based on evidence that such principles facilitate learning and retention of motor routines involved in skilled limb movements (Schmidt, 1991). The empirical support for each approach to treatment is reviewed here.

Enhancing Articulatory Kinematics at the Segmental Level. Several facilitative techniques have been recommended to enhance postural shaping and phasing of the articulators at the segmental and syllable levels and have been described in detail by Wertz, LaPointe, and Rosenbek (1984). These techniques include (1) *phonetic derivation,* which refers to the shaping of speech sounds based on corresponding nonspeech postures, (2) *progressive approximation,* which involves the gradual shaping of targeted speech segments from other speech segments, (3) *integral stimulation and phonetic placement,* which employ visual models, verbal descriptions and physical manipulations to achieve the desired articulatory posture, and movement, and (4) *minimal pairs contrasts,* which requires patients to produce syllable or word pairs in which one member of the pair differs minimally with respect to manner, place, or voicing features from the other member of the pair.

Several early studies examined, in isolation or in various combinations, the effects of these facilitative techniques on speech production, and reported positive treatment responses (Rosenbek et al., 1973; Holtzapple and Marshall, 1977; Deal and Florance, 1978; Thompson and Young, 1983; LaPointe, 1984; Wertz, 1984). However, most of these studies suffered from methodological limitations, including inadequate subject selection criteria, nonreplicable treatment protocols, and pre-experimental research designs, which precluded firm conclusions regarding the validity and generalizability of the reported treatment effects. Contemporary investigations have addressed these methodological shortcomings and support earlier findings regarding the positive effects of treatment techniques aimed at enhancing articulatory kinematic aspects of speech at the sound, syllable, and word levels.

Specifically, in a series of investigations using single-subject experimental designs Wambaugh and colleagues examined the effects of a procedurally explicit treatment protocol employing the facilitative techniques of integral stimulation, phonetic placement, and minimal pair contrasts in 11 well-described subjects with AOS (Wambaugh et al., 1996, 1998, 1999; Wambaugh, West, and Doyle, 1998; Wambaugh and Cort, 1998; Wambaugh, 2000). These studies revealed positive treatment effects on targeted phonemes in trained and untrained words for all subjects across all studies, and positive maintenance effects of targeted sounds at 6 weeks post-treatment. In addition, two subjects showed positive generalization of trained sounds to novel stimulus contexts (i.e., untrained phrases), and one subject showed positive generalization to untrained sounds within the same sound class (voiced stops). These results provide initial experimental evidence that treatment strategies designed to enhance postural shaping and phasing of the articulators are efficacious in improving sound production of treated and untreated words. Further, there is limited evidence that for some patients and some sounds, generalization to untrained contexts may be expected.

Enhancing Segmental Sequencing of Longer Speech Units. Several facilitative techniques have been recommended to improve speech production in persons with AOS, based on the premise that the sequencing and coordination of movement parameters required for the production of longer speech units (and other complex motor behaviors) are governed by internal oscillatory mechanisms (Gracco, 1990) and temporal constraints (Kent and Adams, 1989). Treatment programs and tactics grounded in this framework employ techniques designed to reduce or control speech rate while enhancing the natural rhythm and stress contours of the targeted speech unit. The effects of several such specific facilitative techniques have been studied. These include metronomic pacing (Shane and Darley, 1978; Dworkin, Abkarian, and Johns, 1988; Dworkin and Abkarian, 1996; Wambaugh and Martinez, 1999), prolonged speech (Southwood, 1987), vibrotactile stimulation (Rubow et al., 1982), and intersystemic facilitation (i.e., finger counting) (Simmons, 1978). In addition, the effects of similarly motivated treatment programs, melodic intonation therapy (Sparks, 2001) and surface prompts (Square, Chumpelik, and Adams, 1985), have also been reported.

As with studies examining the effects of techniques designed to enhance articulatory kinematic aspects of speech at the segmental level, the empirical evidence supporting the facilitative effects of rhythmic pacing, rate control, and stress manipulations on the production of longer speech units in adults with AOS is limited. That is, among the reports cited, only five subjects were studied under conditions that permit valid conclusions to be drawn regarding the relationship between application of the facilitative technique and the dependent measures reported (Southwood, 1987; Dworkin et al., 1988; Dworkin and Abkarian, 1996; Wambaugh et al., 1999). Whereas each of these studies reported positive results, it is difficult to compare them because of differences in the severity of the disorder, in the frequency, duration, and context in which the various facilitative techniques were applied, in the behaviors targeted for intervention, and in the extent to which important aspects of treatment effectiveness (i.e., generalized effects) were evaluated. As such, the limited available evidence suggests that techniques that reduce the rate of articulatory movements and highlight rhythmic and prosodic aspects of speech production may be efficacious in improving segmental coordination in longer speech units. However, until these findings can be systematically replicated, their generalizability remains unknown.

General Principles of Motor Learning. The contemporary explication of AOS as a disorder of motor planning and programming has given rise to a call for the application of motor learning principles in the treatment of AOS (McNeil et al., 1997, 2000; Ballard, 2001). The habituation, transfer, and retention of skilled movements (i.e., motor learning) and their controlling variables have been studied extensively in limb systems from the perspective of schema theory (Schmidt, 1975). This research has led to the specification of several principles regarding the structure of practice and feedback that were found to enhance retention of skilled limb movements post-treatment, and greater transfer of treatment effects to novel movements (Schmidt, 1991). Three such principles are particularly relevant to the treatment of AOS: (1) the need for intensive and repeated practice of the targeted skilled movements, (2) the order in which targeted movements are practiced, and (3) the nature and schedule of feedback.

With respect to the first of these principles, clinical management of AOS has long espoused intensive drill of targeted speech behaviors (Rosenbek, 1978; Wertz et al., 1984). However, no studies have examined the effects of manipulating the number of treatment trials on the acquisition and retention of speech targets in AOS, and little attention has been paid to the structure of drills used in treatment. That is, research on motor learning in limb systems has shown that practicing several different skilled actions in random order within training sessions facilitates greater retention and transfer of targeted actions than does blocked practice of skilled movements (Schmidt, 1991). This finding has been replicated by Knock et al. (2000) in two adult subjects with AOS in the only study to date to experimentally manipulate random versus blocked practice to examine acquisition, retention, and transfer of speech movements.

The final principle to be discussed concerns the nature and schedule of feedback employed in the training of skilled movements. Two types of feedback have been studied, knowledge of results (KR) and knowledge of performance (KP). KR provides information only with respect to whether the intended movement was performed accurately or not. KP provides information regarding aspects of the movement that deviate from the intended action and how the intended action is to be performed. Schmidt and Lee (1999) argue that KP is most beneficial during the early stages of training but that KR administered at low response frequencies promotes greater retention of skilled movements. Both types of feedback are frequently employed in the treatment of AOS. Indeed, the facilitative techniques of integral stimulation and phonetic placement provide the type of information that is consistent with the concept of KP. However, these facilitative techniques are most frequently used as antecedent conditions to enhance target performance, and response-contingent feedback frequently takes the form of KR. The effects of the nature, schedule, and timing of performance feedback have not been systematically investigated in AOS.

In summary, AOS is a treatable disorder of motor planning and programming. Studies examining the effects of facilitative techniques aimed at improving postural shaping and phasing of the articulators at the segmental level and sequencing and coordination of segments into long utterances have reported positive outcomes. These studies are in need of carefully controlled systematic replications before generalizability can be inferred. Further, the effects of motor learning principles (Schmidt and Lee, 1999) on the habituation, maintenance, and transfer of speech behaviors require systematic evaluation in persons with AOS.

—*Patrick J. Doyle and Malcolm R. McNeil*

References

Ballard, K. J. (2001). *Principles of motor learning and treatment for AOS.* Paper presented at the biennial Motor Speech Conference, Williamsburg, VA.

Darley, F. L. (1968). *Apraxia of speech: 107 years of terminological confusion.* Paper presented at the annual convention of the American Speech and Hearing Association, Denver, CO.

Deal, J. L., and Florance, C. L. (1978). Modification of the eight-step continuum for treatment of apraxia of speech in adults. *Journal of Speech and Hearing Disorders, 43,* 89–95.

Dworkin, J. P., and Abkarian, G. G. (1996). Treatment of phonation in a patient with apraxia and dysarthria secondary to severe closed head injury. *Journal of Medical Speech-Language Pathology, 4,* 105–115.

Dworkin, J. P., Abkarian, G. G., and Johns, D. F. (1988). Apraxia of speech: The effectiveness of a treatment regime. *Journal of Speech and Hearing Disorders, 53,* 280–294.

Gracco, V. L. (1990). Characteristics of speech as a motor control system. In G. E. Hammond (Ed.), *Cerebral control of speech and limb movements.* Amsterdam: North-Holland.

Holtzapple, P., and Marshall, N. (1977). The application of multiphonemic articulation therapy with apraxic patients. In R. H. Brookshire (Ed.), *Clinical Aphasiology Conference proceedings* (pp. 46–58). Minneapolis: BRK.

Kent, R. D., and Adams, S. G. (1989). The concept and measurement of coordination in speech disorders. In S. A. Wallace (Ed.), *Advances in psychology: Perspectives on the coordination of movement* (pp. 415–450). New York: Elsevier.

Knock, T. R., Ballard, K. J., Robin, D. A., and Schmidt, R. (2000). Influence of order of stimulus presentation on speech motor learning: A principled approach to treatment for apraxia of speech. *Aphasiology, 14,* 653–668.

LaPointe, L. L. (1984). Sequential treatment of split lists: A case report. In J. Rosenbek, M. McNeil, and A. Aronson (Eds.), *Apraxia of speech: Physiology, acoustics, linguistics, management* (pp. 277–286). San Diego, CA: College-Hill Press.

McNeil, M. R., Doyle, P. J., and Wambaugh, J. (2000). Apraxia of speech: A treatable disorder of motor planning and programming. In S. E. Nadeau, L. J. Gonzalez-Rothi, and B. Crosson (Eds.), *Aphasia and language: From theory to practice* (pp. 221–265). New York: Guilford Press.

McNeil, M. R., Robin, D. A., and Schmidt, R. A. (1997). Apraxia of speech: Definition, differentiation, and treatment. In M. R. McNeil (Ed.), *Clinical management of sen-*

sorimotor speech disorders (pp. 311–344). New York: Thieme.

Rosenbek, J. C. (1978). Treating apraxia of speech. In D. F. Johns (Ed.), *Clinical Management of neurogenic communicative disorders* (pp. 191–241). Boston: Little, Brown.

Rosenbek, J. C., Lemme, M. L., Ahern, M. B., Harris, E. H., and Wertz, R. T. (1973). A treatment for apraxia of speech in adults. *Journal of Speech and Hearing Disorders, 38,* 462–472.

Rubow, R. T., Rosenbek, J. C., Collins, M. J., and Longstreth, D. (1982). Vibrotactile stimulation for intersystemic reorganization in the treatment of apraxia of speech. *Archives of Physical Medicine Rehabilitation, 63,* 150–153.

Schmidt, R. A. (1975). A schema theory of discrete motor skill learning. *Psychological Review, 82,* 225–260.

Schmidt, R. A. (1988). *Motor control and learning: A behavioral emphasis* (2nd ed.). Champaign, IL: Human Kinetics.

Schmidt, R. A. (1991). Frequent augmented feedback can degrade learning: Evidence and interpretations. In R. Requin and G. E. Stelmach (Eds.), *Tutorials in neuroscience.* Dordrecht: Kluwer Academic.

Schmidt, R. A., and Lee, T. D. (1999). *Motor control and learning: A behavioral emphasis* (3rd ed.). Champaign, IL: Human Kinetics.

Shane, H. C., and Darley, F. L. (1978). The effect of auditory rhythmic stimulation on articulatory accuracy in apraxia of speech. *Cortex, 14,* 444–450.

Simmons, N. N. (1978). Finger counting as an intersystemic reorganizer in apraxia of speech. In R. H. Brookshire (Ed.), *Clinical Aphasiology Conference proceedings* (pp. 174–179). Minneapolis: BRK.

Southwood, H. (1987). The use of prolonged speech in the treatment of apraxia of speech. In R. H. Brookshire (Ed.), *Clinical Aphasiology Conference proceedings* (pp. 277–287). Minneapolis: BRK.

Sparks, R. W. (2001). Melodic intonation therapy. In R. Chapey (Ed.), *Language intervention strategies in adult aphasia* (4th ed., pp. 703–717). Baltimore: Lippincott Williams and Wilkins.

Square, P. A., Chumpelik, D., and Adams, S. (1985). Efficacy of the PROMPT system of therapy for the treatment of acquired apraxia of speech. In R. H. Brookshire (Ed.), *Clinical Aphasiology Conference proceedings* (pp. 319–320). Minneapolis: BRK.

Square-Storer, P., and Hayden, D. C. (1989). PROMPT treatment. In P. Square-Storer (Ed.), *Acquired apraxia of speech in aphasic adults* (pp. 190–219). London: Taylor and Francis.

Thompson, C. K., and Young, E. C. (1983). *A phonological process approach to apraxia of speech: An experimental analysis of cluster reduction.* Paper presented at a meeting of the American Speech Language and Hearing Association, Cincinnati, OH.

Van der Merwe, A. (1997). A theoretical framework for the characterization of pathological speech sensorimotor control. In McNeil (Ed.), *Clinical management of sensorimotor speech disorders* (pp. 1–25). New York: Thieme.

Wambaugh, J. L. (2000). *Stimulus generalization effects of treatment for articulatory errors in apraxia of speech.* Poster session presented at the biennial Motor Speech Conference, San Antonio, TX.

Wambaugh, J. L., and Cort, R. (1998). *Treatment for AOS: Perceptual and VOT changes in sound production.* Poster session presented at the biennial Motor Speech Conference, Tucson, AZ.

Wambaugh, J. L., Doyle, P. J., Kalinyak, M., and West, J. (1996). A minimal contrast treatment for apraxia of speech. *Clinical Aphasiology, 24*, 97–108.

Wambaugh, J. L., Kalinyak-Flizar, M. M., West, J. E., and Doyle, P. J. (1998). Effects of treatment for sound errors in apraxia of speech and aphasia. *Journal of Speech Language and Hearing Research, 41*, 725–743.

Wambaugh, J. L., and Martinez, A. L. (1999). Effects of rate and rhythm control on sound production in apraxia of speech. *Aphasiology, 14*, 603–617.

Wambaugh, J. L., Martinez, A. L., McNeil, M. R., and Rogers, M. (1999). Sound production treatment for apraxia of speech: Overgeneralization and maintenance effects. *Aphasiology, 13*, 821–837.

Wambaugh, J. L., West, J. E., and Doyle, P. J. (1998). Treatment for apraxia of speech: Effects of targeting sound groups. *Aphasiology, 12*, 731–743.

Wertz, R. T. (1984). Response to treatment in patients with apraxia of speech. In J. C. Rosenbek, M. R. McNeil, and A. E. Aronson (Eds.), *Apraxia of speech: Physiology, acoustics, linguistics, management* (pp. 257–276). San Diego, CA: College-Hill Press.

Wertz, R. T., LaPointe, L. L., and Rosenbek, J. C. (1984). *Apraxia of speech in adults: The disorder and its management.* Orlando, FL: Grune and Stratton.

Further Readings

Dabul, B., and Bollier, B. (1976). Therapeutic approaches to apraxia. *Journal of Speech and Hearing Disorders, 41*, 268–276.

Freed, D. B., Marshall, R. C., and Frazier, K. E. (1977). The long-term effectiveness of PROMPT treatment in a severely apractic-aphasic speaker. *Aphasiology, 11*, 365–372.

Florance, C. L., Rabidoux, P. L., and McCauslin, L. S. (1980). An environmental manipulation approach to treating apraxia of speech. In R. H. Brookshire (Ed.), *Clinical Aphasiology Conference proceedings* (pp. 285–293). Minneapolis: BRK.

Howard, S., and Varley, R. (1995). EPG in therapy: Using electropalatography to treat severe acquired apraxia of speech. *European Journal of Disorders of Communication, 30*, 246–255.

Keith, R. L., and Aronson, A. E. (1975). Singing as therapy for apraxia of speech and aphasia: Report of a case. *Brain and Language, 2*, 483–488.

Lane, V. W., and Samples, J. M. (1981). Facilitating communication skills in adult apraxics: Application of blisssymbols in a group setting. *Journal of Communication Disorders, 14*, 157–167.

Lee, T. D., and Magill, R. A. (1983). The locus of contextual interference in motor-skill acquisition. *Journal of Experimental Psychology: Learning, Memory, and Cognition, 9*, 730–746.

McNeil, M. R., Prescott, T. E., and Lemme, M. L. (1976). An application of electro-myographic biofeedback to aphasia/apraxia treatment. In R. H. Brookshire (Ed.), *Clinical Aphasiology Conference proceedings* (pp. 151–171). Minneapolis: BRK.

Rabidoux, P., Florance, C., and McCauslin, L. (1980). The use of a Handi Voice in the treatment of a severely apractic nonverbal patient. In R. H. Brookshire (Ed.), *Clinical Aphasiology Conference proceedings* (pp. 294–301). Minneapolis: BRK.

Raymer, A. M., and Thompson, C. K. (1991). Effects of verbal plus gestural treatment in a patient with aphasia and severe apraxia of speech. In T. E. Prescott (Ed.), *Clinical Aphasiology, 20*, 285–298. Austin, TX: Pro-Ed.

Robin, D. A. (1992). Developmental apraxia of speech: Just another motor problem. *American Journal of Speech-Language Pathology: A Journal of Clinical Practice, 1*, 19–22.

Schmidt, R. A., and Bjork, R. A. (1992). New conceptualizations of practice: Common principles in three paradigms suggest new concepts for training. *Psychological Science, 3*, 207–217.

Shea, C. H., and Morgan, R. L. (1979). Contextual interference effects on the acquisition retention, and transfer of a motor skill. *Journal of Experimental Psychology: Human Learning and Memory, 5*, 179–187.

Shea, J. B., and Wright, D. L. (1991). When forgetting benefits motor retention. *Research Quarterly for Exercise and Sport, 62*, 293–301.

Simmons, N. N. (1980). Choice of stimulus modes in treating apraxia of speech: A case study. In R. H. Brookshire (Ed.), *Clinical Aphasiology Conference proceedings* (pp. 302–307). Minneapolis: BRK.

Square, P. A., Chumpelik, D., Morningstar, D., and Adams, S. (1986). Efficacy of the PROMPT system of therapy for the treatment of acquired apraxia of speech: A follow-up investigation. In R. H. Brookshire (Ed.), *Clinical Aphasiology Conference proceedings* (pp. 221–226). Minneapolis: BRK.

Square-Storer, P. (1989). Traditional therapies for AOS: Reviewed and rationalized. In P. Square-Storer (Ed.), *Acquired apraxia of speech in aphasic adults.* London: Taylor and Francis.

Square-Storer, P., and Martin, R. E. (1994). The nature and treatment of neuromotor speech disorders in aphasia. In R. Chapey (Ed.), *Language intervention strategies in adult aphasia* (pp. 467–499). Baltimore: Williams and Wilkins.

Wambaugh, J. L., and Doyle, P. D. (1994). Treatment for acquired apraxia of speech: A review of efficacy reports. *Clinical Aphasiology, 22*, 231–243.

Wulf, G., and Schmidt, R. A. (1994). Feedback-induced variability and the learning of generalized motor programs. *Journal of Motor Behavior, 26*, 348–361.

Aprosodia

Prosody consists of alterations in pitch, stress, and duration across words, phrases, and sentences. These same parameters are defined acoustically as fundamental frequency, intensity, and timing. It is the variation in these parameters that not only provides the melodic contour of speech, but also invests spoken language with linguistic and emotional meaning. Prosody is thus crucial to conveying and understanding communicative intent.

The term "aprosodia" was first used by Monrad-Krohn (1947) to describe loss of the prosodic features of speech. It resurfaced in the 1980s in the work of Ross and his colleagues to refer to the attenuated use of and decreased sensitivity to prosodic cues by right hemisphere damaged patients (Ross and Mesulam, 1979; Ross, 1981; Gorelick and Ross, 1987).

Prosodic deficits in expression or comprehension can accompany a variety of cognitive, linguistic, and psychiatric conditions, including dysarthria and other motor speech disorders, aphasia, chronic alcoholism, schizophrenia, depression, and mania, as well as right hemisphere damage (RHD) (Duffy, 1995; Myers, 1998; Monnot, Nixon, Lovallo, and Ross, 2001). The term *aprosodia*, however, typically refers to the prosodic impairments that can accompany RHD from stroke, head injury, or progressive neurologic disease with a right hemisphere focus. Even the disturbed prosody of other illnesses, such as schizophrenia, may be the result of alterations in right frontal and extrapyramidal areas, areas considered important to prosodic impairment subsequent to RHD (Sweet, Primeau, Fichtner et al., 1998; Ross et al., 2001).

The clinical presentation of expressive aprosodia is a flattened, monotonic, somewhat robotic, stilted prosodic production characterized by reduced variation in prosodic features and somewhat uniform intersyllable pause time. The condition often, but not always, accompanies flat affect, a more general form of reduced environmental responsivity, reduced sensitivity to the paralinguistic features of communication (gesture, body language, facial expression), and attenuated animation in facial expression subsequent to RHD. Aprosodia can occur in the absence of dysarthria and other motor speech disorders, in the absence of depression or other psychiatric disturbances, and in the absence of motor programming deficits typically associated with apraxia of speech. Because it is associated with damage to the right side of the brain, it usually occurs in the absence of linguistic impairments (Duffy, 1995; Myers, 1998).

Expressive aprosodia is easily recognized in patients with flat affect. Deficits in prosodic perception and comprehension are less apparent in clinical presentation. It is important to note that receptive and expressive prosodic processing can be differentially affected in aprosodia.

First observed in the emotional domain, aprosodia has also been found to occur in the linguistic domain. Thus, patients may have problems both *encoding* and *decoding* the tone of spoken messages and the intention behind the message as conveyed through both *linguistic* and *emotional* prosody.

In the acute stage, patients with aprosodia are usually unaware of the problem until it is pointed out to them. Even then, they may deny it, particularly if they suffer from other forms of denial of deficit. Severity of neglect, for example, has been found to correlate with prosodic deficits (Starkstein, Federoff, Price et al., 1994). In rare cases, aprosodia may last for months and even years when other signs of RHD have abated. Patients with persistent aprosodia may be aware of the problem but feel incapable of correcting it.

Treatment of aprosodia is often limited to training patients to adopt compensatory techniques. Patients may be taught to attend more carefully to other forms of emotional expression (e.g., gesture, facial expression) and to signal mood by explicitly stating their mood to the listener. There has, however, been at least one report of successful symptomatic treatment using pitch biofeedback and modeling (Stringer, 1996). Treatment has

been somewhat limited by uncertainty about the underlying mechanisms of aprosodia. It is not clear the extent to which expressive aprosodia is a motor problem, a pragmatic problem, a resource allocation problem, or some combination of conditions. Similarly, it is not clear whether receptive aprosodia is due to perceptual interference in decoding prosodic features, to restricted attention (which may reduce sensitivity to prosodic cues), or to some as yet unspecified mechanism.

Much of the research in prosodic processing has been conducted to answer questions about the laterality of brain function. Subjects with unilateral left or right brain damage have been asked to produce linguistic and emotional prosody in spontaneous speech, in imitation, and in reading tasks at the single word, phrase, and sentence level. In receptive tasks they have been asked to determine the emotional valence of expressive speech and to discriminate between various linguistic forms and emotional content in normal and in filtered-speech paradigms. Linguistic tasks include discriminating between nouns and noun phrases based on contrastive stress patterns (e.g., *green*house versus green *house*); using stress patterns to identify sentence meaning (*Joe* gave Ella flowers versus Joe gave *Ella* flowers); and identifying sentence types based on prosodic contour (e.g., the rising intonation pattern for interrogatives versus the flatter pattern for declaratives).

The emphasis on laterality of function has helped to establish that both hemispheres as well as some subcortical structures contribute to normal prosodic processing. The extensive literature supporting a particular role for the right hemisphere in processing content generated the central hypotheses guiding prosodic laterality research. The first hypothesis suggests that affective or emotional prosody is in the domain of the right hemisphere (Heilman, Scholes, and Watson, 1975; Borod, Koff, Lorch et al., 1985; Blonder, Bowers, and Heilman, 1991). Another hypothesis holds that prosodic cues themselves are lateralized, independent of their function (emotional or linguistic) (Van Lancker and Sidtis, 1992). Finally, lesion localization studies have found that certain subcortical structures, the basal ganglia in particular, play a role in prosodic processing (Cancelliere and Kertesz, 1990; Bradvik, Dravins, Holtas et al., 1991). Cancelliere and Kertesz (1990) speculated that the basal ganglia may be important not only because of their role in motor control, but also because of their limbic and frontal connections which may influence the expression of emotion in motor action.

Research findings have varied as a function of task type, subject selection criteria, and methods of data analysis. Subjects across and within studies may vary in terms of time post-onset, the presence or absence of neglect and dysarthria, intrahemispheric site of lesion, and severity of attentional and other cognitive deficits. With the exception of site of lesion, these variables have rarely been taken into account in research design. Data analysis has varied across studies. In some studies it has been based on perceptual judgments by one or more listeners, which adds a subjective component. In others, data are submitted to acoustic analysis, which affords increased objective control but in some cases may not match listener perception of severity of impairment (Ryalls, Joanette, and Feldman, 1987).

In general, acoustic analyses of prosodic productions by RHD patients supports the theory that prosody is lateralized according to individual prosodic cues rather than according to the function prosody serves (emotional versus linguistic). In particular, pitch cues are considered to be in the domain of the right hemisphere. Duration and timing cues are considered to be in the domain of the left hemisphere (Robin, Tranel, and Damasio, 1990; Van Lancker and Sidtis, 1992; Baum and Pell, 1997).

Research suggests that reduced pitch variation and a somewhat restricted pitch range appear to be significant factors in the impaired prosodic production of RHD subjects (Colsher, Cooper, and Graff-Radford, 1987; Behrens, 1989; Baum and Pell, 1997; Pell, 1999a). RHD patients are minimally if at all impaired in the production of emphatic stress. However, they may have an abnormally flat pitch pattern in declarative sentences, less than normal variation in pitch for interrogative sentences, and may produce emotionally toned sentences with less than normal acoustic variation (Behrens, 1988; Emmory, 1987; Pell, 1999). Pitch variation is crucial to signaling emotions, which may explain why impaired production of emotional prosody appears particularly prominent in aprosodia. Interestingly, in the case of tonal languages (e.g., Chinese, Thai, and Norwegian) in which pitch patterns in individual words serve a semantic role, pitch has been found to be a left hemisphere function (Packard, 1986; Ryalls and Reinvang, 1986; Gandour et al., 1992).

Prosodic perception or comprehension deficits associated with aprosodia tend to follow the pattern found in production. Non-temporal properties such as pitch appear to be more problematic than time-dependent properties such as duration and timing (Divenyi and Robinson, 1989; Robin et al., 1990; Van Lancker and Sidtis, 1992). For example, Van Lancker and Sidtis (1992) found that right- and left-hemisphere-damaged patients used different cues to identify emotional stimuli. Patients with RHD tended to base their decisions on durational cues rather than on fundamental frequency variability while left-hemisphere-damaged patients did the opposite. These data suggest a perceptual, rather than a functional (linguistic versus emotional), impairment. Although a study by Pell and Baum (1997) failed to replicate these results, the data are supported by data from dichotic listening and other studies that have investigated temporal versus time-independent cues such as pitch information (Chobor and Brown, 1987; Sidtis and Volpe, 1988; Divenyi and Robinson, 1989; Robin et al., 1990).

Almost all studies of prosodic deficits have focused on whether unilateral brain damage produces prosodic deficits, rather than describing the characteristics of prosodic problems in patients known to have prosodic deficits. The body of laterality research has established that pro-

sodic deficits can occur in both left as well as right hemisphere damage, and has furthered our understanding of the mechanisms and differences in prosodic processing across the hemispheres. However, the focus on laterality has had some drawbacks for understanding aprosodia per se. The main problem is that while subjects in laterality studies are selected for unilateral brain damage, they are not screened for prosodic impairment. Thus, the data pool on which we rely for conclusions about the nature of RHD prosodic deficits consists largely of subjects with *and subjects without* prosodic impairment. The characteristics of aprosodia, its mechanisms, duration, frequency of occurrence in the general RHD population, and the presence/absence of other RHD deficits that may accompany it have yet to be clearly delineated. These issues will remain unclear until a working definition of aprosodia is established and descriptive studies using that definition as a means of screening patients are undertaken.

See also PROSODIC DEFICITS, RIGHT HEMISPHERE LANGUAGE AND COMMUNICATION FUNCTIONS IN ADULTS; RIGHT HEMISPHERE LANGUAGE DISORDER.

—*Penelope S. Myers*

References

Baum, S. R., and Pell, M. D. (1997). Production of affective and linguistic prosody by brain-damaged patients. *Aphasiology, 11*, 177–198.

Behrens, S. J. (1988). The role of the right hemisphere in the production of linguistic stress. *Brain and Language, 33*, 104–127.

Behrens, S. J. (1989). Characterizing sentence intonation in a right hemisphere-damaged population. *Brain and Language, 37*, 181–200.

Blonder, L. X., Bowers, D., and Heilman, K. M. (1991). The role of the right hemisphere in emotional communication. *Brain, 114*, 1115–1127.

Borod, J. C., Koff, E., Lorch, M. P., and Nicholas, M. (1985). Channels of emotional expression in patients with unilateral brain damage. *Archives of Neurology, 42*, 345–348.

Bradvik, B., Dravins, C., Holtas, S., Rosen, I., Ryding, E., and Ingvar, D. H. (1991). Disturbances of speech prosody following right hemisphere infarcts. *Acta Neurologica Scandinavica, 84*, 114–126.

Cancelliere, A. E. B., and Kertesz, A. (1990). Lesion localization in acquired deficits of emotional expression and comprehension. *Brain and Cognition, 13*, 133–147.

Chobor, K. L., and Brown, J. W. (1987). Phoneme and timbre monitoring in left and right cerebrovascular accident patients. *Brain and Language, 30*, 78–284.

Colsher, P. L., Cooper, W. E., and Graff-Radford, N. (1987). Intonation variability in the speech of right-hemisphere damaged patients. *Brain and Language, 32*, 379–383.

Divenyi, P. L., and Robinson, A. J. (1989). Nonlinguistic auditory compatabilities in aphasia. *Brain and Language, 37*, 290–396.

Duffy, J. R. (1995). *Motor speech disorders.* St. Louis: Mosby.

Emmory, K. D. (1987). The neurological substrates for prosodic aspects of speech. *Brain and Language, 30*, 305–320.

Gandour, J., Ponglorpisit, S., Khunadorn, F., Dechongkit, S., Boongird, P., Boonklam, R., and Potisuk, S. (1992). Lexical tones in Thai after unilateral brain damage. *Brain and Language*, *43*, 275–307.

Gorelick, P. B., and Ross, E. D. (1987). The aprosodias: Further functional-anatomical evidence for the organization of affective language in the right hemisphere. *Journal of Neurology, Neurosurgery, and Psychiatry*, *50*, 553–560.

Heilman, K. M., Scholes, R., and Watson, R. T. (1975). Auditory affective agnosia: Disturbed comprehension of affective speech. *Journal of Neurology, Neurosurgery, and Psychiatry*, *38*, 69–72.

Mohrad-Krohn, G. H. (1947). Dysprosody or altered "melody of language." *Brain*, *70*, 405–415.

Monnot, M., Nixon, S., Lovallo, W., and Ross, E. (2001). Altered emotional perception in alcoholics: Deficits in affective prosody comprehension. *Alcoholism: Clinical and Experimental Research*, *25*, 362–369.

Myers, P. S. (1998). Prosodic deficits. In *Right hemisphere damage: Disorders of communication and cognition* (pp. 73–90). San Diego, CA: Singular.

Packard, J. (1986). Tone production deficits in nonfluent aphasic Chinese speech. *Brain and Language*, *29*, 212–223.

Pell, M. D. (1999a). Fundamental frequency encoding of linguistic and emotional prosody by right hemisphere damaged speakers. *Brain and Language*, *62*, 161–192.

Pell, M. D. (1999b). The temporal organization of affective and non-affective speech in patients with right-hemisphere infarcts. *Cortex*, *35*, 163–182.

Pell, M. D., and Baum, S. R. (1997). Unilateral brain damage, prosodic comprehension deficits, and the acoustic cues to prosody. *Brain and Language*, *57*, 195–214.

Robin, D. A., Tranel, D., and Damasio, H. (1990). Auditory perception of temporal and spectral events in patients with focal left and right cerebral lesions. *Brain and Language*, *39*, 539–555.

Ross, E. D. (1981). The aprosodias: Functional-anatomic organization of the affective components of language in the right hemisphere. *Archives of Neurology*, *38*, 561–569.

Ross, E. D., and Mesulam, M.-M. (1979). Dominant language functions of the right hemisphere? Prosody and emotional gesturing. *Archives of Neurology*, *36*, 144–148.

Ross, E. D., Orbelo, D. M., Cartwright, J., Hansel, S., Burgard, M., Testa, J. A., and Buck, R. (2001). Affective-prosodic deficits in schizophrenia: Profiles of patients with brain damage and comparison with relation schizophrenic symptoms. *Journal of Neurology, Neurosurgery, and Psychiatry*, *70*, 597–604.

Ryalls, J., Joanette, Y., and Feldman, L. (1987). An acoustic comparison of normal and right-hemisphere-damage speech prosody. *Cortex*, *23*, 685–694.

Ryalls, J., and Reinvang, I. (1986). Functional lateralization of linguistic tones: Acoustic evidence from Norwegian. *Language and Speech*, *29*, 389–398.

Sidtis, J. J., and Volpe, B. T. (1988). Selective loss of complex pitch or speech discrimination after unilateral lesion. *Brain and Language*, *34*, 235–245.

Starkstein, S. E., Federoff, J. P., Price, T. R., Leiguarda, R. C., and Robinsn, R. G. (1994). Neuropsychological and neuroradiologic correlates of emotional prosody comprehension. *Neurology*, *44*, 516–522.

Stringer, A. Y. (1996). Treatment of motor aprosodia with pitch biofeedback and expression modelling. *Brain Injury*, *10*, 583–590.

Sweet, L. H., Primeau, M., Fichtner, C. G., Lutz, G. (1998). Dissociation of affect recognition and mood state from blunting in patients with schizophrenia. *Psychiatry Research*, *81*, 301–308.

Van Lancker, D., and Sidtis, J. J. (1992). The identification of affective-prosodic stimuli by left- and right-hemisphere-damaged subjects: All errors are not created equal. *Journal of Speech and Hearing Research*, *35*, 963–970.

Further Reading

Baum, S. R., and Pell, M. D. (1999). The neural bases of prosody: Insights from lesion studies and neuroimaging. *Aphasiology*, *13*, 581–608.

Augmentative and Alternative Communication Approaches in Adults

An augmentative and alternative communication (AAC) system is an integrated group of components used by individuals with severe communication disorders to enhance their competent communication. Competent communication serves a variety of functions, of which we can isolate four: (1) communication of wants and needs, (2) information transfer, (3) social closeness, and (4) social etiquette (Light, 1988). These four functions broadly encompass all communicative interactions. An appropriate AAC system addresses not only basic communication of wants and needs, but also the establishment, maintenance, and development of interpersonal relationships using information transfer, social closeness, and social etiquette.

AAC is considered multimodal, and as such it incorporates the full communication abilities of the adult. It includes any existing natural speech or vocalizations, gestures, formal sign language, and aided communication. "AAC allows individuals to use every mode possible to communicate" (Light and Binger, 1998, p. 1).

AAC systems are typically described as high-technology, low- or light-technology, and no-technology in respect to the aids used in implementation. High-technology AAC systems use electronic devices to support digitized or synthesized communication strategies. Low- or light-technology systems include items such as communication boards (symbols), communication books, and light pointing devices. A no-technology system involves the use of strategies and techniques, such as body movements, gestures, and sign language, without the use of specific aids or devices.

AAC is used to assist adults with a wide range of disabilities, including congenital disabilities (e.g., cerebral palsy, mental retardation), acquired disabilities (e.g., traumatic head injury, stroke), and degenerative conditions (e.g., multiple sclerosis, amyotrophic lateral sclerosis) (American Speech-Language-Hearing Association [ASHA], 1989). Individuals at any point across the life span and in any stage of communication ability may use AAC (see the companion entry, AUGMENTATIVE AND ALTERNATIVE COMMUNICATION APPROACHES IN CHILDREN).

Adults with severe communication disorders benefit from AAC. ASHA (1991, p. 10) describes these people as "those for whom natural gestural, speech, and/or written communication is temporarily or permanently inadequate to meet all of their communication needs." An important consideration is that "although some individuals may be able to produce a limited amount of speech, it is inadequate to meet their varied communication needs" (ASHA, 1991, p. 10). AAC may also be used to support comprehension and cognitive abilities by capitalizing on residual skills and thus facilitating communication.

Many adults with severe communication disorders demonstrate some ability to communicate using natural speech. Natural speech is more time-efficient and linguistically flexible than other modes (involving AAC). Speech supplementation AAC techniques (alphabet and topic supplementation) used in conjunction with natural speech can provide extensive contextual knowledge to increase the listener's ability to understand a message. As the quality of the acoustic signal and the quality of environmental information improve, comprehensibility—intelligibility in context—of messages is enhanced (Lindblom, 1990). Similarly, poor-quality acoustic signals and poor environmental information result in a deterioration in message comprehensibility. When a speaker experiences reduced acoustic speech quality, optimizing any available contextual information through AAC techniques will increase the comprehensibility of the message. "Given that communication effectiveness varies across social situations and listeners, it is important that individuals who use natural speech, speech-supplementation, and AAC strategies learn to switch communication modes depending on the situation and the listener" (Hustad and Beukelman, 2000, p. 103).

The patterns of communication disorders in adults vary from condition to condition. Persons with aphasia, traumatic brain injury, Parkinson's disease, Guillain-Barré syndrome, multiple sclerosis, and numerous motor speech impairments benefit from using AAC (Beukelman and Mirenda, 1998). ACC approaches for a few adult severe communication disorders are described here.

Amyotrophic lateral sclerosis (ALS) is a disease of rapid degeneration involving the motor neurons of the brain and spinal cord that leaves cognitive abilities generally intact. The cause is unknown, and there is no known cure. For those whose initial impairments are in the brainstem, speech symptoms typically occur early in the disease progression. On average, speech intelligibility in this (bulbar) group declines precipitously approximately 10 months after diagnosis. For those whose impairment begins in the lower spine, speech intelligibility declines precipitously approximately 25 months after diagnosis. Some individuals maintain functional speech much longer. Clinically, a drop in speaking rate predicts the onset of the abrupt drop in speech intelligibility (Ball, Beukelman, and Pattee, 2001). As a group, 80% of individuals with ALS eventually require use of AAC. Because the drop in intelligibility is so sudden, intelligibility is not a good measure to use in determining the timing of an AAC evaluation. Rather, because the speaking rate declines more gradually, an AAC evalua-

tion should be completed when an individual reaches 50% of his or her habitual speaking rate (approximately 100 words per minute) on a standard intelligibility assessment (such as the Sentence Intelligibility Test; Yorkston, Beukelman, and Tice, 1996). Frequent objective measurement of speaking rate is important to provide timely AAC intervention. Access to a communication system is increasingly important as ALS advances (Mathy, Yorkston, and Gutmann, 2000).

Traumatic brain injury (TBI) refers to injuries to the brain that involve rapid acceleration and deceleration, whereby the brain is whipped back and forth in a quick motion, which results in compromised neurological function (Levin, Benton, and Grossman, 1982). The goal of AAC in TBI is to provide a series of communication systems and strategies so that individuals can communicate at the level at which they are currently functioning (Doyle et al., 2000). Generally, recovery of cognitive functioning is categorized into phases (Blackstone, 1989). In the early phase, the person is minimally responsive to external stimuli. AAC goals include providing support to respond to one-step motor commands and discriminate one of an array of choices (objects, people, locations). AAC applications during this phase include low-technology pictures and communication boards and choices of real objects to support communication. In the middle phase, the person exhibits improved consistency of responses to external stimuli. It is in this phase that persons who are unable to speak because of severe cognitive confusion become able to speak. If they do not become speakers by the end of this phase, it is likely a result of chronic motor control and language impairments. AAC goals during this phase address providing a way to indicate basic needs and giving a response modality that increases participation in the evaluation and treatment process. AAC intervention strategies usually involve nonelectronic, low-technology, or no-technology interventions to express needs. In the late phase, if the person continues to be nonspeaking, it is likely the result of specific motor or language impairment. AAC intervention may be complicated by co-existing cognitive deficits. Intervention goals address provision of functional ways to interact with listeners in a variety of settings and to assist the individual to participate in social, vocational, educational, and recreational settings. AAC intervention makes use of both low- and high-technology strategies in this phase of recovery.

Brainstem stroke (cerebrovascular accident, or CVA) disrupts the circulation serving the lower brainstem. The result is often severe dysarthria or anarthria, and reduced ability to control the muscles of the face, mouth, and larynx voluntarily or reflexively. Communication symptoms vary considerably with the extent of damage. Some individuals are dysarthric but able to communicate partial or complete messages, while others may be unable to speak. AAC intervention is typically described in five stages (Beukelman and Mirenda, 1998). In stage 1, the person exhibits no functional speech. The goal of intervention is to provide early communication so that the person can respond to yes/no questions, initial choice making, pointing, and introduction of a multipurpose AAC device. In stage 2, the goal is to reestablish speech by working directly to develop control over the respiratory, phonatory, velopharyngeal, and articulatory subsystems. Early in this stage, the AAC system will support the majority of interactions; however, late in this stage persons are able to convey an increasing percentage of messages with natural speech. In stage 3, the person exhibits independent use of natural speech. The AAC intervention focuses on intelligibility, with alphabet supplementation used early, but later only to resolve communication breakdowns. In this stage, the use of AAC may become necessary only to support writing. In stages 4 and 5, the person no longer needs to use an AAC system.

In summary, adults with severe communication disorders are able to take advantage of increased communication through the use of AAC. The staging of AAC interventions is influenced by the individual's communication abilities and the natural course of the disorder, whether advancing, remitting, or stable.

—*Laura J. Ball*

References

American Speech-Language-Hearing Association. (1989). Competencies for speech-language pathologists providing services in augmentative communication. *ASHA, 31,* 107–110.

American Speech-Language-Hearing Association. (1991). Report: Augmentative and alternative communication. *ASHA, 33*(Suppl. 5), 9–12.

Ball, L., Beukelman, D., and Pattee, G. (2001). A protocol for identification of early bulbar signs in ALS. *Journal of Neurological Sciences, 191,* 43–53.

Beukelman, D., and Mirenda, P. (1998). *Augmentative and alternative communication: Management of severe communication disorders in children and adults.* Baltimore: Paul H. Brookes.

Blackstone, S. (1989). For consumer: Societal rehabilitation. *Augmentative Communication News, 2*(3), 1–3.

Doyle, M., Kennedy, M., Jausalaitis, G., and Phillips, B. (2000). AAC and traumatic brain injury: Influence of cognition on system design and use. In K. Yorkston, D. Beukelman, and J. Reichle (Eds.), *Augmentative and alternative communication for adults with acquired neurologic disorders* (pp. 271–304). Baltimore: Paul H. Brookes.

Hustad, K., and Beukelman, D. (2000). Integrating AAC strategies with natural speech in adults. In K. Yorkston, D. Beukelman, and J. Reichle (Eds.), *Augmentative and alternative communication for adults with acquired neurologic disorders* (pp. 83–106). Baltimore: Paul H. Brookes.

Levin, H., Benton, A., and Grossman, R. (1982). *Neurobehavioral consequences of closed head injury.* New York: Oxford University Press.

Light, J. (1988). Interaction involving individuals using augmentative and alternative communication systems: State of the art and future directions. *Augmentative and Alternative Communication, 5*(3), 66–82.

Light, J., and Binger, C. (1998). *Building communicative competence with individuals who use augmentative and alternative communication.* Baltimore: Paul H. Brookes.

Lindblom, B. (1990). On the communication process: Speaker-listener interaction and the development of speech. *Augmentative and Alternative Communication, 6,* 220–230.

Mathy, P., Yorkston, K., and Gutmann, M. (2000). AAC for individuals with amyotrophic lateral sclerosis. In K. Yorkston, D. Beukelman, and J. Reichle (Eds.), *Augmentative and alternative communication for adults with acquired neurologic disorders* (pp. 183–229). Baltimore: Paul H. Brookes.

Yorkston, K., Beukelman, D., and Tice, R. (1996). *Sentence Intelligibility Test.* Lincoln, NE: Tice Technologies.

Further Readings

Beukelman, D., Yorkston, K., and Reichle, J. (2000). *Augmentative and alternative communication for adults with acquired neurologic disorders.* Baltimore: Paul H. Brookes.

Collier, B. (1997). *See what we say: Vocabulary and tips for adults who use augmentative and alternative communication.* North York, Ontario, Canada: William Bobek Productions.

DeRuyter, F., and Kennedy, M. (1991). Augmentative communication following traumatic brain injury. In D. Beukelman and K. Yorkston (Eds.), *Communication disorders following traumatic brain injury: Management of cognitive, language, and motor impairments* (pp. 317–365). Austin, TX: Pro-Ed.

Fried-Oken, M., and Bersani, H. (2000). *Speaking up and spelling it out: Personal essays on augmentative and alternative communication.* Baltimore: Paul H. Brookes.

Garrett, K., and Kimelman, M. (2000). AAC and aphasia: Cognitive-linguistic considerations. In D. Beukelman, K. Yorkston, and J. Reichle (Eds.), *Augmentative and alternative communication for adults with acquired neurologic disorders* (pp. 339–374). Baltimore: Paul H. Brookes.

Klasner, E., and Yorkston, K. (2000). AAC for Huntington disease and Parkinson's disease: Planning for change. In K. Yorkston, D. Beukelman, and J. Reichle (Eds.), *Augmentative and alternative communication for adults with acquired neurologic disorders* (pp. 233–270). Baltimore: Paul H. Brookes.

Ladtkow, M., and Culp, D. (1992). Augmentative communication with the traumatically brain injured population. In K. Yorkston (Ed.), *Augmentative communication in the medical setting* (pp. 139–243). Tucson, AZ: Communication Skill Builders.

Yorkston, K. (1992). *Augmentative communication in the medical setting.* San Antonio, TX: Psychological Corporation.

Yorkston, K., Miller, R., and Strand, E. (1995). *Management of speech and swallowing in degenerative diseases.* Tucson, AZ: Communication Skill Builders.

Augmentative and Alternative Communication Approaches in Children

The acquisition of communication skills is a dynamic, bidirectional process of interactions between speaker and listener. Children who are unable to meet their daily needs using their own speech require alternative systems to support their communication interaction efforts (Reichle, Beukelman, and Light, 2001). An augmentative and alternative communication (AAC) system is an integrated group of components used by a child to enhance or develop competent communication. It includes any existing natural speech or vocalizations, gestures, formal sign language, and aided communication. "AAC allows individuals to use every mode possible to communicate" (Light and Drager, 1998, p. 1).

The goal of AAC support is to provide children with access to the power of communication, language, and literacy. This power allows them to express their needs and wants, develop social closeness, exchange information, and participate in social, educational, and community activities (Beukelman and Mirenda, 1998). In addition, it provides a foundation for language development and facilitates literacy development (Light and Drager, 2001). Timeliness in implementing an AAC system is paramount (Reichle, Beukelman, and Light, 2001). The earlier that graphic and gestural mode supports can be put into place, the greater will be the child's ability to advance in communication development.

Children experience significant cognitive, linguistic, and physical growth throughout their formative years, from preschool through high school. AAC support for children must address both their current communication needs as well as predict future communication needs and abilities, so that they will be prepared to communicate effectively as they mature. Because participation in the general classroom requires many kinds of extensive communication, effective AAC systems that are age appropriate and context appropriate serve as critical tools for academic success (Sturm, 1998, p. 391). Early interventions allow children to develop the linguistic, operational, and social competencies necessary to support their participation in academic settings.

Many young children and those with severe multiple disabilities cannot use traditional spelling and reading skills to access their AAC systems. Very young children, who are preliterate, have not yet developed reading and writing skills, while older children with severe cognitive impairments may remain nonliterate. For individuals who are not literate, messages within their AAC systems must be represented by one or more symbols or codes. With children, early communication development focuses on vocabulary that is needed to communicate essential messages and to develop language skills. Careful analysis of environmental and communication needs is used to develop vocabulary for the child's AAC system. This vocabulary selection assessment includes examination of the ongoing process of vocabulary and message maintenance.

The vocabulary needs of children comprise contextual variations, including *school talk*, in which they speak with relatively unfamiliar adults in order to acquire knowledge. *Home talk* is used with familiar persons to meet needs and develop social closeness, as well as to assist parents in understanding their child. An example of vocabulary needs is exhibited by preschool children, who have been found to use generic small talk for nearly half of their utterances, when in preschool and at home (Ball et al., 1999). Generic small talk refers to messages

that can be used without change in interaction with a variety of different listeners. Examples include "Hello"; "What are you doing?"; "What's that?"; "I like that!"; and "Leave me alone!"

Extensive instructional resources are available to school-age children. In the United States, the federal government has mandated publicly funded education for children with disabilities, in the form of the Individuals with Disabilities Education Act, and provides a legal basis for AAC interventions. Public policy changes have been adopted in numerous other countries to address resources available to children with disabilities.

AAC interventionists facilitate transitions from the preschool setting to the school setting by ensuring comprehensive communication through systematic planning and establishing a foundation for communication. A framework for integrating children into general education programs may be implemented by following the participation model (Beukelman and Mirenda, 1998), which includes four variables that can be manipulated to achieve appropriate participation for any child. Children transitioning from preschool to elementary school, self-contained to departmentalized programs, or school to post-school (vocational) will attain optimal participation when consideration is made for integration, social participation, academic participation, and independence. An AAC system must be designed to support literacy and other academic skill development as well as peer interactions. It must be appealing to children so that they find the system attractive and will continue using it (Light and Drager, 2001).

AAC systems are used by children with a variety of severe communication disorders. *Cerebral palsy* is a developmental neuromuscular disorder resulting from a nonprogressive abnormality of the brain. Children with severe cerebral palsy primarily experience motor control problems that impair their control of their speech mechanisms. The resulting motor speech disorder (dysarthria) may be so severe that AAC technology is required to support communication. Large numbers of persons with cerebral palsy successfully use AAC technology (Beukelman, Yorkston, and Smith, 1985; Mirenda and Mathy-Laikko, 1989). Typically, AAC support is provided to these children by a team of interventionists. In addition to the communication/AAC specialist, the primary team often includes occupational and physical therapists, technologists, teachers, and parents. A secondary support team might include orthotists, rehabilitation engineers, and pediatric ophthalmologists.

Intellectual disability, or mental retardation, is characterized by significantly subaverage intellectual functioning coexisting with limitations in adaptive skills (communication, self-care, home living, social skills, community use, self-direction, health and safety, academics, leisure, and work) that appear before the age of 18 (Luckasson et al., 1992). For children with communication impairments, it is important to engage in AAC instruction and interactions in natural rather than segregated environments. Calculator and Bedrosian noted that "communication is neither any more nor less than a tool that facilitates individuals' abilities to function in the various activities of daily living" (1988, p. 104). Children who are unable to speak because of cognitive limitations, with and without accompanying physical impairments, have demonstrated considerable success using AAC strategies involving high-technology (electronic devices) and low-technology (communication boards and books) options (Light, Collier, and Parnes, 1985a, 1985b, 1985c).

Autism and pervasive developmental disorders are described with three main diagnostic features: (1) impaired social interaction, (2) impaired communication, and (3) restricted, repetitive, and stereotypical patterns of behaviors, interests, and activities (American Psychiatric Association, 1994). These disorders occur as a spectrum of impairments of different causes (Wing, 1996). Children with a pervasive developmental disorder may have cognitive, social/communicative, language, and processing impairments. Early intervention with an emphasis on speech, language, and communication is extremely important (Dawson and Osterling, 1997). A range of intervention approaches has been suggested, and as a result, AAC interventionists may need to work with professionals whose views differ from their own, thus necessitating considerable collaboration (Simeonsson, Olley, and Rosenthal, 1987; Dawson and Osterling, 1997; Freeman, 1997).

Developmental apraxia of speech (DAS) results in language delays, communication problems that influence academic performance, communication problems that limit effective social interaction, and significant speech production disorder. Children with suspected DAS have difficulty performing purposeful voluntary movements for speech (Caruso and Strand, 1999). Their phonological systems are impaired because of their difficulties in managing the intense motor demands of connected speech (Strand and McCauley, 1999). Children with DAS have a guarded prognosis for the acquisition of intelligible speech (Bernthal and Bankson, 1993). DAS-related speech disorders may result in prolonged periods of unintelligibility, particularly during the early elementary grades.

There is ongoing debate over the best way to manage suspected DAS. Some children with DAS have been treated with phonologically based interventions and others with motor learning tasks. Some interventionists support very intense schedules of interventions. These arguments have changed little in the last 20 years. However, the need to provide these children with some means to communicate so that they can successfully participate socially and in educational activities is becoming increasingly accepted. Cumley (1997) studied children with DAS who were provided with AAC technology. He reported that the group of children with lower speech intelligibility scores used their AAC technology more frequently than children with higher intelligibility. When children with DAS with low intelligibility scores used AAC technology, they did not reduce their speech efforts, but rather used the technology to resolve communication breakdowns. The negative effect of reduced speech intelligibility on social and educational participation has been documented extensively (Kent, 1993; Camarata, 1996). The use of AAC strategies to support the communicative interactions of children with such severe DAS that their speech is unintelligible is receiving increased attention (Culp, 1989; Cumley and Swanson, 2000).

In summary, children with severe communication disorders benefit from using AAC systems, from a variety of perspectives. Children with an assortment of clinical disorders are able to take advantage of increased communication through the use of AAC. The provision of AAC intervention is influenced by the child's communication abilities and access to memberships. Membership involves integration, social participation, academic participation, and ultimately independence. A web site (http://aac.unl.edu) provides current information about AAC resources for children and adults.

—Laura J. Ball

References

American Psychiatric Association. (1994). *Diagnostic and statistical manual for mental disorders* (4th ed.). Washington, DC: Author.

Ball, L., Marvin, C., Beukelman, D., Lasker, J., and Rupp, D. (1999). Generic small talk use by preschool children. *Augmentative and Alternative Communication, 15,* 145–155.

Bernthal, J., and Bankson, N. (1993). *Articulation and phonological disorders* (3rd ed.). Englewood Cliffs, NJ: Prentice Hall.

Beukelman, D., and Mirenda, P. (1998). *Augmentative and alternative communication: Management of severe communication disorders in children and adults* (2nd ed.). Baltimore: Paul H. Brookes.

Beukelman, D., Yorkston, K., and Smith, K. (1985). Third-party payer response to requests for purchase of communication augmentation systems: A study of Washington state. *Augmentative and Alternative Communication, 1,* 5–9.

Calculator, S., and Bedrosian, J. (1988). *Communication assessment and intervention for adults with mental retardation.* San Diego, CA: College-Hill Press.

Camarata, S. (1996). On the importance of integrating naturalistic language, social intervention, and speech-intelligibility training. In L. Koegel and R. Koegel (Eds.), *Positive behavioral support: Including people with difficult behavior in the community* (pp. 333–351). Baltimore: Paul H. Brookes.

Caruso, A., and Strand, E. (1999). Motor speech disorders in children: Definitions, background, and a theoretical framework. In A. Caruso and E. Strand (Eds.), *Clinical management of motor speech disorders in children* (pp. 1–28). New York: Thieme.

Culp, D. (1989). Developmental apraxia of speech and augmentative communication: A case example. *Augmentative and Alternative Communication, 5,* 27–34.

Cumley, G. (1997). *Introduction of augmentative and alternative modality: Effects on the quality and quantity of communication interactions of children with severe phonological disorders.* Unpublished doctoral dissertation, University of Nebraska, Lincoln.

Cumley, G., and Swanson, S. (2000). Augmentative and alternative communication options for children with developmental apraxia of speech: Three case studies. *Augmentative and Alternative Communication, 15,* 110–125.

Dawson, G., and Osterling, J. (1997). Early intervention in autism. *Journal of Applied Behavioral Analysis, 24,* 369–378.

Freeman, B. (1997). Guidelines for evaluating intervention programs for children with autism. *Journal of Autism and Developmental Disorders, 27*(6), 641–651.

Kent, R. (1993). Speech intelligibility and communicative competence in children. In A. Kaiser and D. Gray (Eds.), *Enhancing children's communication: Research foundations for intervention.* Baltimore: Paul H. Brookes.

Light, J., Collier, B., and Parnes, P. (1985a). Communication interaction between young nonspeaking physically disabled children and their primary caregivers: Part I. Discourse patterns. *Augmentative and Alternative Communication, 1*(2), 74–83.

Light, J., Collier, B., and Parnes, P. (1985b). Communication interaction between young nonspeaking physically disabled children and their primary caregivers: Part II. Communicative function. *Augmentative and Alternative Communication, 1*(3), 98–107.

Light, J., Collier, B., and Parnes, P. (1985c). Communication interaction between young nonspeaking physically disabled children and their primary caregivers: Part III. Modes of communication. *Augmentative and Alternative Communication, 1*(4), 125–133.

Light, J., and Drager, K. (1998). *Building communicative competence with individuals who use augmentative and alternative communication.* Baltimore: Paul H. Brookes.

Light, J., and Drager, K. (2001, Aug. 2). *Improving the design of AAC technologies for young children.* Paper presented at a meeting of the United States Society of Augmentative and Alternative Communication, St. Paul, MN.

Luckasson, R., Coulter, D., Polloway, E., Reiss, S., Schalock, R., Snell, M., et al. (1992). *Mental retardation: Definition, classification, and systems of support* (9th ed.). Washington, DC: American Association on Mental Retardation.

Mirenda, P., and Mathy-Laikko, P. (1989). Augmentative and alternative communication applications for persons with severe congenital communication disorders: An introduction. *Augmentative and Alternative Communication, 5*(1), 3–14.

Reichle, J., Beukelman, D., and Light, J. (2001). *Exemplary practices for beginning communicators: Implications for AAC* (vol. 2). Baltimore: Paul H. Brookes.

Simeonsson, R., Olley, J., and Rosenthal, S. (1987). Early intervention for children with autism. In M. Guralnick and F. Bennett (Eds.), *The effectiveness of early intervention for at-risk and handicapped children* (pp. 275–293). New York: Academic Press.

Strand, E., and McCauley, R. (1999). Assessment procedures for treatment planning in children with phonologic and motor speech disorders. In A. Caruso and E. Strand (Eds.), *Clinical management of motor speech disorders in children* (pp. 73–108). New York: Thieme.

Sturm, J. (1998). Educational inclusion of AAC users. In D. Beukelman and P. Mirenda (Eds.), *Augmentative and alternative communication: Management of severe communication disorders in children and adults* (2nd ed., pp. 391–424). Baltimore: Paul H. Brookes.

Wing, L. (1996). *The autistic spectrum: A guide for parents and professionals.* London: Constable.

Further Readings

Bedrosian, J. (1997). Language acquisition in young AAC system users: Issues and directions for future research. *Augmentative and Alternative Communication, 13,* 179–185.

Bristow, D., and Fristoe, M. (1988). Effects of test adaptations on test performance. *Augmentative and Alternative Communication, 4,* 171.

Culp, D. E. (1996). *ChalkTalk: Augmentative communication in the classroom.* Anchorage: Assistive Technology Library of Alaska.

Cumley, G., and Swanson, S. (1999). Augmentative and alternative communication options for children with developmental apraxia of speech: Three Case Studies. *Augmentative and Alternative Communication, 15*(2), 110–125.

Dowden, P. (1997). Augmentative and alternative communication decision making for children with severely unintelligible speech. *Augmentative and Alternative Communication, 13,* 48–58.

Elder, P. G. (1996). *Engineering training environments for interactive augmentative communication: Strategies for adolescents and adults who are moderately/severely developmentally delayed.* Solana Beach, CA: Mayer-Johnson.

Goossens, C., Crain, S., and Elder, P. (1992). *Engineering the preschool environment for interactive, symbolic communication.* Birmingham, AL: Southeast Augmentative Communication Conference Publications.

King-Debaun, P. (1993). *Storytime just for fun: Stories, symbols, and emergent literacy activities for young, special needs children.* Park City, UT: Creative Communicating.

Light, J. B. (1998). *Building communicative competence with individuals who use augmentative and alternative communication.* Baltimore: Paul H. Brookes.

Mirenda, P., Iacono, T., and Williams, R. (1990). Communication options for persons with severe and profound disabilities: State of the art and future directions. *Journal of the Association for Persons with Severe Handicaps, 15,* 3–21.

Reichle, J. (1993). *Communication alternatives to challenging behavior: Integrating functional assessment and intervention strategies* (vol. 3). Baltimore: Paul H. Brookes.

Reichle, J., Beukelman, D., and Light, J. (2002). *Exemplary practices for beginning communicators: Implications for AAC* (vol. 2). Baltimore: Paul H. Brookes.

Autism

The term *autism* was first used in 1943 by Leo Kanner to describe a syndrome of "disturbances in affective contact," which he observed in 11 boys who lacked the dysmorphology often seen in mental retardation, but who were missing the social motivation toward communication and interaction that is typically present even in children with severe intellectual deficits. Despite their obvious impairments in social communication, the children Kanner observed did surprisingly well on some parts of IQ tests, leading Kanner to believe they did not have mental retardation.

Kanner's observation about intelligence has been modified by subsequent research. When developmentally appropriate, individually administered IQ testing is administered, approximately 80% of people with autism score in the mentally retarded range, and scores remain stable over time (Rutter et al., 1994). However, individuals with autism do show unusual scatter in their abilities, with nonverbal, visually based performance often significantly exceeding verbal skills; unlike the performance seen in children with other kinds of retardation, whose scores are comparable across all kinds of tasks.

Recent research on the genetics of autism suggests that there are heritable factors that may convey susceptibility (Rutter et al., 1997). This vulnerability may be expressed in a range of social, communicative, and cognitive difficulties expressed in varying degrees in parents, siblings, and other relatives of individuals with autism.

Although genetic factors appear to contribute to some degree to the appearance of autism, the condition can also be associated with other medical conditions. Dykens and Volkmar (1997) reported the following:

- Approximately 25% of individuals with autism develop seizures.
- Tuberous sclerosis (a disease characterized by abnormal tissue growth) is associated with autism with higher than expected prevalence.
- The co-occurrence of autism and fragile X syndrome (the most common heritable form of mental retardation) is also higher than would be expected by chance.

Autism is considered one of a class of disabilities referred to as pervasive developmental disorders, according to the *Diagnostic and Statistical Manual of the American Psychiatric Association* (4th ed., 1994). The diagnostic criteria for autism are more explicitly stated in *DSM-IV* than the criteria for other pervasive developmental disorders. The criteria for autism are the result of a large field study conducted by Volkmar et al. (1994). The field trial showed that the criteria specified in *DSM-IV* exhibit reliability and temporal stability. Similar research on diagnostic criteria for other pervasive developmental disorders is not yet available.

The primary diagnostic criteria for autism include the following:

Early onset. Many parents first become concerned at the end of the first year of life, when a child does not start talking. At this period of development, children with autism also show reduced interest in other people; less use of communicative gestures such as pointing, showing, and waving; and noncommunicative sound making, perhaps including echoing that is far in advance of what can be produced in spontaneous or meaningful contexts. There may also be unusual preoccupations with objects (e.g., an intense interest in vacuum cleaners) or actions (such as twanging rubber bands) that are not like the preoccupations of other children at this age.

Impairment in social interaction. This is the hallmark of the autistic syndrome. Children with autism do not use facial expressions, eye contact, body posture, or gestures to engage in social interaction as other children do. They are less interested in sharing attention to objects and to other people, and they rarely attempt to direct others' attention to objects or events they want to point out. They show only fleeting interest in peers, and often appear content to be left on their own to pursue their solitary preferred activities.

Impairment in communication. Language and communicative difficulties are also core symptoms in autism. Communicative differences in autism include the following:

- Mutism. Approximately half of people with autism never develop speech. Nonverbal communication, too, is greatly restricted (Paul, 1987). The range of communicative intentions expressed is limited to requesting and protesting. Showing off, labeling, acknowledging, and establishing joint attention, seen in normal preverbal children, are absent in this population. Wants and needs are expressed preverbally, but forms for expression are aberrant. Some examples are pulling a person toward a desired object without making eye contact, instead of pointing, and the use of maladaptive and self-injurious behaviors to express desires (Donnellan et al., 1984). Pointing, showing, and turn-taking are significantly reduced.
- For people with autism who do develop speech, both verbal and nonverbal forms of communication are impaired. Forty percent of people with autism exhibit echolalia, an imitation of speech they have heard—either immediate echolalia, a direct parroting of speech directed to them, or delayed echolalia, in which they repeat snatches of language they have heard earlier, from other people or on TV, radio, and so on. Both kinds of echolalia are used to serve communicative functions, such as responding to questions they do not understand (Prizant and Duchan, 1981). Echolalia decreases, as in normal development, with increases in language comprehension.

A significant delay in comprehension is one of the strongest distinctions between people with autism and those with other developmental disabilities (Rutter, Maywood, and Howlin, 1992). Formal aspects of language production are on par with developmental level. Children with autism are similar to mental age–matched children in the acquisition of rule-governed syntax, but language development lags behind nonverbal mental age (Lord and Paul, 1997). Articulation is on par with mental age in children with autism who speak; however, high-functioning adults with autism show higher than expected rates of speech distortions (Shriberg et al., 2001).

Word use is a major area of deficit in those who speak (Tager-Flusberg, 1995). Words are assigned to the same categories that others use (Minshew and Goldsein, 1993), and scores on vocabulary tests are often a strength. However, words may be used with idiosyncratic meanings, and difficulty is seen with deictic terms (i.e., *you/I, here/there*), whose meaning changes, depending on the point of view of the speaker. This was first thought to reflect a lack of self, as evidenced by difficulty with saying *I*. More recent research suggests that the flexibility required to shift referents and difficulty assessing others' state of knowledge are more likely to account for this observation (Lee, Hobson, and Chiat, 1994).

Pragmatic, interpersonal uses of language present the greatest challenges to speakers with autism. The rate of initiation of communication is low (Stone and Caro-Martinez, 1990), and speech is often idiosyncratic and contextually inappropriate (Lord and Paul, 1997). Few references are made to mental states, and people with autism have difficulty inferring the mental states of others (Tager-Flusberg, 1995). Deficits are seen in providing relevant responses or adding new information to established topics; primitive strategies such as imitation are used to continue conversations (Tager-Flusberg and Anderson, 1991).

For individuals at the highest levels of functioning, conversation is often restricted to obsessive interests. There is little awareness of listeners' lack of interest in extended talk about these topics. Difficulty is seen in adapting conversation to take into account *all* participants' purposes. Very talkative people with autism are impaired in their ability to use language in functional, communicative ways (Lord and Paul, 1997), unlike other kinds of children with language impairments, whose language use improves with increased amount of speech.

Paralinguistic features such as voice quality, intonation, and stress are frequently impaired in speakers with autism. Monotonic intonation is one of the most frequently recognized aspects of speech in autism. It is a major contributor to listeners' perception of oddness (Mesibov, 1992). The use of pragmatic stress in spontaneous speech and speech fluency are also impaired (Shriberg et al., 2001).

Stereotypic patterns of behavior. Abnormal preoccupations with objects or parts of objects are characteristic of autism, as is a need for routines and rituals always to be carried out in precisely the same way. Children with autism become exceedingly agitated over small changes in routine. Stereotyped motor behaviors, such as hand flapping, are also typical but are related to developmental level and are likely to emerge in the preschool period.

Delays in imaginative play. Children with autism are more impaired in symbolic play behaviors than in other aspects of cognition, although strengths are seen in constructive play, such as stacking and nesting (Schuler, Prizant, and Wetherby, 1997).

There is no medical or biological profile that can be used to diagnose autism, nor is there one diagnostic test that definitely identifies this syndrome. Current assessment methods make use primarily of multidimensional scales, either interview or observational, that provide separate documentation of aberrant behaviors in each of the three areas that are known to be characteristic of the syndrome: social reciprocity, communication, and restricted, repetitive behaviors. The most widely used for research purposes are the Autism Diagnostic Interview (Lord, Rutter, and Le Conteur, 1994) and the Autism Diagnostic Observation Scale (Lord et al., 2000).

Until recently, autism was thought to be a rare disorder, with prevalence estimates of 4–5 per 10,000 (Lotter, 1966). However, these prevalence figures were based on identifying the disorder in children who, like the classic patients described by Kanner, had IQs within normal range. As it became recognized that the social and communicative deficits characteristic of autism could be found in children along the full range of the IQ spectrum, prevalence estimates rose to 1 per 1000 (Bryson, 1997).

Currently, there is a great deal of debate about incidence and prevalence, particularly about whether incidence is rising significantly. Although clinicians see more children today who receive a label of autism than they did 10 years ago, this is likely to be due to a broadening of the definition of the disorder to include children who show some subset of symptoms without the full-blown syndrome. Using this broad definition, current prevalence estimates range from 1 in 500 to as low as 1 in 300 (Fombonne, 1999). Although there is some debate about the precise ratio, autism is more prevalent in males than in females (Bryson, 1997).

In the vast majority of cases, children with autism grow up to be adults with autism. Only 1%–2% of cases have a fully normal outcome (Paul, 1987). The classic image of the autistic child—mute or echolalic, with stereotypic behaviors and a great need to preserve sameness—is most characteristic of the preschool period. As children with autism grow older, they generally progress toward more, though still aberrant, social involvement. In adolescence, 10%–35% of children with autism show some degree of regression (Gillberg and Schaumann, 1981). Still, with continued intervention, growth in both language and cognitive skills can be seen (Howlin and Goode, 1998).

Approximately 75% of adults with autism require high degrees of support in living, with only about 20% gainfully employed (Howlin and Goode, 1998). Outcome in adulthood is related to IQ, with good outcomes almost always associated with IQs above 60 (Rutter, Greenfield, and Lockyer, 1967). The development of functional speech by age 5 is also a strong predictor of good outcome (DeMyer et al., 1973).

Major changes have taken place in the treatments used to address autistic behaviors. Although a variety of pharmacological agents have been tried, and some are effective at treating certain symptoms (see McDougle, 1997, for a review), the primary forms of treatment for autism are behavioral and educational. Early intervention, when provided with a high degree of intensity (at least 20 hours per week), has proved particularly effective (Rogers, 1996). There is ongoing debate about the best methods of treatment, particularly for lower functioning children. There are proponents of operant applied behavior treatments (Lovaas, 1987), of naturalistic child-centered approaches (Greenspan and Wieder, 1997), and of approaches that are some hybrid of the two (Prizant and Wetherby, 1998). Recent innovations focus on the use of alternative communication systems (e.g., Bondi and Frost, 1998) and on the use of environmental compensatory supports, such as visual calendars, to facilitate communication and learning (Quill, 1998). Although all of these approaches have been shown to be associated with growth in young children with autism, no definitive study has yet compared approaches or measured long-term change.

For higher functioning and older individuals with autism, most interventions are derived from more general strategies used in children with language impairments. These strategies focus on the development of conversational skills, the use of scripts to support communication, strategies for communicative repair, and the use of reading to support social interaction (Prizant et al., 1997). "Social stories," in which anecdotal narratives are encouraged to support social understanding and participation, is a new method that is often used with higher functioning individuals (Gray, 1995).

—Rhea Paul

References

American Psychiatric Association. (1994). *Diagnostic and statistical manual of the American Psychiatric Association* (4th ed.). Washington, DC: Author.

Bondi, A., and Frost, L. (1998). The picture exchange communication system. *Seminars in Speech and Language, 19,* 373–389.

Bryson, S. (1997). Epidemiology of autism: Overview and issues outstanding. In D. Cohen and F. Volkmar (Eds.), *Handbook of autism and pervasive developmental disorders* (pp. 41–46). New York: Wiley.

DeMyer, M., Barton, S., DeMyer, W., Norton, J., Allen, J., and Steele, R. (1973). Prognosis in autism: A follow-up study. *Journal of Autism and Childhood Schizophrenia, 3,* 199–246.

Donnellan, A., Mirenda, P., Mesaros, P., and Fassbender, L. (1984). Analyzing the communicative function of aberrant behavior. *Journal of the Association for Persons with Severe Handicaps, 9,* 202–212.

Dykens, E., and Volkmar, F. (1997). Medical conditions associated with autism. In D. Cohen and F. Volkmar (Eds.), *Handbook of autism and pervasive developmental disorders* (pp. 388–410). New York: Wiley.

Fombonne, E. (1999). The epidemiology of autism: A review. *Psychological Medicine, 29,* 769–786.

Gillberg, C., and Schaumann, H. (1981). Infantile autism and puberty. *Journal of Autism and Developmental Disorders, 11,* 365–371.

Gray, C. (1995). *The original social story book.* Arlington, TX: Future Horizons.

Greenspan, S., and Wieder, S. (1997). An integrated developmental approach to interventions for young children with severe difficulties relating and communicating. *Zero to Three, 18,* 5–17.

Howlin, P., and Goode, S. (1998). Outcome in adult life for people with autism and Asperger syndrome. In F. Volkmar (Ed.), *Autism and pervasive developmental disorders* (pp. 209–241). Cambridge, UK: Cambridge University Press.

Kanner, L. (1943). Autistic disturbances of affective contact. *Nervous Child, 2,* 416–426.

Lee, A., Hobson, R., and Chiat, S. (1994). I, you, me, and autism: An experimental study. *Journal of Autism and Developmental Disorders, 24,* 155–176.

Lord, C., and Paul, R. (1997). Language and communication in autism. In D. Cohen and F. Volkmar (Eds.), *Handbook of autism and pervasive developmental disorders* (pp. 195–225). New York: Wiley.

Lord, C., Risi, S., Lambrecht, L., Cook, E. H., Jr., Leventhal, B. L., DiLavore, P. C., Pickles, A., and Rutter, M. (2000). The Autism Diagnostic Observation Schedule—Generic: A standard measure of social and communication deficits associated with the spectrum of autism. *Journal of Autism and Developmental Disorders, 30*(3), 205–223.

Lord, C., Rutter, M., and Le Conteur, A. (1994). Autism Diagnostic Interview—Revised: A revised version of a diagnostic interview for caregivers of individuals with possible pervasive developmental disorders. *Journal of Autism and Developmental Disorders, 24,* 659–685.

Lotter, V. (1966). Epidemiology of autistic conditions in young children. *Social Psychiatry, 1,* 124–137.

Lovaas, O. (1987). Behavioral treatment and normal educational and intellectual functioning in young autistic children. *Journal of Consulting and Clinical Psychology, 55,* 3–9.

McDougle, C. (1997). Psychopharmocology. In D. Cohen and F. Volkmar (Eds.), *Handbook of autism and pervasive developmental disorders* (pp. 707–729). New York: Wiley.

Mesibov, G. (1992). Treatment issues with high functioning adolescents and adults with autism. In E. Schopler and G. Mesibov (Eds.), *High functioning individuals with autism* (pp. 143–156). New York: Plenum Press.

Minshew, N., and Goldsein, G. (1993). Is autism an amnesic disorder? Evidence from the California Verbal Learning Test. *Neuropsychology, 7,* 261–170.

Paul, R. (1987). Communication. In D. J. Cohen and A. M. Donnellan (Eds.), *Handbook of autism and pervasive developmental disorders* (pp. 61–84). New York: Wiley.

Prizant, B., and Duchan, J. (1981). The functions of immediate echolalia in autistic children. *Journal of Speech and Hearing Disorders, 46,* 241–249.

Prizant, B., and Wetherby, A. (1998). Understanding the continuum of discrete-trial traditional behavioral to social-pragmatic developmental approaches in communication enhancement for young children with autism/PDD. *Seminars in Speech and Language, 19,* 329–354.

Prizant, B., Schuler, A., Wetherby, A., and Rydell, P. (1997). Enhancing language and communication development: Language approaches. In D. Cohen and F. Volkmar (Eds.), *Handbook of autism and pervasive developmental disorders* (pp. 572–605). New York: Wiley.

Quill, K. (1998). Environmental supports to enhance social-communication. *Seminars in Speech and Language, 19,* 407–423.

Rogers, S. (1996). Brief report: Early intervention in autism. *Journal of Autism and Developmental Disorders, 26,* 243–246.

Rutter, M., Bailey, A., Bolton, P., and Le Conteur, A. (1994). Autism and known medical conditions: Myth and substance. *Journal of Child Psychology and Psychiatry and Allied Disciplines, 35,* 311–322.

Rutter, M., Bailey, A., Simonoff, E., Pickles, A. (1997). Genetic influences of autism. In D. Cohen and F. Volkmar (Eds.), *Handbook of autism and pervasive developmental disorders* (pp. 370–387). New York: Wiley.

Rutter, M., Greenfield, D., and Lockyer, L. (1967). A five to fifteen year follow-up study of infantile psychosis: II. Social and behavioral outcome. *British Journal of Psychiatry, 113,* 1183–1199.

Rutter, M., Maywood, L., and Howlin, P. (1992). Language delay and social development. In P. Fletcher and D. Hall (Eds.), *Specific speech and language disorders in children* (pp. 63–78). London: Whurr.

Schuler, A., Prizant, B., and Wetherby, A. (1997). Enhancing language and communication development: Prelinguistic approaches. In D. Cohen and F. Volkmar (Eds.), *Handbook of autism and pervasive developmental disorders* (pp. 539–571). New York: Wiley.

Shriberg, L., Paul, R., McSweeney, J., Klin, A., Cohen, D., and Volkmar, F. (2001). Speech and prosody in high functioning adolescents and adults with autism and Asperger syndrome. *Journal of Speech, Language, and Hearing Research, 44*, 1097–1115.

Stone, W., and Caro-Martinez, L. (1990). Naturalistic observations of spontaneous communication in autistic children. *Journal of Autism and Developmental Disorders, 20*, 437–453.

Tager-Flusberg, H. (1995). Dissociations in form and function in the acquisition of language by autistic children. In H. Tager-Flusberg (Ed.), *Constraints on language acquisition: Studies of atypical children* (pp. 175–194). Hillsdale, NJ: Erlbaum.

Tager-Flusberg, H., and Anderson, M. (1991). The development of contingent discourse ability in autistic children. *Journal of Child Psychology and Psychiatry, 32*, 1123–1143.

Volkmar, F. (1998). *Autism and pervasive developmental disorders.* Cambridge, UK: Cambridge University Press.

Volkmar, F., Klin, A., Siegel, B., Szatmari, P., Lord, C., et al. (1994). Field trial for autistic disorder in DSM-IV. *American Journal of Psychiatry, 151*, 1361–1367.

Further Readings

Baron-Cohen, S. (1995). *Mindblindness.* Cambridge, MA: MIT Press.

Baron-Cohen, S., and Bolton, P. (1993). *Autism: The facts.* Oxford, UK: Oxford University Press.

Bauman, M., and Kempter, T. (1994). *The neurobiology of autism.* Baltimore: Johns Hopkins University Press.

Catalano, R. (1998). *When autism strikes.* New York: Plenum Press.

Cohen, D., and Volkmar, F. (Eds.). (1997). *Handbook of autism and pervasive developmental disorders.* New York: Wiley.

Dawson, G. (1989). *Autism: Nature, diagnosis, and treatment.* New York: Guilford Press.

Donnellan, A. (1985). *Classic readings in autism.* New York: Teachers' College Press.

Frith, U. (1989). *Autism: Explaining the enigma.* Oxford, UK: Blackwell.

Glidden, L. (2000). *International review of research in mental retardation: Autism.* San Diego, CA: Academic Press.

Happe, F. (1995). *Autism: An introduction to psychological theory.* Cambridge, MA: Harvard University Press.

Hogdon, L. (1999). *Solving behavior problems in autism.* Troy, MI: QuirkRoberts Publishing.

Matson, J. (1994). *Autism in children and adults.* Pacific Grove, CA: Brooks/Cole.

Morgan, H. (1996). *Adults with autism.* Cambridge, UK: Cambridge University Press.

Powers, M. (1989). *Children with autism: A parents' guide.* Bethesda, MD: Woodbine House.

Quill, K. (1995). *Teaching children with autism.* Albany, NY: Delmar.

Rimland, B. (1962). *Infantile autism.* New York: Appleton-Century-Crofts.

Rutter, M., and Schopler, M. (1978). *Autism.* New York: Plenum Press.

Schopler, E., and Mesibov, G. (1985–2000). *Current issues in autism* (series). New York: Plenum Press.

Sigman, M., and Capps, L. (1997). *Children with autism.* Cambridge, MA: Harvard University Press.

Sperry, V. (2000). *Fragile success.* Baltimore: Paul H. Brookes.

Wetherby, A., and Prizant, B. (2000). *Autistic spectrum disorders.* Baltimore: Paul H. Brookes.

Wing, L. (1972). *Autistic children.* New York: Brunner/Mazel.

Bilingualism, Speech Issues in

In evaluating the properties of bilingual speech, an anterior question that must be answered is who qualifies as bilingual. Scholars have struggled with this question for decades. Bilingualism defies delimitation and is open to a variety of descriptions and interpretations. For example, Bloomfield (1933) required native-like control of two languages, while Weinreich (1968) and Mackey (1970) considered as bilingual an individual who alternately used two languages. Beatens-Beardsmore (1982), observing a wide range of variations in different contexts, concluded that it is not possible to formulate a single neat definition, and stated that bilingualism as a concept has "open-ended semantics."

It has long been recognized that bilingual individuals form a heterogeneous population in that their abilities in their two languages are not uniform. Although some bilingual speakers may have attained a native-like production in each language, the great majority are not balanced between the two languages. The result is interference from the dominant language. Whether a child becomes bilingual simultaneously (two languages are acquired simultaneously) or successively (one language, generally the home language, is acquired earlier, and the other language is acquired, for example, when the child goes to school), it is impossible to rule out interference. In the former case, this may happen because of different degrees of exposure to the two languages; in the latter, the earlier acquired language may put its imprint on the one acquired later. More children become bilingual successively, and the influence of one language on the other is more evident. Yet even here there is no uniformity among speakers, and the range of interference from the dominant language forms a continuum.

The different patterns that a bilingual child reveals in speech may not necessarily be the result of interference. Bilingual children, like their monolingual counterparts, may suffer speech and/or language disorders. Thus, when children who grow up with more than one language produce patterns that are erroneous with respect to the speech of monolingual speakers, it is crucial to determine whether these nonconforming patterns are due to the influence of the child's other language or are indications of a speech-language disorder.

To be able to make accurate diagnoses, speech-language pathologists must use information from interference patterns, normal and disordered phonological development in general as well as in the two languages, and the specific dialect features. In assessing the phonological development of a bilingual child, both languages should be the focus of attention, and each should be examined in detail, even if the child seems to be a dominant speaker of one of the languages. To this end, all phonemes of the languages should be assessed in different word positions, and phonotactic patterns should be evaluated. Assessment tools that are designed for English, no matter how perfect they are, will not be appropriate for the other language and may be the cause of over- or underdiagnosis.

Certain cases lend themselves to obvious identification of interference. For example, if we encounter in the English language productions of a Portuguese-English bilingual child forms like [tʃiz] for "tease" and [tʃɪp] for "tip," whereby target /t/ turns into [tʃ], we can, with confidence, say that these renditions were due to Portuguese interference, as such substitutions are not commonly observed in developmental phonologies, and the change of /t/ to [tʃ] before /i/ is a rule of Portuguese phonology.

The decision is not always so straightforward, however. For example, substitutions may reflect certain developmental simplification processes that are universally phonetically motivated and shared by many languages. If a bilingual child's speech reveals any such processes, and if the first language of the child does not have the opportunities for such processes to surface, then it would be very difficult to identify the dominant language as the culprit and label the situation as one of interference. For example, if a 6-year-old child bilingual in Spanish and English reveals processes such as final obstruent devoicing (e.g., [bæk] for "bag," [bɛt] for "bed") and/or deletion of clusters that do not follow sonority sequencing ([tap] for "stop," [pɪt] for "spit"), we cannot claim that these changes are due to Spanish interference. Rather, these processes are among the commonly occurring developmental processes that occur in the speech of children in many languages. However, because these common simplification processes are usually suppressed in normally developing children by age 6, this particular situation suggests a delay or disorder. In this case, these processes may not have surfaced until age 6 because none of these patterns are demanded by the structure of Spanish. In other words, because Spanish has no voiced obstruents in final position and no consonant clusters that do not follow sonority sequencing, it is impossible to refer to the first language as the explanation. In such instances we must attribute these patterns to universally motivated developmental processes that have not been eliminated according to the expected timetable.

We may also encounter a third situation in which the seemingly clear distinction between interference and the developmental processes is blurred. This occurs when one or more of the developmental processes are also the patterns followed by the first (dominant) language. An example is final obstruent devoicing in the English language productions of a child with German, Russian, Polish, or Turkish as the first language. Although final obstruent devoicing is a natural process that even occurs in the early speech of monolingual English-speaking children, it is also a feature of the languages listed. Thus, the result is a natural tendency that receives extra impetus from the rule of the primary system. Other examples that could be included in the same category would be consonant cluster reduction in children whose primary language is Japanese, Turkish, or Finnish, and single obstruent coda deletion in children whose primary language is Japanese, Italian, Spanish, or Portuguese.

Besides the interference patterns and common developmental processes, speech-language pathologists must be watchful for some unusual (idiosyncratic) processes that are observed in children (Grunwell, 1987; Dodd, 1993). Processes such as unusual cluster reduction, as in [ren] for *train* (instead of the expected [ten]), fricative gliding, as in [wɪg] for *fig*, frication of stops, as in [væn] for *ban*, and backing, as in [pæk] for *pat*, may occur in children with phonological disorders.

Studies that have examined the phonological patterns in normally developing bilingual children (Gildersleeve, Davis, and Stubbe, 1996) and bilingual children with a suspected speech disorder (Dodd, Holm, and Wei, 1997) indicate that children in both groups exhibit patterns different from matched, monolingual peers. Compared with their monolingual peers, normally developing bilingual children and bilingual children with phonological disorders had a lower overall intelligibility rating, made more errors overall, distorted more sounds, and produced more uncommon error patterns. As for the difference between normally developing bilingual children and bilingual children with phonological disorders, it appears that children with phonological disorders manifest more common simplification patterns, suppress such patterns over time more slowly, and are likely to have uncommon processes.

As speech-language pathologists become more adept at differentiating common and uncommon phonological patterns and interference patterns in bilingual children, they will also need to consider not only the languages of the client, but also the specific dialects of those languages. Just as there are several varieties of English spoken in different countries (e.g., British, American, Australian, South African, Canadian, Indian) and even within one country (New England variety, Southern variety, General American, and African American Vernacular in the United States), other languages also show dialectal variation. Because none of these varieties or dialects of a given language is or can be considered a disordered form of that language, the child's dialectal information is essential. Any assessment of the child's speech must be made with respect to the norm of the particular variety she or he is learning. Not accounting for dialect features may either result in the misdiagnosis of a phonological disorder or escalate the child's severity rating.

Last but definitely not least is the desperate need for information on phonological development in bilingual children and assessment procedures unique to these individuals. Language skills in bilingual persons have almost always been appraised in reference to monolingual standards (Grosjean, 1992). Accordingly, a bilingual child is assessed with two procedures, one for each language, that are designed to evaluate monolingual speakers of these languages. This assumes that a bilingual individual is two monolingual individuals in one person. However, because of the constant interaction of the two languages, each phonological system of a bilingual child may, and in most cases will, not necessarily be acquired in a way identical to that of a monolingual child (Watson, 1991).

In order to characterize bilingual phonology accurately, detailed information on both languages being acquired by the children is indispensable. However, data on the developmental patterns in two languages separately would not be adequate, as information on phonological development in bilingual children is the real key to understanding bilingual phonology. Because bilingual speakers' abilities in the two languages vary immensely from one individual to another, developing assessment tools for phonological development is a huge task, perhaps the biggest challenge for the field.

See also BILINGUALISM AND LANGUAGE IMPAIRMENT.

—Mehmet Yavas

References

Beatens-Beardsmore, H. (1982). *Bilingualism: Basic principles.* Clevedon, UK: Tieto.

Bloomfield, L. (1933). *Language.* New York: Wiley.

Dodd, B. (1993). Speech disordered children. In G. Blanken, J. Dittman, H. Grimm, J. Marshall, and C. Wallesh (Eds.), *Linguistics: Disorders and pathologies* (pp. 825–834). Berlin: De Gruyter.

Dodd, B., Holm, A., and Wei, L. (1997). Speech disorder in preschool children exposed to Cantonese and English. *Clinical Linguistics and Phonetics, 11,* 229–243.

Gildersleeve, C., Davis, B., and Stubbe, E. (1996). *When monolingual rules don't apply: Speech development in a bilingual environment.* Paper presented at the annual convention of the American Speech-Language-Hearing Association, Seattle, WA.

Grosjean, F. (1992). Another view of bilingualism. In R. J. Harris (Ed.), *Cognitive processing in bilinguals* (pp. 51–62). New York: Elsevier.

Grunwell, P. (1987). *Clinical phonology* (2nd ed.). London: Croom Helm.

Mackey, W. (1970). Interference, integration and the synchronic fallacy. In J. Alatis (Ed.), *Bilingualism and language contact.* Washington, DC: Georgetown University Press.

Watson, I. (1991). Phonological processing in two languages. In E. Bialystok (Ed.), *Language processing in bilingual children.* Cambridge, UK: Cambridge University Press.

Weinreich, U. (1968). *Languages in contact.* The Hague: Mouton.

Further Readings

Bernthal, J. E., and Bankson, N. W. (Eds.). (1998). *Articulation and phonological disorders* (4th ed.). Needham Heights, MA: Allyn and Bacon.

Bortolini, U., and Leonard, L. (1991). The speech of phonologically disordered children acquiring Italian. *Clinical Linguistics and Phonetics, 5,* 1–12.

Cheng, L. R. (1987). *Assessing Asian language performance: Guidelines for evaluating limited-English-proficient students.* Rockville, MD: Aspen.

Deuchar, M., and Quay, S. (2000). *Bilingual acquisition.* New York: Oxford University Press.

Ferguson, C. A., Menn, L., and Stoel-Gammon, C. (Eds.). (1992). *Phonological development: Models, research, implications.* Timonium, MD: York Press.

Goldstein, B., and Iglesias, A. (1996a). Phonological patterns in normally developing Spanish speaking 3- and 4-year-olds of Puerto Rican descent. *Language, Speech, and Hearing Services in the Schools, 27,* 82–90.

Goldstein, B., and Iglesias, A. (1996b). Phonological patterns in Puerto Rican Spanish-speaking children with phonological disorders. *Journal of Communication Disorders, 29,* 367–387.

Grunwell, P. (1985). *Phonological assessment of child speech.* London: Nfer-Nelson.

Hodson, B. W. (1986). *Assessment of phonological processes in Spanish.* San Diego, CA: Los Amigos.

Hodson, B. W., and Paden, E. (1991). *Targeting intelligible speech* (2nd ed.). Austin, TX: Pro-Ed.

Keyser, H. (Ed.). (1995). *Bilingual speech-language pathology: An Hispanic focus.* San Diego, CA: Singular Publishing Group.

Magnusson, E. (1983). *The phonology of language disordered children: Production, perception and awareness.* Lund, Sweden: Gleerup.

Mann, D., and Hodson, B. (1994). Spanish-speaking children's phonologies: Assessment and remediation of disorders. *Seminars in Speech and Language, 15,* 137–147.

Mason, M., Smith, M., and Hinshaw, M. (1976). *Medida Espanola de Articulacion.* San Ysidoro, CA: San Ysidoro School District.

Nettelbladt, U. (1983). *Developmental studies of dysphonology in children.* Lund, Sweden: Gleerup.

So, L. (1992). *Cantonese Segmental Phonology Test.* Hong Kong University, Department of Speech and Hearing Sciences.

So, L., and Dodd, B. (1995). The acquisition of phonology by Cantonese speaking children. *Journal of Child Language, 22,* 473–495.

Stoel-Gammon, C., and Dunn, C. (1985). *Normal and disordered phonology in children.* Austin, TX: Pro-Ed.

Toronto, A. (1977). *Southwest Spanish Articulation Test.* Austin, TX: National Education Laboratory Publishers.

Yavas, M. (1998). *Phonology: Development and disorders.* San Diego, CA: Singular Publishing Group.

Yavas, M. (2002). VOT patterns in bilingual phonological development. In F. Windsor, L. Kelly, and N. Hewlett (Eds.), *Investigations in clinical linguistics* (pp. 341–350). Mahwah, NJ: Erlbaum.

Yavas, M., and Goldstein, B. (1998). Speech sound differences and disorders in first and second language acquisition: Theoretical issues and clinical applications. *American Journal of Speech and Language Pathology, 7.*

Yavas, M., Hernandorena, C., and Lamprecht, R. (1991). *Avaliacao fonologica da Crianca* (Phonological assessment tool for Brazilian Portuguese). Porto Alegre, Brazil: Artes Medicas.

Developmental Apraxia of Speech

Developmental apraxia of speech (DAS) is a developmental speech disorder frequently defined as difficulty in programming of sequential speech movements based on presumed underlying neurological differences. Theoretical constructs motivating understanding of DAS have been quite diverse. Motor-based or pre-motor planning speech output deficits (e.g., Hall, Jordon, and

Robin, 1993), phonologically based deficits in representation (e.g., Velleman and Strand, 1993), or deficits in neural tissue with organizational consequences (e.g., Crary, 1984; Sussman, 1988) have been posited. Reflecting these varied views of causality, a variety of terms have been employed: developmental apraxia of speech, developmental verbal dyspraxia, and developmental articulatory dyspraxia. Clinically, DAS has most often been defined by exclusion from functional speech disorder or delay using a complex of behavioral symptoms (e.g., Stackhouse, 1992; Shriberg, Aram, and Kwiatkowski, 1997).

The characterization of DAS was originally derived from apraxia of speech in adults, a disorder category based on acquired brain damage resulting in difficulty in programming speech movements (Broca, 1861). Morley, Court, and Miller (1954) first applied the term dyspraxia to children based on a proposed similarity in behavioral correlates with adult apraxic symptoms. A neurological etiology was implied by the analogy but has not been conclusively delineated, even with increasingly sophisticated instrumental techniques for understanding brain-behavior relations (see Bennett and Netsell, 1999; LeNormand et al., 2000). Little coherence and consensus is available in this literature at present. In addition, despite nearly 40 years of research, differential diagnostic correlates and range of severity levels characterizing DAS remain imprecisely defined. Guyette and Deidrich (1981) have suggested that DAS may not be a theoretically or clinically definable entity, as current empirical evidence does not produce any behavioral symptom not overlapping with other categories of developmental speech disorder or delay. In addition, no currently available theoretical constructs specifically disprove other possible theories for the origins of DAS (see Davis, Jakielski, and Marquardt, 1998). In contrast to developmental disorder categories such as hearing impairment or cleft palate, lack of a link of underlying cause or theoretical base with behavioral correlates results in an "etiological" disorder label with no clearly established basis. Evidence for a neurological etiology for DAS is based on behavioral correlates that are ascribed to a neurological basis, thus achieving a circular argument structure for neural origins (Marquardt, Sussman, and Davis, 2000).

Despite the lack of consensus on theoretical motivation, etiology, or empirical evidence precisely defining behavioral correlates, there is some consensus among practicing clinicians as well as researchers (e.g., Shriberg, Aram, and Kwiatkowski, 1997) that DAS exists. It thus represents an incompletely understood disorder that poses important challenges both to practicing clinicians and to the establishment of a consistent research base for overall understanding. An ethical differential diagnosis for clinical intervention and research investigations should, accordingly, be based on awareness of the current state of empirically established data regarding theories and behavioral correlates defining this disorder. Cautious application of the diagnostic label should be the norm, founded on a clear understanding of positive benefits to the client in discerning long-term prognosis,

appropriate decisions regarding clinical intervention, and valid theory building to understand the underlying nature of the disorder. Use of DAS as an "umbrella term for children with persisting and serious speech difficulties in the absence of obvious causation, regardless of the precise nature of their unintelligibility" (Stackhouse, 1992, p. 30) is to be avoided. Such practice continues to cloud the issue of precise definition of the presence and prevalence of the disorder in child clinical populations.

Accordingly, a review of the range of behavioral correlates presently in use is of crucial importance to careful definition and understanding of DAS. The relationship of behavioral correlates to differential diagnosis from "functional" speech disorder or delay is of primary importance to discriminating DAS as a subcategory of functional speech disorder. If no single defining characteristic or complex of characteristics emerges to define DAS, the utility of the label is seriously questionable for either clinical or research purposes. In every instance, observed behaviors need to be evaluated against developmental behaviors appropriate to the client's *chronological* age. In the case of very young clients, the differential diagnosis of DAS is complicated (Davis and Velleman, 2000). Some listed characteristics may be normal aspects of earliest periods of speech and language development (e.g., predominant use of simple syllable shapes or variability in production patterns at the onset of meaningful speech; see Vihman, 1997, for a review of normal phonetic and phonological development).

Before the clinical symptoms presently employed to define DAS are outlined, specific issues with available research will be reviewed briefly. It should be emphasized that behavioral inclusion criteria are not consistently reported and differing criteria are included across studies. Criteria for inclusion in studies then become recognized symptoms of involvement, achieving a circularity that is not helpful for producing valid characterization of the disorder (Stackhouse, 1992). Subject ages vary widely, from preschoolers (Bradford and Dodd, 1996) to adults (Ferry, Hall, and Hicks, 1975). Some studies include control populations of functional speech disorders for differential diagnosis (Stackhouse, 1992; Dodd, 1995); others do not (Horowitz, 1984). Associated language and praxis behaviors are included as differential diagnostic correlates in some studies (Crary and Towne, 1984), while others explicitly exclude these deficits (e.g., Hall, Jordon, and Robin, 1993). Severity is not reported consistently. When it is reported, the basis for assigning severity judgments is inconsistent across studies. A consequence of this inconsistency is lack of consensus on severity level appropriate to the DAS label. In some reports, the defining characteristic is severe and persistent disorder (e.g., Shriberg, Aram, and Kwiatkowski, 1997). In other reports (e.g., Thoonen et al., 1997), a continuum of severity is explored. In the latter conceptualization, DAS can manifest as mild, moderate, or severe speech disorder.

Despite the foregoing critique, the large available literature on DAS suggests some consensus on behavioral correlates that should be evaluated in establishing a differential diagnosis. The range of expression of these characteristics, although frequently cited, has not been specified quantitatively. Accordingly, these behaviors should not be considered definitive but suggestive of directions for future research as well as guidelines for the practicing clinician based on emerging research.

Exclusionary criteria for a differential diagnosis have been suggested in the areas of peripheral motor and sensory function, cognition, and receptive language. Exclusionary criteria frequently noted include (1) no peripheral organic disorder (e.g., cleft palate), (2) no sensory deficit (i.e., in vision or hearing), (3) no peripheral muscle weakness or dysfunction (e.g., dysarthria, cerebral palsy), (4) normal IQ, and (5) normal receptive language.

Phonological and phonetic correlates have also been listed. Descriptive terminology varies from phonetic (e.g., Murdoch et al., 1995) to phonological (Forrest and Morrisette, 1999; Velleman and Shriberg, 1999) according to the theoretical perspective of the researcher, complicating understanding of the nature of the disorder and comparison across studies. In addition, behavioral correlates have been established across studies with highly varied subject pools and differing exclusionary criteria. The range of expression of symptoms is not established (i.e., what types and severity of suprasegmental errors are necessary or sufficient for the diagnosis?). Some characteristics are in common with functional disorders and thus do not constitute a differential diagnostic characteristic (i.e., how limited does the consonant or vowel repertoire have to be to express DAS?). In addition, not all symptoms are consistently reported as being necessary to a diagnosis of DAS (e.g., not all clients show "groping postures of the articulators"). Long-term persistence of clinical symptoms in spite of intensive therapy has also frequently been associated with DAS. Phonological/phonetic correlates reported include (1) limited consonant and vowel phonetic inventory, (2) predominant use of simple syllable shapes, (3) frequent omission of errors, (4) a high incidence of vowel errors, (5) altered suprasegmental characteristics (including rate, pitch, loudness, and nasality), (6) variability and lack of consistent patterning in speech output, (7) increased errors on longer sequences, (8) groping postures, and (9) lack of willingness or ability to imitate a model.

Co-occurring characteristics of DAS in several related areas have also been mentioned frequently. However, co-occurrence may be optional for a differential diagnosis, because these characteristics have not been consistently tracked across available studies. Co-occurring characteristics frequently cited include (1) delays in gross and fine motor skills, (2) poor volitional oral nonverbal skills, (3) inconsistent diadokokinetic rates, (4) delay in syntactic development, and (5) reading and spelling delays.

Clearly, DAS is a problematic diagnostic category for both research and clinical practice. Although it has long been a focus of research and a subject of intense interest to clinicians, little consensus exists on definition, etiology, and characterization of behavioral or neural correlates. Circularity in the way in which etiology and

behavioral correlates have been described and studied does not lend to precision in understanding DAS. Research utilizing consistent subject selection criteria is needed to begin to link understanding of DAS to ethical clinical practices in assessment and intervention and to elucidate the underlying causes of this disorder.

See also MOTOR SPEECH INVOLVEMENT IN CHILDREN.

—*Barbara L. Davis*

References

Bennett, S., and Netsell, R. W. (1999). Possible roles of the insula in speech and language processing: Directions for research. *Journal of Medical Speech-Language Pathology, 7,* 255–272.

Bradford, A., and Dodd, B. (1996). Do all speech-disordered children have motor deficits? *Clinical Linguistics and Phonetics, 10,* 77–101.

Broca, P. (1861). Remarques sur le siege do la faculte du language articule, suives d'une observation d'aphemie (peste de la parole). *Bulletin de la Societe d'Anatomique, 2nd série, 6,* 330–337.

Crary, M. A. (1984). Phonological characteristics of developmental verbal dyspraxia. *Seminars in Speech and Language, 6*(2), 71–83.

Crary, M. A., and Towne, R. (1984). The asynergistic nature of developmental verbal dyspraxia. *Australian Journal of Human Communication Disorders, 12,* 27–37.

Davis, B. L., Jakielski, K. J., and Marquardt, T. M. (1998). Devlopmental apraxia of speech: Determiners of differential diagnosis. *Clinical Linguistics and Phonetics, 12,* 25–45.

Davis, B. L., and Velleman, S. L. (2000). Differential diagnosis of developmental apraxia of speech in infants and toddlers. *Infant Toddler Intervention, 10*(3), 177–192.

Dodd, B. (1995). Procedures for classification of sub-groups of speech disorder. In B. Dodd (Ed.), *Differential diagnosis and treatment of children with speech disorders.* London: Whurr.

Ferry, P. C., Hall, S. M., and Hicks, J. L. (1975). Dilapidated speech: Developmental verbal dyspraxia. *Developmental Medicine and Child Neurology, 17,* 432–455.

Forrest, K., and Morrisette, M. L. (1999). Feature analysis of segmental errors in children with phonological disorders. *Journal of Hearing, Language, and Speech Research, 42,* 187–194.

Guyette, T. W., and Deidrich, W. M. (1981). A critical review of developmental apraxia of speech. In N. J. Lass (Ed.), *Speech and language advances in basic practice* (No. 11). London: Academic Press.

Hall, P. K., Jordan, L. S., and Robin, D. A. (1993). *Developmental apraxia of speech,* Austin, TX: Pro-Ed.

Horowitz, J. (1984). Neurological findings in developmental verbal apraxia. *Seminars in Speech and Language, 6*(2), 11–18.

LeNormand, M.-T., Vaivre-Douret, L., Payan, C., and Cohen, H. (2000). Neuromotor development and language processing in developmental dyspraxia: A follow-up case study. *Journal of Clinical and Experimental Neuropsychology, 22,* 408–417.

Marquardt, T. M., Sussman, H. M., and Davis, B. L. (2000). Developmental apraxia of speech: Advances in theory and practice. In D. Vogel and M. Cannito (Eds.), *Treating disorders of speech motor control.* Austin, TX: Pro-Ed.

Morley, M. E., Court, D., and Miller, H. (1954). Developmental dysarthria. *British Medical Journal, 1,* 463–467.

Murdoch, B. E., Aqttard, M. D., Ozanne, A. E., and Stokes, P. D. (1995). Impaired tongue strength and endurance in developmental verbal dyspraxia: A physiological analysis. *European Journal of Disorders of Communication, 30,* 51–64.

Shriberg, L. D., Aram, D. M., and Kwiatkowski, J. (1997). Developmental apraxia of speech: I. Descriptive and theoretical perspectives. *Journal of Speech, Language, and Hearing Research, 40,* 273–285.

Stackhouse, J. (1992). Developmental verbal dyspraxia: I. A review and critique. *European Journal of Disorders of Communication, 27,* 19–34.

Sussman, H. M. (1988). The neurogenesis of phonology. In H. Whitaker (Ed.), *Phonological processes and brain mechanisms.* New York: Springer-Verlag.

Thoonen, G., Maasen, B., Gabreels, F., Schreuder, R., and de Swart, B. (1997). Towards a standardized assessment procedure for DAS of speech. *European Journal of Disorders of Communication, 32,* 37–60.

Velleman, S. L., and Shriberg, L. D. (1999). Metrical analysis of the speech of children with suspected developmental apraxia of speech. *Journal of Speech, Language, and Hearing Research, 42,* 1444–1460.

Velleman, S. L., and Strand, K. (1993). Developmental verbal dyspraxia. In J. E. Bernthal and N. W. Bankson (Eds.), *Child phonology: Characteristics, assessment, and intervention with special populations.* New York: Thieme.

Vihman, M. M. (1997). *Phonological development.* Cambridge, UK: Blackwell.

Further Readings

Aram, D. M., and Nelson, J. E. (1982). *Child language disorders.* St. Louis: Mosby.

Bradford, A., and Dodd, B. (1994). The motor planning abilities of phonologically disordered children. *European Journal of Disorders of Communication, 29,* 349–369.

Bridgeman, E., and Snowling, M. (1988). The perception of phoneme sequence: A comparison of dyspraxic and normal children. *British Journal of Communication, 23,* 25–252.

Crary, M. (1993). *Developmental motor speech disorders.* San Diego, CA: Singular Publishing Group.

Croce, R. (1993). A review of the neural basis of apractic disorders with implications for remediation. *Adapted Physical Review Quarterly, 10,* 173–215.

Dewey, D. (1995). What is developmental dyspraxia? *Brain and Cognition, 29,* 254–274.

Dewey, D., Roy, E. A., Square-Storer, P. A., and Hayden, D. (1988). Limb and oral praxic abilities of children with verbal sequencing deficits. *Developmental Medicine and Child Neurology, 30,* 743–751.

Hall, P. K. (1989). The occurrence of developmental apraxia of speech in a mild articulation disorder: A case study. *Journal of Communication Disorders, 22,* 265–276.

Hayden, D. A. (1994). Differential diagnosis of motor speech dysfunction in children. *Clinics in Communication Disorders, 4,* 119–141.

Hodge, M. (1994). Assessment of children with developmental apraxia of speech: A rationale. *Clinics in Communication Disorders, 4,* 91–101.

Kent, R. D. (2000). Research on speech motor control and its disorders: A review and prospective. *Journal of Communication Disorders, 33,* 391–428.

Pollock, K. E., and Hall, P. K. (1991). An analysis of the vowel misarticulations of five children with developmental apraxia of speech. *Clinical Linguistics and Phonetics, 5,* 207–224.

Rosenbek, J. C., and Wertz, R. T. (1972). A review of fifty cases of developmental apraxia of speech. *Language, Speech, and Hearing Services in the Schools, 5,* 23–33.

Shriberg, L. D., Aram, D. M., and Kwiatkowski, J. (1997). Developmental apraxia of speech: III. A subtype marked by inappropriate stress. *Journal of Speech, Language, and Hearing Research, 40,* 313–337.

Skinder, A., Connaghan, K., Strand, E. A., and Betz, S. (2000). Acoustic correlates of perceived lexical stress errors in children with developmental apraxia of speech. *Journal of Medical Speech-Language Pathology, 8,* 279–284.

Skinder, M. S., Strand, E. A., and Mignerey, M. (1999). Perceptual and acoustic analysis of lexical and sentential stress in children with developmental apraxia of speech. *Journal of Medical Speech-Language Pathology, 7,* 133–144.

Square, P. (1994). Treatment approaches for developmental apraxia of speech. *Clinics in Communication Disorders, 4,* 151–161.

Stackhouse, J., and Snowling, M. (1992). Barriers to literacy development: I. Two cases of developmental verbal dyspraxia. *Cognitive Neuropsychology, 9,* 273–299.

Strand, E. A., and Debertine, P. (2000). The efficacy of integral stimulation intervention with developmental apraxia of speech. *Journal of Medical Speech-Language Pathology, 8,* 295–300.

Sussman, H. M., Marquardt, T. P., and Doyle, J. (2000). An acoustic analysis of phonemic integrity and contrastiveness in developmental apraxia of speech. *Journal of Medical Speech-Language Pathology, 8,* 301–313.

Thoonen, G., Maasen, B., Wit, J., Gabreels, F., and Schreuder, R. (1994). Feature analysis of singleton consonant errors in developmental verbal dyspraxia (DVD). *Journal of Speech, Language, and Hearing Research, 37,* 1424–1440.

Thoonen, G., Maasen, B., Wit, J., Gabreels, F., and Schreuder, R. (1996). The integrated use of maximum performance tasks in differential diagnostic evaluations among children with motor speech disorders. *Clinical Linguistics and Phonetics, 10,* 311–336.

Thoonen, G., Maasen, B., Gabreels, F., and Schreuder, R. (1999). Validity of maximum performance tasks to diagnose motor speech disorders in children. *Clinical Linguistics and Phonetics, 13,* 1–23.

Till, J. A., Yorkston, K. M., and Buekelman, D. R. (1994). *Motor speech disorders: Advances in assessment and treatment.* Baltimore: Paul H. Brookes.

Walton, J. H., and Pollock, K. E. (1993). Acoustic validation of vowel error patterns in developmental apraxia of speech. *Clinical Linguistics and Phonetics, 2,* 95–101.

Williams, R., Packman, A., Ingham, R., and Rosenthal, J. (1981). Clinician agreement of behaviors that identify developmental articulatory dyspraxia. *Australian Journal of Human Communication Disorders, 8,* 16–26.

Yorkston, K. M., Buekelman, D. R., Strand, E. A., and Bell, K. R. (1999). *Management of motor speech disorders.* Austin, TX: Pro-Ed.

Dialect, Regional

Dialects or language varieties are a result of systematic, internal linguistic changes that occur within a language. Unlike accents, in which linguistic changes occur mainly at the phonological level, dialects reflect structural changes in phonology, morphology, and syntax, as well as lexical or semantic changes. The degree of mutual intelligibility that a speaker's language has with a designated standard linguistic system is often used to distinguish dialect from language. Mutual intelligibility means that speakers of one dialect can understand speakers of another dialect.

Although the construct of mutual intelligibility is frequently employed to differentiate dialect from language, there are counterexamples. On one hand, speakers may have the same language, but the dialects may not be mutually intelligible. For example, Chinese has a number of dialects, such as Cantonese and Mandarin, each spoken in different geographical regions. Although Cantonese and Mandarin speakers consider these dialects, the two lack mutual intelligibility since those who speak only Cantonese do not easily understand those who speak only Mandarin, and vice versa. On the other hand, speakers may produce different languages but have mutual intelligibility. For instance, Norwegian, Swedish, and Danish are thought of as different languages, yet speakers of these languages can easily understand one another.

A dialect continuum or dialect continua may account for lack of mutual intelligibility in a large territory. A dialect continuum refers to a distribution of sequentially arranged dialects that progressively change speech or linguistic forms across a broad geographical area. Some speech shifts may be subtle, others may be more dramatic. Assume widely dispersed territories are labeled towns A, B, C, D, and E and are serially adjacent to one another, thereby creating a continuum. B is adjacent to A and C, C is adjacent to B and D, and so on. There will be mutual intelligibility between dialects spoken in A and B, between B and C, between C and D, and between D and E. However, the dialects of the two towns at the extremes, A and E, may not be mutually intelligible, owing to the continuous speech and language shifts that have occurred across the region. It is also possible that some of the intermediate dialects, such as B and D, may not be mutually intelligible.

Because different conditions influence dialects, it is not easy to discriminate dialect precisely from language. Using mutual intelligibility as a primary marker of distinction should be considered relative to the territories of interest. For example, in the United States, the concept of mutual intelligibility appears valid, whereas it is not completely valid in many other countries.

Dialects exist in all languages and are often discussed in terms of social or regional varieties. Social dialects represent a speaker's social stratification within a given society or cultural group. Regional dialects are associated with geographical location or where speakers live. Regional and social dialects may co-occur within language patterns of the same speaker. In other words, social and regional dialects are not mutually exclusive.

Regional dialects constitute a unique cluster of language characteristics that are distributed across a specified geographical area. Exploration of regional dialectal systems is referred to as dialectology, dialect geography, or linguistic geography. For many years, dialects spoken in cities were thought of as prestigious. Therefore, in traditional dialect studies, data were mainly collected in rural areas. Surveys, questionnaires, and interview techniques were used as primary mechanisms of data collection. A field worker would visit an area and talk to residents using predetermined elicitation techniques that would encourage the speaker to produce the distinctive items of interest. The field worker would then manually note whether the individual's speech contained the distinctive linguistic features of interest. These methods generated a number of linguistic atlases that contained linguistic maps displaying geographical distributions of language characteristics.

Data were used to determine where a selected set of features was produced and where people stopped using this same set of features. The selected features could include vocabulary, specific sounds, or grammatical forms. Lines, or isoglosses, were drawn on a map to indicate the existence of specific features. When multiple isoglosses, or a bundle of isoglosses, surround a specific region, this is used to designate dialect boundaries. The bundle of isoglosses on a linguistic map would indicate that people on one side produced a number of lexical items and grammatical forms that were different from the speech of those who lived outside the boundary. Theoretically, the dialect was more distinctive, with a greater amount of bundling.

After the 1950s, audio and, eventually, video recordings were made of speakers in designated regions. Recordings allow a greater depth of analysis because they can be repeatedly replayed. Concurrent with these technological advances, there was increased interest in urban dialects, and investigators began to explore diversity of dialects within large cities, such as Boston, Detroit, New York, and London. Technological developments also led to more quantitative studies. Strong statistical analysis (dialectometry) has evolved since the 1970s and allows the investigator to explore large data sets with large numbers of contrasts.

Several factors contribute to the formation of regional dialects. Among these factors are settlement and migration patterns. For instance, regional English varieties began to appear in the United States as speakers immigrated from different parts of Britain. Speakers from the eastern region of England settled in New England, and those from Ulster settled in western New England and in Appalachia. Each contributed different variations to the region in which they settled.

Regional dialect formation may also result from the presence of natural boundaries such as mountains, rivers, and swamps. Because it was extremely difficult to traverse the Appalachian mountain range, inhabitants of the mountains were isolated and retained older English forms that contributes some of the unique characteristics of Appalachian English. For example, the morphological a-prefix in utterances such as "He come a-running" or "She was a-tellin' the story" appears to be a retention from older forms of English that were prevalent in the seventeenth century.

Commerce and culture also play important roles in influencing regional dialects, as can be observed in the unique dialect of people in Baltimore, Maryland. Speakers of "Bawlamerese" live in "Merlin" (Maryland), whose state capitol is "Napolis" (Annapolis), located next to "Warshnin" (Washington, D.C.), and refer to Bethlehem Steel as "Bethlum." Because the "Bethlum" mill, located in Fells Point, has been a primary employer of many individuals, language has evolved to discuss employment. Many will say they work "down a point" or "down a mill," where the boss will "har and far" (hire and fire) people. While most people working "down a point" live in "Dundock" (Dundalk), some may live as far away as "Norf Abnew" (North Avenue), "Habberdy Grace" (Harve de Grace), or even "Klumya" (Columbia).

Two other types of geolinguistic variables are often associated with regional dialects. One variable is a set of linguistic characteristics that are unique to a geographical area or that occur only in that area. For instance, unique to western Pennsylvania, speakers say "youse" (you singular), "yens" (you plural) and "yens boomers" (a group of people). The second variable is the frequency of occurrence of regional linguistic characteristics in a specific geographic area. For example, the expression "take 'er easy" is known throughout the United States, but mainly used in central and western Pennsylvania.

—*Adele Proctor*

Further Readings

Chambers, J. K. (1992). Dialect acquisition. *Language, 68,* 673–705.

Chambers, J. K., and Trudgill, P. (1998). *Dialectology.* New York: Cambridge University Press.

Labov, W. (1994). *Principles of linguistic change. Vol. 1. Internal factors.* Cambridge, MA: Blackwell.

Linn, M. D. (1998). *Handbook of dialects and language variation.* New York: Academic Press.

Romaine, S. (2000). *Language in society: An introduction to sociolinguistics.* New York: Oxford University Press.

Dysarthrias: Characteristics and Classification

The dysarthrias are a group of neurological disorders that reflect disturbances in the strength, speed, range, tone, steadiness, timing, or accuracy of movements necessary for prosodically normal, efficient and intelligible speech. They result from central or peripheral nervous system conditions that adversely affect respiratory, phonatory, resonatory, or articulatory speech movements. They are often accompanied by nonspeech impairments (e.g., dysphagia, hemiplegia), but sometimes they are the only manifestation of neurological disease. Their course can be transient, improving, exacerbating-remitting, progressive, or stationary.

Endogenous or exogenous events as well as genetic influences can cause dysarthrias. Their neurological bases can be present congenitally or they can emerge acutely, subacutely, or insidiously at any time of life. They are associated with many neurological conditions, but vascular, traumatic, and degenerative diseases are their most common cause in most clinical settings; neoplastic, toxic-metabolic, infectious, and inflammatory causes are also possible.

Although incidence and prevalence are not precisely known, dysarthria often is present in a number of frequently occurring neurological diseases, and it probably represents a significant proportion of all acquired neurological communication disorders. For example, approximately one-third of people with traumatic brain injury may be dysarthric, with nearly double that prevalence during the acute phase (Sarno, Buonaguro, and Levita, 1986; Yorkston et al., 1999). Dysarthria probably occurs in 50%–90% of people with Parkinson's disease, with increased prevalence as the disease progresses (Logemann et al., 1978; Mlcoch, 1992), and it can be among the most disabling symptoms of the disease in some cases (Dewey, 2000). Dysarthria emerges very frequently during the course of amyotrophic lateral sclerosis (ALS) and may be among the presenting symptoms and signs in over 20% (Rose, 1977; Gubbay et al., 1985). It occurs in 25% of patients with lacunar stroke (Arboix and Marti-Vilata, 1990). In a large tertiary care center, dysarthria was the primary communication disorder in 46% of individuals with any acquired neurological disease seen for speech-language pathology evaluation over a 4-year period (Duffy, 1995).

The clinical diagnosis is based primarily on auditory perceptual judgments of speech during conversation, sentence repetition, and reading, as well as performance on tasks such as vowel prolongation and alternating motion rates (AMRs; for example, repetition of "puh," "tuh," and "kuh" as rapidly and steadily as possible). Vowel prolongation permits judgments about respiratory support for speech as well as the quality, pitch, and duration of voice. AMRs permit judgments about the rate and rhythm of repetitive movements and are quite useful in distinguishing among certain dysarthria types (e.g., they are typically slow but regular in spastic dysarthria, but irregular in ataxic dysarthria). Visual and physical examination of the speech mechanism at rest and during nonspeech responses (e.g., observations of asymmetry, weakness, atrophy, fasciculations, adventitious movements, pathological oral reflexes) and information from instrumental measures (e.g., acoustic, endoscopic, videofluorographic) often provide confirmatory diagnostic evidence.

Dysarthria severity can be indexed in several ways, but quantitative measures usually focus on intelligibility and speaking rate. The most commonly used intelligibility measures are the Computerized Assessment of Intelligibility in Dysarthric Speakers (Yorkston, Beukelman, and Traynor, 1984) and the Sentence Intelligibility Test (Yorkston, Beukelman, and Tice, 1996), but other measures are available for clinical and research purposes (Enderby, 1983; Kent et al., 1989).

A wide variety of acoustic, physiological, and anatomical imaging methods are available for assessment. Some are easily used clinically, whereas others are primarily research tools. Studies using them have often yielded results consistent with predictions about pathophysiology from auditory-perceptual classification, but discrepancies that have been found make it clear that correspondence between perceptual attributes and physiology cannot be assumed (Duffy and Kent, 2001). Methods that show promise or that already have refined what we understand about the anatomical and physiological underpinnings of the dysarthrias include acoustic, kinematic, and aerodynamic methods, electromyography, electroencephalography, radiography, tomography, computed tomography, magnetic resonance imaging, functional magnetic resonance imaging, positron emission tomography, single-photon emission tomography, and magnetoencephalography (McNeil, 1997; Kent et al., 2001).

The dysarthrias can be classified by time of onset, course, site of lesion, and etiology, but the most widely used classification system in use today is based on the auditory-perceptual method developed by Darley, Aronson, and Brown (1969a, 1969b, 1975). Often referred to as the Mayo Clinic system, the method identifies dysarthria types, with each type representing a perceptually distinguishable grouping of speech characteristics that presumably reflect underlying pathophysiology and locus of lesion. The following summarizes the major types, their primary distinguishing perceptual attributes, and their presumed underlying localization and distinguishing neurophysiological deficit.

Flaccid dysarthria is due to weakness in muscles supplied by cranial or spinal nerves that innervate respiratory, laryngeal, velopharyngeal, or articulatory structures. Its specific characteristics depend on which nerves are involved. Trigeminal, facial, or hypoglossal nerve lesions are associated with imprecise articulation of phonemes that rely on jaw, face, or lingual movement. Vagus nerve lesions can lead to hypernasality or weak pressure consonant production when the pharyngeal branch is affected or to breathiness, hoarseness, diplophonia, stridor, or short phrases when the laryngeal branches are involved. When spinal respiratory nerves are affected, reduced loudness, short phrases, and alterations in breath patterning for speech may be evident. In general, unilateral lesions and lesions of a single nerve produce relatively mild deficits, whereas bilateral lesions or multiple nerve involvement can have devastating effects on speech.

Spastic dysarthria is usually associated with bilateral lesions of upper motor neuron pathways that innervate relevant cranial and spinal nerves. Its distinguishing characteristics are attributed to spasticity, and they often include a strained-harsh voice quality, slow rate, slow but regular speech AMRs, and restricted pitch and loudness variability. All components of speech production are usually affected.

Ataxic dysarthria is associated with lesions of the cerebellum or cerebellar control circuits. Its distinguishing characteristics are attributed primarily to incoordination, and they are perceived most readily in articulation and prosody. Characteristics often include irregular articulatory breakdowns, irregular speech AMRs, inappropriate variations in pitch, loudness, and duration, and sometimes excess and equal stress across syllables.

Hypokinetic dysarthria is associated with basal ganglia control circuit pathology, and its features seem mostly related to rigidity and reduced range of motion. Parkinson's disease is the prototypic disorder associated with hypokinetic dysarthria, but other conditions can also cause it. Its distinguishing characteristics include reduced loudness, breathy-tight dysphonia, monopitch and monoloudness, and imprecise and sometimes rapid, accelerating, or "blurred" articulation and AMRs. Dysfluency and palilalia also may be apparent.

Hyperkinetic dysarthria is also associated with basal ganglia control circuit pathology. Unlike hypokinetic dysarthria, its distinguishing characteristics are a product of involuntary movements that interfere with intended speech movements. Its manifestations vary across several causal movement disorders, which can range from relatively regular and slow (tremor, palatopharyolaryngeal myoclonus), to irregular but relatively sustained (dystonia), to relatively rapid and predictable or unpredictable (chorea, action myoclonus, tics). These movements may be a nearly constant presence, but sometimes they are worse during speech or activated only during speech. They may affect any one or all levels of speech production, and their effects on speech can be highly variable. Distinguishing characteristics usually reflect regular or unpredictable variability in phrasing, voice, articulation, or prosody.

Unilateral upper motor neuron dysarthria has an anatomical rather than pathophysiological label because it has received little systematic study. It most commonly results from stroke affecting upper motor neuron pathways. Because the damage is unilateral, severity usually is rarely worse than mild to moderate. Its characteristics often overlap with varying combinations of those associated with flaccid, spastic, or ataxic dysarthria (Duffy and Folger, 1996; Hartman and Abbs, 1992).

Mixed dysarthrias reflect combinations of two or more of the single dysarthria types. They occur more frequently than any single dysarthria type in many clinical settings. Some diseases are associated only with a specific mix; for example, flaccid-spastic dysarthria is the only mix expected in ALS. Other diseases, because the locus of lesions they cause is less predictable (e.g., multiple sclerosis, traumatic brain injury), may be associated with virtually any mix. The presence of mixed dysarthria is very uncommon or incompatible with some diseases (e.g., myasthenia gravis is associated only with flaccid dysarthria), so sometimes the presence of a mixed dysarthria can make a particular disease an unlikely cause or raise the possibility that more than a single disease is present.

Because of their potential to inform our understanding of the neural control of speech, and because their prevalence in frequently occurring neurological diseases is high and their functional effects are significant, dysarthrias draw considerable attention from clinicians and researchers. The directions of clinical and more basic research are broad, but many current efforts are aimed at the following: refining the differential diagnosis and indices of severity; delineating acoustic and physiological correlates of dysarthria types and intelligibility; more precisely establishing the relationships among perceptual dysarthria types, neural structures and circuitry, and acoustic and pathophysiological correlates; and developing more effective treatments for the underlying impairments and functional limitations imposed by them. Advances are likely to come from several disciplines (e.g., speech-language pathology, speech science, neurology) working in concert to integrate clinical, anatomical, and physiological observations into a coherent understanding of the clinical disorders and their underpinnings.

See also DYSARTHRIAS: MANAGEMENT.

—*Joseph R. Duffy*

References

Arboix, A., and Marti-Vilata, J. L. (1990). Lacunar infarctions and dysarthria. *Archives of Neurology, 47,* 127.

Darley, F. L., Aronson, A. E., and Brown, J. R. (1969a). Differential diagnostic patterns of dysarthria. *Journal of Speech and Hearing Research, 12,* 249–269.

Darley, F. L., Aronson, A. E., and Brown, J. R. (1969b). Clusters of deviant dimensions in the dysarthrias. *Journal of Speech and Hearing Research, 12,* 462–496.

Darley, F. L., Aronson, A. E., and Brown, J. R. (1975). *Motor speech disorders.* Philadelphia: Saunders.

Dewey, R. B. (2000). Clinical features of Parkinson's disease. In C. H. Adler and J. E. Ahlskog (Eds.), *Parkinson's disease and movement disorders* (pp. 77–84). Totowa, NJ: Humana Press.

Duffy, J. R. (1995). *Motor speech disorders: Substrates, differential diagnosis, and management.* St. Louis: Mosby.

Duffy, J. R., and Folger, W. N. (1996). Dysarthria associated with unilateral central nervous system lesions: A retrospective study. *Journal of Medical Speech-Language Pathology, 4,* 57–70.

Duffy, J. R., and Kent, R. D. (2001). Darley's contributions to the understanding, differential diagnosis, and scientific study of the dysarthrias. *Aphasiology, 15,* 275–289.

Enderby, P. (1983). *Frenchay dysarthria assessment.* San Diego, CA: College-Hill Press.

Gubbay, S. S., Kahana, E., Zilber, N., and Cooper, G. (1985). Amyotrophic lateral sclerosis: A study of its presentation and prognosis. *Journal of Neurology, 232,* 295–300.

Hartman, D. E., and Abbs, J. H. (1992). Dysarthria associated with focal unilateral upper motor neuron lesion. *European Journal of Disorders of Communication, 27,* 187–196.

Kent, R. D., Duffy, J. R., Slama, A., Kent, J. F., and Clift, A. (2001). Clinicoanatomic studies in dysarthria: Review, critique, and directions for research. *Journal of Speech, Language, and Hearing Research, 44,* 535–551.

Kent, R. D., Weismer, G., Kent, J. F., and Rosenbek, J. C. (1989). Toward phonetic intelligibility testing in dysarthria. *Journal of Speech and Hearing Disorders, 54,* 482–499.

Logemann, J. A., Fischer, H. B., Boshes, B., and Blonsky, E. (1978). Frequency and cooccurence of vocal tract dysfunction in the speech of a large sample of Parkinson patients. *Journal of Speech and Hearing Disorders, 43,* 47–57.

McNeil, M. R. (Ed.). (1997). *Clinical management of sensorimotor speech disorders.* New York: Thieme.

Mlcoch, A. G. (1992). Diagnosis and treatment of parkinsonian dysarthria. In W. C. Koller (Ed.), *Handbook of Parkinson's disease* (pp. 227–254). New York: Marcel Dekker.

Rose, F. C. (1977). *Motor neuron disease.* New York: Grune and Stratton.

Sarno, M. T., Buonaguro, A., and Levita, E. (1986). Characteristics of verbal impairment in closed head injured patients. *Archives of Physical Medicine and Rehabilitation, 67,* 400–405.

Yorkston, K. M., Beukelman, D. R., Strand, E. A., and Bell, K. R. (1999). *Management of motor speech disorders in children and adults.* Austin, TX: Pro-Ed.

Yorkston, K. M., Beukelman, D. R., and Tice, R. (1996). *Sentence Intelligibility Test.* Lincoln, NE: Tice Technology Services.

Yorkston, K. M., Beukelman, D. R., and Traynor, C. (1984). *Computerized Assessment of Intelligibility of Dysarthric Speech.* Austin, TX: Pro-Ed.

Further Readings

Bunton, K., and Weismer, G. (2001). The relationship between perception and acoustics for a high-low vowel contrast produced by speakers with dysarthria. *Journal of Speech, Language, and Hearing Research, 44,* 1215–1228.

Cannito, M. P., Yorkston, K. M., and Beukelman, D. R. (Eds.). (1998). *Neuromotor speech disorders: Nature, assessment, and management.* Baltimore: Paul H. Brookes.

Duffy, J. R. (1994). Emerging and future concerns in motor speech disorders. *American Journal of Speech-Language Pathology, 3,* 36–39.

Gentil, M., and Pollack, P. (1995). Some aspects of parkinsonian dysarthria. *Journal of Medical Speech-Language Pathology, 3,* 221–238.

Goozee, J. V., Murdoch, B. E., and Theodoros, D. G. (1999). Electropalatographic assessment of articulatory timing characteristics in dysarthria following traumatic brain injury. *Journal of Medical Speech-Language Pathology, 7,* 209–222.

Hammen, V. L., and Yorkston, K. M. (1994). Respiratory patterning and variability in dysarthric speech. *Journal of Medical Speech-Language Pathology, 2,* 253–262.

Kent, R. D., Duffy, J. R., Kent, J. F., Vorperian, H. K., and Thomas, J. E. (1999). Quantification of motor speech abilities in stroke: Time-energy analysis of syllable and word repetition. *Journal of Medical Speech-Language Pathology, 7,* 83–90.

Kent, R. D., Kent, J. F., Duffy, J. R., and Weismer, G. (1998). The dysarthrias: Speech-voice profiles, related dysfunctions, and neuropathology. *Journal of Medical Speech-Language Pathology, 6,* 165–211.

Kent, R. D., Kent, J. F., Duffy, J. R., Weismer, G., and Stuntebeck, S. (2000). Ataxic dysarthria. *Journal of Speech-Language-Hearing Research, 43,* 1275–1289.

Kent, R. D., Kent, J. F., Weismer, G., and Duffy, J. R. (2000). What dysarthrias can tell us about the neural control of speech. *Journal of Phonetics, 28,* 273–302.

Kent, R. D., Kim, H., Weismer, H. G., Kent, J. F., Rosenbek, J., Brooks, B. R., and Workinger, M. (1994). Laryngeal dysfunction in neurological disease: Amyotrophic lateral sclerosis, Parkinson's disease, and stroke. *Journal of Medical Speech-Language Pathology, 2,* 157–176.

Kent, R. D., Weismer, G., Kent, J. F., Vorperian, H. K., and Duffy, J. R. (1999). Acoustic studies of dysarthric speech: Methods, progress, and potential. *Journal of Communication Disorders, 32,* 141–186.

King, J. B., Ramig, L. O., Lemke, J. H., and Horii, Y. (1994). Parkinson's disease: Longitudinal changes in acoustic parameters of phonation. *Journal of Medical Speech-Language Pathology, 2*, 29–42.

Kleinow, J., Smith, A., and Ramig, L. O. (2001). Speech motor stability in IPD: Effects of rate and loudness manipulations. *Journal of Speech, Language, and Hearing Research, 44*, 1041–1051.

LaPointe, L. L. (1999). *Journal of Medical Speech-Language Pathology, 7*(2) (entire issue).

LaPointe, L. L. (2000). *Journal of Medical Speech-Language Pathology, 8*(4) (entire issue).

Lefkowitz, D., and Netsell, R. (1994). Correlation of clinical deficits with anatomical lesions: Post-traumatic speech disorders and MRI. *Journal of Medical Speech-Language Pathology, 2*, 1–14.

Moore, C. A., Yorkston, K. M., and Beukelman, D. R. (Eds.). (1991). *Dysarthria and apraxia of speech: Perspectives on management.* Baltimore: Paul H. Brookes.

Murdoch, B. E., Thompson, E. C., and Stokes, P. D. (1994). Phonatory and laryngeal dysfunction following upper motor neuron vascular lesions. *Journal of Medical Speech-Language Pathology, 2*, 177–190.

Robin, D. A., Yorkston, K. M., and Beukelman, D. R. (Eds.). (1996). *Disorders of motor speech: Assessment, treatment, and clinical characterization.* Baltimore: Paul H. Brookes.

Samlan, R., and Weismer, G. (1995). The relationship of selected perceptual measures of diadochokinesis in speech intelligibility in dysarthric speakers with amyotrophic lateral sclerosis. *American Journal of Speech-Language Pathology, 4*, 9–13.

Solomon, N. P., Lorell, D. M., Robin, D. R., Rodnitzky, R. L., and Luschei, E. S. (1994). Tongue strength and endurance in mild to moderate Parkinson's disease. *Journal of Medical Speech-Language Pathology, 3*, 15–26.

Thompson, E. C., Murdoch, B. E., and Stokes, P. D. (1995). Tongue function in subjects with upper motor neuron type dysarthria following cerebrovascular accident. *Journal of Medical Speech-Language Pathology, 3*, 27–40.

Till, J. A., Yorkston, K. M., and Beukelman, D. R. (Eds.). (1994). *Motor speech disorders: Advances in assessment and treatment.* Baltimore: Paul H. Brookes.

Ziegler, W., and Hartmann, E. (1996). Perceptual and acoustic methods in the evaluation of dysarthric speech. In M. J. Ball and M. Duckworth (Eds.), *Advances in clinical phonetics* (pp. 91–114). Amsterdam: John Benjamins.

Dysarthrias: Management

Dysarthria is a collective term for a group of neurological speech disorders caused by damage to mechanisms of motor control in the central or peripheral nervous system. The dysarthrias vary in nature, depending on the particular neuromotor systems involved. Consequently, a number of issues are considered when devising a management approach for a particular patient. These issues include the type of dysarthria (reflecting the underlying neuromuscular status), the physiological processes involved, severity, and the expected course.

Management of the dysarthrias is generally focused on improving the intelligibility and naturalness of speech, or on helping the speaker convey more communicative intent using speech plus the environment, context, and augmentative aids. *Intelligibility* refers to the degree to which the listener is able to understand the acoustic signal (Kent et al., 1989). *Comprehensibility* refers to the dynamic process by which individuals convey communicative intent, using the acoustic signal plus all information available from the environment (Yorkston, Strand, and Kennedy, 1996). In conversational interaction, listeners take advantage of environmental cues such as facial expression, gestures, the situation, the topic, and so on. As the acoustic speech signal becomes more degraded, contextual information becomes more critical for maintaining comprehensibility.

Decisions regarding whether to focus treatment on intelligibility or on comprehensibility depend largely on the severity of the dysarthria. Management for mildly dysarthric individuals focuses on improving intelligibility and naturalness. Individuals with moderate levels of severity benefit from both intelligibility and comprehensibility approaches. Finally, management of very severe dysarthria often focuses on augmentative communication.

Management focus also depends on whether the dysarthria is associated with a condition in which physiological recovery is likely to occur (e.g., cerebrovascular accident) versus one in which the dysarthria is likely to get progressively worse (e.g., amyotrophic lateral sclerosis [ALS]). For patients with degenerative diseases such as ALS, early treatment may focus on maintaining intelligibility. Later in the disease progression, the focus of treatment is less on the acoustic signal and more on communicative interaction, maximizing listener support and environmental cues, allowing the patient to continue to use speech for a much longer period of time before having to use augmentative and alternative communication. Yorkston (1996) provides a comprehensive review of the treatment efficacy literature for the dysarthrias associated with a number of different neurological disorders.

Intelligibility

Deficits in intelligibility vary according to the type of dysarthria as well as the relative contribution of the basic physiological mechanisms involved in speech: respiration, phonation, resonance, and articulation. Medical (e.g., surgical, pharmacological), prosthetic (e.g., palatal lift), and behavioral interventions are used to improve the function of those physiological systems.

Behavioral intervention for respiratory support focuses on achieving and maintaining a consistent subglottal air pressure level, allowing adequate loudness and length of breath groups (Yorkston et al., 1999). Methods to improve respiratory support (Netsell and Daniel, 1979; Hixon, Hawley, and Wilson, 1982) often involve having the speaker blow and maintain target levels of water pressure (i.e., 5 cm H_2O) for 5 seconds. Sustained phonation tasks are also used, giving the speaker feedback on maintained loudness. Finally, individuals are encouraged to produce sentences with appropriate phrase lengths, focusing on maintaining adequate respiratory pressure. In each case, the clinician works to focus the speaker's attention and effort toward taking in more air and using more force with exhaled air. Occasionally speakers may release too much airflow during speech. Netsell (1995) has suggested the use of inspiratory checking, in which patients are taught to use the inspiratory muscles to counter the elastic recoil forces of the respiratory system. For individuals who exhibit discoordination (e.g., ataxic dysarthria), respiratory treatment is focused on helping the speaker consistently initiate phonation at appropriate inspiratory lung volume levels, taking the next breath at the appropriate phrase boundary, given the expiratory lung volume level.

Laryngeal system impairment frequently results in either hypophonia, in which the vocal folds do not achieve adequate closure for phonation (as in flaccid dysarthria, or the hypokinetic dysarthria that accompanies Parkinson's disease), or hyperphonia, in which the vocal folds exhibit too much closure (as in spastic dysarthria). Individuals with lower motor neuron deficits involving the laryngeal muscles may benefit from surgical intervention either to medialize the vocal fold or to augment the bulk of the fold. The most common procedure for medialization is a type I thyroplasty, often with arytenoid adduction (Isshiki, Okamura, and Ishikawa, 1975; Nasseri and Maragos, 2000). Teflon and autogenous fat are also used to increase the bulk of a paralyzed or atrophied fold (Heikki, 1998). Patients with myasthenia gravis are typically successfully treated with anticholinesterase drugs or with a thymectomy. This medical management usually results in improvement in their voice and vocal fatigue.

Behavioral treatment for hypophonia focuses on increasing glottal closure, but it also requires that the patient maximize respiratory pressures. For mild weakness, exercises to increase the patient's awareness of efficient glottal adduction, without extraneous supraglottic tension, are helpful. Effort closure techniques such as pushing and grunting may maximize vocal fold adduction (Rosenbek and LaPoint, 1985). The Lee Silverman Voice Therapy Program (Ramig et al., 1995, 1996) has been shown to be efficacious for individuals with Parkinson's disease and is a commonly used therapy technique to reduce the hypophonic aspects of their dysarthria.

Treatment of phonation due to laryngeal spasticity is difficult, and behavioral intervention typically is not successful for this group of patients. Techniques to facilitate head and neck relaxation as well as laryngeal relaxation, strategies to maximize efficiency of the respiratory system, and the use of postural control may be helpful. Patients with phonatory deficits due to laryngeal dystonia pose similar problems. Medical management, such as botulinum toxin injection, is frequently used to improve the vocal quality of individuals with spasmodic dysphonia and laryngeal dystonias.

Behavioral approaches to the treatment of resonance problems focus on increasing the strength and function of the soft palate, but researchers and clinicians disagree as to their effectiveness. Kuehn and Wachtel (1994) suggest the use of continuous positive airway pressure in a resistance exercise program to strengthen the velopharyngeal muscles. A common prosthetic approach is to use a palatal lift, which is a rigid appliance that covers the hard palate and extends along the surface of the soft palate, raising it to the pharyngeal wall. Palatal lifts should be considered for patients who are consistently unable to achieve velopharyngeal closure and who have relatively isolated velopharyngeal impairment.

Treatment focused on improving articulation often uses the hierarchical practice of selected syllable, words and phrases (Robertson, 2001). However, because articulatory imprecision may be due to reduced respiratory support, velopharyngeal insufficiency, or rate control, the treatment of articulation is not always focused on improving the place and manner of articulatory contacts. When specific work on improving articulatory function is warranted, behavioral approaches involve focusing the speaker's attention on increased effort for bigger and stronger movements. Compensatory strategies such as using a different place of articulation or exaggerating selected articulatory movements may be used (DeFao and Schaefer, 1983). The use of minimal contrasts (tie/sigh) or intelligibility drills (having the speaker produce a carefully selected set of stimulus words) focus the speaker's attention on making specific sound contrasts salient and clear. Strength training is sometimes advocated, but only when the speaker is habitually generating less force than is necessary for speech and has the capacity to increase strength with effort. Strengthening is most appropriate for speakers with flaccid dysarthria; it is contraindicated for patients with disorders such as myasthenia gravis, in which muscular activity causes increasing weakness, and for patients with degenerative disorders such as ALS.

Surgical and medical management may also improve articulation. Neural anastomosis is sometimes used to improve function to a damaged nerve, usually the seventh cranial nerve (Daniel and Guitar, 1978). Botulinum toxin has been used to improve speech in speakers with orofacial and mandibular dystonias (Schulz and Ludlow, 1991). Although pharmacological treatment is frequently used to decrease limb spasticity, its effects on articulation are less clear (Duffy, 1995). Medications to decrease tremor or chorea sometimes help improve speech by reducing the extraneous movement.

Rate control is frequently the focus of treatment for dysarthric individuals. Yorkston et al. (1999) point out that this variable alone may result in the most dramatic changes in speech intelligibility for some individuals. Rate control is most effective for individuals with hypokinetic or ataxic dysarthria, but it may be appropriate for individuals with other types of dysarthria as well. Rate reduction improves intelligibility by facilitating increased precision of movement through the full range, by facilitating more appropriate breath group units, and by allowing listeners more time to process the degraded acoustic signal.

Behavioral approaches are geared toward slowing the rate by increasing consonant and vowel duration, increasing interword interval durations, and increasing pause time at phrasal boundaries, while working to avoid any diminution in speech naturalness. Instrumentation can also be helpful in rate control. In delayed auditory feedback, the speaker's own voice is fed back to the speaker through earphones after an interval delay. This technique typically slows the rate of speech and improves intelligibility. Visual biofeedback is used to facilitate the speaker's use of pause time and to slow the rate. Oscilloscopes can provide real-time feedback regarding rate over time. Computer screens can be used that cue the speaker to a target rate and mark the location of pauses (Beukelman, Yorkston, and Tice, 1997).

Comprehensibility

When there is evidence that the individual is able to improve respiratory, phonatory, articulatory, or resonating aspects of speech through behavioral, prosthetic, or medical management, intelligibility is the primary focus of management. However, as the severity of dysarthria increases, management focuses more on the communication interaction between the dysarthric speaker and his or her communicative partners. Management strategies are designed to help the listener maximize the use of context to improve ability to understand even a very degraded acoustic signal. Such strategies include being sure to have the listener's attention, making eye contact, providing (or asking for) the topic, signaling topic changes, reducing environmental noise, using simple but complete grammatical constructs, using predictable wording, adding gestures if possible, and using alphabet board supplementation. Also important is to adopt a consistent strategy for communication repair that is agreed upon by both speaker and listener. By working on communication interaction between speaker and listener, the dysarthric individual is often able to continue to use speech as a primary mode of communication.

See also DYSARTHRIAS: CHARACTERISTICS AND CLASSIFICATION.

—*Edythe A. Strand*

References

Beukelman, D. R., Yorkston, K. M., and Tice, R. (1997). *Pacer/tally rate measurement software*. Lincoln, NE: Tice Technology Services.

Daniel, R., and Guitar, B. (1978). EMG feedback and recovery of facial and speech gestures following neural anastomosis. *Journal of Speech and Hearing Disorders, 43*, 9–20.

DeFao, A., and Schaefer, C. (1983). Bilateral facial paralysis in a preschool child: Oral-facial and articulatory characteristics. A case study. In W. Berry (Ed.), *Clinical dysarthria* (pp. 165–190). Autsin, TX: Pro-Ed.

Duffy, J. (1995). *Motor speech disorders: Substrates, differential diagnosis, and management*. St. Louis: Mosby.

Heiki, R. (1998). Vocal fold augmentation by injection of autologous fascia. *Laryngoscope, 108*, 51–54.

Hixon, T., Hawley, J., and Wilson, K. (1982). An around-the-house device for the clinical determination of respiratory driving pressure: A note on making the simple even simpler. *Journal of Speech and Hearing Disorders, 48*, 413–415.

Isshiki, N., Okamura, H., and Ishikawa, T. (1975). Thyroplasty type I (lateral compression) for dysphonia due to vocal cord paralysis or atrophy. *Acta Oto-Laryngologica, 80*, 465–473.

Kent, R., Weismer, G., Kent, J., and Rosenbek, J. (1989). Toward phonetic intelligibility testing in dysarthria. *Journal of Speech and Hearing Disorders, 54*, 482–499.

Kuehn, D., and Wachtel, J. (1994). CPAP therapy for treating hypernasality following closed head injury. In J. A. Till, K. Yorkston, and D. Beukelman (Eds.), *Motor speech disorders: Advances in assessment and treatment* (pp. 207–212). Baltimore: Paul H. Brookes.

Nasseri, S. S., and Maragos, N. E. (2000). Combination thyroplasty and the "twisted larynx": Combined type IV and type I thyroplasty for superior laryngeal nerve weakness. *Journal of Voice, 14*, 104–111.

Netsell, R. (1995). Speech rehabilitation for individuals with unintelligible speech and dysarthria: The respiratory and velopharyngeal systems. *Neurophysiology and Neurogenic Speech Language Disorders, 5*, 6–9.

Netsell, R., and Daniel, B. (1979). Dysarthria in adults: Physiologic approach to rehabilitation. *Archives of Physical Medicine and Rehabilitation, 60*, 502.

Ramig, L., Countryman, S., O'Brien, C., Hoehn, M., and Thompson, L. (1996). Intensive speech treatment for patients with Parkinson's disease: Short- and long-term comparison of two techniques. *Neurology, 47*, 1496–1504.

Ramig, L., Countryman, S., Thompson, L., and Horii, Y. (1995). Comparison of two forms of intensive speech treatment for Parkinson disease. *Journal of Speech and Hearing Research, 38*, 1232–1251.

Robertson, S. (2001). The efficacy of oro-facial and articulation exercises in dysarthria following stroke. *International Journal of Language and Communication Disorders, 36*(Suppl.), 292–297.

Rosenbek, J., and LaPoint, L. (1985). The dysarthrias: Description, diagnosis, and treatment. In D. Johns (Ed.), *Clinical management of neurogenic communication disorders* (pp. 97–152). Boston: Little, Brown.

Schulz, G., and Ludlow, C. (1991). Botulinum treatment for orolingual-mandibular dystonia: Speech effects. In C. Moore, K. Yorkston, and D. Beukelman (Eds.), *Dysarthria and apraxia of speech: Perspectives in management* (pp. 227–242). Baltimore: Paul H. Brookes.

Yorkston, K. (1996). Treatment efficacy in dysarthria. *Journal of Speech, Language, and Hearing Research, 39*, S46–S57.

Yorkston, K. M., Beukelman, D., Strand, E., and Bell, K. (1999). *Clinical management of motor speech disorders*. Boston: Little, Brown.

Yorkston, K., Strand, E., and Kennedy, M. (1996). Comprehensibility of dysarthric speech: Implications for assessment and treatment planning. *American Journal of Speech-Language Pathology, 5*, 55–66.

Further Readings

Adams, S. (1994). Accelerating speech in a case of hypokinetic dysarthria: Descriptions and treatment. In J. Till, K. Yorkston, and D. Beukelman (Eds.), *Motor speech disorders: Advances in assessment and treatment*. Baltimore: Paul H. Brookes.

Aronson, A. E. (1990). *Clinical voice disorders*. New York: Thieme.

Bellaire, K., Yorkston, K., and Beukelman, D. (1986). Modification of breath patterning to increase naturalness of a mildly dysarthric speaker. *Journal of Communicative Disorders, 19,* 271–280.

Cannito, M., Yorkston, K., and Beukelman, D. (1998). *Neuromotor speech disorders.* Baltimore: Paul H. Brookes.

Darley, F., Aronson, A., and Brown, J. (1969a). Differential diagnostic patterns of dysarthria. *Journal of Speech and Hearing Research, 12,* 246–269.

Darley, F., Aronson, A., and Brown, J. (1969b). Clusters of deviant speech dimensions in the dysarthrias. *Journal of Speech and Hearing Research, 12,* 462–496.

Darley, F., Aronson, A., and Brown, J. (1975). *Motor speech disorders.* Philadelphia: Saunders.

Dworkin, J. (1991). *Motor speech disorders: A treatment guide.* St. Louis: Mosby.

Hanson, W., and Metter, E. (1983). DAF speech modification in Parkinson's disease: A report of two cases. In W. Berry (Ed.), *Clinical dysarthria.* Boston: College Hill Press.

Jankovic, J. (1989). Blepharospasm and oromandibular-laryngeal-cervical dystonia: A controlled trial of botulinum A toxin therapy. In S. Fahn (Ed.), *Advances in neurology,* Vol. 50. New York: Raven Press.

Liebson, E., Walsh, M., Jankowiak, J., and Albert, M. (1994). Pharmacotherapy for posttraumatic dysarthria. *Neuropsychiatry, Neuropsychology, and Behavioral Neurology, 7,* 122–124.

McHenry, M., Wilson, R., and Minton, J. (1994). Management of multiple physiologic system deficits following traumatic brain injury. *Journal of Medical Speech-Language Pathology, 2,* 58–74.

McNeil, M. (Ed.). (1997). *Clinical management of sensorimotor speech disorders.* New York: Thieme.

McNeil, M., Rosenbek, J., and Aronson, A. (Eds.). (1984). *The dysarthrias: Physiology, acoustic perception, and management,* San Diego: Singular Publishing Group.

Moore, C., Yorkston, K., and Beukelman, D. (1991). *Dysarthria and apraxia of speech: Perspectives on management.* Baltimore: Paul H. Brookes.

Netsell, R., and Rosenbek, J. (1985). *Treating the dysarthrias: Speech and language evaluation in neurology. Adult Disorders.* New York: Grune and Stratton.

Ramig, L. (1992). The role of phonation in speech intelligibility: A review and preliminary data from patients with Parkinson's disease. In R. Kent (Ed.), *Intelligibility in speech disorders.* Amsterdam: John Benjamin.

Ramig, L., and Dromey, C. (1996). Aerodynamic mechanisms underlying treatment-related changes in vocal intensity in patients with Parkinson's disease. *Journal of Speech and Hearing Research, 39,* 798–807.

Robin, D., Yorkston, K., and Beukelman, D. (1996). *Disorder of motor speech.* Baltimore: Paul H. Brookes.

Rubow, R. (1984). The role of feedback, reinforcement, and compliance on training and transfer in biofeedback-based rehabilitation of motor speech disorders. In M. McNeil, J. Rosenbek, and A. Aronson (Eds.), *The dysarthrias: Physiology, acoustic perception, and management.* San Diego, CA: Singular Publishing Group.

Rubow, R., and Swift, E. (1985). A microcomputer-based wearable biofeedback device to improve transfer of treatment in parkinsonian dysarthria. *Journal of Speech and Hearing Disorders, 49,* 26.

Till, J., Yorkston, K., and Beukelman, D. (1994). *Motor speech disorders: Advances in assessment and treatment.* Baltimore: Paul H. Brookes.

Vogel, D., and Miller, L. (1991). A top down approach to treatment of dysarthric speech. In D. Vogel and M. Cannito (Eds.), *Treating disorders speech motor control: For clinician, by clinicians.* Austin, TX: Pro-Ed.

Yorkston, K., and Beukelman, D. (Eds.). (1989). *Recent advances in clinical dysarthria.* Boston: College-Hill Press.

Yorkston, K., Hammen, V., Beukelman, D., and Traynor, C. (1990). The effect of rate control on the intelligibility and naturalness of dysarthric speech. *Journal of Speech and Hearing Disorders, 55,* 550–561.

Yorkston, K., Honsinger, M., Beukelman, D., and Taylor, T. (1989). The effects of palatal lift fitting on the perceived articulatory adequacy of dysarthric speakers. In K. Yorkston and D. Beukelman (Eds.), *Recent advances in clinical dysarthria.* Boston: College-Hill Press.

Yorkston, K., Miller, R., and Strand, E. (1995). *Management of speech and swallowing in degenerative neurologic disease.* Tucson, AZ: Communication Skill Builders.

Dysphagia, Oral and Pharyngeal

"Dysphagia" is an impaired ability to swallow. Dysphagia can result from anatomic variation or neuromuscular impairment anywhere from the lips to the stomach. Although some investigators choose to consider the voluntary oral preparatory stage of deglutition as a separate stage, swallowing is traditionally described as a three-stage event (oral, pharyngeal, and esophageal). Historically, research as well as evaluation and treatment of dysphagia were directed primarily toward the esophageal stage, which is generally treated by a gastroenterologist. However, over the past few decades, speech-language pathologists have become increasingly responsible for the research in, as well as the diagnosis and treatment of, the oral and pharyngeal aspects of deglutition.

The neuroanatomical substrate of dysphagia reflects lower motor neuron innervation by cranial nerves V, VII, IX, X, and XII. Dysphagia can result from unilateral or bilateral cortical insult. Within the cortex, primary sites that contribute to deglution include the premotor cortex, primary motor cortex, primary somatosensory cortex, insula, and the ventroposterior medial nucleus of the thalamus (Alberts et al., 1992; Daniels, Foundas, Iglesia, et al., 1996; Daniels and Foundas, 1997). Other portions of the cortical system have also been found to be active during swallowing (Hamdy et al., 1999, 2001; Martin et al., 2001).

Dysphagia is associated with an increased risk of developing malnutrition and respiratory complications such as aspiration pneumonia. In a study by Schmidt et al. (1994), the odds ratio that pneumonia would develop was 7.6 times greater for stroke patients who were identified as aspirators than for stroke patients who did not aspirate. Furthermore, the odds ratio of dying was 9.2 times greater for patients who aspirated thickened viscosities than for those who did not aspirate or who aspirated only thin fluids. Davalos et al. (1996) studied the effects of dysphagia on nutritional status in stroke patients who had similar nutritional status at the time of hospital admission. One week after the stroke, 48.3% of patients who developed dysphagia while in the hospi-

Table 1. Clinical Signs Suggestive of Dysphagia in Adults

Difficulty triggering the swallow
Difficulty managing oral secretions, with or without drooling
Abnormal or absent laryngeal elevation during swallow
  attempts
Choking or coughing during or after intake of food or liquid
Wet-sounding cough
Wet, gurgly voice quality
Decreased oral sensation
Weak sign of the cough
Prolonged oral preparation with food
Inability to clear the mouth of food after intake
Absent gag reflex
Food or liquid leaking from a tracheostomy site
Fullness or tightness in the throat (globus sensation)
Food or liquid leaking from the nose
Regurgitation of food
Sensation of food sticking in the throat or sternal region
Xerostomia (dry mouth)
Odynophagia (pain on swallowing)
Repeated incidents of upper respiratory infections with or
  without a diagnosis of aspiration pneumonia
Tightness or pain in the chest, particularly after eating or
  when lying down
Heartburn or indigestion
Unintended weight loss not related to disease

tal were malnourished, while only 13.6% of patients without dysphagia were malnourished. In a study of the nutritional status of patients admitted to a rehabilitation service, 65% of patients admitted with stroke and dysphagia were malnourished (Finestone et al., 1995).

Inadequate nutrition negatively affects the ability of the immune system to fight disease and contributes to the development of respiratory and cardiac insufficiency, the formation of decubitus ulcers, and impaired gastrointestinal function. The already comprised patient can become increasingly comprised, which prolongs the hospital length of stay and increases medical costs.

Certain clinical signs help to alert health care providers to the likely presence of dysphagia. Table 1 lists commonly observed clinical signs that are suggestive of dysphagia in the adult population. The absence of any or all of these signs does *not* indicate that a patient has a safe swallow or that the patient is able to ingest an adequate number of calories by mouth to remain properly nourished. For example, a diminished or absent gag has not been found to distinguish aspirators from non-aspirators (Horner and Massey, 1988). Many of these signs can be indicative of a serious medical illness. Therefore, patients who exhibit these signs and who have not been seen by a physician should be referred for medical examination.

Although clinical indicators have been found to have a relationship to laryngeal penetration, a significant number of patients who aspirate do so with no clinical indication. The incidence of silent aspiration is very high, and the difficulty of detecting it is suggested by the following: (1) Discriminant analysis of 11 clinical indicators resulted in identification of the presence of aspiration in only 66% of patients (Linden, Kuhlemeier, and Patterson, 1993). (2) In a heterogeneous group of 1101

patients with dysphagia, 276 (59%) of the 469 patients who aspirated were found to have silent aspiration (Smith et al., 1999). (3) When 47 stroke patients with mixed sites of lesions were examined, 24 (51%) of the patients were found to aspirate; of those 24 patients, 11 (46%) were silent aspirators (Horner and Massey, 1988). (4) In a study of 107 patients in a rehabilitation facility, 43 (40%) were found to aspirate on videofluoroscopic examination; however, clinical evaluation identified only 18 (42%) of the aspirators (Splaingard et al., 1988). Because of the additional expense encountered in caring for patients with respiratory or nutritional complications, studies such as these support the argument that money, as well as life, can be saved when patients are properly evaluated.

Dysphagia can occur at any age across the life span. Among young adults, traumatic brain injury is a not uncommon cause of acquired dysphagia, whereas elderly individuals are more likely to acquire dysphagia as a result of illness. However, young adults are also susceptible to the same causes of dysphagia as the elderly. Neurological disorders take a particular toll: it has been estimated that 300,000–600,000 persons per year experience dysphagia secondary to neurological disorders, and the greatest percentage of these experience dysphagia secondary to stroke (Doggett et al., 2001). After stroke and neurological disease, the most frequent causes of dysphagia in adults include muscle disease, head and neck surgery, radiation to the head and neck, dementia, motor end-plate disease, traumatic brain injury, systemic disease, cervical spine disease, medication effects, and senescent changes in the sensorimotor system.

Evaluation and Treatment

There are various methods for studying the swallow. The choice of method for a particular patient depends on the information that is sought. When a patient is first seen, the assessment begins with a clinical examination (Perlman et al., 1991). The clinical examination provides important information that assists in the decision-making process, but it is not intended to identify the underlying variables that result in difficulty with oral intake. Furthermore, this examination provides no information relative to the pharyngeal stage of the swallow and does not elicit adequate information to determine proper therapy. Therefore, the clinician will turn to one or more imaging modalities or other specific techniques.

Videofluoroscopy is the most frequently used assessment technique because it provides the most complete body of information. Interpretation of this examination is performed after observation of no less than two dozen events within the oral cavity, pharynx, and larynx. For most patients, this is the only instrumental procedure that will be performed.

Endoscopy permits the examiner to evaluate the status of vocal fold function, the extent of vallecular or pyriform sinus stasis, and the presence of spillover or of delayed initiation of the pharyngeal stage of the swallow (Langmore, Schatz, and Olsen, 1988; Aviv et al., 2000). Additionally, the view of velar function is superior to that obtained with videofluoroscopy. Information relating to the oral stage of deglutition, the extent of elevation of the hyoid bone, or information on the larynx or pharynx during the moment of swallow is not observed with endoscopy.

Ultrasound allows for observation of the motion of the tongue (Sonies, 1991). Additionally, the shadow reflected from the hyoid bone permits the examiner to observe and to measure the displacement of the hyoid. The advantages to using ultrasound for assessing the oral stage of the swallow are the absence of exposure to ionizing radiation and the fact that the parent can hold an infant or small child and feed the child a familiar food while the examination is being performed. The information obtainable with ultrasound is restricted to the oral stage of deglutition. When a small child has a tracheotomy tube, it is often extremely difficult to obtain a good ultrasound image, because the tracheostomy tube prohibits good transducer placement.

Muscle paralysis is best determined with intramuscular electromyography (Cooper and Perlman, 1997; Perlman et al., 1999). In the examination of swallowing, it is advisable to use bipolar hooked wire electrodes, because needle electrodes can cause discomfort and the subject may alter the swallowing pattern.

Respirodeglutometry (RDG) is a method for assessing the coordination of respiration and deglutition (Perlman, Ettema, and Barkmeier, 2000). This technique is presently being investigated to determine the physiological correlates of RDG output and to determine changes in the respiratory-swallowing pattern as a function of age and various medical diagnoses.

Decisions regarding behavioral, medical, or surgical intervention are made once the evaluation has been completed. Therapeutic intervention is determined as a function of the anatomical and physiological observations that were made during the evaluation process. Specific treatments are beyond the scope of this discussion but can be found in textbooks listed in Further Readings.

—Adrienne L. Perlman

References

Alberts, M. J., Horner, J., Gray, L., and Brazer, S. R. (1992). Aspiration after stroke: Lesion analysis by brain MRI. Dysphagia, 7, 170–173.

Aviv, J., Kaplan, S., Thomson, J., Spitzer, J., Diamond, B., and Close, L. (2000). The safety of flexible endoscopic evaluation of swallowing with sensory testing (FEESST): An analysis of 500 consecutive evaluations. Dysphagia, 15, 39–44.

Cooper, D., and Perlman, A. (1997). Electromyography in the functional and diagnostic testing of deglutition. In A. Perlman and K. Schulze-Delrieu (Eds.), Deglutition and its disorders. San Diego, CA: Singular Publishing Group.

Daniels, S., and Foundas, A. (1997). The role of the insular cortex in dysphagia. Dysphagia, 12, 146–156.

Daniels, S., Foundas, A., Iglesia, G., and Sullivan, M. (1996). Lesion site in unilateral stroke patients with dysphagia. Journal of Stroke and Cerebrovascular Disease, 6, 30–34.

Davalos, A., Ricart, W., Gonzalez-Huix, F., Soler, S., Marrugat, J., Molins, A., et al. (1996). Effect of malnutrition after acute stroke on clinical outcome. Stroke, 27, 1028–1032.

Doggett, D., Tappe, K., Mitchell, M., Chapell, R., and Coates, V. (2001). Prevention of pneumonia in elderly stroke patients by systematic diagnosis and treatment of dysphagia: An evidence-based comprehensive analysis of the literature. Dysphagia, 16, 279–295.

Finestone, H., Greene-Finestone, L., Wilson, E., and Teasell, R. (1995). Malnutrition in stroke patients on the rehabilitation service and at follow-up: Prevalence and predictors. Archives of Physical Medicine and Rehabilitation, 76, 310–316.

Hamdy, S., Aziz, Q., Thompson, D., and Rothwell, J. (2001). Physiology and pathophysiology of the swallowing area of the human motor cortex. Neural Plast., 8, 91–97.

Hamdy, S., Mikulis, D., Crawley, A., Xue, S., Lau, H., Henry, S., et al. (1999). Cortical activation during human volitional swallowing: An event-related fMRI study. American Journal of Physiology, 277, G219–G225.

Horner, J., and Massey, E. W. (1988). Silent aspiration following stroke. Neurology, 38, 317–319.

Langmore, S. E., Schatz, K., and Olsen, N. (1988). Fiberoptic endoscopic examination of swallowing safety: A new procedure. Dysphagia, 2, 216–219.

Linden, P., Kuhlemeier, K., and Patterson, C. (1993). The probability of correctly predicting subglottic penetration from clinical observations. Dysphagia, 8, 170–179.

Martin, R. E., Goodyear, B. G., Gati, J. S., and Raiv, S. M. (2001). Cerebral cortical representation of automatic and volitional swallowing in humans. Journal of Neurophysiology, 85, 938–950.

Perlman, A., Ettema, S., and Barkmeier, J. (2000). Respiratory and acoustic signals associated with bolus passage through the pharynx. Dysphagia, 15, 89–94.

Perlman, A. L., Langmore, S., Milianti, F., Miller, R., Mills, H., and Zenner, P. (1991). Comprehensive clinical examination of orophayngeal swallowing function: Veterans Administration procedure. Seminars in Speech and Language, 12, 246–254.

Perlman, A., Palmer, P., McCulloch, T., and VanDaele, D. (1999). Electromyographic activity from human submental, laryngeal, and pharyngeal muscles during swallowing. Journal of Applied Physiology, 86, 1663–1669.

Schmidt, J., Holas, M., Halvorson, K., and Reding, M. (1994). Videofluoroscopic evidence of aspiration predicts pneumonia and death but not dehydration following stroke. Dysphagia, 9, 7–11.

Smith, C. H., Logemann, J. A., Colangelo, L. A., Rademaker, A. W., and Pauloski, B. R. (1999). Incidence and patient characteristics associated with silent aspiration in the acute care setting. Dysphagia, 14, 1–7.

Sonies, B. (1991). Normal and abnormal swallowing: Imaging in diagnosis and therapy. New York: Springer-Verlag.

Splaingard, M. L., Hutchins, B., Sulton, L. D., and Chaundhuri, G. (1988). Aspiration in rehabilitation patients: Videofluoroscopy vs bedside clinical assessment. Archives of Physical Medicine and Rehabilitation, 69, 637–640.

Further Readings

Huckabee, M., and Pelletier, C. (1999). Management of adult neurogenic dysphagia. San Diego, CA: Singular Publishing Group.

Logemann, J. (1998). Evaluation and treatment of swallowing disorders (2nd ed.). Austin, TX: Pro-Ed.

Logemann, J. A. (1999). Behavioral management for oropharyngeal dysphagia. *Folia Phoniatrica et Logopedica, 51,* 199–212.

Lundy, D. S., Smith, C., Colangelo, L., Sullivan, P. A., Logemann, J. A., Lazarus, C. L., et al. (1999). Aspiration: Cause and implications. *Otolaryngology–Head and Neck Surgery, 120,* 474–478.

McHorney, C. A., Bricker, D. E., Robbins, J., Kramer, A. E., Rosenbek, J. C., Chignell, K. A. (2000). The SWAL-QOL outcomes tool for oropharyngeal dysphagia in adults: II. Item reduction and preliminary scaling. *Dysphagia, 15,* 122–133.

Perlman, A., and Schulze-Delrieu, K. (Eds.). (1997). *Deglutition and its disorders.* San Diego, CA: Singular Publishing Group.

Preiksaitis, H., Mayrand, S., Robins, K., and Diamant, N. E. (1992). Coordination of respiration and swallowing: Effect of bolus volume in normal adults. *American Journal of Physiology, 263,* R624–R630.

Rosenbeck, J., Robbins, J., Roecker, J., Coyle, J., and Wood, J. (1996). A penetration-aspiration scale. *Dysphagia, 11,* 93–98.

Sonies, B. (Ed.). (1997). *Instrumental imaging technologies and procedures.* Gaithersburg, MD: Aspen.

Early Recurrent Otitis Media and Speech Development

Otitis media can be defined as inflammation of the middle ear mucosa, resulting from an infectious process (Scheidt and Kavanagh, 1986). When the inflammation results in the secretion of effusion, or liquid, into the middle ear cavity, the terms otitis media with effusion (OME) and middle ear effusion (MEE) are often used. Middle ear effusion may be present during the period of acute inflammation (when it is known as acute otitis media), and it may persist for some time after the acute inflammation has subsided (Bluestone and Klein, 1996a).

The prevalence of OME in young children is remarkably high. OME has been described as one of the most common infectious diseases of childhood (Bluestone and Klein, 1996a) and evidence from several large studies supports this conclusion. For example, in a prospective epidemiologic study of 2253 children enrolled by age 2 months, Paradise et al. (1997) reported that nearly 80% of children had at least one episode of OME by 12 months of age; more than 90% had an episode by age 24 months. The mean cumulative percentage of days with MEE was 20.4% between 2 and 12 months of age, and 16.6% between 12 and 24 months. Low socioeconomic status, male sex, and amount of exposure to other children were associated with an increased prevalence of OME during the first 2 years of life (Paradise et al., 1997).

The literature addressing the hypothesis that early recurrent OME poses a threat to children's speech and language development is large and contentious (for reviews, see Stool et al., 1994; Shriberg, Flipsen, et al., 2000). OME has been reported to result in adverse

effects, no effects, and small beneficial effects (e.g., Shriberg, Friel-Patti, et al., 2000), sometimes within the same study. Substantive methodological differences may account for much of the disparity in findings, with the method by which OME is diagnosed in different studies being critically important. The gold standard for diagnosing OME is an examination of the tympanic membrane via pneumatic otoscopy, after any necessary removal of cerumen, to determine whether indicators of effusion such as bulging, retraction, bubbling, or abnormal mobility are present (Stool et al., 1994; Bluestone and Klein, 1996b). Behavioral symptoms such as irritability are neither sensitive nor specific to the condition, and the validity of parental judgments concerning the frequency or duration of episodes of OME is poor even when repeated feedback is provided (Anteunis et al., 1999). In addition, it is important that OME be documented prospectively rather than via retrospective reports or chart reviews, because a substantial percentage of apparently healthy and symptom-free children are found to have OME on otoscopic assessment (Bluestone and Klein, 1996a).

A second important difference among studies of OME and speech development is the extent to which hearing levels are documented. The hypothesis that OME poses a threat to speech or language development is typically linked to the assumption that effusion causes conductive hearing loss, which prevents children from perceiving and processing speech input in the usual fashion (e.g., K. Roberts, 1997). However, the presence of effusion is a poor predictor of hearing loss. Although hearing thresholds for the majority of children with MEE fall between 21 and 30 dB (mild to moderate degrees of impairment), thresholds from 0 to 50 dB are not uncommon (Bess, 1986). Hearing thresholds must be measured directly to determine whether OME has effects on development independent of its variable effects on hearing (e.g., Shriberg, Friel-Patti, et al., 2000).

Studies also vary with respect to their ability to separate the contribution of OME to poor developmental outcome from the effects of other variables with which OME is known to be associated, such as sex and socioeconomic status. As noted earlier, OME is significantly more prevalent in males than in females, and in children from less privileged backgrounds than in their more privileged counterparts (Paradise et al., 1997; Peters et al., 1997). Statistical procedures are necessary to control for such confounding in order to distinguish the effects of OME from those of other variables. Several recent studies have shown that after controlling for socioeconomic confounds, OME accounts for little if any of the variance in developmental outcome measures (e.g., J. E. Roberts et al., 1998; Paradise et al., 2000).

Finally, studies have also differed substantially in the measures used to document the outcome variable of speech development and in the extent to which effect sizes for significant differences on outcome measures are reported (cf. Casby, 2001). No accepted standard metric for speech delay or disorder currently exists, although the Speech Disorders Classification System developed by

Shriberg et al. (1997) represents an important advance toward meeting this need. Instead, the effects of OME on speech have been sought on a wide range of articulatory and phonological measures, not all of which are known to be predictive of eventual speech outcome (e.g., Rvachew et al., 1999).

When these cautions are borne in mind, the literature on early recurrent otitis media and speech development suggests converging evidence that OME in and of itself has a negligible relationship to early speech development. Several prospective investigations have shown little or no relationship between cumulative duration of otitis media (documented otoscopically) and measures of speech production in otherwise healthy children. In a longitudinal study of 55 low-SES children, J. E. Roberts et al. (1988) found no correlation between OME and number of consonant errors or phonological processes on a single-word test of articulation at ages 3, 4, 5, 6, 7, or 8 years. Shriberg, Friel-Patti, et al. (2000) examined ten speech measures derived from spontaneous speech samples obtained from 70 otherwise healthy, middle to upper middle class 3-year-olds who were classified according to the number of episodes of OME from 6 to 18 months of age; only one significant speech difference was found, in which the group with more OME paradoxically obtained higher intelligibility scores than the group with fewer bouts of OME. Paradise et al. (2000) likewise found no relationship between cumulative duration of MEE and scores on the Percentage of Consonants Correct–Revised measure (PCC-R; Shriberg, 1993) in 241 sociodemographically diverse children at age 3 years. Paradise et al. (2001) reported that PCC-R scores from children with even more persistent MEE from 2 to 36 months of age did not differ significantly from those of children with the less persistent levels of effusion reported by Paradise et al. (2000). Further, children with persistent and substantial MEE who were randomly assigned to undergo prompt tympanostomy tube placement had no better PCC-R scores at age 3 than children who underwent tube placement after a delay of 6–9 months, during which their MEE persisted (Paradise et al., 2001). These findings of little or no relationship between OME and speech development mirror those of several recent reports showing negligible associations between early OME and later oral and written language performance (Peters et al., 1997; Casby, 2001).

By contrast with these negative findings concerning the impact of OME, several studies in which hearing was documented showed poorer speech outcomes for children with elevated hearing thresholds. In a sample of 70 middle to upper middle class 3-year-olds who received otoscopic evaluations every 6 weeks and hearing evaluations every 6 months between 6 and 18 months of age, Shriberg, Friel-Patti, et al. (2000) reported that children with hearing loss, defined as average thresholds $\geq$20 dB (HL) during one evaluation between 6 and 18 months of age, had a significantly increased risk of scoring more than 1.3 standard deviations below the sample mean on several percentage-consonants-correct metrics. Shriberg et al. note the need for some caution in interpreting these findings, given that increased risk was not found across all speech metrics and that confidence intervals for risk estimates were wide. In addition, the results of structural equation modeling suggested that hearing loss did not operate directly to lower speech performance, but rather was mediated significantly by language performance, providing another indication of the need for multifactorial approaches to identifying the factors and pathways involved in normal and abnormal speech development.

Although the best available current evidence suggests that OME itself does not represent a significant risk to speech development in otherwise healthy children, the question of whether OME may contribute independently to outcome when it occurs in conjunction with other risk factors or health conditions (e.g., Wallace et al., 1996; J. E. Roberts et al., 1998; Shriberg, Flipsen, et al., 2000) remains open. Additional investigations that include prospective otoscopic diagnosis of OME; frequent and independent assessments of hearing; valid, reliable assessments of both medical and sociodemographic risk factors; and a multifactorial analytic strategy will be needed to answer this question.

See also OTITIS MEDIA: EFFECTS ON CHILDREN'S LANGUAGE.

—*Christine Dollaghan and Thomas Campbell*

References

Anteunis, L. J. C., Engel, J. A. M., Hendriks, J. J. T., and Manni, J. J. (1999). A longitudinal study of the validity of parental reporting in the detection of otitis media and related hearing impairment in infancy. *Audiology, 38*, 75–82.

Bess, F. H. (1986). Audiometric approaches used in the identification of middle ear disease in children. In J. F. Kavanagh (Ed.), *Otitis media and child development* (pp. 70–82). Parkton, MD: York Press.

Bluestone, C. D., and Klein, J. O. (1996a). Otitis media, atelectasis, and eustachian tube dysfunction. In C. D. Bluestone, S. E. Stool, and M. A. Kenna (Eds.), *Pediatric otolaryngology* (3rd ed., vol. 1, pp. 388–582). Philadelphia: Saunders.

Bluestone, C. D., and Klein, J. O. (1996b). Methods of examination: Clinical examination. In C. D. Bluestone, S. E. Stool, and M. A. Kenna (Eds.), *Pediatric otolaryngology* (3rd ed., vol. 1, pp. 150–164). Philadelphia: Saunders.

Casby, M. W. (2001). Otitis media and language development: A meta-analysis. *American Journal of Speech-Language Pathology, 10*, 65–80.

Paradise, J. L., Dollaghan, C. A., Campbell, T. F., Feldman, H. M., Bernard, B. S., Colborn, D. K., et al. (2000). Language, speech sound production, and cognition in three-year-old children in relation to otitis media in their first three years of life. *Pediatrics, 105*, 1119–1130.

Paradise, J. L., Feldman, H. M., Campbell, T. F., Dollaghan, C. A., Colborn, D. K., Bernard, B. S., et al. (2001). Effect of early or delayed insertion of tympanostomy tubes for persistent otitis media on developmental outcomes at the age of three years. *New England Journal of Medicine, 344*, 1179–1187.

Paradise, J. L., Rockette, H. E., Colborn, D. K., Bernard, B. S., Smith, C. G., Kurs-Lasky, M., et al. (1997). Otitis media in 2253 Pittsburgh-area infants: Prevalence and risk factors during the first two years of life. *Pediatrics, 9,* 318–333.

Peters, S. A. F., Grievink, E. H., van Bon, W. H. J., van den Bercken, J. H. L., and Schilder, A. G. M. (1997). The contribution of risk factors to the effect of early otitis media with effusion on later language, reading and spelling. *Developmental Medicine and Child Neurology, 39,* 31–39.

Roberts, J. E., Burchinal, M. R., Koch, M. A., Footo, M. M., and Henderson, F. W. (1988). Otitis media in early childhood and its relationship to later phonological development. *Journal of Speech and Hearing Disorders, 53,* 416–424.

Roberts, J. E., Burchinal, M. R., Zeisel, S. A., Neebe, E. C., Hooper, S. R., Roush, J., et al. (1998). Otitis media, the caregiving environment, and language and cognitive outcomes at 2 years. *Pediatrics, 102,* 346–354.

Roberts, K. (1997). A preliminary account of the effects of otitis media on 15-month-olds' categorization and some implications for early language learning. *Journal of Speech, Language, and Hearing Research, 40,* 508–518.

Rvachew, S., Slawinski, E. B., Williams, M., and Green, C. L. (1999). The impact of early onset otitis media on babbling and early language development. *Journal of the Acoustical Society of America, 105,* 467–475.

Scheidt, P. C., and Kavanagh, J. F. (1986). Common terminology for conditions of the middle ear. In J. F. Kavanagh (Ed.), *Otitis media and child development* (pp. xv–xvii). Parkton, MD: York Press.

Shriberg, L. D. (1993). Four new speech and prosody-voice measures for genetics research and other studies in developmental phonological disorders. *Journal of Speech and Hearing Research, 36,* 105–140.

Shriberg, L. D., Austin, D., Lewis, B. A., McSweeny, J. L., and Wilson, D. L. (1997). The Speech Disorders Classification System (SDCS): Extensions and lifespan reference data. *Journal of Speech, Language, and Hearing Research, 40,* 723–740.

Shriberg, L. D., Flipsen, P., Thielke, H., Kwiatkowski, J., Kertoy, M. K., Katcher, M. L., et al. (2000). Risk for speech disorder associated with early recurrent otitis media with effusion: Two retrospective studies. *Journal of Speech, Language, and Hearing Research, 43,* 79–99.

Shriberg, L. D., Friel-Patti, S., Flipsen, P., and Brown, R. L. (2000). Otitis media, fluctuant hearing loss, and speech-language outcomes: A preliminary structural equation model. *Journal of Speech, Language, and Hearing Research, 43,* 100–120.

Stool, S. E., Berg, A. O., Berman, S., et al. (1994, July). *Otitis media with effusion in young children: Clinical practice guideline No. 12* (AHCPR Publication No. 94-0622). Rockville, MD: Agency for Health Care Policy and Research.

Wallace, I. F., Gravel, J. S., Schwartz, R. G., and Ruben, R. J. (1996). Otitis media, communication style of primary caregivers, and language skills of 2 year olds: A preliminary report. *Developmental and Behavioral Pediatrics, 17,* 27–35.

Further Readings

Creps, C. L., and Vernon-Feagans, L. (2000). Infant daycare and otitis media: Multiple influences on children's later development. *Journal of Applied Developmental Psychology, 21,* 357–378.

Friel-Patti, S., and Finitzo, T. (1990). Language learning in a prospective study of otitis media with effusion in the first two years of life. *Journal of Speech and Hearing Research, 33,* 188–194.

Roberts, J. E., Wallace, I. F., and Henderson, F. W. (Eds.). (1997). *Otitis media in young children: Medical, develop-*

mental, and educational considerations. Baltimore: Paul H. Brookes.

Teele, D. W., Klein, J. O., Chase, C., Menyuk, P., and Rosner, B. A. (1990). Otitis media in infancy and intellectual ability, school achievement, speech, and language at age 7 years. *Journal of Infectious Diseases, 162,* 685–694.

Teele, D. W., Klein, J. O., Rosner, B. A., and the Greater Boston Otitis Media Study Group. (1984). Otitis media with effusion during the first three years of life and development of speech and language. *Pediatrics, 74,* 282–287.

Laryngectomy

Total laryngectomy is a surgical procedure to remove the larynx. Located in the neck, where it is commonly referred to as the Adam's apple, the larynx contains the vocal folds for production of voice for speech. Additionally, the larynx serves as a valve during swallowing to prevent food and liquids from entering the airway and lungs. When a total laryngectomy is performed, the patient loses his or her voice and must breathe through an opening created in the neck called a tracheostoma.

Total laryngectomy is usually performed to remove advanced cancers of the larynx, most of which arise from prolonged smoking or a combination of tobacco use and alcohol consumption. Laryngeal cancers account for less than 1% of all cancers. About 10,000 new cases of laryngeal cancer are diagnosed each year in the United States, with a male-female ratio approximately 4 to 1 (American Cancer Society, 2000). The Surveillance, Epidemiology and End Results (SEER) program of the National Cancer Institute (Ries et al., 2000) reports that laryngeal cancer rates rise sharply in the fifth, sixth, and first half of the seventh decades of life (Casper and Colton, 1998). The typical person diagnosed with cancer of the larynx is a 60-year-old man who is a heavy smoker with moderate to heavy alcohol intake (Casper and Colton, 1998). Symptoms of laryngeal cancer vary, depending on the exact site of the disease, but persistent hoarseness is common. Other signs include lowered pitch, sore throat, a lump in the throat, a lump in the neck, earache, difficulty swallowing, coughing, difficulty breathing, and audible breathing (National Cancer Institute, 1995). It is estimated that there are 50,000 laryngectomees (laryngectomized people) living in the United States today.

As a treatment of laryngeal cancer, total laryngectomy is a proven technique to control disease. The primary disadvantages of total laryngectomy are the loss of the vocal folds that produce voice for speech and the need for a permanent tracheostomy for breathing. Before the introduction of the extended partial laryngectomy, patients with cancer of the larynx were treated primarily with total laryngectomy (Weber, 1998). Today, early and intermediate laryngeal cancers can be cured with conservation operations that preserve voice, swallowing, and nasal breathing, and total laryngectomy is performed only in cases of very advanced cancers that are bilateral, extensive, and deeply invasive (Pearson, 1998). Radiation therapy is often administered before or after total laryngectomy. In addition, radiation therapy alone and sometimes in combination with chemotherapy has proved to be curative treatment for laryngeal cancer, depending on the site and stage of the disease (Chyle, 1998). Controversy and research continue over nonsurgical versus surgical intervention or a combination of these for advanced laryngeal cancer, weighing the issues of survival, preservation of function, and quality of life (Weber, 1998).

A person with laryngeal cancer and the family members have many questions about survival, treatment options, and the long-term consequences and outcomes of various treatments. An otolaryngologist is the physician who usually diagnoses cancer of the larynx and provides information about possible surgical interventions. A radiation oncologist is a physician consulted for opinions about radiation and chemotherapy approaches to management. If the patient decides to have a total laryngectomy, a speech pathologist meets with the patient and family before the operation to provide information on basic anatomy and physiology of normal breathing, swallowing, and speaking, and how these will change after removal of the larynx (Keith, 1995). Also, the patient is informed that, after a period of recovery and rehabilitation, and with a few modifications, most laryngectomized people return to the same vocational, home, and recreational activities they participated in prior to the laryngectomy.

Besides voicelessness, laryngectomized persons experience other changes. Since the nasal and oral tracts filter the air as well as provide moisture and warmth in normal breathing, laryngectomees often require an environment with increased humidity, and they may wear heat- and moisture-exchanging filters over their tracheostoma to replicate the functions of nasal and oral breathing (Grolman and Schouwenberg, 1998). There is no concern for aspiration of food and liquids into the lungs after total laryngectomy, because the respiratory and digestive tracts are completely separated and no longer share the pharynx as a common tract. Unless the tongue is surgically altered or extensive pharyngeal or esophageal reconstruction beyond total laryngectomy is performed, most laryngectomees return to a normal diet and have few complaints about swallowing other than that it may require additional effort (Logemann, Pauloski, and Rademaker, 1997).

There are nonspeech methods of communicating that can be used immediately after total laryngectomy. These include writing on paper or on a slate, pointing to letters or words or pictures on a speech or communication board, gesturing with pantomimes that are universally recognizable, using e-mail, typing on portable keyboards or speech-generating devices, and using life-line emergency telephone monitoring systems. None of these methods of communicating is as efficient or as personal as one's own speech.

A common fear of the laryngectomee is that he or she will never be able to speak without vocal folds. There are several methods of alaryngeal (without a larynx) speech. Immediately or soon after surgery, a laryngectomized person can make speech movements with the tongue and lips as before the surgery, but without voice. This silent speech is commonly referred to as "mouthing words" or "whispering"; however, unlike a normal whisper, air from the lungs does not move through the mouth after a laryngectomy. The effectiveness of the technique is variable and depends largely on the laryngectomee's ability to precisely articulate speech movements and the ability of others to recognize or "read" them.

Artificial larynges have been used since the first recorded laryngectomy in 1873 (Billroth and Gussenbauer, 1874). Speech with an artificial larynx, also known as an electrolarynx, can be an effective method of communicating after laryngectomy, and many people can use one of these instruments as early as a day or two after surgery. Most modern instruments are battery powered and produce a mechanical tone. Usually the device is pressed against the neck or under the chin at a location where it produces the best sound, and the person articulates this "voice" into speech. If the neck is too swollen after surgery or the skin is hard as a result of radiation therapy, the tone of the artificial larynx may not be conducted into the throat sufficiently for production of speech. In this circumstance it may be possible to use an oral artificial larynx with a plastic tube to place the tone directly into the mouth, where it is articulated into speech. Speech with an artificial larynx has a sound quality that is mechanical, yet a person who uses an artificial larynx well can produce intelligible speech in practically all communication situations, including over the telephone. Most laryngectomized people require training by a speech pathologist to use an artificial larynx optimally.

A laryngectomized person may be able to learn to use esophageal voice, also known as esophageal speech. For this method, commonly known as "burp speech," the person learns to use the esophagus (food tube) to produce voice. First the laryngectomee pumps or sucks air into the esophagus. Sound or "voice" is generated as the air trapped in the upper esophagus moves back up through the narrow junction of the pharynx and esophagus known as the PE segment. Then the voice is articulated into speech by the tongue and lips.

A key to producing successful esophageal speech is getting air into the esophagus consistently and efficiently, followed by immediate sound production for speech. Esophageal speech has distinct advantages over other alaryngeal speech techniques. The esophageal speaker requires no special equipment or devices, and the speaker's hands are not monopolized during conversation. A significant disadvantage of esophageal speech is that it takes a relatively long time to learn to produce voice that is adequate for everyday speech purposes. Additionally, insufficient loudness and a speaking rate that is usually slower than before laryngectomy are common concerns of esophageal speakers. Although some become excellent esophageal speakers, many do not attain a level of fluent speech sufficient for all communicative situations.

Tracheoesophageal puncture with a voice prosthesis is another method of alaryngeal voice production (Singer and Blom, 1980; Blom, 1998). During the surgery to remove the larynx or at a later time, the surgeon makes an opening (puncture) just inside and inferior to the superior edge of the tracheostoma. The opening is a tract through the posterior wall of the trachea and the anterior wall of the esophagus. Usually a catheter is placed in the opening and a prosthesis is placed a few days later. A speech pathologist specially trained in tracheoesophageal voice restoration measures the length of the tract between the trachea and the esophagus, and a silicone tube with a one-way valve—a voice prosthesis— is placed in the puncture site. The prosthesis is nonpermanent and must be replaced periodically. It does not generate voice itself. When the person exhales and the tracheostoma is covered with a thumb, finger, or special valve, air from the lungs moves up the trachea, through the prosthesis, into the upper esophagus, and through the PE segment to produce voice. Because lung air is used to produce voice with a tracheoesophageal puncture, the speech characteristics of pitch and loudness, rate, phrasing, and timing more closely resemble the laryngectomee's presurgical speech qualities than can be achieved with other forms of alaryngeal speech. For many laryngectomees, fluent speech can be achieved soon after placement of a voice prosthesis.

There are disadvantages associated with tracheoesophageal puncture. The laryngectomee may dislike using a thumb or finger to cover the tracheostoma when speaking, and use of a tracheostoma valve for hands-free speaking may not be possible. Expenses associated with tracheoesophageal puncture include those for initial training in the use and maintenance of the prosthesis with a speech pathologist and subsequent clinical visits for modification or replacement of the voice prosthesis, and ongoing costs of prosthesis-related supplies. If the PE segment is hypertonic and the tracheoesophageal voice is not satisfactorily fluent for conversation, or if it requires considerable effort to produce, injection of botulinum neurotoxin, commonly known as Botox, may be required (Hoffman and McCulloch, 1998; Lewin et al., 2001), or myotomy of the pharyngeal constrictor muscles may be considered (Hamaker and Chessman, 1998).

Historically, laryngectomees and speech pathologists have felt strongly about one form of alaryngeal speech being superior to others. In the 1960s, newly laryngectomized persons were discouraged from using artificial larynges, which were thought to delay or interfere with the learning of esophageal speech (Lauder, 1968). Today some think tracheoesophageal speech is superior because many laryngectomees are able to speak fluently and fairly naturally with this method only a few weeks after surgery. Others maintain that esophageal speech, with no reliance on a prosthesis or other devices, is the gold standard against which all other methods should be compared (Stone, 1998). Most believe any form of speech after laryngectomy is acceptable and should be encouraged, since speaking is a fundamental and essential part of being human.

People who undergo total laryngectomy experience the same emotions of shock, fear, stress, loss, depression, and grief as others with life-threatening illnesses. Along with regular medical follow-up to monitor for possible recurrence of cancer and to review all the body systems, laryngectomized persons may benefit from referral to other professionals and resources for psychological, marital, nutritional, rehabilitation, and financial concerns.

The International Association of Laryngectomees and the American Cancer Society provide services to laryngectomized persons. They sponsor peer support groups, provide speech therapy, and distribute educational materials on topics of interest, such as cardiopulmonary resuscitation for neck breathers, smoking cessation, and specialized products and equipment for laryngectomized persons.

See also ALARYNGEAL VOICE AND SPEECH REHABILITATION.

—*Jack E. Thomas*

References

American Cancer Society. (2000). *Cancer facts and figures 2000*. Washington, DC: Author.

Billroth, C. A. T., and Gussenbauer, C. (1874). Über die erste durch Th. Billroth am Menschen ausgeführte Kehlkopf Extirpation und die Anwendung eines kunstlichen Kehlkopes. *Archiv fur die Klinische Chirurgie, 17*, 343–356. Cited by R. L. Keith and J. C. Shanks in Historical highlights: Laryngectomee rehabilitation. In R. L. Keith and F. L. Darley (Eds.), *Laryngectomee rehabilitation* (pp. 1–48). Austin, TX: Pro-Ed.

Blom, E. D. (1998). Evolution of tracheoesophageal voice prosthesis. In E. D. Blom, M. I. Singer, and R. C. Hamaker (Eds.), *Tracheoesophageal voice restoration following total laryngectomy* (pp. 1–8). San Diego, CA: Singular Publishing Group.

Casper, J. K., and Colton, R. H. (1998). *Clinical manual for laryngectomy and head/neck cancer rehabilitation* (2nd ed.). San Diego, CA: Singular/Thomson Learning.

Chyle, V. (1998). Toxicity of primary radiotherapy for early stage cancers of the larynx. In T. Robbins and T. Murry (Eds.), *Head and neck cancer: Organ preservation, function, and rehabilitation* (pp. 19–21). San Diego, CA: Singular Publishing Group.

Grolman, W., and Schouwenberg, P. F. (1998). Postlaryngectomy airway humidification and air filtration. In E. D. Blom, M. I. Singer, and R. C. Hamaker (Eds.), *Tracheoesophageal voice restoration following total laryngectomy* (pp. 109–121). San Diego, CA: Singular Publishing Group.

Hamaker, R. C., and Cheesman, A. D. (1998). Surgical management of pharyngeal constrictor muscle hypertonicity. In E. D. Blom, M. I. Singer, and R. C. Hamaker (Eds.), *Tracheoesophageal voice restoration following total laryngectomy* (pp. 33–39). San Diego, CA: Singular Publishing Group.

Hoffman, H. T., and McCulloch, T. M. (1998). Botulinum neurotoxin for tracheoesophageal voice failure. In E. D. Blom, M. I. Singer, and R. C. Hamaker (Eds.), *Tracheoesophageal voice restoration following total laryngectomy* (pp. 83–87). San Diego, CA: Singular Publishing Group.

Keith, R. L. (1995). *Looking forward: A guidebook for the laryngectomee* (3rd ed.). New York: Thieme.

Lauder, E. (1968). The laryngectomee and the artificial larynx. *Journal of Speech and Hearing Disorders, 33*, 147–157.

Lewin, J. S., Bishop-Leone, J. K., Forman, A. D., and Diaz, E. M. (2001). Further experience with Botox injection for tracheoesophageal speech failure. *Head and Neck, 23*, 456–460.

Logemann, J. A., Pauloski, B. R., and Rademaker, A. W. (1997). Speech and swallowing rehabilitation for head and neck cancer patients. *Oncology, 11*, 651–659.

National Cancer Institute. (1995). *What you need to know about cancer of the larynx* (NIH Publication No. 95-1568). Bethesda, MD: Author.

Pearson, B. W. (1998). Surgical options in laryngeal cancer. In T. Robbins and T. Murry (Eds.), *Head and neck cancer: Organ preservation, function, and rehabilitation* (pp. 37–44). San Diego, CA: Singular Publishing Group.

Ries, L. A. G., Eisner, M. P., Kosary, C., Hankey, B. F., Miller, B. A., Clegg, L., et al. (Eds.). (2000). *SEER cancer statistics review, 1973–1997*. Bethesda, MD: National Cancer Institute.

Singer, M. I., and Blom, E. D. (1980). An endoscopic technique for restoration of voice after laryngectomy. *Annals of Otology, Rhinology, and Laryngology, 89*, 529–533.

Stone, R. E. (1998). Oral communication after laryngectomy. In T. Robbins and T. Murry (Eds.), *Head and neck cancer: Organ preservation, function, and rehabilitation* (pp. 59–71). San Diego, CA: Singular Publishing Group.

Weber, R. S. (1998). Advanced laryngeal cancer: Defining the issues. In T. Robbins and T. Murry (Eds.), *Head and neck cancer: Organ preservation, function, and rehabilitation* (pp. 33–36). San Diego, CA: Singular Publishing Group.

Further Readings

Doyle, P. C. (1994). *Foundations of voice and speech rehabilitation following laryngeal cancer*. San Diego, CA: Singular Publishing Group.

Graham, M. S. (1997). *The clinician's guide to alaryngeal speech therapy*. Boston: Butterworth-Heinemann.

Keith, R. L., and Thomas, J. E. (1995). *A handbook for the laryngectomee* (4th ed.). Austin, TX: Pro-Ed.

Rosenbaum, E. H., and Rosenbaum, I. (1998). *Cancer supportive care: A comprehensive guide for patients and their families*. Toronto: Somerville House Books.

Salmon, S. J., and Mount, K. H. (Eds.). (1998). *Alaryngeal speech rehabilitation: For clinicians by clinicians* (2nd ed.). Austin, TX: Pro-Ed.

Shanks, J. C., and Stone, R. E. (Eds.). (1983). *Help employ laryngectomized persons*. Stillwater, OK: National Clearinghouse of Rehabilitation Disorders, Oklahoma State University.

Mental Retardation and Speech in Children

Mental retardation is defined by the American Association on Mental Retardation as significantly subaverage intellectual functions with related limitations in social and behavioral skills. According to the most recent estimates (Larson et al., 2001), the prevalence of mental retardation in the noninstitutionalized population of the United States is 7.8 people per thousand; if institutionalized individuals are included in the prevalence rates, the number increases to 8.73 per thousand. Mental retardation is associated with limitations in learning and in the ability to communicate, and has a profound effect on a child's ability to learn to talk. At one time it was believed that the language acquisition of all persons with mental retardation represented a slow-motion version of normal language development. This hypothesis has two major flaws: first, patterns of language development vary across types of mental retardation, and second, within a single type of mental retardation, there is considerable heterogeneity.

The majority of research on children with mental retardation has involved children with Down syndrome (or trisomy 21). This syndrome is the most common genetic cause of mental retardation, occurring in approximately one out of every 800 births. Because Down syndrome is identifiable at birth, researchers have been able to trace developmental patterns from the first months of life. The development of speech and language is severely affected in children with Down syndrome, with levels lower than would be expected, given mental age (Miller, 1988). Speech intelligibility is compromised throughout the life span because of problems with articulation, prosody, and voice.

Children with Down syndrome differ from the normal population in respect to a variety of anatomical and physiological features that may affect speech production. These features include differences in the vocal cords, the presence of a high palatal vault and a larger than normal tongue in relation to the oral cavity, weak facial muscles, and general hypotonicity. Although the precise effect of these differences is difficult to determine, they undoubtedly influence speech-motor development and thus the articulatory and phonatory abilities of children with Down syndrome. An additional factor affecting the speech of children with Down syndrome is fluctuating hearing loss associated with otitis media and middle ear pathologies.

Fragile X syndrome, the most common known cause of inherited mental retardation (Down syndrome is more common but is not inherited), has an estimated prevalence of approximately one per 1250 in males and one per 2500 in females, with males exhibiting more severe effects. Little research has been done on the speech of young children with fragile X syndrome. Available reports on older children (Abbeduto and Hagerman, 1997) indicate abnormalities in articulatory development, disfluncies, and the presence of atypical rate and rhythm. These abnormalities may be attributed, in part, to differences in the structure and function of the oral-motor systems of boys with fragile X syndrome, including excessive drooling, hypotonia involving the oral-facial muscles, and the presence of a narrow, high-arched palate. Like their peers with Down syndrome, children with fragile X syndrome have a high incidence of otitis media and intermittent hearing loss.

Autism is a developmental disorder with prevalence estimates ranging from two to five per 10,000 (3:1 males). This disorder is characterized by deficits in social interaction, communication, and play; two out of three children with autism are mentally retarded (Pennington and Bennetto, 1998). Although in phonetic form, the prelinguistic vocalizations are like those of nonretarded infants, social communication skills in the prelinguistic period are atypical. About 50% of autistic children fail to develop spoken language; the other 50% exhibit delays in acquiring language, although not to the same extent as children with Down syndrome do. Speech production is characterized by echolalia and abnormal prosody (see AUTISM).

Williams syndrome, a genetic disorder that includes mental retardation, is relatively rare, occurring in one in 25,000 live births. One of the most striking aspects of Williams syndrome is that, in spite of marked impairments in cognition, linguistic skills appear to be relatively normal (Bellugi, Lai, and Wang, 1997; Mervis and Bertrand, 1997). This dissociation of language and cognition underscores the importance of examining the relationship between mental retardation and speech in a variety of mentally retarded populations.

The foundations for speech development are laid in the first year of life, with the emergence of nonmeaningful vocal types that serve as precursors for the production of words and phrases. Of particular importance is the production of consonant-vowel syllables, such as [baba], which generally appear around age 6–7 months. Phonetically, these "canonical" babbles are similar or even identical to the forms used in first words; thus, the production [mama] may be a nonmeaningful babble at 8 months and a word at 14 months. The difference is recognition of the sound-meaning relationships that are the basis for words. In general, prelinguistic vocal development of infants with mental retardation resembles that of their nonretarded peers in terms of types of vocalizations and schedule for emergence. Infants with retardation begin to produce canonical babble within the normal time frame or with minor delays.

Despite the nearly normal onset of canonical babble, however, the emergence of words is often delayed among infants with mental retardation, particularly those with Down syndrome (Stoel-Gammon, 1997). Research suggests great variability among children in this domain, with a few reports of word use in the second year of life for a few children with Down syndrome but the majority showing first words appearing between 30 and 60 months. The magnitude of the delay cannot be easily predicted from the degree of retardation. Moreover, once words appear, vocabulary growth is relatively slow. Whereas nonretarded children have a vocabulary of 250 words at 24 months, this milestone is not reached until the age of 4–6 years for most children with Down syndrome.

In terms of phonemic development, acquisition patterns for children with mental retardation are similar to those documented for nonretarded children (Rondal and Edwards, 1997). In the early stages, words are "simplified" in terms of their structure: consonant clusters are reduced to single consonants, unstressed syllables are deleted, and consonants at the ends of words may be omitted. Phonemes that are later-acquired in normal

populations, primarily fricatives, affricates, and liquids, also pose difficulties for children with mental retardation. Among nonretarded children acquiring English, correct pronunciation of all phonemes is achieved by the age of 8 years. Some reports suggest that the phonologies of children with Williams syndrome may be relatively adultlike by the (chronological) age of 8.

In contrast, individuals with Down syndrome, even when they have a mental age of 8, exhibit many articulation errors. Moreover, comparisons of phonological development in three populations matched for mental age, Down syndrome, non-Down syndrome with mental retardation, and typically developing, revealed a greater number and variety of error types in the children with Down syndrome (Dodd, 1976). A persistent problem in children with Down syndrome, is that their speech is hard to understand (Kumin, 1994). Parents report low levels of intelligibility through adolescence as a result of speech sound errors, rate of speech, disfluencies, abnormal voice quality, and unusual voice quality. There is some indication that children with fragile X syndrome also suffer from low levels of intelligibility (Abbeduto and Hagerman, 1997).

For many children with mental retardation, delays in the acquisition of speech and language may serve as the first indication of a cognitive delay (except for Down syndrome, which is easily diagnosed at birth). Parents may be the first to raise concerns about atypical patterns of development, and pediatricians and social workers should be aware of the link between linguistic and cognitive development. Once mental retardation has been confirmed, assessment typically adheres to traditional practices in speech-language pathology. In the prelinguistic period, which may be quite protracted for some children, assessment is initially based on unstructured observations and parental report. If language is slow to emerge, it is important to assess hearing and oral-motor function. More formal assessments are done in two ways: by means of standardized tests that focus on the individual sounds and structures of a predetermined set of words (i.e., a normed articulation test) and by analyzing samples of conversational speech to determine intelligibility and overall speech characteristics.

Recommendations for the treatment of speech deficits in children with mental retardation range from intervention directed toward underlying causes such as hearing loss and deficits in speech-motor skills (Yarter, 1980) to programs aimed at modifying parent-to-child speech in order to provide optimal input in the face of delayed language acquisition. Most phonological interventions focus on increasing the phonetic repertoire and reducing the number of errors, using therapy techniques similar to those for children with phonological delay or disorder. In some cases, therapy may occur at home, with the parents, as well as in the clinic (Dodd and Leahy, 1989; Cholmain, 1994).

See also COMMUNICATION SKILLS OF PEOPLE WITH DOWN SYNDROME; MENTAL RETARDATION.

—*Carol Stoel-Gammon*

References

Abbeduto, L., and Hagerman, R. J. (1997). Language and communication in fragile X syndrome. *Mental Retardation and Developmental Disabilities Research Reviews, 3,* 313–322.

Bellugi, U., Lai, Z., and Wang, P. (1997). Language, communication, and neural systems in Williams syndrome. *Mental Retardation and Developmental Disabilities Research Reviews, 3,* 334–342.

Cholmain, C. N. (1994). Working on phonology with young children with Down syndrome. *Journal of Clinical Speech and Language Studies, 1,* 14–35.

Dodd, B. J. (1976). A comparison of the phonological systems of mental age matched normal, severely abnormal and Down's syndrome children. *British Journal of Disorders of Communication, 11,* 27–42.

Dodd, B. J., and Leahy, P. (1989). Phonological disorders and mental handicap. In M. Beveridge, G. Conti-Ramsden, and I. Leudar (Eds.), *Language and communication in mentally handicapped people* (pp. 33–56). London: Chapman and Hall.

Kumin, L. (1994). Intelligibility of speech in children with Down syndrome in natural settings: Parents' perspective. *Perceptual and Motor Skills, 78,* 307–313.

Larson, S. A., Lakin, K. C., Anderson, L., Kwak, N., Lee, J. H., and Anderson, D. (2001). Prevalence of mental retardation and developmental disabilities: Estimates from the 1994/1995 National Health Interview Survey Disability Supplements. *American Journal on Mental Retardation, 106,* 231–252.

Mervis, C. B., and Bertrand, J. (1997). Developmental relations between cognition and language: Evidence from Williams syndrome. In L. B. Adamson and M. A. Romski (Eds.), *Communication and language acquisition: Discoveries from atypical development* (pp. 75–106). Baltimore: Paul H. Brookes.

Miller, J. F. (1998). The developmental asynchrony of language development in children with down syndrome. In L. Nadel (Ed.), *The psychobiology of Down syndrome* (pp. 167–198). Cambridge, MA: MIT Press.

Pennington, B. F., and Bennetto, L. (1998). Toward a neuropsychology of mental retardation. In J. A. Burack, R. M. Hodapp, and E. Zigler (Eds.), *Handbook of mental retardation and development* (pp. 80–114). Cambridge, UK: Cambridge University Press.

Rondal, J., and Edwards, S. (1997). *Language in mental retardation.* London: Whurr.

Stoel-Gammon, C. (1997). Phonological development in Down syndrome. *Mental Retardation and Developmental Disabilities Research Reviews, 3,* 300–306.

Yarter, B. H. (1980). Speech and language programs for the Down's population. *Seminars in Speech, Language and Hearing, 1,* 49–61.

Motor Speech Involvement in Children

Motor speech involvement of unknown origin is a relatively new diagnostic category that is applied when children's speech production deficits are predominantly linked to sensorimotor planning, programming, or execution (Caruso and Strand, 1999). The disorder occurs in the absence of obvious neuromotor causes and often includes concomitant language deficits. This category is broader than and encompasses that of DEVELOPMENTAL APRAXIA OF SPEECH (DAS), which refers specifically to impaired planning, or praxis. Classically, developmental speech production deficits have been categorized as either phonological or DAS. However, recent empirical evidence suggests that a wider range of children (e.g., those with specific language impairment [SLI] or inconsistent speech errors) may exhibit deficits that are influenced by motor variables and, in these cases, may be classified as motor speech involved.

Although the underlying causes of motor speech involvement are unclear, there is general evidence that motor and cognitive deficits often co-occur (Diamond, 2000). Neurophysiological findings support the interaction of cognitive and motor development, most notably in common brain mechanisms in the lateral perisylvian cortex, the neocerebellum, and the dorsolateral prefrontal cortex (Diamond, 2000; Hill, 2001). Apparently, speech motor and language domains co-develop and mutually influence one another across development.

In late infancy, basic movement patterns observed in babbling are linked to emerging intents and words (de Boysson-Bardis and Vihman, 1991; Levelt, Roelofs, and Meyer, 1999). At this level, it is apparent how language and motor levels constrain one another. However, the relations between language and motor levels in later periods of development have not been specified. Language models include categories such as concepts, semantics, syntax, and phonology (Levelt, Roelofs, and Meyer, 1999). Motor systems are discussed in the very different terms of cortical inputs to pattern generators in the brainstem, which in turn provide inputs to motor neuron pools for the generation of muscle activity. Sensory feedback is also a necessary component of motor systems (A. Smith, Goffman, and Stark, 1995). Although it is established that motor and language domains both show a protracted developmental time course, speech production models are not explicit about the nature of the linkages. The general view is that increasingly complex linguistic structures are linked to increasingly complex movements in the course of development. Motor speech deficits occur when movement variables interfere with the acquisition of speech and language production.

A large range of speech and language characteristics have been reported in children diagnosed with motor speech disorders. In the following summary, emphasis is placed on those that are at least partially motor in origin.

Variability. Children with motor speech disorders have been reported to produce highly variable errors, even across multiple productions of the same word (Davis, Jakielski, and Marquardt, 1998). When the deficit involves movement planning, imitation and repetition may not aid performance (Bradford and Dodd, 1996). Although variability is observed in speech motor (A. Smith and Goffman, 1998) and phonetic output of young children who are normally developing, it is extreme and persistent in disordered children. Usually, variability is discussed as a phonetic error type. However, kinematic analysis of lip and jaw movement reveals that children with SLI show movement output that is less stable than that of their normally developing peers, even when producing an accurate phonetic segment (Goffman, 1999). Thus, both phonological and motor factors may contribute. Deficits in planning and implementing spatially and temporally organized movements may influence the acquisition of stable phonological units (Hall, Jordan, and Robin, 1993).

Duration. Increased movement durations are a hallmark of immature motor systems (B. L. Smith, 1978; Kent and Forner, 1980). In children with motor speech involvement, the slow implementation of movement may lead to decreased performance on a nonlinguistic diadochokinetic task (Crary, 1993) as well as increased error rates on longer and more complex utterances. An additional error type that may also be related to timing is poor movement coordination across speech subsystems. Such timing deficits in articulatory and laryngeal coordination may lead to voicing and nasality errors. Hence, these errors may have origins in movement planning and implementation. A decreased speech rate provides the child with time to process, plan, and implement movement (Hall, Jordan, and Robin, 1993), but it may also negatively influence speech motor performance.

Phonetic Movement Organization and Sequencing. As they develop, children produce increasingly differentiated speech movements, both within and across articulatory, laryngeal, and respiratory subsystems (Gibbon, 1999; Moore, 2001). A lack of differentiated and coordinated movement leads to a collapsing of phonetic distinctions. It follows that segmental and syllabic inventories are reduced for children with motor speech deficits (Davis, Jakielski, and Marquardt, 1998). Vowel and consonant errors may be considered in reference to articulatory complexity. Vowel production requires highly specified movements of the tongue and jaw (Pollock and Hall, 1991). Consonant sounds that are early-developing and that are most frequently seen in the phonetic inventories of children with motor speech deficits make relatively few demands on the motor system (Hall, Jordan, and Robin, 1993). Kent (1992) suggests that early-developing stop consonants such as [b] and [d] are produced with rapid, ballistic movements. Fricatives require fine force control and are acquired later. Liquids, which require highly controlled tongue movements, are learned quite late in the developmental process. Using electropalatography, Gibbon (1999) has provided direct evidence that children with speech deficits contact the entire palate with the tongue, not just the anterior region, in their production of alveolar consonants. Such data indicate that motor control of differentiated tongue movements has not developed in these children. Overall, as proposed by Kent (1992), motor variables account for many aspects of the developmental sequence frequently reported in speech- and language-impaired children.

Syllable shapes may also be influenced by motor factors. The earliest consonant-vowel structure seen in babbling is hypothesized to consist of jaw oscillation without independent control of the lips and tongue (MacNeilage and Davis, 2000). More complex syllable structures probably require increased movement control, such as the homing movement for final consonant production (Kent, 1992).

Prosodic Movement Organization and Sequencing. One major aspect of motor development that has been emphasized in motor speech disorders is rhythmicity. Rhythmicity is thought to have origins in prelinguistic babbling (and, perhaps, in early stereotypic movements, such as kicking and banging objects) (e.g., Thelen and Smith, 1994). Rhythmicity underlies the prosodic structure of speech, which is used to convey word and sentence meaning as well as affect. Children with motor speech disorders display particular deficits in prosodic aspects of speech. Shriberg and his colleagues (Shriberg, Aram, and Kwiatkowski, 1997) found that a significant proportion of children diagnosed with DAS demonstrated errors characterized by even or misplaced stress in their spontaneous speech. In a study using direct measures of lip and jaw movement during the production of different stress patterns, Goffman (1999) reported that children with a diagnosis of SLI, who also demonstrated speech production and morphological errors, were poor at producing large and small movements sequentially across different stress contexts. For example, in the problematic weak-strong prosodic sequence, these children had difficulty producing small movements corresponding to unstressed syllables. Overall, the control of movement for the production of stress is a frequently cited deficit in children with motor speech disorders.

General Motor Development. In the clinical literature, general neuromotor status has long been implicated as contributing to even relatively subtle speech and language deficits (Morris and Klein, 1987). Empirical studies have provided evidence that aspects of gross and fine motor (e.g., peg moving, gesture imitation) performance are below expected levels in children with variable speech errors, DAS (Bradford and Dodd, 1996), and many diagnosed with SLI (Bishop and Edmundson, 1987; Hill, 2001). Such findings suggest that many speech production disorders include a general motor component.

As is apparent, an understanding of speech motor contributions to the acquisition of speech and language is in its infancy. However, it is clear that intervention approaches for these children need to incorporate motor as well as language components. Although efficacy studies are scarce, several investigators have proposed techniques for the treatment of motor speech disorders in children. Although the emphasis has been on DAS, these approaches could be tailored to more general motor speech deficits. Major approaches to intervention have focused on motor programming (Hall, Jordan, and Robin, 1993) and tactile-kinesthetic and rhythmic (Square, 1994) deficits. Hierarchical language organization has also been emphasized, supporting the intimate links between linguistic and movement variables (Velleman and Strand, 1994).

New models of speech and language development are needed that integrate motor and language variables in a way that is consistent with recent neurophysiological and behavioral evidence. Further, new methods of recording respiratory, laryngeal, and articulatory behaviors of infants and young children during the production of meaningful linguistic activity should provide crucial data for understanding how language and motor components of development interact across normal and disordered development. Such tools should also help answer questions about appropriate interventions for children whose deficits are influenced by atypical motor control processes.

See also DEVELOPMENTAL APRAXIA OF SPEECH.

—*Lisa Goffman*

References

Bishop, D. V. M., and Edmundson, A. (1987). Specific language impairment as a maturational lag: Evidence from longitudinal data on language and motor development. *Developmental Medicine and Child Neurology, 29,* 442–459.

Bradford, A., and Dodd, B. (1996). Do all speech-disordered children have motor deficits? *Clinical Linguistics and Phonetics, 10,* 77–101.

Caruso, A. J., and Strand, E. A. (1999). *Clinical management of motor speech disorders in children.* New York: Thieme.

Crary, M. A. (1993). *Developmental motor speech disorders.* San Diego, CA: Singular Publishing Group.

Davis, B. L., Jakielski, K. J., and Marquardt, T. M. (1998). Developmental apraxia of speech: Determiners of differential diagnosis. *Clinical Linguistics and Phonetics, 12,* 25–45.

de Boysson-Bardis, B., and Vihman, M. M. (1991). Adaptation to language: Evidence from babbling and first words in four languages. *Language, 67,* 297–318.

Diamond, A. (2000). Close interaction of motor development and cognitive development and of the cerebellum and prefrontal cortex. *Child Development, 71,* 44–56.

Gibbon, F. E. (1999). Undifferentiated lingual gestures in children with articulation/phonological disorders. *Journal of Speech, Language, and Hearing Research, 42,* 382–397.

Goffman, L. (1999). Prosodic influences on speech production in children with specific language impairment and speech deficits. *Journal of Speech, Language, and Hearing Research, 42,* 1499–1517.

Hall, P. K., Jordan, L. S., and Robin, D. A. (1993). *Developmental apraxia of speech: Theory and clinical practice.* Austin, TX: Pro-Ed.

Hill, E. L. (2001). Non-specific nature of specific language impairment: A review of the literature with regard to concomitant motor impairments. *International Journal of Language and Communication Disorders, 36,* 149–171.

Kent, R. D. (1992). The biology of phonological development. In C. A. Ferguson, L. Menn, and C. Stoel-Gammon (Eds.), *Phonological development: Models, research, implications* (pp. 65–90). Timonium, MD: York Press.

Kent, R. D., and Forner, L. L. (1980). Speech segment durations in sentence recitations by children and adults. *Journal of Phonetics, 8,* 157–168.

Levelt, W., Roelofs, A., and Meyer, A. (1999). A theory of lexical access in speech production. *Behavioral and Brain Sciences, 22,* 1–75.

MacNeilage, P. F., and Davis, B. L. (2000). On the origin of internal structure of word forms. *Science, 288,* 527–531.

Moore, C. A. (2001). Physiologic development of speech production. In B. Maasen, W. Hulstijn, R. Kent, H. F. M. Peters, and P. H. M. M. van Lieshout (Eds.), *Speech motor control in normal and disordered speech* (pp. 40–43). Nijmegen, Netherlands: Uitgeverij Vantilt.

Morris, S. E., and Klein, M. D. (1987). *Pre-feeding skills.* Tucson, AZ: Therapy Skill Builders.

Pollock, K., and Hall, P. (1991). An analysis of vowel misarticulations of five children with developmental apraxia of speech. *Clinical Linguistics and Phonetics, 5,* 207–224.

Shriberg, L. D., Aram, D. M., and Kwiatkowski, J. (1997). Developmental apraxia of speech: III. A subtype marked by inappropriate stress. *Journal of Speech, Language, and Hearing Research, 40,* 313–337.

Smith, A., and Goffman, L. (1998). Stability and patterning of speech movement sequences in children and adults. *Journal of Speech, Language, and Hearing Research, 41,* 18–30.

Smith, A., Goffman, L., and Stark, R. E. (1995). Speech motor development. *Seminars in Speech and Language, 16,* 87–99.

Smith, B. L. (1978). Temporal aspects of English speech production: A developmental perspective. *Journal of Phonetics, 6,* 37–67.

Square, P. A. (1994). Treatment approaches for developmental apraxia of speech. *Journal of Communication Disorders, 4,* 151–161.

Thelen, E., and Smith, L. B. (1994). *A dynamic systems approach to the development of cognition and action.* Cambridge, MA: MIT Press.

Velleman, S., and Strand, C. (1994). Developmental verbal dyspraxia. In J. Bernthal and N. Bankson (Eds.), *Child phonology: Characteristics, assessment, and intervention with special populations.* New York: Thieme.

Further Readings

Bernhardt, B., and Stemberger, J. P. (Eds.). (1998). *Handbook of phonological development from the perspective of constraint-based nonlinear phonology.* San Diego, CA: Academic Press.

Dodd, B. (1995). *Differential diagnosis and treatment of children with speech disorder.* San Diego, CA: Singular Publishing Group.

Finan, D. S., and Barlow, S. M. (1998). Intrinsic dynamics and mechanosensory modulation of non-nutritive sucking in human infants. *Early Human Development, 52,* 181–197.

Green, J. R., Moore, C. A., Higashikawa, M., and Steeve, R. W. (2000). The physiologic development of speech motor control: Lip and jaw coordination. *Journal of Speech, Language, and Hearing Research, 43,* 239–255.

Hayden, D. A., and Square, P. A. (1999). *The Verbal Motor Production Assessment for Children.* San Antonio, TX: Psychological Corp.

Hodge, M. (1995). Assessment of children with developmental apraxia of speech: A rationale. *Clinics in Communication Disorders, 4,* 91–101.

Locke, J. (2000). Movement patterns in spoken language. *Science, 288,* 449–450.

Robbins, J., and Klee, T. (1987). Clinical assessment of oropharyngeal motor development in young children. *Journal of Speech and Hearing Research, 52,* 272–277.

Shriberg, L. D., Aram, D. M., and Kwiatkowski, J. (1997). Developmental apraxia of speech: I. Descriptive and theoretical markers. *Journal of Speech, Language, and Hearing Research, 40*, 273–285.

Statholpoulos, E. T. (1995). Variability revisited: An acoustic, aerodynamic, and respiratory kinematic comparison of children and adults during speech. *Journal of Phonetics, 23*, 67–80.

Strand, E. A. (1995). Treatment of motor speech disorders in children. *Seminars in Speech and Language, 16*, 126–139.

Velleman, S., and Shriberg, L. D. (1999). Metrical analysis of speech in children with suspected developmental apraxia of speech. *Journal of Speech, Language, and Hearing Research, 42*, 1444–1460.

Mutism, Neurogenic

Mutism is speechlessness. It can be neurologic or behavioral. Neurogenic mutism is a sign and can result from many developmental or acquired nervous system diseases and conditions. It usually accompanies other signs, but in rare cases it appears in isolation. All levels of the neuroaxis from the brainstem to the cortex have been implicated. Damage to any of the putative processes critical to speech, including intention, motor programming, and execution, as well as linguistic and prelinguistic processes have been invoked to explain mutism's appearance. A reasonably traditional review of the syndromes and conditions of which mutism is a frequent part and traditional and emerging explanations for mutism's appearance are offered here.

Definition. Duffy defines mutism traditionally as "the absence of speech" (1995, p. 282). Von Cramon (1981) adds the inability to produce nonverbal utterances. Lebrun (1990) requires normal or relatively preserved comprehension. Gelabert-Gonzalez and Fernandez-Villa (2001) require "unimpaired consciousness" (p. 111). Each of these definitions has strengths, but none dominates the literature. Therefore, the literature can be a bit of a muddle. The literature is also challenging because of the mutism population's heterogeneity. One response to this heterogeneity has been to classify mutism according to relatively homogeneous subtypes.

Traditionally, groupings of mute patients have been organized according to the putative pathophysiology (Turkstra and Bayles, 1992), by syndrome, by etiology, or by a mix of syndrome and medical etiology (Lebrun, 1990; Duffy, 1995). This last approach guides the organization of the following discussion.

Akinetic Mutism. Akinetic mutism (AM) is a syndrome of speechlessness and general akinesia that exists in the context of residual sensory, motor, and at least some cognitive integrity and a normal level of arousal. The designation *abulic state* may be a synonym (Duffy, 1995), as are *apallic state* and *coma vigil*. Persons with AM often are silent, despite pain or threat. Bilateral and occasionally unilateral left or right anterior cerebral artery occlusion with involvement of the anterior cingulate gyrus or supplementary motor area is frequently implicated (Nicolai, van Putten, and Tavy, 2001). Recent data suggest that the critical areas are the portions of the medial frontal lobes immediately anterior to the supplementary motor area and portions of the anterior cingulate gyrus above the most anterior body of the corpus callosum. These regions appear to be involved in gating intention (plans of action) (Picard and Strick, 1996; Cohen et al., 1999). Lesions of the globus pallidus, thalamus, and other subcortical structures can also result in AM. Schiff and Plum (2000) advocate for a companion syndrome of "hyperkinetic mutism" resulting most frequently from bilateral temporal, parietal, and occipital junction involvement in which the patient is speechless but moving. The cause may be any nervous system–altering condition, including degenerative diseases such as Creutzfeldt-Jacob disease (Otto et al., 1998), that alters what Schiff and Plum (2000) posit to be a series of corticostriatopallidal-thalamocortical (CSPTC) loops. CSPTC loops are critical to triggering or initiating vocalization (Mega and Cohenour, 1997) and to the drive or will to speak. AM is to be differentiated from persistent vegetative state, which reflects extensive damage to all cerebral structures, most critically the thalamus, with preservation of brainstem function (Kinney et al., 1994).

Mutism in Aphasia. Mutism can be a feature of severe global aphasia. Patients with severe anomia, most often in relation to thalamic lesions, may initially exhibit no capacity for spontaneous language and little for naming, but they can repeat. Certain types of transcortical motor aphasia (Alexander, Benson, and Stuss, 1989), most particularly the adynamic aphasia of Luria (1970), may be associated with complete absence of spontaneous speech. However, these patients are reasonably fluent during picture description, and this syndrome likely reflects a prelinguistic disorder involving defective spontaneous engagement of concept representations (Gold et al., 1997).

Mutism in Apraxia. Immediately after stroke, a profound apraxia of speech (called aphemia and by a variety of other names in the world's literature) can cause mutism, as can primary progressive apraxia of speech. In the acute stage of stroke, the mutism is thought to signal an apraxia of phonation. The hypothesis is that mutism due to apraxia reflects a profound failure of motor programming.

Mutism in Dysarthria. Mutism can be the final stage of dysarthria (anarthria) in degenerative diseases such as amyotrophic lateral sclerosis, slowly progressive anarthria (Broussolle et al., 1996), olivopontocerebellar atrophy, Parkinson's disease, Shy-Drager syndrome, striatonigral degeneration, and progressive supranuclear palsy (Nath et al., 2001). Speech movements are impossible because of upper and lower motor neuron destruction. Cognitive changes may hasten the mutism in some of these degenerative diseases. Anarthric mutism can be present at onset and chronically in locked-in syndrome (Plum and Posner, 1966) and the syndrome of bilateral infarction of opercular motor cortex. Relatively recently, a syndrome beginning with mutism and evolving to dysarthria, called temporary mutism followed by dysarthria (TMFD) (Orefice et al., 1999) or mutism and subsequent dysarthria syndrome (MSD) (Dunwoody, Alsagoff, and Yuan, 1997), has been described. Ponto-mesencephalic stroke is one cause.

Mutism in Dementia.   Mutism has been reported in Alzheimer's disease, cerebrovascular dementia, and most frequently and perhaps earliest in frontotemporal dementia (Bathgate et al., 2001). It can also occur in other corticosubcortical degenerative diseases, including corticobasal degeneration. Its occurrence in the late stages of these conditions is predictable, based on the hierarchical organization of cognitive, linguistic, and speech processes. When cognitive processes are absent or severely degraded, speech does not occur.

Mutism Post Surgery.   Mutism can occur after neurosurgery (Pollack, 1997; Siffert et al., 2000). So-called cerebellar mutism can result from posterior fossa surgery, for example. It is hypothesized that disruption of connections between the cerebellum, thalamus, and supplementary motor area causes impaired triggering of vocalization (Gelabert-Gonzalez and Fernandez-Villa, 2001). Mutism may also occur after callosotomy (Sussman et al., 1983), perhaps because of damage to frontal lobe structures and the cingulate gyrus.

Mutism in Traumatic Brain Injury.   Mutism is frequent in traumatic brain injury. Von Cramon (1981) called it the "traumatic midbrain syndrome." He speculated that the mechanism is "temporary inhibition of neural activity within the brain stem vocalization center" (p. 804) within the pontomesencephalic area. Often mutism is followed by a period of whispered speech in this population.

Summary.   Speech depends on myriad general and specific cognitive, motor, and linguistic processes. These processes are widely distributed in the nervous system. However, the frontal lobes and their connections to subcortical and brainstem structures are the most critical. Mutism, therefore, is common, but not inevitable, as an early, late, or chronic sign of damage, regardless of type, to these mechanisms.

—*John C. Rosenbek*

References

Alexander, M. P., Benson, D. F., and Stuss, D. T. (1989). Frontal lobes and language. *Brain and Language, 37,* 656–691.

Bathgate, D., Snowden, J. S., Varma, A., Blackshaw, A., and Neary, D. (2001). Behavior in frontotemporal dementia, Alzheimer's disease and vascular dementia. *Acta Neurologica Scandinavica, 103,* 367–378.

Broussole, E., Bakchine, S., Tommasi, M., Laurent, B., Bazin, B., Cinotti, L., et al. (1996). Slowly progressive anarthria with late anterior opercular syndrome: A variant of frontal cortical atrophy syndromes. *Journal of the Neurological Sciences, 144,* 44–58.

Cohen, R. A., Kaplan, R. F., Moser, D. J., Jenkins, M. A., and Wilkinson, H. (1999). Impairments of attention after cingulotomy. *Neurology, 53,* 819–824.

Duffy, J. R. (1995). *Motor speech disorders: Substrates, differential diagnosis, and management.* St. Louis: Mosby.

Dunwoody, G. W., Alsagoff, Z. S., and Yuan, S. Y. (1997). Cerebellar mutism with subsequent dysarthria in an adult: Case report. *British Journal of Neurosurgery, 11,* 161–163.

Gelabert-Gonzalez, M., and Fernandez-Villa, J. (2001). Mutism after posterior fossa surgery: Review of the literature. *Clinical Neurology and Neurosurgery, 103,* 111–114.

Gold, M., Nadeau, S. E., Jacobs, D. H., Adair, J. C., Gonzalez-Rothi, L. J., and Heilman, K. M. (1997). Adynamic aphasia: A transcortical motor aphasia with defective semantic strategy formation. *Brain and Language, 57,* 374–393.

Kinney, H. C., Korein, J., Panigrahy, A., Dikkes, P., and Goode, R. (1994). Neuropathological findings in the brain of Karen Ann Quinlan: The role of the thalamus in the persistent vegetative state. *New England Journal of Medicine, 21,* 1469–1475.

Lebrun, Y. (1990). *Mutism.* London: Whurr.

Luria, A. R. (1970). *Traumatic aphasia: Its syndromes, psychology and treatment.* The Hague, Paris: Mouton.

Mega, M. S., and Cohenour, R. C. (1997). Akinetic mutism: Disconnection of frontal-subcortical circuits. *Neuropsychiatry, Neuropsychology, and Behavioral Neurology, 10,* 254–259.

Nath, U., Ben-Shlomo, Y., Thomson, R. G., Morris, H. R., Wood, N. W., Lees, A. J., et al. (2001). The prevalence of progressive supranuclear palsy (Steele-Richardson-Olszewski syndrome) in the UK. *Brain, 124,* 1438–1449.

Nicolai, J., van Putten, M. J. A. M., and Tavy, D. L. J. (2001). BIPLEDs in akinetic mutism caused by bilateral anterior cerebral artery infarction. *Clinical Neurophysiology, 112,* 1726–1728.

Orefice, G., Fragassi, N. A., Lanzillo, R., Castellano, A., and Grossi, D. (1999). Transient muteness followed by dysarthria in patients with pontomesencephalic stroke. *Cerebrovascular Diseases, 9,* 124–126.

Otto, A., Zerr, I., Lantsch, M., Weidehaas, K., Riedmann, C., and Poser, S. (1998). Akinetic mutism as a classification criterion for the diagnosis of Creutzfeldt-Jakob disease. *Journal of Neurology, Neurosurgery, and Psychiatry, 64,* 524–528.

Picard, N., and Strick, P. L. (1996). Motor areas of the medial wall: A review of their location and functional activation. *Cerebral Cortex, 6,* 342–353.

Plum, F., and Posner, J. (1966). *Diagnosis of stupor and coma.* Philadelphia: Davis.

Pollack, I. F. (1997). Posterior fossa syndrome. *International Review of Neurobiology, 41,* 411–432.

Schiff, N. D., and Plum, F. (2000). The role of arousal and "gating" systems in the neurology of impaired consciousness. *Journal of Clinical Neurophysiology, 17,* 438–452.

Siffert, J., Poussaint, T. Y., Goumnerova, L. C., Scott, R. M., LaValley, B., Tarbell, N. J., et al. (2000). Neurological dysfunction associated with postoperative cerebellar mutism. *Journal of Neuro-Oncology, 48,* 75–81.

Sussman, N. M., Gur, R. C., Gur, R. E., and O'Connor, M. J. (1983). Mutism as a consequence of callosotomy. *Journal of Neurosurgery, 59*, 514–519.

Turkstra, L. S., and Bayles, K. A. (1992). Acquired mutism: Physiopathy and assessment. *Archives of Physical Medicine and Rehabilitation, 73*, 138–144.

von Cramon, D. (1981). Traumatic mutism and the subsequent reorganization of speech functions. *Neuropsychologia, 19*, 801–805.

Further Readings

Bannur, U., and Rajshekhar, V. (2000). Post operative supplementary motor area syndrome: Clinical features and outcome. *British Journal of Neurosurgery, 14*, 204–210.

Bogen, J. E. (1976). Linguistic performance in the short term following cerebral commissurotomy. In H. A. Whitaker and H. Whitaker (Eds.), *Perspectives in neurolinguistics and psycholinguistics* (vol. 2, pp. 193–224). New York: Academic Press.

Brun, A., Englund, E., Gustafson, L., Passant, U., Mann, D. M. A., Neary, D., et al. (1994). Clinical and neuropathological criteria for frontotemporal dementia. *Journal of Neurology, Neurosurgery, and Psychiatry, 57*, 416–418.

Cairns, H., Oldfield, R. C., Pennybacker, J. D., and Whitteridge, O. (1941). Akinetic mutism with an epidermoid cyst of III ventricle. *Brain, 64*, 273–290.

Catsman-Berrevoets, C. E., Van Dongen, H. R., Mulder, P. G. H., Paz y Geuze, D., Paquier, P. F., and Lequin, M. H. (1999). Tumor type and size are high risk factors for the syndrome of "cerebellar" mutism and subsequent dysarthria. *Journal of Neurology, Neurosurgery, and Psychiatry, 67*, 755–757.

Damasio, A. R., and Geschwind, N. (1984). The neural basis of language. *Annual Review of Neuroscience, 7*, 127–147.

Daniel, S. E., de Bruin, V. M., and Lees, A. J. (1995). The clinical and pathological spectrum of Steele-Richardson-Olszewski syndrome (progressive supranuclear palsy): A reappraisal. *Brain, 118*, 759–770.

Kertesz, A., Martinez-Lage, P., Davidson, W., and Munoz, D. G. (2000). The corticobasal degeneration syndrome overlaps progressive aphasia and frontotemporal dementia. *Neurology, 55*, 1368–1375.

Minagar, A., and David, N. J. (1999). Bilateral infarction in the territory of the anterior cerebral arteries. *Neurology, 52*, 886–888.

Pasquier, F., Lebert, F., Lavenu, I., and Guillaume, B. (1999). The clinical picture of frontotemporal dementia: Diagnosis and follow-up. *Dementia and Geriatric Cognitive Disorders, 10*, 10–14.

Penfield, W., and Roberts, L. (1959). *Speech and brain mechanisms.* Princeton, NJ: Princeton University Press.

Penfield, W., and Welch, K. (1951). The supplementary motor area of the cerebral cortex. *Archives of Neurology, 66*, 289–317.

Rekate, H. L., Grubb, R. L., Aram, D. M., Hahn, J. F., and Ratcheson, R. A. (1985). Muteness of cerebellar origin. *Archives of Neurology, 42*, 697–698.

Shuper, A., Stahl, B., and Mimouni, M. (2000). Transient opercular syndrome: A manifestation of uncontrolled epileptic activity. *Acta Neurologica Scandinavica, 101*, 335–338.

Steele, J. C., Richardson, J. C., and Olszewski, J. (1964). Progressive supranuclear palsy. *Archives of Neurology, 10*, 333–359.

Ure, J., Faccio, E., Videla, H., Caccuri, R., Giudice, F., Ollari, J., et al. (1998). Akinetic mutism: A report of three cases. *Acta Neurologica Scandinavica, 98*, 439–444.

Weller, M. (1993). Anterior opercular cortex lesions cause dissociated lower cranial nerve palsies and anarthria but no aphasia: Foix-Chavney-Marie syndrome and "automatic voluntary dissociation" revisited. *Journal of Neurology, 240*, 199–208.

Van der Nerwe, A. (1997). A theoretical framework for the characterization of pathological speech sensorimotor control. In M. R. McNeil (Ed.), *Clinical management of sensorimotor speech disorders.* New York: Thieme.

Orofacial Myofunctional Disorders in Children

Orofacial myology is the scientific and clinical knowledge related to the structure and function of the muscles of the mouth and face (orofacial muscles) (American Speech-Language-Hearing Association [ASHA], 1993). Orofacial myofunctional disorders are characterized by abnormal fronting of the tongue during speech or swallowing, or when the tongue is at rest. ASHA defines an orofacial myofunctional disorder as "any pattern involving oral and/or orofacial musculature that interferes with normal growth, development, or function of structures, or calls attention to itself" (ASHA, 1993, p. 22). With orofacial myofunctional disorders, the tongue moves forward in an exaggerated way and may protrude between the upper and lower teeth during speech, swallowing, or at rest. This exaggerated tongue fronting is also called a tongue thrust or a tongue thrust swallow and may contribute to malocclusion, lisping, or both (Young and Vogel, 1983; ASHA, 1989).

A tongue thrust type of swallow is normal for infants. The forward tongue posture typically diminishes as the child grows and matures. Orofacial myofunctional disorders may also be due to lip incompetence, which is a "lips-apart resting posture or the inability to achieve a lips-together resting posture without muscle strain" (ASHA, 1993, p. 22). During normal development, the lips are slightly separated in children. With orofacial myofunctional disorders, a lips-apart posture persists.

Orofacial myofunctional disorders may be due to a familial genetic pattern that determines the size of the mouth, the arrangement and number of teeth, and the strength of the lip, tongue, mouth, or face muscles (Hanson and Barrett, 1988). Environmental factors such as allergies may also lead to orofacial myofunctional disorders. For example, an open mouth posture may result from blocked nasal airways due to allergies or enlarged tonsils and adenoids. The open-mouth breathing pattern may persist even after medical treatment for the blocked airway. Other environmental causes of orofacial myofunctional disorders may be excessive thumb or finger sucking, excessive lip licking, teeth clenching, and grinding (Van Norman, 1997; Romero, Bravo, and Perez, 1998). Thumb sucking, for example, may change the shape of a child's upper and lower jaw and teeth, requiring speech, dental, and orthodontic intervention (Umberger and Van Reenen, 1995; Van Norman, 1997).

The severity of the problem depends on how long the habit is maintained.

Typically, a team of professionals, including a dentist, orthodontist, physician, and speech-language pathologist, is involved in the assessment and treatment of children with orofacial myofunctional disorders (Benkert, 1997; Green and Green, 1999; Paul-Brown and Clausen, 1999). Assessment is conducted to diagnose normal and abnormal parameters of oral myofunctional patterns (ASHA, 1997). The dentist focuses on the effect of pressure of the tongue against the gums; this kind of tongue pressure may interfere with the normal process of tooth eruption. An orthodontist may be involved when the tongue pressure interferes with alignment of the teeth and jaw. A physician needs to verify that an airway obstruction is not causing the tongue thrust. Speech-language pathologists assess and treat swallowing disorders, speech disorders, or lip incompetence that result from orofacial myofunctional disorders. As with all other assessment and treatment processes, speech-language pathologists need to have the appropriate training, education, and experience to practice in the area of orofacial myofunctional disorders (ASHA, 2002).

An orofacial myofunctional assessment is typically prompted by referral or a failed speech screening for a child older than 4 years of age. Assessment should be based on orofacial myofunctional abilities and education, vocation, social, emotional, health, and medical status. An orofacial myofunctional assessment by a speech-language pathologist typically includes the following procedures (ASHA, 1997, p. 54):

- Case history
- Review of medical/clinical health history and status (including any structural or neurological abnormalities)
- Observation of orofacial myofunctional patterns
- Instrumental diagnostic procedures
- Structural assessment, including observation of the face, jaw, lips, tongue, teeth, hard palate, soft palate, and pharynx
- Perceptual and instrumental measures to assess oral and nasal airway functions as they pertain to orofacial myofunctional patterns and/or speech production (e.g., speech articulation testing, aerodynamic measures)

Speech may be unaffected by orofacial myofunctional disorders (Khinda and Grewal, 1999). However, some speech sound errors, called speech misarticulations, may be causally related to orofacial myofunctional disorders. The sounds most commonly affected by orofacial myofunctional disorders include s, z, sh, zh, ch, and j. Sound substitutions (e.g., th for s, as in "thun" for "sun") or sound distortions may occur. A weak tongue tip may result in difficulties producing the sounds t, d, n, and l.

Speech-language pathologists evaluate speech sound errors resulting from orofacial myofunctional disorders, as well as lip incompetence and swallowing disorders (ASHA, 1991). The assessment information is used to develop appropriate treatment plans for individuals who

are identified with orofacial myofunctional disorders. Before speech and swallowing treatment is initiated, medical treatment may be necessary if the airway is blocked due to enlarged tonsils and adenoids or allergies. Excessive and persistent oral habits, such as thumb and finger sucking or lip biting, may also need to be eliminated or reduced before speech and swallowing treatments are initiated.

Some speech and swallowing treatment techniques include

- Increasing awareness of mouth and facial muscles.
- Increasing awareness of mouth and tongue postures.
- Completing an individualized oral muscle exercise program to improve muscle strength and coordination. Treatment strategies may include alternation of tongue and lip resting postures and muscle retraining exercises (ASHA, 1997, p. 69).
- Establishing normal speech articulation.
- Establishing normal swallowing patterns. Treatment strategies may include modification of handling and swallowing of solids, liquids, and saliva (ASHA, 1997, p. 69).

The expected outcome of treatment is to improve or correct the patient's orofacial myofunctional swallowing and speech patterns. Orofacial myofunctional treatment may be conducted concurrently with speech treatment.

Oral myofunctional treatment is effective in modifying tongue and lip posture and movement and in improving dental occlusion and a dental open bite or overbite (Christensen and Hanson, 1981; ASHA, 1991; Benkert, 1997). Lip exercises may be successful in treating an open-mouth posture (ASHA, 1989; Pedrazzi, 1997). A combination treatment approach, with a focus on speech correction as well as exercises to treat tongue posture and swallowing patterns, appears to be the optimal way to improve speech and tongue thrust (Umberger and Johnston, 1997). The length of treatment varies according to the severity of the disorder, the age and maturity of the patient, and the timing of treatment in relation to orthodontia. Typically 14–20 sessions or more may occur over a period of 3 months to a year (ASHA, 1989). The value of early treatment is emphasized in the literature (Pedrazzi, 1997; Van Norman, 1997).

ASHA has identified the basic content areas to be covered in university curricula to promote competency in the assessment and treatment of orofacial myofunctional disorders (ASHA, 1989, p. 92), including the following:

1. Oral-facial-pharyngeal structure, development, and function
2. Interrelationships among oral-vegetative functions and adaptations, speech, and dental occlusion, using interdisciplinary approaches
3. Nature of atypical oral-facial patterns and their relationship to speech, dentition, airway competency, and facial appearance

4. Relevant theories such as those involving oral-motor control and dental malocclusion

5. Rationale and procedures for assessment of oral myofunctional patterns, and observation and participation in the evaluation and treatment of patients with orofacial myofunctional disorders

6. Application of current instrumental technologies to document clinical processes and phenomena associated with orofacial myofunctional disorders

7. Treatment options

A Joint Committee of ASHA and the International Association of Orofacial Myology has also delineated the knowledge and skills needed to evaluate and treat persons with orofacial myofunctional disorders (ASHA, 1993). The tasks required include the following:

- Understanding dentofacial patterns and applied physiology pertinent to orofacial myology
- Understanding factors causing, contributing, or related to orofacial myology
- Understanding basic orthodontic concepts
- Understanding interrelationships between speech and orofacial myofunctional disorders
- Demonstrating competence in comprehensive assessment procedures and in identifying factors affecting prognosis
- Demonstrating competence in selecting an appropriate, individualized, criterion-based treatment plan
- Demonstrating a clinical environment appropriate to the provision of professional services
- Demonstrating appropriate documentation of all clinical services
- Demonstrating professional conduct within the scope of practice for speech-language pathology (ASHA, 2001)

Further information on oral myofunction and oral myofunctional disorders is available from ASHA's Special Interest Division on Speech Science and Orofacial Disorders (www.asha.org) and the International Association of Orofacial Myology (www.iaom.com).

—Diane Paul-Brown

References

American Speech-Language-Hearing Association. (1989, November). Report: Ad hoc Committee on Labial-Lingual Posturing Function. *ASHA, 31,* 92–94.

American Speech-Language-Hearing Association. (1991). The role of the speech-language pathologist in management of oral myofunctional disorders. *ASHA, 33*(Suppl. 5), 7.

American Speech-Language-Hearing Association. (1993). Orofacial myofunctional disorders: Knowledge and skills. *ASHA, 35*(Suppl. 10), 21–23.

American Speech-Language-Hearing Association. (1997). *Preferred practice patterns for the profession of speech-language pathology.* Rockville, MD: Author.

American Speech-Language-Hearing Association. (2001). *Scope of practice in speech-language pathology.* Rockville, MD: Author.

American Speech-Language-Hearing Association. (2002). Code of ethics. Rockville, MD: Author.

Benkert, K. K. (1997). The effectiveness of orofacial myofunctional therapy in improving dental occlusion. *International Journal of Orofacial Myology, 23,* 35–46.

Christensen, M., and Hanson, M. (1981). An investigation of the efficacy of oral myofunctional therapy precursor to articulation therapy for pre-first grade children. *Journal of Speech and Hearing Disorders, 46,* 160–165.

Green, H. M., and Green, S. E. (1999). The interrelationship of wind instrument technic, orthodontic treatment, and orofacial myology. *International Journal of Orofacial Myology, 25,* 18–29.

Hanson, M., and Barrett, R. (1988). *Fundamentals of orofacial myology.* Springfield, IL: Charles C Thomas.

Khinda, V., and Grewal, N. (1999). Relationship of tongue-thrust swallowing and anterior open bite with articulation disorders: A clinical study. *Journal of Indian Society of Pedodontia and Preventive Dentistry, 17*(2), 33–39.

Paul-Brown, D., and Clausen, R. P. (1999, July/August). Collaborative approach for identifying and treating speech, language, and orofacial myofunctional disorders. *Alpha Omegan, 92*(2), 39–44.

Pedrazzi, M. E. (1997). Treating the open bite. *Journal of General Orthodontia, 8,* 5–16.

Romero, M. M., Bravo, G. A., and Perez, L. L. (1998). Open bite due to lip sucking: A case report. *Journal of Clinical Pediatric Dentistry, 22,* 207–210.

Umberger, F., and Johnston, R. G. (1997). The efficiency of oral myofunctional and coarticulation therapy. *International Journal of Orofacial Myology, 23,* 3–9.

Umberger, F., and Van Reenen, J. (1995). Thumb sucking management: A review. *International Journal of Orofacial Myology, 21,* 41–45.

Van Norman, R. (1997). Digit sucking: A review of the literature, clinical observations, and treatment recommendations. *International Journal of Orofacial Myology, 22,* 14–33.

Young, L. D., and Vogel, V. (1983). The use of cueing and positive practice in the treatment of tongue thrust swallowing. *Journal of Behavior Therapy and Experimental Psychiatry, 14,* 73–77.

Further Readings

Alexander, S., and Sudha, P. (1997). Genioglossis muscle electrical activity and associated arch dim changes in simple tongue thrust swallow pattern. *Journal of Clinical Pediatric Dentistry, 21,* 213–222.

Andrianopoulos, M. V., and Hanson, M. L. (1987). Tongue thrust and the stability of overjet correction. *Angle Orthodontist, 57,* 121–135.

Bresolin, D., Shapiro, P. A., Shapiro, G. G., Chapko, M. K., and Dassel, S. (1983). Mouth breathing in allergic children: Its relationship to dentofacial development. *American Journal of Orthodontics, 83,* 334–340.

Cayley, A. S., Tindall, A. P., Sampson, W. J., and Butcher, A. R. (2000). Electropalatographic and cephalometric assessment of myofunctional therapy bite subjects. *Australian Orthodontic Journal, 16,* 23–33.

Cayley, A. S., Tindall, A. P., Sampson, W. J., and Butcher, A. R. (2000). Electropalatographic and cephalometric assessment of tongue function in open and non-open bite subjects. *European Journal of Orthodontics, 22,* 463–474.

Christensen, M., and Hanson, M. (1981). An investigation of the efficacy of oral myofunctional therapy as a precursor to articulation therapy for pre-first grade children. *Journal of Speech and Hearing Disorders, 46,* 160–167.

Dworkin, J. P., and Culatta, K. H. (1980). Tongue strength: Its relationship to tongue thrusting, open-bite, and articulatory proficiency. *Journal of Speech and Hearing Disorders, 45,* 277–282.

Gommerman, S. L., and Hodge, M. M. (1995). Effects of oral myofunctional therapy on swallowing and sibilant production. *International Journal of Orofacial Myology, 21,* 9–22.

Hanson, J. L., and Andrianopoulos, M. V. (1982). Tongue thrust and malocclusion. *International Journal of Orthodontics, 29,* 9–18.

Hanson, J. L., and Cohen, M. S. (1973). Effects of form and function on swallowing and the developing dentition. *American Journal of Orthodontics, 64,* 63–82.

Hanson, M. L. (1988). Orofacial myofunctional disorders: Guidelines for assessment and treatment. *International Journal of Orofacial Myology, 14,* 27–32.

Hanson, M. L., and Peachey, G. (1991). Current issues in orofacial myology. *International Journal of Orofacial Myology, 17*(2), 4–7.

Khinda, V., and Grewel, N. (1999). Relationship of tongue-thrust swallowing and anterior open bite with articulation disorders: A clinical study. *Journal of the Indian Society of Pedodontics and Preventive Dentistry, 17*(2), 33–39.

Martin, R. E., and Sessle, B. J. (1993). The role of the cerebral cortex in swallowing. *Dysphagia, 8,* 195–202.

Mason, R. M. (1988). Orthodontic perspectives on orofacial myofunctional therapy. *International Journal of Orofacial Myology, 14*(1), 49–55.

Nevia, F. C., and Wertzner, H. F. (1996). A protocol for oral myofunctional assessment: For application with children. *International Journal of Oral Myology, 22,* 8–19.

Pedrazzi, M. E. (1997). Treating the open bite. *Journal of General Orthodontics, 8,* 5–16.

Pierce, R. B. (1988). Treatment for the young child. *International Journal of Oral Myology, 14,* 33–39.

Pierce, R. B. (1996). Age and articulation characteristics: A survey of patient records on 100 patients referred for "tongue thrust therapy" January 1990–June 1996. *International Journal of Orofacial Myology, 22,* 32–33.

Saito, M. (2001). A study on improving tongue functions of open-bite children mixed dentition period: Modifications of a removable habit-breaker appliance and their sonographic analysis. *Kokubyo Gakkai Zasshi, 68,* 193–207.

Umberger, F. G., Weld, G. L., and Van Rennen, J. S. (1985). Tongue thrust: Attitudes and practices of speech pathologists and orthodontists. *International Journal of Orofacial Myology, 11*(3), 5–13.

Wasson, J. L. (1989). Correction of tongue-thrust swallowing habits. *Journal of Clinical Orthodontics, 12*(1), 27–29.

Phonetic Transcription of Children's Speech

Phonetic transcription entails using special symbols to create a precise written record of an individual's speech. The symbols that are most commonly used are those of the International Phonetic Alphabet (IPA), first developed in the 1880s by European phoneticians. Their goal was to provide a different symbol for each unique sound, that is, to achieve a one-to-one correspondence between sound and symbol. For example, because [s]

and [ʃ] are phonemically distinct in some languages, such as English, they are represented differently in the phonetic alphabet. Thus, the elongated *s* is used for the voiceless *palatoalveolar* fricative, as in [ʃu]), to differentiate it from the voiceless *alveolar* fricative, as in [su].

The IPA has undergone several revisions since its inception but remains essentially unchanged. In the familiar consonant chart, symbols for pulmonic consonants are organized according to place of articulation, manner of articulation, and voicing. Nonpulmonic consonants, such as clicks and ejectives, are listed separately, as are vowels, which are shown in a typical vowel quadrangle. Symbols for suprasegmentals, such as length and tone, are also provided, as are numerous diacritics, such as [s̪] for a dentalized [s].

The most recent version of the complete IPA chart can be found in the *Handbook of the International Phonetic Association* (IPA, 1999) as well as in a number of phonetics books (e.g., Ladefoged, 2001; Small, 1999). Illustrations of the sounds of the IPA are available through various sources, such as Ladefoged (2001) and Wells and House (1995). In addition, training materials and phonetic fonts can be downloaded from the Internet. Some new computers now come equipped with "Unicode" phonetic symbols.

Although extensive, the IPA does not capture all of the variations that have been observed in children's speech. For this reason, some child/clinical phonologists have proposed additional symbols and diacritics (e.g., Bush et al., 1973; Edwards, 1986; Shriberg and Kent, 2003). The extended IPA (extIPA) was adopted by the International Clinical Phonetics and Linguistics Association (ICPLA) Executive Committee in 1994 to assist in and standardize the transcription of atypical speech (e.g., Duckworth et al., 1990). The extIPA includes symbols for sounds that do not occur in "natural" languages, such as labiodental and interdental plosives, as well as many diacritics, such as for denasalized and unaspirated sounds. It also includes symbols for transcribing connected speech (e.g., sequences of quiet speech, fast or slow speech), as well as ways to mark features such as silent articulation. Descriptions and examples can be found in Ball, Rahilly, and Tench (1996) and Powell (2001).

When transcribing child or disordered speech, it is sometimes impossible to identify the exact nature of a segment. In such cases, "cover symbols" may be used. These symbols consist of capital letters to represent major sound classes, modified with appropriate diacritics. Thus, an unidentifiable voiceless fricative can be transcribed with a capital F and a small under-ring for voicelessness (e.g., Stoel-Gammon, 2001).

Relatively little attention has been paid to the transcription of vowels in children's speech (see, however, Pollock and Berni, 2001). Even less attention has been paid to the transcription of suprasegmentals or prosodic features. Examples of relevant IPA and extIPA symbols appear in Powell (2001), and Snow (2001) illustrates special symbols for intonation.

Broad or "phonemic" transcriptions, which capture only the basic segments, are customarily written in slashes (virgules), as in /paɪ/ or /tɛləfon/. "Narrow" or "close" transcriptions, which often include diacritics, are written in square brackets. A narrow transcription more accurately represents actual pronunciation, whether correct or incorrect, as in [pʰaɪ] for *pie*, with aspiration on the initial voiceless stop, or a young child's rendition of *star* as [t=aʊ] or *fish* as [ɸɪs].

How narrow a transcription needs to be in any given situation depends on factors such as the purpose of the transcription, the skill of the transcriber, and the amount of time available. As Powell (2001) points out, basic IPA symbols are sufficient for some clinical purposes, for example, if a client's consonant repertoire is a subset of the standard inventory. A broad transcription is generally adequate to capture error patterns that involve deletion, such as final consonant deletion or cluster reduction, as well as those that involve substitutions of one sound class for another, such as gliding of liquids or stopping of fricatives.

If no detail is included in a transcription, however, the analyst may miss potentially important aspects of the production. For instance, if a child fails to aspirate initial voiceless stops, the unaspirated stops should be transcribed with the appropriate (extIPA) diacritic (e.g., [p=], [t=], as in [p=i] for *pea*). Such stops can easily be mistaken for the corresponding voiced stops and erroneously transcribed as [b], [d], and so on. The clinician might then decide to work on initial voicing, using minimal pairs such as *pea* and *bee*. This could be frustrating for a child who is already making a subtle (but incorrect) contrast, for example, between [p=] and [b].

To give another example, a child who is deleting final consonants may retain some features of the deleted consonants as "marking" on the preceding vowel, for instance, vowel lengthening (if voiced obstruents are deleted) or nasalization (if nasal consonants are deleted). Unless the vowels are transcribed narrowly, the analyst may miss important distinctions, such as between [bi] (*beet*), [bi:] (*bead*), and [bĩ] (*bean*).

Stoel-Gammon (2001) suggests using diacritics only when they provide additional information, not when they represent adultlike use of sounds. For example, if a vowel is nasalized preceding a nasal consonant, the nasalization would not need to be transcribed. However, if a vowel is nasalized in the absence of a nasal consonant, as in the preceding example, or if inappropriate nasalization is observed, a narrow transcription is crucial.

Phonetic transcription became increasingly important for speech-language pathologists with the widespread acceptance of phonological assessment procedures in the 1980s and 1990s. Traditional articulation tests (e.g., Goldman and Fristoe, 1969) did not require much transcription. Errors were classified as substitutions, omissions, or distortions, and only the substitutions were transcribed. Therefore, no narrow transcription was involved.

In order to describe patterns in children's speech, it is necessary to transcribe their errors. Moreover, most phonological assessment procedures require whole word transcription (e.g., Hodson, 1980; Khan and Lewis, 1986), so that phonological processes involving more than one segment, such as assimilation (as in [gʌk] for *truck*), can be more easily discerned. (In fact, Shriberg and Kwiatkowski, 1980, use continuous speech samples, necessitating transcription of entire utterances.)

To facilitate whole word transcription, some clinical phonologists, such as Hodson (1980) and Louko and Edwards (2001), recommend writing out broad transcriptions of target words (e.g., /trʌk/) ahead of time and modifying them "on line" for a tentative live transcription that can be verified or refined by reviewing a tape of the session. Although this makes the transcription process more efficient, it can also lead the transcriber to mishear sounds or to "hear" sounds that are not there (Oller and Eilers, 1975). Louko and Edwards (2001) provide suggestions for counteracting the negative effects of such expectation.

If a speech-language pathologist is going to expend the time and energy necessary to complete a phonological analysis that is maximally useful, the transcription on which it is based must be as accurate and reliable as possible. Ideally, the testing session should be audio- or video-recorded on high-quality tapes and using the best equipment available, and it should take place in a quiet environment, free of distractions (see Stoel-Gammon, 2001). Because some sounds are difficult to transcribe accurately from an audiotape (e.g., unreleased final stops), it is advisable to do some transcribing on-line.

One way to enhance the accuracy of a transcription is to transcribe with a partner or to find a colleague who is willing to provide input on difficult items. "Transcription by consensus" (Shriberg, Kwiatkowski, and Hoffman, 1984), although impractical in some settings, is an excellent way to derive a transcription and to sharpen one's skills. This involves two or more people transcribing a sample at the same time, working independently, then listening together to resolve disagreements.

Sometimes it is desirable to assess the reliability of a transcription. For *intrajudge* reliability, the transcriber relistens to a portion of the sample at some later time and compares the two transcriptions on a sound-by-sound basis, determining a percent of "point-to-point" agreement. The same procedure may be used for determining *interjudge* reliability, except that a second listener's judgments are compared with those of the first transcriber. Reliability rates for children's speech vary greatly, depending on factors such as the type of sample (connected speech or single words) and how narrow the transcription is, with reliability rates being higher for broad transcription (see Cucchiarini, 1996; Shriberg and Lof, 1991). Alternative methods of assessing transcription agreement may sometimes be appropriate. For instance, in assessing the phonetic inventories of young children, Stoel-Gammon (2001) suggests measuring agreement of *features* (place or manner) rather than identity of segments.

People who spend long hours transcribing children's speech often look forward to the day when accurate computer transcription will become a reality. Although computer programs may be developed to make transcription more objective and time-efficient, speech-language pathologists will continue to engage in the transcription process because of what can be learned through carefully listening to and trying to capture the subtleties of a person's speech. Therefore, phonetic transcription is likely to remain an essential skill for anyone engaged in assessing and remediating speech sound disorders.

—*Mary Louise Edwards*

References

Ball, M. J., Rahilly, J., and Tench, P. (1996). *The phonetic transcription of disordered speech*. San Diego, CA: Singular Publishing Group.

Bush, C. N., Edwards, M. L., Luckau, J. M., Stoel, C. M., Macken, M. A., and Peterson, J. D. (1973). *On specifying a system for transcribing consonants in child language.* Unpublished manuscript, Committee on Linguistics, Stanford University, Stanford, CA.

Cucchiarini, C. (1996). Assessing transcription agreement: Methodological aspects. *Clinical Linguistics and Phonetics, 10*, 131–155.

Duckworth, M., Allen, G., Hardcastle, W. J., and Ball, M. J. (1990). Extensions to the International Phonetic Alphabet for the transcription of atypical speech. *Clinical Linguistics and Phonetics, 4*, 273–280.

Edwards, M. L. (1986). *Introduction to applied phonetics: Laboratory workbook.* Needham Heights, MA: Allyn and Bacon.

Goldman, R., and Fristoe, M. (1969). *Goldman-Fristoe Test of Articulation.* Circle Pines, MN: American Guidance Service.

Hodson, B. W. (1980). *The Assessment of Phonological Processes.* Danville, IL: Interstate Printers and Publishers.

International Clinical Phonetics and Linguistics Association Executive Committee. (1994). The extIPA chart. *Journal of the International Phonetic Association, 24*, 95–98.

International Phonetic Association. (1999). *Handbook of the International Phonetic Association: A guide to the use of the International Phonetic Alphabet.* Cambridge, UK: Cambridge University Press.

Khan, L. M. L., and Lewis, N. (1986). *Khan-Lewis phonological analysis.* Circle Pines, MN: American Guidance Service.

Ladefoged, P. (2001). *A course in phonetics* (4th ed.). Fort Worth, TX: Harcourt College Publishers.

Ladefoged, P. (2001). *Vowels and consonants: An introduction to the sounds of languages.* Oxford, UK: Blackwell.

Louko, L. J., and Edwards, M. L. (2001). Issues in collecting and transcribing speech samples. *Topics in Language Disorders, 21*, 1–11.

Oller, D. K., and Eilers, R. E. (1975). Phonetic expectation and transcription validity. *Phonetica, 31*, 288–304.

Pollock, K. E., and Berni, M. C. (2001). Transcription of vowels. *Topics in Language Disorders, 21*, 22–41.

Powell, T. (2001). Phonetic transcription of disordered speech. *Topics in Language Disorders, 21*, 53–73.

Shriberg, L. D., and Kent, R. D. (2003). *Clinical phonetics* (3rd ed.). Needham Heights, MA: Allyn and Bacon.

Shriberg, L. D., and Kwiatkowski, J. (1980). *Natural process analysis.* New York: Wiley.

Shriberg, L. D., Kwiatkowski, J., and Hoffman, K. (1984). A procedure for phonetic transcription by consensus. *Journal of Speech and Hearing Research, 27*, 456–465.

Shriberg, L. D., and Lof, G. L. (1991). Reliability studies in broad and narrow phonetic transcription. *Clinical Linguistics and Phonetics, 5*, 225–279.

Small, L. H. (1999). *Phonetics: A practical guide for students.* Boston: Allyn and Bacon.

Snow, D. (2001). Transcription of suprasegmentals. *Topics in Language Disorders, 21*(4), 42–52.

Stoel-Gammon, C. (2001). Transcribing the speech of young children. *Topics in Language Disorders, 21*(4), 12–21.

Wells, J., and House, J. (1995). *The sounds of the International Phonetic Alphabet.* London: Department of Phonetics and Linguistics, University College London.

Further Readings

Amorosa, H., von Benda, U., and Keck, A. (1985). Transcribing phonetic detail in the speech of unintelligible children: A comparison of procedures. *British Journal of Disorders of Communication, 20*, 281–287.

Ball, M. J. (1991). Recent developments in the transcription of non-normal speech. *Journal of Communication Disorders, 24*, 59–78.

Ball, M. J. (1993). *Phonetics for speech pathology* (2nd ed.). London: Whurr.

Ball, M. J., Code, C., Rahilly, J., and Hazelett, D. (1994). Non-segmental aspects of disordered speech: Developments in transcription. *Clinical Linguistics and Phonetics, 8*, 67–83.

Bernhardt, B., and Ball, M. J. (1993). Characteristics of atypical speech currently not included in the Extension to the IPA. *Journal of the International Phonetic Association, 23*, 35–38.

Bronstein, A. J. (Ed.). (1988). *Conference papers on American English and the International Phonetic Alphabet.* Tuscaloosa, AL: University of Alabama Press.

Compton, A. J., and Hutton, S. (1980). *Phonetics for children's misarticulations.* San Francisco: Carousel House.

Edwards, H. T. (1997). *Applied Phonetics: The Sounds of American English* (2nd ed.). San Diego, CA: Singular Publishing Group.

Grunwell, P., and Harding, A. (1996). A note on describing types of nasality. *Clinical Linguistics and Phonetics, 10*, 157–161.

Johnson, K. (1997). *Acoustic and auditory phonetics.* Oxford, UK: Blackwell.

Ladefoged, P., and Maddieson, I. (1996). *The sounds of the world's languages.* Oxford, UK: Blackwell.

Laver, J. (1994). *Principles of phonetics.* Cambridge, UK: Cambridge University Press.

Lehiste, I. (1970). *Suprasegmentals.* Cambridge, MA: MIT Press.

Louko, L. J., and Edwards, M. L. (Eds.). (2001). *Collecting and transcribing speech samples: Enhancing phonological analysis. Topics in Language Disorders, 21*(4).

Maassen, B., Offerninga, S., Vieregge, W., and Thoonen, G. (1996). Transcription of pathological speech in children by means of extIPA: Agreement and relevance. In T. Powell (Ed.), *Pathologies of speech and language: Contributions of clinical phonetics and linguistics* (pp. 37–43). New Orleans, LA: ICPLA.

Mackay, I. (1987). *Phonetics: The science of speech production* (2nd ed.). Boston: Little, Brown.

Paden, E. P. (1989). *Excercises in phonetic transcription: A programmed workbook* (2nd ed.). Woburn, MA: Butterworth-Heinemann.

PRDS. (1983). *The Phonetic Representation of Disordered Speech: Final report*. London: King's Fund.

Pullum, G. K., and Ladusaw, W. A. (1996). *Phonetic symbol guide* (2nd ed.). Chicago: University of Illinois Press.

Shriberg, L., Hinke, R., and Trost-Steffen, C. (1987). A procedure to select and train persons for narrow phonetic transcription by consensus. *Clinical Linguistics and Phonetics, 1*, 171–189.

Vieregge, W. H., and Maassen, B. (1999). ExtIPA transcriptions of consonants and vowels spoken by dyspractic children: Agreement and validity. In B. Maassen and P. Groenen (Eds.), *Pathologies of speech and language: Advances in clinical phonetics and linguistics* (pp. 275–284). London: Whurr.

On-line Resources

International Phonetic Association (IPA) home page
http://www2.arts.gla.ac.uk/IPA/ipa.html

SIL International home page
http://www.sil.org

IPA learning materials
http://www2.arts.gla.ac.uk/IPA/cassettes.html
http://hctv.humnet.ucla.edu/departments/linguistics/VowelsandConsonants

IPA Fonts
http://www2.arts.gla.ac.uk/IPA/ipafonts.html
http://www.sil.org/computing/fonts/encore-ipa.html
http://www.chass.utoronto.ca/~rogers/fonts.html

Phonological Awareness Intervention for Children with Expressive Phonological Impairments

Phonological awareness refers to an individual's awareness of the sound structure of a language. Results from a number of studies indicate that phonological awareness skills are highly correlated with reading success (see Stanovich, 1980) and that phonological awareness can be enhanced by direct instruction (see Blachman et al., 1994). Some scientists prefer using the terms phonological sensitivity or metaphonology rather than phonological awareness. These three terms are generally considered comparable in meaning, except that metaphonology implies that the awareness is at a more conscious level. A fourth term, phonemic awareness, refers only to phonemes, whereas phonological awareness includes syllables and intrasyllabic units (onset and rime). Phonological processing, the most encompassing of these related terms, includes phonological production, verbal working memory, word retrieval, spelling, and writing, as well as phonological awareness. Among the individuals who have been identified most consistently as being "at risk" for failure to develop appropriate phonological awareness skills, and ultimately literacy,

are children with expressive phonological impairments (EPIs) (Webster and Plante, 1992).

Relationship Between Expressive Phonological Impairment (EPI) and Phonological Awareness. A growing body of evidence indicates that young children with severe EPI go on to experience problems in literacy. As well, results from another line of research indicate that individuals with reading disabilities evidence more phonological production difficulties (e.g., with multisyllabic words) than their peers with typical reading abilities (Catts, 1986). Bird, Bishop, and Freeman (1995) found that the children who had severe EPI experienced greater difficulty with phonological awareness tasks than their ability-matched peers, even when the tasks did not require a verbal response. Clarke-Klein and Hodson (1995) obtained similar results for spelling. Larivee and Catts (1999), who tested children first in kindergarten and again 1 year later, found that expressive phonology (measured by a multisyllabic word and nonword production task) and phonological awareness scores in kindergarten accounted for significant amounts of variance in first-grade reading.

Several investigators (e.g., Bishop and Adams, 1990; Catts, 1993), however, have reported that phonological impairments alone do not have as great an impact on literacy as language impairments do. A possible explanation for this discrepancy may be the level of EPI severity in the participants in their studies.

Severity Considerations. A common practice in the articulation/phonology literature is to report the number of errors on an articulation test. Not all speech sound errors are equal, however. For example, if two children have 16 errors on the same test, some examiners might view them as equal. If, however, one child evidences a lisp for all sibilants and the other has 16 omissions, the impact on intelligibility will be vastly different. Moreover, the child with extensive omissions might be identified as having a language impairment because of the omission of final consonants (which would affect the production of word-final morphemes on an expressive language measure). Some highly unintelligible children who are considered to have a language impairment may, in fact, have a severe phonological impairment with intact receptive language abilities. Typically such children produce final morphemes as they learn the phonological pattern of word-final consonants.

Phonological Awareness Treatment Studies for Children with EPI. Although there have been numerous studies reporting the results of phonological awareness treatment, only a few investigators have focused on children with phonological or language impairments. van Kleeck, Gillam, and McFadden (1998) provided classroom-based phonological awareness treatment (15 minutes twice a week) to 16 children with speech and/or language disorders (8 in a preschool class and 8 in a prekindergarten class). The small-group sessions focused on rhyming during the first semester and on phoneme awareness during the second semester. The treatment groups and a nontreatment comparison group all made substantial gains in rhyming. Children in the treatment groups, however, made markedly greater gains on phonemic awareness tasks than children in the nontreatment group. Information on changes in expressive phonology or language was not provided by the investigators.

Howell and Dean (1994) used their Metaphon program to provide both phonological awareness and production treatment for 13 preschool children with EPI in Scotland. In phase 1 of this program, children progress from the concept/sound (not speech) level to the phoneme level to the word level. Minimal pairs are used extensively during phase 1. In phase 2, the progression is from word level to sentence level. The children attended between 11 and 34 30-minute sessions weekly. Single subject case study results indicated that the children improved on both phonological production and phonological awareness tasks (sentence and phoneme segmentation).

Harbers, Paden, and Halle (1999) provided individual treatment to four preschool children with EPI for 6–9 months that focused on both feature awareness and production for three phonological patterns that the children lacked. All four children targeted /s/ clusters. Three targeted strident singletons, two targeted velars, two targeted liquids, and one targeted final consonants. The investigators used a combination of the Metaphon (Howell and Dean, 1994) and Cycles (Hodson and Paden, 1991) treatment approaches. Improvement in the production of /s/ clusters coincided with gains in recognizing /s/ cluster features for two of the four children targeting /s/ clusters. Both of the children targeting velars also evidenced concomitant gains in production and awareness. For the remaining targets, there was a slight tendency for the two variables (phonological awareness and production) to move in similar directions, but inconsistencies occurred.

Gillon (2000) conducted a phonological awareness treatment study in New Zealand that involved 91 children with "spoken language impairment" between the ages of 5 and 7 years. Twenty-three children participated in an experimental "integrated" treatment program. A second group of 23 children received traditional speech-sound treatment. Two additional groups served as controls. One treatment group of 15 children who received "minimal" intervention, and the other consisted of 30 phonologically normal children. Children in the first treatment group received two 60-minute sessions per week until a total of 20 hours of intervention had been completed. The second group participated in phoneme-oriented sessions for the same amount of time. All of the children continued participating in their regular classroom literacy instruction, which was based on a "Whole Language" model.

The children in the first group did not receive direct production treatment for EPI during the course of the study. Additional stimulus items for children's individual speech sound errors were integrated into some of the activities, however. The phonological awareness treatment focused on the development of skills at the phonemic level and integrated phonological awareness activities with grapheme-phoneme correspondence training. Activities included (a) picture Bingo and oddity games for rhyme awareness, (b) identification of initial and final sounds, and sometimes medial sounds, (c) phoneme segmentation, (d) phoneme blending, and (e) linking speech to print. The children in this group made significantly greater gains in phonological awareness and reading scores than the children in the other groups. Moreover, the children also made greater gains in phonological production than children in the other groups with EPI. The results of this investigation lend support to the contention that it is important to incorporate phonological awareness tasks into treatment sessions for children with EPI.

Enhancing Phonological Awareness Skills. Available tasks range in difficulty from simple "yes-no" judgments regarding whether two words rhyme to complex phonological manipulation activities (e.g., pig Latin, spoonerisms). Moreover, many activities that are commonly used in treatment sessions have phonological awareness components. When children are taught how a sound is produced and how it feels, they develop awareness about place, manner, and voicing aspects of the sounds in their phonological system. One phonological awareness treatment program (Lindamood and Lindamood, 1998) has a component that specifically addresses teaching the articulatory characteristics of phonemes to all children with reading disabilities, even when there are no phonological production problems. Moreover, when children learn about where a sound is located in a word (initial, medial, or final position), they develop awareness about word positions.

One phonological awareness activity that has proved to be particularly effective is the "Say-It-And-Move-It" task, using Elkonin cards (Ball and Blachman, 1991, adapted from Elkonin, 1963). Children are taught to represent the sounds in one- (e.g., *a*), two- (e.g., *up*), or three-phoneme (e.g., *cat*) words by using manipulatives. Initially blank tiles or blocks are used. Tiles with graphemes are incorporated after the child demonstrates recognition of the sounds for the letters. The top half of the paper has a picture of a word. The bottom half has the appropriate number of boxes for the phonemes needed for the word. Children are taught to say each word slowly and to move one manipulative for each sound into the boxes from left to right.

Another phonological awareness activity that is widely used both for assessment and for segmentation practice is categorization. This task requires matching and oddity awareness skills. Typically the child is given four pictures and is to identify the one that does not match the others in some aspect (e.g., rhyme) and thus is the "odd one out." Categorization also is used for individual sounds (e.g., initial consonants).

Learning to blend phonological segments to make words is another important task and one that is extremely difficult for some children. Blending tasks commonly start at the word level with compound words (e.g., *ice* plus *cream*) followed by blending syllables (e.g., *can* plus *dee*; *candy*). Blending intrasyllabic units (e.g., onset and rime, as *sh* plus *eep*; and body and coda, as *shee* plus *p*) should precede blending individual phonemes (e.g., *sh* plus *ee* plus *p*).

Another task that has been found to be highly correlated with success in reading is deletion (e.g., elision task, Rosner and Simon, 1971). As with blending, it is important to begin with the larger segments (e.g., compound words). The child says the word (e.g., *cowboy*), and then, after part of the word is removed (e.g., *boy*), says the new word (*cow*). After a child demonstrates success at the larger unit levels, individual phonemes are deleted (e.g., take away /t/ from *note/*, leaving *no*).

The task that consistently has accounted for the greatest amount of variance in predicting decoding success is manipulation. Children who are most successful performing phoneme manipulation tasks such as spoonerisms typically are the best decoders (Strattman, 2001). Phonological manipulation in "pattern" songs (e.g., "Apples and Bananas") seems to be an extremely enjoyable task for very young children and can help them be more aware of sounds and word structures.

Implications for Best Practices. Because children with EPI appear to be at risk for the development of normal reading and writing skills even after they no longer have intelligibility issues, it seems prudent to incorporate activities to enhance phonological awareness skills while they are receiving treatment for phonological production. Moreover, results from Gillon's (2000) study indicate that enhancing phonological awareness skills leads to improvement in phonological production. Thus, enhancing phonological awareness skills appears to serve a dual purpose for children with expressive phonological impairments.

—*Barbara Hodson and Kathy Strattman*

References

Ball, E., and Blachman, B. (1991). Does phoneme awareness training in kindergarten make a difference in early word recognition and developmental spelling? *Reading Research Quarterly, 26,* 49–66.

Bird, J., Bishop, D. V. M., and Freeman, M. H. (1995). Phonological awareness and literacy development in children with expressive phonological impairments. *Journal of Speech and Hearing Research, 38,* 446–462.

Bishop, D. V. M., and Adams, C. (1990). A prospective study of the relationship between specific language impairment, phonological disorders, and reading retardation. *Journal of Child Psychology and Psychiatry, 31,* 1027–1050.

Blachman, B., Ball, E., Black, R., and Tangle, D. (1994). Kindergarten teachers develop phonemic awareness in low-income, inner-city classrooms. Does it make a difference? *Reading and Writing: An Interdisciplinary Journal, 6,* 1–18.

Catts, H. W. (1986). Speech production/phonological deficits in reading-disordered children. *Journal of Learning Disabilities, 19,* 504–508.

Catts, H. W. (1993). The relationship between speech-language impairments and reading disabilities. *Journal of Speech and Hearing Research, 6,* 948–958.

Clarke-Klein, S., and Hodson, B. (1995). A phonologically based analysis of misspellings by third graders with disordered-phonology histories. *Journal of Speech and Hearing Research, 38,* 839–849.

Elkonin, D. B. (1963). The psychology of mastering the elements of reading. In B. Simon and J. Simon (Eds.), *Educational psychology in the USSR* (pp. 165–179). London: Routledge.

Gillon, G. T. (2000). The efficacy of phonological awareness intervention for children with spoken language impairment. *Language, Speech, and Hearing Services in Schools, 31,* 126–141.

Harbers, H. M., Paden, E. P., and Halle, J. W. (1999). Phonological awareness and production: Changes during intervention. *Language, Speech, and Hearing Services in Schools, 30,* 50–60.

Hodson, B., and Paden, E. (1991). *Targeting intelligible speech* (2nd ed.). Austin, TX: Pro-Ed.

Howell, J., and Dean, E. (1994). *Treating phonological disorders in children* (2nd ed.). London: Whurr.

Larrivee, L. S., and Catts, H. W. (1999). Early reading achievement in children with expressive phonological disorders. *American Journal of Speech-Language Pathology, 8,* 118–128.

Lindamood, P. C., and Lindamood, P. D. (1998). The *Lindamood Phoneme Sequencing program for reading, spelling, and speech (LiPS).* Austin, TX: Pro-Ed.

Rosner, J., and Simon, D. (1971). The auditory analysis test. *Journal of Learning Disabilities, 4,* 384–392.

Stanovich, K. E. (1980). Toward an interactive compensatory model of individual differences in the development of reading fluency. *Reading Research Quarterly, 16,* 32–71.

Strattman, K. (2001). *Predictors of second graders' reading and spelling scores.* Unpublished doctoral dissertation. Wichita State University, Wichita, KS.

van Kleeck, A., Gillam, R. B., and McFadden, T. U. (1998). A study of classroom-based phonological awareness training for preschoolers with speech and/or language disorders. *American Journal of Speech-Language Pathology, 7,* 65–76.

Webster, P., and Plante, A. (1992). Effects of phonological impairment on word, syllable, and phoneme segmentation and reading. *Language, Speech, and Hearing Services in Schools, 23,* 176–182.

Further Readings

Adams, M. J., Foorman, B. R., Lundberg, I., and Beeler, T. (1998). *Phonemic awareness in young children: A classroom curriculum.* Baltimore: Paul H. Brookes.

Badian, N. (Ed.). (2000). *Prediction and prevention of reading failure.* Baltimore: York Press.

Blachman, B. (Ed.). (1997). *Foundations of reading acquisition and dyslexia.* Mahwah, NJ: Erlbaum.

Blachman, B., Ball, E., Black, R., and Tangel, D. (2000). *Road to the code.* Baltimore: Paul H. Brookes.

Catts, H. W., and Kamhi, A. G. (Eds.). (1999). *Language and reading disabilities.* Needham Heights, MA: Allyn and Bacon.

Catts, H., and Olsen, T. (1993). *Sounds abound: Listening, rhyming, and reading.* East Moline, IL: LinguiSystems.

Chafouleas, S., VanAuken, T., and Dunham, K. (2001). Not all phonemes are created equal: The effects of linguistic manipulations on phonological awareness tasks. *Journal of Psychoeducational Assessment, 19,* 216–226.

Cunningham, A. (1990). Explicit vs. implicit instruction in phonological awareness. *Journal of Experimental Child Psychology, 50,* 429–444.

Hatcher, P. (1994). *Sound linkage: An integrated programme for overcoming reading difficulties.* London: Whurr.

Hodson, B. (Ed.). (1994). *From phonology to metaphonology: Issues, assessment, and intervention* [special issue]. *Topics in Language Disorders, 14.*

Hulme, E., and Joshi, R. (Eds.). (1998). *Reading and spelling: Development and disorders.* Mahwah, NJ: Erlbaum.

Lencher, O., and Podhajski, B. (1998). *The sounds abound program.* East Moline, IL: LinguiSystems.

Lonigan, C., Burgess, S., Anthony, J., and Barker, T. (1998). Development of phonological sensitivity in 2- to 5-year-old children. *Journal of Educational Psychology, 90,* 294–311.

Moats, L. C. (2000). *Speech to print.* Baltimore: Paul H. Brookes.

Snow, C., Burns, M., and Griffin, P. (Eds.). (1998). *Preventing reading difficulties in young children.* Washington, DC: National Academy Press.

Spector, C. (1999). *Sound effects: Activities for developing phonological awareness.* Eau Claire, WI: Thinking Publications.

Stackhouse, J., and Wells, B. (1997). *Children's speech and literacy difficulties: A psycholinguistic framework.* London: Whurr.

Stackhouse, J., and Wells, B. (Eds.). (2001). *Children's speech and literacy difficulties: Vol. 2. Identification and intervention.* London: Whurr.

Stackhouse, J., Wells, B., and Pascoe, M. (2002). From phonological therapy to phonological awareness. *Seminars in Speech and Language, 23,* 27–42.

Stanovich, K. (2000). *Progress in understanding reading.* New York: Guilford Press.

Torgesen, J., and Mathes, P. (2000). *A basic guide to understanding, assessing, and teaching phonological awareness.* Austin, TX: Pro-Ed.

Wolf, M. (Ed.). (2001). *Dyslexia, fluency, and the brain.* Timonium, MD: York Press.

Phonological Errors, Residual

Shriberg (1994) has conceptualized developmental phonological disorders as speech disorders that originate during the developmental period. In most cases the cause of such disorders cannot be attributed to significant involvement of a child's speech or hearing processes, cognitive-linguistic functions, or psychosocial processes (Bernthal and Bankson, 1998), but causal origins may be related to genetic or environmental differences (Shriberg, 1994; Shriberg and Kwiatkowski, 1994). Children with developmental phonological disorders are heterogeneous and exhibit a range in the severity of their phonological disorders. Generally, the expected developmental period for speech sound acquisition ends at approximately 9 years of age, thus encompassing birth through the early school years. In sum, it is posited that children who exhibit phonological disorders differ with regard to the etiology and severity of the disorder and include both preschool and school-age children (Deputy and Weston, 1998). Some individuals with developmental phonological disorders acquire normal speech, while others continue to exhibit a phonological disorder throughout the life span, despite having received treatment for the phonological disorder (Shriberg et al., 1997).

Residual phonological errors are a subtype of developmental phonological disorders that persist beyond the expected period of speech-sound development or normalization (Shriberg, 1997). They are present in the speech of older school-age children and adults. Individuals with residual errors can be further classified into subgroups of those with a history of speech delay and those without a history of speech delay (i.e., individuals in whom a speech delay was diagnosed at some time during the developmental period and those who were not so diagnosed). It is postulated that the two groups differ with respect to causal factors. The residual errors of the first group are thought to reflect environmental influences, while nonenvironmental causal factors such as genetic transmission are thought to be responsible for the phonological errors of the second group.

Most residual errors have been identified as distortions (Smit et al., 1990; Shriberg, 1993) of the expected allophones of a particular phoneme. Distortions are variant productions that do not fall within the perceptual boundaries of a specific target phoneme (Daniloff, Wilcox, and Stephens, 1980; Bernthal and Bankson, 1998). It has been hypothesized that distortions reflect incorrect allophonic rules or sensorimotor processing limitations. That is, such productions are either permanent or temporary manifestations of inappropriate allophonic representation and/or the sensorimotor control of articulatory accuracy. It has been suggested that children initially delete and substitute sounds and then produce distortions of sounds such as /r/, /l/, and /s/ when normalizing sound production; however, investigative study has not supported this hypothesis as a generality in children who normalize their phonological skills with treatment (Shriberg and Kwiatkowski, 1988). Ohde and Sharf (1992) provide excellent descriptions of the acoustic and physiologic parameters of common distortion errors.

Smit et al. (1990) conducted a large-scale investigation of speech sound acquisition and reported that the distortion errors noted in the speech of their older test subjects varied with respect to judged clinical impact or severity. Some productions were judged to be minor distortions, while others were designated as clinically significant. Shriberg (1993) also noted such differences in his study of children with developmental phonological disorders. He classified the errors into nonclinical and clinical distortion types. Nonclinical distortions are thought to reflect dialect or other factors such as speech-motor constraints and are not targeted for therapy. Clinical distortions are potential targets for treatment and have been categorized by prevalence into common and uncommon types. The most common and uncommon types are listed in Figure 1. The most common residual errors include distortions of the sound classes of liquids, fricatives, and affricates. Uncommon distortion errors include errors such as weak or imprecise consonant production and difficulty maintaining nasal and voicing features. In most cases, residual errors constitute

Common Distortion Errors

1. Dentalization of voiced/voiceless sibilant fricatives or affricates
2. Derhotacized /r/, /ɝ/, /ɚ/
3. Lateralization of voiced/voiceless sibilant fricatives or affricates
4. Velarized /l/ or /r/
5. Labialized /l/ or /r/

Uncommon Distortion Errors

1. Weak consonant productions
2. Imprecise articulation of consonants and vowels
3. Inability to maintain oral/nasal contrasts
4. Difficulty in maintaining correct voicing contrasts

Figure 1. Common and uncommon distortion errors as reported by Shriberg (1993).

minor involvement of phonological production and do not have a significant impact on intelligibility, but research indicates that normal speakers react negatively to persons with even minor residual errors (Mowrer, Wahl, and Doolan, 1978; Silverman and Paulus, 1989; Crowe Hall, 1991).

Treatment for persons with residual errors is generally carried out using approaches that have been used with younger children. The treatment approaches are based on motor learning or cognitive-linguistic concepts (Lowe, 1994; Bauman-Waengler, 2000); however, in most cases a motor learning approach is utilized (Gierut, 1998). Although most individuals normalize their residual errors with intervention, some individuals do not (Dagenais, 1995; Shuster, Ruscello, and Toth, 1995). The actual number of clients in the respective categories is unknown, but survey data of school practitioners reported by Ruscello (1995a) indicate that a subgroup of clients do not improve with traditional treatment methods. Respondents indicated that children either were unable to achieve correct production of an error sound or achieved correct production but were unable to incorporate the sound into spontaneous speech. The respondents did not list the types of sound errors, but the error sounds reported are in agreement with the residual errors identified by both Shriberg (1993) and Smit et al. (1990).

In some cases, specially designed treatments are necessary to facilitate remediation of residual errors. For example, principles from biofeedback and speech physiology have been incorporated into treatments (Dagenais, 1995; Ruscello, 1995b; Gibbon et al., 1999). Different forms of sensory information other than auditory input have been provided to assist the individual in developing appropriate target productions. Shuster, Ruscello, and Toth (1995) identified two older children with residual /r/ errors who had received traditional long-term phonological treatment without success. A biofeedback treatment utilizing real-time spectrography was implemented for both subjects, and the results indi-

cated that the two subjects were able to acquire correct production of the former residual error.

In summary, residual errors are a distinct subtype of developmental phonological errors that are present in the speech of older children and adults who are beyond the period of normal sound acquisition. Most residual errors are described as distortions, which are sound variations that are not within the phonetic boundaries of the intended target sound. Generally, residual errors are minor in terms of severity and do not interfere with intelligibility, but normal speakers do react negatively to such minor speech variations. An exact estimate of children and adults with residual errors is unknown, but it is thought that there are substantial numbers of individuals with such a phonological disorder.

—*Dennis M. Ruscello*

References

Bauman-Waengler, J. (2000). *Articulatory and phonological impairments: A clinical focus.* Boston: Allyn and Bacon.

Bernthal, J. E., and Bankson, N. W. (1998). *Articulation and phonological disorders* (4th ed.). Boston: Allyn and Bacon.

Crowe Hall, B. J. (1991). Attitudes of fourth and sixth graders toward peers with mild articulation disorders. *Language, Speech and Hearing Services in Schools, 22,* 334–339.

Dagenais, P. A. (1995). Electropalatography in the treatment of articulation/phonological disorders. *Journal of Communication Disorders, 28,* 303–330.

Daniloff, R., Wilcox, K., and Stephens, M. I. (1980). An acoustic-articulatory description of children's defective /s/ productions. *Journal of Communication Disorders, 13,* 347–363.

Deputy, P. N., and Weston, A. D. (1998). A framework for differential diagnosis of developmental phonologic disorders. In B. J. Philips and D. M. Ruscello (Eds.), *Differential diagnosis in speech-language pathology* (pp. 113–158). Boston: Butterworth-Heinemann.

Gibbon, F., Stewart, F., Hardcastle, W. J., and Crampin, L. (1999). Widening access to electropalatography for children with persistent sound system disorders. *American Journal of Speech-Language Pathology, 8,* 319–334.

Gierut, J. A. (1998). Treatment efficacy: Functional phonological disorders in children. *Journal of Speech, Language, and Hearing Research, 41,* S85–S100.

Lowe, R. J. (1994). *Phonology: Assessment and intervention applications in speech pathology.* Baltimore: Williams and Wilkins.

Mowrer, D. E., Wahl, P., and Doolan, S. J. (1978). Effect of lisping on audience evaluation of male speakers. *Journal of Speech and Hearing Disorders, 43,* 140–148.

Ohde, R. N., and Sharf, D. J. (1992). *Phonetic analysis of normal and abnormal speech.* New York: Merrill.

Ruscello, D. M. (1995a). Visual feedback in treatment of residual phonological disorders. *Journal of Communication Disorders, 28,* 279–302.

Ruscello, D. M. (1995b). Speech appliances in the treatment of phonological disorders. *Journal of Communication Disorders, 28,* 331–353.

Shriberg, L. D. (1993). Four new speech and prosody-voice measures for genetics research and other studies in developmental phonological disorders. *Journal of Speech and Hearing Research, 36,* 105–140.

Shriberg, L. D. (1994). Five subtypes of developmental phonological disorders. *Clinics in Communication Disorders, 4,* 38–53.

Shriberg, L. D. (1997). Developmental phonological disorders: One or many? In B. W. Hodson and M. L. Edwards (Eds.), *Perspectives in Applied Phonology* (pp. 105–132). Gaithersburg, MD: Aspen.

Shriberg, L. D., Austin, D., Lewis, B., McSweeny, J. L., and Wilson, D. L. (1997). The speech disorders classification system (SDCS): Extensions and lifespan reference data. *Journal of Speech, Language, and Hearing Research, 40,* 723–740.

Shriberg, L. D., and Kwiatkowski, J. (1988). A follow-up study of children with phonologic disorders of unknown origin. *Journal of Speech and Hearing Disorders, 53,* 144–155.

Shriberg, L. D., and Kwiatkowski, J. (1994). Developmental phonological disorders: I. A clinical profile. *Journal of Speech and Hearing Research, 37,* 1100–1126.

Shuster, L. I., Ruscello, D. M., and Toth, A. (1995). The use of visual feedback to elicit correct /r/. *American Journal of Speech-Language Pathology, 4,* 37–44.

Silverman, F. H., and Paulus, P. G. (1989). Peer reactions to teenagers who substitute /w/ for /r/. *Language, Speech, and Hearing Services in Schools, 20,* 219–221.

Smit, A. B., Hand, L., Freilinger, J. J., Bernthal, J. E., and Bird, A. (1990). The Iowa articulation norms project and its Nebraska replication. *Journal of Speech and Hearing Disorders, 55,* 779–798.

Further Readings

Bankson, N. W., and Bernthal, J. E. (1982). Articulation assessment. In N. J. Lass, L. V. McReynolds, J. L. Northern, and D. E. Yoder (Eds.), *Speech, language, and hearing* (pp. 572–590). Philadelphia: Saunders.

Bleile, K. M. (1995). *Manual of articulation and phonological disorders.* San Diego, CA: Singular Publishing Group.

Flipsen, P., Shriberg, L., Weismer, G., Karlsson, H., and McSweeny, J. (1999). Acoustic characteristics of /s/ in adolescents. *Journal of Speech, Language, and Hearing Research, 42,* 663–677.

Ruscello, D. M., St. Louis, K. O., and Mason, N. (1991). School-aged children with phonologic disorders: Coexistence with other speech/language disorders. *Journal of Speech and Hearing Research, 34,* 236–242.

Shriberg, L. D., and Kwiatkowski, J. (1981). Phonological disorders: I. A diagnostic classification system. *Journal of Speech and Hearing Disorders, 47,* 226–241.

Shriberg, L. D., Tomblin, J. B., and McSweeny, J. L. (1999). Prevalence of speech delay in 6-year-old children and comorbidity with language impairment. *Journal of Speech, Language, and Hearing Research, 42,* 1461–1481.

Phonology: Clinical Issues in Serving Speakers of African-American Vernacular English

Word pronunciation is an overt speech characteristic that readily identifies dialect differences among normal speakers even when other aspects of their spoken language do not. Although regional pronunciation differences in the United States were recognized historically, social dialects were not. Nonprestige social dialects in particular were viewed simply as disordered speech. A case in point is the native English dialect spoken by many African Americans, a populous ethnic minority group. This dialect is labeled in various ways but is referred to here as African American Vernacular English (AAVE). As a result of litigation, legislation, and social changes beginning in the 1960s, best clinical practice now requires speech clinicians to regard social dialect differences in defining speech norms for clinical service delivery. This mandate has created challenges for clinical practices.

One clinical issue is how to identify AAVE speakers. African Americans are racially, ethnically, and linguistically diverse. Not all learn AAVE, and among those who do, the density of use varies. This discussion considers only those African Americans with an indigenous slave history in the United States and ancestral ties to Subsaharan Africa. The native English spoken today is rooted partly in a pidgin-creole origin. Since slavery was abolished, the continuing physical and social segregation of African Americans has sustained large AAVE communities, particularly in southern states.

Contemporary AAVE pronunciation is both like and unlike Standard English (SE). In both dialects, the vowel and consonant sounds are the same (with a few exceptions), but their use in words differs (Wolfram, 1994; Stockman, 1996b). Word-initial single and clustered consonants in AAVE typically match those in SE except for interdental fricatives (e.g., this > /dɪs/). The dialects differ in their distributions of word-final consonants. Some final consonants in AAVE are replaced (cf. ba<u>th</u> and ba<u>the</u> > /f/ and /v/, respectively). Others are absent as single sounds (e.g., ma<u>n</u>) or in consonant clusters (tes<u>t</u> > /tɛs/). Yet AAVE is not an open-syllable dialect. Final consonants are variably absent in predictable or rule-governed ways. They are more likely to be absent or reduced in clusters when the following word or syllable begins with another consonant rather than a vowel (Wolfram, 1994) or when a consonant is an alveolar as opposed to a labial or velar stop (Stockman, 1991). In multisyllabic words, unstressed syllables (e.g., away > /-weɪ/) in any position may be absent, depending on grammatical and semantic factors (Vaughn-Cooke, 1986). Consonants may also be reordered in some words (e.g., ask > /s/), and multiple words may be merged phonetically (e.g., fixing to > finna; suppose to > sposta) to function as separate words. These broadly predictable AAVE pronunciation patterns differ enough from SE to compromise its intelligibility for unfamiliar listeners. Intelligibility can be decreased further by co-occurring dialect differences in prosodic or nonsegmental (rhythmic and vocal pitch) features (Tarone, 1975; Dejarnette and Holland, 1993), coupled with known grammatical, semantic, and pragmatic ones. Consider just the number of grammatical and phonological differences between SE and AAVE in the following example:

SE:	They are not fixing to ask for the car /
AAVE:	They not finna ask for the car /
	the ar nat fɪksɪn tu aesk fɔr thə kaɚ /
	deɪ na fɪnə æks fʌ də ka: /

Enough is known about the complex perceptual judgments of speech intelligibility to predict that the more work listeners have to do to figure out what is being said, the more likely is speech to be judged as unclear.

Identifying atypical AAVE speakers can be difficult, especially if known causes of disordered speech—hearing loss, brain damage, and so on—are absent, as is often the case. Clinicians must know a lot about the dialect to defend a diagnosis. But most clinicians (95%) are not African American and have little exposure to AAVE (Campbell and Taylor, 1992). Misdiagnosing normal AAVE speakers as abnormal is encouraged further by the similarity of their typical pronunciation patterns (e.g., final consonant deletion, cluster reduction, and interdental fricative substitutions) to those commonly observed among immature or disordered SE speakers. However, typically developing African-American speakers make fewer errors on standardized articulation tests as they get older (Ratusnik and Koenigsknecht, 1976; Simmons, 1988; Haynes and Moran, 1989). Still, they make more errors than their predominantly white, age-matched peers (Ratusnik and Koenigsknecht, 1976; Seymour and Seymour, 1981; Simmons, 1988; Cole and Taylor, 1990), and they do so beyond the age expected for developmental errors (Haynes and Moran, 1989). Therefore it is unknown whether the overrepresentation of African Americans in clinical caseloads is due to practitioner ignorance, test bias, or an actual higher prevalence of speech disorders as a result of economic poverty and its associated risks for development in all areas.

The accuracy in identifying articulation/phonological disorders improves when test scores are adjusted for dialect differences (Cole and Taylor, 1990), or when the pronunciation patterns for a child and caregiver are compared on the same test words (Terrell, Arensberg, and Rosa, 1992). However, tests of isolated word pronunciation are not entirely useful, even when nonstandard dialect use is not penalized. They typically provide no contexts for sampling AAVE's variable pronunciation rules, which can cross word boundaries, as in the case of final consonant absence. Although standardized deep tests of articulation (McDonald, 1968) do elicit paired word combinations, they favor the sampling of abutting consonant sequences (e.g., bus fish), which penalize AAVE speakers even more, given their tendency to delete final consonants that precede other consonants as opposed to vowels (Stockman, 1993, 1996b). These issues have encouraged the use of criterion-referenced evaluations of spontaneous speech samples for assessment (see Stockman, 1996a, and Schraeder et al., 1999).

Despite the assessment challenges, it is readily agreed that some AAVE speakers do have genuine phonological/articulatory disorders (Seymour and Seymour, 1981; Taylor and Peters, 1986). They differ from typically developing community peers in both the frequency and patterning of speech sound error. This is true whether the clinical and nonclinical groups are distinguished by the judgments of community informants, such as Head Start teachers (Bleile and Wallach, 1992), other classroom teachers (Washington and Craig, 1992),

or speech-language clinicians (Stockman and Settle, 1991; Wilcox, 1996).

AAVE speakers with disorders can differ from their nondisordered peers on speech sounds that are like SE (Type I error, e.g., word-initial single and clustered consonants). They can also differ on sounds that are not like SE either qualitatively (Type II error, e.g., interdental fricative substitutions) or quantitatively (Type III error, e.g., more frequent final consonant absence in abutting consonant sequences). Wolfram (1994) suggested that these three error categories provide a heuristic for scaling the severity of the pronunciation difficulty and selecting targets for treatment.

Two service delivery tracks are within the scope of practice for speech clinicians. One remediates atypical speech relative to a client's native dialect. The other one expands the pronunciation patterns of normal speakers who want to speak SE when AAVE is judged to be socially or professionally handicapping (Terrell and Terrell, 1983). For both client populations, effective service delivery requires clinician sensitivity to cultural factors that impact (1) verbal and nonverbal interactions with clients, (2) selection of stimuli (e.g., games and objects) for therapy activities, and (3) scheduling of sessions (Seymour, 1986; Proctor, 1994). However, the service delivery goals do differ for these two populations. For abnormal speakers, the goal is to eradicate and replace existing patterns that decrease intelligible speech in the native dialect. This means that the pronunciation of bath/bæθ/ as /baf/ should not be targeted for change, if it conforms to the client's target dialect. But a deviation from this expected pronunciation, such as bath/bæθ/ > /bæt/ or /bæs/, is targeted, if observed at an age when developmental errors are not expected. In contrast, the service delivery goal for normal AAVE speakers is to expand rather than eradicate the existing linguistic repertoire (Taylor, 1986). An additive approach assumes that speakers can learn to switch SE and AAVE codes as the communicative situation demands, just as bilingual speakers switch languages. This means that a speaker's bidialectal repertoire includes both the SE and AAVE pronunciation of "bath" (cf. bath > /baθ/ and /bæf/).

Meeting these two different service goals requires attention to some issues that are not the same. They affect which patterns are targeted and how change is facilitated. For typical AAVE speakers learning SE, second language acquisition principles are relevant. Besides the production practice, service delivery requires contrastive analysis of the two dialects and attention to sociocultural issues that affect code switching. Correct or target productions are judged relative to SE.

In contrast, for speakers with abnormal pronunciation, AAVE should be targeted. Which features to target in therapy and how to model the input become issues, because most clinicians do not speak AAVE. They also may resist modeling a low social prestige dialect because of negative social attitudes towards it. Wolfram (1994) reminded us that AAVE and SE share many of the same target features (e.g., most word-initial consonants). Errors on shared features (Type I) should be targeted first in treatment. They are likely to impair intelligibility even more than the smaller sets of qualitative (Type II) errors, such as stop replacement of interdental fricatives (cf. this /dɪs/ > /bɪs/), or quantitative (Type III) errors, such as final consonant deletion in more than the allowable context number and types. AAVE features should be targeted for treatment only when pronunciation patterns differ from AAVE norms. Articulatory patterns would not be modified if they differed from the clinician's SE-modeled pattern but matched expected AAVE patterns.

Legitimizing social dialects like AAVE in the United States has required researchers and clinicians to (1) broaden the reference point for normalcy and (2) explore alternative strategies for identifying service needs and modifying word pronunciation. The issues singled out in this entry are not unique to phonological/articulatory problems. However, given their typically higher frequency of occurrence relative to other domains of spoken language in all groups, they may turn up more often in clinical work.

See also DIALECT SPEAKERS; DIALECT VERSUS DISORDER; LANGUAGE DISORDERS IN AFRICAN-AMERICAN CHILDREN.

—*Ida J. Stockman*

References

Bleile, K., and Wallach, H. (1992). A sociolinguistic investigation of the speech of African-American preschoolers. *American Journal of Speech-Language Pathology, 1,* 54–62.

Campbell, L., and Taylor, O. (1992). ASHA certified speech-language pathologists: Perceived competency levels with selected skills. *Howard Journal of Communication, 3,* 163–176.

Cole, P., and Taylor, O. (1990). Performance of working-class African-American children on three tests of articulation. *Language, Speech, and Hearing Services in Schools, 21,* 171–176.

Dejarnette, G., and Holland, W. (1993). Voice and voice disorders. In D. Battle (Ed.), *Communication disorders in multicultural populations* (pp. 212–238). Boston: Andover.

Haynes, W., and Moran, M. (1989). A cross-sectional developmental study of final consonant production in southern black children from preschool through third grade. *Language, Speech, and Hearing Services in Schools, 20,* 400–406.

McDonald, E. (1968). *The Screening Deep Test of Articulation.* Pittsburgh, PA: Stanwix House.

Moran, M. (1993). Final consonant deletion in African American children speaking Black English: A closer look. *Language, Speech, and Hearing Services in Schools, 24,* 161–166.

Proctor, A. (1994). Phonology and cultural diversity. In R. J. Lowe (Ed.), *Phonology: Assessment and intervention. Applications in speech pathology* (pp. 207–245). Baltimore: Williams and Wilkins.

Ratusnik, D., and Koenigsknecht, R. (1976). Influence of age on black preschoolers' nonstandard performance of certain phonological and grammatical forms. *Perceptual and Motor Skills, 42,* 199–206.

Schraeder, P., Quinn, M., Stockman, I., and Miller, J. (1999). Authentic assessment as an approach to preschool speech-language screening. *American Journal of Speech-Language Pathology, 8,* 95–200.

Seymour, H. (1986). Clinical principles for language intervention for language disorders among nonstandard speakers of English. In O. Taylor (Ed.), *Treatment of communication disorders in culturally and linguistically diverse populations* (pp. 153–178). San Diego, CA: College-Hill Press.

Seymour, H., and Seymour, C. (1981). Black English and Standard American English contrasts in consonantal development for four- and five-year-old children. *Journal of Speech and Hearing Disorders, 46,* 276–280.

Simmons, J. O. (1988). Fluharty Preschool and Language Screening Test: Analysis of construct validity. *Journal of Speech and Hearing Disorders, 53,* 168–174.

Stockman, I. (1991, November). *Constraints on final consonant deletion in Black English.* Poster presented at the annual convention of the American Speech-Language-Hearing Association, Atlanta, GA.

Stockman, I. (1993). Variable word initial and medial consonant relationships in children's speech sound articulation. *Perceptual and Motor Skills, 76,* 675–689.

Stockman, I. (1996a). The promises and pitfalls of language sample analysis as an assessment tool for linguistic minority children. *Language, Speech, and Hearing Services in Schools, 27,* 355–366.

Stockman, I. (1996b). Phonological development and disorders in African American children. In A. Kamhi, K. Pollock, and J. Harris (Eds.), *Communication development and disorders in African American children: Research, assessment and intervention.* Baltimore: Paul H. Brookes.

Stockman, I., and Settle, S. (1991, November). *Initial consonants in young black children's conversational speech.* Poster presented at the annual convention of the American Speech-Language-Hearing Association, Atlanta, GA.

Tarone, E. (1975). Aspects of intonation in Black English. *American Speech, 48,* 29–36.

Taylor, O. (1986). Teaching English as a second dialect. In O. Taylor (Ed.), *Treatment of communication disorders in culturally and linguistically diverse populations* (pp. 153–178). San Diego, CA: College-Hill Press.

Taylor, O., and Peters, C. (1986). Speech and language disorders in blacks. In O. Taylor (Ed.), *The nature of communication disorders in culturally and linguistically diverse populations* (pp. 157–180). San Diego, CA: College-Hill Press.

Terrell, S., Arensberg, K., and Rosa, M. (1992). Parent-child comparative analysis: A criterion-referenced method for the nondiscriminatory assessment of a child who spoke a relatively uncommon dialect of English. *Language, Speech, and Hearing Services in Schools, 23,* 34–42.

Terrell, S., and Terrell, F. (1983). Effects of speaking Black English on employment opportunities. *ASHA, 25,* 27–29.

Vaughn-Cooke, F. (1986). Lexical diffusion: Evidence from a decreolizing variety of Black English. In M. Montgomery and G. Bailey (Eds.), *Language variety in the South* (pp. 111–130). Tuscaloosa: University of Alabama Press.

Washington, J., and Craig, H. (1992). Articulation test performances of low-income, African-American preschoolers with communication impairments. *Language, Speech, and Hearing Services in Schools, 23,* 203–207.

Wilcox, D. L. (1996). *Distinguishing between phonological difference and disorder in children who speak African-American English.* Unpublished master's thesis, Indiana University, Bloomington.

Wolfram, W. (1994). The phonology of a sociocultural variety: The case of African American vernacular English. In J. Bernthal and N. Bankson (Eds.), *Child phonology: Characteristics, assessment, and intervention with special populations* (pp. 227–244). New York: Thieme.

Further Readings

Bailey, G. (1999). *Phonological characteristics of African American Vernacular English.* In S. S. Mufwene, J. R. Rickford, G. Bailey, and J. Baugh (Eds.), *Structure of African American vernacular English.* New York: Routledge.

Battle, D. E. (1998). *Communication disorders in multicultural populations.* Boston: Butterworth-Heinemann.

Baugh, J. (1983). *Black street speech: Its history, structure and survival.* Austin, TX: University of Texas Press.

Dillard, J. L. (1972). *Black English: Its history and usage in the United States.* New York: Random House.

Fasold, R. W., and Shuy, R. W. (1970). *Teaching Standard English in the inner city.* Washington, DC: Center for Applied Linguistics.

Fasold, R. W. (1981). The relation between black and white speech in the South. *American Speech, 56,* 163–189.

Fudala, J. B. (1974). *Arizona Articulation Proficiency Scale* (2nd ed.). Los Angeles: Western Psychological Services.

Goldman, R., and Fristoe, M. (1986). *Goldman-Fristoe Test of Articulation.* Circle Pines, MN: American Guidance Service.

Labov, W. (1972). *Language in the inner city.* Philadelphia: University of Pennysylvania Press.

Luelsdorff, P. A. (1975). *A segmental phonology of Black English.* The Hague: Mouton.

Mowrer, D., and Burger, S. (1991). A comparative analysis of phonological acquisition of consonants in the speech of $2^1/_2$- to 6-year-old Xhosa- and English-speaking children. *Clinical Linguistics and Phonetics, 5,* 139–164.

Myers-Jennings, C. C. (2000). Phonological disorders in culturally diverse populations. In T. J. Coleman (Ed.), *Clinical management of communication disorders in culturally diverse children* (pp. 173–196). Boston: Allyn and Bacon.

Newman, P. W., and Craighead, N. A. (1989). Assessment of articulatory and phonological disorders. In N. Craighead, P. Newman, and W. Secord (Eds.), *Assessment and remediation of articulatory and phonological disorders.* Columbus, OH: Merrill.

Seymour, H., Green, L., and Huntley, R. (1991). *Phonological patterns in the conversational speech of African-American Children.* Poster presented at the national convention of the American Speech-Language-Hearing Association, Atlanta, GA.

Seymour, H., and Ralabate, P. (1985). The acquisition of a phonologic feature of Black English. *Journal of Communication Disorders, 18,* 139–148.

Stockman, I., and Stephenson, L. (1981). Children's articulation of medial consonant clusters: Implications for syllabification. *Language and Speech, 24,* 185–204.

Taylor, O. L. (Ed.). (1986). *Nature of communication disorders in culturally and linguistically diverse populations.* San Diego, CA: College-Hill Press.

Taylor, O. (Ed.). (1986). *Treatment of communication disorders in culturally and linguistically diverse populations.* San Diego, CA: College-Hill Press.

Tull, B. M. (1973). *Analysis of selected prosodic features in the speech of black and white children.* Unpublished dissertation, Ohio State University, Columbus.

Van Keulen, J. E., Weddington, G. T., and Debose, C. E. (1998). *Speech, language, learning and the African American child.* Boston: Allyn and Bacon.

Vaughn-Cooke, F. (1976). The implementation of a phonological change: The case for re-syllabification in Black English. *Dissertation Abstracts International, 38*(01), 234A. (University Microfilms No. AAC7714537)

Vaughn-Cooke, F. (1987). Are black and white vernaculars diverging? *American Speech, 62,* 12–32.

Wolfram, W. (1989). Structural variability in phonological development: Final nasals in vernacular Black English. In R. Fasold and D. Schiffren (Eds.), *Current issues in linguistic theory: Language change and variation* (pp. 301–332). Amsterdam: John Benjamins.

Wolfram, W., and Schilling-Estes, N. (1998). *American English: Dialects and variation.* Malden, MA: Blackwell Publishers.

Psychosocial Problems Associated with Communicative Disorders

Individuals who study communicative disorders have long been interested in the psychosocial difficulties associated with these problems. This interest has taken different faces over the years as researchers and clinicians have focused on various aspects of the relationship between communicative impairment and psychological and social difficulties. For example, relatively early in the development of the profession of speech-language pathology, some investigators approached specific communicative disorders, such as stuttering, as manifestations of underlying psychological dysfunction (e.g., Travis, 1957). More recent approaches have moved away from considering psychiatric dysfunction as the basis for most speech and language impairment (an exception is alexithymia). Despite this reorientation, there is still considerable interest in the psychosocial aspects of communicative disorders. The literature is both extensive and wide-ranging, and much of it focuses on specific types of impairment (e.g., stuttering, language impairment). There are two general areas of study, however, that are of particular interest. The first is the frequent co-occurrence of speech and language impairment and socioemotional problems. A great deal of research has been directed toward exploring this relationship as well as toward determining what mechanisms might underlie this comorbidity. A second area of interest concerns the long-term outcomes of communicative problems across various areas of psychosocial development (e.g., peer relations, socioemotional status). Both of these lines of work are briefly discussed here.

Co-occurrence of Disorders. Numerous investigators have reported a high level of co-occurrence between communicative disorders and socioemotional problems. This high level of co-occurrence has been observed in various groups of children, including both those with a primary diagnosis of speech and language impairment and those with a primary diagnosis of psychiatric impairment or behavior disorder. Illustrative of these findings is the work of Baker and Cantwell (1987). These researchers performed psychiatric evaluations on 600 consecutive patients seen at a community speech, language, and hearing clinic. Children were divided into three subgroups of communication problems: speech (children with disorders of articulation, voice, and fluency), language (children with problems in language expression, comprehension, and pragmatics), and a speech and language group (children with a mixture of problems). Of these children, approximately 50% were diagnosed as having a psychiatric disorder. These problems were categorized into two general groups of behavior disorder and emotional disorder.

Several researchers have speculated on the basis for this high level of co-occurrence between communication and socioemotional disorders. For example, Beitchman, Brownlie, and Wilson (1996) proposed several potential relationships, including the following: (1) impaired communicative skills lead to socioemotional impairment, (2) impaired communicative skills result in academic problems, which in turn lead to behavioral problems, (3) other variables (e.g., socioeconomic status) explain, in part or in whole, the relationship between communicative problems and socioemotional difficulties, and (4) an underlying factor (e.g., neurodevelopmental status) accounts for both types of problems.

Further research is needed to clarify the relationship between speech and language ability and socioemotional status. One approach to this problem has been to investigate various child factors that may contribute to developmental risk. For example, Tomblin et al. (2000) reported that reading disability is a key mediating factor predicting whether children with language impairment demonstrate behavioral difficulties.

Of particular interest is the relationship between social competence, communicative competence, and socioemotional functioning. It is clear that speech and language skills play a critical role in social interaction and that children who have difficulty communicating are likely to have difficulty interacting with others. The way in which various components of behavior interact, however, is not as straightforward as might initially be thought. For example, Fujiki et al. (1999) found that children with language impairment were more withdrawn and less sociable than their typical peers, consistent with much of the existing literature. More specific evaluation revealed that these differences were based on particular types of withdrawal (reticence, solitary active withdrawal). Further, severity of language impairment, at least as measured by a formal test of language, was not related to severity of withdrawal. Further clarification is needed to determine how these areas of development interact to produce social outcomes, and what factors may exacerbate or moderate socioemotional status.

Long-Term Consequences. A related line of work has focused on the long-term psychosocial and sociobehavioral consequences of speech and language impairment. In summarizing numerous studies looking at the outcomes of communication disorders, Aram and Hall (1989) stated that children with language impairment have frequently been found to have high rates of persistent social and behavioral problems. Children with speech impairment tend to have more favorable long-term outcomes.

The work of Beitchman and colleagues provides one example of a research program examining long-term psychosocial outcomes of individuals with communicative impairment. These researchers followed children with speech impairment and language impairment and their typical controls longitudinally over a 14-year period (Beitchman et al., 2001). At age 5, the children in the group with speech impairment and the group with language impairment had a higher rate of behavioral problems than the control group. At age 12, socioemotional status was closely linked to status at age 5. At age 14 years and at age 19 years, individuals in the group with language impairment had significantly higher rates of psychiatric involvement than the control group. Children in the group with speech impairment did not differ from the controls.

A few studies have examined the long-term psychosocial outcomes of individuals with speech and/or language impairment as they enter adulthood. For example, Records, Tomblin, and Freese (1992) examined quality of life in a group of 29 young adults (mean age, 21.6 years) with specific language impairment and 29 controls. The groups did not significantly differ on reported personal happiness or life satisfaction. Additionally, differences were not observed with respect to satisfaction in relation to specific aspects of life, such as employment or social relationships.

Howlin, Mawhood, and Rutter (2000) reported a bleaker picture. They reexamined two groups of young men, 23–24 years of age, who had first been evaluated at 7–8 years of age. One group was identified with autism and the other with language impairment. At follow-up, the group with language impairment showed fewer social and behavioral problems than the group with autism. The two groups had converged over the years, however, and differences between the two were not qualitative. The young men with language impairment showed a high incidence of social difficulties, including problems with social interaction, limited social contacts, and difficulty establishing friendships. Most still lived with their parents and had unstable employment histories in manual or unskilled jobs. Neither childhood language ability nor current language ability predicted social functioning in adulthood. Howlin et al. (2000) concluded that in language impairment, "as in autism, a broader deficit underlies both the language delay and the social impairments" (p. 573).

Given some of the data cited above, it would appear that children with speech difficulties achieve better psychosocial outcomes than children with language difficulties (see also Toppelberg and Shapiro, 2000). Although this may generally be the case, generalizations across individuals with different types of speech impairment must be made with caution. Some types of speech problems, such as stuttering, are likely to have important psychosocial implications, but also have relatively low incidence rates. Thus, in large group design studies where individuals are categorized together under the general heading of "speech," the unique psychosocial difficulties associated with such disorders may be masked by the psychosocial profiles associated with more commonly occurring communication problems.

It should also be noted that speech impairments may vary from having no outward manifestations aside from those involved in talking to relatively severe physical or cognitive deficits. The impact of associated problems on the psychosocial development of children with differing types of communicative impairment is difficult to summarize briefly. Illustrative of the complexity even within a specific category of speech impairment are children with cleft lip and palate. These children may have articulation problems and hypernasality secondary to specific physical anomalies. These physical anomalies may be resolved, to various degrees, with surgery. Speech may also vary considerably. No specific personality type has been associated with children with cleft palate (Richman and Eliason, 1992). Individual studies, however, have found these children to exhibit higher than expected rates of both internalizing and externalizing behavior (Richman and Millard, 1997). It appears that factors such as family support, degree of disfigurement, and self-appraisal interact in complex ways to produce psychosocial outcomes in children with cleft lip and palate.

In summary, it is clear that individuals with communicative disorders often have difficulty with aspects of psychosocial behavior and that these problems can have long-term implications. There is also evidence that children with language impairment have more psychosocial difficulties than children with speech impairment. It must be remembered, however, that speech problems differ by type of impairment, severity, and other variables. Thus, generalizations must be made with caution. Given the accumulated evidence, there is good reason to believe that parents, educators, and clinicians working with children with speech and language impairment should give serious consideration to psychosocial status in planning a comprehensive intervention program.

See also POVERTY: EFFECTS ON LANGUAGE; SOCIAL DEVELOPMENT AND LANGUAGE IMPAIRMENT.

—*Martin Fujiki and Bonnie Brinton*

References

Aram, D. M., and Hall, N. E. (1989). Longitudinal follow-up of children with preschool communication disorders: Treatment implications. *School Psychology Review, 18,* 487–501.

Baker, L., and Cantwell, D. P. (1987). Comparison of well, emotionally disordered, and behaviorally disordered children with linguistic problems. *Journal of the American Academy of Child Adolescent Psychiatry, 26,* 193–196.

Beitchman, J. H., Brownlie, E. B., and Wilson, B. (1996). Linguistic impairment to psychiatric disorder: Pathways to outcome. In J. H. Beitchman, N. Cohen, M. M. Konstantareas, and R. Tannock (Eds.), *Language, learning, and behavior disorders: Developmental, biological, and clinical perspectives* (pp. 493–514). New York: Cambridge University Press.

Beitchman, J. H., Wilson, B., Johnson, C. J., Atkinson, L., Young, A., Adlaf, E., et al. (2001). Fourteen-year follow-up of speech/language-impaired and control children: Psychi-

atric outcome. *Journal of the American Academy of Child and Adolescent Psychiatry, 40,* 75–82.

Fujiki, M., Brinton, B., Morgan, M., and Hart, C. H. (1999). Withdrawn and sociable behavior of children with specific language impairment. *Language, Speech, and Hearing Services in Schools, 30,* 183–195.

Howlin, P., Mawhood, L., and Rutter, M. (2000). Autism and developmental receptive language disorder: A follow-up comparison in early adult life. II. Social, behavioural, and psychiatric outcomes. *Journal of Child Psychology and Psychiatry and Allied Disciplines, 41,* 561–578.

Richman, L. C., and Eliason, M. J. (1992). Disorders of communication: Developmental language disorders and cleft palate. In C. E. Walker and M. C. Roberts (Eds.), *Handbook of clinical child psychology* (2nd ed., pp. 537–552). New York: Wiley.

Richman, L. C., and Millard, T. (1997). Brief report: Cleft lip and palate: Longitudinal behavior and relationships of cleft conditions to behavior and achievement. *Journal of Pediatric Psychology, 22,* 487–494.

Records, N. L., Tomblin, J. B., and Freese, P. R. (1992). The quality of life of young adults with histories of specific language impairment. *American Journal of Speech-Language Pathology, 1,* 44–53.

Tomblin, J. B., Zhang, X., Buckwalter, P., and Catts, H. (2000). The association of reading disability, behavioral disorders, and language impairment among second-grade children. *Journal of Child Psychology and Psychiatry, 41,* 475–482.

Toppelberg, C. O., and Shapiro, T. (2000). Language disorders: A 10-year research update review. *Journal of the American Academy of Child and Adolescent Psychiatry, 39,* 143–152.

Travis, L. E. (1957). The unspeakable feelings of people with special reference to stuttering. In L. E. Travis (Ed.), *Handbook of speech pathology* (pp. 916–946). New York: Appleton-Century-Crofts.

Further Readings

Aram, D. M., Ekelman, B., and Nation, J. (1984). Preschoolers with language disorders: 10 years later. *Journal of Speech and Hearing Research, 27,* 232–244.

Baker, L., and Cantwell, D. P. (1982). Psychiatric disorder in children with different types of communication disorders. *Journal of Communication Disorders, 15,* 113–126.

Baker, L., and Cantwell, D. P. (1987). A prospective psychiatric follow-up of children with speech/language disorders. *Journal of the American Academy of Child and Adolescent Psychiatry, 26,* 546–553.

Beitchman, J. H., Cohen, N. J., Konstantareas, M. M., and Tannock, R. (1996). *Language, learning, and behavior disorders: Developmental, biological, and clinical perspectives.* New York: Cambridge University Press.

Beitchman, J. H., Nair, R., Clegg, M. A., Ferguson, B., and Patel, P. G. (1986). Prevalence of psychiatric disorders in children with speech and language disorders. *Journal of the American Academy of Child Psychiatry, 25,* 528–535.

Beitchman, J. H., Wilson, B., Brownlie, B., Walters, H., Inglis, A., and Lancee, W. (1996). Long-term consistency in speech/language profiles: II. Behavioral, emotional, and social outcomes. *Journal of the American Academy of Child and Adolescent Psychiatry, 35,* 815–825.

Benasich, A. A., Curtiss, S., and Tallal, P. (1993). Language, learning behavioral disturbances in childhood: A longitudinal perspective. *Journal of the American Academy of Child and Adolescent Psychiatry, 32,* 585–594.

Cantwell, D., and Baker, L. (1988). Clinical significance of childhood communication disorders: Perspectives from a longitudinal study. *Journal of Child Neurology, 2,* 257–264.

Cochrane, V. M., and Slade, P. (1999). Appraisal and coping in adults with cleft lip: Associations with well-being and social anxiety. *British Journal of Medical Psychology, 72,* 485–503.

Cohen, N. J., Menna, R., Vallance, D., Barwick, M. A., Im, N., and Horodezky, N. B. (1998). Language, social cognitive processing, and behavioral characteristics of psychiatrically disturbed children with previously identified and unsuspected language impairments. *Journal of Child Psychology and Psychiatry and Allied Disciplines, 39,* 853–864.

Felsenfeld, S., Broen, P. A., and McGue, M. (1992). A 28-year follow-up of adults with a history of moderate phonological disorder: Linguistic and personality results. *Journal of Speech and Hearing Research, 35,* 1114–1125.

Johnson, C. L., Beitchman, J. H., Young, A., Escobar, M., Atkinson, L., Wilson, B., et al. (1999). Fourteen year follow-up of children with and without speech/language impairments: Speech/language stability and outcomes. *Journal of Speech, Language, and Hearing Research, 42,* 744–760.

Mawhood, L., Howlin, P., and Rutter, M. (2000). Autism and developmental receptive language disorder: A comparative follow-up in early adult life. I. Cognitive and language outcomes. *Journal of Child Psychology and Psychiatry and Allied Disciplines, 41,* 547–559.

Noterdaeme, M., and Amorosa, H. (1999). Evaluation of emotional and behavioral problems in language impaired children using the Child Behavior Checklist. *European Child and Adolescent Psychiatry, 8,* 71–77.

Paul, R., and Kellogg, L. (1997). Temperament in late talkers. *Journal of Child Psychology and Psychiatry and Allied Disciplines, 38,* 803–811.

Rapin, I. (1996). Practitioner review: Developmental language disorder: A clinical update. *Journal of Child Psychology and Psychiatry, 6,* 643–655.

Speech and Language Disorders in Children: Computer-Based Approaches

Computers can be used effectively in the assessment of children's speech and language. Biofeedback instrumentation allows the clinician to obtain relatively objective measures of certain aspects of speech production. For example, measures of jitter and shimmer can be recorded, along with perceptual judgments about a client's pitch and intensity perturbations (Case, 1999). Acoustic analyses (Kent and Read, 1992) can be used to supplement the clinician's perceptions of phonological contrasts (Masterson, Long, and Buder, 1998). For the evaluation of a client suspected of having a fluency disorder, recent software developments allow the clinician to gather measures of both the number and type of speech disfluencies and to document signs of effort, struggle, or disruption of airflow and phonation (Bakker, 1999a). Hallowell (1999) discusses the use of instrumentation for detecting and measuring eye movements for the purpose of comprehension assessment. This exciting tool allows the clinician to evaluate comprehen-

sion in a client for whom traditional response modes, such as speaking or even pointing, are not possible.

Computers can also be used to administer or score a formal test (Cochran and Masterson, 1995; Hallowell and Katz, 1999; Long, 1999). Computer-based scoring systems allow the input of raw scores, which are then converted to profiles or derived scores of interest (Long, 1999). The value of such programs is inversely related to the ease of obtaining the derived scores by hand. If the translation of raw scores to derived scores is tedious and time-consuming, clinicians might find the software tools worth their investment in time and money.

Although few computerized tests are currently available, the potential for such instruments is quite high. Hallowell and Katz (1999) point out that computerized test administration could allow tighter standardization of administration conditions and procedures, tracking of response latency, and automated interfacing with alternative response mode systems. Of particular promise are the computerized tests that adapt to a specific client's profile. That is, stimuli are presented in a manner that is contingent on the individual's prior responses (Letz, Green, and Woodard, 1996). The type of task or specific items that are administered can be automatically determined by a client's ongoing performance (e.g., Masterson and Bernhardt, 2001), which makes individualized assessment more feasible than ever. Incorporation of some principles from artificial intelligence also makes the future of computers in assessment exciting. For example, Masterson, Apel, and Wasowicz (2001) developed a tool for spelling assessment that employs complex algorithms for parsing spelling words into target orthographic structures and then aligning a student's spelling with the appropriate correct forms. Based on the type of misspellings exhibited by each individual student, the system identifies related skills that need testing, such as phonological awareness or morphological knowledge. This system makes possible a comprehensive description of a student's spelling abilities that would otherwise be prohibitive because of the time required to perform the analyses by hand and administer the individualized follow-ups.

Computerized language and phonological sample analysis (CL/PSA) has been in use since the 1980s (Evans and Miller, 1999; Long, 1999; Masterson and Oller, 1999; Long and Channell, 2001). These programs allow researchers and clinicians to perform complex, in-depth analyses that would likely be impossible without the technology. They provide instant analysis of a wide range of phonological and linguistic measures, and some provide tools that reduce and simplify the time-consuming process of transcribing samples (Long, 1999). Many of the CL/PSA programs also include comparison databases of language samples from both typical and clinical populations (Evans and Miller, 1999). Despite the power of CL/PSA programs, their use in clinical settings remains limited, for unclear reasons. It is possible that funding for software and hardware is insufficient; however, data from recent surveys (McRay and Fitch, 1996; ASHA, 1997) do not support this conjecture, since most respondents do report owning and using computers for other purposes. Lack of use is more likely related to insufficient familiarity with many of the measures derived from language sample analysis and failure to recognize the benefits of these measures for treatment planning (Cochran and Masterson, 1995; Fitch and McRay, 1997). In an effort to address this problem, Long established the Computerized Profiling Website (http://www.computerizedprofiling.org) in 1999. Clinicians can visit the web site and obtain free versions of this CL/PSA software as well as instructional materials regarding its use and application.

Computer software for use in speech and language intervention has progressed significantly from the early versions, which were based primarily on a drill-and-practice format. Cochran and Nelson (1999) cite literature that confirms what many clinicians knew intuitively: software that allows the child to be in control and to independently explore based on personal interests is more beneficial than computer programs based on the drill-and-practice model. Improvements in multimedia capacities and an appreciation for maximally effective designs have resulted in a proliferation of software packages that can be effectively used in language intervention with young children. As with any tool, the focus must remain on the target linguistic structures rather than the toys or activities that are used to elicit or model productions. In addition to therapeutic benefits, computers offer reasonable compensatory strategies for older, school-age students with language-learning disabilities (Wood and Masterson, 1999; Masterson, Apel, and Wood, 2002). For example, word processors with text-to-speech capabilities allow students to check their own work by listening to as well as reading their text. Spell and grammar checkers can be helpful, as long as students have been sufficiently trained in the optimal use of these tools, including an appreciation of their limitations. Speech recognition systems continue to improve, and perhaps someday they will free writers with language disorders from the burden of text entry, which requires choices regarding spelling, and spelling can be so challenging for students with language disorders that it interferes with text construction. Currently, speech recognition technology remains limited in recognition accuracy for students with language disorders (Wetzel, 1996). Even when accuracy improves to an acceptable level, students will still need specific training in the optimal use of the technology. Optimal writing involves more than a simple, direct translation of spoken language to written form. Students who employ speech recognition software to construct written texts will need focused instruction regarding the differences between the styles of spoken and written language. Finally, the Internet provides not only a context for language intervention, but a potential source of motivation as well. The percentage of school-age children who use the Internet on a daily basis for social as well as academic purposes continues to increase, and it is likely that speech-language pathologists will capitalize on this trend.

Computers add a new twist to an old standard in phonological treatment. Instead of having to sort and carry numerous picture cards from one treatment session to the next, clinicians can choose one of several software packages that allow access and display of multimedia stimuli on the basis of phonological characteristics (Masterson and Rvachew, 1999). New technologies, such as the palatometer, provide clients with critical feedback for sound production when tactile or kinesthetic feedback has not been sufficient. Similarly, computer programs can be used to provide objective feedback regarding the frequency of stutterings, which might be considered less confrontational than feedback provided by the clinician (Bakker, 1999b). One particularly promising technology, the Speech Enhancer, incorporates real-time processing of an individual's speech production and selectively boosts energy only in those frequencies necessary for maximum intelligibility. Cariski and Rosenbek (1999) collected data from a single subject and found that intelligibility scores were higher when using the Speech Enhancer than when using a high-fidelity amplifier. The authors suggested that their results supported the notion that the device did indeed do more than simply amplify the speech output.

The decision to use computers in both assessment and treatment activities will continue to be based on the clinician's judgment as to the added value of the technology application. If a clinician can do an activity just as well without a computer, it is unlikely that she or he will go to the expense in terms of time and money to invest in the computer tool. On the other hand, for those tasks that cannot be done as well or even at all, clinicians will likely turn to the computer if they are convinced that the tasks themselves are worth it.

See also APHASIA TREATMENT: COMPUTER-AIDED REHABILITATION.

—*Julie J. Masterson*

References

American Speech-Language-Hearing Association. (1997). *Omnibus Survey Results: 1997 edition*. Rockville, MD: Author.

Bakker, K. (1999a). Clinical technologies for the reduction of stuttering and enhancement of speech fluency. *Seminars in Speech and Language, 20*, 271–280.

Bakker, K. (1999b). Technical solutions for quantitative and qualitative assessments of speech fluency. *Seminars in Speech and Language, 20*, 185–196.

Cariski, D., and Rosenbek, J. (1999). The effectiveness of the Speech Enhancer. *Journal of Medical Speech-Language Pathology, 7*, 315–322.

Case, J. L. (1999). Technology in the assessment of voice disorder. *Seminars in Speech and Language, 20*, 169–184.

Cochran, P., and Masterson, J. (1995). Not using a computer in language assessment/intervention: In defense of the reluctant clinician. *Language, Speech, and Hearing Services in Schools, 26*, 260–262.

Cochran, P. S., and Nelson, L. K. (1999). Technology applications in intervention for preschool-age children with language disorders. *Seminars in Speech and Language, 20*, 203–218.

Evans, J. L., and Miller, J. (1999). Language sample analysis in the 21st century. *Seminars in Speech and Language, 20,* 101–116.

Fitch, J. L., and McRay, L. B. (1997). Integrating technology into school programs. *Language, Speech, and Hearing Services in Schools, 28,* 134–136.

Hallowell, B. (1999). A new way of looking at auditory linguistic comprehension. In Becker, W., Deubel, H., and Mergner, T. (Eds.). *Current oculomotor research: Physiological and psychological aspects* (pp. 287–291). New York: Plenum Press.

Hallowell, B., and Katz, R. C. (1999). Technological applications in the assessment of acquired neurogenic communication and swallowing disorders in adults. *Seminars in Speech and Language, 20,* 149–167.

Kent, R., and Read, C. (1992). *The acoustic analysis of speech.* San Diego, CA: Singular Publishing Group.

Letz, R., Green, R. C., and Woodard, J. L. (1996). Development of a computer-based battery designed to screen adults for neuropsychological impairment. *Neurotoxicology and Teratology, 18,* 365–370.

Long, S. H. (1999). Technology applications in the assessment of children's language. *Seminars in Speech and Language, 20,* 117–132.

Long, S. H., and Channell, R. W. (2001). Accuracy of four language analysis procedures performed automatically. *American Journal of Speech-Language Pathology, 10,* 180–188.

Masterson, J., Apel, K., and Wasowicz, J. (in press). Spelling Evaluation for Language and Literacy (SPELL) [computer software]. Evanston, IL: Learning by Design.

Masterson, J., Apel, K., and Wood, L. (2002). Linking software and hardware applications to what we know about literacy development. In K. Butler and E. Silliman (Eds.), *Speaking, reading, and writing in children with language-learning disabilities: New paradigms for research and practice* (pp. 273–293). Mahwah, NJ: Erlbaum.

Masterson, J., and Bernhardt, B. (2001). Computerized Articulation and Phonology Evaluation System (CAPES) [computer software]. San Antonio, TX: Psychological Corporation.

Masterson, J., Long, S., and Buder, E. (1998). Instrumentation in clinical phonology. In J. Bernthal and N. Bankson (Eds.), *Articulation and phonological disorders* (4th ed., pp. 378–406). Englewood Cliffs, NJ: Prentice-Hall.

Masterson, J. J., and Oller, D. K. (1999). Use of technology in phonological assessment: Evaluation of early meaningful speech and prelinguistic vocalizations. *Seminars in Speech and Language, 20,* 133–148.

Masterson, J. J., and Rvachew, S. (1999). Use of technology in phonological intervention. *Seminars in Speech and Language, 20,* 233–250.

McRay, L. B., and Fitch, J. L. (1996). A survey of computer use of public school speech-language pathologists. *Language, Speech, and Hearing Services in Schools, 27,* 40–47.

Wetzel, K. (1996). Speech-recognizing computers: A written-communication tool for students with learning disabilities? *Journal of Learning Disabilities, 29,* 371–380.

Wood, L. A., and Masterson, J. J. (1999). The use of technology to facilitate language skills in school-age children. *Seminars in Speech and Language, 20,* 219–232.

Further Readings

American Guidance Service. (1997). PPVT-III ASSIST [Computer software]. Circle Pines, MN: Author.

Case, J. L. (1999). Technology in the treatment of voice disorders. *Seminars in Speech and Language, 20,* 281–295.

Farrall, J. L., and Parsons, C. L. (1992). A comparison of a traditional test format vs. a computerized administration of the Carrow-Woolfolk Test for Auditory Comprehension of Language. *Australian Journal of Human Communication Disorders, 20,* 33–48.

Fitch, J. L., and McRay, L. B. (1997). Integrating technology into school programs. *Language, Speech, and Hearing Services in Schools, 28,* 134–136.

Friel-Patti, S., DesBarres, K., and Thibodeau, L. (2001). Case studies of children using Fast ForWord. *Journal of Speech-Language Pathology, 10,* 203–215.

Jamieson, D. G., and Rvachew, S. (1992). Remediation of speech production errors with sound identification training. *Journal of Speech-Language Pathology and Audiology, 16,* 201–210.

Katz, R. C., and Hallowell, B. (1999). Technological applications in the treatment of acquired neurogenic communication and swallowing disorders in adults. *Seminars in Speech and Language, 20,* 251–269.

Long, S. H., and Channell, R. W. (2001). Accuracy of four language analysis procedures performed automatically. *American Journal of Speech-Language Pathology, 10,* 180–188.

Long, S. H., Fey, M. E., and Channell, R. W. (1998). Computerized Profiling (CP) (Version 9.0) (MS-DOS) [Computer program]. Cleveland, OH: Department of Communication Sciences, Case Western Reserve University.

MacWhinney, B. (1998). *The CHILDES project: Computational tools for analyzing talk.* Mahwah, NJ: Erlbaum.

Masterson, J., and Crede, L. (1999). Learning to spell: Implications for assessment and intervention. *Language, Speech, and Hearing Services in Schools, 30,* 243–254.

Masterson, J., and Perrey, C. (1999). Training analogical reasoning skills in children with language disorders. *American Journal of Speech-Language Pathology, 8,* 53–61.

Masterson, J., Wynne, M., Kuster, J., and Stierwalt, J. (1999). New and emerging technologies: Going where we've never gone before. *ASHA, 41,* 16–20.

Matesich, J., Porch, B., and Katz, R. (1996). PICApad PC [Computer software]. Scottsdale, AZ: Sunset Software.

Miller, J., Freiberg, C., Rolland, M.-B., and Reeves, M. (1992). Implementing computerized language sample analysis in the public school. C. Dollaghan (Ed.), *Topics in language disorders.* Rockville, MD: Aspen Press.

Miller, J. F., and Chapman, R. S. (1998). Systematic analysis of language transcripts (SALT) (Version 4.0, MS-DOS) [Computer program]. Madison, WI: Language Analysis Laboratory, Waisman Center on Mental Retardation and Human Development, University of Wisconsin.

Nelson, L., and Masterson, J. (1999). Using microcomputer technology to advance assessment and intervention for children with language disorders. *Topics in Language Disorders, 19,* 68–86.

Rvachew, S. (1994). Speech perception training can facilitate sound production learning. *Journal of Speech and Hearing Research, 37,* 347–357.

Tye-Murray, N. (1992). Laser videodisc technology in the aural rehabilitation setting: Good news for people with severe and profound hearing impairments. *American Journal of Audiology, 1,* 33–36.

Wilkinson, G. S. (1993). Wide Range Achievement Test 3 (WRAT3) Scoring Program [Computer software]. Odessa, FL: Psychological Assessment Resources.

Woodcock, R. W. (1998). Woodcock Scoring and Interpretive Program [Computer software]. Itasca, IL: Riverside.

Speech and Language Issues in Children from Asian-Pacific Backgrounds

Asian-Pacific Americans originate from Pacific Asia or are descendants of Asian-Pacific island immigrants. Numbering 10,477,000 in the United States, Asian-Pacific Americans are the fastest-growing segment of the U.S. population, representing 3.8% of the nation's population and 10% of California's population (Population Reference Bureau, 2001). By the year 2020, Asian-American children in U.S. schools will total about 4.4 million.

The recent Asian influx represents a diverse group from Southeast Asia, China, India, Pakistan, Malaysia, Indonesia, and other Pacific Rim areas. In general, Pacific Asia is divided into the following regions: East Asia (China, Taiwan, Japan, and Korea), Southeast Asia (Philippines, Vietnam, Cambodia, Laos, Malaysia, Singapore, Indonesia, Thailand), the Indian subcontinent, or South Asia (India, Pakistan, Bangladesh, Sri Lanka), and the Pacific islands (Polynesia, Micronesia, Melanesia, New Zealand, and Australia). Asian-Pacific populations speak many languages, and their English is influenced by various dialects and languages.

Asian-Pacific Americans are extremely diverse in all aspects of life, including attitudes toward disability and treatment, childrearing practices, languages, and culture. The Asian-Pacific island cultures, however, have interacted with and influenced each other for many generations, and therefore share many similarities. The following information is presented to provide an understanding of Asian-Pacific Americans in order to assist speech-language pathologists and audiologists in providing services to these culturally and linguistically diverse populations. Recommended assessment procedures and intervention strategies are provided.

Attitudes Toward Disability and Treatment Methods. What constitutes a disability depends on the values of the cultural group. In general, Eastern cultures may view a disabling condition as the result of wrongdoing of the individual's ancestors, resulting in guilt and shame. Disabilities may be explained by a variety of spiritual or cultural beliefs, such as an imbalance in inner forces, bad wind, spoiled foods, gods, demons, or spirits, hot or cold forces, or fright. Some believe disability is caused by karma (fate) or a curse. All over the world, people use different methods to treat illnesses and diseases, including consulting with priests, healers, herbalists, Qi-Gong specialists, clansmen, shamans, elders, and physicians. Among the Hmong, for example, surgical intervention is viewed as invasive and harmful.

Childrearing Practices. Childrearing practices and expectations of children vary widely from culture to culture (Westby, 1990; Van Kleeck, 1994). There are differences in how parents respond to their children's language, who interacts with children, and how parents

Table 1. Cultural Differences Between Asian-Pacific Americans and Western Groups

Eastern Tendencies	Western Tendencies
A person is not autonomous.	A person is autonomous.
A person is part of society.	A person is unique and individualistic.
A person needs to maintain relationships and have constraints.	A person makes rational choices.
A person is oriented toward harmony.	A person is active in decision making.
A person is a partner in the community where people are mutually responsible for behaviors and consequences.	A person is responsible for own actions and takes the consequences.
A person needs to be humble, improve, and master skills.	A person is different, unique, and special.
A person needs to endure hardships and persevere.	A person needs to feel good about self.
A person needs to self-reflect.	A person needs to toot own horn.

and families encourage children to initiate and continue a verbal interaction. However, socioeconomic and individual differences must always be considered.

Languages. The hundreds of different languages and dialects that are spoken in East and Southeast Asia and the Pacific islands can be classified into five major families: (1) Malayo-Polynesian (Austronesian), including Chamorro, Ilocano, and Tagalog; (2) Sino-Tibetan, including Thai, Yao, Mandarin, and Cantonese; (3) Austro-Asiatic, including Khmer, Vietnamese, and Hmong; (4) Papuan, including New Guinean; and (5) Altaic, including Japanese and Korean (Ma, 1985). Additionally, there are 15 major languages in India from four language families, Indo-Aryan, Dravidian, Austro-Asiatic, and Tibeto-Burman (Shekar and Hegde, 1995).

Cultural Tendencies. Cultural tendencies of Asian-Pacific Americans may be quite different from those of individuals born and raised in a Western culture. Table 1 provides a sampling of these differences. However, caution should be taken not to overgeneralize this information in relation to a particular client or family.

Recommended Assessment Procedures

The following assessment guidelines are often referred to as the RIOT (review, interview, observe, test) protocol (Cheng, 1995, 2002). They are adapted here for Asian-Pacific American populations:

1. *Review* all pertinent documents and background information. Many Asian countries do not have medical records or cumulative school records. Oral reports are sometimes unreliable. A cultural informant or an interpreter is generally needed to obtain this information because of the lack of English language proficiency of the parents or guardians. Pregnancy and delivery records

might not have been kept, especially if the birth was a home birth or in a refugee camp.

2. *Interview* teachers, peers, family members, and other informants and work with them to collect data regarding the client and the home environment. The family can provide valuable information about the communicative competence of the client at home and in the community, as well as historical and comparative data on the client's language development. The clinician needs information regarding whether or not the client is proficient in the home language. The family's home language, its proficiency in different languages, the patterns of language usage, and the ways the family spends time together are some areas for investigation. Interview questions are available from multiple sources (Cheng, 1990, 1991, 2002; Langdon and Saenz, 1996). Questions should focus on obtaining information on how the client functions in his or her natural environment in relation to age peers who have had the same or similar exposure to their home language or to English.

3. *Observe* the client over time in multiple contexts with multiple communication partners. Observe interactions at school, both in and outside the classroom, and at home. This cognitive-ecological-functional model takes into account the fact that clients often behave differently in different settings (Cheng, 1991). Direct observation of social behavior with multiple participants allows the evaluator to observe the ways members of different cultures view their environment and organize their behavior within it.

4. *Test* the client using informal and dynamic assessment procedures in both the school language and the home language. Use the portfolio approach by keeping records of the client's performance over time. Interact with the client, being sensitive to his or her needs to create meaning based on what is perceived as important, the client's frame of reference, and experiences.

What clinicians learn from the assessment should be integrated into their intervention strategies. Intervention should be constructed based on what is most productive for promoting communication and should incorporate the client's personal and cultural experiences. Salient and relevant features of the client's culture should be highlighted to enhance and empower the client.

There are many challenges professionals face in working with the Asian-Pacific American populations. The discourse styles in effect in American homes and schools may differ from those that are practiced in Asian classrooms. Clinicians need to be doubly careful and not interpret these differences as deficient, disordered, aberrant, and undesirable. Behaviors that can be easily misunderstood include the following (Cheng, 1999):

- Delay or hesitation in response
- Frequent topic shifts and poor topic maintenance
- Confused facial expressions, such as a frown signaling concentration rather than displeasure
- Short responses
- Use of a soft-spoken voice
- Taking few risks

- Lack of participation and lack of volunteering information
- Different nonverbal messages
- Embarrassment over praise
- Different greeting rituals, which may appear impolite, such as looking down when the teacher approaches
- Use of Asian-language-influenced English, such as the deletion of plural and past tense

These are just a few examples of the observed behaviors that may be misinterpreted. Asian-Pacific American children may be fluent in English but use the discourse styles of their home culture, such as speaking softly to persons in authority, looking down or away, and avoiding close physical contact. Surface analysis of linguistic and pragmatic functions is not sufficient to determine the communicative competence of children and might even misguide the decision-making process.

Sociol and psychological difficulties arise in the conflict of culture, language, and ideology between Asian students, their parents, and the American educational system. These difficulties can include the background of traditions, religions, and histories of the Asian-Pacific population, problems of acculturation, the understanding of social rules, contrasting influences from home and the classroom, confusion regarding one's sense of identity relating to culture, society, and family, the definition of disability, and the implications of receiving special education services.

Intervention activities and materials can be selected based on the client's family and cultural background, using activities that are culturally and socially relevant. In addition to traditional intervention techniques of modeling and expansion, speech-language pathologists can include activities such as those discussed by Cheng (1989).

Alternative strategies should be offered when clients or caregivers are reluctant to accept the treatment program recommended by the speech-language pathologist or audiologist. Inviting them to special classes or speech and language sessions is a useful way to provide the needed information. Seeking assistance from community leaders and social service providers may also be necessary to convince the clients of the importance of therapy or recommended programs. The clients or caregivers may also be asked to talk with other Asian-Pacific Americans who have experiences with treatment programs. Other individuals can be effective in sharing their personal stories about their experiences with therapy. The clinician should be patient with the clients, letting them think through a problem and waiting for them to make the decision to participate in the treatment program.

Following are some suggestions to create an optimal language learning environment and to reduce difficult communication (Cheng, 1996):

- Make no assumptions about what students know or do not know.
- Anticipate their needs and greatest challenges.
- Expect frustration and possible misunderstanding.

- Encourage students to join social activities such as student government, clubs, and organizations to increase their exposure to different types of discourse, as language is a social tool and should be used for fulfilling multiple social needs and requirements.
- Facilitate the transition into mainstream culture through such activities as role-playing (preparing scripts for commonly occurring activities, using culturally unique experiences as topics for discussions) and conducting social/pragmatic activities (Cheng, 1989), such as a birthday party and a Thanksgiving celebration.
- Nurture bicultural/multicultural identity. Introduce multicultural elements not only in phonology, morphology, and syntax, but also in pragmatics, semantics, and ritualized patterns.

Providing speech-language and hearing services to Asian-Pacific Americans is challenging. Preassessment information on the language, culture, and personal history of the individual lays a solid foundation to further explore the client's strengths and weaknesses. Assessment procedures need to be guided by the general principles of being fair to the culture and nonbiased. The results of assessment should take into consideration the cultural and pragmatic variables of the individual. Intervention can be extremely rewarding when culturally relevant and appropriate approaches are used. The goals of intervention must include the enhancement of appropriate language and communication behaviors, home language, and literacy. Clinicians need to be creative and sensitive in their intervention to provide comfortable, productive, and enriching services for all clients. Some publishers that have developed materials for use with Asian-Pacific American populations include Academic Communications Associates (Oceanside, CA), Communication Skill Builders (Tucson, AZ), Thinking Publications (Eau Claire, WI), Newbury House (Rowley, MA).

—*Li-Rong Lilly Cheng*

References

Cheng, L. L. (1989). Service delivery to Asian/Pacific LEP children: A cross-cultural framework. *Topics in Language Disorders*, 9, 1–14.

Cheng, L. L. (1990). The identification of communicative disorders in Asian-Pacific students. *Journal of Child Communicative Disorders*, 13, 113–119.

Cheng, L. L. (1991). *Assessing Asian language performance: Guidelines for evaluating LEP students.* Oceanside, CA: Academic Communication Associates.

Cheng, L. L. (1995, July). *The bilingual language-delayed child: Diagnosis and intervention with the older school-age bilingual child.* Paper presented at the Israeli Speech and Hearing Association International Symposium on Bilingualism, Haifa, Israel.

Cheng, L. L. (1996). Beyond bilingualism: A quest for communicative competence. *Topics in Language Disorders*, 16, 9–21.

Cheng, L. L. (1999). Sociocultural adjustment of Chinese-American students. In C. C. Park and M. Chi (Eds.), *Asian-American education*. London: Bergin and Garvey.

Cheng, L. L. (2002). Asian and Pacific American cultures. In D. E. Battle (Ed.), *Communication disorders in multicultural populations*. Boston, MA: Butterworth-Heinemann.

Langdon, H. W., and Saenz, T. I. (1996). *Language Assessment and Intervention with Multicultural Students: A Guide for Speech-Language-Hearing Professionals.* Oceanside, CA: Academic Communication Associates.

Ma, L. J. (1985). Cultural diversity. In A. K. Dutt (Ed.), *Southeast Asia: Realm of contrast*, Boulder, CO: Westview Press.

Population Reference Bureau. (2001). On-line. Washington, DC: U.S. Bureau of the Census.

Shekar, C., and Hegde, M. N. (1995). India: Its people, culture, and languages. In L. L. Cheng (Ed.), *Integrating language and learning for inclusion*. San Diego, CA: Singular Publishing Group.

Van Kleeck, A. (1994). Potential bias in training parents as conversational partners with their children who have delays in language development. *American Journal of Speech-Language Pathology*, 3, 67–68.

Westby, C. (1990). Ethnographic interviewing: Asking the right questions to the right people in the right way. *Journal of Childhood Communication Disorders*, 13, 101–111.

On-line Resources

http://www.krysstal.com/langfams.html
http://www.travlang.com/languages
http://www.zompist.com/lang8.html

Speech Assessment, Instrumental

The instrumental analysis of speech can be approached through the three main stages of the speech chain: articulatory, acoustic, and auditory phonetics. This entry reviews the instrumentation used to assess the articulatory and acoustic phases. Auditory phonetic techniques are covered elsewhere in this volume.

Although speech planning in the brain (neurophonetics) lies outside the traditional tripartite speech chain, the neurological aspects of both speech production and perception can be studied through the use of brain imaging techniques. Speech articulation proper is deemed here to begin with the movement of muscles required to produce aerodynamic changes resulting in the flow of an airstream (see Laver, 1994; Ball and Rahilly, 1999). Of course, muscle movements also occur throughout articulation. This area has been investigated using electromyography (EMG). In EMG, electrodes of different types (surface, needle, and hooked wire) are used to gather data on electrical activity within target muscles, and these data are matched with a simultaneously recorded speech signal (Stone, 1996; Gentil and Moore, 1997). In this way the timing of muscle activity in relation to different aspects of speech can be investigated. This technique has been used to examine both normal and disordered speech. Areas studied include

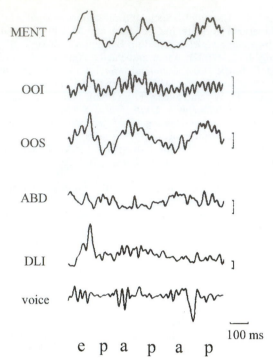

Figure 1. Averaged integrated EMG signals for the mentalis muscle (MENT), orbicularis oris inferior (OOI), orbicularis oris superior (OOS), anterior belly of the digastric (ABD), and the depressor labii inferior (DLI) for a patient with Friedreich's ataxia uttering /epapap/. (Courtesy of Michèle Gentil.)

the respiratory and laryngeal muscles, muscle groups in the lips, tongue, and soft palate, and various disorders, including disorders of voice and fluency, and certain acquired neurological problems. Figure 1 shows EMG traces from a patient with Friedreich's ataxia.

Aerodynamic activity in speech is studied through aerometry. A variety of devices have been used to measure speech aerodynamics (Zajac and Yates, 1997). Many systems have employed an airtight mask that is placed over the subject's face and attached to a pneumotachograph. The mask contains sensors to measure pressure changes and airflow at the nose and mouth, and generally also a microphone to record the speech signal, against which the airflow can be plotted. If the focus of attention is lung volume changes, then a plethysmograph may be employed. This is an airtight box that houses the subject, and any changes to the air pressure within the box (caused by changes in the subject's lung volume) are recorded. A simpler plethysmograph (the respitrace; see Stone, 1996) consists of a wire band placed around the subject's chest that measures changes in cross-sectional area during inhalation and exhalation.

In normal pulmonic egressive speech, airflow from the lungs passes through the larynx, where a variety of phonation types may be implemented. The study of laryngeal activity (more particularly, of vocal fold activity) can be direct or indirect. In direct study, a rigid or flexible endoscope connected to a camera is used to view the

movements of the folds. This technology is often coupled to a stroboscopic light source, as stroboscopic endoscopy allows the viewer to see individual movements of the folds (see Abberton and Fourcin, 1997). Endoscopy, however, is invasive, and use of a rigid endoscope precludes normal speech. Indirect investigation of vocal fold activity is undertaken with electroglottography (EGG), also termed electrolaryngography (see Stone, 1996; Abberton and Fourcin, 1997). This technique allows vocal fold movement to be extrapolated from measuring the varying electrical resistance across the larynx. Both approaches have been used in the investigation of normal and disordered voice.

Velic action and associated differences in oral and nasal airflow (and hence in nasal resonance) can also be measured directly or indirectly. The velotrace is an instrument designed to indicate directly the height of the velum (see Bell-Berti et al., 1993), while nasometric devices of varying sophistication measure oral versus nasal airflow (see Zajac and Yates, 1997). The velotrace is invasive, as part of the device must be inserted into the nasal cavity to sit on the roof of the velum. Nasometers measure indirectly using, for example, two external microphones to measure airflow differences. Figure 2 shows a trace from the Kay Elemetrics nasometer of hypernasal speech.

The next step in the speech production chain is the articulation of sounds. Most important here is the placement of the individual articulators, and electropalatography (EPG) has proved to be a vital development in this area of study. Hardcastle and Gibbon

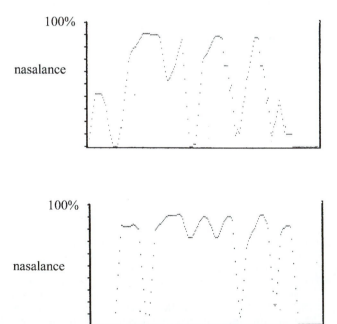

Figure 2. Trace adapted from a Kay Elemetrics nasometer showing normal and hypernasal versions of "eighteen, nineteen, twenty."

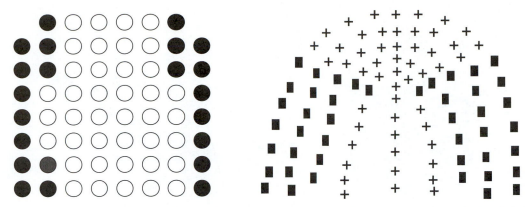

Figure 3. Reading EPG3 system stylized palate diagram (left) showing misarticulated /s/ with wide channel; Kay Palatometer stylized system palate diagram (right) showing target /s/ articulated at the postalveolar region.

(1997) describe this technique. A thin acrylic artificial palate is made to fit the subject. This palate has a large number of electrodes embedded in it (from 62 to 96, depending on the system employed) to cover important areas for speech (e.g., the alveolar region). When the tongue touches these electrodes, they fire, and the resultant tongue-palate contact patterns can be shown on a computer screen. The electrodes are normally sampled 100 times per second, and the patterns are displayed in real time. This allows the technique to be used both for research and for feedback in therapy. EPG has been used to study normal speech and a wide range of disordered speech patterns. Figure 3 shows tongue-palate contact patterns in a stylized way for two different EPG systems.

Other ways of examining articulation (and indeed a whole range of speech-related activity) can be subsumed under the overall heading of speech imaging (see Stone, 1996; Ball and Gröne, 1997). The oldest of these techniques is x-radiography. A variety of different x-ray techniques have been used in speech research, among them videofluorography, which uses low doses of radiation to give clear pictures of the vocal tract, and x-ray microbeam imaging, in which the movements of pellets attached to relevant points of the tongue and palate are tracked. Because of the dangers of radiation, alternative imaging techniques have been sought. Among these is ultrasound, which uses the time taken for sound waves to bounce off a structure and return to a receiver to map structures in the vocal tract. Because ultrasound waves do not travel through the air, mapping of the tongue (from below) is possible, but mapping of tongue–palate distances is not, as the palate cannot be mapped through the air space of the oral cavity. Electromagnetic articulography (EMA) is another tracking technique. In this technique the subject is placed within alternating magnetic fields generated by transmitter coils in a helmet assembly. Small receiver coils are placed at articulatorily important sites (e.g., tongue tip, tongue body). The movements of the receiver coils through the alternating

magnetic fields are measured and recorded by computer. As with x-ray microbeam imaging, the tracked points can be used to infer the shape and movements of articulators within the vocal tract.

The final imaging technique to be considered is magnetic resonance imaging (MRI). The imager surrounds a subject with electromagnets, creating an electromagnetic field. This field causes hydrogen protons (abundant in human tissue) to align but also to precess, or wobble. If a brief radio pulse is introduced at the same frequency as the precessing, the protons are moved out of alignment and then back again. As they realign, they emit weak radio signals, which can be used to construct an image of the tissue involved. MRI can provide good images of the vocal tract but currently not at sufficient frequency to allow analysis of continuous speech. All of these imaging techniques have been used to study aspects of both normal and disordered speech. Figure 4 shows ultrasound diagrams for two vowels and two consonants.

Acoustic analyses via sound spectrography are now easily undertaken with a range of software programs on personal computers as well as on dedicated hardware-software configurations such as the Kay Elemetrics Sonagraph. Reliable analysis depends on good recordings (see Tatham and Morton, 1997). Spectrographic analysis packages currently allow users to analyze temporal, frequency, amplitude, and intensity aspects of a speech signal (see Baken and Daniloff, 1991; Farmer, 1997). For example, a waveform displays amplitude versus time; a wideband spectrogram displays frequency versus time using a wideband pass filter (around 200–300 Hz), giving good time resolution but poor frequency resolution; a narrow-band spectrogram shows frequency versus time using a narrowband pass filter (around 29 Hz), which provides good frequency resolution but poor time resolution; and spectral envelopes show frequency versus intensity at a point in time (produced either by fast Fourier transform or linear predictive coding). Speech analysis research has generally concentrated on wideband spectrograms and spectral envelopes. These

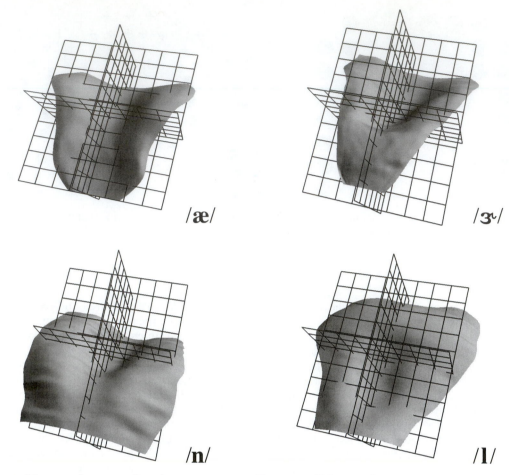

Figure 4. Ultrasound images of two vowels and two consonants. (Courtesy of Maureen Stone.)

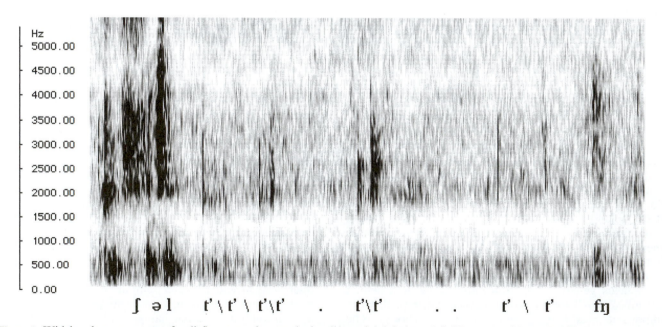

Figure 5. Wideband spectrogram of a disfluent speaker producing "(provin)cial t(owns)." (Courtesy of Joan Rahilly.)

both show formant frequencies (bands of high intensity at certain frequency levels), which are useful in the identification of and discrimination between vowels and other sonorants. Fricatives are distinguishable from the boundaries of the broad areas of frequency seen clearly on a spectrogram, while plosives can be noted from the lack of acoustic activity during the closure stage and the coarticulatory effects on the formants of neighboring sounds. Segment duration can easily be measured from spectrograms in modern analysis packages. Various pitch extraction algorithms are provided for the investigation of intonation. Farmer (1997) provides an extensive review of acoustic analysis work in a range of disorders: voice, fluency, aphasia, apraxia and dysarthria, child speech disorders, and the speech of the hearing-impaired. Figure 5 shows a wideband spectrogram of disfluent speech.

—*Martin J. Ball*

References

Abberton, E., and Fourcin, A. (1997). Electrolaryngography. In M. J. Ball and C. Code (Eds.), *Instrumental clinical phonetics* (pp. 119–148). London: Whurr.

Baken, R., and Daniloff, R. (1991). *Readings in clinical spectrography of speech*. San Diego, CA: Singular Publishing Group.

Ball, M. J., and Gröne, B. (1997). Imaging techniques. In M. J. Ball and C. Code (Eds.), *Instrumental clinical phonetics*, (pp. 194–227). London: Whurr.

Ball, M. J., and Rahilly, J. (1999). *Phonetics: The science of speech*. London: Arnold.

Bell-Berti, F., Krakow, R., Ross, D., and Horiguchi, S. (1993). The rise and fall of the soft palate: The velotrace. *Journal of the Acoustical Society of America*, 93, 2416A.

Farmer, A. (1977). Spectrography. In M. J. Ball and C. Code (Eds.), *Instrumental clinical phonetics* (pp. 22–63). London: Whurr.

Gentil, M., and Moore, W. H., Jr. (1997). Electromyography. In M. J. Ball and C. Code (Eds.), *Instrumental clinical phonetics* (pp. 64–86). London: Whurr.

Hardcastle, W., and Gibbon, F. (1997). Electropalatography and its clinical applications. In M. J. Ball and C. Code (Eds.), *Instrumental clinical phonetics* (pp. 149–193). London: Whurr.

Laver, J. (1994). *Principles of phonetics*. Cambridge, UK: Cambridge University Press.

Stone, M. (1996). Instrumentation for the study of speech physiology. In N. J. Lass (Ed.), *Principles of experimental phonetics* (pp. 495–524). St. Louis: Mosby.

Tatham, M., and Morton, K. (1997). Recording and displaying speech. In M. J. Ball and C. Code (Eds.), *Instrumental clinical phonetics* (pp. 1–21). London: Whurr.

Zajac, D., and Yates, C. (1997). Speech aerodynamics. In M. J. Ball and C. Code (Eds.), *Instrumental clinical phonetics* (pp. 87–118). London: Whurr.

Further Readings

Atal, B., Miller, J., and Kent, R. D. (Eds.). (1991). *Papers in speech communication: Speech processing*. Woodbury, NY: Acoustical Society of America.

Baken, R., and Orlikoff, R. (2000). *Clinical measurement of speech and voice* (2nd ed.). San Diego, CA: Singular Publishing Group.

Ball, M. J., Gracco, V., and Stone, M. (2001). Imaging techniques for the investigation of normal and disordered speech production. *Advances in Speech-Language Pathology*, 3, 13–24.

Ball, M. J., and Lowry, O. (2001). *Methods in clinical phonetics*. London: Whurr.

Borden, G., Harris, K., and Raphael, L. (1994). *Speech science primer: Physiology, acoustics and perception of speech* (3rd ed.). Philadelphia: Lippincott Williams and Wilkins.

Dagenais, P. (1995). Electropalatography in the treatment of articulation/phonological disorders. *Journal of Communication Disorders*, 28, 303–329.

Gentil, M. (1990). EMG analysis of speech production of patients with Friedreich disease. *Clinical Linguistics and Phonetics*, 4, 107–120.

Hardcastle, W. (1976). *Physiology of speech production*. London: Academic Press.

Hardcastle, W., Gibbon, F., and Nicolaidis, K. (1991). EPG data reduction methods and their implications for studies of lingual coarticulation. *Journal of Phonetics*, 19, 251–266.

Hardcastle, W., and Laver, J. (Eds.). (1997). *The handbook of phonetic sciences*. Oxford, UK: Blackwell.

Hirano, M., and Bless, D. (1993). *Videostroboscopy of the larynx*. London: Whurr.

Kent, R. D., Atal, B., and Miller, J. (Eds.). (1991). *Papers in speech communication: Speech production*. Woodbury, NY: Acoustical Society of America.

Kent, R. D., and Read, C. (2002). *The acoustic analysis of speech*. San Diego, CA: Singular Publishing Group.

Lass, N. (Ed.). (1996). *Principles of experimental phonetics*. St. Louis: Mosby.

Lieberman, A. (1996). *Speech: A special code*. Cambridge, MA: MIT Press.

Masaki, S., Tiede, M., Honda, K., Shimada, Y., Fujimoto, I., Nakamura, Y., et al. (1999). MRI-based speech production study using a synchronized sampling method. *Journal of the Acoustical Society of Japan*, 20, 375–379.

Miller, J., Kent, R. D., and Atal, B. (Eds.). (1991). *Papers in speech communication: Speech perception*. Woodbury, NY: Acoustical Society of America.

Perkell, J., Cohen, M., Svirsky, M., Matthies, M., Garabieta, I., and Jackson, M. (1992). Electro-magnetic midsagittal articulometer (EMMA) systems for transducing speech articulatory movements. *Journal of the Acoustical Society of America*, 92, 3078–3096.

Rothenburg, M. (1977). Measurement of airflow in speech. *Journal of Speech and Hearing Research*, 20, 155–176.

Rothenburg, M. (1992). A multichannel electroglottograph. *Journal of Voice*, 6, 36–43.

Speaks, C. (1999). *Introduction to sound* (3rd ed.). San Diego, CA: Singular Publishing Group.

Stevens, K. (1998). *Acoustic phonetics*. Cambridge, MA: MIT Press.

Stone, M. (1990). A three-dimensional model of tongue movement based on ultrasound and x-ray microbeam data. *Journal of the Acoustical Society of America*, 87, 2207–2217.

Stone, M., and Lundberg, A. (1996). Three-dimensional tongue surface shapes of English consonants and vowels. *Journal of the Acoustical Society of America*, 99, 1–10.

Westbury, J. (1991). The significance and measurement of head position during speech production experiments using the x-ray microbeam system. *Journal of the Acoustical Society of America*, 89, 1782–1791.

Speech Assessment in Children: Descriptive Linguistic Methods

Descriptive linguistic methods have long been used in the analysis of fully developed primary languages. These same methods are also well-suited to the study of language development, particularly the analysis of children's speech sound systems. Descriptive methods are a preferred analytic tool because they are designed to gather evidence that reveals the hallmark and defining characteristics of a sound system, independent of theoretical orientation, age, or population of study. The defining properties of descriptive linguistic analyses of children's sound systems are discussed in this article.

The Phonetic Inventory. A phonetic inventory comprises all sounds produced or used by a child, regardless of whether those sounds are correct relative to the intended (adult) target. In the acquisition literature, the conventional criterion for determining the phonetic status of sounds is a two-time occurrence independent of the target or context; that is, any sound produced twice is included in a child's phonetic repertoire (Stoel-Gammon, 1985). Children's phonetic inventories reflect the range of individual variability expected in development. As such, complementary methods have been designed to further depict developmental variation, including the phone tree methodology (Ferguson and Farwell, 1975) and the typology of phonetic complexity (Dinnsen, 1992). For children with speech sound disorders, the phonetic inventory may be quite large despite errors of production, and may consist of sounds that do not occur in the ambient language.

The Phonemic Inventory. Phonemes are used to signal meaning differences in a language. Phonemes are conventionally determined by the occurrence of minimal pairs. A minimal pair is defined as two words identical except for one sound, for example "pat" and "bat" or "cap" and "cab." Here, the consonants /p/ and /b/ are the only point of difference in each pair of words; therefore, these would be said to function as phonemes in the differentiation of meaning. For children, the phonemic inventory is generally smaller than the phonetic inventory (Gierut, Simmerman, and Neumann, 1994). Gaps in the phonemic repertoire often affect the sound classes of fricatives, affricates, and liquids. From a linguistic perspective, the nonoccurrence of these sound classes in children's speech parallels markedness. Markedness defines lawful relationships among sound categories that have been found to hold universally across languages of the world. One type of markedness is implicational in nature, such that the occurrence of property X in a language implies property Y, but not vice versa. The implying property X is taken to be marked, and is presumably more difficult to acquire, whereas the implied property Y is unmarked and predictably easier to learn. In development, then, phonemic gaps in the inventory correspond to more marked (difficult) structures of lan-

guage. In linguistic terminology, these gaps would be characterized as a type of phonotactic constraint (Dinnsen, 1984).

The Distribution of Sounds. Distribution refers to where sounds (phones or phonemes) occur in words and is determined by examining context. For children, sounds may be used in all word positions, initial, intervocalic, and final, or they may be limited to certain contexts. In development, obstruent stops commonly occur word-initially but not postvocalically; whereas fricatives and liquids commonly occur postvocalically but not word-initially (Smith, 1973). As with the phonemic inventory, restrictions on the distribution of sounds correspond to markedness, with children having a tendency toward unmarked as opposed to marked structure.

Rule-Governed Alternations. Asymmetries in the distribution of sounds may be further indicative of systematic rule-governed alternations in sound production (Kenstowicz, 1994). Rule-governed alternations occur when morphologically related words are produced in different ways, for example, "electric" but "electricity." Alternations are typically sampled by adding either a prefix or suffix to a base word in order to change the context in which a sound occurs. There are two general types of rule-governed change: allophonic variation and neutralization. Allophonic variation occurs when a single phoneme has multiple corresponding phonetic outputs that vary by context. An example is /t/ produced as aspirated in word-initial position "tap," as flap in intervocalic position "bitter," and as unreleased in word-final position "it." In each case, the target sound is /t/, but the phonetic characteristics of the output differ predictably by word position. Thus, there is a one-to-many mapping between phoneme and phones in allophonic variation. Neutralization occurs when two or more phonemes are merged into one phonetic output in a well-defined context. An example is /t/ and /d/ both produced as flap in intervocalic position "writer" and "rider." In neutralization, the contrast between phonemes is no longer apparent at the phonetic (surface) level. Consequently, there is a many-to-one mapping between phonemes and phone. In children, the emergence of target-appropriate morphophonemics occurs later in language development. For children with speech sound disorders, nontarget allophonic variation and neutralization have been observed and parallel the rules of fully developed languages of the world (Camarata and Gandour, 1984).

Together, these four properties define the most basic elements of a sound system at a segmental level of structure. In addition to examining these properties, descriptive linguistic methods may evaluate prosodic levels of structure by examining units larger than the sound, such as permissible syllable types and combinations and the overlay of primary and secondary stress on these in the formation of words and phrases (Lleó and Prinz, 1996; Kehoe and Stoel-Gammon, 1997). As with segmental structure, children typically use unmarked prosodic structure, with preferences for open syllables and trochaic (strong-weak) stress assignment.

For children with speech sound disorders, there are other methods of analysis that may be relevant to a comprehensive characterization of the sound system (Fey, 1992; see SPEECH SOUND DISORDERS IN CHILDREN: DESCRIPTION AND CLASSIFICATION). Relational analyses establish a one-to-one correspondence between a child's errored outputs and intended target sounds. These analyses are intended to capture the patterns of a child's errors, and to descriptively label these patterns as phonological processes. Four main categories of phonological processes characterize children's commonly occurring developmental errors (Ingram, 1989). These categories are substitution processes, involving different manners or places of production than the target; syllable shape processes, involving different canonical (consonant-vowel) shapes than the target; assimilatory processes, involving sounds produced more alike in a word than in the target; and other processes, such as reversals in the sequencing of sounds or articulatory differences in sound production such as lisping. Children with speech sound errors are likely to use other unusual phonological processes and to persist in their use of these processes for longer durations than are typical (Leonard, 1992).

Supplementary clinical methods have also been designed to evaluate perceptual or metalinguistic skills, as these skills may affect a child's knowledge of the ambient sound system. The Speech Production-Perception Task is one clinical technique that establishes a child's ability to perceptually differentiate target sounds from their corresponding substitutes (Locke, 1980). Other metalinguistic procedures employ categorization tasks that evaluate a child's judgment of the similarity of target sounds and their substitutes (Klein, Lederer, and Cortese, 1991). Although these methods may have clinical utility in isolating the source of breakdown and in designing appropriate intervention for a child's speech disorder, they are considered external (not primary) evidence in conventional linguistic analyses of sound systems (Anderson, 1981), because these skills lie outside the domain of phonology in particular and language in general.

Finally, one of the most central aspects of a descriptive linguistic analysis of a sound system is the interpretation or theoretical account of the data. A number of theories have been advanced to account for the fundamental properties of sound systems. Each relies on a unique set of assumptions about the structure, function, and organization of sounds in a speaker's mental lexicon. Among the most recognized frameworks are linear phonology, including standard generative and natural frameworks; nonlinear phonology, including autosegmental, metrical, underspecification, and feature geometry frameworks (Goldsmith, 1995); and, most recently, optimality theory (Prince and Smolensky, 1997). Any formal theory of language must account for the facts of acquisition, including those pertinent to children with speech sound disorders. Acquisition data present unique challenges for linguistic theory because of the inherent variability within and across children's sound systems within and across points in time (Chomsky, 1999). These challenges have been handled in different ways by different linguistic theories, but at the core, they have served to outline a well-defined set of research issues about children's speech sound development that as of yet remain unresolved. Central questions bear on the nature of children's mental (internal) representation of sound, the relationship between perception and production in speech sound development, and the contribution of innateness and maturation to language acquisition.

—*Judith A. Gierut*

References

Anderson, S. R. (1981). Why phonology isn't natural. *Linguistic Inquiry*, 12, 493–539.

Camarata, S. M., and Gandour, J. (1984). On describing idiosyncratic phonologic systems. *Journal of Speech and Hearing Disorders*, 49, 262–266.

Chomsky, N. (1999). On the nature, use, and acquisition of child language. In W. Ritchie and T. Bhatia (Eds.), *Handbook of child language acquisition* (pp. 33–54). New York: Academic Press.

Dinnsen, D. A. (1984). Methods and empirical issues in analyzing functional misarticulation. In M. Elbert, D. A. Dinnsen, and G. Weismer (Eds.), *Phonological theory and the misarticulating child* (pp. 5–17). Rockville, MD: American Speech-Language-Hearing Association.

Dinnsen, D. A. (1992). Variation in developing and fully developed phonologies. In C. A. Ferguson, L. Menn, and C. Stoel-Gammon (Eds.), *Phonological development: Models, research, implications* (pp. 191–210). Timonium, MD: York Press.

Ferguson, C. A., and Farwell, C. B. (1975). Words and sounds in early language acquisition: English initial consonants in the first fifty words. *Language*, 51, 419–439.

Fey, M. E. (1992). Articulation and phonology: Inextricable constructs in speech pathology. *Language, Speech and Hearing Services in Schools*, 23, 225–232.

Gierut, J. A., Simmerman, C. L., and Neumann, H. J. (1994). Phonemic structures of delayed phonological systems. *Journal of Child Language*, 21, 291–316.

Goldsmith, J. A. (Ed.). (1995). *The handbook of phonological theory*. Cambridge, MA: Blackwell.

Ingram, D. (1989). *Phonological disability in children*. London: Cole and Whurr.

Kehoe, M., and Stoel-Gammon, C. (1997). The acquisition of prosodic structure: An investigation of current accounts of children's prosodic development. *Language*, 73, 113–144.

Kenstowicz, M. (1994). *Phonology in generative grammar*. Cambridge, MA: Blackwell.

Klein, H. B., Lederer, S. H., and Cortese, E. E. (1991). Children's knowledge of auditory/articulatory correspondences: Phonologic and metaphonologic. *Journal of Speech and Hearing Research*, 34, 559–564.

Leonard, L. B. (1992). Models of phonological development and children with phonological disorders. In C. A. Ferguson, L. Menn, and C. Stoel-Gammon (Eds.), *Phonological development: Models, research, implications* (pp. 495–508). Timonium, MD: York Press.

Lleó, C., and Prinz, M. (1996). Consonant clusters in child phonology and the directionality of syllable structure assignment. *Journal of Child Language*, 23, 31–56.

Locke, J. L. (1980). The inference of speech perception in the phonologically disordered child: Part II. Some clinically novel procedures, their use, some findings. *Journal of Speech and Hearing Disorders, 45,* 445–468.

Prince, A., and Smolensky, P. (1997). Optimality: From neural networks to universal grammar. *Science, 275,* 1604–1610.

Smith, N. V. (1973). *The acquisition of phonology: A case study.* Cambridge, UK: Cambridge University Press.

Stoel-Gammon, C. (1985). Phonetic inventories, 15–24 months: A longitudinal study. *Journal of Speech and Hearing Research, 28,* 505–512.

Further Readings

Barlow, J. A. (Ed.). (2001). Clinical forum: Recent advances in phonological theory and treatment. *Language, Speech, and Hearing Services in Schools, 32,* 225–297.

Barlow, J. A., and Gierut, J. A. (1999). Optimality theory in phonological acquisition. *Journal of Speech, Language, and Hearing Research, 42,* 1482–1498.

Bernhardt, B. H., and Stemberger, J. P. (1998). *Handbook of phonological development from the perspective of constraint-based non-linear phonology.* San Diego, CA: Academic Press.

Bernhardt, B., and Stoel-Gammon, C. (1994). Nonlinear phonology: Introduction and clinical application. *Journal of Speech and Hearing Research, 37,* 123–143.

Chin, S. B., and Dinnsen, D. A. (1991). Feature geometry in disordered phonologies. *Clinical Linguistics and Phonetics, 5,* 329–337.

Donegan, P. J., and Stampe, D. (1979). The study of natural phonology. In D. A. Dinnsen (Ed.), *Current approaches to phonological theory* (pp. 126–173). Bloomington: Indiana University Press.

Edwards, M. L., and Shriberg, L. D. (1983). *Phonology: Applications in communicative disorders.* San Diego, CA: College-Hill Press.

Gandour, J. (1981). The nondeviant nature of deviant phonological systems. *Journal of Communication Disorders, 14,* 11–29.

Gerken, L. (1996). Prosodic structure in young children's language production. *Language, 72,* 683–712.

Gierut, J. A. (1999). Syllable onsets: Clusters and adjuncts in acquisition. *Journal of Speech, Language, and Hearing Research, 42,* 708–726.

Gierut, J. A., Elbert, M., and Dinnsen, D. A. (1987). A functional analysis of phonological knowledge and generalization learning in misarticulating children. *Journal of Speech and Hearing Research, 30,* 462–479.

Goad, H., and Ingram, D. (1987). Individual variation and its relevance to a theory of phonological acquisition. *Journal of Child Language, 14,* 419–432.

Grunwell, P. (1985). *Phonological assessment of child speech.* Windsor, UK: NFER-Nelson.

Haas, W. (1963). Phonological analysis of a case of dyslalia. *Journal of Speech and Hearing Disorders, 28,* 239–246.

Ingram, D. (1981). *Procedures for the phonological analysis of children's language.* Baltimore: University Park Press.

Jakobson, R. (1968). *Child language, aphasia and phonological universals.* The Hague, Netherlands: Mouton.

Kent, R. D., and Ball, M. J. (Eds.). (1997). *The new phonologies: Developments in clinical linguistics.* San Diego, CA: Singular Publishing Group.

Kiparsky, P., and Menn, L. (1977). On the acquisition of phonology. In J. MacNamara (Ed.), *Language Learning and Thought* (pp. 47–78). New York: Academic Press.

Locke, J. L. (1983). *Phonological acquisition and change.* New York: Academic Press.

Macken, M. A. (1980). The child's lexical representation: The "puzzle-puddle-pickle" evidence. *Journal of Linguistics, 16,* 1–17.

McGregor, K. K., and Schwartz, R. G. (1992). Converging evidence for underlying phonological representations in a child who misarticulates. *Journal of Speech and Hearing Research, 35,* 596–603.

Schwartz, R. G. (1992). Clinical applications of recent advances in phonological theory. *Language, Speech and Hearing Services in Schools, 23,* 269–276.

Stemberger, J. P., and Stoel-Gammon, C. (1991). The underspecification of coronals: Evidence from language acquisition and performance errors. In C. Paradis and J.-F. Prunet (Eds.), *Phonetics and phonology: Vol. 2: The Special Status of Coronals* (pp. 181–199). San Diego, CA: Academic Press.

Velten, H. (1943). The growth of phonemic and lexical patterns in infant speech. *Language, 19,* 281–292.

Vihman, M. M. (1996). *Phonological development: The origins of language in the child.* Cambridge, MA: Blackwell.

Speech Development in Infants and Young Children with a Tracheostomy

A tracheostomy is a permanent opening of the trachea to outside air. It most often requires a surgical procedure for closure. The primary reason for performing a surgical tracheostomy is for long-term airway management in cases of chronic upper airway obstruction or central or obstructive sleep apnea, or to provide long-term mechanical ventilatory support. The use of assisted ventilation for more than 1 month in the first year of life has been considered to constitute a chronic tracheostomy (Bleile, 1993). Most of the estimated 900–2,000 infants and children per year who need a tracheostomy, a ventilator, or both for a month or more are, in fact, less than a year old (Singer et al., 1989). Although the mortality associated with a chronic tracheostomy in young children is twice that in adults, the procedure is invaluable for acute and long-term airway management (Fry et al., 1985).

When a tracheostomy or mechanical ventilation is used over a long period, the impact on communication and feeding behavior can be significant. Oral communication in children occurs in tandem with growth and maturation of the structures of the speech apparatus. Neuromuscular or biomechanical difficulties resulting from altered patterns of growth or structural problems can negatively affect the development of oral communication. In particular, the respiratory, laryngeal, and articulatory subsystems of the speech apparatus are at risk for pathological changes affecting the development of speech.

The respiratory subsystem of the speech apparatus comprises the lower airways, rib cage, diaphragm, and abdominal structures. The lower airways consist of the trachea, the right and left mainstem bronchi, and the lungs. The tracheobronchial tree is much smaller in children than in adults, and differs in shape and biomechanics as well. The trachea in young children has been described as the size of a soda straw, and is highly malleable (Fry et al., 1985). The infant tracheal diameter is approximately 0.5 cm, whereas adult tracheal diameters are 1.5–2.5 cm. C-shaped cartilage rings joined by connective tissue help to keep the trachea from collapsing against the flow of air during breathing. Because the membranes of the infant trachea are soft and fragile, there is a risk of tracheal compromise secondary to a tracheostomy. Complications may include reactive granulation at the site of cannula, edema and scaring, chronic irritation of the tracheal lumen, and tracheal collapse as a result of increased negative pressure pulling air through a compromised structure (Fry et al., 1985).

During the first several years of life, significant changes occur in the structure and mechanics of the respiratory system. The airways increase in radius and length and the lungs increase in size and weight. The thoracic cavity enlarges and changes in shape, and overall chest wall compliance decreases with upright posture. Airway resistance decreases, and pleural pressure becomes more subatmospheric (Beckerman, Brouillette, and Hunt, 1992). Tidal volume, inspiratory capacity, vital capacity, and minute ventilation increase with age.

Besides providing phonation, the larynx, along with the epiglottis and soft palate, protects the lower airway. The infant larynx is located high in the neck, close to the base of the tongue. The thyroid cartilage is located directly below the hyoid bone, whereas the cricoid cartilage is the lowest part of the laryngeal structure. Because of its location and size, the infant larynx, like the trachea, is susceptible to trauma during airway management procedures. The laryngeal structures become less susceptible to injury as they change shape and descend during the first year of life.

The articulatory subsystem, composed of the pharynx, mouth, and nose, also undergoes significant changes in growth and function during infancy and early childhood. The pharynx plays a critical role in both respiration and swallowing. The infant pharynx lacks a rigid framework and can collapse if external suction is applied within the airway. If the airway-maintaining muscles are weak or paralyzed, normal negative pressures associated with inspiratory efforts also can cause airway collapse at the level of the pharynx (Thach, 1992). Movement of the pharyngeal walls, elevation of the soft palate, and elevation of posterior portion of the tongue are important maneuvers for achieving velopharyngeal closure. The infant tongue is proportionately larger in relation to mouth size than the adult's; thus, tongue retraction can cause upper airway blockage and respiratory distress. Various craniofacial abnormalities may result in structural or neurological situations that require airway management interventions, including tracheostomy.

The decision to use long-term airway maintenance in the form of a tracheostomy requires consideration of many factors. Even the type of incision can make a difference in overall outcome for the infant or young child (Fry et al., 1985). Other information is needed to select the appropriate tracheostomy tube. Driver (2000) has compiled a list of the critical factors in tracheostomy tube selection. These factors include the child's respiratory requirements, age and weight, tracheal diameter, distance from the tracheal opening to the carina, and anatomical features of the neck for selection of a neck plate or flange. In addition, decisions must be made regarding whether or not there should be an inner cannula, the flexibility of the cannula, whether or not there should be a cuff (an air-inflatable outer bladder used to create a seal against the outer wall of the tracheal tube and trachea), and what external adapters might be used (Driver, 2000).

Tracheostomy tubes are selected primarily on the basis of the ventilatory needs of the infant or young child. Tracheostomy tubes will be larger in diameter and may have a cuff in the event the child needs high ventilator pressures with frequent suctioning. However, because of a young child's susceptibility to trauma of the speech apparatus, it is optimal to have a smaller-diameter, flexible tube without a cuff. When a smaller tube is selected, air leakage around the tube and through the upper airway will be available to the infant for voicing.

Many pediatric upper airway management problems can be successfully addressed with a tracheostomy alone. However, chronic respiratory failure will require some form of mechanical ventilation. The type of mechanical ventilation support required will depend on the type of disorder, the degree of respiratory dependence, and whether the child will ultimately be weaned from ventilatory support. There are two types of mechanical ventilation systems commonly used with children. Negative pressure ventilation is noninvasive and uses negative (below atmospheric) pressure by exerting suction on the outside of the chest and abdomen. As a result, intrathoracic pressure is reduced and induces airflow into the lungs. Expiration is accomplished by passive recoil of the lungs. Negative pressure ventilators work well with children who have relatively normal airways and compliant chest walls. Negative pressure ventilators are associated with fewer complications than positive pressure ventilators and do not require a tracheostomy (Splaingard et al., 1983). However, they are cumbersome and are not adequate for children with severe respiratory disease or rigid chest walls (Driver, 2000). Positive pressure ventilation is invasive and applies positive (above atmospheric) pressure to force air into the lungs via a ventilator connected to a tracheostomy tube (for long-term use). Expiration is accomplished by passive recoil of the lungs. The primary advantages are the flexibility to individualize respiratory support and to deliver various concentrations of oxygen (Metz, 1993). There are two major types of positive pressure ventilators, volume ventilators and pressure ventilators. In addition, ventilators are set in a mode (e.g., assist-control, synchronized intermittent mandatory ventilation) to deliver a certain number of breaths per minute, based on the tidal volume and minute ventilation.

Infants and young children with tracheostomies can become oral communicators if oral motor control is sufficient, the velopharynx is competent, the upper airway is in reasonably good condition (i.e., there is no significant vocal fold paresis or paralysis and no significant airway obstruction), the ability to deliver airflow and pressure to the vocal folds and supporting larngeal structures is sufficient, and chest wall muscular support for speech breathing is sufficient (not a prerequisite for ventilator-supported speech). If oral communication is possible, then the type of tracheostomy tube and the various valve configurations must be selected on the basis of both effective airway management and oral communication criteria. Driver (2000) suggests that the best results for oral communication are achieved if the smallest, simplest tracheostomy tube is selected. The size and nature (fenestrated vs. non-fenestrated) of the tracheostomy tube also will affect the effort required to move gas across the airway (Hussey and Bishop, 1996). Respiratory effort to breathe will impact on the additional effort required to vocalize and speak. The most efficient tracheostomy tube is one that has flow characteristics similar to those of the upper respiratory system for the maintenance of respiratory homeostasis, but with some trade-off for air leakage necessary for vocalization (Mullins et al., 1993). When tracheostomy tubes have a cuff, extreme caution should be taken to ensure that cuff deflation is accomplished prior to any attempts to support oral communication. Tracheostomy tubes with cuffs are not recommended for infants and very young children because of increased risk of tracheal wall trauma.

When a sufficient air leak around the tracheostomy tube exists, then a unidirectional speaking valve can be attached to the hub of the tube. When the child inspires, air enters through a diaphragm that closes on expiration, thus forcing air to exit through the upper airway. The same effect can be accomplished by manually occluding the hub of the tracheostomy tube. Speaking valves can be used with ventilator-assisted breathing as well.

Several factors should be considered when selecting a pediatric speaking valve. These factors include the type of diaphragm construction (bias open or bias closed), the amount of resistance inherent in the valve type, and the amount of air loss during vocalization and speech production. First, speaking valves can be either bias open or bias closed at atmospheric pressure. A biased closed valve remains closed until negative air pressure is applied during inspiration. In this case, the valve will open during inspiration and close during expiration. A bias open valve remains open and only closes during the expiratory phase of the breath cycle. A bias closed valve may require greater effort to achieve airflow (Zajac, Fronataro-Clerici, and Roop, 1999). Differences in resistance have been found among valve types, especially during low flows (.450 liters/sec), however, all valves recently tested have resistances in the range of nasal resistance reported for normal adults. Whereas speaking valves have similar resistances, bias-open valves consistently show air loss during the rise in pressure associated with the /p/ consonant (Zajac, Frontaro-Clerici, and Roop, 1999).

Introducing a speaking valve to a young child can be challenging. The valve changes the sensation of breathing probably due to increases in resistance on both inspiration and expiration. Extra effort from expiratory muscles during phonation also must be generated to force air around the tracheostomy tube to the vocal folds. Finally, young children may not be familiar with coughing up secretions through the oral cavities and show distress until this skill is acquired (McGowan et al., 1993). Initially, the young child may be able to tolerate the speaking valve for only 5 minutes at a time. With encouragement and appropriate reinforcement, the child will likely tolerate the speaking valve for increasing amounts of time. When a speaking valve is placed in line with mechanical ventilation, various volume or pressure adjustments may be made to maximize the timing of phonation and the natural characteristics of the breathing and speaking cycles. Only a few general guidelines on mechanical ventilation and speech in infants and young children have been published (e.g., Lohmeier and Boliek, 1999).

A chronic tracheostomy interferes with the development of oral motor skills and experimentation with sound production by limiting movements of the jaw, tongue, and lips. In addition, long-term intubation may result in a significantly high-vaulted palate and vocal cord injury (Driver, 2000). Adequate breath support for speech also may be affected because of neuromuscular weakness, hypotonia, hypertonia, or paralysis. Consequently, infants and young children may have one or several issues affecting the speech mechanism. Infants and young children who need mechanical ventilation may not vocalize until near the end of the first year of life and may not be able to appropriately time their vocalizations to ventilator cycle until well after 12 months of age (Lohmeier and Boliek, 1999). The speech characteristics of infants and children with tracheostomies, using speaking valves or manual occlusion, include a smaller lung volume initiations, terminations, and excursions, fewer syllables per breath group, variable chest wall configurations during vocalization including rib cage or abdomen paradoxical movements, breathy or pressed voice quality that reflects available airflow and tracheal pressures, intermittent voice stoppages, hypernasality, and poor intelligibility (Lohmeier and Boliek, 1999). In addition, experimentation with vocal play, feeding, and oral-motor exploration may be limited during a sensitive period for speech and language acquisition. Therefore, all efforts should be made to support phonation and other communicative opportunities.

Only a handful of group and single case studies have assessed the developmental outcomes of speech and language following the long-term use of a tracheostomy or mechanical ventilation. These studies suffer from problems such as sample heterogeneity and the prelinguistic or linguistic status of the child at the time the intervention is performed, but they do suggest some general trends and outcomes. Fairly obviously, these children are at risk for delay in speech and language development (Simon and Handler, 1981; Simon, Fowler, and Handler, 1983; Kaslon and Stein, 1985; Simon and Mc-

Gowan, 1989; Bleile and Miller, 1994). Major gains in the development of speech and language can sometimes be made during and after decannulation with total communication intervention approaches. However, the data suggest that residual effects of long-term tracheostomy can be measured long after decannulation. Most reported delays seem to be articulatory in nature; voice and respiratory dysfunction are rarely reported in children after decannulation (Singer, Wood, and Lambert, 1985; Singer et al., 1989; Hill and Singer, 1990; Kamen and Watson, 1991; Kertoy et al., 1999). Taken together, these studies indicate possible residual effects of long-term tracheostomy on the speech mechanism. These effects appear unrelated to the time of intervention (i.e., prelinguistic or linguistic) but may be related to length of cannulation and the general constellation of medical conditions associated with long-term tracheostomy use.

—*Carol A. Boliek*

References

Beckerman, R. C., Brouillette, R. T., and Hunt, C. E. (1992). *Respiratory control disorders in infants and children.* Baltimore: Williams and Wilkins.

Bleile, K. M. (1993). Children with long-term tracheostomies. In K. M. Bleile (Ed.), *The care of children with long-term tracheostomies* (pp. 3–19). San Diego, CA: Singular Publishing Group.

Bleile, K. M., and Miller, S. A. (1994). Toddlers with medical needs. In J. E. Bernthal and N. W. Bankson (Eds.), *Child phonology: Characteristics, assessment, and intervention with special populations* (pp. 81–108). New York: Thieme.

Driver, L. E. (2000). Pediatric considerations. In D. C. Tippett (Ed.), *Tracheostomy and ventilator dependency* (pp. 193–235). New York: Thieme.

Fry, T. L., Jones, R. O., Fischer, N. D., and Pillsbury, H. C. (1985). Comparisons of tracheostomy incisions in a pediatric model. *Annals of Orolaryngology, Rhinology, and Laryngology, 94,* 450–453.

Hill, B. P., and Singer, L. T. (1990). Speech and language development after infant tracheostomy. *Journal of Speech and Hearing Research, 55,* 15–20.

Hoit, J. D., Shea, S. A., and Banzett, R. B. (1994). Speech production during mechanical ventilation in tracheostomized individuals. *Journal of Speech and Hearing Research, 37,* 53–63.

Hussey, J. D., and Bishop, M. J. (1996). Pressures required to move gas through the native airway in the presence of a fenestrated vs a nonfenestrated tracheostomy tube. *Chest, 110,* 494–497.

Kamen, R. S., and Watson, B. C. (1991). Effects of long-term tracheostomy on spectral characteristics of vowel production. *Journal of Speech and Hearing Research, 34,* 1057–1065.

Kaslon, K., and Stein, R. (1985). Chronic pediatric tracheostomy: Assessment and implication for habilitation of voice, speech and language in young children. *International Journal of Pediatric Otorhinolaryngology, 6,* 37–50.

Kertoy, M. K., Guest, C. M., Quart, E., and Lieh-Lai, M. (1999). Speech and phonological characteristics of individual children with a history of tracheostomy. *Journal of Speech, Language, and Hearing Research, 42,* 621–635.

Lohmeier, H. L., and Boliek, C. A. (1999). *Infant respiration and speech production on a ventilator: A case study.* Paper presented at the Annual Meeting of the American Speech-Language and Hearing Association, San Francisco, November 1999.

McGowan, J. S., Bleile, K. M., Fus, L., and Barnas, E. (1993). Communication disorders. In K. M. Bleile (Ed.), *The care of children with long-term tracheostomies* (pp. 113–137). San Diego, CA: Singular Publishing Group.

Metz, S. (1993). Ventilator assistance. In K. M. Bleile (Ed.), *The care of children with long-term tracheostomies* (pp. 41–55). San Diego, CA: Singular Publishing Group.

Mullins, J. B., Templer, J. W., Kong, J., Davis, W. E., and Hinson, J., Jr. (1993). Airway resistance and work of breathing in tracheostomy tubes. *Laryngoscope, 103,* 1367–1372.

Simon, B. M., Fowler, S. M., and Handler, S. D. (1983). Communication development in young children with long-term tracheostomies: Preliminary report. *International Journal of Pediatric Otorhinolaryngology, 6,* 37–50.

Simon, B. M., and Handler, S. D. (1981). The speech pathologist and management of children with tracheostomies. *Journal of Otolaryngology, 10,* 440–448.

Simon, B. M., and McGowan, J. (1989). Tracheostomy in young children: Implications for assessment and treatment of communication and feeding disorders. *Infants and Young Children, 1,* 1–9.

Singer, L. T., Kercsmar, C., Legris, G., Orlowski, J. P., Hill, B., and Doershuk, C. (1989). Developmental sequelae of long-term infant tracheostomy. *Developmental Medicine and Child Neurology, 31,* 224–230.

Singer, L. T., Wood, R., and Lambert, S. (1985). Developmental follow-up of long-term tracheostomy: A preliminary report. *Developmental and Behavioral Pediatrics, 6,* 132–136.

Splaingard, M. L., Frates, R. C., Jr., Jefferson, L. S., Rosen, C. L., and Harrison, D. M. (1983). Home negative pressure ventilation: Report of 20 years of experience in patients with neuromuscular disease. *Archives of Physical Medicine and Rehabilitation, 66,* 239–242.

Thach, B. T. (1992). Neuromuscular control of the upper airway. In R. C. Beckerman, R. T. Brouillette, and C. E. Hunt (Eds.), *Respiratory control disorders in infants and children* (pp. 47–60). Baltimore: Williams and Wilkins.

Zajac, D. J., Fronataro-Clerici, L., and Roop, T. A. (1999). Aerodynamic characteristics of trachcostomy speaking valves: An updated report. *Journal of Speech, Language, and Hearing Research, 42,* 92–100.

Further Readings

Adamson, L. B., and Dunbar, B. (1991). Communication development of young children with tracheostomies. *Augmentative and Alternative Communication, 7,* 275–283.

Ahman, E., and Lipski, K. (1991). Early intervention for technology dependent infants and young children. *Infants and Young Children, 3,* 67–77.

Brodsky, L., and Volk, M. (1993). The airway and swallowing. In J. C. Arvedson and L. Brodsky (Eds.), *Pediatric swallowing and feeding assessment and management.* San Diego, CA: Singular Publishing Group.

Citta-Pietrolungo, T. J., Alexander, M. A., Cook, S. P., and Padman, R. (1993). Complications of tracheostomy and decannulation in pediatric and young patients with traumatic brain injury. *Archives of Physical Medicine and Rehabilitation, 74,* 905–909.

Cox, J. Z., and VanDeinse, S. D. (1997). Special needs of the prelinguistic ventilator-assisted child. In L. E. Driver, V. S.

Nelson, and S. A. Warschausky (Eds.), *The ventilator-assisted child: A practical resource guide*. San Antonio, TX: Communication Skill Builders.

Eliachar, I. (2000). Unaided speech in long-term tube free tracheostomy. *Laryngoscope, 110*, 749–760.

Leder, S. B. (1994). Perceptual rankings of speech quality produced with one-way tracheostomy speaking valves. *Journal of Speech and Hearing Research, 37*, 1308–1312.

Leder, S. B. (1990). Verbal communication for the ventilator dependent patient: Voice intensity with the portex "Talk" tracheostomy tube. *Laryngoscope, 100*, 1116–1121.

Leder, S. B., and Traquina, D. N. (1989). Voice intensity of patients using a communi-trach I cuffed speaking tracheostomy tube. *Laryngoscope, 99*, 744–747.

Lichtman, S. W., Birnbaum, I. L., Sanfilippo, M. R., Pellicone, J. T., Damon, W. J., and King, M. L. (1995). Effect of a tracheostomy speaking valve on secretions, arterial oxygenation, and olfaction: A quantitative evaluation. *Journal of Speech and Hearing Research, 38*, 549–555.

Line, W. S., Jr., Hawkins, D. B., Kahlstrom, E. J., McLaughlin, E., and Ensley, J. (1986). Tracheostomy in infants and young children: The changing perspective. *Laryngoscope, 96*, 510–515.

Manley, S. B., Frank, E. M., Melvin, C. F. (1999). Preparation of speech-language pathologist to provide services to patients with a tracheostomy tube: A survey. *American Journal of Speech-Language Pathology, 8*, 171–180.

McGowan, J. S., Kerwin, M. L., and Bleile, K. M. (1993). Oral-motor and feeding problems. In K. M. Bleile (Ed.), *The care of children with long-term tracheostomies*. San Diego, CA: Singular Publishing Group.

Nash, M. (1988). Swallowing problems in the tracheostomized patient. *Otolaryngology Clinics of North America, 21*, 701–709.

Ramsey, A. M., and Grady, E. A. (1997). Long-term airway management for the ventilator-assisted child. In L. E. Driver, V. S. Nelson, and S. A. Warschausky (Eds.), *The ventilator-assisted child: A practical resource guide*. San Antonio, TX: Communication Skill Builders.

Thompson-Henry, S., Braddock, B. (1995). The modified Evan's blue dye procedure fails to detect aspiration in the tracheostomized patient: Five case reports. *Dysphagia, 10*, 172–174.

Tippett, D. C., and Siebens, A. A. (1995). Reconsidering the value of the modified Evan's blue dye test: A comment on Thompson-Henry and Braddock (1995). *Dysphagia, 11*, 78–81.

VanDeinse, S. D., and Cox, J. Z. (1997). Feeding and swallowing issues in the ventilator-assisted child. In L. E. Driver, V. S. Nelson, and S. A. Warschausky (Eds.), *The ventilator-assisted child: A practical resource guide*. San Antonio, TX: Communication Skill Builders.

Speech Disfluency and Stuttering in Children

Childhood stuttering (also called developmental stuttering) is a communication disorder that is generally characterized by interruptions, or *speech disfluencies*, in the smooth forward flow of speech. Speech disfluencies can take many forms, and not all are considered to be atypical. Disfluencies such as *interjections* ("um", "er"),

phrase repetitions ("I want—I want that"), and *revisions* ("I want—I need that"), which are relatively common in the speech of normally developing children, represent normal aspects of the speaking process. These disfluencies arise when a speaker experiences an error in language formulation or speech production or needs more time to prepare a message. Other types of disfluencies, which occur relatively infrequently in the speech of normally developing children, may be indicative of a developing stuttering disorder. These disfluencies, often called "atypical" disfluencies, "stuttered" disfluencies, or "stutter-like" disfluencies, include *whole-word repetitions* ("I-I-I want that") and, particularly, fragmentations within a word unit, such as *part-word repetitions* ("li-li-like this"), *sound prolongations* ("lllllike this"), and *blocks* ("l—ike this") (Ambrose and Yairi, 1999).

Stuttered speech disfluencies can also be accompanied by affective, behavioral, and cognitive reactions to the difficulties with speech production. These reactions are distinct from the speech disfluencies themselves but are part of the overall stuttering disorder (Yaruss, 1998). Examples of behavioral reactions, which rapidly become incorporated into the child's stuttering pattern, include physical tension and struggle in the speech mechanism as children attempt to control their speech. Affective and cognitive reactions include feelings of anxiety, embarrassment, and frustration. As stuttering continues, children may develop shame, low self-esteem, and avoidance of words, sounds, or speaking situations. These negative reactions can lead to increased stuttering severity and greatly exacerbate the child's communication problems.

Etiology. Numerous theories about the etiology of stuttering have been proposed (Bloodstein, 1993). Historically, these theories tended to focus on single causes acting in isolation. Examples include psychological explanations based on supposed neuroses, physiological explanations involving muscle spasms, neurological explanations focusing on ticlike behaviors, and environmental explanations suggesting that normal disfluency was misidentified as stuttering. None of these theories has proved satisfactory, though, for the phenomenology of stuttering is complex and highly individualized. As a result, current theories focus on multiple etiological factors that interact in complex ways for different children who stutter (e.g., Smith and Kelly, 1997). These interactions involve not only genetic and environmental factors, but also various aspects of the child's overall development.

Pedigree and twin studies have shown a genetic component to childhood stuttering—a family history of stuttering can be identified for approximately 60%–70% of children who stutter (Ambrose, Yairi, and Cox, 1993). The precise nature of that genetic inheritance is not fully understood, however, and studies are currently under way to evaluate different models of genetic transmission. It is also likely that environmental factors, such as the model the child hears when learning to speak and the demands placed on the child to speak quickly or precisely, may play a role in determining whether stuttering will be expressed in a particular child (e.g., Starkweather and Givens-Ackerman, 1997).

There are several aspects of children's overall development that affect children's speech fluency and the development of childhood stuttering. For example, children are more likely to be disfluent when producing longer, more syntactically complex sentences (Yaruss, 1999). It is not clear whether this increase is associated with greater demands on the child's language formulation abilities or speech production abilities; however, it is likely that stuttering arises due to the interaction between linguistic and motoric functions. As a group, children who stutter have been shown to exhibit language formulation and speech production abilities that are slightly lower than their typically fluent peers; however, these differences do not generally represent clinically identifiable deficits in speech or language development (Bernstein Ratner, 1997a). Finally, temperament, and specifically the child's sensitivity to stimuli in the environment as well as to speaking mistakes, has been implicated as a factor contributing to the likelihood that a child will react negatively to speech disfluencies (Conture, 2001).

Onset, Development, and Distribution. The onset of childhood stuttering typically occurs between the ages of 2½ and 5, though later onset is sometimes reported. Stuttering can develop gradually (with increasing frequency of disfluency and growing severity of individual instances of disfluency), or it can appear relatively suddenly (with the rapid development of more severe stuttering behaviors). Stuttering often begins during a period of otherwise normal or possibly even advanced speech-language development, although many children who stutter exhibit concomitant deficits in other aspects of speech and language development. For example, 30%–40% of preschool children who stutter also exhibit a disorder of speech sound production (articulation or phonological disorder), though the exact nature of the relationship between these communication disorders is not clear (Yaruss, LaSalle, and Conture, 1998).

The lifetime incidence of stuttering may be as high as 5%, although the prevalence is only approximately 1%, suggesting that the majority of young children who stutter—perhaps as many as 75%—recover from stuttering and develop normal speech fluency (Yairi and Ambrose, 1999). Children who recover typically do so within the first several months after onset; however, recovery is also common within the first 2 years after onset (Yairi and Ambrose, 1999). After this time, natural or unaided recovery is less common, and children appear to be significantly less likely to experience a complete recovery if they have been stuttering for longer than 2 to 3 years, or if they are still stuttering after approximately age 7 (Andrews and Harris, 1964). Boys are affected more frequently than girls: in adults, the male to female ratio is approximately 4 or 5 to 1, though at onset, the ratio is closer to 2 to 1, suggesting that girls are more

likely to experience recovery than boys. This is particularly true for girls who have other females in their family with a history of recovery from stuttering (Ambrose, Yairi, and Cox, 1997).

Diagnosis and Assessment. The high rate of recovery from early stuttering indicates a positive prognosis for many preschool children who stutter; however, it also complicates the diagnostic process and makes it difficult to evaluate the efficacy of early intervention. There is general agreement among practitioners that it is best to evaluate young children soon after the onset of stuttering to estimate the likelihood of recovery. Often, however, it is difficult to make this determination, and there is considerable disagreement about whether it is best to enroll children in treatment immediately or wait to see whether they will recover without intervention (e.g., Bernstein Ratner, 1997b; Curlee and Yairi, 1997).

Based on the understanding that the etiology of childhood stuttering involves multiple interacting factors, the diagnostic assessment of a preschool child who stutters involves evaluation of several aspects of the child's speech, language, and overall development, as well as selected aspects of the child's environment. Specifically, a complete diagnostic assessment includes the following: (1) a detailed interview with parents or caregivers about factors such as family history of stuttering, the family's reactions to the child's speaking difficulties, the child's reactions to stuttering, the speech and language models the child is exposed to at home, and any other information about communication or other stressors the child may be experiencing, such as competition for talking time with siblings; (2) assessment of the observable characteristics of the child's fluency, including the frequency, duration, and type of disfluencies and a rating of stuttering severity; (3) assessment of the child's speaking abilities, including an assessment of speech sound production/phonological development and oral-motor skills; (4) assessment of the child's receptive and expressive language development, including morphological structures, vocabulary, syntax, and pragmatic interaction; and, increasingly, (5) assessment of the child's temperament, including sensitivity to stimuli in the environment and concerns about speaking difficulties.

Together, these factors can be used to estimate the likelihood that the child will recover from early stuttering without intervention or whether treatment is indicated. Although it is impossible to determine with certainty which children will recover from stuttering without intervention, some diagnostic signs that may indicate an increased risk of continued stuttering and the need for treatment include a family history of chronic stuttering, significant physical tension or struggle during stuttered or fluent speech, concomitant disorders of speech or language, and a high degree of concern about speaking difficulties on the part of the child or the family (e.g., Yairi et al., 1996). Importantly, some practitioners also recommend treatment even in cases where the estimated risk for continued stuttering is low, either in an attempt to speed up the natural recovery process or to help concerned parents reduce their worries about their child's fluency.

Treatment.   As theories about stuttering have changed, so too have preferred treatment approaches, particularly for older children and adults who stutter. At present, there are two primary approaches to treatment for young children who stutter, traditionally labeled "indirect" and "direct" therapy. Indirect therapy is based on the notion that children's fluency is affected by specific characteristics of their speech, such as speaking rate, time allowed for pausing between words and phrases, and the length and complexity of utterances. Specifically, it appears that children are less likely to stutter if they speak more slowly, allow more time for pausing, or use shorter, simpler utterances. If children can learn to use these "fluency facilitating" strategies, they are more likely to be fluent and, presumably, less likely to develop a chronic stuttering disorder.

A key assumption underlying the indirect treatment approach is that these parameters of children's speech are influenced by the communication model of the people in the child's environment. Thus, in indirect therapy, clinicians teach parents and caregivers to use a slower rate of speech, to increase their rate of pausing, and, in some instances, to modify the length and complexity of their utterances, although there is increasing concern among some researchers that restricting the language input children receive may have unintended negative consequence for children's overall language development (e.g., Bernstein Ratner and Silverman, 2000). Furthermore, although it is clear that children do learn certain aspects of communication from their environment, there is relatively little empirical support for the notion that changing parents' speech characteristics directly influences children's speech characteristics or their speech fluency. Even in the absence of clear efficacy data, however, the indirect approach is favored by many clinicians who are hesitant to draw attention to the child's speech or increase the child's concerns about their speech fluency.

In recent years, a competing form of treatment for preschool children who stutter has gained popularity (Harrison and Onslow, 1999). This behavioral approach is based on parent-administered intermittent reinforcement of fluent speech and occasional, mild, supportive correction of stuttered speech. Specifically, when a child stutters, the parent labels the stuttering as "bumpy" speech and encourages the child to repeat the sentence "without the bumps." Efficacy data indicate that this form of treatment is highly successful at reducing the observable characteristics of stuttering, although questions remain about the mechanism responsible for this improved fluency.

Regardless of the approach used in the preschool years, clinicians generally shift from indirect to more direct forms of treatment as children grow older and their awareness of their speaking difficulties increases. Direct treatment strategies include specifically teaching children to use a slower speaking rate or reduced physical tension to smooth out their speech and helping them learn to modify individual instances of stuttering so they are less disruptive to communication (Ramig and Bennett, 1997). Other direct approaches include operant treatments based on reinforcing fluent speech in a hierarchy of utterances of increasing syntactic complexity and length (Bothe, 2002).

A critical component of treatment for older children who stutter, for whom complete recovery is less likely—and even for preschool children who are concerned about their speech or who have significant risk factors indicating a likelihood of continued stuttering (Logan and Yaruss, 1999)—is learning to accept stuttering and to minimize the impact of stuttering in daily activities. As children learn to cope with their stuttering, they are less likely to develop the negative reactions that characterize more advanced stuttering, so the disorder is less likely to become debilitating for them. In addition to pursuing treatment, many older children and families of children who stutter also find meaningful support through self-help groups, and clinicians are increasingly recommending support group participation for their young clients and their families.

Summary.   Stuttering is a complex communication disorder involving the production of certain types of speech disfluencies, as well as the affective, behavioral, and cognitive reactions that may result. There is no one known cause of stuttering. Instead, childhood stuttering appears to arise because of a complex interaction among several factors that are both genetically and environmentally determined, such as the child's linguistic abilities, motoric abilities, and temperament. Therefore, diagnostic evaluations of preschoolers who stutter must examine the child's environment and several aspects of child's development. Treatment options include both indirect and direct approaches designed not only to minimize the occurrence of speech disfluencies, but also to minimize the impact of those disfluencies on the lives of children who stutter.

See also LANGUAGE IN CHILDREN WHO STUTTER; STUTTERING.

—*J. Scott Yaruss*

References

Ambrose, N., and Yairi, E. (1999). Normative disfluency data for early childhood stuttering. *Journal of Speech, Language, and Hearing Research, 42,* 895–909.

Ambrose, N., Yairi, E., and Cox, N. (1993). Genetic aspects of early childhood stuttering. *Journal of Speech, Language, and Hearing Research, 36,* 701–706.

Ambrose, N., Yairi, E., and Cox, N. (1997). The genetic basis of persistence and recovery in stuttering. *Journal of Speech, Language, and Hearing Research, 40,* 567–580.

Andrews, G., and Harris, M. (1964). *The syndrome of stuttering.* London: Heinman Medical Books.

Bernstein Ratner, N. (1997a). Stuttering: A psycholinguistic perspective. In R. F. Curlee and G. M. Siegel (Eds.), *Nature and treatment of stuttering: New directions* (2nd ed., pp. 99–127). Needham Heights, MA: Allyn and Bacon.

Bernstein Ratner, N. (1997b). Leaving Las Vegas: Clinical odds and individual outcomes. *American Journal of Speech-Language Pathology, 6,* 29–33.

Bernstein Ratner, N., and Silverman, S. (2000). Parental perceptions of children's communicative development at stuttering onset. *Journal of Speech, Language, and Hearing Research, 43*, 1252–1263.

Bloodstein, O. (1993). *Stuttering: The search for a cause and a cure.* Needham Heights, MA: Allyn and Bacon.

Bothe, A. (2002). Speech modification approaches to stuttering treatment in schools. *Seminars in Speech and Language, 23*, 181–186.

Conture, E. G. (2001). *Stuttering: Its nature, assessment, and treatment.* Needham Heights, MA: Allyn and Bacon.

Curlee, R., and Yairi, E. (1997). Early intervention with early childhood stuttering: A critical examination of the data. *American Journal of Speech-Language Pathology, 6*, 8–18.

Harrison, E., and Onslow, M. (1999). Early intervention for stuttering: The Lidcombe program. In R. F. Curlee (Ed.), *Stuttering and Related Disorders of Fluency* (2nd ed., pp. 65–79). New York: Thieme.

Logan, K. J., and Yaruss, J. S. (1999). Helping parents address attitudinal and emotional factors with young children who stutter. *Contemporary Issues in Communication Science and Disorders, 26*, 69–81.

Ramig, P. R., and Bennett, E. M. (1997). Clinical management of children: Direct management strategies. In R. F. Curlee and G. M. Siegel (Eds.), *Nature and treatment of stuttering: New directions* (2nd ed., pp. 292–312). Needham Heights, MA: Allyn and Bacon.

Smith, A., and Kelly, E. (1997). Stuttering: A dynamic, multifactorial model. In R. F. Curlee and G. M. Siegel (Eds.), *Nature and treatment of stuttering: New directions* (2nd ed., pp. 204–217). Needham Heights, MA: Allyn and Bacon.

Starkweather, C. W., and Givens-Ackerman, J. (1997). *Stuttering*, Austin, TX: Pro-Ed.

Yairi, E., and Ambrose, N. (1999). Early childhood stuttering: I. Persistence and recovery rates. *Journal of Speech, Language, and Hearing Research, 42*, 1098–1112.

Yairi, E., Ambrose, N., Paden, E. P., and Throneburg, R. N. (1996). Predictive factors of persistence and recovery: Pathways of childhood stuttering. *Journal of Communication Disorders, 29*, 51–77.

Yaruss, J. S. (1998). Describing the consequences of disorders: Stuttering and the International Classification of Impairments, Disabilities, and Handicaps. *Journal of Speech, Language, and Hearing Research, 49*, 249–257.

Yaruss, J. S. (1999). Utterance length, syntactic complexity, and childhood stuttering. *Journal of Speech, Language, and Hearing Research, 42*, 329–344.

Yaruss, J. S., LaSalle, L. R., and Conture, E. G. (1998). Evaluating stuttering in young children: Diagnostic data. *American Journal of Speech-Language Pathology, 7*, 62–76.

Further Readings

Bloodstein, O. (1993). *Stuttering: The search for a cause and a cure.* Needham Heights, MA: Allyn and Bacon.

Bloodstein, O. (1995). *A handbook on stuttering* (5th ed.). San Diego, CA: Singular Publishing Group.

Conture, E. G. (2001). *Stuttering: Its nature, assessment, and treatment.* Needham Heights, MA: Allyn and Bacon.

Curlee, R. F. (1999). *Stuttering and related disorders of fluency.* New York: Thieme.

Curlee, R. F., and Siegel, G. M. (Eds.). (1997). *Nature and treatment of stuttering: New directions* (2nd ed.). Needham Heights, MA: Allyn and Bacon.

Guitar, B. (1998). *Stuttering: An integrated approach to its nature and treatment* (2nd ed.). Baltimore: Williams and Wilkins.

Manning, W. H. (2001). *Clinical decision making in fluency disorders* (2nd ed.). San Diego, CA: Singular Publishing Company.

Shapiro, D. A. (1999). *Stuttering intervention: A collaborative journey to fluency freedom.* Austin, TX: Pro-Ed.

Starkweather, C. W., and Givens-Ackerman, J. (1997). *Stuttering.* Austin, TX: Pro-Ed.

Speech Disorders: Genetic Transmission

Advances in behavioral and molecular genetics over the past decade have made it possible to investigate genetic factors that may contribute to speech sound disorders. These speech sound disorders of unknown etiology were often considered to be "functional" or learned. Mounting evidence suggests that at least some speech sound disorders may in part be genetic in origin. However, the search for a genetic basis of speech sound disorders has been complicated by definitional and methodological problems. Issues that are critical to understanding the genetic transmission of speech disorders include prevalence data, phenotype definitions, sex as a risk factor, familial aggregation of disorders, and behavioral and molecular genetic findings.

Prevalence Estimates. Prevalence estimates of speech sound disorders are essential in conducting behavioral and molecular genetic studies. They are used to calculate an individual's risk of having a disorder as well as to test different genetic models of transmission. Prevalence rates for speech disorders may vary based on the age and sex of the individual, the type of disorder, and the comorbid conditions associated with it. In an epidemiological sample, Shriberg and Austin (1998) reported the prevalence of speech delay in 6-year-old children to be 3.8%. Speech delay was approximately 1.5 times more prevalent in boys than in girls. Shriberg and Austin (1998) also found that children with speech involvement have a two to three times greater risk for expressive language problems than for receptive language problems. Estimates of the comorbidity of receptive language disorders with speech disorders ranged from 6% to 21%, based on whether receptive language was assessed by vocabulary, grammar, or both. Similarly, estimates of comorbidity of expressive language disorders with speech disorders ranged from 38% to 62%, depending on the methods used to assess expressive skills.

Phenotype Definitions. Phenotype definitions (i.e., the behavior that is under study) are also crucial for genetic studies of speech disorders. Phenotype definitions may be broadly or narrowly defined, according to the hypothesis to be tested. A broad phenotype may include language as well as speech disorders and sometimes related language learning difficulties such as reading and spelling disorders (Tallal, Ross, and Curtiss, 1989). An

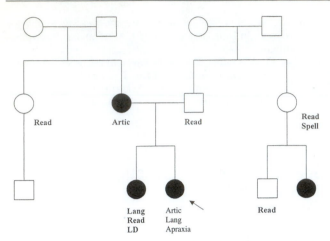

Figure 1. A typical family pedigree of a child with a speech disorder. The arrow indicates the proband child. Male family members are represented by squares and female family members are represented by circles. Individuals who are affected with speech disorders are shaded in black. Other disorders are coded as follows: Read = reading disorder, Spell = spelling disorder, Lang = language disorder, LD = learning disability, Apraxia = apraxia of speech, Artic = articulation disorder.

individual exhibiting a single disorder or a combination of disorders is considered to be affected. Such a broad phenotype may test a general verbal trait deficit hypothesis which holds that there is a common underlying genetic and cognitive basis for speech and language disorders that is expressed differently in individual family members (i.e., variable expression). An alternative explanation is that each disorder has a unique underlying genetic and cognitive basis. Some investigators have narrowly defined the phenotype as a specific speech disorder, such as phonology (Lewis, Ekelman, and Aram, 1989). Even if the proband (i.e., the child with a disorder from whom other family members are identified) is selected by a well-defined criterion, nuclear family members often present a varied spectrum of disorders. Some studies, while narrowly defining the phenotype for the proband, have used a broad phenotype definition for family members. Since older siblings and parents often do not demonstrate speech sound errors in their conversational speech, researchers have relied on historical reports, rather than direct observations of the speech disorder. Figure 1 shows a typical family pedigree of a child with a speech disorder.

Narrow phenotype definitions may examine subtypes of phonology disorders with postulated distinct genetic bases. One schema for the subtyping of phonology disorders may be based on whether or not the phonology disorder is accompanied by more pervasive language disorders (Lewis and Freebairn, 1997). Children with isolated phonology disorders experience fewer academic difficulties than children with phonology disorders accompanied by other language disorders (Aram and Hall, 1989). Shriberg et al. (1997) propose at least two forms of speech sound disorders of unknown origin: those with speech delay and those with questionable

residual errors. These two subtypes may have different genetic or environmental causes.

Sex as a Risk Factor.   A robust finding in studies of familial speech and language disorders has been a higher prevalence of disorders in males than in females, ranging from a 2:1 to a 3:1 ratio (Neils and Aram, 1986; Tallal et al., 1989; Tomblin, 1989; Lewis, 1992). Explanations for this increased prevalence in males include referral bias (Shaywitz et al., 1990), immunoreactive theories (Robinson, 1991), differences in rates and patterns of neurological maturation (Plante, 1996), variation in cognitive phenotypes (Bishop, North, and Donlan, 1995), and differences in genetic transmission of the disorders. An X-linked mode of transmission of speech and language disorders has not been supported by pedigree studies (Lewis, 1992; Beitchman, Hood, and Inglis, 1992). However, a sex-specific threshold hypothesis that proposes that girls have a higher threshold for expression of the disorder, and therefore require a higher genetic loading (more risk genes) before the disorder is expressed, has been supported (Tomblin, 1989; Lewis, 1992; Beitchman, Hood, and Inglis, 1992). Consistent with this hypothesis, a higher percentage of affected relatives are reported for female (38%) than for male probands (26%). Differing sex ratios may be found for various subtypes of phonology disorders (Shriberg and Austin, 1998). Hall, Jordan, and Robin (1993) reported a 3:1 male to female ratio for developmental apraxia of speech. Similarly, boys with phonology disorders were found to have a higher rate of comorbid language disorders than girls with phonology disorders (Shriberg and Austin, 1998). Lewis et al. (1999) found that probands with phonology disorders alone demonstrated a more equal sex ratio (59% male and 41% female) than probands with phonology disorders with language disorders (71% male and 29% female).

Familial Aggregation.   Familial aggregation refers to the percentage of family members demonstrating a disorder. Familial aggregation or family resemblance may be due to heredity, shared family environment, or both. Research has supported the conclusion that speech and language disorders aggregate within families (Neils and Aram, 1986; Tallal, Ross, and Curtiss, 1989; Tomblin, 1989; Gopnik and Crago, 1991; Lewis, 1992; Felsenfeld, McGue, and Broen, 1995; Lahey and Edwards, 1995; Spitz et al., 1997; Rice, Haney, and Wexler, 1998). Reports indicate that 23%–40% of first-degree family members of individuals with speech and language disorders are affected. Differences in reported rates of affected family members again may be attributed to differences in definitional criteria for probands and family members.

Two studies specifically examined familial aggregation of phonology disorders (Lewis, Ekelman, and Aram, 1989; Felsenfeld, McGue, and Broen, 1995). Both studies reported 33% of first-degree family members (nuclear family members) to have had speech-language difficulties. Brothers were most frequently affected.

Behavioral and Molecular Genetic Studies. The twin study paradigm has been employed to identify genetic and environmental contributions to speech and language disorders. Twin studies compare the similarity (concordance) of identical or monozygotic twins to fraternal or dizygotic twins. If monozygotic twins are more concordant than dizygotic twins, a genetic basis is implied. To date, a twin study specifically examining speech sound disorders has not been conducted. Rather, twin studies have employed a broad phenotype definition that includes both speech and language disorders. Twin studies of speech and language disorders (Lewis and Thompson, 1992; Bishop, North, and Donlan, 1995; Tomblin and Buckwalter, 1998) have consistently reported higher concordance rates for monozygotic than for dizygotic twin pairs, confirming a genetic contribution to these disorders. Concordance rates for monozygotic twins range from .70 (Bishop, North, and Donlan, 1995) to .86 (Lewis and Thompson, 1992) and .96 (Tomblin and Buckwalter, 1998). Concordance rates reported for dizygotic twin pairs are as follows: .46 (Bishop, North, and Donlan, 1995), .48 (Lewis and Thompson, 1992), and .69 (Tomblin and Buckwalter, 1998). A large twin study (3000 pairs of twins) suggested that genetic factors may exert more influence at the lower extreme of language abilities, whereas environmental factors may influence normal language abilities more (Dale et al., 1998). These studies, while supporting a genetic contribution to speech and language skills, also indicate a moderate environmental influence. Environmental factors working with genetics may determine speech and language impairment in an individual.

Consistent with these findings, an adoption study by Felsenfeld and Plomin (1997) demonstrated that a history of speech and language disorders in the biological parent best predicted whether or not a child was affected. This relationship was not found when the family history of the adoptive parents was considered. As with twin studies, a broad phenotype definition that encompassed both speech and language disorders was employed. Adoption studies have not been conducted for speech sound disorders alone.

Segregation analyses examine the mode of transmission of the disorder within a family. Segregation analyses have confirmed familial aggregation of speech and language disorders and supported both a major locus model and a polygenic model of transmission of the disorder (Lewis, Cox, and Byard, 1993). The failure to define a definitive mode of transmission may be due to genetic heterogeneity (i.e., more than a single underlying genetic basis).

Only a single study to date has reported a molecular genetic analysis of a family with apraxia of speech and other language impairments. Genetic studies of a single large pedigree, known as the K.E. family, revealed linkage to a region of chromosome 7 (Vargha-Khadem et al., 1995; Fisher et al., 1998). Subsequently, the *FOXP2* gene that is postulated to result in the development of abnormal neural structures for speech and language was identified (Lai et al., 2001). Neuroimaging of family members indicated abnormalities in regions of the frontal lobe and associated motor systems. This was the first study that provided direct evidence for a genetic basis for a speech sound disorder associated with a neurological abnormality. It was the initial step in the application of molecular genetic techniques to the study of speech and language disorders. Further studies are needed to determine if *FOXP2* is found in other families with speech disorders.

See also SPEECH DISORDERS IN CHILDREN: DESCRIPTIVE LINGUISTIC APPROACHES; DEVELOPMENTAL APRAXIA OF SPEECH; PHONOLOGICAL ERRORS, RESIDUAL.

—*Barbara A. Lewis*

References

Aram, D. M., and Hall, N. E. (1989). Longitudinal follow-up of children with preschool communication disorders: Treatment implications. *School Psychology Review, 19,* 487–501.

Bishop, D. V. M., North, T., and Donlan, C. (1995). Nonword repetition as a phenotypic marker for inherited language impairment: Evidence from a twin study. *Journal of Child Psychology and Psychiatry, 37,* 391–403.

Beitchman, J. H., Hood, J., and Inglis, A. (1992). Familial transmission of speech and language impairment: A preliminary investigation. *Canadian Journal of Psychiatry, 37,* 151–156.

Dale, P. S., Simonoff, E., Bishop, D. V. M., Eley, T., Oliver, B., Price, T. S., et al. (1998). Genetic influence on language delay in two-year-old children. *Nature Neuroscience, 1,* 324–328.

Felsenfeld, S., McGue, M., and Broen, P. A. (1995). Familial aggregation of phonological disorders: Results from a 28-year follow-up. *Journal of Speech and Hearing Research, 38,* 1091–1107.

Felsenfeld, S., and Plomin, R. (1997). Epidemiological and offspring analyses of developmental speech disorders using data from the Colorado Adoption Project. *Journal of Speech and Hearing Research, 40,* 778–791.

Fisher, S. E., Vargha-Khadem, F., Watkins, K. E., Monacol, A., and Pembrey, M. E. (1998). Localization of a gene implicated in a severe speech and language disorder. *Nature Genetics, 18,* 168–170.

Gopnik, M., and Crago, M. (1991). Familial aggregation of a developmental language disorder. *Cognition, 39,* 1–50.

Hall, P. K., Jordan, L. S., and Robin, D. A. (1993). *Developmental dyspraxia of speech: Theory and clinical practice.* Austin, TX: Pro-Ed.

Lahey, M., and Edwards, J. (1995). Specific language impairment: Preliminary investigation of factors associated with family history and with patterns of language performance. *Journal of Speech and Hearing Research, 38,* 643–657.

Lai, C. S. L., Fisher, S. E., Hurst, J. A., Vargha-Khadem, F., and Monaco, P. (2001). A forkhead-domain gene is mutated in a severe speech and language disorder. *Nature, 413,* 519–523.

Lewis, B. A. (1992). Pedigree analysis of children with phonology disorders. *Journal of Learning Disabilities, 25,* 586–597.

Lewis, B. A., Cox, N. J., and Byard, P. J. (1993). Segregation analyses of speech and language disorders. *Behavior Genetics, 23,* 291–297.

Lewis, B. A., Ekelman, B. L., and Aram, D. M. (1989). A familial study of severe phonological disorders. *Journal of Speech and Hearing Research, 32,* 713–724.

Lewis, B. A., and Freebairn, L. (1997). Subgrouping children with familial phonology disorders. *Journal of Communication Disorders, 30,* 385–402.

Lewis, B. A., Freebairn, L. A., and Taylor, H. G. (1999). School-age follow-up of children with familial phonology disorders. Paper presented at the annual convention of the American Speech, Language, and Hearing Association. November 1999, San Francisco, CA.

Lewis, B. A., and Thompson, L. A. (1992). A study of developmental speech and language disorders in twins. *Journal of Speech and Hearing Research, 35*, 1086–1094.

Neils, J., and Aram, D. M. (1986). Family history of children with developmental language disorders. *Perceptual and Motor Skills, 63*, 655–658.

Plante, E. (1996). Phenotypic variability in brain-behavior studies of specific language impairment. In M. Rice (Ed.), *Toward a genetics of language.* Mahwah, NJ: Erlbaum.

Rice, M. L., Haney, K. R., and Wexler, K. (1998). Family histories of children with SLI who show extended optional infinitives. *Journal of Speech, Language, and Hearing Research, 41*, 419–432.

Robinson, R. J. (1991). Causes and associations of severe and persistent specific speech and language disorders in children. *Developmental Medicine and Child Neurology, 33*, 943.

Shaywitz, S. E., Shaywitz, B. A., Fletcher, J. M., and Escobar, M. D. (1990). Prevalence of reading disability in boys and girls. *JAMA, 264*, 998–1002.

Shriberg, L. D., and Austin, D. (1998). Comorbidity of speech-language disorders: Implications for a phenotype marker for speech delays. In R. Paul (Ed.), *The speech/language connection.* Baltimore: Paul H. Brookes.

Shriberg, L. D., Austin, D., Lewis, B. A., McSweeny, J. L., and Wilson, D. L. (1997). The percentage of consonants correct (PCC) metric: Extensions and reliability data. *Journal of Speech and Hearing Research, 40*, 708–722.

Spitz, R., Tallal, P., Flax, J., and Benasich, A. A. (1997). Look who's talking: A prospective study of familial transmission of language impairments. *Journal of Speech and Hearing Research, 40*, 990–1001.

Tallal, P., Ross, R., and Curtiss, S. (1989). Familial aggregation in specific language impairment. *Journal of Speech and Hearing Disorders, 54*, 167–173.

Tomblin, J. B. (1989). Familial concentration of developmental language impairment. *Journal of Speech and Hearing Disorders, 54*, 287–295.

Tomblin, J. B., and Buckwalter, P. (1998). The heritability of poor language achievement among twins. *Journal of Speech and Hearing Research, 41*, 188–199.

Vargha-Khadem, F., Watkins, K., Alcock, K., Fletcher, P., and Passingham, R. (1995). Praxic and nonverbal cognitive deficits in a large family with a genetically transmitted speech and language disorder. *Proceedings of the National Academy of Sciences of the United States of America, 92*, 930–933.

Speech Disorders in Adults, Psychogenic

The human communication system is vulnerable to changes in the individual's emotional or psychological state. Several studies show the human voice to be a sensitive indicator of different emotions (Aronson, 1991). Psychiatrists routinely evaluate vocal (intensity, pitch), prosodic (e.g., rhythm, rate, pauses), and other features of communication to diagnosis neurotic states (Brodnitz, 1981). Speech-language pathologists also consider the contributions of psychopathology in the evaluation and management of acquired adult speech disorders (Sapir and Aronson, 1990). This is important because depression and/or anxiety are common in stroke, traumatic brain injury, and progressive neurological disease (Giannoti, 1972). Depression frequently occurs after a laryngectomy and may interfere with rehabilitation efforts (Rollin, 1987). Individuals subjected to prolonged stress may speak with excessive tension in the vocal mechanism. When misuse of the vocal apparatus occurs for a long period of time, it can lead to the formation of vocal fold lesions (e.g., nodules) and long-term dysphonia (Aronson, 1991; Case, 1991). One of the responsibilities of the speech-language pathologist is to determine if and how psychogenic components contribute to acquired speech disorders in adults secondary to structural lesions and neurological disease to enhance differential diagnosis and to plan appropriate intervention (Sapir and Aronson, 1990).

In general, some degree of psychopathology is present in most acquired adult speech disorders. It is reasonable that persons who previously communicated normally would be affected psychologically when their ability to communicate was disrupted. In such cases, psychopathology (e.g., depression and anxiety) contributes to and possibly exacerbates the speech disorder, but it is not the cause of the disorder. Therefore, while the speech-language pathologist must be alert to the role of psychopathology in assessment and management of these cases, these disorders are not "purely" psychogenic in nature.

Purely psychogenic speech disorders, the subject of this chapter, are rare in clinical practice. With psychogenic speech disorders, the communication breakdown stems from a conversion disorder. Conversion disorders are included within a larger family of psychiatric disorders, somatoform illnesses. These tend to be associated with pathologic beliefs and attitudes on the part of the patient that results in somatic symptoms. The American Psychiatric Association (1987) defines a conversion disorder as "an alteration or loss of physical functioning that suggests a physical disorder, that actually represents an expression of a psychological conflict or need." An example might be a woman who suddenly loses her voice because she cannot face the psychological conflict of a spouse's affair. Here the symptom (voice loss) constitutes a lesser threat to her psychological equilibrium than confronting the husband with his infidelity. A partial list of psychogenic speech disorders includes partial (dysphonia) or complete (aphonia) loss of voice (Andersson and Schalen, 1998), dysarthria (Kallen, Marshall, and Casey, 1986), mutism (Kalman and Granet, 1981), and stuttering (Wallen, 1961; Deal, 1982). There are a few reports that indicate patients can also develop psychogenic language disorders, specifically aphasia (Iddings and Wilson, 1981; Sevush and Brooks, 1983) and dyslexia and dysgraphia (Master and Lishman, 1984). Reports of psychogenic swallowing disorders (dysphagia) also exist (Carstens, 1982).

Diagnosis

Before proceeding with the evaluation and treatment of a patient with a suspected psychogenic speech disorder (PSD), the speech-language pathologist should be sure that the patient has been seen by the appropriate medical specialist to rule out an organic cause of the problem. Usually this is not a problem because the PSD patient will have sought care from several specialists, sometimes simultaneously, and may have a complicated medical history in which multiple diagnoses are tenable (Case, 1991). Therefore, definitive diagnosis of a speech disorder as "psychogenic" is an inexact process relying greatly on the examiner's skill, experience, and ability to synthesize information from the clinical interview and examination.

Interview and History

The PSD patient often has a history of other conversion disorders and prior psychological stress unrelated to the symptom (Pincus and Tucker, 1974). PSD onset is sudden and tends to be linked to a specific traumatic event (e.g., surgery) or painful emotional experiences (e.g., death of a family member). In the patient interview, the speech-language pathologist determines what the patient might gain from the presenting speech disorder. *Primary gain* refers to the reduction of anxiety, tension, and conflict provided by the speech disorder. This could be related to a breakdown in communication between the patient and some person of importance, such as a spouse, a boss, or parent. Here the speech problem constitutes a lesser dilemma for the individual than the interpersonal problems from which it arose. *Secondary gain* refers to those benefits received by the individual from the external environment. This could take the form of monetary compensation, attention, and sympathy from others over perceived distress, being given fewer responsibilities (e.g., work, child care), release from social obligations, and satisfaction of dependency needs. Sometimes secondary gains reinforce the PSD and prolong its duration (Morrison and Rammage, 1994). Unlike individuals with acquired adult communication disorders resulting from structural damage or neurological disease, the PSD patient may show unusual calmness and lack of concern over the speech disorder, a phenomenon called *la belle indifférence*. It should be understood, however, that PSD patients do not consciously produce the symptom affecting communication but truly believe they are ill. As a consequence, many PSD patients display excessive concern about their bodies and overreact to normal somatic stimuli.

Clinical Examination

Results of the oral-peripheral and laryngeal examination are often normal or fail to account for the PSD patient's symptoms. Instrumental measures have limited value in assessment and diagnosis of assessing the individual with a PSD, since these contribute to the patient's fixation that his or her problem is organically based. The most

valuable diagnostic information is gleaned from the clinical examination and the interview. PSD symptoms fluctuate widely across patients and within the same patient. Examples of PSDs affecting voice include conversion aphonia (no voiced but articulated air stream), conversion dysphonia (some voice but abnormal pitch, loudness, or quality), and conversion muteness (no voice but moving of the lips as though articulating) (Case, 1991). Individual PSD patients may report speaking better in some situations than others. The patient may even exhibit variability in symptoms within the context of the clinical examination (Case, 1991). Aphonic or dysphonic patients may vocalize normally when laughing, coughing, or clearing of the throat (Morrison and Rammage, 1994). Further, distraction techniques such as asking the patient to hum, grunt, or say "uh-huh" as an affirmation might produce a normal-sounding voice. PSD patients may react unfavorably when it is pointed out that he or she has produced a normal-sounding voice and insist that the examiner identify a physical cause of the problem.

Intervention

After the examining physician has ruled out an organic cause for the speech disorder and the problem definitively diagnosed as psychogenic, an appropriate intervention plan can be selected. Intervention approaches for the patient with a PSD vary widely and largely depend on the work setting, skill, training, and philosophy of the clinician (see also NEUROGENIC MUTISM, LARYNGECTOMY). For the most part, interventions used by speech-language pathologists focus on removal of the symptoms (e.g., aphonia, dysphonia, dysarthria) found to be abnormal in the evaluation, and give limited attention to psychological or psychiatric issues.

Several studies report results of successful interventions for PSD patients (Aronson, 1969; Marshall and Watts, 1975; Kalman and Granet, 1981; Carstens, 1982; Kallen, Marshall, and Casey, 1986; Andersson and Schalen, 1998). These usually begin with the clinician acknowledging the patient's distress and assuring the patient that there is no known organic reason for the problem. Potential factors that might contribute to the patient's distress are discussed in a nonthreatening manner. Here the focus of attention is on how the symptom or symptoms are disrupting communication. Individually designed intervention programs are then initiated and typically proceed in small steps or behavioral increments. For example, a sequence of intervention steps for a patient with psychogenic aphonia may include the following: (1) eliciting a normal vocal tone with a cough, grunt, or hum; (2) prolonging the normal vocalization into a vowel; (3) turning the vowel into a VC word; (4) linking two VC words together; (5) producing sentences using several VC words; and so forth. Relaxation exercises, patient education, and counseling may be included in the intervention programs for some PSD patients. In general, symptomatic interventions are successful with two to 10 sessions of treatment.

Three factors—duration of time elapsing between onset of symptoms and beginning of therapy, severity of the speech disorder, and the degree to which the patient's speech disorder is distinguishable from the emotional disturbance—are related to intervention success (Case, 1991). Generally, intervention is more apt to be successful if the time between the onset of symptoms and the start of intervention is short, if the problem is severe, and if a speech disorder is clearly distinguishable from the emotional disturbance responsible for the problem (Case, 1991). However, certain patients may be more anxious for help and receptive to therapy if they have been without voice for a considerable period of time before consulting a speech-language pathologist (Freeman, 1986). In addition, patients who react unfavorably to intervention success or refuse to accept or acknowledge their "improved communicative status" do not respond well to behavioral treatments and have a poor prognosis for symptom-based interventions. In such cases the speech-language pathologist must refer the patient to the psychologist or the psychiatrist.

—*Robert C. Marshall*

References

American Psychiatric Association. (1987). *Diagnostic and statistical manual of mental disorders* (3rd ed., rev.). Washington, DC: American Psychiatric Press.

Andersson, K., and Schalen, L. (1998). Etiology and treatment of psychogenic voice disorder: Results of a follow-up study of thirty patients. *Journal of Voice, 12,* 96–106.

Aronson, A. E. (1969). Speech pathology and symptom therapy in the interdisciplinary treatment of psychogenic aphonia. *Journal of Speech and Hearing Disorders, 34,* 324–341.

Aronson, A. E. (1991). *Clinical voice disorders.* New York: Thieme.

Brodnitz, F. E. (1981). Psychological considerations in vocal rehabilitation. *Journal of Speech and Hearing Disorders, 4,* 21–26.

Carstens, C. (1982). Behavioral treatment of functional dysphagia in a 12-year-old boy. *Psychomatics, 23,* 195–196.

Case, J. E. (1991). *Clinical management of voice disorders.* Austin, TX: Pro-Ed.

Deal, J. L. (1982). Sudden onset of stuttering: A case report. *Journal of Speech and Hearing Disorders, 47,* 301–304.

Freeman, M. (1986). Psychogenic voice disorders. In M. Fawcus (Ed.), *Voice disorders and their management* (pp. 204–207). London: Croom-Helm.

Gianotti, G. (1972). Emotional behavior and side of lesion. *Cortex, 8,* 41–55.

Iddings, D. T., and Wilson, L. G. (1981). Unrecognized anomic aphasia in an elderly woman. *Psychosomatics, 22,* 710–711.

Kallen, D., Marshall, R. C., and Casey, D. E. (1986). Atypical dysarthria in Munchausen syndrome. *British Journal of Disorders of Communication, 21,* 377–380.

Kalman, T. P., and Granet, R. B. (1981). The written interview in hysterical mutism. *Psychosomatics, 22,* 362–364.

Marshall, R. C., and Watts, M. T. (1975). Behavioral treatment of functional aphonia. *Journal of Behavioral Therapy and Experimental Psychiatry, 6,* 75–78.

Master, D. R., and Lishman, W. A. (1984). Seizures, dyslexia, and dysgraphia of psychogenic origin. *Archives of Neurology, 41,* 889–890.

Morrison, M., and Rammage, L. (1994). *Management of voice disorders.* San Diego, CA: Singular.

Pincus, J. H., and Tucker, G. (1974). *Behavioral neurology.* New York: Oxford Press.

Rollin, W. J. (1987). *The psychology of communication disorders in individuals and their families.* Englewood Cliffs, NJ: Prentice-Hall.

Sapir, S., and Aronson, A. E. (1990). The relationship between psychopathology and speech and language disorders in neurological patients. *Journal of Speech and Hearing Disorders, 55,* 503–509.

Sevush, S., and Brooks, J. (1983). Aphasia versus functional disorder: Factors in differential diagnosis. *Psychosomatics, 24,* 847–848.

Wallen, V. (1961). Primary stuttering in a 28-year-old adult. *Journal of Speech and Hearing Disorders, 26,* 394–395.

Further Readings

Aronson, A. E., Peterson, H. W., Jr., and Liten, E. M. (1964). Voice symptomatology in functional dysphonia. *Journal of Speech and Hearing Disorders, 29,* 367–380.

Aronson, A. E., Peterson, H. W., Jr., and Liten, E. M. (1966). Psychiatric symptomatology in functional dysphonia and aphonia. *Journal of Speech and Hearing Disorders, 31,* 115–127.

Bangs, J. L., and Freidiinger, A. (1950). A case of hysterical dysphonia in an adult. *Journal of Speech and Hearing Disorders, 15,* 316–323.

Boone, D. (1966). Treatment of functional aphonia in a child and an adult. *Journal of Speech and Hearing Disorders, 31,* 69–74.

Dickes, R. A. (1974). Brief therapy of conversion reactions: An in-hospital technique. *American Journal of Psychiatry, 131,* 584–586.

Elias, A., Raven, R., and Butcher, P. (1989). Speech therapy for psychogenic voice disorder: Survey of current practice and training. *British Journal of Disorders of Communication, 24,* 61–76.

Gray, B. F., England, G., and Mahoney, J. (1965). Treatment of benign vocal nodules by reciprocal inhibition. *Behavior Research and Therapy, 3,* 187–193.

Guze, S. B., Woodruff, R. A., and Clayton, P. J. (1971). A study of conversion symptoms in psychiatric outpatients. *American Journal of Psychiatry, 128,* 135–138.

Helm, N. A., Butler, R. B., and Benson, D. F. (1978). Acquired stuttering. *Neurology, 28,* 1159–1165.

Horsley, I. A. (1982). Hypnosis and self-hypnosis in the treatment of psychogenic dysphonia: A case report. *American Journal of Clinical Hypnosis, 24,* 277–283.

Kintzl, J., Biebl, W., and Rauchegger, H. (1988). Functional aphonia: Psychological aspects of diagnosis and therapy. *Folia Phoniatrica, 40,* 131–137.

Koon, R. E. (1983). Conversion dysphagia in children. *Psychomatics, 24,* 182–184.

Mace, C. J. (1994). Reversible cognitive impairment related to conversion disorder. *Journal of Nervous and Mental Diseases, 182,* 186–187.

Marshall, R. C., and Starch, S. A. (1984). Behavioral treatment of acquired stuttering. *Australian Journal of Human Communication Disorders, 12,* 17–24.

Matas, M. (1991). Psychogenic voice disorders: Literature review and case report. *Canadian Journal of Psychiatry, 36,* 363–365.

Neelman, J., and Mann, A. H. (1993). Treatment of hysterical aphonia with hypnosis and prokaletic therapy. *British Journal of Psychiatry, 163,* 816–819.

Oberfield, R. A., Reuben, R. N., and Burkes, L. J. (1983). Interdisciplinary approach of conversion disorders in adolescent girls. *Psychomatics, 24,* 983–989.

Schalen, L., and Andersson, K. (1992). Differential diagnosis of psychogenic dysphonia. *Clinical Otolaryngology, 35,* 225–230.

Teitelbaum, M. L., and Kettl, P. (1985). Psychiatric consultation with a noncooperative, depressed stroke patient. *Psychomatics, 26,* 145–146.

Walton, D. A., and Black, H. (1959). The application of modern learning theory to the treatment of aphonia. *Journal of Psychosomatic Research, 3,* 303–311.

Speech Disorders in Children: A Psycholinguistic Perspective

The terminology used to describe speech problems is rooted in classificatory systems derived from different academic disciplines. In order to understand the rationale behind the psycholinguistic approach, it is helpful to examine other approaches and compare how speech problems have been classified from different perspectives. Three perspectives that have been particularly influential are the medical, linguistic, and psycholinguistic perspectives.

In a medical perspective, speech and language problems are classified according to clinical entity. Commonly used labels include dyspraxia, dysarthria, and stuttering. Causes of speech difficulties can be identified (e.g., cleft palate, hearing loss, neurological impairment) or an associated medical condition is known (e.g., autism, learning difficulties, Down syndrome).

Viewing speech and language disorders from a medical perspective can be helpful in various ways. First, through the medical exercise of constructing a differential diagnosis, a condition may be defined when symptoms commonly associated with that condition are identified; two examples are dyspraxia and dysarthria. Second, for some conditions, medical management can contribute significantly to the prevention or remediation of the speech or language difficulty, such as by insertion of a cochlear implant to remediate hearing loss or by surgical repair of a cleft palate. Third, the medical perspective may be helpful when considering the prognosis for a child's speech and language development, such as when a progressive neurological condition is present.

However, the medical approach has major limitations as a basis for the principled remediation of speech problems in individual children. A medical diagnosis cannot always be made. More often the term "specific speech and/or language impairment" is used once all other possible medical labels have been ruled out. Moreover, even if a neuroanatomical correlate or genetic basis for a speech and language impairment can be identified, the medical diagnosis does not predict with any precision the speech and language difficulties that an individual child will experience, so the diagnosis will not significantly affect the details of a day-to-day intervention program. To plan appropriate therapy, the medical model needs to be supplemented by a linguistic approach.

The linguistic perspective is primarily concerned with the description of language behavior at different levels of analysis. If a child is said to have a *phonetic or articulatory* difficulty, the implication is that the child has problems with the *production* of speech sounds. A *phonological* difficulty refers to inability to *use* sounds contrastively to convey meaning. For example, a child may use [t] for [s] at the beginning of words, even though the child can produce a [s] sound in isolation perfectly well. Thus, the child fails to distinguish between target words (e.g., "sea" versus "tea") and is likely to be misunderstood by the listener. The cause of this difficulty may not be obvious.

The linguistic sciences have provided an indispensable foundation for the assessment of speech and language difficulties (Ingram, 1976; Grunwell, 1987). However, this assessment is still a description and not an explanation of the disorder. Specifically, a linguistic analysis focuses on the child's speech output but does not take account of underlying cognitive processes. For this, a psycholinguistic approach is needed.

The psycholinguistic approach attempts to make good some of the shortcomings of the other approaches by viewing children's speech problems as being derived from a breakdown in an underlying speech processing system. This assumes that the child receives information of different kinds (auditory, visual) about an utterance, remembers it, and stores it in a variety of *lexical representations* (a means for keeping information about words, which may be semantic, grammatical, phonological, motor, or orthographic) within the *lexicon* (a store of words), then selects and produces spoken and written words. Figure 1 illustrates the basic essentials of a psycholinguistic model of speech processing. On the left there is a channel for the input of information via the ear and on the right a channel for the output of information through the mouth. The lexical representations at the top of the model store previously processed information. In psycholinguistic terms, top-down processing refers to an activity whereby previously stored information (i.e., in the lexical representations) is helpful and used, for example, in naming objects in pictures. A bottom-up processing activity requires no such prior knowledge and can be completed without accessing stored linguistic knowledge from the lexical representations; an example is repeating sounds.

A number of models have been developed from this basic structure (e.g., Dodd, 1995; Stackhouse and Wells, 1997; Hewlett, Gibbon, and Cohen-McKenzie, 1998; Chiat, 2000). Although these models differ in their presentation, they share the premise that children's speech

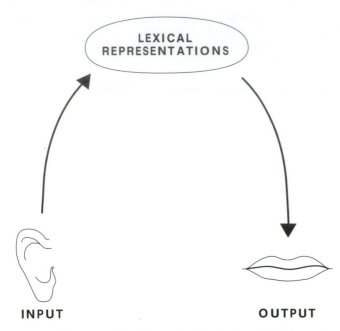

Figure 1. The essentials of a psycholinguistic model of speech processing. (From Stackhouse, J., and Wells, B. [1997]. *Children's speech and literacy difficulties 1: A psycholinguistic framework*. London: Whurr. Reproduced with permission.)

difficulties arise from one or more points in a faulty speech processing system. The aim of the psycholinguistic approach is to find out exactly where a child's speech processing skills are breaking down and how these deficits might be compensated for by coexisting strengths. The investigative procedure to do so entails generating hypotheses, normally from linguistic data, about the levels of breakdown that give rise to disordered speech output. These hypotheses are then tested systematically through carefully constructed tasks that provide sufficient data to assemble a child's profile of speech processing strengths and weaknesses (Stackhouse and Wells, 1997; Chiat, 2000).

Collation of these profiles shows that some children with speech difficulties have problems only on the output side of the model. However, many children with persisting speech problems have pervasive speech processing difficulties (in input, output, and lexical representations) that impede progress. For example, when rehearsing new words for speech or spelling, it is usual to repeat them verbally. An inconsistent or distorted output, normally the result of more than one level of breakdown, may in turn affect auditory processing skills, memory, and the developing lexicon. It is therefore not surprising that children with dyspraxic speech difficulties often have associated input (Bridgeman and Snowling, 1988) and spelling difficulties (Clarke-Klein and Hodson, 1995; McCormick, 1995).

The case study research of children with developmental speech disorders, typical of the psycholinguistic approach, has shown that not only are children unintelligible for different reasons but also that different facets of unintelligibility in an individual child can be related to different underlying processing deficits (Chiat, 1983, 1989; Stackhouse and Wells, 1993). Extending the psycholinguistic approach to word finding difficulties, Constable (2001) has discovered that such difficulties are long-term consequences of underlying speech processing problems that affect how the lexical representations are stored, and in particular how the phonological, semantic, and motor representations are interconnected.

The psycholinguistic approach has also been used to investigate the relationship between spoken and written language and to predict which children may have long-term difficulties (Dodd, 1995; Stackhouse, 2001). Those children who fail to progress to a level of consistent speech output, age-appropriate phonological awareness, and letter knowledge skills are at risk for literacy problems, particularly when spelling. Psycholinguistic analysis of popular phonological awareness tasks (e.g., rhyme, syllable/sound segmentation and completion, blending, spoonerisms) has shown that the development of phonological awareness skills depends on an intact speech processing system (Stackhouse and Wells, 1997). Thus, children with speech difficulties are disadvantaged in school, since developing phonological awareness is a necessary stage in dealing with alphabetic scripts such as English. Further, these phonological awareness skills are needed not just for an isolated activity, such as a rhyme game, but also to participate in the interactions typical of phonological intervention sessions delivered by a teacher or clinician (Stackhouse et al., 2002).

An individual child's psycholinguistic profile of speech processing skills provides an important basis for planning a targeted remediation program (Stackhouse and Wells, 2001). There is no prescription for delivering this program, nor is there a bag of special activities. All intervention materials have the potential to be used in a psycholinguistic way if analyzed appropriately. Principled intervention is based on setting clear aims (Rees, 2001a). Tasks are chosen or designed for their psycholinguistic properties and manipulated to ensure appropriate targeting and monitoring of intervention. To this end, each task is analyzed into its components, as follows:

Task = Materials + Procedure + Feedback ± Technique

Rees (2001b) presents seven questions for examining these four components. She demonstrates how altering any one of them can change the nature of the task and thus the psycholinguistic demands made on the child.

In summary, a psycholinguistic approach to intervention puts the emphasis first on the rationale behind the design and selection of tasks for a particular child, and then on the order in which the tasks are to be presented to a child so that strengths are exploited and weaknesses supported (Vance, 1997; Corrin, 2001a, 2001b; Waters, 2001). The approach tackles the issues of *what* to do, with *whom, why, when,* and *how.*

In a review of psycholinguistic models of speech development, Baker et al. (2001) present both box-

and-arrow and connectionist models as new ways of conceptualizing speech impairment in children. This discussion has focused on the former, since to date, box-and-arrow models have arguably had the most impact on clinical practice by adding to our repertoire of assessment and treatment approaches, and also by promoting communication and collaboration between teachers and clinicians (Popple and Wellington, 2001). The success of the psycholinguistic approach may lie in the fact that it targets the underlying sources of difficulties rather than the symptoms alone (Holm and Dodd, 1999). Although it is true that the outcome of intervention depends on more than a child's speech processing profile (Goldstein and Geirut, 1998), the development of targeted therapy through the setting of realistic aims and quantifiable objectives should make a contribution to the measurement of the efficacy of intervention.

—*Joy Stackhouse*

References

Baker, E., Croot, K., Mcleod, S., and Paul, R. (2001). Psycholinguistic models of speech development and their application to clinical practice. *Journal of Speech, Language, and Hearing Research, 44,* 685–702.

Bridgeman, E., and Snowling, M. (1988). The perception of phoneme sequence: A comparison of dyspraxic and normal children. *British Journal of Disorders of Communication, 23,* 245–252.

Chiat, S. (1983). Why Mikey's right and my key's wrong: The significance of stress and word boundaries in a child's output system. *Cognition, 14,* 275–300.

Chiat, S. (1989). The relation between prosodic structure, syllabification and segmental realization: Evidence from a child with fricative stopping. *Clinical Linguistics and Phonetics, 3,* 223–242.

Chiat, S. (2000). *Understanding children with language problems.* Cambridge, UK: Cambridge University Press.

Clarke-Klein, S., and Hodson, B. (1995). A phonologically based analysis of misspellings by third graders with disordered phonology histories. *Journal of Speech and Hearing Research, 38,* 839–849.

Constable, A. (2001). A psycholinguistic approach to word finding difficulties. In J. Stackhouse and B. Wells (Eds.), *Children's speech and literacy difficulties: Vol. 2. Identification and intervention.* London: Whurr.

Corrin, J. (2001a). From profile to programme: Steps 1–2. In J. Stackhouse and B. Wells (Eds.), *Children's speech and literacy difficulties: Vol. 2. Identification and intervention.* London: Whurr.

Corrin, J. (2001b). From profile to programme: Steps 3–6. In J. Stackhouse and B. Wells (Eds.), *Children's speech and literacy difficulties: Vol. 2. Identification and intervention.* London: Whurr.

Dodd, B. (1995). *Differential diagnosis and treatment of children with speech disorder.* London: Whurr.

Goldstein, H., and Geirut, J. (1998). Outcomes measurement in child language and phonological disorders. In M. Frattali (Ed.), *Measuring outcomes in speech-language pathology.* New York: Thiene.

Grunwell, P. (1987). *Clinical phonology* (2nd ed.). London: Croom Helm.

Hewlett, N., Gibbon, F., and Cohen-McKenzie, W. (1998). When is a velar an alveolar? Evidence supporting a revised psycholinguistic model of speech production in children. *International Journal of Language and Communication Disorders, 2,* 161–176.

Holm, A., and Dodd, B. (1999). An intervention case study of a bilingual child with phonological disorder. *Child Language Teaching and Therapy, 15,* 139–158.

Ingram, D. (1976). *Phonological disability in children.* London: Edward Arnold.

McCormick, M. (1995). The relationship between the phonological processes in early speech development and later spelling strategies. In B. Dodd (Ed.), *Differential diagnosis and treatment of children with speech disorder.* London: Whurr.

Popple, J., and Wellington, W. (2001). Working together: The psycholinguistic approach within a school setting. In J. Stackhouse and B. Wells (Eds.), *Children's speech and literacy difficulties: Vol. 2. Identification and intervention.* London: Whurr.

Rees, R. (2001a). Principles of psycholinguistic intervention. In J. Stackhouse and B. Wells (Eds.), *Children's speech and literacy difficulties: Vol. 2. Identification and intervention.* London: Whurr.

Rees, R. (2001b). What do tasks really tap? In J. Stackhouse and B. Wells (Eds.), *Children's speech and literacy difficulties: Vol. 2. Identification and intervention.* London: Whurr.

Stackhouse, J. (2001). Identifying children at risk for literacy problems. In J. Stackhouse and B. Wells (Eds.), *Children's speech and literacy difficulties: Vol. 2. Identification and intervention.* London: Whurr.

Stackhouse, J., and Wells, B. (1993). Psycholinguistic assessment of developmental speech disorders. *European Journal of Disorders of Communication, 28,* 331–348.

Stackhouse, J., and Wells, B. (1997). *Children's speech and literacy difficulties 1: A psycholinguistic framework.* London: Whurr.

Stackhouse, J., and Wells, B. (Eds.). (2001). *Children's speech and literacy difficulties 2: Identification and intervention.* London: Whurr.

Stackhouse, J., Wells, B., Pascoe, M., and Rees, R. (2002). From phonological therapy to phonological awareness. *Seminars in Speech and Language: Updates in Phonological Intervention, 23,* 27–42.

Vance, M. (1997). Christopher Lumpship: Developing phonological representations in a child with auditory processing deficit. In S. W. Chiat, J. Law, and J. Marshall (Eds.), *Language disorders in children and adults.* London: Whurr.

Waters, D. (2001). Using input processing strengths to overcome speech output difficulties. In J. Stackhouse and B. Wells (Eds.), *Children's speech and literacy difficulties: Vol. 2. Identification and intervention.* London: Whurr.

Further Readings

Bishop, D. V. M. (1997). *Uncommon understanding: Development and disorders of language comprehension in children.* Hove, UK: Psychology Press.

Bishop, D. V. M., and Leonard, L. (2000). *Speech and language impairments in children: Causes, characteristics, intervention, and outcome.* Hove, UK: Psychology Press.

Chiat, S., Law, J., and Marshall, J. (1997). *Language disorders in children and adults: Psycholinguistic approaches to therapy.* London: Whurr.

Constable, A., Stackhouse, J., and Wells, B. (1997). Developmental word-finding difficulties and phonological processing:

The case of the missing handcuffs. *Applied Psycholinguistics*, *18*, 507–536.

Dent, H. (2001). Electropalatography: A tool for psycholinguistic therapy. In J. Stackhouse and B. Wells (Eds.), *Children's speech and literacy difficulties: Vol. 2. Identification and intervention*. London: Whurr.

Ebbels, S. (2000). Psycholinguistic profiling of a hearing impaired child. *Child Language Teaching and Therapy*, *16*, 3–22.

Hodson, B., and Edwards, M. L. (1997). *Perspectives in applied phonology*. Gaithersburg, MD: Aspen.

Lees, J. (1993). *Children with acquired aphasias*. London: Whurr.

Simpson, S. (2000). Dyslexia: A developmental language disorder. *Child Care, Health and Development*, *26*, 355–380.

Snowling, M. (2000). *Dyslexia* (2nd ed.). Oxford: Blackwell.

Snowling, M., and Stackhouse, J. (1996). *Dyslexia, speech language: A practitioner's handbook*. London: Whurr.

Williams, P., and Stackhouse, J. (2000). Rate, accuracy and consistency: Diadochokinetic performance of young, normally developing children. *Clinical Linguistics and Phonetics*, *14*, 267–293.

Wood, J., Wright, J. A., and Stackhouse, J. (2000). *Language and literacy: Joining together—An early years training package*. Reading, UK: British Dyslexia Association.

Speech Disorders in Children: Behavioral Approaches to Remediation

Speech disorders in children include articulation and phonological disorders, stuttering, cluttering, developmental apraxia of speech, and a variety of disorders associated with organic conditions such as brain injury (including cerebral palsy), cleft palate, and genetic syndromes. Despite obvious linguistic influences on the analysis, classification, and theoretical understanding of speech disorders in children, most current treatment methods use behavioral techniques. The effectiveness of behavioral treatment techniques in remediating speech disorders in children has been well documented (Onslow, 1993; Bernthal and Bankson, 1998; Hegde, 1998, 2001; Pena-Brooks and Hegde, 2000). Behavioral techniques that apply to all speech discords—and indeed to most disorders of communication—include positive reinforcement and reinforcement schedules, negative reinforcement, instructions, demonstrations, modeling, shaping, prompting, fading, corrective feedback to reduce undesirable responses, and techniques to promote generalized productions and response maintenance.

A basic procedure in implementing behavioral intervention is establishing the baserates of target behaviors. Baserates, or baselines, are systematically measured values of specified behaviors or skills in the absence of planned intervention. Baserates are the natural rates of response when nothing special (such as modeling or explicit positive reinforcement) is programmed. Baserates help establish a stable and reliable response rate against which the effects of a planned intervention or an experimental treatment can be evaluated. The baserate of any parameter should be determined by at least three measures to establish their stability. For instance, to establish the baserates of stuttering in a child, the clinician should measure stuttering in at least three consecutive speech samples. Baserates also should sample responses adequately. For instance, to establish the baserate of production of a phoneme in a child, 15–20 words, phrases, or sentences that contain the target phoneme should be used. Baserates also may be established for different settings, such as the clinic, classroom, and home. In each setting, multiple measurements would be made.

Positive Reinforcement and Reinforcement Schedules. *Positive reinforcement* is a powerful method of shaping new behaviors or increasing the frequency of low-frequency but desired behaviors. It is a method of selecting and strengthening an individual's behaviors by arranging for certain consequences to occur immediately follow the behavior (Skinner, 1953, 1969, 1974). In using positive reinforcement, the clinician arranges a *behavioral contingency*, which is an interdependent relationship between a response made in the context of a stimulus array and the consequence that immediately follows it. Therefore, technically, behavioral contingency is the heart of behavioral treatment.

Positive reinforcers are specific events or objects that, following a behavior, increase the future probability of that behavior. Speech-language pathologists routinely use a variety of positive reinforcers in teaching speech skills to children and adults. Praise is a common positive reinforcer. Other positive reinforces include tokens, given for correct responses, that may be exchanged for small gifts. Biofeedback or computer feedback as to the accuracy of response are other forms of positive reinforcement.

Positive reinforcers are initially offered for every correct response, resulting in a *continuous reinforcement schedule*. When the new response or skill has somewhat stabilized, the reinforcer may be offered for every *n*th response, resulting in a fixed ratio (FR) schedule. For instance, a child may receive reinforcer for every fifth correct phoneme production (an FR5). Gradually reducing the number of reinforcers with the use of progressively larger ratios will help maintain a skill taught in clinical settings.

Antecedent Control of Target Behaviors. A standard behavioral method is to carefully set the stage for a skill to be taught in treatment sessions. This technique, known as antecedent control, increases the likelihood of a target response by providing stimuli that evoke it. Stimulus manipulations include a variety of procedures, such as modeling, shaping, prompting, and fading.

Modeling. In modeling, the clinician produces the target response, which is then expected to be followed by at least an attempt to produce the same response by the client. The clinician's behavior is the model, which the client attempts to imitate (response). In most cases, modeling is preceded by instructions to the client on how to produce a response, and demonstrations of target responses. Although instructions and demonstrations are part of behavioral treatment procedures, much formal research has focused on modeling as a special stimulus to help establish a new target response.

A child's initial attempt to imitate a target response modeled by the clinician may be more or less correct; nonetheless, the clinician might wish to reinforce all attempts in the right direction. In gradual steps, the clinician may then require responses that are more like the modeled response. To achieve this final result of an imitated response that matches the modeled stimulus, shaping is often used.

Shaping. Whereas straightforward positive reinforcement is effective in increasing the frequency of a low-frequency response, shaping is necessary to create skills that are absent. Shaping, also known as successive approximations, is a procedure to teach new responses in gradual steps. The entire procedure typically includes instructions, demonstrations, modeling, and positive reinforcement. A crucial aspect of shaping is specifying the individual components of a complex response and teaching the components sequentially in a manner that will result in the final target response. For instance, in teaching the correct production of /s/ to a child who has an articulation disorder, the clinician may identify such simplified components of the response as raising the tongue tip to the alveolar ridge, creating a groove along the tongue tip, approximating the two dental arches, blowing air through the tongue-tip groove, and so forth. The child's production of each component response is positively reinforced and practiced several times. Finally, the components are put together to produce the approximation of /s/. Subsequently, and in progressive steps, better approximations of the modeled sound production are reinforced, resulting in an acceptable form of the target response. To further strengthen a newly learned response, the clinician may use the prompting procedure.

Prompting. The probability of a target response that has just emerged with assistance from the previously described procedures may fluctuate from moment to moment. The child may appear unsure and the response rate may be inconsistent. In such cases, prompting will help stabilize that response and increase its frequency. *Prompting* is a special cue or a stimulus that will help evoke a response from an unsure client. Such cues take various verbal and nonverbal forms. Examples of verbal prompts include such statements as "What do you say to this picture?" "The word starts with a /p/" (both prompt a correct naming or articulatory response). Nonverbal prompts include a variety of facial and hand gestures that suggest a particular target response; the meaning of some gestures may first have to be taught to the child. For instance, a clinician might tell a child who stutters that his or her speech should be slowed down when a particular hand gesture is made. In prompting the production of a phone such as /p/, the clinician may press the two lips together, which may lead to the correct

production. Eventually, the influence of such special stimuli as prompts is reduced by a technique called fading.

Fading. Fading is a technique used to gradually withdraw a special stimulus, such as models or prompts, while still maintaining the correct response rate. Abrupt withdrawal of a controlling stimulus will result in failure to respond. In fading, a modeled stimulus or prompt may be reduced in various ways. For instance, a modeling such as "Say I *see sun*" (in training the production of phoneme /s/) may be shortened by the clinician to "Say I see . . ."; or the vocal intensity of the prompter or modeler may be reduced such that the modeling becomes progressively softer and eventually inaudible, with only articulatory movements (e.g., correct tongue position) being shown.

Corrective Feedback. Various forms of corrective feedback may be provided to reduce the frequency of incorrect responses. Verbal feedback such as "that is not correct," "that was bumpy speech" (to correct stuttering in young children), "that was too fast," and so forth is part of all behavioral treatment programs. Additional corrective procedures include token loss for incorrect responses (tokens earned for correct responses and lost for incorrect ones), and time-out, which includes a brief period of no interaction made contingent on incorrect responses. For instance, every stuttering may be followed by a signal to stop talking for 5 seconds.

Generalization and Maintenance. Behavioral techniques to promote generalized production of speech skills in natural environments and maintenance of those skills over time are important in all clinical work. Teaching clients to self-monitor the production of their newly acquired skills and training significant others to prompt and reinforce those skills at home are among the most effective of the generalization and maintenance techniques.

—*M. N. Hegde*

References

Bernthal, J. E., and Bankson, N. W. (1998). *Articulation and phonological disorders* (4th ed.). Boston: Allyn and Bacon.

Hegde, M. N. (1998). *Treatment procedures in communicative disorders* (3rd ed.). Austin, TX: Pro-Ed.

Hegde, M. N. (2001). *Hegde's pocketguide to treatment in speech-language pathology* (2nd ed.). San Diego, CA: Singular Publishing Group.

Pena-Brooks, A., and Hegde, M. N. (2000). *Assessment and treatment of articulation and phonological disorders in children.* Austin, TX: Pro-Ed.

Onslow, M. (1996). *Behavioral management of stuttering.* San Diego, CA: Singular Publishing Group.

Skinner, B. F. (1953). *Science and human behavior.* New York: Macmillan.

Skinner, B. F. (1969). *Contingencies of reinforcement: A theoretical analysis.* New York: Appleton-Century-Crofts.

Skinner, B. F. (1974). *About behaviorism.* New York: Vintage Books.

Further Readings

Axelrod, S., and Hall, R. V. (1999). *Behavior modification* (2nd ed.). Austin, TX: Pro-Ed.

Maag, J. W. (1999). *Behavior management*. San Diego, CA: Singular Publishing Group.

Martin, G., and Pear, J. (1999). *Behavior modification: What it is and how to do it* (6th ed.). Upper Saddle River, NJ: Prentice-Hall.

Speech Disorders in Children: Birth-Related Risk Factors

The youngest clients who receive services from speech-language pathologists are neonates with medical needs. This area of care came into being during the last several decades as the survival rate of infants with medical needs improved and it became apparent that developmental delays would likely be prevalent among the survivors. Since 1970, for example, the survival rate of infants in some low birth weight categories jumped from 30% to 75%; among the survivors the occurrence of mental retardation is 22%–24% (Bernbaum and Hoffman-Williamson, 1991).

The prevalence of developmental delay among previously medically needy neonates resulted in federal and state laws that give these children legal rights to developmental services (Kern, Delaney, and Taylor, 1996). These laws identify the physical and mental conditions and the biological and environmental factors present at birth that are most likely to result in future developmental delay. The purpose in making this identification is to permit an infant to receive intervention services early in life, when brain development is most active and before the negative social consequences of having a developmental delay, including one in the speech domain, can occur (Bleile and Miller, 1994).

The most important federal legal foundation for developmental services for young children with medical needs is the Individuals with Disabilities Education Act (IDEA). This law gives individual states the authority to determine which conditions and factors present at birth place a child at sufficient risk for future developmental delay that the child qualifies for education services. Examples of conditions and factors that the act indicates place an infant at risk for future developmental delay are listed in Table 1. A single child might have several conditions and risk factors. For example, a child born with Down syndrome might also experience respiratory distress as a consequence of the chromosomal abnormality, as well as an unrelated congenital infection.

Many populations of newborn children with medical needs are at high risk for future speech disorders. In part this is because developmental speech disorders are common among all children (Slater, 1992). However, the medical condition or factor itself may contribute to the child having a speech disorder, as occurs with children with cerebral palsy, a tracheotomy, or cleft palate (Bleile, 1993), and the combination of illness and long-

Table 1. Conditions and Factors Present at Birth or Shortly Thereafter with a High Probability of Resulting in Future Developmental Delay

Chromosomal abnormalities such as Down syndrome
Genetic or congenital disorders
Severe sensory impairments, including hearing and vision
Inborn errors of metabolism
Disorders reflecting disturbance of the development of the nervous system
Intracranial hemorrhage
Hyperbilirubinemia at levels exceeding the need for exchange transfusion
Major congenital anomalies
Congenital infections
Disorders secondary to exposure to toxic substances, including fetal alcohol syndrome
Low birth weight
Respiratory distress
Lack of oxygen
Brain hemorrhage
Nutritional deprivation

term stays in the hospital may limit opportunities for learning, including in the speech domain.

Children with hearing impairment and those with Down syndrome are two relatively large populations with birth-related conditions and factors that are likely to experience future speech disorders (see MENTAL RETARDATION AND SPEECH IN CHILDREN). Two additional relatively large populations of newborn children likely to experience future speech disorders are those born underweight and those whose mother engaged in substance abuse during pregnancy.

In the United States, approximately 8.5% of infants are born underweight (Guyer et al., 1995). The major birth weight categories are low birth weight, very low birth weight, extremely low birth weight, and micropremie. Birth weight categories as measured in grams and pounds are shown in Table 2. As the category of micropremie suggests, many low birth weight children are born prematurely. A typical pregnancy lasts 40 weeks from first day of the last normal menstrual cycle; a preterm birth is defined as one occurring before the completion of 37 weeks of gestation. The co-occurrence of low birth weight and prematurity varies by country; in the United States, 70% of low birth weight babies are also born prematurely.

Approximately 36%–41% of women in the United States abuse illicit drugs, alcohol, or nicotine sometime during pregnancy (Center on Addiction and Substance Abuse, 1996). Illicit drugs account for 11% of this

Table 2. Birth Weight Categories, in Grams and Pounds

Categories	Grams	Pounds
Low birth weight	<2,500	5.5
Very low birth weight	<1,500	3.3
Extremely low birth weight	<1,000	2.2
Micropremies	<800	1.76

substance abuse, and heavy use of alcohol or nicotine accounts for the other 25%–30%. Approximately three-quarters of pregnant women who abuse one substance also abuse other substances (Center on Addiction and Substance Abuse, 1996). For example, a pregnant woman who abuses cocaine might also drink heavily. When alcohol is an abused substance, more severely affected children are considered to have fetal alcohol syndrome. The hallmarks of fetal alcohol syndrome are mental retardation and physical deformities (Streissguth, 1997). Children with milder cognitive impairments and without physical deformities are considered to have fetal alcohol effect or alcohol-related neurodevelopmental disorder.

Regardless of the specific cause of the disorder, speech-disordered clients with birth-related conditions and factors receive services similar to those given other children. The clinician's primary responsibility is to provide evaluation and intervention services appropriate to the child's developmental abilities. A difference in care provision is that the child's speech disorder is likely to occur as part of a larger picture of medical problems and developmental delay. This may make it difficult to diagnose and treat the speech disorder, especially when the child is younger and medical problems may predominate. In addition to having thorough training in typical speech and language development, a speech-language clinician working with these children should possess the following:

- Basic knowledge of medical concepts and terminology
- Ability to access and understand information about unfamiliar conditions and factors as need arises
- Knowledge of safety procedures and health precautions
- Ability to work well with teams that include the child's caregivers and professionals

A neonate identified as at risk for future developmental delay typically first receives developmental services in a hospital intensive care unit. Medical and developmental services are provided by a team of health care professionals. Often, a primary role of the speech-language clinician is to assess the oral mechanism to determine readiness to feed. Such evaluations are particularly important for clients at risk for aspiration. These include children with neurological and physical handicaps, as well as those born prematurely, whose immature systems of neurological control often do not allow orally presented food to be managed safely. The speech-language pathologist may also counsel the child's caregivers and offer suggestions about ways to facilitate communication development.

An early intervention program is initiated shortly after the child is born and the risk factor has been identified. The exception is a child born prematurely, whose nervous system may not yet be able to manage environmental stimulation. Such a child typically receives minimal stimulation until the time he or she would have been born if the pregnancy had been full term. Early intervention typically includes a package of services, including occupational and physical therapy, social services, and speech-language pathology. The role of the speech-language pathologist includes assessing communication development and implementing an early intervention program to facilitate the child's communication abilities. Interacting with the child's caregivers assumes increasing importance as medical issues resolve, allowing the family to give greater attention to developmental concerns.

The vast majority of children born with medical needs grow to possess the cognitive and physical capacity for speech. For higher functioning children, the clinician's role includes providing the evaluation and treatment services to facilitate speech and language development. The speech disorders of many high-functioning children resolve by the end of the preschool years or during the early grade school years. Such children are at risk for future reading problems and other learning difficulties, and their progress in communication should continue to be monitored even after the speech disorder has resolved. Speech may prove challenging for children with more extensive developmental problems. A general clinical rule of thumb is that a child who will speak typically will do so by 5 years of age (Bleile, 1995). Children with more limited speech potential may be taught to communicate through a combination of speech and non-oral options. Lower functioning children might be taught to communicate through an alternative communication system (see AUGMENTATIVE AND ALTERNATIVE COMMUNICATION APPROACHES IN CHILDREN). Some useful web sites for further information include www.asha.org; www.autism.org; www.cdc.gov; www.intelehealth.com; www.mayohealth.org; www.med.harvard.cdu; www .modimes.org; www.ncbi.nlm.nih.gov/PubMed/; www .ndss.org; and www.nih.gov.

—*Ken Bleile and Angela Burda*

References

Bernbaum, J., and Hoffman-Williamson, M. (1991). *Primary care of the preterm infant*. St. Louis: Mosby–Year Book.

Bleile, K. (1993). Children with long-term tracheostomies. In K. Bleile (Ed.), *The care of children with long-term tracheostomies*. San Diego, CA: Singular Publishing Group.

Bleile, K. (1995). *Manual of articulation and phonological disorders*. San Diego, CA: Singular Publishing Group.

Bleile, K., and Miller, S. (1994). Toddlers with medical needs. In J. Bernthal and N. Bankson (Eds.), *Child phonology: Characteristics, assessment, and intervention with special populations* (pp. 81–109). New York: Thieme.

Center on Addiction and Substance Abuse. (1996). *Substance abuse and the American woman*. New York: Columbia University.

Guyer, B., Strobino, D., Ventura, S., et al. (1995). Annual summary of vital statistics: 1994. *Pediatrics, 96*, 1029–1039.

Kern, L., Delaney, B., and Taylor, B. (1996). Laws and issues concerning education and related services. In L. Kurtz, P. Dowrick, S. Levy, and M. Batshaw (Eds.), *Handbook of developmental disabilities* (pp. 218–228). Gaithersburg, MD: Aspen.

Slater, S. (1992). Portrait of the professions. *ASHA, 34*, 61–65.

Streissguth, A. (1997). *Fetal alcohol syndrome: A guide for families and communities*. Baltimore: Paul H. Brookes.

Further Readings

Batshaw, M. (1997). *Children with disabilities* (4th ed.). Baltimore: Paul H. Brookes.

Bernbaum, J., and Hoffman-Williamson, M. (1991). *Primary care of the preterm infant*. St. Louis: Mosby–Year Book.

Kurtz, L., Dowrick, P., Levy, S., and Batshaw, M. (Eds.). (1996). *Handbook of developmental disabilities*. Gaithersburg, MD: Aspen.

Streissguth, A. (1997). *Fetal alcohol syndrome: A guide for families and communities*. Baltimore: Paul H. Brookes.

Speech Disorders in Children: Cross-Linguistic Data

Since the 1960s, the term *articulation disorder* has been replaced in many circles by the term *phonological disorder*. This shift has been driven by the recognition that children with articulation disorders show general patterns in their speech that are not easily identified by an articulatory defect approach. Further, these patterns appear similar to those used by younger, typically developing children. The notion of phonological versus articulatory impairment, however, has not been examined in depth through comparisons of typically developing children and children with phonological impairment across a range of languages. Such comparisons would provide the most revealing evidence in support of one view over the other. If articulatory factors are behind children's phonological impairment, children with such impairments should show patterns somewhat independent of their linguistic environment. They should look more like one another than like their linguistically matched peers. If there is a linguistic basis to phonological impairment, such children should look more like their typically developing linguistic peers than like children with phonological delay in other linguistic environments. The basic structure of this research line is presented below, using English and Italian children as examples (TD = typically developing, PI = phonologically impaired):

Cross-Linguistic Predictions

Articulatory Deficit

English TD + Italian TD = different
English PI + Italian PI = same
English TD + English PI = different
Italian TD + Italian PI = different

Linguistic Deficit

English TD + Italian TD = different
English PI + Italian PI = different
English TD + English PI = same
Italian TD + Italian PI = same

The pursuit of this line of research requires two steps. First, it needs to be verified that there are indeed cross-linguistic differences in phonological acquisition between typically developing children. The truth of this claim is not self-evident. Locke (1983), for example, has argued that children will be similar cross-linguistically until some point after the acquisition of the first 50 words. Elsewhere, however, it has been argued that such cross-linguistic differences are evident at the very earliest stages of phonological development (Ingram, 1989). Resolution of this issue will require extensive research into early typical phonological development in a range of languages. To date, the data support early cross-linguistic differences.

The second, critical step is to determine whether children with phonological delay look like their typically developing peers or like children with phonological impairment in other linguistic communities. The data on this issue are even more sparse than for the first step, but some preliminary data exist, and those data support the linguistic account of phonological delay over the articulatory one.

These two steps can be summarized as follows:

Step 1: Verify that typically developing children vary cross-linguistically.

Step 2: Determine whether children with a phonological impairment look like their typically developing peers or like children with phonological impairments in other linguistic communities.

Examination of a range of studies on early phonological development shows that children in different linguistic environments converge in their acquisition toward a basic or core phonetic inventory of speech sounds that is different for each language. This is demonstrated here by examining the production of word-initial consonants in English, French, K'iche', and Dutch.

Below is an inventory of the English consonants typically used in the early stage of phonological acquisition (Ingram, 1981). English-speaking children show early acquisition of three place features, a voicing contrast among stops, and a series of voiceless consonants.

English

m n
b d g
p t k
f s h
w

French shows some similarities to English, but also two striking differences, based on my analysis of selected diary studies. French-speaking children tend to acquire velar consonants later, yet show an early use of /l/, a sound that appears later in English.

French

m
b d
p t
f s
   l

K'iche' (formerly spelled Quiché) is a Mayan language spoken in Guatemala. K'iche' children (Pye, Ingram, and List, 1987) show an early /l/, as in French, and an affricate, /tʃ/, which is one of the most frequent early sounds acquired. The first fricative tends to be the velar /x/, despite the fact that the language has both /s/ and /ʃ/.

K'iche'

```
m   n
p   t   tʃ      ?
            x
w   l
```

Lastly, below is an intermediate stage in Dutch, based on data in Beers (1994). The Dutch inventory shows early use of the velar fricative /x/, as in K'iche', but also the full range of Dutch fricatives, which appear at more or less the same time.

Dutch

```
m   n
p   t       k
f   s       x   h
w       j
```

Data such as these from English, French, K'iche', and Dutch show the widely different ways that children may acquire their early consonantal inventories. It has been proposed that these differences result from the varying roles these consonants play in the phonologies of the languages discussed (Ingram, 1989). The more frequently a consonant is used in a wide range of words, the more likely it is that it will be in the early inventory.

The question now is, what do the inventories of children with phonological impairment look like when comparisons like those above are done? The limited evidence to date indicates that they look like their same language typically developing peers. Data from Italian, Turkish, and Swedish suggest that this is the case.

The first language examined here is Italian, using the data reported in Bortolini, Ingram, and Dykstra (1993). Typically developing Italian children use the affricate /tʃ/ and the fricative /v/, both later acquisitions for English-speaking children. Italian-speaking children with phonological impairment have an inventory that is a subset of the one used by typically developing children. They do not have the affricate but do show the early acquisition of /v/. The early use of /v/ can be traced back to the fact that the voiced labiodental fricative is a much more common sound in the vocabulary of Italian-speaking children than it is in the vocabulary of their English-speaking peers.

Italian

Typically Developing				Phonologically Impaired			
p	t	tʃ	k	p	t		k
b	d		g	b	d		
f	s			f	s		
v				v			

Topbas (1992) provides data on Turkish for both typically developing children and children with phonological impairment. The Turkish inventory of the typically developing children is noteworthy for its lack of early fricatives, despite a system of eight fricatives, both voiced and voiceless, in the adult language. For English-speaking children, the lack of fricatives is often a sign of phonological impairment, but this appears to be expected for typically developing Turkish-speaking children. The data on phonological impairment are from a single child at age 6 years, 0 months. This child shows the same lack of fricatives and the early affricate, just as in the typically developing data.

Turkish

Typically Developing				Phonologically Impaired			
m	n			m	n		
b	d			b	d		
p	t	tʃ	k	p	t	tʃ	
	j				j		

Lastly, Swedish data are available to pursue this issue further (Magnussen, 1983; Nettelbladt, 1983). The data on typically developing Swedish children are based on a case study of a child at age 2 years, 2 months. This child lacked the velar stop and the voiced fricative /v/. The voiced stops were also missing in a group of ten children with phonological impairment; however, these children did show early use of /v/, just as the Italian-speaking children did.

Swedish

Typically Developing				Phonologically Impaired			
m	n			m	n		
p	t			p	t		
b	d			b	d		
f	ɵ	h		f	s		h
				v		j	

Thus, preliminary data from a range of languages support the phonological rather than the articulatory account of phonological impairment. This results in two preliminary conclusions: (1) Typically developing children show early phonological inventories unique to their linguistic environment. (2) Children with phonological impairment show systems more similar to those of their typically developing peers in their own linguistic environment than to those of children with phonological impairment in other language environments.

—David Ingram

References

Beers, M. (1994, May). *Classification of phonological problems: Comparison of segmental inventories*. Paper presented at the European Symposium on Child Language Disorders, Garderen, the Netherlands.

Bortolini, U., Ingram, D., and Dykstra, K. (1993, May). The acquisition of the feature [voice] in normal and phonologically delayed Italian children. Paper presented at the

Symposium on Research in Child Language Disorders, University of Wisconsin, Madison.

Ingram, D. (1981). *Procedures for the phonological analysis of children's language*. Baltimore, MD: University Park Press.

Ingram, D. (1989). *First language acquisition: Method, description, and explanation*. Cambridge, UK: Cambridge University Press.

Locke, J. (1983). *Phonological acquisition and change*. New York: Academic Press.

Magnusson, E. (1983). *The phonology of language disordered children: Production, perception, and awareness*. Travaux de l'Institut de Linguistique de Lund, 17. Lund, Sweden: Gleerup.

Nettelbladt, U. (1983). *Developmental studies of dysphonology in children*. Travaux de l'Institut de Linguistique de Lund, 19. Lund, Sweden: Gleerup.

Pye, C., Ingram, D., and List, H. (1987). A comparison of initial consonant acquisition in English and Quiché. In K. E. Nelson and A. van Kleeck (Eds.), *Children's language* (vol. 6). Hillsdale, NJ: Erlbaum.

Topbas, S. (1992, August). *A pilot study of phonological acquisition by Turkish children and its implications for phonological disorders*. Paper presented at the 6th International Conference on Turkish Linguistics, Anadolu University, Turkey.

Speech Disorders in Children: Descriptive Linguistic Approaches

Linguistic approaches to treating children's speech disorders are motivated by the fact that a phonology is a communication system (Stoel-Gammon and Dunn, 1985; Ingram, 1990; Grunwell, 1997). Within this system, patterns are detectable within and among various subcomponents: (1) syllable and word shapes (phonotactic repertoire), (2) speech sounds (phonetic repertoire), (3) the manner in which sounds contrast with each other (phonemic repertoire), and (4) the behaviors of different sounds in different contexts (phonological processes). Each of these subcomponents may influence the others; each may interfere with successful communication. Therefore, individual sound or structure errors are treated within the context of the child's whole phonological system rather than one by one; remediation begins at the level of communicative function—the word.

The assumption underlying this type of treatment is that the child's phonological system—his or her (subconscious) mental organization of the sounds of the language—is not developing in the appropriate manner for the child's language or at a rate appropriate for the child's age. The goal is for the child to adjust his or her phonological system in the needed direction. Initiating a change in one part of the phonological system is expected to have a more general impact on the whole system.

The sounds of a language are organizable into various categories according to their articulatory or acoustic features. The consonants /p, t, k, b, d, g/, for example,

are all members of the category stops. They are noncontinuant because the airflow is discontinued in the oral cavity during their production. Some stops also have the feature voiceless because they are produced without glottal vibration. Each speech sound can be categorized in different ways according to such features. These features are called distinctive because they differentiate each sound from all others in the language. The (implicit) knowledge of distinctive features is presumed to be one organizational basis for phonological systems.

Distinctive features therapy (McReynolds and Engmann, 1975) focuses on features that a child's system lacks. A child who produces no fricatives lacks the continuant feature, so distinctive features therapy would focus on this feature. In theory, establishing a continuant in any place of articulation (e.g., [s]) would lead to the child's generalization of the feature to other, untrained fricatives. Once the feature is included in the child's feature inventory, it can be combined with other features (e.g., voice, palatal) to yield the remaining English fricatives.

The function of distinctive features is to provide communicative contrast. The more features we use, the more lexical distinctions we make and the more meanings we express. A child who produces several target phonemes identically (e.g., all fricatives as [f]) will have too many homonyms. Therapy will focus on using more distinctive features, for example, producing different target phonemes distinctively. Williams (2000a, 2000b) recommends simultaneously contrasting all target sounds with the overgeneralized phoneme. In some disordered phonologies, features are noncontrastive because they are used in limited positions. For a child who uses voiced stops only in initial position and voiceless stops only in final position, for example, "bad," "bat," "pad," and "pat" are homonyms because they are all pronounced as [bæt]. Conversely, some children with disordered phonology may maintain a contrast, but without the expected feature. A child who does not voice final stops may lengthen the preceding vowel to indicate voicing; "bat" as [bæt] and "bad" as [bæ:t]. Such a child has phonological "knowledge" of the contrast and may independently develop voicing skills. Therefore, Elbert and Gierut (1986) suggest that features of which children have little knowledge are a higher priority for intervention. In other studies (e.g., Rvachew and Nowak, 2001), however, subjects have made more progress when mostknowledge features were addressed first.

Often, distinctive features are remediated with an emphasis on contrast, through *minimal pair therapy*. Treatment focuses on words differing by one distinctive feature. For example, the continuant feature could be taught by contrasting "tap" versus "sap" and "met" versus "mess." Typically the sound that the child substitutes for the target sound (e.g., [t] for /s/) is compared to the target sound ([s]). Therapy may begin with discrimination activities; the child indicates the picture that corresponds to the word produced by the clinician (e.g., a hammer for "tap" versus an oozing tree for "sap"). This highlights the confusion that may result if the wrong sound is used. Communication-oriented production activities are designed to encourage the child to produce the feature that had been missing from his system (e.g., to say "mess" rather than "met"). (See PHONOLOGICAL AWARENESS INTERVENTION FOR CHILDREN WITH EXPRESSIVE PHONOLOGICAL IMPAIRMENTS for a discussion of approaches in which the contrastive role of phonological features and structures is even more explicitly addressed.)

Gierut (1990) has tested the use of *maximal pair therapy*, in which the contrasting sounds differ on many features (e.g., [s] versus [m]). She has found that children may be able to focus better on the missing feature (e.g., continuant) when it is not contrasted with the substituting feature (e.g., noncontinuant) than when it is.

Markedness is another phonological concept with implications for remediation of sounds. Markedness reflects ease of production and perception: [θ] is marked, due to low perceptual salience; [b] is unmarked because it is easy to produce and to perceive. Children typically acquire the least marked sound classes (e.g., stops) and structures (e.g., open CV syllables) of their languages first (Dinnsen et al., 1990). It is unusual for a child to master a more marked sound or structure before a less marked one. Gierut's (1998) research suggests that targeting a more marked structure or sound in therapy facilitates the acquisition of the less marked one "for free." However, other researchers (e.g., Rvachew and Nowak, 2001) report more success addressing less marked sounds first.

Therapy based on *nonlinear phonology* stresses the importance of syllable and word structures as well as segments (Bernhardt, 1994). Minimal pair therapy is often used to highlight the importance of structure (e.g., "go" versus "goat," "Kate" versus "skate," "monkey" versus "monk"). The goal of this therapy is to expand the child's phonotactic repertoire. For example, a child who previously omitted final consonants may or may not produce the correct final consonant in a given word, but will produce some final consonant. Structural and segmental deficits often interact in such a way that a child can produce a sound in certain positions but not others (Edwards, 1996).

The approaches described above focus primarily on what's missing from the child's phonological system. Another set of approaches focuses on what's happening instead of the target production. For example, a child whose phonological system lacks the /θ, ð, s, z/ fricative phonemes may substitute stops (stopping), substitute labial fricatives ([f, v]; fronting), substitute palatal fricatives ([ʃ, ʒ]; backing or palatalization), or omit /θ, ð, s, z/ in various word positions (initial consonant deletion, final consonant deletion, consonant cluster reduction). These patterns are referred to as phonological processes in speech-language pathology.

Phonological process therapy addresses three types of error patterns:

- Substitution processes: sounds with a certain feature are substituted by sounds with a different feature (e.g., fricatives produced as stops, in stopping; liquids produced as glides, in gliding).
- Phonotactic processes: sounds or syllables are omitted, added, or moved. The process changes the shape of the word or syllable. As examples, a CVC word becomes CV; a CCVC word becomes CVC, CVCVC, or CVCC; "smoke" becomes [moks].
- Assimilation processes: two sounds or two syllables become more alike. For example, a child who does not typically front velar consonants in words such as "go" may nonetheless say [dɔd] for "dog." The final velar consonant becomes alveolar in accord with the initial consonant. Similarly, a two-syllable word such as "popcorn" may be reduplicated as [kɔkɔ]; the first syllable changes to match the second.

As in distinctive feature therapy, in phonological process therapy classes of sounds or structures that pattern together are targeted together. Again, either the entire class can be directly addressed in therapy or some representative members of the class may be selected for treatment, in the expectation that treatment effects will generalize to the entire class. The goal is to reduce the child's use of that process, with resultant changes in her phonological system. For example, if the child's phonological system is expanded to include a few final consonants, it is expected that she or he will begin to produce a variety of final consonants, not just those that were targeted in therapy.

Some therapists use traditional production activities (beginning at the word level) to decrease a child's use of a phonological process; others use a minimal pair approach, comparing the targeted class (e.g., velars) with the substituting class (e.g., alveolars). The *cycles approach* (Hodson and Paden, 1991) to process therapy has some unique features. First, each session includes a period of auditory bombardment, during which the child listens (passively) to a list of words that contain the targeted sound class or structure. Second, each pattern is the focus for a predetermined length of time, regardless of progress. Then, treatment moves on to another pattern. Hodson and Paden argue that cycling is more similar to the phonological development of children without phonological disorders.

In summary, the goal of linguistically based approaches to phonological therapy is to make as broad an impact as possible on the child's phonological system, making strategic choices of treatment goals that will trigger changes in untreated as well as treated sounds or structures.

—*Shelley L. Velleman*

References

Bernhardt, B. (1994). Phonological intervention techniques for syllable and word structure development. *Clinics in Communication Disorders, 4*, 54–65.

Dinnsen, D. A., Chin, S. B., Elbert, M., and Powell, T. (1990). Some constraints on functionally disordered phonologies: Phonetic inventories and phonotactics. *Journal of Speech and Hearing Research, 33*, 28–37.

Edwards, M. L. (1996). Word position effects in the production of fricatives. In B. Bernhardt, J. Gilbert, and D. Ingram (Eds.), *UBC International Conference on Phonological Acquisition* (pp. 149–158). Vancouver, BC: Cascadilla Press.

Elbert, M., and Gierut, J. (1986). *Handbook of clinical phonology: Approaches to assessment and treatment.* San Diego, CA: College-Hill Press.

Gierut, J. (1990). Differential learning of phonological oppositions. *Journal of Speech and Hearing Research, 33,* 540–549.

Gierut, J. A. (1998). Treatment efficacy for functional phonological disorders in children. *Journal of Speech, Language and Hearing Research, 41,* S85–S100.

Grunwell, P. (1997). Developmental phonological disability: Order in disorder. In B. W. Hodson and M. L. Edwards (Eds.), *Perspectives in applied phonology* (pp. 61–103). Gaithersburg, MD: Aspen.

Hodson, B. W., and Paden, E. P. (1991). *Targeting intelligible speech: A phonological approach to remediation* (2nd ed.). Austin, TX: Pro-Ed.

Ingram, D. (1990). *Phonological disability in children* (2nd ed.). San Diego, CA: Singular Publishing Group.

McReynolds, L. V., and Engmann, D. (1975). *Distinctive feature analysis of misarticulations.* Baltimore: University Park Press.

Rvachew, S., and Nowak, M. (2001). The effect of target-selection strategy on phonological learning. *Journal of Speech Language and Hearing Research, 44,* 610–623.

Stoel-Gammon, C., and Dunn, C. (1985). *Normal and disordered phonology in children.* Austin, TX: Pro-Ed.

Williams, A. L. (2000a). Multiple oppositions: Theoretical foundations for an alternative contrastive intervention framework. *American Journal of Speech-Language Pathology, 9,* 282–288.

Williams, A. L. (2000b). Multiple oppositions: Case studies of variables in phonological intervention. *American Journal of Speech-Language Pathology, 9,* 289–299.

Further Readings

Ball, M. J., and Kent, R. D. (Eds.). (1997). *The new phonologies: Developments in clinical linguistics.* San Diego, CA: Singular Publishing Group.

Barlow, J. A. (1996). Variability and phonological knowledge. In T. W. Powell (Ed.), *Pathologies of speech and language: Contributions of clinical phonetics and linguistics* (pp. 125–133). New Orleans, LA: International Clinical Phonetics Association.

Bernhardt, B. (1992). Developmental implications of nonlinear phonological theory. *Clinical Linguistics and Phonetics, 6,* 259–282.

Bernhardt, B., and Stemberger, J. P. (1998). *Handbook of phonological development: From the perspective of constraint-based nonlinear phonology.* San Diego, CA: Academic Press.

Bernthal, J. E., and Bankson, N. W. (1998). *Articulation and phonological disorders* (4th ed.). Needham Heights, MA: Allyn and Bacon.

Bleile, K. M. (1995). *Manual of articulation and phonological disorders: Infancy through adulthood.* San Diego, CA: Singular Publishing Group.

Chin, S. B., and Dinnsen, D. A. (1992). Consonant clusters in disordered speech: Constraints and correspondence patterns. *Journal of Child Language, 19,* 259–286.

Ferguson, C. A., Menn, L., and Stoel-Gammon, C. (Eds.). (1992). *Phonological development: Models, research, implications.* Timonium, MD: York Press.

Gierut, J. (1992). The conditions and course of clinically induced phonological change. *Journal of Speech and Hearing Research, 35,* 1049–1063.

Hodson, B. W., and Edwards, M. L. (1997). *Perspectives in applied phonology.* Gaithersburg, MD: Aspen.

McLeod, S., van Doorn, J., and Reed, V. A. (1997). Realizations of consonant clusters by children with phonological impairments. *Clinical Linguistics and Phonetics, 11,* 85–113.

Pena-Brooks, A., and Hegde, M. N. (2000). *Assessment and treatment of articulation and phonological disorders in children.* Austin, TX: Pro-Ed.

Schwartz, R. G., Leonard, L. B., Froem-Loeb, D., and Swanson, L. A. (1987). Attempted sounds are sometimes not: An expanded view of phonological selection and avoidance. *Journal of Child Language, 14,* 411–418.

Stackhouse, J., and Wells, B. (1997). *Children's speech and literacy difficulties: A psycholinguistic framework.* London: Thomson International.

Stoel-Gammon, C., and Herrington, P. (1990). Vowel systems of normally developing and phonologically disordered children. *Clinical Linguistics and Phonetics, 4,* 145–160.

Stoel-Gammon, C., and Stone, J. R. (1991). Assessing phonology in young children. *Clinics in Communication Disorders, 1,* 25–39.

Velleman, S. L. (1998). *Making phonology functional: What do I do first?* Boston: Butterworth-Heinemann.

Velleman, S. L. (Ed.). (2002). Updates in phonological intervention [Special issue]. *Seminars in Speech and Language, 23*(1).

Vihman, M. M. (1993). Variable paths to early word production. *Journal of Phonetics, 21,* 61–82.

Yavas, M. (Ed.). (1994). *First and second language phonology.* San Diego, CA: Singular Publishing Group.

Yavas, M. (Ed.). (1998). *Phonology: Development and disorders.* San Diego, CA: Singular Publishing Group.

Speech Disorders in Children: Motor Speech Disorders of Known Origin

By definition, children with a communication diagnosis of motor speech disorder have brain dysgenesis or have sustained pre-, peri-, or postnatal damage or disease to the central or peripheral nervous system or to muscle tissue that impairs control of speech production processes and subsequent actions of the muscle groups used to speak (respiratory, laryngeal, velopharyngeal, jaw, lip, and tongue) (Hodge and Wellman, 1999). This impairment may manifest with one or more of the following: weakness, tone alterations (hypertonia, hypotonia), reduced endurance and coordination, and involuntary movements of affected speech muscle groups (dysarthria), or as difficulty in positioning muscle groups and sequencing their actions to produce speech that cannot be explained by muscle weakness and tone abnormalities (apraxia of speech). Disturbances affecting higher mental processes of speech motor planning and programming underlie the motor speech diagnosis, apraxia of speech. To date, apraxia of speech of known origin in childhood is rare. Conditions in which it may appear are seizure disorders (e.g., Landau-Kleffner syndrome; Love and Webb, 2001), focal ischemic events (Murdoch, Ozanne, and Cross, 1990), and traumatic brain injury. In these cases the speech apraxia is typically accompanied by expressive and receptive language deficits. Oropharyngeal apraxia and mutism have been reported following posterior fossa tumor resection in children (Dailey and McKhann, 1995). Depending on the severity and duration of the neurological insult, signs of childhood-acquired apraxia of speech remit and may disappear.

Disturbances affecting the execution of speech actions are diagnosed as dysarthrias, with subtypes identified by site of lesion, accompanying pathophysiological signs, and effects on speech production. Dysarthrias are the more common type of childhood motor speech disorder. A known neurological condition affecting neuromuscular function, including that of muscles used in speech, is a key factor leading to the diagnosis of dysarthria. A useful taxonomy of subtypes of childhood dysarthrias (with associated sites of lesion) was described by Love (2000) and includes spastic (upper motor neuron), dyskinetic (basal ganglia control circuit), ataxic (cerebellar control circuit), flaccid (lower motor neuron and associated muscle fibers), and mixed (two or more sites in the previous categories); the mixed type is the most common.

Limited research has been published on the nature of neuromuscular impairment in the various childhood dysarthrias and how this correlates with perceived speech abnormalities (Workinger and Kent, 1991). Solomon and Charron (1998) reviewed the literature on speech breathing in children with cerebral palsy. Love (2000) summarized the literature on respiratory, laryngeal, velopharyngeal, tongue, jaw, and lip impairment in children with dysarthria. It is difficult to generalize from the literature to individual cases because of the relatively small numbers of children studied and the range of individual differences in children with neurogenic conditions, even when they share the same neurological diagnosis. Furthermore, it cannot be assumed that because a neurological diagnosis has implicated a certain site of lesion (e.g., cranial nerve or muscle group), other muscle groups are not also impaired. Murdoch, Johnson, and Theodoros (1997) described the case of a child with Möbius syndrome (commonly held to result from damage to cranial nerves VI and VII) and also identified impaired function at the level of the velopharyngeal, laryngeal, and respiratory subsystems using perceptual and instrumental evaluation. However, a reduction in maximal range of performance of speech muscle groups, persistent dependencies between muscle groups (e.g., lip with jaw, jaw with tongue, tongue body with tongue tip), and reductions in speed, precision, and consistency of speech movements are common themes in the literature on the nature of impairment in childhood motor speech disorders.

The effects of most childhood motor speech disorders are to reduce the rate and quality of affected children's speech development, frequency of speech use, speech intelligibility, speaking rate, and overall speech acceptability. The speech disorder can range from mild to so severe that the child never gains sufficient control over speech muscles to produce voice or recognizable speech sounds. These children's psychosocial development is also at risk because of limitations imposed by the speech disorder on social interactions, which in turn may limit their academic progress because of fewer opportunities to gain experience using language (Hodge and Wellman, 1999).

When the cause of a childhood motor speech disorder is known, it is typically because a physician specializing in pediatric neurology has diagnosed it. If this neurological diagnosis (e.g., cerebral palsy, Möbius syndrome, muscular dystrophy) is made during the prelinguistic period, there is some expectation that if neuromuscular dysfunction was observed in earlier nonspeech activities (e.g., sucking, chewing, swallowing, control of saliva, facial expressions) of muscle groups that are involved in speech production, speech development will also be delayed and disrupted (Love, 2000). Congenital suprabulbar paresis, or Worster-Drought syndrome, which has been classified by Clark et al. (2000) as a mild spastic quadriplegic type of cerebral palsy resulting from damage to the perisylvian areas of the cortex, often is not diagnosed until the child is older, if at all. Early diagnosis of this condition is important to speech-language pathologists (Crary, 1993; Clark et al., 2000) because it is predominantly characterized by persisting signs of abnormal neuromuscular dysfunction in oropharyngeal muscles during infants' feeding and swallowing and later control of speech movements. Closer examination of children with congenital suprabulbar paresis also reveals evidence of persisting neuromuscular abnormalities affecting gross and fine motor development and learning difficulties. These children need coordinated, multidisciplinary services like those afforded children with other subtypes of cerebral palsy.

In other cases of childhood motor speech disorders, no abnormal neurological signs are observed in the child's early development, and signs of the motor speech disorder may be the first or only indication of neurological abnormality (Arvedson and Simon, 1998). In some of these cases, subsequent neurological investigation with electromyography, electroencephalography, neural imaging procedures such as magnetic resonance imaging, and metabolic testing identifies a neurological condition or lesion as the cause of the speech disturbance (e.g., seizures and brain dysmorphology in the bilateral perisylvian region, infection, tumor, progressive conditions such as facioscapulohumeral muscular dystrophy) (Hodge and Wellman, 1999). In rare cases, a motor speech disorder may result from treatment for another medical condition, such as surgery for cerebellar tumors or drug treatment for a debilitating movement disorder such as Tourette's syndrome. In still other cases neurological investigation reveals no identifiable cause.

Many conditions that result in childhood motor speech disorders (e.g., cerebral palsy, traumatic brain injury, chromosomal abnormalities) also affect other areas of brain function. Therefore, children may show a mixed dysarthria or characteristics of both dysarthria and apraxia of speech, and they have a high probability of comorbidities affecting higher cognitive functions of language, thought, attention, and memory, sensory-perceptual processes and control of other motor systems (e.g., eyes, limbs, trunk, head).

Multidisciplinary assessment by members of a pediatric rehabilitation team is accepted clinical practice to determine the presence and severity of comorbid conditions that may negatively affect the child's development. Specific to the motor speech disorder, assessment goals may include one or more of the following: establishing a differential diagnosis; identifying the nature and severity of impaired movement control in each of the muscle groups used to produce speech; describing the nature and extent of limitations imposed by the impairment on the child's speech function in terms of articulatory adequacy, prosody and voice, and speech intelligibility, quality, and rate; determining the child's ability to use speech, together with other modes, to communicate with others in various contexts of daily life; and making decisions about appropriate short- and long-term management (Hodge and Wellman, 1999; Yorkston et al., 1999; Love, 2000). At young ages or in severe cases, making a differential diagnosis can be difficult if the child has insufficient speech behaviors to analyze and lacks the attentional, memory, and cognitive abilities to execute tasks that are classically used to differentiate dysarthria from praxis disturbances. Hodge (1991) summarized strategies for assessing speech motor function in children 0–3 years old. Love and Webb (2001) reviewed primitive and oropharyngeal reflexes that may signal abnormal motor development at young ages. Hayden and Square (1999) developed a standardized, normed protocol to aid in the systematic assessment of neuromotor integrity of the motor speech system at rest and when engaged in vegetative and volitional nonspeech and speech tasks for children ages 3–12 years. Their protocol was designed to identify and differentially diagnose childhood motor speech disorders and is built on their seven-stage hierarchical model of speech motor development and control. Thoonen et al. (1999) described the use of several maximal performance tasks (diadochokinetic rates for repeated mono- and trisyllables, sustained vowel and fricatives) in a decision tree model to identify and diagnose motor speech disorders; they normed their model on children age 6 years and older.

Assessment of impairment should include evaluation of the integrity of structural as well as functional aspects of the speech mechanism, because abnormal resting postures and actions of oropharyngeal muscles can lead to abnormalities in the dental arches, poor control of oral secretions, and an increased risk for middle ear infections. The use of detailed, comprehensive protocols to guide assessment of speech mechanism impairment and interpretation of findings is recommended (e.g., Dworkin and Culatta, 1995; St. Louis and Ruscello, 2000). Instrumental procedures that assess the function of the various speech subsystems (respiratory, laryngeal, velopharyngeal, and oral articulatory) also help to determine the nature and severity of impairment if child

cooperation allows (Murdoch, Johnson, and Theodoros, 1997). Procedures for assessing various aspects of speech function (e.g., phonological system and phonetic adequacy, intelligibility, prosody) and speech ability that can be repeated across time to index change are described in Hodge and Wellman (1999) and Yorkston et al. (1999). In addition to perceptual measures, acoustic measures such as second formant onset and extent and vowel area have been shown to be sensitive to both effective and ineffective compensatory articulation strategies used by children with motor speech disorders (e.g., Nelson and Hodge, 2000).

When making decisions about intervention, the clinician also needs to assess the child's feeding behavior, cognitive and receptive and expressive language skills, hearing, psychosocial status and motivation to speak and communicate, gross and fine motor skills, general health and stamina, and the child's family situation, including family members' goals and perspectives. A multidisciplinary team approach to assessment and intervention planning, with ongoing involvement of the family in selecting, coordinating, and evaluating treatment service options, is critical to the successful management of children with motor speech disorders (Mitchell and Mahoney, 1995).

At present, most childhood motor speech disorders are considered to be chronic because they are the result of brain damage or dysgenesis, for which there is no cure. It is expected that the neurological diagnosis associated with the motor speech disorder will be chronic and may affect the child's academic, social, and vocational future. However, appropriate and sufficient treatment can significantly improve these children's communication effectiveness (Hodge and Wellman, 1999; Love, 2000). The overall goal of treatment is to help these children communicate in the most successful and independent manner possible and includes helping them become desirable communication partners. It is unrealistic to expect that these children will be provided with or benefit from continuous treatment from infancy to adulthood. Families have identified the preschool and early school years, and school transitions (i.e., change in schools due to family relocation, elementary to junior high, junior to senior high, and then to college), as times when the knowledge and support of speech-language pathologists is particularly needed. Children with a congenital or early-onset condition that results in a motor speech disorder must learn how to produce the phonological system of their language with reduced control of the muscle groups used to produce and shape the sound contrasts that signal meaning to their listeners. Explicit, goal-directed opportunities for extensive practice in producing and combining speech sounds in meaningful utterances are typically required for these children to attain their potential for learning their phonological system, its phonetic realization, and making their speech intelligible. In addition to speech development, the child's language, cognitive, and social development is also at risk because of the important role that speech plays in development. Children who suffer neurological insult after the primary period of speech development has occurred (e.g., after 3–4 years of age) are faced with the task of relearning a system that has been acquired with normal speech motor control, so they have internal models of their phonological-phonetic system in place. For these children, the focus is on relearning these, and then monitoring and providing support as needed for acquisition of new spoken language skills that had not been acquired at the time of the neurological insult.

Treatment planning for all children with motor speech disorders should include a team approach that promotes active family involvement in making decisions and implementing treatment, attention to principles of motor learning at a level that is developmentally appropriate to the child (Hodge and Wellman, 1999), consideration of a variety of service delivery forms, and a holistic view of the child with a motor speech problem (Mitchell and Mahoney, 1995). Training tasks need to be goal-directed and should actively engage and involve the child as a problem solver. Because learning is context-specific, training activities should simulate real-world tasks as much as possible and be enjoyed by the child. Training goals should build on previously learned skills and behaviors. The child must have multiple opportunities to practice attaining each goal, and should have knowledge of results.

A combination of treatment approaches that address multiple levels of the communication disorder (impairment, speech functional impairment, and ability to communicate in various contexts) is typically used in management programs for children with motor speech disorders. The particular approaches change with the child's and family's needs and as the child's abilities change. Possible approaches include the following (Hodge and Wellman, 1999; Yorkston et al., 1999; Love, 2000):

General

- Educate family members, other caregivers, and peers about the nature of the child's speech disorder and ways to communicate effectively with the child.
- Augment speech with developmentally appropriate alternative communication modes.
- Provide receptive and expressive language treatment (both spoken and written) as appropriate, and integrate this with speech training activities when possible.
- Address related issues as necessary, including management of any interfering behaviors (e.g., attention, lack of motivation), control of oral secretions and swallowing, oral-dental status, and sensory (auditory-visual) status.

Speech-Specific

- Increase the child's physiological support for speech by increasing spatiotemporal control and coordination of speech muscle groups (respiratory, laryngeal, velopharyngeal, lips, tongue, jaw). The objective is to increase movement control for speech production, and the selection, implementation, and evaluation of these techniques must be made relative to their effect on in-

creasing speech intelligibility and quality. This includes working with other members of pediatric rehabilitation teams to optimize the child's seating and positioning for speech production (Solomon and Charron, 1998; Love, 2000).
- Develop the child's phonological and phonetic repertoire with attention to level of development as well as the specific profile of muscle group impairment; also, develop the child's phonological awareness and pre-literacy and literacy skills.
- Improve vocal loudness and quality through behavioral training.
- Increase speech intelligibility and naturalness through prosodic training.
- Use behavioral training to maximize the effects of drug treatments, prosthetic compensation (e.g., palatal lift), or surgery (e.g., pharyngoplasty).
- Identify and promote the use of effective speech production compensatory behaviors.

Communication Effectiveness

- Teach the effective use of interaction enhancement strategies.
- Model and promote the use of effective conversational repair strategies and speech production self-monitoring skills.
- Teach effective cognitive strategies so the child can use word choice and syntactic structure to maximize listeners' comprehension.
- Promote maintenance of speech production skills that have been established and self-monitoring of communication skills.
- Implement strategies to increase the child's self-esteem and self-confidence in initiating and participating in communication interactions.

See also DEVELOPMENTAL APRAXIA OF SPEECH; DYSARTHRIAS: CHARACTERISTICS AND CLASSIFICATION; MOTOR SPEECH INVOLVEMENT IN CHILDREN.

—*Megan M. Hodge*

References

Arvedson, J., and Simon, D. (1998). Acquired neurologic deficits in young children: A diagnostic journey with Dora. *Seminars in Speech and Language, 19*, 71–80.

Clark, M., Carr, L., Reilly, S., and Neville, B. (2000). Worster-Drought syndrome, a mild tetraplegic perisylvian cerebral palsy: Review of 47 cases. *Brain, 123*, 2160–2170.

Crary, M. (1993). *Developmental motor speech disorders.* San Diego, CA: Singular Publishing Group.

Dailey, A., and McKhann, G. (1995). The pathophysiology of oral pharyngeal apraxia and mutism following posterior fossa tumor resection in children. *Journal of Neurosurgery, 83*, 467–475.

Dworkin, J., and Culatta, R. (1995). *Dworkin-Culatta Oral Mechanism Exam—Treatment (D-COME-T).* Nicholasville, KY: Edgewood Press.

Hayden, D., and Square, P. (1999). *Verbal motor production assessment for children.* Toronto: Psychological Corporation.

Hodge, M. (1991). Assessing early speech motor function. *Clinics in Communication Disorders, 1*, 69–85.

Hodge, M., and Wellman, L. (1999). Clinical management of children with dysarthria. In A. Caruso and E. Stand (Eds.), *Clinical management of children with motor speech disorders* (pp. 209–280). New York: Thieme.

Love, R. J. (2000). *Childhood motor speech disability* (2nd ed.). Toronto: Allyn and Bacon.

Love, R. J., and Webb, W. G. (2001). *Neurology for the speech-language pathologist* (4th ed.). Boston: Butterworth-Heinemann.

Mitchell, P., and Mahoney, G. (1995). Team management for young children with motor speech disorders. *Seminars in Speech and Language, 16,* 159–172.

Murdoch, B., Ozanne, A., and Cross, J. (1990). Acquired childhood motor speech disorders: Dysarthria and dyspraxia. In B. Murdoch (Ed.), *Acquired neurological speech/language disorders in childhood* (pp. 308–342). London: Taylor and Francis.

Murdoch, B. E., Johnson, B. M., and Theodoros, D. G. (1997). Physiological and perceptual features of dysarthria in Moebius syndrome: Directions for treatment. *Pediatric Rehabilitation, 1,* 83–97.

Nelson, M., and Hodge, M. (2000). Effects of facial paralysis and audiovisual information on stop place identification. *Journal of Speech, Language, and Hearing Research, 43,* 158–171.

Solomon, N., and Charron, S. (1998). Speech breathing in able-bodied children and children with cerebral palsy: A review of the literature and implications for clinical intervention. *American Journal of Speech-Language Pathology, 7,* 61–78.

St. Louis, K. O., and Ruscello, D. M. (2000). *Oral Speech Mechanism Screening Examination—Third Edition (OSME-3).* Austin, TX: Pro-Ed.

Thoonen, G., Maassen, B., Gabreels, F., and Schreuder, R. (1999). Validity of maximum performance tasks to diagnose motor speech disorders in children. *Clinical Linguistics and Phonetics, 13,* 1–23.

Workinger, M., and Kent, R. (1991). Perceptual analysis of the dysarthrias in children with athetoid and spastic cerebral palsy. In C. Moore, K. Yorkston, and D. Beukelman (Eds.), *Dysarthria and apraxia of speech: Perspectives on management* (pp. 109–126). Baltimore: Paul H. Brookes.

Yorkston, K., Beukelman, D., Strand, E., and Bell, K. (1999). *Management of motor speech disorders in children and adults* (2nd ed.). Austin, TX: Pro-Ed.

Further Readings

Chapman-Bahr, D. (2001). *Oral motor assessment and treatment: Ages and stages.* Needham Heights, MA: Allyn and Bacon.

Foley, B. (1993). The development of literacy in individuals with severe congenital speech and motor impairments. *Topics in Language Disorders, 13,* 16–22.

Goldblatt, D., and Williams, D. (1986). "I an sniling": Moebius syndrome inside and out. *Journal of Child Neurology, 1,* 71–78.

Gordon, N. (2001). Mutism: Elective, selective, and acquired. *Brain and Development, 23,* 83–87.

Hardy, J. (1983). *Cerebral palsy.* Englewood Cliffs, NJ: Prentice-Hall.

Hayden, D., and Square, P. (1994). Motor speech treatment hierarchy: A systems approach. *Clinics in Communication Disorders, 4,* 162–174.

Hodge, M. (1999). Relationship between F2/F1 vowel quadrilateral area and speech intelligibility in a child

with progressive dysarthria. *Canadian Acoustics, 27,* 84–85.

Horton, S., Murdoch, B., Theodoros, D., and Thompson, E. (1997). Motor speech impairment in a case of childhood basilar artery stroke: Treatment directions derived from physiological and perceptual assessment. *Pediatric Rehabilitation, 1,* 163–177.

Kent, R. (1997). The perceptual sensorimotor examination for motor speech disorders. In M. R. McNeil (Ed.), *Clinical management of sensorimotor speech disorders* (pp. 27–48). New York: Thieme.

Law, M. (1993). Perspectives on understanding and changing the environments of children with disabilities. *Physical and Occupational Therapy in Pediatrics, 13,* 1–17.

Mitchell, P. (1995). A dynamic-interactive developmental view of early speech and language production: Application to clinical practice in motor speech disorders. *Seminars in Speech and Language, 16,* 100–109.

Murdoch, B., and Hudson-Tennant, L. (1994). Speech disorders in children treated for posterior fossa tumors: Ataxic and developmental features. *European Journal of Disorders of Communication, 29,* 379–397.

Redmond, S., and Johnston, S. (2001). Evaluating the morphological competence of children with severe speech and physical impairments. *Journal of Speech, Language, and Hearing Research, 44,* 1362–1375.

Thompson, C. (1988). Articulation disorders in children. In N. Lass, L. McReynolds, J. Northern, and D. Yoder (Eds.), *Handbook of speech pathology and audiology* (pp. 548–590). Toronto: B.C. Decker.

Van Mourik, M., Catsman-Berrevoets, C., van Dongen, H., and Neville, B. (1997). Complex orofacial movements and the disappearance of cerebellar mutism: Report of five cases. *Developmental Medicine and Child Neurology, 39,* 686–690.

Speech Disorders in Children: Speech-Language Approaches

Children with speech disorders often display difficulty in other domains of language, suggesting that they experience difficulty with the language learning process in general. A theoretical shift from viewing children's speech disorders as articulatory-based to viewing them from a linguistic perspective was precipitated by the application of phonological theories and principles to the field of speech pathology, beginning in the late 1970s. Implicit in this shift was the recognition that acquisition of a linguistic system is a gradual, primarily auditory-perceptually based process involving the development of receptive knowledge first (Hodson and Paden, 1991; Ingram, 1997). Another implication from research on normal phonological acquisition is that linguistic input should demonstrate a sound's contrastive role in the ambient phonology because what children are developing is phonological oppositions. As a result of applying a linguistic model to intervention, speech-language approaches have flourished in the past two decades for treating children's speech disorders. These approaches are characterized by: (1) an emphasis on the function of the phonological system to support communication, and thus on the pragmatic limitations of unintelligible speech; (2) a focus on the contrastive nature of phonemes and the use of minimal pair contrast training to facilitate reorganization of the system; (3) the use of phonological analysis and description to identify error patterns; (4) the selection of error patterns for elimination and of sound classes and features for acquisition; and (5) the use of a small set of sounds as exemplars of those patterns/features for acquisition. What separates speech-language approaches from other articulation approaches is the use of phonological analysis to identify error patterns affecting sound classes and sequences rather than the selection of isolated sounds to be trained in each word position. Speech-language approaches differ from articulation approaches in their focus on modifications of groups of sounds via a small set of exemplars (e.g., /f, s/ to represent all fricatives) and their emphasis on contrastivity for successful communication in a social context.

As such, minimal pair contrast treatment is a speech-language approach that highlights the semantic confusion caused when the child produces a sound error that results in a pair of homonyms (e.g., "sun" and "ton" both produced as /tʌn/). This technique involves contrasting a pair of words in which one word contains the child's error production and the other contains the target production (with phonemes differing by only one feature). In minimal pair approaches, the child is instructed to make perceptual and productive contrasts involving the target sound and his or her error. The goal of treatment is to help the child learn to produce the target sound in the word pair to signal a difference in meaning between the two words. Minimal pair contrast interventions have been shown to be effective in eliminating error patterns and increasing the accuracy of target and related error sounds (Ferrier and Davis, 1973; Elbert, Rockman, and Saltzman, 1980; Blache, Parsons, and Humphreys, 1981; Weiner, 1981; Elbert, 1983; Tyler, Edwards, and Saxman, 1987; Saben and Ingham, 1991). Minimal pair approaches that involve solely perception of word contrasts, however, have not resulted in as much change as when production practice with models and phonetic cues is also included (Saben and Ingham, 1991).

Minimal pair contrasts are used somewhat differently in Metaphon (Howell and Dean, 1994; Dean et al., 1995), a "cognitive-linguistic" approach. This approach is considered cognitive-linguistic because it facilitates conceptual development and cognitive reorganization of linguistic information. Its aim is to increase, at the metalinguistic level, awareness and understanding of sound class differences primarily through classification techniques, with little emphasis on production. For example, to contrast alveolars and velars, the concepts of front and back are introduced and applied first to nonspeech sorting and classification activities. Next, these concepts are transferred to the speech domain by having the child listen to minimal pairs and judge whether or not words begin with front or back sounds. Dean et al. (1995) present evidence from several children suggesting that this approach effectively reduced the application of selected phonological processes.

The cycles approach, proposed by Hodson and Paden's (1991), involves a goal attack strategy that capitalizes on observations concerning the gradual manner in which normally developing children acquire their phonological systems. Groups of sounds affected by an error pattern are introduced for only 1 or 2 weeks, then a new error pattern is introduced. Thus, the criterion for advancement to a new goal or target is time-based rather than accuracy-based. A cycle can range from 5 to 15 weeks, depending on the number of deficient patterns, and once completed, the sequence is recycled for the error patterns that still remain in the child's speech. Hodson and Paden's cycle approach involves auditory bombardment and production practice in the form of picture- and object-naming activities, and reportedly eliminates most of a child's phonological error patterns in 1–2 years of intervention (Tyler, Edwards, and Saxman, 1987; Hodson and Paden, 1991; Hodson, 1997).

In contrast to the three approaches just described, which focus on speech within a linguistic framework, there are language-based approaches in which little attention may be drawn to sound errors and these errors may not be specific targets of intervention. Instead, the entire language system (syntax, semantic, phonology, pragmatics) is targeted as a tool for communication, and improvements in phonology are expected from a process of "whole to part learning" (Norris and Hoffman, 1990; Hoffman, 1992). Phonological changes might be expected to occur because phonemes are practiced as parts of larger wholes within the script for an entire event. Language-based approaches involve a variety of naturalistic, conversationally embedded techniques such as scaffolding narratives, focused stimulation in the form of expansions and recasts, and elicited production devices such as forced-choice questions, cloze tasks, and preparatory sets.

Norris and Hoffman's (1990, 1993) language-based approach focuses on scaffolding narratives in the form of expansions, expatiations, and turn assistance devices to help the child talk about picture sequences with higher levels of discourse and semantic complexity. Hoffman, Norris, and Monjure (1990) contrasted their scaffolded narrative approach to a phonological process approach in two brothers with comparable phonological and language deficits. The narrative intervention facilitated gains in phonology that were similar to the phonological approach, and greater gains in syntactic, semantic, and pragmatic performance.

Other language-based approaches reported in the literature have focused primarily on morphosyntactic goals (e.g., finite morphemes, pronouns, complex sentences) using focused stimulation designed to provide multiple models of target morphosyntactic structures in a natural communicative context. Procedures have involved recasts and expansions of child utterances, and opportunities to use target forms in response to forced-choice questions, sentence fill-ins, requests for elaboration, or false assertions in pragmatically appropriate contexts

(Cleave and Fey, 1997). Researchers have been interested in the cross-domain effects of these procedures on improvement in children's speech disorders. Fey et al. (1994) examined the effects of language intervention in 25 children with moderate to severe language and speech impairments who were randomly assigned to a clinician treatment group, a parent treatment group, or a delayed-treatment control group. The treatment groups made large gains in grammar after 5 months of intervention, but improvement in speech was no greater than that achieved by the control group. Tyler and Sandoval (1994) examined the effects of treatment focused only on speech, only on morphosyntax, and on both domains in six preschool children. The two children who received morphosyntactic intervention showed improvements in language but negligible improvement in phonology.

In contrast to these findings that language-based intervention focused on morphosyntax does not lead to gains in speech, Tyler, Lewis, Haskill, and Tolbert (2002) found that a morphosyntax intervention addressing finite morphemes led to improvement in speech in comparison to a control group. Tyler et al. (2002) investigated the efficacy and cross-domain effects of both a morphosyntax and a phonological intervention. Ten preschool children were assigned at random to an intervention of two 12-week blocks, beginning with either a block focused on speech first or a block focused on morphosyntax first. Treatment efficacy was evaluated after one block in the sequence was applied. Not only was the morphosyntax intervention effective in promoting change in morphemes marking tense and agreement in comparison to the no-treatment control group, but it led to improvement in speech that was similar to that achieved by the phonology intervention. Thus, for children who received language intervention, the amount of speech improvement was significantly greater than that observed for the control group. In a similar study, Matheny and Panagos (1978) examined the effect of highly structured interventions focused on syntax only and articulation only in children with deficits in both domains, compared with a control group. Each group made significant gains in the treated domain in comparison with the control group, but also made improvements in the untreated domain. Thus, a language-based intervention focused on complex sentence structures led to improved speech.

Findings regarding the effects of language intervention on speech are equivocal, particularly results from methodologically rigorous studies with control groups (Matheny and Panagos, 1978; Fey et al., 1994; Tyler et al., 2002). One variable that may account for these differing results is the use of different measures to document change. Matheny and Panagos used before and after standardized test scores, whereas Fey et al. used Percent of Consonants Correct (PCC; Shriberg and Kwiatkowski, 1982), a general measure of consonant accuracy, and Tyler et al. used a more discrete measure of target and generalization phoneme accuracy. Nonetheless, the collective findings from studies of the effects of different language-based approaches on speech suggest that some children, especially those with both speech and language impairments, will show improvement in speech when the intervention focuses on language. Determining exactly who these children are is difficult. Preliminary evidence suggests that children whose phonological systems are highly inconsistent may be good candidates for a language-based approach (Tyler, 2002). Finally, service delivery restrictions may dictate the use of language-based approaches in classroom or collaborative settings. These approaches deserve further investigation for their possible benefit in remediating both speech and language difficulties.

In summary, a variety of speech-language approaches have been shown to be effective in improving speech intelligibility and reducing the number and severity of error patterns in children with speech disorders. Although these approaches employ different teaching methods, they originate in a linguistic model and share an emphasis on the function of the phonological system to support communication, and on the contrastive nature of phonemes to reduce the pragmatic limitations of unintelligible speech.

—*Ann A. Tyler*

References

Blache, S. E., Parsons, C. L., and Humphreys, J. M. (1981). A minimal-word-pair model for teaching the linguistic significance of distinctive feature properties. *Journal of Speech and Hearing Disorders, 46,* 291–296.

Cleave, P., and Fey, M. (1997). Two approaches to the facilitation of grammar in children with language impairments: Rationale and description. *American Journal of Speech-Language Pathology, 6,* 22–32.

Dean, E. C., Howell, J., Waters, D., and Reid, J. (1995). Metaphon: A metalinguistic approach to the treatment of phonological disorder in children. *Clinical Linguistics and Phonetics, 9,* 1–19.

Elbert, M. (1983). A case study of phonological acquisition. *Topics in Language Disorders, 3,* 1–9.

Elbert, M., Rockman, B. K., and Saltzman, D. (1980). *Contrasts: The use of minimal pairs in articulation training.* Austin, TX: Exceptional Resources.

Ferrier, E., and Davis, M. (1973). A lexical approach to the remediation of sound omissions. *Journal of Speech and Hearing Disorders, 38,* 126–130.

Fey, M., Cleave, P. L., Ravida, A., Long, S. H., Dejmal, A. E., and Easton, D. L. (1994). Effects of grammar facilitation on the phonological performance of children with speech and language impairments. *Journal of Speech and Hearing Research, 37,* 594–607.

Hodson, B. W. (1997). Disordered phonologies: What have we learned about assessment and treatment? In B. W. Hodson and M. L. Edwards (Eds.), *Perspectives in applied phonology* (pp. 197–224). Gaithersburg, MD: Aspen.

Hodson, B. W., and Paden, E. P. (1991). *Targeting intelligible speech: A phonological approach to remediation* (2nd ed.). Austin, TX: Pro-Ed.

Hoffman, P. R. (1992). Synergistic development of phonetic skill. *Language, Speech, and Hearing Services in Schools, 23,* 254–260.

Hoffman, P. R., Norris, J. A., and Monjure, J. (1990). Comparison of process targeting and whole language treatment for phonologically delayed preschool children. *Language, Speech, and Hearing Services in Schools, 21,* 102–109.

Howell, J., and Dean, E. (1994). *Treating phonological disorders in children: Metaphon—theory to practice* (2nd ed.). London: Whurr.

Ingram, D. (1997). The categorization of phonological impairment. In B. W. Hodson and M. L. Edwards (Eds.), *Perspectives in applied phonology* (pp. 19–41). Gaithersburg, MD: Aspen.

Matheny, N., and Panagos, J. M. (1978). Comparing the effects of articulation and syntax programs on syntax and articulation improvement. *Language, Speech, and Hearing Services in Schools, 9,* 57–61.

Norris, J. A., and Hoffman, P. R. (1990). Language intervention within naturalistic environments. *Language, Speech, and Hearing Services in Schools, 21,* 72–84.

Norris, J. A., and Hoffman, P. R. (1993). *Language intervention for school-age children.* San Diego, CA: Singular Publishing Group.

Saben, C. B., and Ingham, J. C. (1991). The effects of minimal pairs treatment on the speech-sound production of two children with phonologic disorders. *Journal of Speech and Hearing Research, 34,* 1023–1040.

Shriberg, L. D., and Kwiatkowski, J. (1982). Phonological disorders: III. A procedure for assessing severity of involvement. *Journal of Speech and Hearing Disorders, 17,* 256–270.

Tyler, A. A. (2002). Language-based intervention for phonological disorders. *Seminars in Speech and Language, 23,* 69–81.

Tyler, A. A., Edwards, M. L., and Saxman, J. H. (1987). Clinical application of two phonologically based treatment procedures. *Journal of Speech and Hearing Disorders, 52,* 393–409.

Tyler, A. A., and Sandoval, K. T. (1994). Preschoolers with phonologic and language disorders: Treating different linguistic domains. *Language, Speech, and Hearing Services in Schools, 25,* 215–234.

Tyler, A. A., Lewis, K., Haskill, A., and Tolbert, L. (2002). Efficacy and cross-domain effects of a morphosyntax and a phonology intervention. *Language, Speech, and Hearing Services in Schools, 33,* 52–66.

Weiner, F. F. (1981). Treatment of phonological disability using the method of meaningful minimal contrast: Two case studies. *Journal of Speech and Hearing Disorders, 46,* 97–103.

Further Readings

Chaney, C. (1990). Evaluating the whole language approach to language arts: The pros and cons. *Language, Speech, and Hearing Services in Schools, 21,* 244–249.

Crystal, D. (1987). Towards a "bucket" theory of language disability: Taking account of interaction between linguistic levels. *Clinical Linguistics and Phonetics, 1,* 7–22.

Dinnsen, D. A., and Elbert, M. (1984). On the relationship between phonology and learning. In M. Elbert, D. A. Dinnsen, and G. Weismer (Eds.), *Phonological theory and the misarticulating child* (pp. 59–68). (ASHA Monograph No. 22.) Rockville, MD: American Speech-Language-Hearing Association.

Edwards, M. L. (1983). Selection criteria for developing therapy goals. *Journal of Childhood Communication Disorders, 7,* 36–45.

Elbert, M., Dinnsen, D. A., and Powell, T. W. (1984). On the prediction of phonologic generalization learning pat-

terns. *Journal of Speech and Hearing Disorders, 49,* 309–317.

Elbert, M., and McReynolds, L. V. (1985). The generalization hypothesis: Final consonant deletion. *Language and Speech, 28,* 281–294.

Fey, M. (1992). Articulation and phonology: Inextricable constructs in speech pathology. *Language, Speech, and Hearing Services in Schools, 23,* 225–232.

Gierut, J. A. (1989). Maximal opposition approach to phonological treatment. *Journal of Speech and Hearing Disorders, 54,* 9–19.

Gierut, J. A. (1998). Treatment efficacy: Functional phonological disorders in children. *Journal of Speech, Language, and Hearing Research, 41,* S85–S100.

Hodson, B. W. (1986). *The Assessment of Phonological Processes—Revised.* Austin, TX: Pro-Ed.

Kelman, M. E., and Edwards, M. L. (1994). *Phonogroup: A practical guide for enhancing phonological remediation.* Eau Claire, WI: Thinking Publications.

Locke, J. L. (1993). *The child's path to spoken language.* Cambridge, MA: Harvard University Press.

Monahan, D. (1986). Remediation of common phonological processes: Four case studies. *Language, Speech, and Hearing Services in Schools, 17,* 199–206.

Olswang, L. B., and Bain, B. (1994). Data collection: Monitoring children's treatment progress. *American Journal of Speech-Language Pathology, 3,* 55–66.

Paul, R., and Shriberg, L. D. (1982). Associations between phonology and syntax in speech-delayed children. *Journal of Speech and Hearing Research, 25,* 536–547.

Powell, T. W. (1991). Planning for phonological generalization: An approach to treatment target selection. *American Journal of Speech-Language Pathology, 1,* 21–27.

Schwartz, R. G. (1992). Clinical applications of recent advances in phonological theory. *Language, Speech, and Hearing Services in Schools, 23,* 269–276.

Tyler, A. A. (1997). Evidence of linguistic interactions in intervention. *Topics in Language Disorders, 17,* 23–40.

Tyler, A. A., and Watterson, K. (1991). Effects of phonological versus language intervention in preschoolers with both phonological and language impairment. *Child Language Teaching and Therapy, 7,* 141–160.

Wilcox, K. A., and Morris, S. E. (1995a). Speech intervention in a language-focused curriculum. In M. Rice and K. Wilcox (Eds.), *Building a language-focused curriculum for the preschool classroom: A foundation for lifelong communication* (pp. 73–89). Baltimore: Paul H. Brookes.

Wilcox, K. A., and Morris, S. E. (1995b). Speech outcomes of the language-focused curriculum. In M. Rice and K. Wilcox (Eds.), *Building a language-focused curriculum for the preschool classroom: A foundation for lifelong communication* (pp. 171–180). Baltimore: Paul H. Brookes.

Speech Disorders Secondary to Hearing Impairment Acquired in Adulthood

Hearing loss is very common in the general population, with a prevalence of 82.9 per 1000 (U.S. Public Health Service, 1990). It becomes more common with age as a result of noise exposure, vascular disease, ototoxic agents, and other otological diseases. After arthritis and hypertension, hearing loss is the third most common chronic condition in persons over 65 (National Center for Health Statistics, 1982). In a study of 3556 adults from Beaver Dam, Wisconsin, Cruickshanks et al. (1998) found prevalence rates for hearing loss of 21% in adults ages 48–59 years, 44% for those ages 60–69, 66% for those ages 70–79, and 90% for those ages 80–92. The prevalence of perceived hearing handicap, however, is lower than the true prevalence of hearing loss. By age 70, approximately 30% of the population perceives themselves as hearing impaired, and by 80 years, 50% report being hearing impaired (Desai et al., 2001). There is also some indication that the prevalence of hearing impairment in persons 45–69 years old is increasing, especially among men (Wallhagen et al., 1997).

The typical hearing loss configuration in adults is a bilateral high-frequency sensory loss with normal or near normal hearing in the low frequencies (Moscicki et al., 1985; Cruickshanks et al., 1998). Men tend to have more hearing loss than women, and white individuals report greater hearing impairment than African Americans (Cruickshanks et al., 1998; Desai et al., 2001).

Although hearing loss is common in the general population, its effects on speech production are most pronounced in individuals who have congenital hearing loss or hearing losses acquired in early childhood. For individuals who acquire hearing loss as adults, the impact on speech production is limited and usually does not result in any perceptible speech differences (Goehl and Kaufman, 1984). The preservation of speech in most adults with hearing loss likely is a consequence of residual hearing sufficient for auditory feedback.

Speech differences have, however, been reported for some persons with complete loss or nearly complete loss of hearing. These individuals tend to remain intelligible, although the speaking rate may be reduced by about a third when compared with normal-hearing speakers (Leder, Spitzer, Kirchner, et al., 1987). A decreased speaking rate is reflected in increased sentence and pause durations as well as increased word, syllable, and vowel durations (Kirk and Edgerton, 1983; Leder et al., 1986; Leder, Spitzer, Kirchner, et al., 1987; Waldstein, 1990; Lane et al., 1998). Movement durations associated with articulatory gestures also are prolonged in some adventitiously deafened adults (Matthies et al., 1996), and it has been suggested that this overall decrease in rate contributes to a reduction in speech quality and communication effectiveness (Leder, Spitzer, Kirchner, et al., 1987).

Changes in respiratory and vocal control have been noted, as evidenced by abnormal airflow, glottal aperture, and air expenditure per syllable as well as frequent encroachment on respiratory reserve (Lane et al., 1991, 1998). Adventitiously deafened adults also tend to exhibit increased breathiness, vocal intensity, and mean fundamental frequency (Leder, Spitzer, and Kirchner, 1987; Leder, Spitzer, Milner, et al., 1987; Lane et al., 1991; Lane and Webster, 1991; Perkell et al., 1992). In addition, the fundamental frequency tends to be more variable, particularly on stressed vowels (Lane and Webster, 1991).

Reduced phonemic contrast also characterizes the speech of some adventitiously deafened adults. Lane et al. (1995) observed that voice-onset time tends to decrease for both voiced and voiceless stop consonants, while Waldstein (1990) observed this effect only with voiceless stop consonants. Vowel, plosive, and sibilant spectra become less distinct, and vowel formant spacing for some speakers becomes more restricted and centralized (Waldstein, 1990; Lane and Webster, 1991; Matthies et al., 1994, 1996; Lane et al., 1995). The first vowel formant commonly is elevated, with some speakers also exhibiting a reduction in second formant frequency (Perkell et al., 1992; Kishon-Rabin et al., 1999). A greater overlap in articulator postures and placements has also been observed, with a tendency for the consonant place of articulation to be displaced forward and vowel postures to be neutralized (Matthies et al., 1996). Fricatives and affricates appear particularly prone to deterioration with profound hearing loss (Lane and Webtser, 1991; Matthies et al., 1996). Many of these changes, although subtle in many cases and variable in expression across this population, are consistent with the speech differences common to speakers with prelingual hearing loss. Although the evidence is limited, owing to the small numbers of subjects examined, the data across studies suggest that the effects of hearing loss on speech production are most pronounced if the hearing loss occurs in the teens and early twenties than if it occurs in later adulthood.

The primary management procedure for adults with acquired hearing loss severe enough to compromise speech is to restore some degree of auditory feedback. The initial intervention typically consists of fitting traditional amplification in the form of hearing aids. For first-time hearing aid wearers, postfitting rehabilitation consisting of counseling and AUDITORY TRAINING improves auditory performance and retention of the hearing aid, although secondary benefit in respect to speech production in adults has not been studied systematically (Walden et al., 1981).

A sensory implant often is recommended for adults who do not receive sufficient benefit from hearing aids or who cannot wear hearing aids (see COCHLEAR IMPLANTS). Individuals with an intact auditory nerve and a patent cochlea are usually candidates for a cochlear implant. Persons who cannot be fitted with a cochlear implant, such as persons with severed auditory nerves or ossified cochleae, may be candidates for a device that stimulates the auditory system intracranially, such as a brainstem implant. As with hearing aids, adult patients receiving sensory implants benefit from pre- and postfitting counseling and frequent monitoring. With current technologies, many patients show substantial improvement in auditory and speech function within months of device activation with little or no additional intervention, although normalization of all speech parameters may never occur or may take years to achieve (Kishon-Rabin et al., 1999). Some speech parameters, such as vocal intensity and fundamental frequency, show some degree of reversal when an implant is temporarily turned off and then on, but the extent and time course of overall recovery after initial activation vary with the individual. The variability in speech recovery after initial implant activation appears to result from a number of factors, among them age at onset of hearing loss, improvement in auditory skills after implant activation, extent of speech deterioration prior to activation, and the speech parameters affected (Perkell et al., 1992; Lane et al., 1995, 1998; Kishon-Rabin et al., 1999; Vick et al., 2001). As a result, some patients may benefit from behavioral intervention to facilitate recovery. In particular, persons with poor speech quality prior to receiving an implant, as well as persons with central auditory deficits and compromised devices, might benefit from systematic auditory, speech, and communication skills training, although the relationship between speech recovery and behavioral treatment has received little investigation in these patients.

See also AUDITORY TRAINING; COCHLEAR IMPLANTS; HEARING LOSS SCREENING: THE SCHOOL-AGE CHILD; NOISE-INDUCED HEARING LOSS; OTOTOXIC MEDICATIONS; PRESBYCUSIS; SPEECHREADING TRAINING AND VISUAL TRACKING.

—*Sheila Pratt*

References

Cruickshanks, K., Wiley, T., Tweed, T., Klein, B., Klein, R., Mares-Perlman, J., et al. (1998). Prevalence of hearing loss in older adults in Beaver Dam, Wisconsin. *American Journal of Epidemiology, 148,* 879–886.

Desai, M., Pratt, L., Lentzner, H., and Robinson, K. (2001). *Trends in vision and hearing among older Americans. Aging Trends, 2.* Hyattsville, MD: National Center of Health Statistics.

Goehl, H., and Kaufman, D. (1984). Do the effects of adventitious deafness include disordered speech? *Journal of Speech and Hearing Disorders, 49,* 58–64.

Kirk, K., and Edgerton, B. (1983). The effects of cochlear implant use on voice parameters. *Otolaryngologic Clinics of North America, 16,* 281–292.

Kishon-Rabin, L., Taitelbaum, R., Tobin, Y., and Hildesheimer, M. (1999). The effect of partially restored hearing on speech production of postlingually deafened adults with multichannel cochlear implants. *Journal of the Acoustical Society of America, 106,* 2843–2857.

Lane, H., Perkell, J., Svirsky, M., and Webster, J. (1991). Changes in speech breathing following cochlear implant in postlingually deafened adults. *Journal of Speech and Hearing Research, 34,* 526–533.

Lane, H., Perkell, J., Wozniak, J., Mansella, J., Guiod, P., Matthies, M., et al. (1998). The effect of changes in hearing status on speech sound level and speech breathing: A study conducted with cochlear implant users and NF-2 patients. *Journal of the Acoustical Society of America, 104,* 3059–3069.

Lane, H., and Webster, J. W. (1991). Speech deterioration in postlingually deafened adults. *Journal of the Acoustical Society of America, 89,* 859–866.

Lane, H., Wozniak, J., Matthies, M., Svirsky, M., and Perkell, J. (1995). Phonemic resetting versus postural adjustments in the speech of cochlear implant users: An exploration

of voice-onset-time. *Journal of the Acoustical Society of America, 98,* 3096–3106.

Leder, S., Spitzer, J., and Kirchner, J. (1987). Speaking fundamental frequency of postlingually profoundly deaf adult men. *Annals of Otology, Rhinology, and Laryngology, 96,* 322–324.

Leder, S., Spitzer, J., Kirchner, J. C., Flevaris-Phillips, C., Milner, P., and Richardson, F. (1987). Speaking rate of adventitiously deaf male cochlear implant candidates. *Journal of the Acoustical Society of America, 82,* 843–846.

Leder, S., Spitzer, J., Milner, P., Flevaris-Phillips, C., Kirchner, J., and Richardson, F. (1987). Voice intensity of prospective cochlear implant candidates and normal-hearing adult males. *Laryngoscope, 97,* 224–227.

Leder, S., Spitzer, J., Milner, P., Flevaris-Phillips, C., Richardson, F., and Kirchner, J. (1986). Reacquisition of contrastive stress in an adventitiously deaf speaker using a single-channel cochlear implant. *Journal of the Acoustical Society of America, 79,* 1967–1974.

Matthies, M., Svirsky, M., Lane, H., and Perkell, J. (1994). A preliminary study of the effects of cochlear implants on the production of sibilants. *Journal of the Acoustical Society of America, 96,* 1367–1373.

Matthies, M., Svirsky, M., Perkell, J., and Lane, H. (1996). Acoustic and articulatory measures of sibilant production with and without auditory feedback from a cochlear implant. *Journal of Speech and Hearing Research, 39,* 936–946.

Moscicki, E., Elkins, E., Baum, H., and McNamara, P. (1985). Hearing loss in the elderly: An epidemiologic study of the Framingham Heart Study cohort. *Ear and Hearing, 6,* 184–190.

National Center for Health Statistics. (1982). Hearing ability of persons by sociodemographic and health characteristics: United States. *Vital and Health Statistics* (Series 10, No. 140, DHS Publication No. PHS 82-1568). Washington, DC: U.S. Public Health Service.

Perkell, J., Lane, H., Svirsky, M., and Webster, J. (1992). Speech of cochlear implant patients: A longitudinal study of vowel production. *Journal of the Acoustical Society of America, 91,* 2961–2978.

U.S. Public Health Service. (1990). *Healthy People 2000.* Washington, DC: U.S. Government Printing Office.

Vick, J. C., Lane, H., Perkell, J. S., Matthies, M. L., Gould, J., and Zandipour, M. (2001). Covariation of cochlear implant users' perception and production of vowel contrasts and their identification by listeners with normal hearing. *Journal of Speech, Language, and Hearing Research, 44,* 1257–1267.

Walden, B., Erdman, S., Montgomery, A., Schwartz, D., and Prosek, R. (1981). Some effects of training on speech recognition by hearing-impaired adults. *Journal of Speech and Hearing Research, 24,* 207–216.

Waldstein, R. (1990). Effects of postlingual deafness on speech production: Implications for the role of auditory feedback. *Journal of the Acoustical Society of America, 88,* 2099–2114.

Wallhagen, M., Strawbridge, W., Cohen, R., and Kaplan, G. (1997). An increasing prevalence of hearing impairment and associated risk factors over three decades of the Alameda County study. *American Journal of Public Health, 87,* 440–442.

Further Readings

Bennie, C., Daniloff, R., and Buckingham, H. (1982). Phonetic disintegration in a five-year old following sudden hearing loss. *Journal of Speech and Hearing Disorders, 47,* 181–189.

Cowie, R., Douglas-Cowie, E., Phil, D., and Kerr, A. (1982). Speech changes following reimplantation from a single-channel to a multichannel cochlear implant. *Journal of Laryngology and Otology, 96,* 101–112.

Economou, A., Tartter, V., Chute, P., and Hellman, S. (1992). Speech changes following reimplantation from a single-channel to a multichannel cochlear implant. *Journal of the Acoustical Society of America, 92,* 1310–1323.

Lane, H., and Tranel, B. (1971). The Lombard sign and the role of hearing in speech. *Journal of Speech and Hearing Research, 14,* 677–709.

Langereis, M., Bosman, A., van Olphen, A., and Smoorenburg, G. (1997). Changes in vowel quality in post-lingually deafened cochlear implant users. *Audiology, 36,* 279–297.

Langereis, M., Bosman, A., van Olphen, A., and Smoorenburg, G. (1998). Effect of cochlear implantation on voice fundamental frequency in post-lingually deafened adults. *Audiology, 37,* 219–230.

Plant, G. (1984). The effects of an acquired profound hearing loss on speech production. *British Journal of Audiology, 18,* 39–48.

Pratt, S., and Tye-Murray, N. (1997). Speech impairment secondary to hearing loss. In M. R. McNeil (Ed.), *Clinical Management of Sensorimotor Speech Disorders* (pp. 345–387). New York: Thieme.

Smyth, V., Murdoch, B., McCormack, P., and Marshall, I. (1991). Objective and subjective evaluation of subjects fitted with the cochlear multi-channel cochlear prostheses: 3 studies. *Australian Journal of Human Communication Disorders, 19,* 32–52.

Spir, S., and Canter, G. (1991). Postlingual deaf speech and the role of audition in speech production: Comments on Waldstein's paper. *Journal of the Acoustical Society of America, 90,* 1672–1678.

Svirsky, M., Lane H., Perkell, J., and Wozniak, J. (1992). Effects of short-term auditory deprivation on speech production in adult cochlear implant users. *Journal of the Acoustical Society of America, 92,* 1284–1300.

Svirsky, M., and Tobey, E. (1991). Effect of different types of auditory stimulation on vowel formant frequencies in multichannel cochlear implant users. *Journal of the Acoustical Society of America, 89,* 2895–2904.

Zimmermann, G., and Rettaliata, P. (1981). Articulatory patterns of an adventitiously deaf speaker: Implications for the role of auditory information in speech production. *Journal of Speech and Hearing Research, 24,* 169–178.

Speech Issues in Children from Latino Backgrounds

Research into English phonological development in typically developing children and children with phonological disorders has been occurring since the 1930s (e.g., Wellman et al., 1931; Hawk, 1936). There is limited information on phonological development in Latino children, particularly those who are monolingual Spanish speakers and bilingual (Spanish and English) speakers. Over the past 15 years, however, phonological information collected on monolingual Spanish speakers and bilingual (Spanish-English) speakers has increased greatly.

This entry summarizes information on phonological development and disorders in Latino children, focusing on those who are Spanish-speaking. Spanish phonology and phonological development in typically developing Spanish-speaking children, Spanish-speaking children with phonological disorders, typically developing bilingual (Spanish-English) children, and bilingual (Spanish-English) children with phonological disorders will be reviewed.

There are five primary vowels in Spanish, the two front vowels, /i/ and /e/, and the three back vowels, /u/, /o/, and /a/. There are 18 phonemes in General Spanish (Núñez-Cedeño and Morales-Front, 1999): the voiceless unaspirated stops, /p/, /t/, and /k/; the voiced stops, /b/, /d/, and /g/; the voiceless fricatives, /f/, /x/, and /s/; the affricate, /tʃ/; the glides, /w/ and /j/; the lateral, /l/; the flap /ɾ/, the trill /r/; and the nasals, /m/, /n/, and /ɲ/. The three voiced stops /b, d, g/ are in complementary distribution with the spirants [β] (voiced bilabial), [ð] (voiced interdental), and [ɣ] (voiced velar), respectively. The spirant allophones most generally occur intervocalically both within and across word boundaries (e.g., /dedo/ (finger) → [deðo]; /la boka/ (the mouth) → [la βoka]) and in word internal consonant clusters (e.g., /ablaɾ/ (to talk) → [aβlaɾ]).

The phonetic inventory of Spanish differs from that of English. Spanish contains some sounds that are not part of the English phonetic system, including the voiced palatal nasal [ɲ], as in [niɲo] (boy), the voiceless bilabial fricative [ɸ], as in [emɸermo] (sick), the voiceless velar fricative [x], as in [relox] (watch), the voiced spirants [β], as in [klaβo] (nail), and [ɣ], as in [laɣo] (lake), the alveolar trill [r], as in [pero] (dog), and the voiced uvular trill [R], as in [Roto] (broken).

As in English, there are a number of dialectal varieties associated with Spanish. In the United States, the two most prevalent dialect groups of Spanish are Southwestern United States (e.g., Mexican Spanish) and Caribbean (e.g., Puerto Rican Spanish) (Iglesias and Goldstein, 1998). Unlike English, in which dialectal variations are generally defined by alterations in vowels, Spanish dialectal differences primarily affect consonants. Specifically, fricatives and liquids (in particular /s/, /ɾ/, and /r/) tend to show more variation than stops, glides, or the affricate.

Common dialectal variations include deletion and/or aspiration of /s/ (e.g., /dos/ (two) → [do] or [doʰ]); deletion of /ɾ/ (e.g., /koɾtar/ (cut) → [kottaɾ]); substitution of [l] or [i] for /ɾ/ (e.g., /koɾtar/ → [koltaɾ/[koitaɾ]); and substitution of [x] or [R] for /r/ (e.g., /pero/ (dog) → [pexo/peRo]. It should be noted that not every feature is always evidenced in the same manner and that not every speaker of a particular dialect uses each and every dialectal feature.

Phonological Development in Monolingual Spanish-Speaking Children. Most of the developmental phonological data on Spanish have been collected from typically developing, monolingual children. Data from segment-based studies suggest that typically developing, preschool, Spanish-speaking children accurately produce most segments by age 3½ years (Maez, 1981). By 5 years, the following phonemes were found *not* to be mastered (produced accurately at least 90% of the time): /g/, /f/, /s/, /ɲ/, /ɾ/, and /r/ (e.g., de la Fuente, 1985; Anderson and Smith, 1987; Acevedo, 1993). By the time Spanish-speaking children reached first grade, there were only a few specific phones on which typically developing children were likely to show any errors at all: the fricatives [x], [s], and [ð], the affricate [tʃ], the flap [ɾ], the trill [r], the lateral [l], and consonant clusters (Evans, 1974; M. M. Gonzalez, 1978; Bailey, 1982).

Studies examining phonological processes indicate that Spanish-speaking children have suppressed (i.e., are no longer productively using) the majority of phonological processes by the time they reach 3½ years of age (e.g., A. Gonzalez, 1981; Mann et al., 1992; Goldstein and Iglesias, 1996a). Commonly occurring phonological processes (percentages of occurrence greater than 10%) included postvocalic singleton omission, stridency deletion, tap/trill /r/, consonant sequence reduction, and final consonant deletion. Less commonly occurring processes (percentages of occurrence greater than 10%) were fronting (both velar and palatal), prevocalic singleton omission, assimilation, and stopping.

Although there have been quite a number of studies characterizing phonological patterns in typically developing Spanish-speaking children, this information remains sparse for Spanish-speaking children with phonological disorders. Goldstein and Iglesias (1993) examined consonant production in Spanish-speaking preschoolers with phonological disorders and found that all stops, the fricative [f], the glides, and the nasals were produced accurately more than 75% of the time. The spirants [β] and [ð], the affricate, the flap [ɾ], the trill [r], and the lateral [l] were produced accurately 50%–74% of the time. Finally, the fricative [s], the spirant [ɣ], and clusters were produced accurately less than 50% of the time.

Phonological development in Spanish-speaking preschool children with phonological disorders has also been examined (Meza, 1983; Goldstein and Iglesias, 1996b). Meza (1983) found that these children showed errors on liquids, stridents, and bilabials in more than 30% of possible occurrences. Goldstein and Iglesias (1996b) found that low-frequency phonological processes (percentages of occurrence less than 15%) were palatal fronting, final consonant deletion, assimilation, velar fronting, and weak syllable deletion. Moderate frequency processes (percentages of occurrence between 15% and 30% for three processes) were initial consonant deletion, liquid simplification, and stopping. The high-frequency process (percentages of occurrence greater than 30%) was cluster reduction. Other error types exhibited by children with phonological disorders that were not usually observed in typically developing, Spanish-speaking children were deaffrication, lisping, and backing.

Phonological Development in Bilingual (Spanish-English) Children. There is increasing evidence that the phonological systems of bilingual (English-Spanish) speakers develop somewhat differently from the phonological system of monolingual speakers of either language. Gildersleeve, Davis, and Stubbe (1996) and Gildersleeve-Neumann and Davis (1998) found that in English, typically developing, bilingual preschoolers showed an overall lower intelligibility rating, made more errors overall (on both consonants and vowels), distorted more sounds, and produced more uncommon error patterns than monolingual children of the same age. Gildersleeve, Davis, and Stubbe (1996) and Gildersleeve-Neumann and Davis (1998) also found higher percentages of occurrence (7%–10% higher) for typically developing, bilingual children (in comparison to their monolingual peers) on a number of phonological processes, including cluster reduction, final consonant deletion, and initial voicing. This discrepancy between monolingual and bilingual speakers, however, does not seem to be absolute across the range of phonological processes commonly exhibited in children of this age. Goldstein and Iglesias (1999) examined English and Spanish phonological skills in 4-, 5-, and 6-year-old, typically developing bilingual children and found that some phonological patterns (e.g., initial consonant deletion and deaffrication) were exhibited at somewhat lower rates in bilingual children with phonological disorders than has been reported for monolingual, Spanish-speaking children with phonological disorders (Goldstein and Iglesias, 1996b). Thus, although the average percentage-of-occurrence difference is not large between monolingual and bilingual speakers, the results indicate that bilingual children will not always exhibit higher percentages of occurrence on phonological processes than monolingual children.

Goldstein and Washington (2001) indicated that the phonological skills of 4-year-old bilingual children were similar to their monolingual counterparts; however, the substitution patterns used for the target sounds flap /ɾ/ and trill /r/ did vary somewhat between bilingual and monolingual speakers. For example, in bilingual children [l] was a common substitute for the trill, but it was a relatively rare substitute for the trill in monolingual children. All four studies also found that bilingual children exhibited error patterns found in both languages (e.g., cluster reduction) as well as those, like liquid gliding, that were typical in one language (English) but atypical in the other (Spanish).

Data from bilingual children with phonological disorders indicate that they exhibit more errors, lower rates of accuracy on consonants, and higher percentages of occurrence for phonological processes than either typically developing, bilingual children (Goldstein and Iglesias, 1999) or monolingual, Spanish-speaking children with phonological disorders (Goldstein and Iglesias, 1996b). The types of errors exhibited by the children, however, are similar regardless of target language (i.e., Spanish versus English). Specifically, bilingual children with phonological disorders showed higher error rates on clusters, fricatives, and liquids than other classes of sounds. Finally, percentages of occurrence for phonological processes were higher overall for bilingual children with phonological disorders than for monolingual, Spanish-speaking children with phonological disorders.

The number of Latino children who speak Spanish continues to increase. Developmental phonological data collected from typically developing, monolingual Latino children who speak Spanish indicate that by age 3½, they use the dialectal features of their speech community and have mastered the majority of sounds in the language. The phonological development of typically developing, bilingual (Spanish-English) speakers is somewhat different from that of monolingual speakers of either language.

—Brian Goldstein

References

Acevedo, M. A. (1993). Development of Spanish consonants in preschool children. *Journal of Childhood Communication Disorders, 15,* 9–15.

Anderson, R., and Smith, B. (1987). Phonological development of two-year-old monolingual Puerto Rican Spanish-speaking children. *Journal of Child Language, 14,* 57–78.

Bailey, S. (1982). *Normative data for Spanish articulatory skills of Mexican children between the ages of six and seven.* Unpublished master's thesis, San Diego State University, San Diego, CA.

de la Fuente, M. T. (1985). *The order of acquisition of Spanish consonant phonemes by monolingual Spanish speaking children between the ages of 2.0 and 6.5.* Unpublished doctoral dissertation, Georgetown University, Washington, DC.

Evans, J. S. (1974). Word pair discrimination and imitation abilities of preschool Spanish-speaking children. *Journal of Learning Disabilities, 7,* 573–580.

Gildersleeve, C., Davis, B., and Stubbe, E. (1996). *When monolingual rules don't apply: Speech development in a bilingual environment.* Paper presented at the annual convention of the American Speech-Language-Hearing Association, Seattle, WA.

Gildersleeve-Neumann, C., and Davis, B. (1998). *Learning English in a bilingual preschool environment: Change over time.* Paper presented at the annual convention of the American Speech-Language-Hearing Association, San Antonio, TX.

Goldstein, B., and Iglesias, A. (1993). *Phonological patterns in speech-disordered Spanish-speaking children.* Paper presented at a convention of the American Speech-Language-Hearing Association, Anaheim, CA.

Goldstein, B., and Iglesias, A. (1996a). Phonological patterns in normally developing Spanish-speaking 3- and 4-year-olds of Puerto Rican descent. *Language, Speech, and Hearing Services in the Schools, 27,* 82–90.

Goldstein, B., and Iglesias, A. (1996b). Phonological patterns in Puerto Rican Spanish-speaking children with phonological disorders. *Journal of Communication Disorders, 29,* 367–387.

Goldstein, B., and Iglesias, A. (1999, February). *Phonological patterns in bilingual (Spanish-English) children.* Seminar presented at the 1999 Texas Research Symposium on Language Diversity, Austin, TX.

Goldstein, B., and Washington, P. (2001). An initial investigation of phonological patterns in 4-year-old typically developing Spanish-English bilingual children. *Language, Speech, and Hearing Services in the Schools, 32,* 153–164.

Gonzalez, A. (1981). *A descriptive study of phonological development in normal speaking Puerto Rican preschoolers.* Unpublished doctoral dissertation, Pennsylvania State University, State College, PA.

Gonzalez, M. M. (1978). *Cómo detectar al niño con problemas del habla* (Identifying speech disorders in children). México: Editorial Trillas.

Hawk, S. (1936). Speech defects in handicapped children. *Journal of Speech Disorders, 1,* 101–106.

Iglesias, A., and Goldstein, B. (1998). Language and dialectal variations. In J. Bernthal and N. Bankson (Eds.), *Articulation and phonological disorders* (4th ed., pp. 148–171). Needham Heights, MA: Allyn and Bacon.

Maez, L. (1981). *Spanish as a first language.* Unpublished doctoral dissertation, University of California, Santa Barbara.

Mann, D. P., Kayser, H., Watson, J., and Hodson, B. (1992, November). *Phonological systems of Spanish-speaking Texas preschoolers.* Paper presented at the annual convention of the American Speech-Language-Hearing Association, San Antonio, TX.

Meza, P. (1983). *Phonological analysis of Spanish utterances of highly unintelligible Mexican-American children.* Unpublished master's thesis, San Diego State University, San Diego, CA.

Núñez-Cedeño, R., and Morales-Front, A. (1999). *Fonología generativa contemporánea de la lengua española* (Contemporary generative phonology of the Spanish language). Washington, DC: Georgetown University Press.

Wellman, B., Case, I., Mengert, I., and Bradbury, D. (1931). *Speech sounds of young children* (University of Iowa Studies in Child Welfare No. 5). Iowa City: University of Iowa Press.

Further Readings

Cotton, E., and Sharp, J. (1988). *Spanish in the Americas.* Washington, DC: Georgetown University Press.

Dalbor, J. (1980). *Spanish pronunciation: Theory and practice* (2nd ed.). New York: Holt, Rinehart and Winston.

Eblen, R. (1982). A study of the acquisition of fricatives by three-year-old children learning Mexican Spanish. *Language and Speech, 25,* 201–220.

Fantini, A. (1985). *Language acquisition of a bilingual child: A sociolinguistic perspective (to age 10).* San Diego, CA: College-Hill Press.

Goldstein, B. (1995). Spanish phonological development. In H. Kayser (Ed.), *Bilingual speech-language pathology: An Hispanic focus* (pp. 17–38). San Diego, CA: Singular Publishing Group.

Goldstein, B. (1996). The role of stimulability in the assessment and treatment of Spanish-speaking children. *Journal of Communication Disorders, 29,* 299–314.

Goldstein, B. (2000). *Cultural and linguistic diversity resource guide for speech-language pathology.* San Diego, CA: Singular Publishing Group.

Goldstein, B. (2001). Assessing phonological skills in Hispanic/Latino children. *Seminars in Speech and Language, 22,* 39–49.

Goldstein, B., and Cintron, P. (2001). An investigation of phonological skills in Puerto Rican Spanish-speaking 2-year-olds. *Clinical Linguistics and Phonetics, 15,* 343–361.

Goldstein, B., and Pollock, K. (2000). Vowel errors in Spanish-speaking children with phonological disorders: A retrospective, comparative study. *Clinical Linguistics and Phonetics, 14,* 217–234.

Gonzalez, G. (1983). The acquisition of Spanish sounds in the speech of two-year-old Chicano children. In R. Padilla (Ed.), *Theory technology and public policy on bilingual education* (pp. 73–87). Rosslyn, VA: National Clearinghouse for Bilingual Education.

Macken, M. (1978). Permitted complexity in phonological development: One child's acquisition of Spanish consonants. *Lingua, 44*, 219–253.

Macken, M., and Barton, D. (1980). The acquisition of the voicing contrast in Spanish: A phonetic and phonological study of word-initial stop consonants. *Journal of Child Language, 7*, 433–458.

Mann, D., and Hodson, B. (1994). Spanish-speaking children's phonologies: Assessment and remediation of disorders. *Seminars in Speech and Language, 15*, 137–147.

Oller, D. K., and Eilers, R. (1982). Similarity of babbling in Spanish- and English-learning babies. *Child Language, 9*, 565–577.

Pandolfi, A. M., and Herrera, M. O. (1990). Producción fonologica diastratica de niños menores de tres años (Phonological production in children less than three years old). *Revista Teorica y Aplicada, 28*, 101–122.

Perez, E. (1994). Phonological differences among speakers of Spanish-influenced English. In J. Bernthal and N. Bankson (Eds.), *Child phonology: Characteristics, assessment, and intervention with special populations* (pp. 245–254). New York: Thieme.

Poplack, S. (1978). Dialect acquisition among Puerto Rican bilinguals. *Language in Society, 7*, 89–103.

Terrell, T. (1981). Current trends in the investigation of Cuban and Puerto Rican phonology. In J. Amastae and L. Elías-Olivares (Eds.), *Spanish in the United States: Sociolinguistic aspects* (pp. 47–70). Cambridge, UK: Cambridge University Press.

Vaquero, M. (1996). Antillas. In M. Alvar (Ed.), *Manual de dialectología Hispánica* (Manual of Hispanic dialectology) (pp. 51–67). Barcelona, Spain: Ariel.

Watson, I. (1991). Phonological processing in two languages. In E. Bialystok (Ed.), *Language processing in bilingual children* (pp. 25–48). Cambridge, UK: Cambridge University Press.

Yavas, M., and Goldstein, B. (1998). Phonological assessment and treatment of bilingual speakers. *American Journal of Speech-Language Pathology, 7*, 49–60.

Speech Sampling, Articulation Tests, and Intelligibility in Children with Phonological Errors

Children who have speech sound disorders can reasonably be separated into two distinct groups. One group comprises children for whom intelligibility is a primary issue and who tend to use many phonological processes, especially deletion processes. These children are generally in the preschool age range. The second group includes children who have residual errors, that is, substitution and distortion errors that are relatively few in number. These children are typically of school age, and intelligibility is better than in the first group. The first group, namely children with phonological difficulties, is the focus of this entry.

In most cases, when we assess speech production in a preschool child, the purposes of the assessment are to describe the child's phonological system and make decisions about management, if needed. A good audio- or video-recorded speech sample from play interactions with parents or the clinician can capture all of the primary data needed to describe the system, or it can be supplemented with a single-word test instrument. Typically, we define an adequate conversational speech sample as one that includes at least 100 different words (Crystal, 1982). Additionally, these words should not be direct or immediate repetitions of an adult model. Finally, for children with poor intelligibility, it is helpful for the examiner to repeat what he believes the child said after each utterance so that this spoken gloss is also recorded on the tape.

Once the recording has been made, the next task is for the examiner to gloss and transcribe the speech sample, ideally using narrow transcription (Edwards, 1986; Shriberg and Kent, 2003). Professionals who frequently do extensive transcription may wish to use a computer-based system. (See Masterson, Long, and Buder, 1998, for an excellent review of such software.) However, such systems are only as good as the clinician's memory for the symbols and diacritics and her memory of their location on the keyboard; consequently, doing transcription by hand may be the more reliable way to go about this task if one does not do it frequently.

With the transcript in hand, the clinician now has a choice of types of analyses. First of all, one can undertake both independent and relational analyses (Stoel-Gammon and Dunn, 1985). Independent analyses treat the child's system as self-contained, that is, with no reference to the adult system. They include a phonetic inventory for consonants and perhaps for vowels, as well as tallies of syllable or word shapes. Relational analyses, on the other hand, explicitly compare the child's production to that of the adult, including a segmental (phonemic) inventory for consonants and perhaps for vowels and a list of the phonological processes that the child uses.

Independent analyses are appropriate for children who are very young, or who have very poor intelligibility, or who appear to use few differentiated speech sounds. Clinicians typically devise their own forms for these analyses, although some of the software mentioned above permits certain of these independent analyses to be done automatically. Frequency of use is an issue in independent analyses, so the various phones and syllable structures that appear in the transcript should be tallied on the inventory form. It is helpful to structure these forms into major consonant classes and major vowel classes, as well as syllable position—syllable-initial, syllable-final, and intervocalic. In addition, for some types of analysis, separate inventories should be done for one-, two-, and three-syllable utterances or words.

One kind of relational analysis, the segmental or phonemic inventory, which compares the child's production to the adult target, is more familiar to clinicians because it resembles typical published tests of articulation and phonology. Phonological process analysis is also considered to be relational in nature. If clinicians are working from a transcript of conversational speech, all of the software mentioned earlier can provide at least a list of phonological processes. Alternatively, clinicians may again devise their own forms for the segmental inventories and the list of phonological processes. Typically, the list of phonological processes will include the 8–10 processes commonly listed in texts and tests of phonology, as well as any unique or idiosyncratic processes that the child uses. The examiner then goes through the transcript noting what the child produces for each adult form. These productions are also tallied.

One other important measure that is relational in nature is the Percentage of Consonants Correct (PCC; Shriberg and Kwiatkowski, 1982). The number of adult targets that the child attempts is tallied, using the standards of colloquial speech, and the number of targets that the child produces acceptably is also tallied. Simple division of these tallies results in the PCC. The PCC is considered to be a measure of severity. It is a useful measure for assessing change over long periods of treatment, such as 6 months.

Tests of Phonology.   Several tests published commercially permit analysis of children's use of phonological processes on the basis of single-word naming of objects or pictures. They include the Bernthal-Bankson Test of Phonology (BBTOP; Bernthal and Bankson, 1990), the Khan-Lewis Phonological Analysis (KLPA; Khan and Lewis, 1986), and the Smit-Hand Articulation and Phonology Evaluation (SHAPE; Smit and Hand, 1997), all of which are based on pictures or photos, and the Assessment of Phonological Processes–Revised (APP-R; Hodson, 1986), which is based on object naming.

Tests of phonology can complement analyses of the conversational sample. One of their virtues is that for the phonological processes that are assessed, they incorporate multiple exemplars of each process, so that there is some assurance that the child's use of the process is not happenstance. For some extremely unintelligible children, tests of phonology may be the only way to figure out the child's patterns because the clinician at least knows what the intended word should be. Some of these tests (BBTOP, KLPA, and SHAPE) also permit comparisons to be made between the child's performance and normative data.

On the other hand, if a test of phonology becomes the primary assessment tool, the clinician needs to be aware that measures derived from single-word naming may differ from measures derived from conversation. The conversational speech of disordered children generally includes more nonadult productions than does single-word naming. In addition, tests of phonology tend to deal with a very circumscribed set of phonological processes, and they do not deal at all with vowel productions. Consequently, if the child uses important but idiosyncratic processes, such as glottal replacement, or has systematic vowel errors, they may not be picked up.

(However, SHAPE has an extensive list of potential idiosyncratic processes in an appendix, along with instructions for determining the frequency of use of these processes.)

Specialized testing using single-word stimuli may be required for specific treatment orientations. For example, in order to carry out a generative analysis, Elbert and Gierut (1986) have developed a test with more than 300 items in which bound morphemes, such as *re-* (meaning *again*) or the diminutive *-y* or *-ie*, are added to the word at either end. The purpose is to determine whether the child changes an error production of the first consonant or the last consonant in the presence of the morphological addition and changes it in a way that clarifies the child's underlying representation.

Another example of specialized testing using either single words or connected speech is the elicitation of data needed for nonlinear analysis (Bernhardt and Stoel-Gammon, 1994). Nonlinear approaches deal with the hierarchies of representation of words, for example, at the segmental level, the syllable level, the foot level, and so on. Productions of multisyllabic words with varying stress patterns are needed to complete these analyses. In most cases these multisyllabic words must be elicited by imitation or picture naming.

Finally, an altogether different type of specialized testing is the determination of stimulability. A child is said to be stimulable for an error sound if the clinician can elicit an acceptable production using models, cues, or phonetic placement instructions. This part of the assessment is often performed informally and usually for just a few error sounds. However, Perrine, Bain, and Weston (2000) have devised a systematic way to assess stimulability based on a hierarchy of cues and models that is helpful in planning intervention.

Intelligibility.   Intelligibility refers to how well the child's words can be understood by others. There are at least two measures of intelligibility that are based on counts of intelligible words, as well as many scales for making perceptual judgments of intelligibility. The most straightforward numerical measure, Percent of Intelligible Words (PIW), has been described by Shriberg and Kwiatkowski (1982). To determine this measure, a person who does not know the child listens to the conversational speech sample but does not hear the clinician's comments. This person attempts to gloss the sample. The number of words correctly glossed by the listener is divided by the total number of words to obtain the PIW.

A second measure based on counts, the Preschool Intelligibility Measure, has been developed by Morris, Wilcox, and Schooling (1995). The child is asked to imitate a series of one- or two-syllable words that are selected randomly from a large database of words, and her productions are recorded. Then the audiotape is played for listeners, who see 12 foils for each word and circle the one they think the child said. This measure is better suited for documenting changes in intelligibility over time than it is for initial evaluation.

Other scales of intelligibility involve judgments on the part of the clinician or significant others in the child's environment about how well the child communicates. For example, teachers might be asked to rate how well they understand the child on a 6-point scale, with 1 representing "all the time" and 6 representing "never." Or a parent might be asked to rate the difficulty that family members have in understanding the child.

Treatment Decisions and Prognosis. Decisions about whether to treat and how often the child should be seen are made primarily on the basis of severity and secondarily on the basis of stimulability. Although there is little research on the topic of appropriate treatment decisions, severity appears to have universal acceptance among speech-language pathologists as the most important variable in deciding for or against treatment.

With respect to prognosis, until recently there has been little research about how children normalize (achieve age-appropriate phonology) and how long it takes. However, work by Shriberg, Gruber, and Kwiatkowski (1994) and by Gruber (1999) suggests that some children who receive intervention normalize by about 6 years of age, and that the outer limit for normalization is about 8.5 years. However, the predictors of normalization are not yet known.

—Ann Bosma Smit

References

Bernhardt, B., and Stoel-Gammon, C. (1994). Nonlinear phonology: Introduction and clinical application. *Journal of Speech and Hearing Research, 37,* 123–143.

Bernthal, J., and Bankson, N. (1990). *Bernthal-Bankson Test of Phonology (BBTOP)*. Chicago, IL: Riverside Press.

Crystal, D. (1982). *Profiling linguistic disability*. London: Edward Arnold.

Edwards, M. L. (1986). *Introduction to applied phonetics: Laboratory workbook*. San Diego, CA: College-Hill Press.

Elbert, M., and Gierut, J. (1986). *Handbook of clinical phonology: Approaches to assessment and treatment*. San Diego, CA: College-Hill Press.

Gruber, F. A. (1999). Probability estimates and paths to consonant normalization in children with speech delay. *Journal of Speech, Language, and Hearing Research, 42,* 448–459.

Hodson, B. (1986). *Assessment of Phonological Processes–Revised (APP-R)*. Danville, IL: Interstate Publishers and Printers.

Khan, L., and Lewis, N. (1986). *The Khan-Lewis Phonological Analysis (KLPA)*. Circle Pines, MN: American Guidance Service.

Masterson, J., Long, S., and Buder, E. (1998). Instrumentation in clinical phonology. In J. E. Bernthal and N. W. Bankson (Eds.), *Articulation and phonological disorders* (4th ed., pp. 378–406). Boston: Allyn and Bacon.

Morris, S. R., Wilcox, K. A., and Schooling, R. L. (1995). The Preschool Intelligibility Measure. *American Journal of Speech-Language Pathology, 4,* 22–28.

Perrine, S. L., Bain, B. A., and Weston, A. D. (2000). *Dynamic assessment of phonological stimulability: Construct validation of a cueing hierarchy*. Paper presented at the annual convention of the American Speech-Language-Hearing Association, Washington, DC, Nov. 16, 2000.

Shriberg, L. D., Gruber, F. A., and Kwiatkowski, J. (1994). Developmental disorders: III. Long-term speech-sound normalization. *Journal of Speech, Language, and Hearing Research, 37,* 1151–1177.

Shriberg, L. D., and Kent, R. D. (2003). *Clinical phonetics* (3rd ed.). Boston: Allyn and Bacon.

Shriberg, L. D., and Kwiatkowski, J. (1982). Phonological disorders: III. A procedure for assessing severity of involvement. *Journal of Speech and Hearing Disorders, 47,* 256–270.

Smit, A., and Hand, L. (1997). *Smit-Hand Articulation and Phonology Evaluation (SHAPE)*. Los Angeles, CA: Western Psychological Services.

Stoel-Gammon, C., and Dunn, C. (1985). *Normal and disordered phonology in children*. Austin, TX: Pro-Ed.

Further Readings

Bauman-Waengler, J. (2000). *Articulatory and phonological impairments: A clinical focus*. Boston, MA: Allyn and Bacon.

Bernthal, J. E., and Bankson, N. W. (1998). *Articulation and phonological disorders* (4th ed.). Boston: Allyn and Bacon.

Perrine, S. L., Bain, B. A., and Weston, A. D. (2000). Dynamic assessment of phonological stimulability: Construct validation of a cueing hierarchy. Paper presented at the annual convention of the American Speech-Language-Hearing Association, Washington, DC, Nov. 16, 2000.

Shriberg, L. D. (1994). Five subtypes of developmental phonological disorders. *Clinics in Communication Disorders, 4,* 38–53.

Shriberg, L. D., and Kent, R. D. (2003). *Clinical phonetics* (3rd ed.). Allyn and Bacon.

Shriberg, L. D., and Kwiatkowski, J. (1982). Phonological disorders III: A procedure for assessing severity of involvement. *Journal of Speech and Hearing Disorders, 47,* 256–270.

Smit, A., Hand, L., Freilinger, J., Bernthal, J., and Bird, A. (1990). The Iowa Articulation Norms Project and its Nebraska replication. *Journal of Speech and Hearing Disorders, 55,* 779–798.

Stoel-Gammon, C., and Dunn, C. (1985). *Normal and disordered phonology in children*. Austin, TX: Pro-Ed.

Tomblin, J. B., Morris, H. L., and Spriestersbach, D. C., (Eds.). (2000). *Diagnosis in speech-language pathology* (2nd ed.). San Diego, CA: Singular Publishing Group.

Speech Sampling, Articulation Tests, and Intelligibility in Children with Residual Errors

Children who have speech sound errors that have persisted past the preschool years are considered to have residual errors (Shriberg, 1994). Typically, these school-age children have substitution and distortion errors rather than deletions, and intelligibility is not usually a primary issue. Children with residual errors generally have acquired the sound system of their language, but they have errors that draw attention to the speaking pattern. The assumption is usually made that they are having difficulty with the articulatory movements needed to produce the acceptable sound and with embedding that sound into the stream of speech. It should be noted, however, that in the early days of studying communication disorders, authorities such as Van Riper (1978) assumed that the child's difficulty was first of all perceptual.

Until recently, there has been little research about how residual speech sound errors develop, even though some of the earliest research and intervention in communication disorders focused on children with residual errors. The profession has uncovered bits and pieces of information about development after the preschool period, but no coherent picture has emerged to assist in predicting which children will actually make needed changes without intervention. The question is an important one, because if we fail to treat a child at age 6 who is not going to change spontaneously, and instead we wait until age 9, the child has 3 additional years of practice on an error phoneme, and remediation will likely be more difficult. Certain information that can be obtained from speech sampling may provide insight into the prediction question:

- Most residual errors affect a subset of the phonemes of English ("the big 10"): /s z ʃ ʒ tʃ dʒ θ ð v r/ (Winitz, 1969). These are typically late-acquired phonemes, but most of them are used correctly by 90% of children by age 8 (Smit et al., 1990).
- The phoneme in error may make a difference. Reanalysis of the Smit et al. (1990) cross-sectional data suggests that children may be less likely to self-correct the alveolar and palatal fricatives and affricates than they are the /r/ and the /θ ð/ (Smit, unpublished).
- The nature and allophonic distribution of the error may make a difference. Stephens, Hoffman, and Daniloff (1986) showed that children with lateral productions of alveolopalatal fricatives and children who substituted back sounds for these fricatives generally did not improve spontaneously, whereas about half of the children with dental errors corrected them. Hoffman, Schuckers, and Daniloff (1980) showed that children who produced the consonantal /r/ allophone correctly some of the time were likely to achieve the other /r/-allophones spontaneously.
- The length of time that the child has made the error may make a difference. It is reasonable to assume that if a child's production of a phoneme has not changed at all in several years, then spontaneous change is unlikely.
- The child's developmental history may make a difference. Shriberg (1994) has pointed out that some children had phonological errors as preschoolers, while others did not. On logical grounds, children who had phonological problems earlier are less likely to change without intervention because they have already demonstrated difficulties in learning the sound system of their native language.
- The pattern of change in the child's errors may be important. Recent research by Gruber (1999) into the time taken for children who are receiving intervention to normalize (achieve age-appropriate phonology) has

provided some clues about prognosis. For example, it appears that if the child reduces substitutions and omissions while increasing distortions, that child will take longer to normalize than the child who decreases all types of errors.

Speech Sampling. Speech-language pathologists typically elicit a speech sample using a published test of articulation, supplemented with a conversational speech sample. For a school-age child, the conversational sample should be audio- or video-recorded, with careful attention to the quality of the recording. This sample should include at least 100 different words and 3 minutes of child talking time. If the child has a relatively large number of errors, this speech sample can be transcribed phonetically for further analysis. If the child has just a few sounds in error, then the clinician may decide not to transcribe the entire speech sample. Instead, he tallies all instances of a target phoneme in the sample, determines how many were acceptably produced, and derives a percentage of correctly produced sounds. When these counts are based on a 3-minute sample, this procedure results in a TALK sample (Diedrich, 1971), which is a probe of conversational speech.

Articulation Tests. Some of the first tests that were commercially available in communication disorders were tests of articulation and were designed to assess the development of speech sounds. Typically, tests of this type are based on the single-word naming of pictures without a model from the examiner. Most tests of articulation assess production of all English consonant phonemes in word-initial and word-final position, and possibly English consonant clusters as well. Scoring sheets usually allow explicit comparisons between adult targets and the children's productions. Most articulation tests result in a summary numerical score that can be compared to normative data. Some currently used tests of articulation include the Templin-Darley Tests of Articulation (Templin and Darley, 1969), the Goldman-Fristoe Test of Articulation—2 (Goldman and Fristoe, 2000), the Smit-Hand Articulation and Phonology Evaluation (SHAPE; Smit and Hand, 1997), and the Photo Articulation Test—Third Edition (Lippke et al., 1987).

Most of the inventory tests do not require that the clinician use narrow transcription, the exception being SHAPE. Rather, broad transcription is generally used, even when the test requires only a notation of "correct," "substitution," "omission," or "distortion."

The error sounds identified on an inventory test are often examined in light of "ages of acquisition" for those sounds. The age of acquisition is the age at which 75% or 90% of children typically say the sound correctly (Templin, 1957; Smit et al., 1990). The guidelines used by many school districts to determine caseload make reference to these ages of acquisition.

There are other types of tests of articulation besides inventory tests. In particular, there are several tests of contextual variation, among them the McDonald Deep Test of Articulation (McDonald, 1964), the Contextual

Test of Articulation (Aase et al., 2000), and the Secord Contextual Articulation Tests (S-CAT; Secord and Shine, 1997). Contextual variation is a way of manipulating the phonetic environment of a target sound in order to see if the client can produce the target sound acceptably in one or more of these novel phonetic environments. If the child is able to do so, then the clinician can use these facilitating contexts in the first few treatment sessions.

Still another kind of assessment involves determining stimulability. Stimulability refers to the ability to elicit an acceptable production of a speech sound or structure, such as a consonant cluster, from the child by presenting instructions, cues, and models. A systematic way to assess stimulability has been proposed by Perrine, Bain, and Weston (2000). The implications of stimulability have been addressed by numerous researchers, but that research can be summed up in a few statements:

1. The child who is not stimulable for a specific phoneme target is the child who should have the highest priority for intervention.
2. If a child is stimulable for a target phoneme, the child may or may not improve without intervention.
3. Stimulable phonemes are likely to bring about quick success in intervention.

Finally, the clinician may assess inconsistency. Inconsistency refers to variations in the child's productions of a given phoneme. If the child's production is characterized by "inconsistency with hits" (correct productions), then the context of the hits can be determined. Just as in the case for contextual variation, a hit can serve as an entrée into intervention. To look for inconsistencies, the clinician may catalogue the productions of the target that are heard in the conversational speech sample. Alternatively, she can administer the Story-Telling Probes of Articulation Competence from the S-CAT (Secord and Shine, 1997).

Intelligibility.   Intelligibility is defined as a listener's ability to understand a speaker's words. Although intelligibility of speech can be reduced in children who have residual errors, the reduction often is not substantial. One exception is the child who may have a few distortions of phonemes but who has particular difficulty in stringing sounds together in multisyllabic utterances. This difficulty may manifest itself as weak or imprecise articulations of sounds, along with deletions of some consonants. In such cases, the examining clinician may want to repeat what she understood the child to say immediately afterward, so that her gloss is also recorded on the tape when the conversational speech sample is recorded.

The standard way to assess intelligibility in a numerical way is to have a person who is not familiar with the child listen to the audio recording of the conversational sample, but without hearing the examiner's speech. This person writes down the child's words. This gloss is compared to the one generated by the examining clinician,

and a Percent of Intelligible Words is calculated (Shriberg and Kwiatkowski, 1982).

For children with residual speech sound errors, a more salient issue than intelligibility may be that their errors call attention to their speech, that is, to the medium rather than the message. Listeners may consider their speech to be babyish, bizarre, or odd. The clinician can develop questionnaires and rating scales and can ask persons familiar with the child to fill them out in order to document this perception, in addition to asking the child about the content of any teasing that may occur.

Interpreting the Data.   Decisions about whether to provide intervention are often based on multiple factors. These include the child's age relative to the age of acquisition for the child's error phonemes, whether or not the child is stimulable for correct production, intelligibility, and the degree to which the child and significant others consider the speech to be a problem. There is little research other than that of Gruber (1999) to go by in establishing prognosis. However, a reasonable assumption is that the older the child who has residual errors, the longer it will take to achieve normalization in a treatment program.

—*Ann Bosma Smit*

References

Aase, D., Hovre, C., Krause, K., Schelfhout, S., Smith, J., and Carpenter, L. J. (2000). *Contextual Test of Articulation.* Eau Claire, WI: Thinking Publications.

Diedrich, W. (1971). Procedures for counting and charting a target phoneme. *Language, Speech, and Hearing Services in Schools, 18*–32.

Goldman, R., and Fristoe, M. (2000). *Goldman-Fristoe Test of Articulation—2.* Circle Pines, MN: American Guidance Service.

Gruber, F. A. (1999). Probability estimates and paths to consonant normalization in children with speech delay. *Journal of Speech, Language, and Hearing Research, 42,* 448–459.

Hoffman, P. R., Schuckers, G. H., and Daniloff, R. G. (1980). Developmental trends in correct /r/ articulation as a function of allophone type. *Journal of Speech and Hearing Research, 23,* 746–755.

Lippke, B. A., Dickey, S. E., Selmar, J. W., and Soder, A. L. (1987). *Photo Articulation Test—Third Edition.* Los Angeles, CA: Western Psychological Services.

McDonald, E. (1964). *A Deep Test of Articulation.* Pittsburgh, PA: Stanwix House.

Perrine, S. L., Bain, B. A., and Weston, A. D. (2000). *Dynamic assessment of phonological stimulability: Construct validation of a cueing hierarchy.* Paper presented at the annual convention of the American Speech-Language-Hearing Association, Washington, DC, Nov. 16, 2000.

Secord, W. A., and Shine, R. E. (1997). *Secord Contextual Articulation Tests.* Salt Lake City, UT: Red Rock Publishing.

Shriberg, L. D. (1994). Five subtypes of developmental phonological disorders. *Clinics in Communication Disorders, 4,* 38–53.

Shriberg, L. D., and Kwiatkowski, J. (1982). Phonological disorders: III. A procedure for assessing severity of involvement. *Journal of Speech and Hearing Disorders, 47,* 256–270.

Smit, A., and Hand, L. (1997). *Smit-Hand Articulation and Phonology Evaluation*. Los Angeles, CA: Western Psychological Services.

Smit, A., Hand, L., Freilinger, J., Bernthal, J., and Bird, A. (1990). The Iowa Articulation Norms Project and its Nebraska replication. *Journal of Speech and Hearing Disorders, 55*, 779–798.

Stephens, I., Hoffman, P., and Daniloff, R. (1986). Phonetic characteristics of delayed /s/ development. *Journal of Phonetics, 14*, 247–256.

Templin, M. C. (1957). *Certain language skills in children*. Westport, CT: Greenwood Press.

Templin, M., and Darley, F. (1969). *The Templin-Darley Tests of Articulation*. Iowa City: University of Iowa, Bureau of Education Research and Service.

Van Riper, C. (1978). *Speech correction: Principles and methods* (6th ed.). Englewood Cliffs, NJ: Prentice-Hall.

Winitz, H. (1969). *Articulatory acquisition and behavior*. Englewood Cliffs, NJ: Prentice-Hall, Inc.

Further Readings

See the list for SPEECH SAMPLING, ARTICULATION TESTS, AND INTELLIGIBILITY IN CHILDREN WITH PHONOLOGICAL ERRORS.

Speech Sound Disorders in Children: Description and Classification

Children with speech sound disorders form a heterogeneous group whose problems differ in severity, scope, etiology, course of recovery, and social consequences. Beyond manifest problems with speech production and use, their problems can include reduced intelligibility, risk for broader communication disorders, and academic difficulties, as well as social stigma.

Because of the heterogeneity of children's speech sound disorders, the description and classification of these disorders have been attempted from a variety of perspectives, with persisting controversy as a predictable result. Nonetheless, one distinction that has garnered relatively universal support is the division of children's speech disorders into those that are developmental (with onset in early or middle childhood, e.g., before age 9) and those that are nondevelopmental (occurring after that time period and resulting from known causes). Developmental disorders have received substantially more research attention to date.

A second widely accepted distinction separates developmental disorders with known causes from those without. For developmental speech disorders of known causes in children, the terminology has been relatively stable and has typically referenced etiological factors (e.g., speech disorders due to mental retardation, cleft palate). In contrast, the terminology for children's speech disorders of unknown origin is less stable, reflecting uncertainty about their nature and origin. During the past 30 years, commonly used terms have included functional articulation disorders, phonological disorders (Locke, 1983), articulation and phonological disorders (Bernthal and Bankson, 1998), and persistent sound system disorders (Shelton, 1993).

Proposed classifications of child speech disorders have been advanced along descriptive, predictive, and clinical grounds (Shriberg, 1994). Three classifications currently warrant particular attention either because of empirical support (those associated with Shriberg and Dodd) or practical significance (the *Diagnostic and Statistical Manual of Mental Disorders-IV-TR*; American Psychiatric Association, 2000).

Currently, the most comprehensive and rigorously studied classification is the Speech Disorders Classification System, developed through a 20-year program of research by Shriberg and his colleagues (Shriberg, 1994, 1999; Shriberg and Kwiatkowski, 1982, 1994a, 1994b, 1994c; Shriberg et al., 1997). This evolving classification is designed to provide a framework for identifying and describing subtypes and testing etiological hypotheses. At this time, it is primarily a research tool.

Within this classification, children's speech sound disorders of unknown origin are divided into speech delay and residual error categories. Speech delay, with an estimated prevalence of 3.8% among 6-year-olds (Shriberg, Tomblin, and McSweeney, 1999), is characterized by reduced intelligibility and increased risk for broader communication and academic difficulties. It encompasses more severe forms of speech disorder. Residual speech errors, with a tentatively estimated prevalence of 5% among individuals older than age 9 (Shriberg, 1994), is characterized by the presence of at least one speech sound error (often involving distortion of a sibilant fricative or liquid) that persists past the developmental period. Although the category of residual speech errors encompasses less severe forms of speech disorder that are associated with neither reduced intelligibility nor broader communication difficulties, disorders in this category remain of interest for theoretical reasons (i.e., genetic versus environmental origin) and for their potential social and vocational costs, which for some individuals can continue throughout life.

Within the Speech Disorders Classification System, the major categories of speech delay and residual speech errors are further divided according to suspected etiological factors or developmental pattern. Five subtypes of speech delay are postulated in relation to the following possible causes: genetic transmission, early history of recurrent otitis media with effusion (Shriberg et al., 2000), motor speech involvement associated with developmental apraxia of speech (Shriberg, Aram, and Kwiatkowski, 1997), motor speech involvement associated with mild dysarthria, and developmental psychosocial involvement. In each case the etiological factor is considered dominant in a mechanism that is suspected to be multifactorial in nature. Two subtypes of residual speech errors are proposed, those found in association with a documented history of speech delay (residual error-A) and those for which no previous history of speech disorder was reported (residual error-B) (e.g., Shriberg et al., 2001). Ongoing research is aimed at increasing understanding of the causal, developmental, and cognitive processing mechanisms underlying each of these five subtypes.

The classification description described by Dodd (1995) is well motivated from theoretical perspectives and based on processing accounts of child speech disorders, but has been less thoroughly validated than the Speech Disorders Classification System. Nontheless, Dodd's classification system has been supported by studies that examine characteristics of clinical populations (Dodd, 1995), error patterns across languages (e.g., Fox and Dodd, 2001), bilingual children's generalization patterns (Holm and Dodd, 2001), and treatment efficacy (Dodd and Bradford, 2000). Thus, its empirical support is growing rapidly. It is intended primarily to be used to aid in differential diagnosis and clinical management, and was proposed as a system that uniquely combined four historical approaches to classifying speech disorders. These four approaches were based on age at onset, severity, causal and maintenance factors, and description of symptoms, respectively.

Dodd's classification system recognizes five subtypes: articulation disorder, delayed phonological acquisition, consistent deviant disorder, inconsistent disorder, and other. Within this system, an articulation disorder is defined as inability to produce an undistorted version of a speech sound or sounds that are expected, given the child's age. English sounds that are often affected in such disorders include /s/, /r/, and the interdental fricatives. This label is applied regardless of whether the cause is an anatomical anomaly or is unknown. Delayed phonological acquisition is defined in cases where a child's speech errors are consistent with those seen in younger, normally developing children. Consistent deviant disorder is the label applied when a child demonstrates a reduced variety of syllable structure use as well as errors that are atypical of those seen in normal development.

Inconsistent disorder is identified when a child's productions are inconsistent in ways that cannot be explained by complex phonological rules or the effects of linguistic load on production. Ozanne (1995) described a study suggesting that inconsistent disorder represents one subgroup associated with developmental verbal dyspraxia (the condition referred to by Shriberg and others as developmental [or childhood] apraxia of speech). Inconsistent disorder is operationally defined using a 25-item word list. The child is asked to produce each word three times, with inconsistency noted when the child produces at least ten of the words differently on two of the three elicited productions. Dodd's "other" category encompasses suspected motor speech disorders.

The *DSM-IV-TR* (American Psychiatric Association, 2000) classification represents the most streamlined classification of children's speech disorders and one that is perhaps more familiar than others to a broad range of speech pathologists, who use it for billing purposes, and non-speech-language pathologists who come in contact with children with childhood speech disorders. Within this classification, Phonological Disorders 315.39 (formerly Developmental Articulation Disorders) is nested within Communication Disorders. Communication Disorders, in turns, falls under the relatively large category Disorders Usually First Diagnosed in Infancy, Childhood, or Adolescence. This category includes, among others, mental retardation, learning disorders (learning disabilities), and pervasive developmental disorders.

In the most recent *DSM-IV* classification, phonological disorders is defined by the failure to use speech sounds that are expected given the child's age and dialect. Although subtypes are not described, the American Psychiatric Association's description of the category phonological disorders acknowledges that errors may reflect difficulties in peripheral production as well as more abstract difficulties in the child's representation and use of the sound system of the target language. Under comments on differential diagnosis, phonological disorders is described as a possible secondary diagnosis when speech errors in excess of expectations are noted in association with disorders that might be considered known causes for speech difficulties (viz., mental retardation, hearing impairment or other sensory deficit, speech motor deficit, and severe environmental deprivation). Speech difficulties that may be associated with the term "Developmental (or Childhood) Apraxia of Speech" are addressed neither in the *DSM-IV* criteria nor as a subclassification, although that term is described as a possible label for some forms of phonological disorder in *DSM-IV-TR*—a revision designed to increase the currency of the *DSM* without changing the actual classificatory categories.

Classifications of children's speech disorders are encumbered by demands that they address numerous audiences and unresolved controversies. Among the current audiences to be served are clinicians, researchers, and administrators. Each of the three classifications described here addresses those audiences to a different degree. One of the unresolved controversies that has been addressed to some degree by each is the status of clinically postulated entities such as developmental or childhood apraxia of speech. A second controversy, and one that is being addressed by Shriberg and colleagues, relates to how child speech sound disorders should be conceptualized in relation to other communication disorders that frequently co-occur, but are associated with causal mechanisms that are more ill-defined than those for conditions that fall under child speech disorders with known causes (e.g., hearing loss, cleft palate). Two that are of particular interest are specific language impairment (Shriberg, Tomblin, and McSweeney, 1999) and stuttering (Guitar, 1998). In addition, classifications are ideally consistent with developmental as well as psychological processing accounts of the manifest behaviors associated with child speech disorders. The accounts of Shriberg, Dodd, and their colleagues appear to be pursuing these challenging issues.

—*Rebecca J. McCauley*

References

American Psychiatric Association. (1994). *Diagnostic and statistical manual of mental disorders—Fourth edition*. Washington, DC: Author.

American Psychiatric Association. (2000). *Diagnostic and statistical manual of mental disorders—Fourth edition, Text revision (DSM-IV-TR)*. Washington, DC: American Psychiatric Publishing.

Bernthal, J. E., and Bankson, N. W. (1998). *Articulation and phonological disorders*. Boston: Allyn and Bacon.

Dodd, B. (1995). Procedures for classification of subgroups of speech disorder. In B. Dodd (Ed.), *Differential diagnosis and treatment of children with speech disorders* (pp. 49–64). San Diego, CA: Singular Publishing Group.

Dodd, B., and Bradford, A. (2000). A comparison of three therapy methods for children with different types of developmental phonological disorders. *International Journal of Language and Communication Disorders, 35,* 189–209.

Fox, A., and Dodd, B. (2001). Phonologically disordered German-speaking children. *American Journal of Speech-Language Pathology, 10,* 291–307.

Guitar, B. (1998). *Stuttering: An integrated approach to its nature and treatment* (2nd ed.). Baltimore: Williams and Wilkins.

Holm, A., and Dodd, B. (2001). Comparison of cross language generalisation following speech therapy. *Folia Phoniatrica et Logopaedica, 53,* 166–172.

Locke, J. L. (1983). Clinical phonology: The explanation and treatment of speech sound disorders. *Journal of Speech and Hearing Disorders, 48,* 339–341.

Ozanne, A. (1995). The search for developmental verbal dyspraxia. In B. Dodd (Ed.), *Differential diagnosis and treatment of children with speech disorders* (pp. 231–247). San Diego, CA: Singular Publishing Group.

Shelton, R. L. (Ed.). (1993). Persistent sound system disorder: Nature and treatment. *Seminars in Speech and Language, 14.*

Shriberg, L. D. (1994). Five subtypes of developmental phonological disorders. *Clinics in Communication Disorders, 4,* 38–53.

Shriberg, L. D. (1999). *Emerging profiles for five phonological disorders.* Presented at the Child Phonology Conference, Bangor, Wales.

Shriberg, L. D., Aram, D., and Kwiatkowski, J. (1997a). Developmental apraxia of speech: I. Descriptive perspectives. *Journal of Speech, Language, and Hearing Research, 40,* 273–285.

Shriberg, L. D., Aram, D., and Kwiatkowski, J. (1997b). Developmental apraxia of speech: II. Toward a diagnostic marker. *Journal of Speech, Language, and Hearing Research, 40,* 286–312.

Shriberg, L. D., Aram, D., and Kwiatkowski, J. (1997c). Developmental apraxia of speech: III. A subtype marked by inappropriate stress. *Journal of Speech, Language, and Hearing Research, 40,* 313–337.

Shriberg, L. D., Austin, D., Lewis, B. A., McSweeny, J. L., and Wilson, D. L. (1997). The Speech Disorders Classification System (SDCS): Extensions and lifespan reference data. *Journal of Speech, Language, and Hearing Research, 40,* 723–740.

Shriberg, L. D., Flipsen, P., Jr., Karlsson, H. B., and McSween, J. L. (2001). Acoustic phenotypes for speech-genetic studies: An acoustic marker for residual /er/ distortions. *Clinical Linguistics and Phonetics, 15,* 631–650.

Shriberg, L. D., Friel-Patti, S., Flipsen, P., Jr., and Brown, R. L. (2000). Otitis media, fluctuant hearing loss, and speech-language outcomes: A preliminary structural equation model. *Journal of Speech, Language, and Hearing Research, 43,* 100–120.

Shriberg, L. D., and Kwiatkowski, J. (1982). Phonological disorders: II. A diagnostic classification system. *Journal of Speech and Hearing Disorders, 47,* 226–241.

Shriberg, L. D., and Kwiatkowski, J. (1994a). Developmental phonological disorders: I. A clinical profile. *Journal of Speech and Hearing Research, 37,* 1100–1126.

Shriberg, L. D., and Kwiatkowski, J. (1994b). Developmental phonological disorders: II. Short-term speech-sound normalization. *Journal of Speech and Hearing Research, 37,* 1127–1150.

Shriberg, L. D., and Kwiatkowski, J. (1994c). Developmental phonological disorders: II. Long-term speech-sound normalization. *Journal of Speech and Hearing Research, 37,* 1151–1177.

Shriberg, L. D., Tomblin, J. B., and McSweeney, J. L. (1999). Prevalence of speech delay in 6-year-old children and comorbidity with language impairment. *Journal of Speech, Language, and Hearing Research, 42,* 1461–1481.

Further Readings

Felsenfeld, S., Broen, P. A., and McGue, M. (1992). A 28-year follow-up of adults with a history of moderate phonological disorder: Linguistic and personality results. *Journal of Speech and Hearing Research, 35,* 1114–1125.

Felsenfeld, S., Broen, P. A., and McGue, M. (1994). A 28-year follow-up of adults with a history of moderate phonological disorder: Educational and occupational results. *Journal of Speech and Hearing Research, 37,* 1341–1353.

Goodyer, I. M. (2001). Language difficulties and psychopathology. In D. V. M. Bishop and L. B. Leonard (Eds.), *Speech and language impairments in children: Causes, characteristics, intervention, and outcome* (pp. 227–244). Philadelphia: Taylor and Francis.

Holm, A., and Dodd, B. (1999). An intervention case study of a bilingual child with phonological disorder. *Child Language Teaching and Therapy, 15,* 139–158.

Holm, A., Ozanne, A., and Dodd, B. (1997). Efficacy of intervention for a bilingual child making articulation and phonological errors. *International Journal of Bilingualism, 1,* 55–69.

So, L., and Dodd, B. (1994). Phonologically disordered Cantonese-speaking children. *Clinical Linguistics and Phonetics, 8,* 235–255.

Stackhouse, J., and Wells, B. (1997). *Children's speech and literacy difficulties.* London: Whurr.

Zhu, H., and Dodd, B. (2000). Putonghua (modern standard Chinese)-speaking children with speech disorders. *Clinical Linguistics and Phonetics, 14,* 15–191.

Stuttering

Stuttering is a developmental disorder of communication that affects approximately 5% of children born in the United States and Western Europe. Children are at highest risk for beginning to stutter between their second and fourth birthdays. The risk decreases gradually thereafter, with few onsets occurring after 9 or 10 years of age (Andrews and Harris, 1964). The percentage of older children, adolescents, and adults who stutter is much lower, about 0.5%–1.0% (Andrews, 1984; Bloodstein, 1995), and the discrepancy between the percentage of children affected (i.e., incidence) and the percentage of older children and adults who stutter (i.e., prevalence) indicates that 75%–90% of the children who begin to stutter stop. Complete, untreated remissions of stuttering are most likely to occur within 2 years of onset (Andrews and Harris, 1964; Yairi and Ambrose, 1999; Mansson, 2000), with decreasing frequency after that.

Most of the data on the epidemiology of stuttering have been obtained from cross-sectional surveys that asked informants if they or family members currently stutter or had ever stuttered. The credibility of such data is compromised by a number of methodological weaknesses (Yairi, Ambrose, and Cox, 1996). Prospective, longitudinal studies employing trained examiners have been completed in England (Andrews and Harris, 1964) and Denmark (Mansson, 2000). The incidence (5.0%) and remission rate (>75%) reported by both studies were remarkably similar, despite substantial differences in their designs and the populations studied.

The incidence, prevalence, and remission or persistence of stuttering are affected by sex and family histories of stuttering. More than two-thirds of the children who stutter have first-, second-, or third-degree relatives who currently or once stuttered (Ambrose, Yairi, and Cox, 1993). Like most speech-language disorders, stuttering affects more males than females, with about twice as many young male preschoolers affected as females, a ratio that increases to four or more males to every female among adults (Ambrose, Yairi, and Cox, 1993). Similar ratios have been reported in other countries and cultures (Bloodstein, 1995; Ambrose, Cox, and Yairi, 1997; Mansson, 2000). The increase in male-female ratio with age reflects, in part, higher rates of remission among females (Ambrose, Cox, and Yairi, 1997), whereas family histories of remission and persistence are linked, respectively, to untreated remissions of stuttering within 2 years of onset or its persistence for 3 or more years (Ambrose, Cox, and Yairi, 1997).

Findings from family pedigree studies are consistent with the vertical transmission (i.e., generation to generation) of a genetic susceptibility or predisposition to stutter but are inconsistent with autosomal dominant, recessive, or sex-linked transmissions (Kidd, Heimbuch, and Records, 1981; Yairi, Ambrose, and Cox, 1996). Twin studies have found that stuttering occurs in both members of monozygotic twin pairs much more often than in same-sex, dizygotic twins (e.g., Howie, 1981); however, the lack of concordance of stuttering in some monozygotic twin pairs indicates that both genetic and environmental factors are involved in some, if not all, cases. Segregation analyses suggest that a single major locus is a primary contributor to stuttering phenotypes but that other genes are involved in determining whether or not stuttering persists (Ambrose, Cox, and Yairi, 1997). Research centers in the United States and Europe are currently engaged in linkage analyses designed to identify the specific genes involved.

Current etiological theories reflect diverse beliefs about the nature of stuttering, its origins, and the levels of description that will provide the most useful scientific explanation. However, no theory of origin has achieved general acceptance in the field. There are, for example, cognitive theories, such as Bloodstein's (1997) anticipatory struggle theory, which hypothesizes that a child's belief that speech is difficult elicits tension that causes stuttering when he or she tries to speak; psycholinguistic theories (e.g., Ratner, 1997), which propose that the lin-

guistic processes responsible for everyday speech errors are also responsible for developmental stuttering; motor control theories, which link stuttering to sensorimotor or speech motor processes (e.g., Neilson and Neilson, 1987); and multifactor theories, which attribute stuttering to an interplay of the cognitive, linguistic, motor, and affective processes involved in spoken language (e.g., Perkins, Kent, and Curlee, 1991; Smith and Kelly, 1997).

Adult stuttering typically involves various behaviors and affective-cognitive reactions that affect, in varying degrees, interpersonal communication, vocational opportunities, and personal-social adjustment. Frequent repetitions and prolongations of sounds and syllables and blockages of speech occur that cannot be readily controlled (Perkins, 1990). These speech disruptions are often accompanied by facial grimaces and tremors, disrhythmic phonation, and extraneous bodily movements that seem to involve muscle tension and excessive effort.

Stuttering does not occur randomly, but as if constrained by various linguistic variables (Ratner, 1997). For example, it occurs more often than chance would suggest on initial words of phrases, clauses, and sentences, on stressed syllables, and on longer, less familiar words. With the exception of the sentence-initial position, these are the same loci that attract the speech errors of nonstuttering speakers (Fromkin, 1993), suggesting that the same linguistic variables affect both groups' speech.

The frequency and severity of adults' stuttering may vary substantially across time, social settings, and contexts, but it often occurs on specific words (e.g., the person's name) and in situations where stuttering has frequently occurred in the past (Bloodstein, 1995). Thus, adults' prior stuttering experiences may lead them to avoid specific words and speaking situations and to develop attitudes and beliefs about speaking, stuttering, and themselves that can be more disabling or handicapping than their stuttered speech.

Stuttering is substantially reduced, sometimes eliminated, in a number of verbal activities (Bloodstein, 1995). For example, most adults stutter little or not at all when singing, speaking while alone or with pets or infants, reading or reciting in unison with others, pacing speech with a rhythmical stimulus, and reading or speaking with auditory masking. Stuttering reappears, however, as soon as such activities end.

Much of what is known about adults who stutter has been obtained by studies that compared stuttering and nonstuttering speakers' motor, sensory, perceptual, and cognitive abilities, as well as the two groups' affective and personality characteristics. A variety of differences have been found, but usually with substantial overlaps in the data of the two groups. In addition, it is seldom clear if or how such differences might be functionally related to stuttering. A comprehensive review of this work led Bloodstein (1995) to conclude that the two groups are similar, for the most part, except when they speak. Recent advances in brain imaging technology, however, have allowed investigators to compare the brain activity patterns of the two groups while the subjects read aloud, and the brain activity of stuttering speakers during stuttered and fluent speech.

There are no reliable differences in cerebral blood flow of stuttering and nonstuttering adult men when they are not speaking (Ingham et al., 1996; Braun et al., 1997). A series of $H_2^{15}O$ positron emission tomography (PET) of the two speaker groups during solo and choral reading conditions found greater right than left hemisphere activity in the supplementary motor and premotor areas (BA 6), anterior insula, and cerebellum and reduced activity in primary auditory areas (BA 41/42) of stuttering speakers in the solo condition, but exactly the opposite pattern of activity in nonstuttering speakers (Ingham, 2001). These differences decreased, however, when fluent speech was induced in stuttering speakers by having them read aloud in unison (i.e., choral reading) with a recording.

A follow-up PET study of subsets of the same two groups was conducted while subjects imagined they were reading aloud (Ingham et al., 2000). Stuttering subjects were instructed to imagine they were stuttering in the solo condition and fluent in the choral condition. The patterns of activity that had occurred when each group read aloud were similar to those observed when speakers merely imagined they were reading. As such studies continue, a much better understanding of the brain-behavior substrates of stuttered and stutter-free or normal speech may be achieved.

Adults who have been stuttering most of their lives often develop various situational fears, social anxieties, lowered expectations, diminished self-esteem, and an array of escape and avoidance behaviors. Prior to initiating treatment, clinicians should obtain a thorough history of an adult's stuttering and prior treatment, including major current concerns, treatment expectations, and goals, and should assess attitudes, affective reactions and behaviors, and self-concepts that may require treatment. Analyses of samples recorded in various speaking situations document the type, frequency, duration, and overall severity of stuttering. Such information allows clinicians to select appropriate treatment strategies, track progress, and determine when treatment objectives have been achieved. Current treatment strategies focus either on modifying adults' affective, cognitive, and behavioral reactions to stuttering (e.g., Prins, 1993; Manning, 1996) or on learning speech production techniques (i.e., fluency training) to reduce or eliminate stuttering (e.g., Neilson and Andrews, 1993; Onslow, 1996). Most clinicians apparently prefer a combined strategy to manage the constellation of speech, affective, and cognitive symptoms commonly presented by adults who stutter. No well-controlled clinical trials of stuttering treatments have been reported, but some relapse in treatment gains is common. It is generally agreed, therefore, that complete, permanent recovery from chronic stuttering is rare when stuttering persists into adult life, regardless of the treatment employed. Consequently, local self-help groups of the National Stuttering Association, which promote sharing of experience, information, and support among members, have become an increasingly important component to successful, long-term management of stuttering in adults in the United States.

See also SPEECH DISFLUENCY AND STUTTERING IN CHILDREN.

—*Richard F. Curlee*

References

Ambrose, N., Yairi, E., and Cox, N. (1993). Genetic aspects of early childhood stuttering. *Journal of Speech and Hearing Research, 36,* 701–706.

Ambrose, N., Cox, N., and Yairi, E. (1997). The genetic basis of persistence and recovery in stuttering. *Journal of Speech, Language, and Hearing Research, 40,* 567–580.

Andrews, G. (1984). The epidemiology of stuttering. In R. F. Curlee and W. H. Perkins (Eds.), *Nature and treatment of stuttering: New directions* (1st ed.). San Diego, CA: College-Hill Press.

Andrews, G., and Harris, M. (1964). *The syndrome of stuttering. Clinics in Developmental Medicine, 17.*

Bloodstein, O. (1995). *A handbook on stuttering* (5th ed.). San Diego, CA: Singular Publishing Group.

Bloodstein, O. (1997). Stuttering as an anticipatory struggle reaction. In R. F. Curlee and G. M. Siegel (Eds.), *Nature and treatment of stuttering: New directions* (2nd ed.). Boston: Allyn and Bacon.

Braun, A. R., Varga, M., Stager, S., Schulz, G., Selbie, S., Maisog, J. M., et al. (1997). Altered patterns of cerebral activity during speech and language production in developmental stuttering. An $H_2^{15}O$ positron emission tomography study. *Brain, 120,* 761–784.

Fromkin, V. (1993). Speech production. In J. Berko Gleason and N. Bernstein Ratner (Eds.), *Psycholinguistics.* Austin, TX: Harcourt, Brace and Jovanovich.

Howie, P. (1981). Concordance for stuttering in monozygotic and dizygotic twin pairs. *Journal of Speech and Hearing Research, 24,* 317–321.

Ingham, R. J. (2001). Brain imaging studies of developmental stuttering. *Journal of Communication Disorders, 34,* 493–516.

Ingham, R. J., Fox, P. T., Ingham, J. C., and Zamarripa, F. (2000). Is overt stuttering a prerequisite for the neural activations associated with chronic developmental stuttering? *Brain and Language, 75,* 163–194.

Ingham, R. J., Fox, P. T., Ingham, J. C., Zamarripa, F., Jerabek, P., and Cotton, J. (1996). A functional lesion investigation of developmental stuttering using positron emission tomography. *Journal of Speech and Hearing Research, 39,* 1208–1227.

Kidd, K., Heimbuch, R., and Records, M. (1981). Vertical transmission of susceptibility to stuttering with sex-modified expression. *Proceedings of the National Academy of Science, 78,* 606–610.

Manning, W. H. (1996). *Clinical decision making in the diagnosis and treatment of fluency disorders.* Albany, NY: Delmar.

Mansson, H. (2000). Childhood stuttering: Incidence and development. *Journal of Fluency Disorders, 25,* 47–57.

Neilson, M., and Andrews, G. (1993). Intensive fluency training of chronic stutterers. In R. F. Curlee (Ed.), *Stuttering and related disorders of fluency.* New York: Thieme.

Neilson, M. D., and Neilson, P. D. (1987). Speech motor control and stuttering: A computational model of adaptive sensory motor processing. *Speech Communication, 6,* 325–333.

Onslow, M. (1996). *Behavioral management of stuttering*. San Diego, CA: Singular Publishing Group.

Perkins, W. H. (1990). What is stuttering? *Journal of Speech and Hearing Disorders, 55*, 370–382.

Perkins, W. H., Kent, R. D., and Curlee, R. F. (1991). A theory of neuropsycholinguistic function in stuttering. *Journal of Speech and Hearing Research, 34*, 734–752.

Prins, D. (1993). Management of stuttering: Treatment of adolescents and adults. In R. F. Curlee (Ed.), *Stuttering and related disorders of fluency*. New York: Thieme.

Ratner, N. (1997). Stuttering: A psycholinguistic perspective. In R. F. Curlee and G. M. Siegel (Eds.), *Nature and treatment of stuttering: New directions* (2nd ed.). Boston: Allyn and Bacon.

Smith, A., and Kelly, E. (1997). Stuttering: A dynamic, multifactorial model. In R. F. Curlee and G. M. Siegel (Eds.), *Nature and treatment of stuttering: New directions* (2nd ed.). Boston: Allyn and Bacon.

Yairi, E., and Ambrose, N. (1999). Early childhood stuttering: I. Persistence and recovery rates. *Journal of Speech, Language, and Hearing Research, 42*, 1097–1112.

Yairi, E., Ambrose, N., and Cox, N. (1996). Generics of stuttering: A critical review. *Journal of Speech and Hearing Research, 39*, 771–784.

Further Readings

Adams, M. R. (1990). The demands and capacities model: I. Theoretical elaborations. *Journal of Fluency Disorders, 15*, 135–141.

Boberg, E., and Kully, D. (1994). Long-term results of an intensive treatment program for adults and adolescents who stutter. *Journal of Speech and Hearing Research, 37*, 1050–1059.

Brady, J. P. (1991). The pharmacology of stuttering: A critical review. *American Journal of Psychiatry, 148*, 1309–1316.

Caruso, A. J., Chodzko-Zajko, W. J., Bidinger, D. A., and Sommers, R. K. (1994). Adults who stutter: Responses to cognitive stress. *Journal of Speech and Hearing Research, 37*, 746–754.

Cordes, A. K. (1998). Current status of the stuttering treatment literature. In A. K. Cordes and R. J. Ingham (Eds.), *Treatment efficacy research: A search for empirical bases*. San Diego, CA: Singular Publishing Group.

Cox, N. (1988). Molecular genetics: The key to the puzzle of stuttering? *ASHA, 4*, 36–40.

DeNil, L. F., Kroll, R. M., Kapur, S., and Houle, S. (1998). A positron emission tomography study of silent and oral single word reading in stuttering and nonstuttering adults. *Journal of Speech, Language, and Hearing Research, 43*, 1038–1053.

Denny, M., and Smith, A. (1997). Respiratory and laryngeal control in stuttering. In R. F. Curlee and G. M. Siegel (Eds.), *Nature and treatment of stuttering: New directions* (2nd ed.). Boston: Allyn and Bacon.

Folkins, J. W. (1991). Stuttering from a speech motor control perspective. In H. F. Peters, W. Hulstijn, and C. W. Starkweather (Eds.), *Speech motor control and stuttering*. Amsterdam: Elsevier.

Fox, P. T., Ingham, R. J., George, M. S., Mayberg, H., Ingham, J. C., Roby, J., et al. (1997). Imaging human intracerebral connectivity by PET during TMS. *NeuroReport, 8*, 2787–2791.

Fox, P. T., Ingham, R. J., Ingham, J. C., Zamarripa, F., Xing, J.-H., and Lancaster, J. (2000). Brain correlates of stuttering and syllable production: A PET performance-correlation analysis. *Brain, 123*, 1985–2004.

Gregory, H. (1997). The speech-language pathologist's role in stuttering self-help groups. *Seminars in Speech and Language, 18*, 401–409.

Hedges, D. W., Umar, F., Mellon, C. D., Herrick, L. C., Hanson, M. L., and Wahl, M. J. (1995). Direct comparison of the family history method and the family study method using a large stuttering pedigree. *Journal of Fluency Disorders, 20*, 25–33.

Ingham, R. J. (1993). Stuttering treatment efficacy: Paradigm dependent or independent? *Journal of Fluency Disorders, 18*, 133–149.

Ingham, R. J., Fox, P. T., Ingham, J. C., Collins, J., and Pridgen, S. (2000). TMS in developmental stuttering and Tourette's syndrome. In M. S. George and R. H. Belmaker (Eds.), *Transcranial magnetic stimulation (TMS) in neuropsychiatry*. New York: American Psychiatric Press.

Janssen, P., Kraaiment, F., and Brutten, G. (1990). Relationship between stutterers' genetic history and speech-associated variables. *Journal of Fluency Disorders, 15*, 39–48.

Kolk, H., and Postma, A. (1997). Stuttering as a covert repair phenomenon. In R. F. Curlee and G. M. Siegel (Eds.), *Nature and treatment of stuttering: New directions* (2nd ed.). Boston: Allyn and Bacon.

Kully, D., and Langevin, M. J. (1999). Intensive treatment for stuttering adolescents. In R. F. Curlee (Ed.), *Stuttering and related disorders of fluency* (2nd ed.). New York: Thieme.

Ludlow, C., and Braun, A. (1993). Research evaluating the use of neuropharmacological agents for treating stuttering: Possibilities and problems. *Journal of Fluency Disorders, 18*, 169–182.

Onslow, M., and Packman, A. (1997). Designing and implementing a strategy to control stuttered speech in adults. In R. F. Curlee and G. M. Siegel (Eds.), *Nature and treatment of stuttering: New directions* (2nd ed.). Boston: Allyn and Bacon.

Prins, D. (1991). Theories of stuttering as event and disorder: Implications for speech production processes. In H. F. M. Peters, W. Hulstijn, and C. W. Starkweather (Eds.), *Speech motor control and stuttering*. Amsterdam: Elsevier.

Prins, D. (1993). Models for treatment efficacy studies of adult stutterers. *Journal of Fluency Disorders, 18*, 333–349.

Salmelin, R., Schnitzler, A., Schmitz, F., and Freund, H. J. (2000). Single word reading in developmental stutterers and fluent speakers. *Brain, 123*, 1184–1202.

Sandak, R., and Fiez, J. L. (2000). Stuttering: A view from neuroimaging. *Lancet, 356*, 445–446.

Webster, W. G. (1993). Hurried hands and tangled tongues. Implications of current research for the management of stuttering. In E. Boberg (Ed.), *Neuropsychology of stuttering*. Edmonton: University of Alberta Press.

Transsexualism and Sex Reassignment: Speech Differences

According to the *Random House Dictionary*, a transsexual individual is "A person having a strong desire to assume the physical characteristics and gender role of the opposite sex; a person who has undergone hormone treatment and surgery to attain the physical characteristics of the opposite sex" (Flexner, 1987). Brown and

Rounsley (1996) explain, "Transsexuals are individuals who strongly feel that they are, or ought to be, the opposite sex. The body they were born with does not match their own inner conviction and mental image of who they are or want to be.... This dilemma causes them intense emotional distress and anxiety and often interferes with their day-to-day functioning" (p. 6).

Historically, examples of transsexualism existed in Greek and Roman times, during the Middle Ages, and in the Renaissance (Doctor, 1988). However, the first documented sex reassignment surgery is thought to have been performed around 1923. It involved a man who married at 20 but came to believe he should have been a woman, and took the name of Lili (Hoyer, 1933). The most celebrated case in the United States was that of Christine Jorgensen, who grew up in New York City as a male and had transsexual reassignment surgery performed in Denmark in 1952 (Jorgensen, 1967).

The prevalence of transsexualism is difficult to determine. The United States does not have a national registry to collect information from all possible sources that may deal with the transsexual person. Furthermore, some individuals may remain undiagnosed or may wish to remain "closeted," or they may travel to foreign countries for sex reassignment surgery.

Data from other countries suggest that one in 30,000 adult males and one in 100,000 adult females seek sex reassignment surgery. However, the overall prevalence figures are greater if one includes transsexuals who do not elect sex reassignment surgery. In the United States, it is estimated that 6000–10,000 transsexuals had undergone sex reassignment surgery by 1988 (Brown and Rounsley, 1996). Spencer (1988) reported that in 1979, more than 4000 U.S. citizens had undergone sex reassignment surgery and about 50,000 were thought to be awaiting surgery. Estimates vary greatly concerning the number of male-to-female transsexuals compared to the number of female-to-male transsexuals, although all estimates indicate that the number of male-to-female transsexuals exceeds the number of female-to-male transsexuals by as much as 3 or 4 to 1 (Oates and Dacakis, 1983; Doctor, 1988; Spencer, 1988; Wolfe et al., 1990).

The transsexual individual (also referred to as a transgendered individual) who seeks therapy and possibly surgery is often referred to a clinic specializing in the treatment of gender dysphoria. Programs that are offered through these clinics include psychological counseling, hormone treatments, and other nonsurgical procedures, which may then lead to the final surgical reassignment surgery. Male-to-female surgery generally requires a single operation and is less expensive than female-to-male surgery, which requires at least three operations, is considerably more expensive, and is not associated with as good aesthetic and functional results as male-to-female surgery (Brown and Rounsley, 1988).

The literature on therapy for the male-to-female transsexual and the female-to-male transsexual represents two extremes. Therapy for the male-to-female transsexual has focused on voice therapy as a major component. Voice therapy for the female-to-male transsexual is virtually nonexistent. In fact, there appears to be considerable agreement among researchers studying the treatment of the transsexual that voice therapy for the female-to-male transsexual is unnecessary because lowering of the fundamental frequency occurs automatically as a result of androgens administered to the female-to-male transsexual (Spencer, 1988; Colton and Casper, 1996). Van Borsel et al. (2000) conducted a two-part study of the voice problems of the female-to-male transsexual. Part 1 was a survey of 16 individuals who had been treated with androgens for at least 1 year by the Gent University Gender Team in Belgium. Questionnaires indicated that 14 of the 16 respondents had experienced a "lower" or "heavier" voice. The remaining two reported that they had a lower-pitched voice before treatment started. Only one of the subjects was not pleased with his voice because of what he perceived as strain in speaking at a lower pitch. Fourteen indicated that voice change was as important as sex reassignment surgery, although 11 of the 16 did not consider the need for speech therapy important. The study confirmed the view that pitch is lowered as a result of androgen treatment and appears to result in an acceptable male voice. Part 2 was a longitudinal study of the voice change of two female-to-male transsexuals who were administered androgens. Acoustic measures of fundamental frequency, jitter, and shimmer were made of the sustained vowel production of /a/ and the reading of a standard paragraph. The measures for one subject were made over 17 months and for the other subject over 13 months. The results confirmed that the fundamental frequency was substantially reduced for sustained vowel production and reading, although not by more than one octave. Measures of jitter and shimmer were relatively unchanged over time.

The administration of hormones for the male-to-female transsexual has little effect on voice. Some studies have examined the male-to-female transsexual's changes in fundamental frequency and its relationship to the identification of the voice as a female voice (Bradley et al., 1978; Spencer, 1988; Dacakis, 2000; Gelfer and Schofield, 2000). Although there is some agreement that fundamental frequency is most often perceived as a female voice at 155–160 Hz and above, it is not sufficient alone to identify the male-to-female transsexual as a female speaker (Bradley et al., 1978; Gelfer and Schofield, 2000). Mount and Salmon (1988) conducted a long-range study of a 63-year-old male-to-female transsexual who had undergone sex reassignment surgery. The individual was able to increase her speaking fundamental frequency after 4 months of therapy. However, she was not perceived as a female speaker until formant frequencies had increased, particularly F2 values. This was achieved through the modification of resonance and articulation. Gelfer and Schofeld (2000) conducted a study of 15 male-to-female transsexuals with a control group of six biological females and three biological males. All subjects recorded the Rainbow Passage and produced the isolated vowels /a/ and /i/. Twenty undergraduate psychology majors served as listeners. The only significant differences among subjects were that the "Subjects perceived as female had a higher SFF [speaking fundamental frequency] and a higher upper limit of SFF than subjects perceived as male" (p. 30). Although formant frequencies for /a/ and /i/ were not significantly different between the male-to-female transsexuals perceived as male and those perceived as female, the mean formant frequencies for the perceived female speakers were all higher than those of the transsexual speakers judged to be male. Gunzburger (1995) had six male-to-female transsexual speakers record a list of Dutch words that were also combined into prose. Subjects were asked to read the material in a female manner and a male manner. Acoustic analyses indicated that the central frequency of F3 was systematically higher in the female version. Recordings of two male-to-female speakers that were representative of a male speaker and a female speaker were played to 31 male and female naive listeners, who were asked to identify the sex of the speaker. The perceptual judgments supported the results of the acoustic analyses. It appeared that the male-to-female transsexual speakers judged to be female had F3 formants more like those associated with the female voice. The shorter vocal tract typically found in females produces higher F3 formants than those of males, with a longer vocal tract (Peterson and Barney, 1952; Fant, 1960). Gunzburger (1995) attributed these changes to a decreased vocal cavity length in the perceived female male-to-female transsexual and pointed out that shortening the vocal tract can be accomplished through changes in articulation and retracting the corners of the mouth (p. 347).

According to Stemple, Glaze, and Gerdeman (1995), the male-to-female transsexual not only has to increase her fundamental frequency while being careful not to damage the vocal folds, but also has to learn to modify the resonance, inflection, and intonation to make articulation more precise, and to modify coughing, vocalized pauses, and throat clearing (p. 204).

Therapy for the female-to-male transsexual appears to be less of an issue than therapy for the male-to-female transsexual. Many of the textbooks on voice disorders include a discussion of the therapy needs for the male-to-female transsexual but do not provide any details on procedures, techniques, or concerns for the clinician to consider in the therapy process. De Bruin, Coerts, and Greven (2000) provide the clinician with a detailed approach, including specific goals and subgoals, to follow in therapy for the male-to-female transsexual. Among the major goals are minimizing chest resonance; modifying intonation patterns, articulation, intensity, and rate; and feminizing laughing and coughing. In addition, they address other verbal and nonverbal aspects of feminine communication such as gestures, movements, greetings, shaking hands, dress, and hairdo. The authors briefly discuss laryngeal surgery but conclude that it only results in raising the fundamental frequency (which is not in itself sufficient to guarantee a feminine voice) and that the results of this surgery are not predictable. Batin

(1983) includes vocabulary and language forms and uses videotapes of the male-to-female transsexual to teach the individual how to walk, sit down, and enter a room. Chaloner (1991) provides case histories, and uses role playing in group therapy to help the male-to-female transsexual become more successful in "living the female role" (p. 330). Future research on the assessment and treatment of transgendered individuals should provide the clinician with a larger repertoire of approaches to assist the transsexual individual in making the transition to a different sexual role.

—*John M. Pettit*

References

Batin, R. R. (1983). Treatment of the transsexual voice. In W. Perkins (Ed.), *Voice disorders: Current therapy of communication disorders* (pp. 63–66). New York: Thieme-Stratton.

Bradley, R. C., Bull, G. L., Gore, C. H., and Edgerton, M. T. (1978). Evaluation of vocal pitch in male transsexuals. *Journal of Communication Disorders, 11*, 443–449.

Brown, M. L., and Rounsley, C. A. (1996). *True selves.* San Francisco: Jossey-Bass.

Chaloner, J. (1991). The voice of the transsexual. In M. Fawcus (Ed.), *Voice disorders and their management* (2nd ed., pp. 314–332). London: Chapman and Hall.

Colton, R. H., and Casper, J. K. (1996). *Understanding voice problems* (2nd ed., pp. 281–282). Baltimore: Lippincott, Williams and Wilkins.

Dacakis, G. (2000). Long-term maintenance of fundamental frequency increases in male-to-female transsexuals. *Journal of Voice, 14*, 549–556.

de Bruin, M. D., Coerts, M. J., and Greven, A. J. (2000). Speech therapy in the management of male-to-female transsexuals. *Folia Phoniatrica, 52*, 220–227.

Doctor, R. F. (1988). *Transvestites and transsexuals: Toward a theory of cross-gender behavior.* New York: Plenum Press.

Fant, G. (1960). *Acoustic theory of speech production.* The Hague: Mouton.

Flexner, S. B. (Ed.). (1987). *Random House Dictionary of the English Language, Unabridged* (2nd ed.). New York: Random House.

Gelfer, M. P., and Schofield, K. J. (2000). Comparison of acoustic and perceptual measures of voice in male-to-female transsexuals perceived as female versus those perceived as male. *Journal of Voice, 14*, 22–33.

Gunzburger, D. (1995). Acoustic and perceptual implications of the transsexual voice. *Archives of Sexual Behavior, 24*, 339–348.

Hoyer, N. (1933). *Man into woman: An authentic record of a change of sex.* New York: Dutton.

Jorgenson, C. (1967). *Christine Jorgensen: A personal autobiography.* New York: Bantam Books.

Mount, K. H., and Salmon, S. J. (1988). Changing the vocal characteristics of a postoperative transsexual patient: A longitudinal study. *Journal of Communication Disorders, 21*, 229–238.

Oates, J. M., and Dacakis, G. (1983). Speech pathology considerations in the management of transsexualism: A review. *British Journal of Disorders of Communication, 18*, 139–151.

Peterson, G., and Barney, H. (1952). Control methods used in the study of the vowels. *Journal of the Acoustical Society of America, 24*, 175–184.

Spencer, L. E. (1988). Speech characteristics of male-to-female transsexuals: A perceptual and acoustic study. *Folia Phoniatrica, 40,* 31–42.

Stemple, J. C., Glaze, L. E., and Gerdeman, B. K. (1995). *Clinical voice pathology: Theory and management* (2nd ed.). San Diego, CA: Singular Publishing Group.

Van Borsel, J., DeCuypere, G., Rubens, R., and Destaerke, B. (2000). Voice problems in female-to-male transsexuals. *International Journal of Language and Communication Disorders, 35,* 427–442.

Wolfe, V. I., Ratusnik, D. L., Smith, F. H., and Northrop, G. (1990). Intonation and fundamental frequency in male-to-female transsexuals. *Journal of Speech and Hearing Disorders, 55,* 43–50.

Further Readings

Andrews, M. L., and Schmidt, C. P. (1997). Gender presentation: Perceptual and acoustical analyses of voice. *Journal of Voice, 11,* 307–313.

Boone, D. R., and McFarlane, S. C. (2000). *The voice and voice therapy* (6th ed.). Boston: Allyn and Bacon.

Brown, M., Perry, A., Cheesman, A. D., and Pring, T. (2000). Pitch change in male-to-female transsexuals: Has phonosurgery a role to play? *International Journal of Language and Communication Disorders, 35,* 129–136.

Case, J. L. (1991). *Clinical management of voice disorders* (2nd ed.). Austin, TX: Pro-Ed.

Chivers, M. L., and Bailey, J. M. (2000). Sexual orientation of female-to-male transsexuals: A comparison of homosexual and nonhomosexual types. *Archives of Sexual Behavior, 29,* 259–278.

Donald, P. J. (1982). Voice change surgery in the transsexual. *Head and Neck Surgery, 4,* 433–437.

Feinbloom, D. H. (1976). *Transvestites and transsexuals: Mixed views.* New York: Delecorte Press.

Gross, M. (1999). Pitch-raising surgery in male-to-female transsexuals. *Journal of Voice, 13,* 246–250.

Gunzburger, D. (1993). An acoustic analysis and some perceptual data concerning voice change in male-to-female transsexuals. *European Journal of Disorders of Communication, 28,* 13–21.

Kunachak, S., Prakunhungsit, S., and Sujjalak, K. (2000). Thyroid cartilage and vocal fold reduction: A new phonosurgical method for male-to-female transsexuals. *Annals of Otology, Rhinology, and Laryngology, 109,* 10826–10829.

Rogers, A. (1993). Legal implications of transsexualism. *Lancet, 341,* 1085–1086.

Ventilator-Supported Speech Production

When breathing becomes difficult or impossible, it may be necessary to use a ventilator to sustain life. Usually the need for a ventilator is temporary, such as during a surgical procedure. However, if breathing difficulty is chronic, ventilatory support may be required for an extended period, sometimes a lifetime. The main indications for ventilatory support are respiratory insufficiency resulting in hypoventilation (not enough gas moving into and out of the lungs), hypoxemia (not enough oxygen in the arterial blood), or hypercapnea (too much carbon dioxide in the blood). Many medical conditions can cause severe respiratory insufficiency requiring ventilatory support. Examples include cervical spinal cord injury (rostral enough to impair diaphragm function), muscular dystrophy, amyotrophic lateral sclerosis, and chronic obstructive pulmonary disease.

Several types of ventilator systems are available for individuals with respiratory insufficiency, including positive-pressure ventilators, negative-pressure ventilators, phrenic nerve pacers, abdominal pneumobelts, and rocking beds (Banner, Blanch, and Desautels, 1990; Hill, 1994; Levine and Henson, 1994). Positive-pressure ventilators operate by "pushing" air into the pulmonary system for inspiration, whereas negative-pressure ventilators work to lower the pressure around the respiratory system and expand it for inspiration. Phrenic nerve pacers stimulate the phrenic nerves and cause the diaphragm to contract to generate inspiration. Abdominal pneumobelts displace the abdomen inward (by inflation of a bladder) to push air out of the pulmonary system for expiration, and then allow the abdomen to return to its resting position (by deflation of the bladder) for inspiration. Rocking beds are designed to move an individual upward toward standing and downward toward supine to drive inspiration and expiration, respectively, using gravitational force to displace the abdomen and diaphragm. All of these systems are currently used (Make et al., 1998); however, the most commonly used one today and the one that the speech-language pathologist is most likely to encounter in clinical practice is the positive-pressure ventilator (Spearman and Sanders, 1990).

The positive-pressure ventilator uses a positive-pressure pump to drive air through a tube into the pulmonary system. The tube can be routed through (1) the larynx (in this case, it is called an endotracheal tube), such as during surgery or acute respiratory failure; (2) the upper airway, via a nose mask, face mask, or mouthpiece (this is called noninvasive ventilation); or (3) a tracheostoma (a surgically fashioned entry through the anterior neck to the tracheal airway). The latter two modes of delivery are used in individuals who need long-term ventilatory support. With noninvasive positive-pressure ventilation, speech is produced in a relatively normal manner. That is, after inspiratory air from the ventilator flows into the nose and/or mouth, expiration begins and speech can be produced until the next inspiration is delivered. The situation is quite different, however, when inspiratory air is delivered via a tracheostoma. In some cases it is not possible to produce speech with the ventilator-delivered air because the air is not allowed to reach the larynx. This occurs when the tracheostomy tube, which is secured in the tracheostoma and provides a connection to the ventilator's tubing, is configured so as to block airflow to the larynx. This is done by inflating a small cuff that surrounds the tube where it lies within the trachea. However, if the cuff is deflated (or if there is no cuff), it is possible to speak using the ventilator-delivered air. Because the air from the ventilator enters below the larynx, speech can be

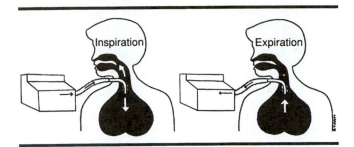

Figure 1. Inspiration and expiration during positive-pressure ventilation with a deflated tracheostomy tube cuff. (From Hoit, J. D., and Banzett, R. B. [1997]. Simple adjustments can improve ventilator-supported speech. *American Journal of Speech-Language Pathology*, 6, 87–96, adapted from Tippett, D. C., and Siebens, A. A. [1995]. Preserving oral communication in individuals with tracheostomy and ventilator dependency. *American Journal of Speech-Language Pathology*, 4, 55–61, Fig. 7. Reproduced with permission.)

produced during both the inspiratory and the expiratory phase of the ventilator cycle (Fig. 1). During the inspiratory phase, speech production competes with ventilation because the ventilator-delivered air that flows through the larynx to produce speech is routed away from the pulmonary system, where gas exchange takes place (i.e., oxygen is exchanged for carbon dioxide). For this and other reasons, the act of speaking with a tracheostomy and positive-pressure ventilator is challenging, and the resultant speech often is quite abnormal.

Positive-pressure ventilators can be adjusted to meet each individual's ventilatory needs. These adjustments typically are determined by the pulmonologist and executed by the respiratory therapist. The most basic adjustments involve setting the tidal volume and breathing rate, the product of which is the minute ventilation (the amount of air moved into or out of the pulmonary system per minute). These parameters are adjusted primarily according to the client's body size and breathing comfort, and their appropriateness is confirmed by blood gas measurements. Most ventilators allow adjustment of other parameters, such as inspiratory duration, magnitude and pattern of inspiratory flow, fraction of inspired oxygen, and pressure at end-expiration (called positive end-expiratory pressure, or PEEP), among others. How these parameters are adjusted influences ventilation and can also have a substantial influence on speech production.

The speech produced with a tracheostomy and positive-pressure ventilator is usually abnormal. Some of its common features are short utterances, long pauses, and variable loudness and voice quality (Hoit, Shea, and Banzett, 1994). The mechanisms underlying these speech features are most easily explained by relating them to the tracheal pressure waveform associated with ventilator-supported speech. This waveform is shown schematically in Figure 2, along with a waveform associated with normal speech production. Whereas tracheal pressure dur-

ing normal speech production is positive (i.e., above atmospheric pressure), generally low in amplitude (i.e., in the range of 5–10 cm H_2O), and relatively unchanging throughout the expiratory phase of the breathing cycle, tracheal pressure during ventilator-supported speech production is generally fast-changing (i.e., rapidly rising during the inspiratory phase of the ventilator cycle and rapidly falling during the expiratory phase of the cycle), high-peaked (approximately 35 cm H_2O in the figure), and not always above atmospheric pressure (i.e., during the latter 2 s of the cycle in the figure). These waveforms can also be examined relative to the minimum pressure required to maintain vibration of the vocal folds for phonation (labeled Threshold Pressure in the figure). From this comparison, it is clear that the tracheal pressure associated with normal speech production exceeds this threshold pressure throughout the cycle (expiratory phase), whereas the pressure associated with the ventilator-supported speech production is below the threshold pressure for nearly half the cycle. This latter observation largely explains why ventilator-supported speech is characterized by short utterances and long pauses. The periods during which the pressure is above the voicing threshold pressure are relatively short (compared with normal speech-related expirations) and the periods during which the pressure is below that threshold are relatively long (compared with normal speech-related inspirations). The reason why ventilator-supported speech is variable in loudness and voice quality has to do with the fast-changing nature of the tracheal pressure waveform. The rapid rate at which the pressure rises and falls makes it impossible for the larynx to make the adjustments necessary to produce a steady voice loudness and quality.

There are several strategies for improving ventilator-supported speech. One set of strategies is mechanical in nature and involves modifying the tracheal pressure waveform. Specifically, speech can be improved if the tracheal pressure stays above the voicing threshold

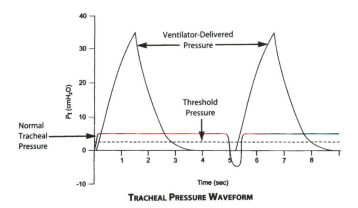

Figure 2. Schematic representation of tracheal pressure during normal speech production and ventilator-supported speech production. The dashed line indicates the minimum pressure required to vibrate the vocal folds. (From Hoit, J. D. [1998]. *Speak to me. International Ventilator Users Network News, 12,* 6. Reproduced with permission.)

pressure for a longer portion of the ventilator cycle (to increase utterance duration and decrease pause duration) and if it changes less rapidly and does not peak as highly (to decrease variability of loudness and voice quality). The tracheal pressure waveform can be modified by adjusting certain parameters on the ventilator (such as those mentioned earlier) or by adding external valves to the ventilator system (e.g., Dikeman and Kazandjian, 1995; Hoit and Banzett, 1997). Ventilator-supported speech can also be improved using behavioral strategies. Such strategies include the use of linguistic manipulations designed to hold the floor during conversation (e.g., breaking for obligatory pauses at linguistically inappropriate junctures) and the incorporation of another sound source to supplement the laryngeal voicing source (e.g., buccal or pharyngeal speech).

Evaluation and management of the speech of a client with a tracheostomy and positive-pressure ventilator involves a team approach, with the team usually consisting of a speech-language pathologist working in collaboration with a pulmonologist and a respiratory therapist. Such collaboration is critical because speech production and ventilation are highly interdependent in a client who uses a ventilator. An intervention designed to improve speech will almost certainly influence ventilation, and an adjustment to ventilation will most likely alter the quality of the speech. As an example, a speech-language pathologist might request that a client be allowed to deflate his cuff so that he can speak. Cuff deflation should not compromise ventilation as long as tidal volume is increased appropriately (Bach and Alba, 1990). By understanding the interactions between speech production and ventilation, clinicians can implement interventions that optimize spoken communication without compromising ventilation, thereby improving the overall quality of life in clients who use ventilators.

—*Jeannette D. Hoit*

References

Bach, J. R., and Alba, A. S. (1990). Tracheostomy ventilation: A study of efficacy with deflated cuffs and cuffless tubes. *Chest, 97,* 679–683.

Banner, M. J., Blanch, P., and Desautels, D. A. (1990). Mechanical ventilators. In R. R. Kirby, M. J. Banner, and J. B. Downs (Eds.), *Clinical applications of ventilatory support* (pp. 401–503). New York: Churchill Livingstone.

Dikeman, K. J., and Kazandjian, M. S. (1995). *Communication and swallowing management of tracheostomized and ventilator-dependent adults.* San Diego, CA: Singular Publishing Group.

Hill, N. S. (1994). Use of the rocking bed, pneumobelt, and other noninvasive aids to ventilation. In M. J. Tobin (Ed.), *Principles and practice of mechanical ventilation* (pp. 413–425). New York: McGraw-Hill.

Hoit, J. D., and Banzett, R. B. (1997). Simple adjustments can improve ventilator-supported speech. *American Journal of Speech-Language Pathology, 6,* 87–96.

Hoit, J. D., Shea, S. A., and Banzett, R. B. (1994). Speech production during mechanical ventilation in tracheostomized individuals. *Journal of Speech and Hearing Research, 37,* 53–63.

Levine, S., and Henson, D. (1994). Negative pressure ventilation. In M. J. Tobin (Ed.), *Principles and practice of mechanical ventilation* (pp. 393–411). New York: McGraw-Hill.

Make, B. J., Hill, N. S., Goldberg, A. I., Bach, J. R., Criner, G. J., Dune, P. E., et al. (1998). Mechanical ventilation beyond the intensive care unit: Report of a consensus conference of the American College of Chest Physicians. *Chest, 113,* 289S–344S.

Spearman, C. B., and Sanders, H. G., Jr. (1990). Physical principles and functional designs of ventilators. In R. R. Kirby, M. J. Banner, and J. B. Downs (Eds.), *Clinical applications of ventilatory support* (pp. 63–104). New York: Churchill Livingstone.

Further Readings

American Speech-Language-Hearing Association, Ad Hoc Committee on Use of Specialized Medical Speech Devices. (1993). Position statement and guidelines for the use of voice prostheses in tracheostomized persons with or without ventilatory dependency. *ASHA, 35*(Suppl. 10), 17–20.

Bach, J. R. (1992). Ventilator use by Muscular Dystrophy Association patients. *Archives of Physical Medicine and Rehabilitation, 73,* 179–183.

Bloch-Salisbury, E., Shea, S. A., Brown, R., Evans, K., and Banzett, R. B. (1996). Air hunger induced by acute increase in Pco_2 adapts to chronic elevation of Pco_2 in ventilated humans. *Journal of Applied Physiology, 81,* 949–956.

Gilgoff, I. (1991). Living with a ventilator. *Western Journal of Medicine, 154,* 619–622.

Hoit, J. D., Banzett, R. B., and Brown, R. (1997). *Improving ventilator-supported speech.* TELEROUNDS No. 39 Live Satellite Transmission (Dec. 10, 1997). Tucson, AZ: National Center for Neurogenic Communication Disorders. [Videotape available.]

Hoit, J. D., and Shea, S. A. (1996). Speech production and speech with a phrenic nerve pacer. *American Journal of Speech-Language Pathology, 5,* 53–60.

Isaki, E., and Hoit, J. D. (1997). Ventilator-supported communication: A survey of speech-language pathologists. *Journal of Medical Speech-Language Pathology, 5,* 263–272.

Kirby, R. R., Banner, M. J., and Downs, J. B. (Eds.). (1990). *Clinical applications of ventilatory support.* New York: Churchill Livingstone.

Mason, M. (Ed.). (1993). *Speech pathology for tracheostomized and ventilator dependent patients.* Newport Beach, CA: Voicing!

Reeve, C. (1998). *Still me.* New York: Random House.

Shea, S. A., Hoit, J. D., and Banzett, R. B. (1998). Competition between gas exchange and speech production in ventilated subjects. *Biological Psychology, 49,* 9–27.

Sparker, A. W., Robbins, K. T., Nevlud, G. N., Watkins, C., and Jahrsdoerfer, R. (1987). A prospective evaluation of speaking tracheostomy tubes for ventilator dependent patients. *Laryngoscope, 97,* 89–92.

Sternburg, L. L. (1982). *Some adaptive compensations in speech control achieved after respiratory paralysis: Four cases.* Unpublished doctoral dissertation, Brandeis University, Waltham, MA.

Sternburg, L. L., and Sternburg, D. (1986). *View from the seesaw.* New York: Dodd, Mead.

Tippett, D. C. (Ed.). (2000). *Tracheostomy and ventilator dependency: Management of breathing, speaking, and swallowing.* New York: Thieme.

Tobin, M. J. (Ed.). (1994). *Principles and practice of mechanical ventilation.* New York: McGraw-Hill.

Part III: Language

Agrammatism

Agrammatism is a disorder that leads to difficulties with sentences. These difficulties can relate both to the correct comprehension and the correct production of sentences. That these difficulties occur at the sentence level is evident from the fact that word comprehension and production can be relatively spared.

Agrammatism occurs in many clinical populations. In patients with Wernicke's aphasia, for instance, agrammatism has been established both for comprehension (Lukatela, Schankweiler, and Crain, 1995) and for production (Haarmann and Kolk, 1992). Agrammatic comprehension has been demonstrated in patients with Parkinson's disease (Grossman et al., 2000), Alzheimer's disease (Waters, Caplan, and Rochon, 1995), and in children with specific language disorders (Van-der-Lely and Dewart, 1986). Agrammatic comprehension has even been demonstrated in normal subjects processing under stressfull conditions (Dick et al., 2001). However, agrammatism has been studied most systematically in patients with Broca's aphasia, and it is this group this review will focus on.

Symptoms of agrammatic comprehension are typically assessed by presenting a sentence to the subject and asking the subject to pick from a number of pictures the one depicting the proper interpretation of the sentence. Another procedure is to ask subjects to act out the meaning of the sentence with the help of toy figures. The main symptoms thus established are the following: (1) Sentences in which the two thematic roles can be reversed (e.g., "The cat is chasing the dog") are substantially harder to understand than their nonreversible counterparts ("The cat is drinking milk") (Caramazza and Zurif, 1976; Kolk and Friederici, 1985). Roughly speaking, thematic roles specify who is doing what to whom. (2) Sentences with noncanonical ordering of thematic roles around the verb are harder to comprehend than ones with canonical ordering. In English, the order of the active sentence is considered to be canonical: agent-action-patient (or subject-verb-object). Sentences with a word order deviating from this pattern are relatively difficult to understand. Thus, passive constructions are harder to understand than active ones (Schwartz, Saffran, and Marin, 1980; Kolk and van Grunsven 1985), and object relative sentences ("The boy whom the girl pushed was tall") are harder than subject relative sentences ("The boy who pushed the girl was tall") (Lukatela, Schankweiler, and Crain, 1995; Grodzinsky, 1999), to mention the most frequently studied contrasts. (3) Sentences with a complex—more deeply branched—phrase structure are harder to understand than their simple counterparts, even if they have canonical word order. For instance, a locative construction (e.g., "The letter is on the book") is harder to understand than a simple active construction ("The sailor is kissing the girl"), even if subjects are able to comprehend the locative proposition as such (Schwartz, Saffran, and Marin, 1980; Kolk and van Grunsven, 1985). Furthermore,

sentences with embedded clauses ("The man greeted by his wife was smoking a pipe") are harder to comprehend than sentences with two conjoined sentences ("The man was greeted by his wife and he was smoking a pipe") (Goodglass et al., 1979; Caplan and Hildebrandt, 1988).

Agrammatic production has attracted much less attention than agrammatic comprehension. Symptoms of agrammatic production have traditionally been assessed by analyzing spontaneous speech (Goodglass and Kaplan, 1983; Rochon, Saffran, Berndt, and Schwartz, 2000). Four types of symptoms of spontaneous speech have been established. (1) Reduced variety of grammatical form. If sentences are produced at all, they have little subordination or phrasal elaboration. (2) Omission of function words (articles, pronouns, auxiliaries, prepositions, and the like) and inflections. (3) Omission of main verbs. (4) A slow rate of speech. Whereas these symptoms have been established in English-speaking subjects, similar symptoms occur in many other languages (Menn and Obler, 1990). A number of studies have attempted to elicit production of grammatical morphology and word order in agrammatic patients. A complicating factor is that there are systematic differences between spontaneous speech and elicited speech. In particular, function word omission is less frequent in elicited speech and function word substitution is more frequent (Hofstede and Kolk, 1994). The following symptoms have been observed on elicitation tests. (1) Grammatical word order is impaired (Saffran, Schwartz, and Marin, 1980). (2) It is more impaired in embedded clauses than in main clauses (Kolk and van Grunsven, 1985). (3) Inflection for tense is harder than inflection for agreement (Friedmann and Grodzinsky, 1997). (4) Sentences with noncanonical ordering of thematic roles appear harder to produce than their canonical counterparts (Caplan and Hanna, 1998; Bastiaanse and van Zonneveld, 1998; but see also Kolk and van Grunsven, 1985).

The localization of agrammatism is variable. With respect to both production and comprehension, agrammatism is associated with lesions across the entire left perisylvian cortex.

Theories of agrammatism abound. Some researchers claim that differences between patients are so great that a unitary theory will not be possible (Miceli et al., 1989). Extant theories pertain either to comprehension or to production. This is justified by the fact that agrammatic production and comprehension can be dissociated (Miceli et al., 1983). The most important approaches are the following. The TRACE DELETION HYPOTHESIS about agrammatic comprehension holds that traces, or empty elements resulting from movement transformations according to generative linguistic theories, are lacking (Grodzinsky, 2000). The mapping hypothesis maintains that it is not a defect in the structural representation that is responsible for these difficulties but a defect in the procedures by which these representations are employed to derive thematic roles (Linebarger, Schwartz, and Saffran, 1983). Finally, a number of hypotheses claim a processing limitation to be the bottleneck. The limitation may relate to working memory capacity (Caplan and Waters, 1999), altered weights or increased noise in a distributed neural network (Dick et al., 2001), or a slowdown in syntactic processing (Kolk and van Grunsven, 1985). With respect to production, the tree truncation hypothesis maintains that damage to a particular node in the syntactic tree leads to the impossibility of processing any structure higher than the damaged node (Friedmann and Grodzinsky, 1997). Finally, the adaptation theory of agrammatic speech (Kolk and van Grunsven, 1985) maintains that the underlying deficit is a slowing down of the syntactic processor. A second claim is that the actual slow, telegraphic output results from the way patients adapt to this deficit.

Treatment programs for agrammatism vary from theoretically neutral syntax training programs (Helms-Estabrooks, Fitzpatrick, and Barresi, 1981), to programs motivated by the mapping hypothesis (Schwartz et al., 1994) or by the trace deletion hypothesis (Thompson et al., 1996). The reduced syntax therapy proposed by Springer and Huber (2000) takes a compensatory approach to treatment and fits well with the adaptation theory.

—*Herman Kolk*

References

Bastiaanse, R., and van Zonneveld, R. (1998). On the relation between verb inflection and verb position in Dutch agrammatic subjects. *Brain and Language, 64,* 165–181.

Caplan, D., and Hanna, J. E. (1998). Sentence production by aphasic patients in a constrained task. *Brain and Language, 63,* 159–183.

Caplan, D., and Hildebrandt, N. (1988). *Disorders of syntactic comprehension.* Cambridge, UK: Bradford Books.

Caplan, D., and Waters, G. (1999). Verbal working memory and sentence comprehension. *Behavioral and Brain Sciences, 22,* 77–94.

Caramazza, A., and Zurif, E. G. (1976). Dissociation of algorithmic and heuristic processes in sentence comprehension: Evidence from aphasia. *Brain and Language, 3,* 572–582.

Dick, F., Bates, E., Wulfeck, B., Utman, J., Dronkers, N., and Gernsbacher, M. (2001). Language deficits, localization, and grammar: Evidence for a distributive model of language breakdown in aphasic patients and neurologically intact individuals. *Psychological Review, 108,* 759–788.

Friedmann, N., and Grodzinsky, Y. (1997). Tense and agreement in agrammatic production: Pruning the syntactic tree. *Brain and Language, 56,* 397–425.

Goodglass, H., Blumstein, S. E., Gleason, J. B., Hyde, M. R., Green, E., and Stadlender, S. (1979). The effects of syntactic encoding on sentence comprehension in aphasia. *Brain and Language, 7,* 201–209.

Goodglass, H., and Kaplan, E. (1983). *The assessment of aphasia and related disorders* (2nd ed.). Philadelphia: Lea and Febiger.

Grodzinsky, Y. (2000). The neurology of syntax: Language use without Broca's area. *Behavioral and Brain Sciences, 23,* 1–92.

Grossmann, M., Kalmanson, J., Bernhardt, N., Morris, J., Stern, M. B., and Hurtig, H. I. (2000). Cognitive resource limitations in Parkinson's disease. *Brain and Language, 73,* 1–16.

Haarmann, H. J., and Kolk, H. H. J. (1992). The production and comprehension of grammatical morphology in Broca's and Wernicke's aphasics: Speed and accuracy factors. *Cortex, 28,* 97–112.

Helms-Estabrooks, N., Fitzpatrick, P. M., and Barresi, B. (1981). Response of an agrammatic patient to a syntax stimulation program for aphasia. *Journal of Speech and Hearing Disorders, 46,* 422–427.

Hofstede, B. T. M., and Kolk, H. H. J. (1994). The effects of task variation on the production of grammatical morphology in Broca's aphasia: A multiple case study. *Brain and Language, 46,* 278–328.

Kolk, H. H. J., and Friederici, A. D. (1985). Strategy and impairment in sentence understanding by Broca's and Wernicke's aphasics. *Cortex, 21,* 47–67.

Kolk, H. H. J., and van Grunsven, M. F. (1985). Agrammatism as a variable phenomenon. *Cognitive Neuropsychology, 2,* 347–384.

Linebarger, M. C., Schwartz, M., and Saffran, E. (1983). Sensitivity to grammatical structure in so-called agrammatic aphasia. *Cognition, 13,* 361–392.

Lukatela, K., Schankweiler, D., and Crain, S. (1995). Syntactic processing in agrammatic aphasia by speakers of a Slavic language. *Brain and Language, 49,* 50–76.

Menn, L., and Obler, L. (1990). *Agrammatic aphasia: A cross-language narrative source book.* Amsterdam: Benjamins.

Miceli, G., Mazzuchi, A., Menn, L., and Goodglass, H. (1983). Contrasting cases of Italian agrammatic aphasia without comprehension disorder. *Brain and Language, 35,* 24–65.

Miceli, G., Silveri, M. C., Romani, C., and Caramazza, A. (1989). Variation in the pattern of omissions and substitutions of grammatical morphemes in the spontaneous speech of so-called agrammatic patients. *Brain and Language, 26,* 447–492.

Rochon, E., Saffran, E. M., Berndt, R. S., and Schwartz, M. F. (2000). Quantitative analysis of aphasic sentence production: Further development and new data. *Brain and Language, 72,* 193–218.

Saffran, E., Schwartz, and Marin, O. (1980). The word order problem in agrammatism: II. Production. *Brain and Language, 10,* 263–280.

Schwartz, M. F., Saffran, E. M., and Marin, O. (1980). The word order problem in agrammatism: I. Comprehension. *Brain and Language, 10,* 249–262.

Schwartz, M. F., Saffran, E. M., Fink, R. B., Meyers, J. L., and Martin, N. (1994). Mapping therapy: a treatment program for agrammatism. *Aphasiology, 8,* 9–54.

Springer, L., and Huber, W. (2000). Agrammatism: Deficit or compensation? Consequences for aphasia therapy. *Neuropsychological Rehabilitation, 10,* 279–309.

Thompson, C. K., Shapiro, L. P., Tait, M. E., Jacobs, B. J., and Schneider, S. L. (1996). Training *Wh*-question production in agrammatic aphasia: Analysis of argument and adjunct movement. *Brain and Language, 52,* 175–228.

Van-der-Lely, H., and Dewart, H. (1986). Sentence comprehension strategies in specifically language impaired children. *British Journal of Disorders of Communication, 21,* 291–306.

Waters, G. S., Caplan, D., and Rochon, E. (1995). Processing capacity and sentence comprehension in patients with Alzheimer's disease. *Cognitive Neuropsychology, 12,* 1–30.

Further Readings

Badecker, W., and Caramazza, A. (1985). On considerations of method and theory governing the use of clinical categories in neurolinguistics and cognitive neuropsychology: The case against agrammatism. *Cognition, 20,* 97–125.

Beretta, A. (2001). Linear and structural accounts of theta role assignment in agrammatic aphasia. *Aphasiology*, *15*, 515–531.

Berndt, R. S., and Haendiges, A. N. (2000). Grammatical class in word and sentence production: Evidence from an aphasic patient. *Journal of Memory and Language*, *43*, 249–273.

Berndt, R. S., Mitchum, C. C., and Haendiges, A. N. (1996). Comprehension of reversible sentences in "agrammatism": A meta-analysis. *Cognition*, *58*, 289–308.

Crain, S., Ni, W., and Shankweiler, D. (2001). Grammatism. *Brain and Language*, *77*, 294–304.

Druks, J., and Marshall, J. C. (1995). When passives are harder than actives: Two case studies of agrammatic comprehension. *Cognition*, *55*, 311–331.

Friederici, A. D., and Frazier, L. (1992). Thematic analysis in agrammatic comprehension: Thematic structure and task demands. *Brain and Language*, *42*, 1–29.

Friederici, A. D., and Gorrell, P. (1998). Structural prominence and agrammatic theta-role assignment: A reconsideration of linear strategies. *Brain and Language*, *65*, 253–275.

Friedmann, N. (2001). Agrammatism and the psychological reality of the syntactic tree. *Journal of Psycholinguistic Research*, *30*, 71–90.

Haarmann, H. J., Just, M. A., and Carpenter, P. A. (1997). Aphasic sentence comprehension as a resource deficit: A computational approach. *Brain and Language*, *59*, 76–120.

Hagiwara, H. (1995). The breakdown of functional categories and the economy of derivation. *Brain and Language*, *50*, 92–116.

Hartsuiker, R. J., and Kolk, H. J. (1998). Syntactic facilitation in agrammatic sentence production. *Brain and Language*, *62*, 221–254.

Hickok, G., Zurif, E., and Canseco-Gonzalez, E. (1993). Structural description of agrammatic comprehension. *Brain and Language*, *45*, 371–395.

Hillis, A. E., and Caramazza, A. (1995). Representation of grammatical categories of words in the brain. *Journal of Cognitive Neuroscience*, *7*, 396–407.

Kolk, H. H. J. (1995). A time-based approach to agrammatic production. *Brain and Language*, *50*, 282–303.

Linebarger, M. C., Schwartz, M. F., Romania, J. R., Kohn, S. E., and Stephens, D. L. (2000). Grammatical encoding in aphasia: Evidence from a "processing prosthesis." *Brain and Language*, *75*, 416–427.

Luzatti, C., Toraldo, A., Guasti, M., Ghirardi, G., Lorenzi, L., and Guarnaschelli, C. (2001). Comprehension of reversible active and passive sentences in agrammatism. *Aphasiology*, *15*, 419–442.

Marslen-Wilson, W. D., and Tyler, L. K. (1997). Dissociating types of mental computation. *Nature*, *387*, 592–594.

Martin, R. C., and Romani, C. (1994). Verbal working memory and sentence comprehension: A multiple-components view. *Neuropsychology*, *8*, 506–523.

Mauner, G., Fromkin, V. A., and Cornell, T. L. (1993). Comprehension and acceptability judgments in agrammatism: Disruptions in the syntax of referential dependency. *Brain and Language*, *45*, 340–370.

Miyake, A., Carpenter, P. A., and Just, M. A. (1995). Reduced resources and specific impairments in normal and aphasic sentence comprehension. *Cognitive Neuropsychology*, *12*, 651–679.

Nespoulous, J. L., Dordain, M., Perron, C., Ska, B., Bub, D., Caplan, D., Mehler, J., and Lecours, A. R. (1988). Agrammatism in sentence production without comprehension deficits: Reduced availability of syntactic structures and/or of

grammatical morphemes? A case study. *Brain and Language*, *33*, 273–295.

Pulvermueller, F. (1995). Agrammatism: Behavioral description and neurobiological explanation. *Journal of Cognitive Neuroscience*, *7*, 165–181.

Saffran, E. M., Schwartz, M. F., and Linebarger, M. C. (1998). Semantic influences on thematic role assignment: Evidence from normals and aphasics. *Brain and Language*, *62*, 255–279.

Schwartz, M., Linebarger, M. C., Saffran, E., and Pate, D. (1987). Syntactic transparency and sentence interpretation in aphasia. *Language and Cognitive Processing*, *2*, 85–113.

Swaab, T. Y., Brown, C., and Hagoort, P. (1998). Understanding ambiguous words in sentence contexts: Electrophysiological evidence for delayed contextual selection in Broca's aphasia. *Neuropsychologia*, *36*, 737–761.

Swinney, D., Zurif, E., Prather, P., and Love, T. (1996). Neurological distribution of processing resources underlying language comprehension. *Journal of Cognitive Neuroscience*, *8*, 174–184.

Agraphia

Agraphia (or dysgraphia) is the term used to describe an acquired impairment of writing. The impairment may result from damage to any of the cognitive, linguistic, or sensorimotor processes that normally support the ability to spell and write. These procedures can be conceptualized within the framework of a cognitive model of language processing such as that shown in Figure 1 (Ellis, 1988; Shallice, 1988; Rapcsak and Beeson, 2000). According to the model, the writing process can be divided into central and peripheral components. The central components are linguistic in nature and are responsible for the retrieval of appropriate words and provision of information about their correct spelling. Peripheral procedures serve to translate spelling knowledge into handwriting, and to guide the motor control for appropriate movements of the hand.

When the system is working normally and an individual wants to write a familiar word, the relevant concepts in the semantic system activate representations in the memory store for learned spellings (i.e., the orthographic output lexicon). Access to this lexicon via the semantic system is referred to as the lexical-semantic spelling route. In contrast, when the individual attempts to spell unfamiliar words or pronounceable nonwords (such as *flig*), reliance on knowledge of sound-to-letter correspondences allows the assembly of plausible spellings by a process referred to as phoneme-grapheme conversion. This alternative means of spelling is depicted in Figure 1 by the arrow from the phonological buffer (where phonological information is held) to the graphemic buffer (where the assembled spelling is held). Spelling in this manner is considered a nonlexical process, because spellings are not retrieved as whole words from the lexicon. Spellings generated by the lexical-semantic and nonlexical spelling routes are subsequently processed in the graphemic buffer. This buffer serves as an interface between central spelling processes and the

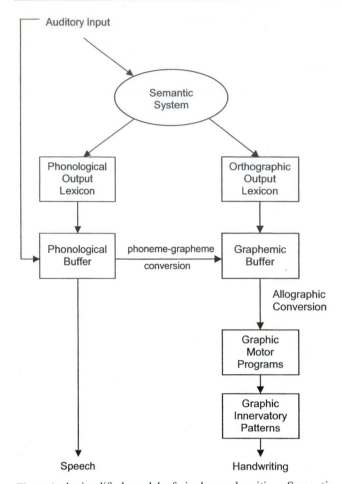

Figure 1. A simplified model of single-word writing. Semantic system refers to knowledge of word meanings. Orthographic output lexicon refers to memory store of learned spellings. Phoneme-grapheme conversion is the process of spelling by converting units of sound to corresponding letters. Graphemic buffer denotes a working memory system that temporarily stores orthographic representations while they are being converted into output for handwriting (or typing or oral spelling). Allographic conversion is the process by which abstract orthographic representations are converted into appropriate physical letter shapes. Graphic motor programs are spatiotemporal codes for writing movements that contain information about the sequence, position, direction, and relative size of the strokes necessary to create different letters. Graphic innervatory patterns are motor commands to specific muscle systems specifying the appropriate force, speed, and amplitude of movement. Phonological output lexicon is the memory store of sound patterns for familiar words used in speech production. Phonological buffer is a working memory system for phonological information.

peripheral procedures that support the production of handwriting. Peripheral writing procedures are accomplished through a series of hierarchically organized stages that include letter selection (referred to as allographic conversion), motor programming, and the generation of graphic innervatory patterns.

Clinical assessment of spelling and writing provides an understanding of the nature and degree of impairment to specific processes as well as the availability of residual abilities (Kay, Lesser, and Coltheart, 1992; Beeson and Hillis, 2001; Beeson and Rapcsak, 2002). Damage to specific components of the spelling process may result in identifiable agraphia syndromes with relatively predictable lesion sites (Roeltgen, 1993, 1994; Rapcsak and Beeson, 2000, 2002). *Central agraphia syndromes* reflect damage to the lexical-semantic or nonlexical spelling routes, or the graphemic buffer, and result in similar impairments across different modalities of output (e.g., written spelling, oral spelling, typing). Central agraphia syndromes include lexical agraphia, phonological agraphia, deep agraphia, and graphemic buffer agraphia. *Peripheral agraphia syndromes* reflect damage to writing processes that are distal to the graphemic buffer. Dysfunction primarily affects the selection or production of letters in handwriting. These syndromes include allographic disorders, apraxic agraphia, and nonapraxic disorders of neuromuscular execution (Roeltgen, 1993; Rapcsak, 1997; Rapcsak and Beeson, 2000). An individual may have impairment to multiple components of the writing process so that the agraphia profile does not conform to a recognized syndrome.

Lexical agraphia (also called surface agraphia) is a central agraphia syndrome that results from damage to the lexical-semantic spelling route. It is characterized by the loss or unavailability of orthographic knowledge, so that spelling is accomplished by phoneme-grapheme conversion and words are spelled as they sound. Spelling accuracy is strongly influenced by orthographic regularity in that regular words (e.g., *bake*) and nonwords are spelled correctly, but attempts to spell words with irregular sound-to-spelling relationships result in phonologically plausible errors (e.g., *cough—coff*). Low-frequency, irregular words are especially vulnerable to error. In addition, if the semantic influence on spelling is impaired, there is difficulty writing homophonic words that cannot be spelled correctly without reference to meaning (e.g., *dear—deer*). Lexical agraphia is typically seen following damage to left extrasylvian temporoparietal regions. The syndrome has also been described in patients with Alzheimer's disease and in semantic dementia.

Phonological agraphia and *deep agraphia* are central agraphia syndromes attributable to dysfunction of the nonlexical spelling route. In both syndromes, spelling is accomplished primarily via a lexical-semantic strategy, and individuals have difficulty using phoneme-grapheme conversion to spell unfamiliar words or nonwords. In phonological agraphia, the spelling of familiar words, both regular and irregular, may be relatively spared;

however, in deep agraphia, there is concomitant impairment of the lexical-semantic spelling route, so that semantic errors are prevalent (e.g., *boy—girl*). In both syndromes, spelling accuracy is better for highly frequent, concrete words (e.g., *house*) than for low-frequency, abstract words (e.g., *honor*). There is also an influence of grammatical word class in that nouns are easier to spell than function words such as prepositions, pronouns, and articles. Other spelling errors may include morphological errors (*talked—talking*) and functor substitutions (*as—with*). As in any of the central agraphia syndromes, patients may recall only some of the letters of the target word, reflecting partial orthographic knowledge. Phonological and deep agraphia are associated with damage to the perisylvian language areas, including Broca's area, Wernicke's area, and the supramarginal gyrus. Deep agraphia in patients with extensive left hemisphere lesions may reflect reliance on the right hemisphere for writing (Rapcsak, Beeson, and Rubens, 1991).

Graphemic buffer agraphia reflects impairment of the ability to retain orthographic representations in short-term memory as the appropriate graphic motor programs are selected and implemented. Damage to the graphemic buffer leads to abnormally rapid decay of information relevant to the order and identity of stored graphemes. Spelling accuracy is notably affected by word length because each additional grapheme increases the demand on limited storage capacity. In contrast to other central agraphia syndromes, spelling in graphemic buffer agraphia is not significantly influenced by lexical status (words versus nonwords), lexical-semantic features (frequency, concreteness, grammatical class), or orthographic regularity. Characteristic spelling errors include letter substitutions, additions, deletions, and transpositions (e.g., *garden—garned*). These errors are observed in all spelling tasks and across all modalities of output (writing, oral spelling, typing). Lesion sites in patients with graphemic buffer agraphia have been variable, but left parietal and frontal cortical involvement is common.

Allographic disorders are peripheral writing impairments that reflect the breakdown of procedures by which orthographic representations are mapped to letter-specific graphic motor programs. Allographic disorders are characterized by an inability to activate or select appropriate letter shapes, whereas oral spelling is preserved. Patients may have difficulty that is specific to writing upper- or lowercase letters, or they may produce case-mixing errors (e.g., *pApeR*). Other patients produce well-formed letter substitution errors that bear physical similarity to the target. Allographic disorders are usually associated with damage to the left parieto-occipital region.

Apraxia agraphia is a peripheral writing impairment caused by damage to graphic motor programs, or it may reflect an inability to translate information contained in these programs into specific motor commands. Apraxic agraphia is characterized by poor letter formation that cannot be attributed to sensorimotor impairment (i.e.,

weakness, deafferentation) or damage to the basal ganglia (i.e., tremor, rigidity) or cerebellum (i.e., ataxia, dysmetria). Typical errors of letter morphology include spatial distortions and stroke omissions or additions, which may result in illegible handwriting. Spelling by other modalities (e.g., oral spelling) is typically spared. In right-handers, apraxic agraphia is associated with damage to a left hemisphere cortical network dedicated to the motor programming of handwriting movements. The major functional components of this neural network include posterior-superior parietal cortex (including the region of the intraparietal sulcus), dorsolateral premotor cortex, and the supplementary motor area (SMA). Callosal lesions in right-handers may be accompanied by unilateral apraxic agraphia of the left hand.

Writing disorders attributable to *impaired neuromuscular execution* are caused by damage to motor systems involved in generating graphic innervatory patterns. Poor motor control results in defective control of writing force, speed, and amplitude. Such writing disorders reflect the specific underlying disease or locus of damage. In the case of Parkinson's disease, micrographia results from reduced force and amplitude of movements of the hand. In patients with cerebellar dysfunction, movements of the pen may be disjointed and erratic. Breakdown of graphomotor control in these neurological conditions suggests that the basal ganglia and the cerebellum, working in concert with dorsolateral premotor cortex and the SMA, are critically involved in the selection and implementation of kinematic parameters for writing movements. Obviously, patients with hemiparesis often have weakness and spasticity of the hand and limb that markedly impairs their ability to write with the preferred hand.

Behavioral treatments for agraphia may target central or peripheral components of the writing process (Behrmann and Byng, 1992; Carlomagno, Iavarone, and Colombo, 1994; Hillis and Caramazza, 1994; Patterson, 1994; Beeson and Hillis, 2001; Beeson and Rapcsak, 2002). Treatments for central agraphias may be directed toward the lexical-semantic or nonlexical spelling procedures. In contrast, treatments for peripheral agraphias are designed to improve the selection and implementation of graphic motor programs for writing. In general, agraphia treatments are designed to strengthen damaged processes and take advantage of residual abilities.

See also ALEXIA; PHONOLOGICAL ANALYSIS OF LANGUAGE DISORDERS IN APHASIA; PHONOLOGY AND ADULT APHASIA.

—*Pelagie M. Beeson and Steven Z. Rapcsak*

References

Beeson, P. M., and Hillis, A. E. (2001). Comprehension and production of written words. In R. Chapey (Ed.), *Language intervention strategies in adult aphasia* (4th ed., pp. 572–604). Baltimore: Lippincott, Williams and Wilkins.

Beeson, P. M., and Rapcsak, S. Z. (2002). Clinical diagnosis and treatment of spelling disorders. In A. E. Hillis (Ed.), *Handbook on adult language disorders: Integrating cognitive neuropsychology, neurology, and rehabilitation* (pp. 101–120). Philadelphia: Psychology Press.

Behrmann, M., and Byng, S. (1992). A cognitive approach to the neurorehabilitation of acquired language disorders. In D. I. Margolin (Ed.), *Cognitive neuropsychology in clinical practice* (pp. 327–350). New York: Oxford University Press.

Carlomagno, S., Iavarone, A., and Colombo, A. (1994). Cognitive approaches to writing rehabilitation: From single case to group studies. In M. J. Riddoch and G. W. Humphreys (Eds.), *Cognitive neuropsychology and cognitive rehabilitation* (pp. 485–502). Hillsdale, NJ: Erlbaum.

Ellis, A. W. (1988). Normal writing processes and peripheral acquired dysgraphias. *Language and Cognitive Processes, 3*, 99–127.

Hillis, A. E., and Caramazza, A. (1994). Theories of lexical processing and rehabilitation of lexical deficits. In M. J. Riddoch and G. W. Humphreys (Eds.), *Cognitive neuropsychology and cognitive rehabilitation* (pp. 1–30). Hillsdale, NJ: Erlbaum.

Kay, J., Lesser, R., and Coltheart, M. (1992). *Psycholinguistic assessments of language processing in aphasia (PALPA)*. East Sussex, England: Erlbaum.

Patterson, K. (1994). Reading, writing, and rehabilitation: A reckoning. In M. J. Riddoch and G. W. Humphreys (Eds.), *Cognitive neuropsychology and cognitive rehabilitation* (pp. 425–447). Hillsdale, NJ: Erlbaum.

Rapcsak, S. Z. (1997). Disorders of writing. In L. J. G. Rothi and K. M. Heilman (Eds.), *Apraxia: The neuropsychology of action* (pp. 149–172). Hove, England: Psychology Press.

Rapcsak, S. Z., and Beeson, P. M. (2000). Agraphia. In L. J. G. Rothi, B. Crosson, and S. Nadeau (Eds.), *Aphasia and language: Theory and practice* (pp. 184–220). New York: Guilford Press.

Rapcsak, S. Z., and Beeson, P. M. (2002). Neuroanatomical correlates of spelling and writing. In A. E. Hillis (Ed.), *Handbook on adult language disorders: Integrating cognitive neuropsychology, neurology, and rehabilitation* (pp. 71–99). Philadelphia: Psychology Press.

Rapcsak, S. Z., Beeson, P. M., and Rubens, A. B. (1991). Writing with the right hemisphere. *Brain and Language, 41*, 510–530.

Roeltgen, D. P. (1993). Agraphia. In K. M. Heilman and E. Valenstein (Eds.), *Clinical neuropsychology* (3rd ed., pp. 63–89). New York: Oxford University Press.

Roeltgen, D. P. (1994). Localization of lesions in agraphia. In A. Kertesz (Ed.), *Localization and neuroimaging in neuropsychology* (pp. 377–405). San Diego, CA: Academic Press.

Shallice, T. (1988). *From neuropsychology to mental structure*. Cambridge, U.K.: Cambridge University Press.

Alexia

Alexia, or acquired impairment of reading, is extremely common after stroke, dementia, or traumatic brain injury. Reading can be affected in a variety of different ways, leading to a number of different clinical syndromes or types of alexia. To understand these alexic syndromes, it is necessary to appreciate the cognitive processes underlying the task of reading words. Reading aloud a familiar word, such as *leopard*, normally entails at the very least seeing and perceiving the entire written letter string,

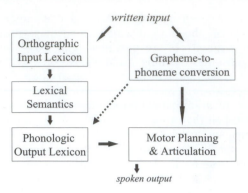

Figure 1. The cognitive processes underlying reading.

recognizing the word as a known word (by accessing a stored representation of the learned spelling of the word, in the orthographic input lexicon), accessing its meaning (or semantic representation), and accessing the pronunciation (the stored sound of the word, in the phonological output lexicon), as well as activating motor speech mechanisms for articulating the word. Even the first of these components, seeing and perceiving the entire written letter string, requires complex visual-perceptual skills, including computation of several levels of spatial representation, before the stored representations can be accessed. Furthermore, reading an unfamiliar word—say, an unfamiliar surname—entails access to print-to-sound conversion, or grapheme-to-phoneme conversion (GPC), mechanisms. Familiar words can also be read via GPC mechanisms, but the accuracy of pronunciation will depend on the "regularity" of the word—the extent to which the word conforms to typical GPC rules. For example, *sail* but not *yacht* can be read accurately via GPC mechanisms.

These components underlying the reading process are schematically depicted in Figure 1 (see Hillis and Caramazza, 1992, or Hillis, 2002, for a review of the evidence for various components of this model). Various features of this model are controversial, such as the precise nature and arrangement of the components, the degree to which they interact, and whether the various levels of representation are accessed in parallel or serially (Shallice, 1988; Hillis and Caramazza, 1991; Plaut and Shallice, 1993; Hillis, 2002). Nevertheless, most models of naming include most of the components depicted in Figure 1. Neurological impairment can selectively impair any one or more of these components of the reading process, with different consequences in terms of the types of errors produced and the types of stimuli that are affected. In addition, because several of the components of reading are cognitive mechanisms that are also involved in other tasks, damage to one of these shared components will have predictable consequences for reading *and* other tasks. For example, impairment at the level of semantics, or word meaning, will affect not only the reading of familiar irregular words but also the naming and comprehension of words. Thus, it is possible to identify what component of the reading system is impaired by considering the types of errors produced by the individual, the types of words that elicit errors, and the accuracy of performance across other language tasks, such as spoken naming and comprehension. The consequences of damage to each level of the reading process are discussed here.

Visual Attention and Perception. To read a familiar or unfamiliar word, the string of letters must be accurately perceived in the correct order and converted to a series of graphemes (abstract letter identities, without a particular case or font). Perception of the printed word can break down when there is (1) poor visual acuity or visual field cut, (2) impairment in distinguishing individual letters or symbols in a string (attentional dyslexia; Shallice, 1988), or (3) impairment in perception of more than one object or feature at a time (called simultagnosia; Parkin, 1996). An individual with simultagnosia might read the word *chair* as "h" or "i". Finally, individuals with damage to the nondominant (usually right) hemisphere of the brain often fail to perceive the side of a visual stimulus like a word that is contralateral to the brain damage. Such an impairment, known as neglect dyslexia, results in reading errors such as *chair* → "fair," *spool* → "pool," and *love* → "glove," errors that entail substitution, deletion, or insertion of letters on the left side (or initial letters) of words (Kinsbourne and Warrington, 1962; see papers in Riddoch, 1991, for reviews). Depending on the level of spatial representation affected, reading accuracy is sometimes improved by moving the printed word to the unaffected side of space or by spelling the word aloud to the person (see Hillis and Caramazza, 1995, for a discussion of various types of neglect dyslexia resulting from damage to distinct levels of spatial representation that are computed prior to accessing a stored graphemic representation). All types of reading stimuli are likely to be affected in neglect dyslexia, although words that have final letter strings in common with other words often elicit the most errors. For example, the words *light, fight, might, right, tight, sight, blight, bright, slight,* and so on are all likely to be read as the same word, since only the final letters are perceived and used to access the stored graphemic representation for recognition. Pseudo-words also elicit comparable errors (e.g., *glamp* → "lamp" or "damp"). An individual with impairment in computing one or more levels of spatial representation will usually also make errors in perceiving the left side of nonlinguistic visual stimuli (Hillis and Caramazza, 1995), although exceptional cases of pure neglect dyslexia, without other features of hemispatial neglect, have been reported (Costello and Warrington, 1987; Patterson and Wilson, 1990).

Orthographic Input Lexicon. Impairment at the level of accessing learned spellings of familiar words, or stored graphemic representations that constitute the "orthographic input lexicon," results in impaired recognition of written words despite accurate perception of the letters. The individual with this impairment will often fail to distinguish familiar from unfamiliar words, or pseudo-words (e.g., *glamp*), in a task known as *lexical decision.* Sometimes such an individual will read each letter in the string aloud serially, which seems to facilitate access to the orthographic input lexicon (resulting in letter-by-letter reading; see papers in Coltheart, 1998). If GPC mechanisms are intact, these mechanisms may be used to read even familiar words, resulting in "regularization" of irregular words (e.g., *one* → "own"). Other errors are predominantly visually similar words (e.g., *though* → "touch"). Oral reading of all types of words may be affected, although very familiar words—those frequently encountered in reading—may be relatively spared. Since the orthographic input lexicon is not involved in other linguistic tasks, damage to this cognitive process does not cause errors in other tasks. Therefore, individuals with impairment of this component are said to have pure alexia.

Semantic System. Disruption of semantic representations is often incomplete, such that the meanings that are accessed are often impoverished, and only certain categories of words are affected. For example, an alexic patient may read *dog* as "cat" if an incomplete semantic representation of dog is accessed that specifies only ⟨animal⟩, or ⟨mammal⟩, ⟨domesticated⟩, ⟨quadraped⟩, etc., without information about what differentiates a dog from a cat. Thus, most errors are semantically related words, such as *robin* → "cardinal" or *robin* → "bird" (errors called semantic paralexias). However, if GPC mechanisms are available, these may be used to read all types of words, or used to block semantic paralexias. Or GPC mechanisms may be combined with partial semantic information to access the correct phonological representation in the output lexicon, so that the individual can read aloud words better than he or she can understand words (Hillis and Caramazza, 1991). Often there is especially incomplete semantic information to distinguish abstract words, so that abstract words are read less accurately than concrete words. Similarly, functors are read least accurately, often with one functor substituted for another (e.g., *therefore* → "because"); verbs are read less accurately than adjectives; and adjectives are read less accurately than nouns (Coltheart, Patterson, and Marshall, 1980). If GPC mechanisms are also impaired (a commonly co-occurring deficit), pseudo-words and unfamiliar words cannot be read. Since the semantic system is shared by the tasks of naming and comprehension, semantic errors are also made in oral and written naming and in comprehension of spoken and written words (Hillis et al., 1990).

Phonological Output Lexicon. Impairment in accessing phonological representations for output results in poor oral reading despite accurate comprehension of printed words. For example, *gray* might be read as "blue" but defined as "the color of hair when you get old" (from Caramazza and Hillis, 1990). Again, if GPC mechanisms are available, these mechanisms may be used to

Table 1. Characteristics of Reported Individuals with Surface Alexia (Compensatory Use of GPC Mechanisms)

	PS*	JJ*	HG*
Error types (example of errors)	Regularization (*bear* → "beer")	Regularization (*were* → "we're")	Regularization (*one* → "own")
Lexical decision	Impaired	Intact	Intact
Written word comprehension	Impaired (e.g., *shoe* understood as "show")	Impaired (e.g., *shoe* understood as sock)	Intact[†]
Spoken word comprehension	Intact	Impaired (e.g., "shoe" understood as sock)	Intact[†]
Oral naming	Intact	Impaired (e.g., a shoe named as "sock")	Impaired (e.g., shoe named as "glove")
GPC mechanisms	Intact	Intact	Intact
Level of deficit	Orthographic input lexicon	Semantic system	Phonological output lexicon

*PS is described in Hillis (1993); JJ is described in Hillis and Caramazza (1991); HG is described in Hillis (1991).

[†] HG also had a semantic impairment for certain categories of words; this table describes her performance for categories for which she had intact comprehension, such as numbers and clothing. PS also had a mild semantic impairment in the categories of animals and vegetables; this table describes his performance for categories for which he had intact comprehension.

read aloud all types of words, resulting in regularization errors on irregular words. Otherwise, errors may be semantically related (e.g., *fork* → "spoon"), or phonologically related to the target (e.g., *choir* → "queer"). Phonological representations of words that are used more frequently may be more accessible than other words, so that high-frequency words are read more accurately than low-frequency words. Since the phonological output lexicon is also essential for oral naming and spontaneous speech, the person will make similar errors on these tasks as in reading.

Types of Alexia

A number of alexic syndromes consisting of a particular pattern of frequently co-occurring symptoms in reading have been described. (These types of alexia are also known as acquired dyslexia.) Individuals with a particular alexic syndrome may have different underlying deficits, however. To identify which component of the reading process is impaired it is necessary to know not only the error types and the types of words that are misread, but also the individual's pattern of performance on other lexical tasks, such as naming and comprehension.

Surface alexia or surface dyslexia refers to a pattern of reading that reflects use of GPC mechanisms to read both familiar and unfamiliar words, so that irregular words are often read as regularization errors (e.g., *bear* → "beer"; see papers in Patterson, Coltheart, and Marshall, 1985). Regular words, which can be read accurately via GPC mechanisms, are more likely to be read correctly than irregular words. Comprehension of homophones, such as *eight* and *ate*, may be confused. Oral reading of pseudo-words is accurate. This pattern can be seen with damage to any level of the reading system that requires reliance on GPC mechanisms to bypass the damaged component. For example, Table 1 describes features of three patients with surface alexia who

each had impairment at different levels of lexical representation but had intact GPC mechanisms.

Phonological alexia or phonological dyslexia refers to impairment in use of GPC mechanisms, so that the reader is unable to compose a plausible pronunciation of unfamiliar words or pseudo-words. In addition, occasional semantic paralexias or functor substitutions are produced, presumably because these errors are not blocked by GPC mechanisms (see Beauvois and Derouesne, 1979; Goodglass and Budin, 1988; Shallice, 1988).

Deep alexia or deep dyslexia is a pattern that arises when there is damage to both GPC mechanisms and another component of the "semantic route" of reading: the semantic system and/or the phonological output lexicon (see Coltheart, Patterson, and Marshall, 1980). Semantic paralexias and functor substitutions are invariably produced, although visually similar word errors and derivational errors (e.g., *write* → "writer"; *predicted* → "prediction") are also common. Concrete words are read more accurately than abstract words, and there is the following grammatical category effect: nouns > adjectives > verbs > functors (nouns most accurate). Table 2 characterizes patterns of performance across tasks in patients with deep dyslexia with damage to different components of the semantic route. It has been argued that the pattern of reading errors reflects reliance on the nondominant hemisphere's rudimentary language capabilities (Coltheart, 1980), although direct evidence for this proposal is lacking.

Neglect dyslexia, attentional dyslexia, and pure alexia were described under impairments of specific components.

Neurological disease or focal brain damage can disrupt one or more relatively distinct cognitive mechanisms that underlie the task of reading, resulting in different patterns of reading impairment. It is generally possible to identify the impaired components by determining the types of errors made, the types of stimuli that

Table 2. Characteristics of Reported Individuals with Deep Alexia (Compensatory Use of GPC Mechanisms)

	KE*	RGB*
Error types (example of errors)	Semantic paralexias (e.g., *peach* → apple), derivational errors (e.g., *walked* → "walk"), functor substitutions (e.g., *in* → "for")	Semantic paralexias (e.g., *hope* → "faith"), derivational errors (e.g., *crime* → "criminal"), functor substitutions (e.g., *toward* → "shall")
Written word comprehension	Impaired (e.g., *shoe* understood as "mitten")	Intact (e.g., *six* read as "seven," but defined as "half a dozen")
Spoken word comprehension	Impaired (e.g., "shoe" understood as mitten)	Intact
Oral naming	Impaired (e.g., shoe named as "mitten")	Impaired (e.g., mittens named as "socks")
GPC mechanisms	Impaired	Impaired
Levels of deficit	Semantic system and GPC mechanisms	Phonological output lexicon and GPC mechanisms

*KE is described in Hillis et al. (1990); RGB is described in Caramazza and Hillis (1990).

are misread, and the accuracy of performance on related tasks, such as word comprehension and naming. The various components of the reading system have distinct neural substrates, so that damage to different parts of the brain results in different patterns of alexia (see Black and Behrmann, 1994, and Hillis et al., 2002, for reviews).

—*Argye E. Hillis*

References

Beauvois, M. F., and Derouesne, J. (1979). Phonological alexia: Three dissociations. *Journal of Neurology, Neurosurgery, and Psychiatry*, 42, 1115–1124.

Black, S., and Behrmann, M. (1994). Localization in alexia. In A. Kertesz (Ed.), *Localization and neuroimaging in neuropsychology* (pp. 152–184). San Diego, CA: Academic Press.

Caramazza, A., and Hillis, A. E. (1990). Where do semantic errors come from? *Cortex*, 26, 95–122.

Coltheart, M. (1980). Deep dyslexia: A right hemisphere hypothesis. In M. Coltheart, K. E. Patterson, and J. C. Marshall (Eds.), *Deep dyslexia* (pp. 326–380). London: Routledge and Kegan Paul.

Coltheart, M. (Ed.) (1998). Pure alexia (letter-by-letter reading) [Special issue]. *Cognitive Neuropsychology*, 15, 1–238.

Coltheart, M., Patterson, K., and Marshall, J. C. (Eds.). (1980). *Deep dyslexia*. London: Routledge and Kegan Paul.

Costello, A. de L., and Warrington, E. K. (1987). Dissociation of visuo-spatial neglect and neglect dyslexia. *Journal of Neurology, Neurosurgery, and Psychiatry*, 50, 1110–1116.

Goodglass, H., and Budin, C. (1988). Category and modality specific dissociations in word comprehension and concurrent phonological dyslexia. *Neuropsychologia*, 26, 67–78.

Hillis, A. E. (1991). Effects of a separate treatments for distinct impairments within the naming process. In T. Prescott (Ed.), *Clinical aphasiology* (vol. 19, pp. 255–265). Austin, TX: Pro-Ed.

Hillis, A. E. (1993). The role of models of language processing in rehabilitation of language impairments. *Aphasiology*, 7, 5–26.

Hillis, A. E. (2002). The cognitive processes underlying reading. In A. E. Hillis (Ed.), *Handbook of adult language disorders: Integrating cognitive neuropsychology, neurology, and rehabilitation*. Philadelphia: Psychology Press.

Hillis, A. E., and Caramazza, A. (1991). Mechanisms for accessing lexical representations for output: Evidence from a category-specific semantic deficit. *Brain and Language*, 40, 106–144.

Hillis, A. E., and Caramazza, A. (1992). The reading process and its disorders. In D. I. Margolin (Ed.), *Cognitive neuropsychology in clinical practice* (pp. 229–261). New York: Oxford University Press.

Hillis, A. E., and Caramazza, A. (1995). A framework for interpreting distinct patterns of hemispatial neglect. *Neurocase*, 1, 189–207.

Hillis, A. E., Kane, A., Barker, P., Beauchamp, N., and Wityk, R. (2001). Neural substrates of the cognitive processes underlying reading: Evidence from magnetic resonance perfusion imaging in hyperacute stroke. *Aphasiology*, 15, 919–931.

Hillis, A. E., Rapp, B. C., Romani, C., and Caramazza, A. (1990). Selective impairment of semantics in lexical processing. *Cognitive Neuropsychology*, 7, 191–244.

Kinsbourne, M., and Warrington, E. K. (1962). A variety of reading disability associated with right hemisphere lesions. *Journal of Neurology, Neurosurgery, and Psychiatry*, 25, 334–339.

Parkin, A. J. (1996). *Explorations in cognitive neuropsychology*. Oxford, U.K.: Blackwell.

Patterson, K., and Wilson, B. (1990). A ROSE is a ROSE or a NOSE: A deficit in initial letter identification. *Cognitive Neuropsychology*, 7, 447–477.

Patterson, K. E., Coltheart, M., and Marshall, J. C. (1985). *Surface dyslexia*. London: LEA.

Plaut, D., and Shallice, T. (1993). Deep dyslexia: A case study of connectionist neuropsychology. *Cognitive Neuropsychology*, 10, 377–500.

Riddoch, M. J. (Ed.). (1991). *Neglect and the peripheral dyslexias*. Hove, U.K.: Erlbaum.

Shallice, T. (1988). *From neuropsychology to mental structure*. Cambridge, U.K.: Cambridge University Press.

Further Readings

Benson, D. F., and Geschwind, N. (1969). The alexias. In P. J. Vinken and G. W. Bruyn (Eds.), *Handbook of clinical neuropsychology* (vol. 4). Amsterdam: North Holland.

Coltheart, M., and Funnell, E. (1987). Reading and writing: One lexicon or two? In D. A. Allport, D. G. Mackay, W. Prinz, and E. Scheerer (Eds.), *Language perception and production: Shared mechanisms in listening, reading, and writing*. London: Academic Press.

Friedman, R. B., and Alexander, M. P. (1984). Pictures, images, and pure alexia: A case study. *Cognitive Neuropsychology*, 1, 9–23.

Marshall, J. C., and Newcombe, F. (1966). Syntactic and semantic errors in paralexia. *Neuropsychologia, 4,* 169–176.

Marshall, J. C., and Newcombe, F. (1973). Patterns of paralexia: A psycholinguistic approach. *Journal of Psycholinguistic Research, 2,* 175–199.

Rapcsak, S. Z., Gonzalez Rothi, L., and Heilman, K. M. (1987). Phonologic alexia with optic and tactile anomia: A neuropsychological and anatomic study. *Brain and Language, 31,* 109–121.

Rapp, B., Folk, J. R., Tainturier, M. (2001). Word reading. In B. Rapp (Ed.), *The handbook of cognitive neuropsychology.* Philadelphia: Psychology Press.

Reuter-Lorenz, P. A., and Brunn, J. L. (1990). A prelexical basis for letter-by-letter reading: A case study. *Cognitive Neuropsychology, 7,* 1–20.

Alzheimer's Disease

Alzheimer's disease (AD) is a neurodegenerative condition that results in insidiously progressive cognitive decline. According to widely recognized clinical diagnostic criteria for AD (McKhann et al., 1984), these patients have language processing impairments as well as difficulty with memory, visual perceptual-spatial processing, and executive functioning. The language impairment changes as the disease progresses (Bayles et al., 2000), and one profound consequence of language difficulty in AD is that this deficit strongly reflects clinical decline and the need for additional skilled nursing support (Chan et al., 1995). This article briefly summarizes the studies showing that AD patients' language deficit includes difficulty with comprehension and expression of the sounds/letters, words, and sentences that are used to communicate in day-to-day circumstances. Work relating these language deficits to a specific neuroanatomical distribution of disease is also reviewed.

We may consider first the semantic impairment in AD. This deficit limits the comprehension and expression of concepts represented by single words and sentences. In expression, for example, a significant word-finding deficit is a prominent and early clinical feature of AD (Bayles, Tomoeda, and Trosset, 1990; White-Devine et al., 1996; Cappa et al., 1998). This is seen in spontaneous speech as well as on measures of confrontation naming. Naming difficulty due to a semantic impairment often is manifested as semantic paraphasic errors, such as the substitution of "chair" for the intended target "table." As the condition progresses, AD patients' spontaneous speech becomes limited to the use of overlearned phrases and ultimately becomes quite empty of content, while they fail to provide any responses during confrontation naming.

Semantic deficits are also prominent in comprehension. More than 50% of AD patients differ significantly from healthy seniors in their performance on simple category judgment tasks. For example, many AD patients are impaired when shown a word or a picture and asked, "Is this a vegetable?" (Grossman et al., 1996). Priming is a relatively automatic measure of semantic

integrity: AD patients have relatively preserved priming for high-frequency lexical associates such as "cottage-cheese" that have little semantic relationship (Nebes, 1989; Ober et al., 1991), but they are impaired in their priming for coordinates taken from the same semantic category, such as "peach-banana" (Glosser and Friedman, 1991; Glosser et al., 1998). Item-by-item analyses show reduced priming for words that are difficult to understand and name (Chertkow, Bub, and Seidenberg, 1989). The unity of impairment across comprehension and expression is emphasized by the observation of the greatest naming difficulty in patients with significant semantic comprehension deficits (Chertkow and Bub, 1990; Hodges, Salmon, and Butters, 1992). The basis for this pattern of impaired semantic memory has been an active focus of investigation. Some studies associate the semantic comprehension impairment in AD with the degradation of knowledge about a word and its associated concept (Gonnerman et al., 1997; Garrard et al., 1998; Conley, Burgess, and Glosser, 2001). A category-specific deficit understanding or naming natural kinds such as "animals" compared with manufactured artifacts such as "implements" may emerge in AD (Silveri et al., 1991). Other recent work suggests that difficulty understanding words and pictures in AD is related to an impairment in the categorization process that is so crucial to understanding concepts. In particular, AD patients appear to have difficulty implementing rule-based processes for understanding the critical features of words that determine category membership (Grossman, Smith, et al., submitted) or for learning the category membership of new concepts (Koenig et al., 2001).

The comprehension and expression of concepts often requires appreciating the long-distance relationships among several words in a sentence. Some early work attributes sentence processing difficulty in AD to a grammatical deficit. Paragrammatic errors such as "mices" and "catched" can be observed in speech, oral reading, and writing. Other studies relate impaired comprehension to difficulty with the grammatical features of phrases and a deficit in understanding grammatically complex sentences such as those containing a center-embedded clause (Emery and Breslau, 1989; Kontiola et al., 1990; Grober and Bang, 1995; Croot, Hodges, and Patterson, 1999). Essentially normal performance during on-line studies of sentence comprehension cast doubt on this claim (Kempler et al., 1998; Grossman and Rhee, 2001). More recently, considerable evidence indicates that sentence processing difficulty is related to a limitation in the working memory resources often needed to support sentence processing. Although the precise nature of the limited cognitive resource(s) remains to be established, AD patients' grammatical comprehension deficit can be brought out by experimental manipulations that stress cognitive resources such as working memory, inhibitory control, and information processing speed. Studies demonstrate working memory limitations through the use of verbs featuring unusual syntactic-thematic mapping in a sentence comprehension task (Grossman and White-Devine, 1998), concurrent performance of a secondary task during sentence comprehension (Waters, Caplan, and Rochon, 1995; Waters, Rochon, and Caplan, 1998), and limited inhibition of the context-inappropriate meaning of a polysemous word (Faust et al., 1997).

Semantic memory and sentence processing appear to be preserved in some AD patients. Nevertheless, this cohort of AD patients may have a different language impairment profile. Many of these patients, despite preserved single-word and sentence comprehension, are impaired in retrieving words from the mental lexicon. This kind of naming difficulty is marked by changes in the sounds contributing to a word, such as omissions and substitutions (Biassou et al., 1995). This limitation in lexical retrieval appears to be equally evident on oral lexical retrieval tasks and in writing. AD patients appear to be quite accurate at discriminating between speech sounds that vary in the place of articulation or voice onset timing, but phonemic (single-sound) substitutions can also be heard in their speech.

Alzheimer's disease is a focal neurodegenerative condition. Functional neuroimaging studies obtained at rest with modalities such as single-photon emission computed tomography, positron emission tomography, and functional magnetic resonance imaging (fMRI) (Foster et al., 1983; Friedland, Brun, and Budinger, 1985; DeKosky et al., 1990; Johnson et al., 1993; Alsop, Detre, and Grossman, 2000) and histopathological studies of autopsied brains (Brun and Gustafson, 1976; Arnold et al., 1991; Braak and Braak, 1995) show that specific brain regions are compromised in AD. The neuroanatomical distribution of disease revealed by these studies includes gross defects such as atrophy and microscopic abnormalities such as neuritic plaques and neurofibrillary tangles in the temporal, parietal, and frontal association cortices of the brain. The neural basis for the language difficulties in AD is investigated most commonly through brain-behavior correlation studies, although occasional functional neuroimaging reports describe defects in regional brain activation during language challenges. Early correlation studies relate sentence comprehension difficulty to reduced resting activity in posterior temporal and inferior parietal regions of the left hemisphere (Haxby et al., 1985; Grady et al., 1988). More recent work associates difficulty understanding single words and impaired confrontation naming with left temporoparietal cortex (Desgranges et al., 1998). Moreover, the defect in this brain region is significantly greater in AD patients with a semantic memory impairment than in AD patients with relatively preserved semantic memory (Grossman et al., 1997), and a comparative study demonstrates the specificity of this correlative pattern in AD relative to patients with a frontotemporal form of dementia (Grossman et al., 1998). By comparison, only very modest correlations show a relationship between grammatical comprehension and left inferior frontal cortex in AD.

A handful of functional neuroimaging studies report monitoring the regional cortical responses of AD patients during language challenges. One study shows limited activation of middle and inferior frontal regions in AD patients that had been recruited during a category membership semantic decision in healthy seniors (Saykin et al., 1999). More recently, a BOLD fMRI study of semantic judgments described limited activation of left temporoparietal cortex and frontal cortex in AD patients compared to healthy seniors, and AD patients recruited brain regions adjacent to the activated areas seen in elderly control subjects for specific categories of knowledge such as "animals" and "implements" (Grossman, Koenig, et al., in press).

AD patients thus have prominent deficits at several levels of language processing. This includes impaired semantic memory, manifested in measures of comprehension and expression. There is also difficulty with lexical retrieval in reading and writing, although perceptual judgments of speech sounds are relatively preserved. The neural basis for these language impairments appears to be a defect in temporoparietal association cortex of the left hemisphere, although a defect in left frontal association cortex also may contribute to the language impairments in AD.

See also DEMENTIA.

Acknowledgments

Work was supported in part by U.S. Public Health Service grants AG15116, AG17586, and NS35867.

—Murray Grossman

References

Alsop, D. C., Detre, J., and Grossman, M. (2000). Assessment of cerebral blood flow in Alzheimer's disease by arterial spin labelling fMRI. *Annals of Neurology, 47,* 93–100.

Arnold, S. E., Hyman, B. T., Flory, J., Damasio, A. R., and van Hoesen, G. W. (1991). The topographic and neuroanatomical distribution of neurofibrillary tangles and neuritic plaques in the cerebral cortex of patients with Alzheimer's disease. *Cerebral Cortex, 1,* 103–116.

Bayles, K. A., Tomoeda, C. K., Cruz, R. F., and Mahendra, N. (2000). Communication abilities of individuals with late-stage Alzheimer disease. *Alzheimer Disease and Associated Disorders, 14,* 176–182.

Bayles, K. A., Tomoeda, C. K., and Trosset, M. W. (1990). Naming and categorical knowledge in Alzheimer's disease: The process of semantic memory deterioration. *Brain and Language, 39,* 498–510.

Biassou, N., Grossman, M., Onishi, K., Mickanin, J., Hughes, E., Robinson, K. M., et al. (1995). Phonological processing deficits in Alzheimer's disease. *Neurology, 45,* 2165–2169.

Braak, H., and Braak, E. (1995). Staging of Alzheimer's disease-related neurofibrillary changes. *Neurobiology of Aging, 16,* 271–278.

Brun, A., and Gustafson, L. (1976). Distribution of cerebral degeneration in Alzheimer's disease: A clinico-pathologic study. *Archives für Psychiatrik Nervenkrasse, 223,* 15–33.

Cappa, S. F., Binetti, G., Pezzini, A., Padovani, A., Rozzini, L., and Trabucchi, M. (1998). Object and action naming in Alzheimer's disease and fronto-temporal dementia. *Neurology, 50,* 351–355.

Chan, A. S., Salmon, D. P., Butters, N., and Johnson, S. A. (1995). Semantic network abnormality predicts rate of cognitive decline in patients with probable Alzheimer's disease. *Journal of the International Neuropsychological Society, 1*, 297–303.

Chertkow, H., and Bub, D. N. (1990). Semantic memory loss in dementia of the Alzheimer's type: What do the various measures measure? *Brain, 113*, 397–417.

Chertkow, H., Bub, D. N., and Seidenberg, M. (1989). Priming and semantic memory loss in Alzheimer's disease. *Brain and Language, 36*, 420–446.

Conley, P., Burgess, C., and Glosser, G. (2001). Age vs. Alzheimer's: A computational model of changes in representation. *Brain and Cognition, 46*, 86–90.

Croot, K., Hodges, J. R., and Patterson, K. (1999). Evidence for imapired sentence comprehension in early Alzheimer's disease. *Journal of the International Neuropsychological Society, 5*, 393–404.

DeKosky, S. T., Shih, W. J., Schmitt, F. A., Coupal, J., and Kirkpatrick, C. (1990). Assessing utility of single photon emission computed tomography (SPECT) scan in Alzheimer's disease: Correlation with cognitive severity. *Alzheimer Disease and Associated Disorders, 4*, 14–23.

Desgranges, B., Baron, J.-C., de la Sayette, V., Petit-Taboue, M. C., Benali, K., Landeau, B., et al. (1998). The neural substrates of memory systems impairment in Alzheimer's disease: A PET study of resting brain glucose utilization. *Brain, 121*, 611–631.

Emery, O. B., and Breslau, L. D. (1989). Language deficits in depression: Comparisons with SDAT and normal aging. *Journal of Gerontology, 44*, M85–M92.

Faust, M., Balota, D. A., Duchek, J. M., Gernsbacher, M. A., and Smith, S. (1997). Inhibitory control during sentence comprehension in individuals with dementia of the Alzheimer type. *Brain and Language, 57*, 225–253.

Foster, N. L., Chase, T. N., Fedio, P., Patronas, N. J., Brooks, R. A., and DiChiro, G. (1983). Alzheimer's disease: Focal cortical changes shown by positron emission tomography. *Neurology, 33*, 961–965.

Friedland, R., Brun, A., and Budinger, T. (1985). Pathological and positron emission tomographic correlations in Alzheimer's disease. *Lancet, 1*, 288.

Garrard, P., Patterson, K., Watson, P. C., and Hodges, J. R. (1998). Category specific semantic loss in dementia of Alzheimer's type: Functional-anatomic correlations from cross-sectional analyses. *Brain, 121*, 633–646.

Glosser, G., and Friedman, R. (1991). Lexical but not semantic priming in Alzheimer's disease. *Psychology and Aging, 6*, 522–527.

Glosser, G., Friedman, R., Grugan, P. K., Lee, J. H., and Grossman, M. (1998). Lexical semantic and associative priming in Alzheimer's disease. *Neuropsychology, 12*, 218–224.

Gonnerman, L. M., Andersen, E. S., Devlin, J. T., Kempler, D., and Seidenberg, M. S. (1997). Double dissociation of semantic categories in Alzheimer's disease. *Brain and Language, 57*, 254–279.

Grady, C. L., Haxby, J. V., Horwitz, B., and Sundaram, M. (1988). Longitudinal study of the early neuropsychological and cerebral metabolic changes in dementia of the Alzheimer type. *Journal of Clinical and Experimental Neuropsychology, 10*, 576–596.

Grober, E., and Bang, S. (1995). Sentence comprehension in Alzheimer's disease. *Developmental Neuropsychology, 11*, 95–107.

Grossman, M., D'Esposito, M., Hughes, E., Onishi, K., Biassou, N., White-Devine, T., et al. (1996). Language comprehension difficulty in Alzheimer's disease, vascular dementia, and fronto-temporal degeneration. *Neurology, 47*, 183–189.

Grossman, M., Koenig, P., Glosser, G., DeVita, C., Moore, P., Rhee, J., et al. (in press). Semantic memory difficulty in Alzheimer's disease: An fMRI study. *Brain.*

Grossman, M., Payer, F., Onishi, K., D'Esposito, M., Morrison, D., Sadek, A., and Alavi, A. (1998). Language comprehension and regional cerebral defects in frontotemporal degeneration and Alzheimer's disease. *Neurology, 50*, 157–163.

Grossman, M., and Rhee, J. (2001). Cognitive resources during sentence processing in Alzheimer's disease. *Neuropsychologia, 39*, 1419–1431.

Grossman, M., Smith, E. E., Koenig, P., Glosser, G., Rhee, J., and Dennis, K. (submitted). Categorization of object descriptions in Alzheimer's disease and frontotemporal dementia: Limitation in rule-based processing.

Grossman, M., and White-Devine, T. (1998). Sentence comprehension in Alzheimer's disease. *Brain and Language, 62*, 186–201.

Grossman, M., White-Devine, T., Payer, F., Onishi, K., D'Esposito, M., Robinson, K. M., et al. (1997). Constraints on the cerebral basis for semantic processing from neuroimaging studies of Alzheimer's disease. *Journal of Neurology, Neurosurgery, and Psychiatry, 63*, 152–158.

Haxby, J. V., Duara, R., Grady, C., Cutler, N., and Rapoport, S. (1985). Relations between neuropsychological and cerebral metabolic asymmetries in early Alzheimer's disease. *Journal of Cerebral Blood Flow and Metabolism, 5*, 193–200.

Hodges, J. R., Salmon, D. P., and Butters, N. (1992). Semantic memory impairment in Alzheimer's disease: Failure of access or degraded knowledge. *Neuropsychologia, 30*, 301–314.

Johnson, K. A., Kijewski, M. F., Becker, J. A., Garada, B., Satlin, A., and Holman, B. L. (1993). Quantitative brain SPECT in Alzheimer's disease and normal aging. *Journal of Nuclear Medicine, 34*, 2044–2048.

Kempler, D., Almor, A., Tyler, L. K., Andersen, E. S., and MacDonald, M. C. (1998). Sentence comprehension deficits in Alzheimer's disease: A comparison of off-line vs. on-line sentence processing. *Brain and Language, 64*, 297–316.

Koenig, P., Smith, E. E., Rhee, J., Moore, P., Petock, L., and Grossman, M. (2001). Categorization of novel animals in Alzheimer's disease. *Neurology, 56*, A56–A57.

Kontiola, P., Laaksonen, R., Sulkava, R., and Erkinjuntti, T. (1990). Pattern of language impairment is different in Alzheimer's disease and multi-infarct dementia. *Brain and Language, 38*, 364–383.

McKhann, G., Drachman, D., Folstein, M., Katzman, R., Price, D., and Stadian, E. M. (1984). Clinical diagnosis of Alzheimer's disease: Report on the NINCDS-ADRDA work group under the auspices of the Department of Health and Human Services Task Force on Alzheimer's disease. *Neurology, 34*, 939–944.

Nebes, R. D. (1989). Semantic memory in Alzheimer's disease. *Psychological Bulletin, 106*, 377–394.

Ober, B. A., Shenaut, G. K., Jagust, W. J., and Stillman, R. C. (1991). Automatic semantic priming with various category relations in Alzheimer's disease and normal aging. *Psychology and Aging, 6*, 647–660.

Saykin, A. J., Flashman, L. A., Frutiger, S. A., Johnson, S. C., Mamourian, A. C., Moritz, C. H., et al. (1999). Neuroanatomic substrates of semantic memory impairment in Alzheimer's disease: Patterns of functional MRI activation. *Journal of the International Neuropsychological Society, 5*, 377–392.

Silveri, M. C., Daniele, A., Giustolisi, L., and Gainotti, G. (1991). Dissociation between living and nonliving things in dementia of the Alzheimer type. *Neurology, 41,* 545–546.

Waters, G. S., Caplan, D., and Rochon, E. (1995). Processing capacity and sentence comprehension in patients with Alzheimer's disease. *Cognitive Neuropsychology, 12,* 1–30.

Waters, G. S., Rochon, E., and Caplan, D. (1998). Task demands and sentence comprehension in patients with dementia of the Alzheimer's type. *Brain and Language, 62,* 361–397.

White-Devine, T., Robinson, K. M., Onishi, K., Seidl, A., Biassou, N., D'Esposito, M., et al. (1996). Verb confrontation naming and word-picture matching in Alzheimer's disease. *Neuropsychology, 10,* 495–503.

Aphasia, Global

Global aphasia is an acquired language disorder characterized by severe loss of comprehension with concomitant deficits in expressive abilities (Peach, 2001). Unlike other syndromes of aphasia, few distinctions are found between preserved and impaired components of these patients' language. The outlook for recovery from global aphasia tends to be bleak (Kertesz and McCabe, 1977). For this reason, the term global may be more prognostic than descriptive.

Several isolated areas of relatively preserved comprehension have been identified in global aphasia. These include recognition of specific word categories (Wapner and Gardner, 1979) and famous personal and geographic names (Yasuda and Ono, 1998). Globally aphasic subjects also show relatively better comprehension for personally relevant information (Van Lancker and Nicklay, 1992).

Globally aphasic patients are most severely impaired in their expressive abilities. The verbal output of many patients with global aphasia consists primarily of stereotypic recurring utterances or speech automatisms. Recurrent utterances have been described as being either nondictionary verbal forms (unrecognizable) consisting of consonant-vowel (CV) syllables (for example, do-do-do or ma-ma-ma) or dictionary forms (word or sentence) (Alajouanine, 1956). Blanken, Wallesch, and Papagno (1990) investigated the relationship between the nondictionary forms of recurrent utterances and comprehension disturbances in global aphasia. Although recurrent utterances are frequently associated with comprehension disturbances, the overall variability in language comprehension suggests that speech stereotypes cannot be used to infer the presence of severe comprehension deficits.

Patients with global aphasia give the impression of having more preserved communicative abilities than is actually the case because of their use of the suprasegmental aspects of speech. To investigate this, deBlesser and Poeck (1985) analyzed the spontaneous utterances of a group of globally aphasic subjects with output limited to CV recurrences. They concluded that the length and pitch of these utterances were stereotypical and that the prosody of these patients did not seem to reflect communicative intent. The contributions to conversation that are credited to these patients, therefore, may be the result of the communicative partners' need for informative communication rather than the patients' use of prosodic elements to convey intent.

The efficiency of communication following global aphasia depends on the type of question that is asked (Herrmann et al., 1989). Better performance is observed for responses to yes/no questions than for responses to interrogative pronoun questions and narrative requests. Patients with global aphasia mostly use gesture in their responses to yes/no questions. The other types of questioning require increased verbal output and thus create the need for more complex communicative responses.

Patients with global aphasia rarely take the initiative to communicate or expand on shared topics (Herrmann et al., 1989). Their most frequent communication strategies are those that enable them to secure comprehension (e.g., indicating comprehension problems, requesting support for establishing comprehension). Although these individuals rely most heavily on nonverbal strategies, the efficiency of their communication may approximate that of less impaired aphasic patients while imposing nearly as low a burden on the communication partner (Marshall, Freed, and Phillips, 1997).

Global aphasia results most commonly from a cerebrovascular event in the middle cerebral artery at a level inferior to the point of branching. The majority of lesions producing global aphasia are extensive and involve both prerolandic and postrolandic areas of the left hemisphere. These include Broca's (posterior frontal) and Wernicke's (superior temporal) areas and may extend to subcortical areas, including the basal ganglia, internal capsule, and thalamus (Murdoch et al., 1986). Occasionally, the lesion is confined to anterior, posterior, or deep cortical and subcortical regions (Mazzocchi and Vignolo, 1979). Global aphasia has also been described in patients with lesions restricted to subcortical regions, including the basal ganglia, internal capsule, periventricular white matter, temporal isthmus, and thalamus (Alexander, Naeser, and Palumbo, 1987).

Ferro (1992) investigated the influence of lesion site on recovery from global aphasia. The lesions in his subjects with global aphasia were grouped into five types with differing outcomes. Type 1 included patients with large pre- and postrolandic middle cerebral artery infarcts. These patients had a very poor prognosis. The remaining four groups were classified as follows: type 2, prerolandic; type 3, subcortical; type 4, parietal, and type 5, double frontal and parietal lesion. Patients in these latter groups demonstrated variable outcomes, improving generally to Broca's or transcortical aphasia. Complete recovery was observed in some patients with type 2 and 3 infarcts. In contrast, Basso and Farabola (1997) investigated recovery in three cases of aphasia based on the patients' lesion patterns. One patient had global aphasia from a large lesion involving both the anterior and posterior language areas, while two other patients had Broca's and Wernicke's aphasia from lesions restricted to either the anterior or posterior language areas, respectively. The patient with global aphasia recovered better than his two aphasic counterparts and had an outstanding outcome. Basso and Farrabola concluded that group recovery patterns based on aphasia severity and site of lesion may not be able to account for the improvement that is occasionally observed in individual patients.

Global aphasia has the lowest recovery rate of all the aphasias (Kertesz and McCabe, 1977). When assessing the language recovery that does occur, comprehension is found to improve more than expression (Prins, Snow, and Wagenaar, 1978). Differences have been reported in the temporal patterns of recovery depending on whether the subjects were receiving speech and language treatment. For globally aphasic patients not receiving treatment, improvement appears to be greatest during the first 6 months after onset (Pashek and Holland, 1988).

Globally aphasic patients receiving treatment demonstrate substantial improvements during the first 3–6 months but also continue to improve during the period between 6 and 12 months or more after onset. Sarno and Levita (1981) observed the most accelerated improvement between 6 and 12 months after stroke. Nicholas et al. (1993) found different patterns of recovery for language and nonlanguage skills during the first year. Substantial improvements in praxis and oral-gestural expression were noted only in the first 6 months after onset, while similar improvements in auditory and reading comprehension were observed only between 6 and 12 months after onset.

The majority of patients with global aphasia will not recover to less severe forms of the disorder. Some patients, however, will improve such that the condition evolves into other aphasia syndromes, including Broca's, transcortical motor, mixed nonfluent, conduction, anomic, and Wernicke's aphasias. Occasionally, patients make a complete recovery to normal language. One apparent explanation for the variability among these patients might be the greater instability of language scores (and therefore aphasia classifications) obtained during the first 4 weeks after stroke versus those obtained after the first month post onset. McDermott, Horner, and DeLong (1996) found greater magnitudes of change in scores and frequencies of aphasia type evolution in subjects tested during the first 30 days after onset than in subjects tested in the second 30 days after onset. Aphasia tends to be more severe during the acute stage, giving observers an initial impression of global aphasia. However, globally aphasic patients who do progress to some other form of aphasia may demonstrate changes that extend into the first months after onset (Pashek and Holland, 1988). In some cases, the global aphasia may not begin to evolve until after the first month has passed. The discrepancies in these studies, therefore, do not appear to be simply the result of the time at which the initial language observations were recorded. Apparently, evolution from global aphasia is the result of a complex interaction among a number of heretofore incompletely understood variables.

Several factors have been investigated for their prognostic significance with regard to global aphasia. The patient's age appears to have an impact on recovery: the younger the patient, the better the prognosis (Holland, Swindell, and Forbes, 1985). However, numerous exceptions to this trend have been described. Age may also relate to the type of aphasia at 1 year post stroke. In the study by Holland, Swindell, and Forbes (1985), younger globally aphasic patients evolved to a nonfluent Broca's aphasia while older patients evolved to increasingly severe fluent aphasias with advancing age. The oldest patients remained globally aphasic.

Absence of hemiparesis with global aphasia may be a positive indicator for recovery. Tranel et al. (1987) described globally aphasic patients with dual discrete lesions (anterior and posterior cerebral) that spared the primary motor area. Global aphasia improved significantly in this group within the first 10 months after onset. These conclusions are tempered by the results of Keyserlingk et al. (1997), who found that chronic globally aphasic patients with no history of hemiparesis did not fare any better with regard to language outcome than did their globally aphasic counterparts with hemiparesis from the time of onset.

The radiologic findings of patients with global aphasia have also been studied to determine whether lesion patterns found on computed tomography may provide prognostic information. Although the findings have been generally mixed, Naeser et al. (1990) were able to show significantly better recovery of auditory comprehension for a group of globally aphasic subjects whose damage did not include Wernicke's area (i.e., the lesions were limited to the subcortical temporal isthmus).

Finally, it appears that a lack of variability between auditory comprehension scores and other language scores may be viewed as a negative indicator (Mark, Thomas, and Berndt, 1992). The more performance differs among language tasks, the better the outlook. Within auditory comprehension scores, globally aphasic patients who produce yes/no responses to simple questions, regardless of their accuracy, seem to have a better outcome at 1 year post onset than those who cannot grasp the yes/no format.

—*Richard K. Peach*

References

Alajouanine, M. S. (1956). Verbal realization in aphasia. *Brain*, *79*, 1–28.

Alexander, M. P., Naeser, M. A., and Palumbo, C. L. (1987). Correlations of subcortical CT lesion sites and aphasia profiles. *Brain*, *110*, 961–991.

Basso, A., and Farrabola, M. (1997). Comparison of improvement of aphasia in three patients with lesions in anterior, posterior, and antero-posterior language areas. *Neuropsychological Rehabilitation*, *7*, 215–230.

Blanken, G., Wallesch, C. W., and Papagno, C. (1990). Dissociations of language functions in aphasics with speech automatisms (recurring utterances). *Cortex*, *26*, 41–63.

deBlesser, R., and Poeck, K. (1985). Analysis of prosody in the spontaneous speech of patients with CV-recurring utterances. *Cortex, 21,* 405–416.

Ferro, J. M. (1992). The influence of infarct location on recovery from global aphasia. *Aphasiology, 6,* 415–430.

Herrmann, M., Koch, U., Johannsen-Horbach, H., and Wallesch, C. W. (1989). Communicative skills in chronic and severe nonfluent aphasia. *Brain and Language, 37,* 339–352.

Holland, A. L., Swindell, C. S., and Forbes, M. M. (1985). The evolution of initial global aphasia: Implications for prognosis. *Clinical Aphasiology, 15,* 169–175.

Kertesz, A., and McCabe, P. (1977). Recovery patterns and prognosis in aphasia. *Brain, 100,* 1–18.

Keyserlingk, A. G., Naujokat, C., Niemann, K., Huber, W., and Thron, A. (1997). Global aphasia—with and without hemiparesis. *European Neurology, 38,* 259–267.

Mark, V. W., Thomas, B. E., and Berndt, R. S. (1992). Factors associated with improvement in global aphasia. *Aphasiology, 6,* 121–134.

Marshall, R. C., Freed, D. B., and Phillips, D. S. (1997). Communicative efficiency in severe aphasia. *Aphasiology, 11,* 373–385.

Mazzocchi, F., and Vignolo, L. A. (1979). Localization of lesions in aphasia: Clinical CT scan correlations in stroke patients. *Cortex, 15,* 627–654.

McDermott, F. B., Horner, J., and DeLong, E. R. (1996). Evolution of acute aphasia as measured by the Western Aphasia Battery. *Clinical Aphasiology, 24,* 159–172.

Murdoch, B. E., Afford, R. J., Ling, A. R., and Ganguley, B. (1986). Acute computerized tomographic scans: Their value in the localization of lesions and as prognostic indicators in aphasia. *Journal of Communication Disorders, 19,* 311–345.

Naeser, M. A., Gaddie, A., Palumbo, C. L., and Stiassny-Eder, D. (1990). Late recovery of auditory comprehension in global aphasia: Improved recovery observed with subcortical temporal isthmus lesion vs. Wernicke's cortical area lesion. *Archives of Neurology, 47,* 425–432.

Nicholas, M. L., Helm-Estabrooks, N., Ward-Lonergan, J., and Morgan, A. R. (1993). Evolution of severe aphasia in the first two years post onset. *Archives of Physical Medicine and Rehabilitation, 74,* 830–836.

Pashek, G. V., and Holland, A. L. (1988). Evolution of aphasia in the first year post-onset. *Cortex, 24,* 411–423.

Peach, R. K. (2001). Clinical intervention for global aphasia. In R. Chapey (Ed.), *Language intervention strategies in aphasia and related neurogenic communication disorders* (4th ed., pp. 487–512). Philadelphia: Lippincott Williams and Wilkins.

Prins, R. S., Snow, E., and Wagenaar, E. (1978). Recovery from aphasia: Spontaneous speech versus language comprehension. *Brain and Language, 6,* 192–211.

Sarno, M. T., and Levita, E. (1981). Some observations on the nature of recovery in global aphasia after stroke. *Brain and Language, 13,* 1–12.

Tranel, D., Biller, J., Damasio, H., Adams, H. P., and Cornell, S. H. (1987). Global aphasia without hemiparesis. *Archives of Neurology, 44,* 304–308.

Van Lancker, D., and Nicklay, C. K. H. (1992). Comprehension of personally relevant (PERL) versus novel language in two globally aphasic patients. *Aphasiology, 6,* 37–61.

Wapner, W., and Gardner, H. (1979). A note on patterns of comprehension and recovery in global aphasia. *Journal of Speech and Hearing Research, 29,* 765–772.

Yasuda, K., and Ono, Y. (1998). Comprehension of famous personal and geographical names in global aphasic subjects. *Brain and Language, 61,* 274–287.

Further Readings

Alexander, M. P., and Loverso, F. L. (1993). A specific treatment for global aphasia. *Clinical Aphasiology, 21,* 277–289.

Collins, M. J. (1997). Global aphasia. In L. L. LaPointe (Ed.), *Aphasia and related neurogenic language disorders* (2nd ed., pp. 133–150). New York: Thieme.

Conlon, C. P., and McNeil, M. R. (1991). The efficacy of treatment for two globally aphasic adults using visual action therapy. *Clinical Aphasiology, 19,* 185–195.

Forde, E., and Humphreys, G. W. (1995). Refractory semantics in global aphasia: On semantic organisation and the access-storage distinction in neuropsychology. *Memory, 3,* 265–307.

Gold, B. T., and Kertesz, A. (2000). Preserved visual lexico-semantics in global aphasia: A right-hemisphere contribution? *Brain and Language, 75,* 359–375.

Hanlon, R. E., Lux, W. E., Dromerick, A. W. (1999). Global aphasia without hemiparesis: Language profiles and lesion distribution. *Journal of Neurology, Neurosurgery, and Psychiatry, 66,* 365–369.

Helm, N. A., and Barresi, B. (1980). Voluntary control of involuntary utterances: A treatment approach for severe aphasia. *Clinical Aphasiology, 10,* 308–315.

Helm-Estabrooks, N., Fitzpatrick, P. M., and Barresi, B. (1982). Visual action therapy for global aphasia. *Journal of Speech and Hearing Disorders, 47,* 385–389.

Masand, P., and Chaudhary, P. (1994). Methylphenidate treatment of poststroke depression in a patient with global aphasia. *Annals of Clinical Psychiatry, 6,* 271–274.

McCall, D., Shelton, J. R., Weinrich, M., and Cox, D. (2000). The utility of computerized visual communication for improving natural language in chronic global aphasia: Implications for approaches to treatment in global aphasia. *Aphasiology, 14,* 795–826.

Naeser, M. A., Baker, E. H., Palumbo, C. L., Nicholas, M., Alexander, M. P., Samaraweera, R., et al. (1998). Lesion site patterns in severe, nonverbal aphasia to predict outcome with a computer-assisted treatment program. *Archives of Neurology, 55,* 1438–1448.

Sarno, M. R., and Levita, E. (1979). Recovery in treated aphasia during the first year post-stroke. *Stroke, 10,* 663–670.

Van Lancker, D., and Klein, K. (1990). Preserved recognition of familiar personal names in global aphasia. *Brain and Language, 39,* 511–529.

Weinrich, M., Steele, R., Carlson, G. S., Kleczewska, M., Wertz, R. T., and Baker, E. H. (1989). Processing of visual syntax in a globally aphasic patient. *Brain and Language, 36,* 391–405.

Weinrich, M., Steele, R., Kleczewska, M., Carlson, G. S., Baker, E. H., and Wertz, R. T. (1989). Representation of "verbs" in a computerized visual communication system. *Aphasiology, 3,* 501–512.

Aphasia, Primary Progressive

The clinical syndrome of primary progressive aphasia is a diagnostic category applied to conditions in which individuals exhibit at least a 2-year history of progressive language deterioration not accompanied by other cognitive symptoms and not attributable to any vascular, neoplastic, metabolic, or infectious diseases. The disease is considered to be a focal cortical atrophy syndrome, as neuronal cell death is, at least initially, limited to circumscribed cortical regions and symptoms are isolated to specific abilities and behaviors subserved by the affected region (Polk and Kertesz, 1993; Black, 1996). Primary progressive aphasia (PPA) is characterized by the gradual worsening of language dysfunction in the context of preserved memory, judgment, insight, visuospatial skills, and overall comportment, at least until the later stages of the disease. Historically viewed as an atypical presentation of dementia, the isolated deterioration of language in the context of degenerative disease has been reported for more than 100 years. PPA was first recognized as a distinct clinical entity by Mesulam in 1982. Mesulam and Weintraub (1992) distinguished PPA from other degenerative neurological conditions such as Alzheimer's disease (AD) by its gradual progression of language dysfunction in the absence of more widespread cognitive or behavioral disturbances for a period of at least 2 years. In some cases, the syndrome may later become associated with cognitive and behavioral disturbances similar to those seen in frontal lobe or frontotemporal dementia or with motor speech disorders (dysarthria, apraxia of speech), as observed in corticobasal degeneration or upper motor neuron disease (e.g., primary lateral sclerosis) (Kertesz and Munoz, 1997). In other cases, the symptoms remain limited to the dissolution of language production and comprehension abilities throughout the duration of the affected individual's life.

The diagnosis of PPA is typically made based on a 2-year history of progressive language deterioration that emerges in the absence of any marked disturbance of other cognitive function and is not associated with any vascular, neoplastic, metabolic, or infectious disease (Duffy and Petersen, 1992; Mesulam and Weintraub, 1992). In addition to neurological examination, medical assessment typically includes neuroimaging and neuropsychological testing. During the first few years, computed tomographic and magnetic resonance imaging results typically are negative or reveal mild to moderate atrophy of the left perisylvian region. Metabolic neuroimaging (e.g., positron emission tomography) typically reveals left perisylvian hypometabolism and is sensitive to abnormalities earlier than structural neuroimaging methods (e.g., Kempler et al., 1990; McDaniel, Wagner, and Greenspan, 1991). Neuropsychological assessment typically reveals relative preservation of nonverbal cognitive function (e.g., abstract reasoning, visual short-term memory, visuoperceptual organization) in conjunction with below-normal performance on tests requiring verbal processing, such as immediate verbal recall, novel verbal learning, and verbal fluency (e.g., Sapin, Anderson, and Pulaski, 1989; Weintraub, Rubin, and Mesulam, 1990). Additionally, many studies have reported the presence of nonlinguistic sequelae known to frequently co-occur in nonprogressive forms of aphasia, such as acalculia, dysphagia, depression, limb apraxia, and apraxia of speech (Rogers and Alarcon, 1999).

At present, the cause of PPA is unknown. It is similarly unclear whether PPA is related to a distinct neuropathological entity. Investigations of the neuropathology associated with PPA yield heterogeneous findings (Black, 1996). Most case studies that include histological data report nonspecific neuronal loss in the left perisylvian region accompanied by spongiform changes in the superficial cortical layers (Snowden et al., 1992; Scheltens, Ravid, and Kamphorst, 1994). Other cases have been reported of individuals who initially presented with progressive language disturbances but eventually were diagnosed with AD (Pogacar and Williams, 1984; Kempler et al., 1990), Pick's disease (Holland et al., 1985; Graff-Radford et al., 1990; Scheltens et al., 1990; Kertesz et al., 1994), and Creutzfeldt-Jakob disease (Shuttleworth, Yates, and Paltan-Ortiz, 1985; Mandell, Alexander, and Carpenter, 1989). However, most of these cases do not meet the diagnostic criteria for PPA according to Mesulam's definition. Furthermore, it is possible that the onset of neuropathophysiological changes related to AD develop sometime after the onset of the focal cortical degeneration associated with PPA, thus explaining the initial appearance of isolated language symptoms, followed by the onset of more widespread cognitive involvement. Thus, autopsy findings of pathology associated with AD do not preclude the possibility that two distinct disease processes may co-occur within the same individual. Although PPA is recognized as a distinct clinical entity, the issue of whether it is a distinct pathological entity remains unresolved.

The course of the disease is quite varied. After a 2-year history of isolated language symptoms, some proportion of individuals diagnosed with PPA eventually exhibit more widespread cognitive involvement consistent with a diagnosis of dementia (i.e., deterioration in two or more cognitive areas such as memory, personality changes, and the ability to independently carry out activities of daily living due to cognitive as opposed to physical impairments). Mesulam (1982) suggested waiting 5 years after the onset of symptoms before trying to predict the course of cognitive involvement. However, there is no indication from the literature that after 5 years, individuals are less likely to develop dementia (Rogers and Alarcon, 1999). Estimates vary concerning the percentage of individuals who, after initially presenting with a 2-year history of isolated language dissolution, eventually exhibit widespread cognitive involvement. These estimates range from 30% to 50% (Duffy and Petersen, 1992; Mesulam and Weintraub, 1992; Rogers and Alarcon, 1999). Thus it is likely that between 50% and 70% of individuals diagnosed with PPA experience only the consequences of declining speech, language, and communication for many years. These individuals continue to drive, manage their own finances, and in all respects other than speech, language, and communication maintain baseline levels of performance on repeated testing over many years. Thus, the course is variable, with some patients progressing rapidly, but for others, the course can be quite prolonged, typically taking 6 or 7 years before they develop severe aphasia or mutism. For these individuals, the global cognitive deterioration does not occur as early in the disease process or to the same extent as seen in AD.

Researchers have attempted to identify clinical symptoms that could serve as reliable predictors of eventual cognitive status. The profile of speech and language dysfunction has been investigated as a prognostic indicator of whether an individual is likely to develop generalized dementia. The hypothesis that a language profile consistent with fluent aphasia as opposed to nonfluent aphasia predicts a course of earlier cognitive decline has been investigated through case study (e.g., Snowden et al., 1992) and systematic review of the literature (Duffy and Petersen, 1992; Mesulam and Weintraub, 1992; Rogers and Alarcon, 1999). The fluency dimension in aphasia refers to a dichotomous classification based on the nature of the spoken language disturbance. Individuals with fluent aphasia produce speech at normal to fast rates with normal to long phrase length and few, if any, phonological speech errors. Verbal output in fluent aphasia is characterized as logorrheic (running on and on) and neologistic (novel words), and it tends to be empty (devoid of meaningful content). Disturbances of auditory comprehension and anomia (i.e., word retrieval difficulties) were the primary symptoms in most cases of fluent PPA reviewed by Rogers and Alarcon (1999). Hodges and Patterson (1996) found these to be the primary presenting complaints in the individuals with fluent PPA that they labeled semantic dementia. Unlike individuals with AD, individuals with semantic dementia or fluent PPA have relatively spared episodic (both recent and old autobiographical) memory but exhibit loss of semantic memory, especially as concerns mapping concepts to their spoken form (Kertesz and Munoz, 1997).

A nonfluent profile is characterized by effortful speech, sparse output with decreased phrase length, impaired access to phonological word-form information, infrequent use of grammatical markers, and disturbed prosody, and is frequently associated with apraxia of speech. Auditory comprehension, while affected, generally deteriorates later than expressive language skills. Nonfluent spontaneous speech and the production of phonemic paraphasias in naming have been proposed as important characteristics distinguishing PPA from the aphasia-like symptoms in AD. However, the language disorder evinced by individuals with PPA rarely fits neatly and unambiguously into the fluency typology. Snowden et al. (1992) described a group of individuals with PPA who exhibited expressive and receptive disruptions of phonology and semantics. Be'land and Ska (1992) described an individual with PPA who presented with "a syntactic deficit as in Broca's ... auditory comprehension deficits of the Wernicke's aphasia type ... and phonemic approximations as found in conduction aphasia" (p. 358). Although there is no accepted classification for individuals exhibiting this profile, the term "mixed aphasia" has been applied (e.g., Snowden et al., 1992). Although reliable sorting of aphasia in PPA into the fluent or nonfluent classes has not been established, the hypothesis that individuals with a fluent profile are more likely to develop generalized cognitive involvement than those with a nonfluent profile has received much attention (e.g., Weintraub, Rubin, and Mesulam, 1990; Duffy and Peterson, 1992; Snowden et al., 1992; Rogers and Alarcon, 1999).

The hypothesis that the profile of language impairment may predict the course of generalized cognitive involvement has been investigated primarily through systematic review of the literature. Duffy and Peterson (1992) reviewed 28 reports, published between 1977 and 1990, describing 54 individuals with PPA. Approximately half of the 54 individuals developed generalized dementia, but none of the 12 patients identified with nonfluent profiles evinced generalized cognitive involvement. This finding was interpreted as supporting the hypothesis that a nonfluent profile may predict a longer duration of isolated language symptoms, or perhaps a lower probability of developing widespread cognitive involvement. Mesulam and Weintraub (1992) reviewed 63 cases of PPA. The average duration of isolated language symptoms was 5.2 years, and six individuals exhibited isolated language symptoms for more than 10 years. They reported that, compared to either probable or pathologically confirmed AD, the PPA group contained more males, a higher incidence of onset before age 65, and a greater incidence of nonfluent aphasia. A nonfluent profile was never observed in the AD group, whereas the distribution of fluent and nonfluent profiles in the PPA group was balanced (48% fluent, 44% nonfluent). According to Mesulam and Weintraub (1992), not all individuals with probable AD exhibit aphasic disturbances, but those who do, exhibit only the fluent aphasia subtype.

Rogers and Alarcon (1999) reviewed 57 articles published between 1982 and 1998 describing 147 individuals with relatively isolated deterioration of speech and language for at least 2 years. Thirty-seven patients had fluent PPA, 88 had nonfluent PPA, and in 22 cases the type of aphasia was indeterminate. Among the individuals with fluent PPA, 27% exhibited dementia at the time of the published report. Among the nonfluent PPA group, 37% were reported to have developed generalized dementia. Of the 22 individuals with an undetermined type of aphasia, 73% exhibited clinical symptoms of dementia. The average duration of isolated language symptoms among the 77 individuals who developed generalized dementia was 5 years (6.6 years in fluent PPA, 4.3 years in nonfluent PPA, and 3.7 years among those with an undetermined type of aphasia). The aggregate data in this review did not support the hypothesis that individuals with a nonfluent profile are less likely to develop generalized cognitive involvement than those with a fluent profile. Furthermore, the data did not support the hypothesis that a nonfluent profile predicts a longer duration of isolated language symptoms. Despite the unequal number of patients in each of the fluency groups, the lack of control regarding the time post onset across cases, and the possibility that there may be considerable impetus to report PPA in individuals who do not exhibit generalized dementia, it does not appear that the fluency profile is a reliable predictor of eventual cognitive status.

The initial symptoms of PPA vary from individual to individual, but anomia is the most commonly reported presenting complaint in patients with both fluent and nonfluent PPA (Mesulam, 1987; Rogers and Alarcon, 1999). Another early symptom, particularly in nonfluent PPA, is slow, hesitant speech, frequently punctuated by long pauses and filler words ("um," "uh"). Although this may represent simply one of many manifestations of anomia, it also portends the language formulation difficulties that later render the speech of these individuals telegraphic (reduced mean length of utterance consisting primarily of content words). Impaired access to phonologic form is frequently associated with later-emerging spelling difficulties, although partial access to initial letters and syllable structure may be retained for many years (Rogers and Alarcon, 1998, 1999). Difficulties with phonologic encoding have also been reported in cases of fluent PPA. Tyler et al. (1997) described the anomic difficulties of one individual with fluent PPA as impaired mapping between the semantic lexicon and output phonology. More typically, individuals who eventually exhibit fluent PPA initially complain of difficulties understanding spoken language (Hodges and Patterson, 1996), whereas individuals with nonfluent PPA typically exhibit preserved language comprehension in the early stages (Karbe, Kertesz, and Polk, 1993). Some individuals with a nonfluent presentation of PPA initially exhibit motor symptoms consistent with a diagnosis of dysarthria or apraxia of speech. The initial symptom of progressive speech apraxia has been reported by Hart, Beach, and Taylor (1997). Dysarthria and orofacial apraxia have been reported as initial symptoms in a variation of PPA labeled slowly progressive anarthria (Broussolle et al., 1996). The relationships between and among nonfluent PPA, primary progressive apraxia, slowly progressive anarthria, corticobasal degeneration, primary lateral sclerosis, and Parkinson's disease is of interest, because these conditions exhibit considerable clinical overlap and in some cases share similar pathophysiology. In the later stages of all of these syndromes, individuals lose the ability to communicate by speech and are uniformly described as "mute," despite apparent differences regarding the underlying nature of the specific impairment precluding the production of spoken language.

Regardless of the subtype of PPA, the progressive loss of language need not result in the total cessation of all communication, as there are augmentative and alternative communication tools and strategies that can be proactively established so that the individual with PPA can maximize communication competency at every stage, despite the relentless deterioration in speech and language (Rogers, King, and Alarcon, 2000).

—*Margaret A. Rogers*

References

Be'land, R., and Ska, B. (1992). Interaction between verbal and gestural language in progressive aphasia: A longitudinal case study. *Brain and Language, 43,* 355–385.

Black, S. E. (1996). Focal cortical atrophy syndromes. *Brain and Cognition, 31,* 188–229.

Broussolle, E., Serge, B., Tommasi, M., Laurent, B., Bazin, B., Cinotti, L., et al. (1996). Slowly progressive anarthria with late opercular syndrome: A variant form of frontal cortical atrophy syndromes. *Journal of the Neurological Sciences, 144,* 44–58.

Duffy, J. R., and Peterson, R. C. (1992). Primary progressive aphasia. *Aphasiology, 6,* 1–13.

Graff-Radford, N. R., Damasio, A. R., Hyman, B. T., Hart, M. N., Tranel, D., Damasio, H., et al. (1990). Progressive aphasia in a patient with Pick's disease: A neuropsychological, radiologic, and anatomic study. *Neurology, 40,* 620–626.

Hart, R. P., Beach, W. A., and Taylor, J. R. (1997). A case of progressive apraxia of speech and non-fluent aphasia. *Aphasiology, 11,* 73–82.

Hodges, J. R., and Patterson, K. (1996). Nonfluent progressive aphasia and semantic dementia: A comparative neuropsychological study. *Journal of the International Neuropsychological Society, 2,* 511–524.

Holland, A. L., McBurney, D. H., Moossy, J., and Reinmuth, O. M. (1985). The dissolution of language in Pick's disease with neurofibrillary tangles: A case study. *Brain and Language, 24,* 36–58.

Karbe, H., Kertesz, A., and Polk, M. (1993). Profiles of language impairment in primary progressive aphasia. *Archives of Neurology, 50,* 193–200.

Kempler, D., Metter, E. J., Riege, W. H., Jackson, C. A., Benson, D. F., and Hanson, W. R. (1990). Slowly progressive aphasia: Three cases with language, memory, CT and PET data. *Journal of Neurology, Neurosurgery, and Psychiatry, 53,* 987–993.

Kertesz, A., Hudson, L., Mackenzie, I. R. A., and Munoz, D. G. (1994). The pathology and nosology of primary progressive aphasia. *Neurology, 44,* 2065–2072.

Kertesz, A., and Munoz, D. G. (1997). Primary progressive aphasia. *Clinical Neuroscience, 4*(2), 95–102.

Mandell, A. M., Alexander, M. P., and Carpenter, S. (1989). Creutzfeld-Jacob disease presenting as isolated aphasia. *Neurology, 39,* 55–58.

McDaniel, K. D., Wagner, M. T., and Greenspan, B. S. (1991). The role of brain single photon emission computed tomography in the diagnosis of primary progressive aphasia. *Archives of Neurology, 48,* 1257–1260.

Mesulam, M. M. (1982). Slowly progressive aphasia without generalized dementia. *Annals of Neurology, 11,* 592–598.

Mesulam, M. M. (1987). Primary progressive aphasia: Differentiation from Alzheimer's disease. *Annals of Neurology, 22,* 533–534. Editorial.

Mesulam, M. M., and Weintraub, S. (1992). Spectrum of primary progressive aphasia. In M. N. Rossor (Ed.), *Unusual dementias. Bailliere's Clinical Neurology, 1*(3), 583–609.

Pogacar, S., and Williams, R. S. (1984). Alzheimer's disease presenting as slowly progressive aphasia. *Rhode Island Medical Journal, 67,* 181–185.

Polk, M., and Kertesz, A. (1993). Music and language in degenerative disease of the brain. *Brain and Cognition, 22,* 98–117.

Rogers, M. A., and Alarcon, N. B. (1998). Dissolution of spoken language in primary progressive aphasia. *Aphasiology, 12,* 635–650.

Rogers, M. A., and Alarcon, N. B. (1999). Characteristics and management of primary progressive aphasia. *Neurophysiology and Neurogenic Speech and Language Disorders Newsletter, 9*(4), 12–26.

Rogers, M. A., King, J. M., and Alarcon, N. B. (2000). Proactive management of primary progressive aphasia. In D. Beukelman, K. Yorkston, and J. Reichle (Eds.), *Augmentative Communication for Adults with Neurogenic and Neuromuscular Disabilities* (pp. 305–337). Baltimore: Paul H. Brookes.

Sapin, L. R., Anderson, F. H., and Pulaski, P. D. (1989). Progressive aphasia without dementia: Further documentation. *Annals of Neurology, 25,* 411–413.

Scheltens, P., Hazenberg, G. J., Lindeboom, J., Valk, J., and Wolters, E. C. (1990). A case of progressive aphasia without dementia: "temporal" Pick's disease? *Journal of Neurology, Neurosurgery, and Psychiatry, 53,* 79–80.

Scheltens, P., Ravid, R., and Kamphorst, W. (1994). Pathologic finding in a case of primary progressive aphasia. *Neurology, 44,* 279–282.

Shuttleworth, E. C., Yates, A. J., and Paltan-Ortiz, J. D. (1985). Creutzfeld-Jacob disease presenting as progressive aphasia. *Journal of the National Medical Association, 77,* 649–655.

Snowden, J. S., Neary, D., Mann, D. M. A., Goulding, P. J., and Testa, H. J. (1992). Progressive language disorder due to lobar atrophy. *Annals of Neurology, 31,* 174–183.

Tyler, L. K., Moss, H. F., Patterson, K., and Hodges, J. (1997). The gradual deterioration of syntax and semantics in a patient with progressive aphasia. *Brain and Language, 56,* 426–476.

Weintraub, S., Rubin, N., and Mesulam, M. (1990). Primary progressive aphasia: Longitudinal course, neuropsychological profile, and language features. *Archives of Neurology, 47,* 1329–1335.

Aphasia: The Classical Syndromes

Aphasia is an acquired disorder of language subsequent to brain damage that affects auditory comprehension, reading, oral-expressive language, and writing. Early observations by Broca (1861a, 1861b) and Wernicke (1874) suggested that aphasia might be classified into a variety of syndromes, or types, based on differences in auditory comprehension and oral-expressive language behaviors. Moreover, different syndromes were believed to result from different sites of brain damage. Revisions of early classification systems yield a contemporary taxonomy that comprises seven syndromes: global, Broca's, transcortical motor, Wernicke's, transcortical sensory, conduction, and anomic (Benson, 1988; Kertesz, 1979). Classification is based on the aphasic person's auditory comprehension, oral-expressive fluency (phrase length and syntax), spoken repetition, and naming abilities. The seven syndromes can be divided into nonfluent, those with short phrase length and impaired morphosyntax (global, Broca's, and transcortical motor), and fluent, those with longer phrase length and apparent preservation of syntactic structures (Wernicke's, transcortical sensory, conduction, and anomic). An aphasic person's syndrome may be determined by informal examination or by administering a standardized test, for example, the Western Aphasia Battery (WAB) (Kertesz, 1982) or the Boston Diagnostic Aphasia Examination (BDAE) (Goodglass and Kaplan, 1983). The following describes each syndrome and the assumed site of lesion associated with each.

Global Aphasia. This nonfluent syndrome is associated with a large left hemisphere lesion that may involve the frontal, temporal, and parietal lobes, insula, and underlying white matter, including the arcuate fasciculus (Dronkers and Larsen, 2001). It is the most severe of all of the syndromes. Auditory comprehension is markedly reduced and may be limited to inconsistent comprehension of single words. Oral-expressive language is sparse, often limited to a recurring intelligible—"bees, bees, bees"—or unintelligible—"doobe, doobe, doobe"—stereotype. Other automatic expressions, including profanity and counting, may also be preserved. Globally aphasic patients are unable to repeat words, and no naming ability is present. Reading and writing abilities are essentially absent.

Broca's Aphasia. This nonfluent syndrome receives its name from the early reports by Paul Broca (1861a, 1861b). Classical localization of the lesion resulting in Broca's aphasia is damage in the left, inferior frontal gyrus—Broca's area (Brodmann's areas 44 and 45) (Damasio, 1992). However, both historical (Marie, 1906) and contemporary (Mohr, 1976; Dronkers et al., 1992) reports question the classical lesion localization. Patients have been described who have lesions in Broca's area without Broca's aphasia, and other patients have Broca's aphasia but their lesion does not involve Broca's area. Auditory comprehension is relatively good for single words and short sentences. However, comprehension of grammatically complex sentences is impaired. Their phrase length is short, and they produce halting, telegraphic, agrammatic speech that contains, primarily, content words. For example, describing how he spent the weekend, a patient with Broca's aphasia related, "Ah, frat, no Saturday, ah, frisk, no, fishing, son." Repetition of words and sentences is poor. Naming ability is disrupted, and reading and writing show a range of impairment.

Transcortical Motor Aphasia. Lichtheim (1885) provided an early description of this nonfluent syndrome, and he observed that the site of lesion spared the perisylvian language region. Currently, it is believed that the lesion resulting in transcortical motor aphasia is smaller than that causing Broca's aphasia and is in the left anterior-superior frontal lobe (Alexander, Benson, and Stuss, 1989). With one exception, language behaviors are similar to those in Broca's aphasia: good auditory comprehension for short, noncomplex sentences; short, halting, agrammatic phrase production; disrupted naming ability; and impaired reading and writing. The exception is relatively preserved ability to repeat phrases and sentences. Essentially, patients with transcortical motor aphasia repeat much better than would be predicted from their disrupted, volitional productions.

Wernicke's Aphasia.   This fluent syndrome received its name from the early report by Carl Wernicke (1874). The traditional belief is that Wernicke's aphasia results from a lesion in Wernicke's area (posterior Brodmann's area 22) in the left hemisphere auditory-association cortex (Damasio, 1992), with extension into Brodmann's areas 37, 39, and 40. However, Basso et al. (1985) have reported cases of Wernicke's aphasia resulting from exclusively anterior lesions, and Dronkers, Redfern, and Ludy (1995) have found Wernicke's aphasia in patients whose lesions also spared Wernicke's area. Spoken phrase length averages six or more words, and a semblance of syntax is present. However, the oral-expressive behavior includes phonological errors and jargon. One patient with Wernicke's aphasia described where he went to college, Washington and Lee University, by relating, "There was the old one, ah Frulich, and the young one, young hunter, ah, Frulich and young hunter or Brulan." A salient sign in Wernicke's aphasia is impaired auditory comprehension. These patients understand little of what is said to them, and the deficit cannot be explained by reduced auditory acuity. In addition, verbal repetition and naming abilities are impaired, and there is a range of reading and writing deficits.

Transcortical Sensory Aphasia.   This fluent syndrome may result from lesions surrounding Wernicke's area, posteriorly or inferiorly (Damasio, 1992). Oral-expressive language is similar to that seen in Wernicke's aphasia: longer phrase length and relatively good syntax. Auditory comprehension is impaired, similar to that in Wernicke's aphasia, and naming, reading, and writing deficits are present. The salient sign in transcortical sensory aphasia is preserved verbal repetition ability for words and, frequently, long and complex sentences. Essentially, transcortical sensory aphasia patients repeat better than one would predict based on their impaired auditory comprehension.

Conduction Aphasia.   Wernicke (1874) described this fluent syndrome. Lesion localization has been controversial. Geschwind (1965) proposed that conduction aphasia results from a lesion in the arcuate fasciculus that disrupts connections between the posterior language comprehension area and the anterior motor speech area. Damasio (1992) suggested that conduction aphasia results from damage in the left hemisphere supramarginal gyrus (Brodmann's area 40), with or without extension to the white matter beneath the insula, or damage in the left primary auditory cortices (Brodmann's areas 41 and 42), the insula, and the underlying white matter. Dronkers et al. (1998) reported that all of their patients with conduction aphasia had a lesion that involved the posterior-superior temporal gyrus, often extending into the inferior parietal lobule. The salient sign in conduction aphasia is impaired ability to repeat phrases and sentences in the presence of relatively good auditory comprehension and oral-expressive abilities. Although auditory comprehension is relatively good, it is not perfect. And, while oral-expressive language is fluent (longer phrase length and a semblance of syntax), patients with conduction aphasia make numerous phonological errors and replace intended words with words that sound similar. Naming, reading, and writing abilities are disrupted to some extent.

Anomic Aphasia.   This fluent syndrome is the least severe. Anomia—word-finding difficulty—is present in all aphasic syndromes; thus, localization of the lesion that results in anomic aphasia is not precise. It can be found subsequent to anterior or posterior lesions (Dronkers and Larsen, 2001), and Kreisler et al. (2000) report anomic aphasia resulting from a lesion in the thalamus; medial temporal area; or frontal cortex, insula, and anterior part of the temporal gyri. Patients with anomic aphasia display longer phrase length and preserved syntax; mild, if any, auditory comprehension deficits; good repetition ability; and mild reading and writing impairment. Frequently, the anomic patient will substitute synonyms for the intended words or replace the desired word with a generalization, for example, "thing" or "stuff."

Cautions

The classification of aphasia into the classical syndromes is not exempt from controversy. Some (Caramazza, 1984; Caplan, 1987) have challenged its validity. Darley (1982) suggested that aphasic people differ on the basis of severity or the presence of a coexisting communication disorder, frequently apraxia of speech. He advocated viewing aphasia unmodified by adjectives. The relationship between the site of lesion and the corresponding syndrome is also controversial. The classical sites of lesion for most aphasic syndromes are challenged by exceptions (Basso et al., 1985; Murdoch, 1988; Dronkers and Larsen, 2001). Some of the inconsistency may result from the time post onset when behavioral observations are made. Improvement in aphasia over time results in approximately 50% of aphasic patients changing from one syndrome to another (Kertesz and McCabe, 1977). Thus, an acutely aphasic patient with an inferior left frontal gyrus lesion may display the expected Broca's aphasia; however, at 6 months after onset, the same patient's language characteristics may resemble anomic aphasia. Confusion may also result from the methods employed to classify the aphasias. For example, classifications made with the WAB do not always agree with those made with the BDAE (Wertz, Deal, and Robinson, 1984). Finally, controversy and confusion may result from misuse of the term syndrome (Benson and Ardila, 1996). The behavioral profile that constitutes a specific aphasic "syndrome" is characterized by a range of impairment and not by identical performance among all individuals within a specific syndrome. In many, certainly not all, aphasic people, impaired behavioral features—fluency, auditory comprehension, verbal repetition, naming—tend to result in different clusters that represent different profiles. These have led to the development and use of the classical syndromes in aphasia.

—Robert T. Wertz, Nina F. Dronkers, and Jennifer Ogar

References

Alexander, M. P., Benson, D. F., and Stuss, D. T. (1989). Frontal lobes and language. *Brain and Language, 37,* 656–691.

Basso, A., Lecours, A. R., Moraschini, S., and Vanier, M. (1985). Anatomical correlations of the aphasias as defined through computerized tomography: Exceptions. *Brain and Language, 26,* 201–229.

Benson, D. F. (1988). Classical syndromes of aphasia. In F. Boller and J. Grafman (Eds.), *Handbook of neuropsychology* (vol. 1, pp. 269–280). Amsterdam: Elsevier.

Benson, D. F., and Ardila, A. (1996). *Aphasia: A clinical perspective.* New York: Oxford University Press.

Broca, P. (1861a). Remarques sur le siège de la faculté du langage articulé, suivies d'une observation d'aphémie (perte de la parole). *Bulletins de la Société d'Anatomie* (Paris), 2e série, *6,* 330–357.

Broca, P. (1861b). Nouvelle observation d'aphémie produite par une lésion de la troisième circonvolution frontale. *Bulletins de la Société d'Anatomie* (Paris), 2e série, *6,* 398–407.

Caplan, D. (1987). *Neurolinguistics and linguistic aphasiology.* Cambridge, U.K.: Cambridge University Press.

Caramazza, A. (1984). The logic of neuropsychological research and the problem of patient classification in aphasia. *Brain and Language, 21,* 9–20.

Damasio, A. R. (1992). Aphasia. *New England Journal of Medicine, 326,* 531–539.

Darley, F. L. (1982). *Aphasia.* Philadelphia: Saunders.

Dronkers, N. F., and Larsen, J. (2001). Neuroanatomy of the classical syndromes of aphasia. In R. S. Berndt (Ed.), *Handbook of neuropsychology* (2nd ed., vol. 3). Amsterdam: Elsevier.

Dronkers, N. F., Redfern, B. B., and Ludy, C. A. (1995). Lesion localization in chronic Wernicke's aphasia. *Brain and Language, 51,* 62–65.

Dronkers, N. F., Redfern, B. B., Ludy, C., and Baldo, J. (1998). Brain regions associated with conduction aphasia and echoic rehearsal. *Journal of the International Neuropsychological Society, 4,* 23–24.

Dronkers, N. F., Shapiro, J. K., Redfern, B., and Knight, R. T. (1992). The role of Broca's area in Broca's aphasia. *Journal of Clinical and Experimental Neuropsychology, 14,* 52–53.

Geschwind, N. (1965). Disconnection syndromes in animals and man. *Brain, 88,* 237–294.

Goodglass, H., and Kaplan, E. (1983). *The Boston Diagnostic Aphasia Examination.* Philadelphia: Lea and Febiger.

Kertesz, A. (1979). *Aphasia and associated disorders: Taxonomy, localization, and recovery.* New York: Grune and Stratton.

Kertesz, A. (1982). *The Western Aphasia Battery.* New York: Grune and Stratton.

Kertesz, A., and McCabe, P. (1977). Recovery patterns and prognosis in aphasia. *Brain, 100,* 1–18.

Kreisler, A., Godefroy, O., Dalmaire, C., Debachy, B., Leclercq, M., Pruvo, J.-P., et al. (2000). The anatomy of aphasia revisited. *Neurology, 54,* 1117–1122.

Lichtheim, L. (1885). On aphasia. *Brain, 7,* 433–484.

Marie, P. (1906). Revision de la question de l'aphasie: La troisieme circonvolution frontale gauche ne joue aucun role special dans la fonction du langage. *Semaine Medicale, 26,* 241–247.

Mohr, J. P. (1976). Broca's area and Broca's aphasia. In H. Whitaker and H. Whitaker (Eds.), *Studies in neurolinguistics* (vol. 1, pp. 201–233). New York: Academic Press.

Murdoch, B. E. (1988). Computerized tomographic scanning: Its contributions to the understanding of the neuroanatomical basis of aphasia. *Aphasiology, 2,* 437–462.

Wernicke, C. (1874). *Der aphasische Symptomencomplex.* Breslau, Poland: Kohn and Weigert.

Wertz, R. T., Deal, J. L., and Robinson, A. J. (1984). Classifying the aphasias: A comparison of the Boston Diagnostic Aphasia Examination and the Western Aphasia Battery. In R. H. Brookshire (Ed.), *Clinical Aphasiology Conference proceedings* (pp. 40–47). Minneapolis: BRK.

Further Readings

Alexander, M. P. (1997). Aphasia: Clinical and anatomic aspects. In T. E. Feinberg and M. J. Farah (Eds.), *Behavioral neurology and neuropsychology* (pp. 133–149). New York: McGraw-Hill.

Bogen, J. E., and Bogen, G. M. (1976). Wernicke's region: Where is it? *Annals of the New York Academy of Sciences, 280,* 834–843.

Caplan, D., Hildebrandt, N., and Marlies, N. (1996). Location of lesions in stroke patients with deficits in syntactic processing in sentence comprehension. *Brain, 119,* 933–949.

Damasio, H., and Damasio, A. R. (1989). *Lesion analysis in neuropsychology.* New York: Oxford University Press.

Dronkers, N. F. (1996). A new brain region for coordinating speech articulation. *Nature, 384,* 159–161.

Freedman, M., Alexander, M. P., and Naeser, M. A. (1984). Anatomic basis of transcortical motor aphasia. *Neurology, 34,* 409–417.

Geschwind, N. (1972). Language and the brain. *Scientific American, 226,* 76–83.

Godefroy, O., Duhamel, A., Leclerc, X., Saint Michel, T., Henon, H., and Leys, D. (1998). Brain-behavior relationships: Models for the study of brain damaged patients. *Brain, 121,* 1545–1556.

Goodglass, H. (1993). *Understanding aphasia.* San Diego, CA: Academic Press.

Kertesz, A., Sheppard, A., and MacKenzie, R. (1982). Localization in transcortical sensory aphasia. *Archives of Neurology, 39,* 475–478.

Kirshner, H. S., Alexander, M., Lorch, M. P., and Wertz, R. T. (1999). Disorders of speech and language. *Continuum: Lifelong Learning in Neurology, 5,* 1–237.

Naeser, M. A., and Hayward, R. W. (1978). Lesion localization in aphasia with computed tomography and the Boston Diagnostic Aphasia Exam. *Neurology, 28,* 545–551.

Palumbo, C. L., Alexander, M. P., and Naeser, M. A. (1992). CT scan lesion sites associated with conduction aphasia. In K. Se (Ed.), *Conduction aphasia* (pp. 51–75). Hillsdale, NJ: Erlbaum.

Sarno, M. E. (Ed.). (1998). *Acquired aphasia* (3rd ed.). San Diego, CA: Academic Press.

Stemmer, B., and Whitaker, H. A. (Eds.). (1998). *Handbook of neurolinguistics.* San Diego, CA: Academic Press.

Vignolo, L. A., Boccardi, E., and Caverni, L. (1986). Un-expected CT-scan findings in global aphasia. *Cortex*, *22*, 55–69.

Wertz, R. T. (1983). Classifying the aphasias: Commodious or chimerical? In R. H. Brookshire (Ed.), *Clinical Aphasiology Conference proceedings* (pp. 296–303). Minneapolis: BRK.

Willmes, K., and Poeck, K. (1998). To what extent can aphasic syndromes be localized? *Brain*, *116*, 1527–1540.

Aphasia, Wernicke's

A new concept in aphasiology was created when Wernicke (1874/1977) described ten patients with different forms of aphasia, and showed that two of the patients had fluent but paraphasic speech with poor comprehension (i.e., sensory aphasia). At autopsy of another patient, a lesion was found in the left posterior temporal lobe. This type of aphasia has been called by many names, including receptive, impressive, sensory, or more generally fluent aphasia. In most of the current classification systems, this type of syndrome is called Wernicke's aphasia. It affects 15%–25% of all patients with aphasia (Laska et al., 2001).

Although the exact boundaries of Wernicke's area are controversial, the typical lesion associated with Wernicke's aphasia is most often located in the posterior temporal area. The middle and superior temporal lobe posterior to the primary auditory cortex are affected in almost all cases. The primary auditory cortex is also often affected, as are the white matter subjacent to the posterior temporal lobe, the angular gyrus, and the supramarginal gyrus. In rare cases, restricted subcortical lesions may result in Wernicke's aphasia and hemiplegia, the latter being uncommon in cases with cortical lesions. Recent studies have not changed these classical views of the clinico-anatomical relations of initial aphasia.

Patients with Wernicke's aphasia are usually older than patients with Broca's aphasia. However, some rare cases of children with acquired fluent aphasia and a posterior temporal lesion have been described (Paquier and Van Dongen, 1991). Ferro and Madureira (1997) have attributed the age difference between patients with fluent aphasia and those with nonfluent aphasia to the higher prevalence of posterior infarcts in older patients. The most common etiological factor in vascular Wernicke's aphasia is cardiac embolus, which more often affects the temporal area, whereas carotid atherosclerotic infarctions are in most cases located in the frontoparietal area (Harrison and Marshall, 1987; Knepper et al., 1989). Coppens (1991), however, points to a higher mortality rate in older patients with stroke, which might cause a selection bias in studies showing a relationship between age and type of aphasia.

The typical clinical signs of Wernicke's aphasia include poor comprehension of spoken and written language and fluent but paraphasic (phonemic and semantic) speech. In some cases, neologistic jargon may occur. Naming is also severely affected, and phonemic or semantic prompting is of no help. Poor repetition distinguishes Wernicke's aphasia from transcortical sensory aphasia. Writing mirrors the speech output. Handwriting is usually well formed, but the text is without content, and jargonagraphia may occur. Because of posterior lesions, hemiparesis is present in rare cases, but visual field defects are more common. Many patients also show signs of anosognosia, especially during the acute stage of the illness. In most cases, the use of gestural communication or pantomime is affected as well.

Patients not traditionally classified as having aphasia may also show language disturbances resembling Wernicke's aphasia, such as patients with schizophrenia, dementia, or semantic dementia, a fluent form of primary progressive aphasia.

Some authors suggest that Wernicke's aphasia is not a uniform entity but includes many variants. Forms of neologistic, semantic, and phonemic jargon and pure word deafness may all be grouped under Wernicke's aphasia. Pure word deafness is a rare disorder characterized by severe difficulties in speech comprehension and repetition with preservation of other language functions, including the comprehension of nonverbal sounds and music (Kirshner, Webb, and Duncan, 1981). However, when Buchman et al. (1986) reviewed 34 published cases, they were unable to find any really pure cases—that is, cases without any other more generalized perceptual disorders that could be classified as acoustic agnosia or mild language disorders such as paraphasia, naming difficulties, and reading and writing disorders. Most of the patients with "pure" word deafness have had bilateral temporal lesions, but some patients with unilateral left hemisphere lesions have been described (Takahashi et al., 1992).

Personality factors may play a role in the clinical expression of aphasia. In some views, jargon aphasia is not solely a linguistic deficit. Rochford (1974) suggested that a pathological arousal mechanism and lack of control were crucial to jargon aphasia. Weinstein and Lyerly (1976) suggested that jargon aphasia could emanate from abnormal adaptation to the aphasic speech disorder. They found a significant difference in premorbid personality between patients with jargon aphasia and those without jargon aphasia. Most of their patients with jargon aphasia had a strong premorbid tendency to deny illness or openly expressed fear of illness, indicating the importance of anosognosic features in jargon aphasia.

Linguistically, patients with Wernicke's aphasia speak with normal fluency and prosody without articulatory distortions. They often provide long and fluent answers (logorrhoea) to simple questions. In fact, patients with Wernicke's aphasia produce an equal number of words as persons without aphasia in spontaneous speech. However, they show less lexical variety, a high proportion of repetitions, and empty speech (Bates et al., 2001). This may give an impression of grammatically correct speech, but the meaning of the utterances is lost because of a high proportion of paraphasias and neologisms (Lecours and Lhermitte, 1983). This type of speech error is called paragrammatism. Patients with Wernicke's aphasia show morphological errors, but less so than patients with Broca's aphasia (Bates et al., 2001). However, there is some evidence that in highly inflected languages such as Finnish, the number of errors is higher on inflected words than on the lexical stems (Niemi, Koivuselkä-Sallinen, and Laine, 1987). At least in spontaneous speech, distorted sentence structure in utterances of patients with Wernicke's aphasia is related to the lexical-semantic difficulties rather than to morphosyntactic problems (Helasvuo, Klippi, and Laakso, 2001). The same has been found in sentence comprehension. Patients with Wernicke's aphasia performed correctly only on sentences that did not require semantic operations (Pinango and Zurif, 2001). According to these findings, the deficit in phonemic hearing does not explain the nature of comprehension problems in patients with Wernicke's aphasia.

Most patients show skill in pragmatic abilities, such as using gaze direction and other nonverbal actions in conversation. Unawareness of one's own speech errors usually occurs initially in Wernicke's aphasia, but some degree of auditory self-monitoring develops after onset, and patients then begin to use various self-repair strategies to manage conversation (Laakso, 1997). In contrast to self-repair sequences in nonaphasic speakers, these sequences are very lengthy and often unsuccessful.

The initial severity of the aphasia is considered the most important single factor in predicting recovery from aphasia. Wernicke's aphasia is usually tantamount to severe aphasia. In a study by Ross and Wertz (2001), of all patients with aphasia, those with Wernicke's aphasia and global aphasia showed the most severe impairment in language functions and communication. These patients showed only limited recovery when measured at the impairment level by the Boston Diagnostic Aphasia Examination (BDAE) and at the disability level by CADL. In addition to initial severity of aphasia, supramarginal and angular gyri involvements seem to relate to poor recovery in comparison with cases without extension to the posterior superior temporal gyrus (Kertesz, Lau, and Polk, 1993).

Patients who have recovered from Wernicke's aphasia have shown a clear increase in activation in the right perisylvian area, suggesting a functional reorganization of the language with the help of the right hemisphere (Weiller et al., 1995). However, Karbe et al. (1998) reported that increased activity in the right hemisphere was present in patients with poor recovery and reflected the large lesions in the left hemisphere. Patients with good recovery showed increased activation in the left hemisphere surrounding the damaged area.

The classification of aphasia depends strongly on the methods used in the assessment. The major diagnostic tests, such as the BDAE, the Western Aphasia Battery (WAB), or the Aachener Aphasie Test (AAT), have slightly different criteria for classification. For example, whereas the WAB assigns all patients to some aphasia classification, up to 70% of patients examined with the BDAE might be designated as having unclassified aphasia. Another issue that confuses classification is the time after onset at which the evaluation is done. Depending on the sample studied, more than half of patients with aphasia will show evolution to another type of aphasia during the first year after the onset of illness (Ross and Wertz, 2001). Patients with initial Wernicke's aphasia will usually evolve to have a conduction or transcortical type of aphasia, and may evolve further to have anomic aphasia (Pashek and Holland, 1988). On the other hand, the condition of elderly patients with initial global aphasia tends to evolve to Wernicke's aphasia during the recovery period, and the condition of younger patients evolves to Broca's aphasia. This could explain why only one-third of patients with fluent aphasia and lesions in Wernicke's area have a persisting aphasia, and only slightly more than half of patients with chronic Wernicke's aphasia have lesions in Wernicke's area (Dronkers, 2000).

—*Matti Lehtihalmes*

References

Bates, E., Reilly, J., Wulfeck, B., Dronkers, N., Opie, M., Fenson, J., et al. (2001). Differential effects of unilateral lesions on language production in children and adults. *Brain and Language*, 79, 223–265.

Buchman, A. S., Garron, D. C., Trost-Cardamone, J. E., Wichter, M. D., and Schwartz, M. (1986). Word deafness: One hundred years later. *Journal of Neurology, Neurosurgery, and Psychiatry*, 49, 489–499.

Coppens, P. (1991). Why are Wernicke's aphasia patients older than Broca's? A critical view of the hypotheses. *Aphasiology*, 5, 279–290.

Dronkers, N. F. (2000). The pursuit of brain–language relationships. *Brain and Language*, 71, 59–61.

Ferro, J. M., and Madureira, S. (1997). Aphasia type, age and cerebral infarct localisation. *Journal of Neurology*, 244, 505–509.

Harrison, M. J. G., and Marshall, J. (1987). Wernicke aphasia and cardiac embolism. *Journal of Neurology, Neurosurgery, and Psychiatry*, 50, 938–939.

Helasvuo, M.-L., Klippi, A., and Laakso, M. (2001). Grammatical structuring in Broca's and Wernicke's aphasia in Finnish. *Journal of Neurolinguistics*, 14, 231–254.

Karbe, H., Thiel, A., Weber-Luxenburger, G., Herholz, K., Kessler, J., and Heiss, W. D. (1998). Brain plasticity in poststroke aphasia: What is the contribution of the right hemisphere? *Brain and Language*, 64, 215–230.

Kertesz, A., Lau, W. K., and Polk, M. (1993). The structural determinants of recovery in Wernicke's aphasia. *Brain and Language*, 44, 153–164.

Kirshner, H. S., Webb, W. G., and Duncan, G. W. (1981). Word deafness in Wernicke's aphasia. *Journal of Neurology, Neurosurgery, and Psychiatry*, 44, 197–201.

Knepper, L. E., Biller, J., Tranel, D., Adams, H. P., and Marsh, E. E., III (1989). Etiology of stroke in patients with Wernicke's aphasia. *Stroke*, 20, 1730–1732.

Laakso, M. (1997). *Self-initiated repair by fluent aphasic speakers in conversation* (Studia Fennica Linguistica 8). Helsinki: Finnish Literature Society.

Laska, A. C., Hellbom, A., Murray, V., Kahan, T., and von Arbin, M. (2001). Aphasia in acute stroke and relation to outcome. *Journal of Internal Medicine*, 249, 413–422.

Lecours, A. R., and Lhermitte, F. (1983). Clinical forms of aphasia. In A. R. Lecours, F. Lhermitte, and B.

Bryans (Eds.), *Aphasiology* (pp. 76–108). London: Baillière Tindall.

Niemi, J., Koivuselkä-Sallinen, P., and Laine, M. (1987). Lexical deformations are sensitive to morphosyntactic factors in posterior aphasia. *Aphasiology, 1*, 53–57.

Paquier, P., and Van Dongen, H. R. (1991). Two contrasting cases of fluent aphasia in children. *Aphasiology, 5*, 235–245.

Pashek, G. V., and Holland, A. L. (1988). Evolution of aphasia in the first year post-onset. *Cortex, 24*, 411–424.

Pinango, M. M., and Zurif, E. B. (2001). Semantic operations in aphasic comprehension: Implications for the cortical organization of language. *Brain and Language, 79*, 297–308.

Rochford, G. (1974). Are jargon dysphasics dysphasic? *British Journal of Disorders of Communication, 9*, 35–44.

Ross, K. B., and Wertz, R. T. (2001). Type and severity of aphasia during the first seven months poststroke. *Journal of Medical Speech-Language Pathology, 9*, 31–53.

Takahashi, N., Kawamura, M., Shonotou, H., Hirayama, K., Kaga, K., and Shindo, M. (1992). Pure word deafness due to left hemisphere damage. *Cortex, 28*, 295–303.

Weiller, C., Isensee, C., Rijntjes, M., Huber, W., Müller, S., Bier, D., et al. (1995). Recovery from Wernicke's aphasia: A positron emission tomographic study. *Annals of Neurology, 37*, 723–732.

Weinstein, E. A., and Lyerly, O. G. (1976). Personality factors in jargon aphasia. *Cortex, 12*, 122–133.

Wernicke, C. (1874). Der Aphatische Symptomencomplex: Eine psychologische Studie auf anatomischer Basis. Breslau: Cohn and Weigert. (English translation by Gertrude H. Eggert, in G. H. Eggert [1977]. *Wernicke's works on aphasia: A sourcebook and review* [pp. 91–145]. The Hague: Mouton.)

Further Readings

Best, W., and Howard, D. (1994). Word sound deafness resolved. *Aphasiology, 8*, 223–256.

Blanken, G., Dittmann, J., and Sinn, H. (1994). Old solutions to new problems: A contribution to today's relevance of Carl Wernicke's theory of aphasia. *Aphasiology, 8*, 207–221.

Cooper, W. E., and Zurif, E. B. (1983). Aphasia: Information processing in language production and reception. In B. Butterworth (Ed.), *Language production Vol. 2: Development, writing and other language processes* (pp. 225–256). London: Academic Press.

Garrard, P., and Hodges, J. R. (1999). Semantic dementia: Implications for the neural basis of language and meaning. *Aphasiology, 13*, 609–623.

Godefroy, O., Dubois, C., Debachy, B., Leclerc, M., and Kreisler, A. (2002). Vascular aphasias: Main characteristics of patients hospitalised in acute stroke units. *Stroke, 33*, 702–705.

Graham-Keegan, L., and Caspari, I. (1997). Wernicke's aphasia. In L. L. LaPointe (Ed.), *Aphasia and related neurogenic language disorders* (2nd ed., pp. 42–62). New York: Thieme.

Hickok, G., and Poeppel, D. (2000). Towards a functional neuroanatomy of speech perception. *Trends in Cognitive Sciences, 4*, 131–138.

Kertesz, A. (1983). Localization of lesions in Wernicke's aphasia. In A. Kertesz (Ed.), *Localization in neuropsychology* (pp. 209–230). New York: Academic Press.

Kertesz, A., Appell, J., and Fisman, M. (1986). The dissolution of language in Alzheimer's disease. *Canadian Journal of Neurological Sciences, 13*, 415–418.

Mackenzie, C. (2000). The relevance of education and age in the assessment of discourse comprehension. *Clinical Linguistics and Phonetics, 14*, 151–161.

Maneta, A., Marshall, J., and Lindsay, J. (2001). Direct and indirect therapy for sound deafness. *International Journal of Language and Communication Disorders, 36*, 91–106.

Marshall, J., Pring, T., Chiat, S., and Robson, J. (1995/6). Calling a salad a federation: An investigation of semantic jargon. Part 1. Nouns. *Journal of Neurolinguistics, 9*, 237–250.

Marshall, J., Chiat, S., Robson, J., and Pring, T. (1995/6). Calling a salad a federation: An investigation of semantic jargon. Part 2. Verbs. *Journal of Neurolinguistics, 9*, 251–260.

Niemi, J., and Laine, M. (1989). The English language bias in neurolinguistics: New languages give new perspectives. *Aphasiology, 3*, 155–159.

Obler, L. K., Albert, M. L., Goodglass, H., and Benson, D. F. (1978). Aphasia type and aging. *Brain and Language, 6*, 318–322.

Peterson, L. N., and Kirshner, H. S. (1981). Gestural impairment and gestural ability in aphasia. *Brain and Language, 14*, 333–348.

Portnoff, L. A. (1982). Schizophrenia and semantic aphasia: A clinical comparison. *International Journal of Neuroscience, 16*, 189–197.

Simmons, N. N., and Buckingham, H. W., Jr. (1992). Recovery in jargonaphasia. *Aphasiology, 6*, 403–414.

Van Dongen, H. R., Loonen, M. C. B., and Van Dongen, K. J. (1985). Anatomical basis for acquired fluent aphasia in children. *Annals of Neurology, 17*, 306–309.

Aphasia Treatment: Computer-Aided Rehabilitation

The role of technology in treating clinical aphasiology has been evolving since studies first demonstrated the feasibility of using computers in the treatment of aphasic adults. This journey began with remote access to treatment in rural settings using large computer systems over the telephone. There followed the introduction and widespread use of personal computers and portable computers, with the subsequent development of complex software and multimedia programs. This changing course is not simply the result of technological progress but represents greater understanding by clinicians and researchers of the strengths and limitations of computer-aided treatment for aphasia and related disorders.

Four common types of treatment activities are appropriate for presentation on a computer: stimulation, drill and practice, simulations, and tutorials. *Stimulation* activities offer the participant numerous opportunities to respond quickly and usually correctly over a relatively long period of time for the purpose of maintaining and stabilizing the underlying processes or skills, rather than simply learning a new set of responses. It is easy to design computer programs that contain a large database of stimuli, and then to control variables (e.g., word length) as a function of the participant's response accuracy. *Drill and practice* exercises teach specific information so that the participant can function more independently. Stimuli are selected for a particular participant and goal, and therefore authoring or editing options are required to modify stimuli and target responses. A limited number of stimuli are presented and are replaced with new items when a criterion is reached. Because response accuracy is the focus of the task, the program should present an intervention or cues to help shape the participant's response toward the target response. Drill and practice programs are convergent tasks. *Simulations* ("microworlds") create a structured environment in which a problem is presented and possible solutions are offered. Simulations may be simple, such as presenting a series of text describing a problem, followed by a list of possible solutions. Complex programs more closely simulate real-life situations by using pictures and sound. Simulations provide the opportunity to design divergent treatment tasks that more fully recruit real-life problem-solving strategies than those addressed by more traditional, convergent computer tasks, for example, by including several alternative but equally correct solutions. Whether computer simulations can improve communicative behavior in real-life settings remains to be tested. *Tutorials* offer valuable information regarding communication and quality of life to the family, friends, and others who can influence the aphasic patient's world for the better. Computer tutorials present information commonly found in patient information pamphlets but in an interactive, self-paced, format. Tutorials can incorporate features of an *expert system*, in which information is provided in response to a patient/family profile.

Computers can be incorporated into treatment in three fundamentally different ways. *Computer-only treatment* (COT) software is designed to allow patients, as part of clinician-provided treatment programs, to practice alone at the computer, without the simultaneous supervision or direct assistance from clinicians. The operation of COT programs should be familiar and intuitive for the patients, particularly those who cannot read lengthy or complex text. The program may alter in a limited way elements of the task in response to patient performance, such as reducing the number of stimuli or presenting predetermined cues in response to errors (e.g., Seron et al., 1980; Katz and Nagy, 1984). As all possible cues and therapeutic strategies that may be helpful to every patient cannot be anticipated, intervention is commonly simplistic, inflexible, or nonexistent. Consequently, COT programs are usually convergent tasks (e.g., drills) with simple, obvious goals and, if effective, increase treatment efficiency as supplementary tasks designed to reinforce or help generalize recently learned skills.

Computer-assisted treatment (CAT) software is presented on a computer as the patient and clinician work together on the program. The role for the computer is limited to supportive functions (e.g., presenting stimuli, storing responses, summarizing performance). The clinician retains responsibility for the most therapeutically critical components, particularly designing, administering, monitoring, and modifying the intervention in re-

sponse to the patient's particular needs. This relation between clinician and computer permits considerable flexibility, thus compensating for limitations inherent in the COT approach. In addition to treatment programs written specifically for use with clinicians (e.g., Loverso, Prescott, and Selinger, 1992; Van de Sandt-Koenderman, 1994), other software, such as COT word processing or a variety of video game programs, and even some web-based activities, can be used in this manner as long as clinicians provide patients with the additional information needed to perform the task.

Augmentative communication devices (ACDs) in aphasia treatment usually refer to small computers functioning as sophisticated "electronic pointing boards." Unlike devices used by patients with severe dysarthria or other speech problems, patients with aphasia and other disorders affecting language cannot type the words they are unable to speak. ACDs designed for these individuals may incorporate digitized speech, pictures, animation, and a minimum of text. To facilitate both expression and comprehension, some devices are designed to permit both communication partners to exchange messages. Although ACDs vary in design and organization, some devices allow modification of the organization and semantic content in response to the particular needs and abilities of each patient. Researchers such as Aftonomos, Steele, and Wertz (1997) claim that for some patients with aphasia, treatment utilizing ACDs results in improved performance on standardized tests and in "natural language" (speaking, listening, etc.).

A speech-language pathologist educated in communication theory and sufficiently experienced in the clinic and in real life can create an infinite number of novel and relevant treatment activities and evaluate and modify these activities in response to unique and idiosyncratic patient behavior, even when those behaviors are unanticipated, for example, resulting from previously unacknowledged associations. In contrast, computer-provided treatment is based on a finite set of rules that are stated explicitly to evoke specific response that are (at best) likely to occur at particular points during a future treatment session, as in a game of chess. However, unlike chess, many elements of language, communication, and rehabilitation are not well delineated or universally recognized.

In describing four interrelated properties of computers and programming, Bolter (1984) helped aphasiologists better understand the relation between computers and treatment. (1) Computers deal with *discrete* (or *digital*) units of data, typically unambiguous numbers or other values, but many fundamental and recurrent aspects of communication are not clearly defined or understood. Whether during treatment or real-life, purposeful interactions, language and communication units are often incomplete, emanate (simultaneously and sequentially) from various modalities, and depend on context and past experiences. (2) Computers are *conventional*, that is, they apply predetermined rules to symbols that have no effect on the rules. Regardless of the value of the symbols, the sophistication of the program ("complex branching algorithms") or the outcome of the program, the rules never change (e.g., Katz and Nagy, 1984). In aphasia treatment, all the rules of treatment are not known and those that are may not be correct for all conditions, requiring clinicians to monitor and sometimes modify rules for each patient. Unlike clinician-provided treatment, computer-provided treatment does not modify the rules of the treatment it applies; therefore, computers do not respond adequately to the dynamics of patient performance. (3) Computers are *finite*. Their rules and symbols are defined within the program. Except in a limited way for artificial intelligence software, unanticipated responses do not result in the creation of new rules and symbols. Therapy demands a different approach. Not all therapeutically relevant behaviors have been identified, and those that have often vary in relevance among patients and situations. Treatment software that incorporates artificial intelligence (e.g., Guyard, Masson, and Quiniou, 1990) only roughly approximates this approach, usually by reducing the scope of the task. (4) Computers are *isolated* from real-world experience. Problems and their solutions exist within the boundaries of the program and frequently have little to do with reality. Problems are created with the intention that they can be solved by manipulating symbols in a predetermined, finite series of steps. This lack of "world knowledge" is perhaps the most significant obstacle to comprehensive computer-provided treatment, as it limits the ability of programs to present real-world problems with multiple options and practical, flexible solutions.

In an extensive review of the literature, Robinson (1990) reported that the efficacy of computer-aided treatment for aphasia and for other cognitive disorders had not been demonstrated. The research studies reviewed suffered from inappropriate experimental designs, insufficient statistical analyses, and other deficiencies. Robinson stated that some researchers obscured the basic question by asking what works with whom under what conditions (see Darley, 1972).

There is no substitute for carefully controlled, randomized studies, the documentation of which has become the scientific foundation of aphasiology. Research reported over the last 15 years has assessed the effect of particular computerized interventions (e.g., Crerar, Ellis, and Dean, 1996) and incorporated increasingly sophisticated designs and greater numbers of subjects to assess the efficacy of computer-aided aphasia treatment, from simple A-B-A designs and comparisons of pre- and posttreatment testing (Mills, 1982) to large, randomly assigned single-subject studies (Loverso, Prescott, and Selinger, 1992) and group studies incorporating several conditions (Katz and Wertz, 1992, 1997). The efficacy of computerized aphasia treatment is being addressed one study at a time.

See also SPEECH AND LANGUAGE DISORDERS IN CHILDREN: COMPUTER-BASED APPROACHES.

—*Richard C. Katz*

References

Aftonomos, L. B., Steele, R. D., and Wertz, R. T. (1997). Promoting recovery in chronic aphasia with an interactive technology. *Archives of Physical Medicine, 78,* 841–846.

Bolter, J. D. (1984). *Turing's man: Western culture in the computer age.* Chapel Hill: University of North Carolina Press.

Crerar, M. A., Ellis, A. W., and Dean, E. C. (1996). Remediation of sentence processing deficits in aphasia using a computer-based microworld. *Brain and Language, 52,* 229–275.

Darley, F. L. (1972). The efficacy of language rehabilitation in aphasia. *Journal of Speech and Hearing Research, 37,* 3–21.

Guyard, H., Masson, V., and Quiniou, R. (1990). Computer-based aphasia treatment meets artificial intelligence. *Aphasiology, 4,* 599–613.

Katz, R. C., and Nagy, V. T. (1984). An intelligent computer-based task for chronic aphasic patients. In R. H. Brookshire (Ed.), *Clinical aphasiology: 1984 conference proceedings* (pp. 159–165). Minneapolis: BRK.

Katz, R. C., and Wertz, R. T. (1992). Computerized hierarchical reading treatment in aphasia. *Aphasiology, 6,* 165–177.

Katz, R. C., and Wertz, R. T. (1997). The efficacy of computer-provided reading treatment for chronic aphasic adults. *Journal of Speech, Language, and Hearing Research, 40,* 493–507.

Loverso, F. L., Prescott, T. E., and Selinger, M. (1992). Microcomputer treatment applications in aphasiology. *Aphasiology, 6,* 155–163.

Mills, R. H. (1982). Microcomputerized auditory comprehension training. In R. H. Brookshire (Ed.), *Clinical aphasiology: 1982 conference proceedings* (pp. 147–152). Minneapolis: BRK.

Robinson, I. (1990). Does computerized cognitive rehabilitation work? A review. *Aphasiology, 4,* 381–405.

Seron, X., Deloche, G., Moulard, G., and Rouselle, M. (1980). A computer-based therapy for the treatment of aphasic subjects with writing disorders. *Journal of Speech and Hearing Disorders, 45,* 45–58.

Van de Sandt-Koenderman, M. (1994). Multicue, a computer program for word finding in aphasia, *1. International Congress Language-Therapy-Computers,* Graz, Austria: University of Graz.

Further Readings

Bengston, V. L. (1973). Self-determination: A social psychologic perspective on helping the aged. *Geriatrics, 28,* 1118–1130.

Colby, K. M., and Kraemer, H. C. (1975). An objective measurement of nonspeaking children's performance with a computer-controlled program for the stimulation of language behavior. *Journal of Autism and Childhood Schizophrenia, 5,* 139–146.

Crerar, M. A., and Ellis, A. W. (1995). Computer-based therapy for aphasia: Towards second generation clinical tools. In C. Code and D. Müller (Eds.), *Treatment of aphasia: From theory to practice* (pp. 223–250). London: Whurr.

Dean, E. C. (1987). Microcomputers and aphasia. *Aphasiology, 1,* 267–270.

Delouche, G., Dordain, M., and Kremin, H. (1993). Rehabilitation of confrontational naming in aphasia: Relations between oral and written modalities. *Aphasiology, 7,* 201–216.

Enderby, P. (1987). Microcomputers in assessment, rehabilitation and recreation. *Aphasiology, 1,* 151–166.

Glisky, E. L., Schlacter, D. L., and Tuving, E. (1986). Learning and retention of computer-related vocabulary in memory-impaired patients: Method of vanishing cues. *Journal of Clinical and Experimental Neuropsychology*, 8, 292–312.

Katz, R. C. (1986). *Aphasia treatment and microcomputers*. San Diego, CA: College-Hill Press.

Katz, R. C. (1987). Efficacy of aphasia treatment using microcomputers. *Aphasiology*, 1, 141–150.

Katz, R. C. (1990). Intelligent computerized treatment or artificial aphasia therapy. *Aphasiology*, 4, 621–624.

Katz, R. C., and Hallowell, B. (1999). Computer applications in treatment of acquired neurogenic communication disorders in adults. *Seminars in Speech and Language*, 20, 251–269.

Loverso, F. L. (1987). Unfounded expectations: Computers in rehabilitation. *Aphasiology*, 1, 157–160.

Loverso, F. L., Prescott, T. E., Selinger, M., and Riley, L. (1988). Comparison of two modes of aphasia treatment: Clinician and computer-clinician assisted. *Clinical Aphasiology*, 18, 297–319.

Lucas, R. W. (1977). A study of patients' attitudes to computer interrogation. *International Journal of Man-Machine Studies*, 9, 69–86.

Odor, J. P. (1988). Student models in machine-mediated learning. *Journal of Mental Deficiency Research*, 32, 247–256.

Petheram, B. (1988). Enabling stroke victims to interact with a minicomputer—comparison of input devices. *International Disabilities Studies*, 10, 73–80.

Rushakoff, G. E. (1984). Clinical applications in communication disorders. In A. H. Schwartz (Ed.), *Handbook of microcomputer applications in communication disorders* (pp. 148–171). San Diego, CA: College-Hill Press.

Scott, C., and Byng, S. (1989). Computer-assisted remediation of a homophone comprehension disorder in surface dyslexia. *Aphasiology*, 3, 301–320.

Steele, R. D., Weinrich, M., Kleczewska, M. K., Wertz, R. T., and Carlson, G. S. (1987). Evaluating performance of severely aphasic patients on a computer-aided visual communication system. In R. H. Brookshire (Ed.), *Clinical aphasiology: 1987 conference proceedings* (pp. 46–54). Minneapolis: BRK.

Vaughn, G. R., Amster, W. W., Bess, J. C., Gilbert, D. J., Kearrns, K. P., Rudd, A. K., et al. (1987). Efficacy of remote treatment of aphasia by TEL-communicology. *Journal of Rehabilitative Research and Development*, 25, 446–447.

Weinrich, M., McCall, D., Weber, C., Thomas, K., and Thornburg, L. (1995). Training on an iconic communication system for severe aphasia can improve natural language production. *Aphasiology*, 9, 343–364.

Wertz, R. T., Dronkers, N. F., Knight, R. T., Shenaut, G. K., and Deal, J. L. (1987). Rehabilitation of neurogenic communication disorders in remote settings. *Journal of Rehabilitative Research and Development*, 25, 432–433.

Aphasia Treatment: Pharmacological Approaches

For over a century, clinicians have sought to use pharmacological agents to remediate aphasia and/or to help compensate for it, but without much success (Small, 1994). However, in several limited areas, the use of drug treatment as an adjunct to traditional (behavioral) speech therapy has shown some promise. Furthermore, the future for pharmacological and other biological treatments is bright (Small, 2000).

In this brief article, we restrict our attention to the subacute and chronic phases of aphasia, rather than the treatments for acute neurological injury. Much of this work has focused on a class of neurotransmitters, the catecholamines, which occur throughout the brain. Two important catecholamines are dopamine, produced by the substantia nigra, and norepinephrine, produced by the locus coeruleus. Since the catecholamines do not cross the blood-brain barrier, typical therapy involves agents that increase catecholamine concentrations. Dextro-amphetamine is the most popular agent of this sort, acting nonspecifically to increase the concentrations of all the catecholamines at synaptic junctions. In the early studies, a single dose of dextro-amphetamine led to accelerated recovery in a beam-walking task in rats with unilateral motor cortex ablation (Feeney, Gonzalez, and Law, 1982). By contrast, a single dose of haloperidol, a dopamine antagonist, blocked the amphetamine effect. When given alone, haloperidol delays spontaneous recovery, whereas phenoxybenzamine, an α_1-adrenergic antagonist, reproduces the deficits in animals that have recovered. Similar results have now been obtained in several species and in motor and visual systems (Feeney and Sutton, 1987; Feeney, 1997).

The role of antidepressant medications in stroke recovery, including selective serotonin reuptake inhibitors (SSRIs) and the less selective tricyclics, is not straightforward. Neither fluoxetine (an SSRI) nor direct administration of serotonin seems effective in improving motor function in a rat model (Boyeson, Harmon, and Jones, 1994), whereas the tricyclics have produced mixed effects (Boyeson and Harmon, 1993; Boyeson, Harmon, and Jones, 1994).

The role of the inhibitory transmitter γ-aminobutyric acid (GABA) has been investigated in several studies. Intracortical infusion of GABA exacerbates the hemiparesis produced by a small motor cortex lesion in rats (Schallert et al., 1992). The short-term administration of diazepam, a benzodiazepine and indirect GABA agonist, can permanently impede sensory cortical recovery. Furthermore, phenobarbital, which may have some GABA agonist effects, also impedes recovery (Hernandez and Holling, 1994).

A number of early studies were conducted with limited success and are summarized in two recent reviews (Small, 1994; Small, 2001). Modern studies of pharmacological treatment of aphasia have focused on neurotransmitter systems, particularly catecholaminergic systems. A number of studies have been conducted, not all well designed. At present, no drug has been adequately shown to help aphasia recovery to the degree that would be necessary to recommend its general use. Several biological approaches that have been tested for aphasia recovery have been shown to be ineffective (e.g., meprobamate, hyperbaric oxygen) or very poorly supported by published results (e.g., amobarbital, selegiline).

Several studies have examined the role of dopamine. Albert et al. (1988) described a case suggesting that the dopamine agonist bromocriptine helped restore speech fluency in a patient with transcortical motor aphasia resulting from stroke. Another case report failed to find a similar benefit in a similar patient (MacLennan et al., 1991). Two additional patients improved in speech fluency but not in other aspects of language function (Gupta and Mlcoch, 1992). Another open-label study suggested some effect in moderate but not severe aphasia (Sabe, Leiguarda, and Starkstein, 1992).

Dextro-amphetamine is perhaps the most widely studied biological treatment for the chronic effects of stroke, including aphasia (Walker-Batson, 2000), yet both its clinical efficacy and mode of action remain unclear (Goldstein, 2000). Nonetheless, evidence from both animal model systems and humans make this a somewhat promising drug for the treatment of aphasia.

In a study of motor rehabilitation from stroke, more than half of a group of 88 elderly patients who had been classified as rehabilitation failures because of poor progress in physical therapy benefited from dextroamphetamine as an adjunct to physical therapy (Clark and Mankikar, 1979). A double-blind placebo-controlled study replicated this finding (Crisostomo et al., 1988) in eight patients with ischemic stroke.

An early study of aphasia pharmacotherapy with methylphenidate (similar to amphetamine) and chlordiazepoxide (a benzodiazepine) revealed no effects (Darley, Keith, and Sasanuma, 1977). A recent prospective double-blind study of motor recovery with methylphenidate found a significant difference in motor and depression scores on some measures but not others (Grade et al., 1998). Methylphenidate may play a role in the treatment of post-stroke depression (Lazarus et al., 1992).

Walker-Batson et al. (1991) have reported a study of six aphasic patients with ischemic cerebral infarction. Each patient took dextro-amphetamine every 4 days, about an hour prior to a session of speech and language therapy, for a total of ten sessions. When evaluated after this period, the patients performed at significantly above expected levels.

Of potential significance, the studies showing beneficial effects of dextro-amphetamine, that is, the study by Walker-Batson et al. (1991), a motor study by the same group (Walker-Batson et al., 1995), and the other study of motor rehabilitation (Crisostomo et al., 1988), share the common feature of evaluating the drug as an enhancement to behavioral or physical therapy rather than as a monotherapeutic panacea.

Piracetam is a GABA derivative that acts as a nootropic agent on the central nervous system (CNS) and facilitates cholinergic and excitatory amine neurotransmission (Giurgea, Greindl, and Preat, 1983; Vernon and Sorkin, 1991). A large multicenter trial (De Deyn et al., 1997) showed no effect on the primary outcome measure of neurological status at 4 weeks. Another study showed improvement at 12 weeks that was no longer present at 24 weeks (Enderby et al., 1994). A later study (Huber et al., 1997) showed that improvement occurred on only one subtest (written language) of a large battery.

A crucial issue that must be addressed as part of aphasia rehabilitation is depression, since it can adversely affect language recovery. Following stroke, patients with depression have more cognitive impairment than patients with comparable lesions but no depression (Downhill and Robinson, 1994). Furthermore, in stroke patients matched for severity and lesion localization, patients with depression experience a poorer recovery than their nondepressed counterparts in functional status and cognitive performance (Morris, Raphael, and Robinson, 1992).

Growth factors have been advocated for a variety of purposes in the treatment of stroke, particularly in the acute phase of ischemic brain injury (Zhang et al., 1999), but also as neuroprotective agents useful in the chronic phase of recovery from brain injury (Olson et al., 1994). Gene transfer into the CNS might ultimately play a role in delivering trophins or other agents to damaged brain areas and thus to help stimulate recovery or increased synaptic connectivity.

Neural stem cells are multipotential precursors to neurons and glia. Attempts have been made to induce differentiation into neurons and glial cells, and further into specific types of such cells. Specifically with regard to stroke and the treatment of cortical lesions, fetal neocortical cells have been successfully transplanted into the site of cortical lesions (Johansson, 2000), and have even been shown to migrate selectively into areas of experimental cell death (Macklis, 1993; Snyder et al., 1997).

One important consequence of this research into the pharmacology of aphasia is the realization that drugs are not only potential therapeutic adjuncts but can also serve as inhibitors of successful recovery. The first study of this type, by Porch and colleagues (1985), showed that patients taking certain medicines performed more poorly on an aphasia battery than those who were not taking medicines.

In a formal retrospective (chart review) study, patients with motor deficits after stroke were divided into one group taking a number of specific drugs at the time of stroke (clonidine, prazosin, any dopamine receptor antagonist [e.g., neuroleptics], benzodiazepines, phenytoin, or phenobarbital) and another group that was not (Goldstein, 1995). Statistical analysis revealed that whereas patient demographics and stroke severity were similar between groups, motor recovery time was significantly shorter in the patients who were not taking one of these drugs.

This work has profound relevance to aphasia rehabilitation. To maximize functional recovery, it is important not only to ensure adequate behavioral treatment, but also to ensure the appropriate neurobiological substrate for this treatment (or, more concretely, to ensure that this substrate is not pharmacologically inhibited from responding to the therapy). It is thus advisable for patients in aphasia therapy to avoid drugs that might interfere with catecholaminergic or GABAergic function or that are thought to delay recovery by empirical study.

Current knowledge suggests a potential beneficial effect of increased CNS catecholamines on human motor recovery and aphasia rehabilitation. Although pharmacotherapy cannot be used as a replacement for speech and language therapy, it might play a role as an adjunct, and other biological therapies, such as cell transplantation, might play a role in concert with carefully designed, adaptive learning approaches. In the published cases where pharmacotherapy improved language functioning in people with aphasia, it was used adjunctively, not alone. It is very likely that pharmacotherapy has a valuable role to play as an adjunct to behavioral rehabilitation to decrease performance variability and to improve mean performance in patients with mild to moderate language dysfunction from cerebral infarctions.

Acknowledgments

Research was supported by the National Institute of Deafness and Other Communication Disorders, National Institutes of Health, under grant NIH DC R01-3378.

—Steven L. Small

References

Albert, M. L., Bachman, D. L., Morgan, A., and Helm-Estabrooks, N. (1988). Pharmacotherapy for aphasia. Neurology, 38, 877–879.

Boyeson, M. G., and Harmon, R. L. (1993). Effects of trazodone and desipramine on motor recovery in brain-injured rats. American Journal of Physical Medicine and Rehabilitation, 72, 286–293.

Boyeson, M. G., Harmon, R. L., and Jones, J. L. (1994). Comparative effects of fluoxetine, amitriptyline and serotonin on functional motor recovery after sensorimotor cortex injury. American Journal of Physical Medicine and Rehabilitation, 73, 76–83.

Clark, A. N. G., and Mankikar, G. D. (1979). d-Amphetamine in elderly patients refractory to rehabilitation procedures. Journal of the American Geriatrics Society, 27, 174–177.

Crisostomo, E. A., Duncan, P. W., Propst, M., Dawson, D. V., and Davis, J. N. (1988). Evidence that amphetamine with physical therapy promotes recovery of motor function in stroke patients. Annals of Neurology, 23, 94–97.

Darley, F. L., Keith, R. L., and Sasanuma, S. (1977). The effect of alerting and tranquilizing drugs upon the performance of aphasic patients. Clinical Aphasiology, 7, 91–96.

De Deyn, P. P., Reuck, J. D., Deberdt, W., Vlietinck, R., and Orgogozo, J. M. (1997). Treatment of acute ischemic stroke with piracetam. Members of the Piracetam in Acute Stroke Study (PASS) Group. Stroke, 28, 2347–2352.

Downhill, J. R., Jr., and Robinson, R. G. (1994). Longitudinal assessment of depression and cognitive impairment following stroke. Journal of Nervous and Mental Disease, 182, 425–431.

Enderby, P., Broeckx, J., Hospers, W., Schildermans, F., and Deberdt, W. (1994). Effect of piracetam on recovery and rehabilitation after stroke: A double-blind, placebo-controlled study. Clinical Neuropharmacology, 17, 320–331.

Feeney, D. M. (1997). From laboratory to clinic: noradrenergic enhancement of physical therapy for stroke or trauma patients. Advances in Neurology, 73, 383–394.

Feeney, D. M., Gonzalez, A., and Law, W. A. (1982). Amphetamine, haloperidol, and experience interact to affect rate of recovery after motor cortex injury. Science, 217, 855–857.

Feeney, D. M., and Sutton, R. L. (1987). Pharmacotherapy for recovery of function after brain injury. Critical Reviews in Neurobiology, 3, 135–197.

Giurgea, C. E., Greindl, M. G., and Preat, S. (1983). Nootropic drugs and aging. Acta Psychiatrica Belgium, 83, 349–358.

Goldstein, L. B. (1995). Common drugs may influence motor recovery after stroke. The Sygen in Acute Stroke Study Investigators [see comments]. Neurology, 45, 865–871.

Goldstein, L. B. (2000). Effects of amphetamines and small related molecules on recovery after stroke in animals and man. Neuropharmacology, 39, 852–859.

Grade, C., Redford, B., Chrostowski, J., Toussaint, L., and Blackwell, B. (1998). Methylphenidate in early post-stroke recovery: A double-blind, placebo-controlled study. Archives of Physical Medicine and Rehabilitation, 79, 1047–1050.

Gupta, S. R., and Mlcoch, A. G. (1992). Bromocriptine treatment of nonfluent aphasia. Archives of Physical Medicine and Rehabilitation, 73, 373–376.

Hernandez, T. D., and Holling, L. C. (1994). Disruption of behavioral recovery by the anti-convulsant phenobarbital. Brain Research, 635, 300–306.

Huber, W., Willmes, K., Poeck, K., Van Vleymen, B., and Deberdt, W. (1997). Piracetam as an adjuvant to language therapy for aphasia: A randomized double-blind placebo-controlled pilot study. Archives of Physical Medicine and Rehabilitation, 78, 245–250.

Johansson, B. B. (2000). Brain plasticity and stroke rehabilitation. The Willis Lecture. Stroke, 31, 223–230.

Lazarus, L. W., Winemiller, D. R., Lingam, V. R., Neyman, I., Hartman, C., Abassian, M., et al. (1992). Efficacy and side effects of methylphenidate for poststroke depression [see comments]. Journal of Clinical Psychiatry, 53, 447–449.

Macklis, J. D. (1993). Transplanted neocortical neurons migrate selectively into regions of neuronal degeneration produced by chromophore-targeted laser photolysis. Journal of Neuroscience, 13, 3848–3863.

MacLennan, D. L., Nicholas, L. E., Morley, G. K., and Brookshire, R. H. (1991). The effects of bromocriptine on speech and language function in a man with transcortical motor aphasia. Clinical Aphasiology, 21, 145–155.

Morris, P. L., Raphael, B., and Robinson, R. G. (1992). Clinical depression is associated with impaired recovery from stroke. Medical Journal of Australia, 157, 239–242.

Olson, L., Backman, L., Ebendal, T., Eriksdotter-Jonhagen, M., Hoffer, B., Humpel, C., et al. (1994). Role of growth factors in degeneration and regeneration in the central nervous system: Clinical experiences with NGF in Parkinson's and Alzheimer's diseases. *Journal of Neurology, 242* (Suppl. 1), S12–S15.

Porch, B., Wyckes, J., and Feeney, D. M. (1985). *Haloperidol, thiazides, and some antihypertensives slow recovery from aphasia.* Paper presented at the Annual Meeting of the Society for Neuroscience.

Sabe, L., Leiguarda, R., and Starkstein, S. E. (1992). An open-label trial of bromocriptine in nonfluent aphasia. *Neurology, 42,* 1637–1638.

Schallert, T., Jones, T., Weaver, M., Shapiro, L., Crippens, D., and Fulton, R. (1992). Pharmacologic and anatomic considerations in recovery of function. *Physical Medicine and Rehabilitation, 6,* 375–393.

Small, S. L. (1994). Pharmacotherapy of aphasia: A critical review. *Stroke, 25,* 1282–1289.

Small, S. L. (2000). The future of aphasia treatment. *Brain and Language, 71,* 227–232.

Small, S. L. (2001). Biological approaches to the treatment of aphasia. In A. Hillis (Ed.), *Handbook on adult language disorders: Integrating cognitive neuropsychology, neurology, and rehabilitation* (in press). Philadelphia: Psychology Press.

Snyder, E. Y., Yoon, C., Flax, J. D., and Macklis, J. D. (1997). Multipotent neural precursors can differentiate toward replacement of neurons undergoing targeted apoptotic degeneration in adult mouse neocortex. *Proceedings of National Academy of Sciences of the United States of America, 94,* 11663–11668.

Vernon, M. W., and Sorkin, E. M. (1991). Piracetam. An overview of its pharmacological properties and a review of its therapeutic use in senile cognitive disorders. *Drugs and Aging, 1,* 17–35.

Walker-Batson, D. (2000). Use of pharmacotherapy in the treatment of aphasia. *Brain and Language, 71,* 252–254.

Walker-Batson, D., Devous, M. D., Curtis, S., Unwin, D. H., and Greenlee, R. G. (1991). Response to amphetamine to facilitate recovery from aphasia subsequent to stroke. *Clinical Aphasiology, 21,* 137–143.

Walker-Batson, D., Smith, P., Curtis, S., Unwin, H., and Greenlee, R. (1995). Amphetamine paired with physical therapy accelerates motor recovery after stroke. Further evidence. *Stroke, 26,* 2254–2259.

Zhang, W. R., Kitagawa, H., Hayashi, T., Sasaki, C., Sakai, K., Warita, H., et al. (1999). Topical application of neurotrophin-3 attenuates ischemic brain injury after transient middle cerebral artery occlusion in rats. *Brain Research, 842,* 211–214.

Aphasia Treatment: Psychosocial Issues

Although researchers are developing a useful understanding of aphasia as a neurocognitive condition, the world we experience is a social and interactive one. The social aspects of life contribute to quality of life, although quality of life has been difficult to characterize scientifically and in ways that have clinical utility (Hilari et al., in press).

Psychosocial refers to the social context of emotional experience. Most emotions are closely associated with social interactions. Aphasia has implications for the individual's whole social network, especially the immediate family. The value dimensions in our lives, such as health, sexuality, career, creativity, marriage, intelligence, money, and family relations, contribute to quality of life and are markedly affected for the aphasic person (Hinckley, 1998) and that person's relatives. All may expect considerable disruption of professional, social, and family life, reduced social contact, depression, loneliness, frustration, and aggression (Herrmann and Wallesch, 1989).

Recovery and response to rehabilitation in aphasia are also significantly influenced by emotional and psychosocial factors. The aphasic person's family and other caregivers need to be involved as much as possible in intervention, and this involvement extends beyond discharge. The experienced disability rather than the impairment itself is the focus of rehabilitation. Rehabilitation increasingly includes community-based work and support from not-for-profit organizations and self-help groups.

Whereas intervention during the acute stages of aphasia is largely based on the medical model, adjustment to aphasia is set more broadly within a social approach. Several broad psychosocial and quality-of-life areas have been incorporated into rehabilitation: dealing with depression and other emotions, social reintegration, and the development of autonomy and self-worth. Autonomy involves cooperating with others to achieve ends, whereas independence implies acting alone and may not be an achievable goal. These areas provide a basis for developing broad-ranging programs.

Emotion

We need to distinguish the *direct* effects of damage on the neurophysical substrate of emotion and the *indirect* effects, which are natural reactions to catastrophic personal circumstances (Code, Hemsley, and Herrmann, 1999). Our understanding of these factors is improving. Three different forms of depression can follow damage: catastrophic reaction, major post-stroke depression, and minor post-stroke depression. There is little research separating reactive from direct effects but Herrmann, Bartels, and Wallesch (1993) found significantly higher ratings for physical signs of depression, generally considered direct effects, during the acute stage.

Some view depression accompanying aphasia within the framework of the grief model (Tanner and Gerstenberger, 1988). In this view, individuals grieve for the loss of communication, moving through the stages of denial, anger, bargaining, depression, and acceptance. Whether people do in fact go through these stages has not been investigated, but it has served as a framework for counseling. Determining denial, bargaining, acceptance, and so on is problematic but has been investigated interpretively with personal construct therapy techniques by Brumfitt (1985), who argues that aphasia affects a person's core role constructs, with grief for the essential element of *self* as a speaker.

A further problem is that the symptoms of depression, such as changes in sleep and eating, restlessness, and crying, can also be caused by physical illness, anxiety, hospitalization, and factors unrelated to mood state. Language impairment plays a special role in the problem of identifying and measuring mood, and one approach has been to use the nonverbal Visual Analogue Mood Scale (VAMS), substituting schematic faces for words (Stern, 1999).

Åström et al. (1993) found major depression in 25% of stroke survivors, which rose to 31% at 3 months post onset, fell to 16% at 12 months, and increased again over the next 2 years to 29%. Some workers take the position that drugs should be avoided, but others suggest incorporating drugs and psychotherapy, with drugs perhaps being more appropriate at early stages to counter direct effects and psychotherapy and counseling more appropriate later, when the individual is more ready to deal with the future. Individual and group counseling are effective, and aphasic people themselves have recently become involved as counselors.

Social Reintegration and Self-Esteem

Self-esteem and self-worth are complex constructs, tied to social activity, that workers suggest should be central to psychosocial rehabilitation. The importance of self has been examined by Brumfitt (1993) using personal construct techniques. Facilitating participation in the community entails passing responsibility to the individual gradually so that the individual can develop autonomy, develop greater self-esteem, and take greater ownership of the issues that they face. The importance of involving the aphasic individual fully has been addressed by Parr et al. (1997).

Hersh (1998) argues that particularly at discharge from formal therapy, an account of the ongoing management of psychosocial adjustment is needed. Simmons-Mackie (1998) argues that the traditional concept of a plateau being reached, where linguistic progress slows down for many, is not relevant when considering the social consequences of aphasia. The aim should be to prepare and assist clients to integrate into a community. Social affiliation is stressed as a means of maintaining and developing self-identity.

Not-for-profit organizations and centers such as the Pat Orato Aphasia Center in Ontario and the Aphasia Center in Oakland, California, provide community-based programs for aphasic people and their families, including the training of relatives and professionals as better conversation partners. Through such programs, the psychosocial well-being of both aphasic participants and their families is improved (Hoen, Thelander, and Worsley, 1997). Training volunteers as communication partners results in gains in psychological well-being and communication among aphasic participants, caregivers, and the communication partners themselves. In philosophy and approach, these centers resemble United Kingdom charities such as Speakability and Connect. Organizations like these are increasingly offering more long-term and psychosocially oriented programs. Many use volunteers, who figure increasingly in social reinte-

gration, providing a valuable resource and helping to establish, facilitate, and maintain groups.

The efficacy of self-help groups in which the aphasic members decide on the group's purpose, take responsibility for running the group, and serve as officers of the group (e.g., chair, secretary) is being evaluated, particularly in relation to the development of independence and autonomy. Structured support groups are of benefit. The self-help groups in the United Kingdom attract mainly younger and less severely impaired individuals and use little in the way of statutory resources (Code et al., 2001).

Wahrborg et al. (1997) have reported benefits from integrating aphasic people into educational programs and organizations, and Elman (1998) has introduced adult education instructors into an aphasia center.

Work and other purposeful activity is an important value dimension central in the development and maintenance of self-worth and autonomy. Returning to work remains a constant concern of many aphasic people. Ramsing, Blomstrand, and Sullivan (1991) explored prognostic factors for return to work, but there has been little follow-up to this research. Parr et al. (1997) report that only one person in their study who was working at the time of the stroke returned to the same employment. A few found part-time work, and the rest became unemployed or retired. Garcia, Barrette, and Laroche (2000) studied perceived barriers to work and found that therapists focused on personal and social barriers, employers focused on organizational ones, and aphasic people focused on barriers of all types. The groups also suggested strategies for reducing barriers to work.

Family therapy, to include people close to the aphasic person, is generally beneficial and can lead to positive changes (Nichols, Varchevker, and Pring, 1996).

Conclusions

A psychosocial approach to improving quality of life aims to aid social reintegration in such a way that the individual is able to maintain identity, develop self-esteem and purpose, and become socially reaffiliated. Significant others, professionals, and volunteers are involved. This approach offers a challenge to clinicians, as it extends their role and requires a more comprehensive approach to management. There remains a lack of evidence-based approaches to managing psychosocial adjustment, but it is clear that volunteers, organizations, charities, and community-based centers are contributing. The challenge facing clinical aphasiology is to evaluate the benefits of psychosocial support for aphasic people and its impact on quality of life.

Acknowledgments

The first author was a Fellow at the Hanse Institute of Advanced Study, Delmenhorst, Germany, when this chapter was completed.

—Chris Code and Dave J. Muller

References

Åström, M., Adolfsson, R., and Asplund, K. (1993). Major depression in stroke patients: A 3-year longitudinal study. *Stroke, 24,* 976–982.

Brumfitt, S. (1985). The use of repertory grids with aphasic people. In N. Beail (Ed.), *Repertory grid techniques and personal constructs.* London: Croom Helm.

Brumfitt, S. (1993). Losing your sense of self: What aphasia can do. *Aphasiology, 7,* 569–574.

Code, C., Hemsley, G., and Herrmann, M. (1999). The emotional impact of aphasia. *Seminars in Speech and Language, 20,* 19–31.

Code, C., Eales, C., Pearl, G., Conan, M., Cowin, K., and Hickin, J. (2001). Profiling the membership of self-help groups for aphasic people. *International Journal of Language and Communication Disorders, Supplement, 36,* 41–45.

Elman, R. (1998). Memories of the "plateau": Health care changes provide an opportunity to redefine aphasia treatment and discharge. *Aphasiology, 12,* 227–231.

Garcia, L. J., Barrette, J., and Laroche, C. (2000). Perceptions of the obstacles to work reintegration for persons with aphasia. *Aphasiology, 14,* 269–290.

Herrmann, M., Bartels, C., and Wallesch, C. W. (1993). Depression in acute and chronic aphasia: Symptoms, pathoanatomo-clinical correlations, and functional implications. *Journal of Neurology, Neurosurgery, and Psychiatry, 56,* 672–678.

Herrmann, M., and Wallesch, C.-W. (1989). Psychosocial changes and adjustment with chronic and severe nonfluent aphasia. *Aphasiology, 3,* 513–526.

Hersh, D. (1998). Beyond the "plateau": Discharge dilemmas in chronic aphasia. *Aphasiology, 12,* 207–218.

Hilari, K., Wiggins, R. D., Roy, P., Byng, S., and Smith, S. C. (in press). Predictors of health-related quality of life (HRQOL) in people with chronic aphasia. *Aphasiology.*

Hinckley, J. J. (1998). Investigating the predictors of lifestyle satisfaction among younger adults with chronic aphasia. *Aphasiology, 12,* 509–518.

Hoen, B., Thelander, M., and Worsley, J. (1997). Improvement in psychosocial well-being of people with aphasia and their families: Evaluation of a community-based programme. *Aphasiology, 11,* 681–691.

Kagan, A. (1998). Supported conversation for adults with aphasia: Methods and resources for training conversation partners. *Aphasiology, 9,* 816–831.

Nichols, F., Varchevker, A., and Pring, T. (1996). Working with people with aphasia and their families: An exploration of the use of family therapy techniques. *Aphasiology, 10,* 767–781.

Parr, S., Byng, S., Gilpin, S., and Ireland, C. (1997). *Talking about aphasia.* Buckingham, U.K.: Open University Press.

Ramsing, S., Blomstrand, C., and Sullivan, M. (1991). Prognostic factors for return to work in stroke patients with aphasia. *Aphasiology, 5,* 583–588.

Simmons-Mackie, N. (1998). A solution to the discharge dilemma in aphasia: Social approaches to aphasia management. *Aphasiology, 12,* 231–239.

Stern, R. (1999). Assessment of mood states in aphasia. *Seminars in Speech and Language, 20,* 33–50.

Tanner, D. C., and Gerstenberger, D. L. (1988). The grief response in neuropathologies of speech and language. *Aphasiology, 2,* 79–84.

Wahrborg, P., Borenstein, P., Linell, S., Hedberg-Borenstein, E., and Asking, A. (1997). Ten year follow-up of young aphasic participants in a 34-week course at a Folk High School. *Aphasiology, 11,* 709–715.

Further Readings

Borenstein, P., Linell, S., and Wahrborg, P. (1987). An innovative therapeutic programme for aphasic patients and their relatives. *Scandinavian Journal of Rehabilitation Medicine, 19,* 51–56.

Carnworth, T. C. M., and Johnson, D. A. W. (1987). Psychiatric morbidity among spouses of patients with stroke. *British Medical Journal, 294,* 409–411.

Christensen, A. (1997). Communication in relation to self-esteem. *Aphasiology, 11,* 727–734.

Code, C. (Ed.). (1996). *The impact of neurogenic communication disorders: Beyond the impairment. Disability and Rehabilitation, 18.* [Special issue]

Code, C. (Ed.). (1999). Management of psychosocial issues in aphasia. *Seminars in Speech and Language, 20.* [Special issue]

Elman, R., and Bernstein-Ellis, E. (1999). Psychosocial aspects of group communication treatment: Preliminary findings. *Seminars in Speech and Language, 20,* 65–72.

Gainotti, G. (Ed.). (1997). Emotional, psychological and psychosocial problems of aphasic patients. *Aphasiology, 11.* [Special issue]

Lapointe, L. L. (1999). Quality of life in aphasia. *Seminars in Speech and Language, 20,* 5–17.

Müller, D. J. (1992). Psychosocial aspects of aphasia. In G. Blanken, J. Dittmann, H. Grimm, J. C. Marshall, and C.-W. Wallesch (Eds.), *Linguistic disorders and pathologies: An international handbook.* Berlin: Walter de Gruyter.

Parr, S. (2001). Psychosocial aspects of aphasia: Whose perspectives? *Folia Phoniatrica et Logopaedica, 53,* 266–288.

Parr, S., Pound, C., Syng, S., and Long, B. (1999). *The aphasia handbook.* Woodhouse Eves, U.K.: Ecodistribution.

Rice, B., Paull, A., and Müller, D. J. (1987). An evaluation of a social support group for spouses and aphasic adults. *Aphasiology, 1,* 247–256.

Sarno, M. T. (Ed.). (1995). Aphasia recovery: Family-consumer issues. *Topics in Stroke Rehabilitation, 2.* [Special issue]

Sarno, M. T. (1997). Quality of life in aphasia in the first post-stroke year. *Aphasiology, 11,* 665–679.

Wahrborg, P. (1991). *Assessment and management of emotional and psychosocial reactions to brain damage and aphasia.* London: Whurr.

Aphasic Syndromes: Connectionist Models

Connectionist models of aphasic syndromes first emerged in the late nineteenth century. Broca (1861) described a patient, Leborgne, whose speech was limited to the monosyllable *tan* but whose ability to understand spoken language and nonverbal cues and ability to express himself through gestures and facial expressions were normal. Leborgne's brain contained a lesion whose center was in the posterior portion of the inferior frontal convolution of the left hemisphere, now known as Broca's area. Broca claimed that Leborgne had lost "the faculty of articulate speech" and that this brain region was the neural site of the mechanism involved in speech production. In 1874, Karl Wernicke described a patient with a speech disturbance that was very different from that seen in Leborgne. Wernicke's patient was fluent, but his speech contained words with sound errors, other errors of word forms, and words that were semantically inappropriate. Unlike Leborgne, Wernicke's patient did not understand spoken language. Wernicke related the two impairments—one of speech production and one of comprehension—by arguing that the patient had sustained damage to "the storehouse of auditory word forms," leading to speech containing the types of errors that were seen and impaired comprehension. By extrapolation from a similar case he had not personally examined, Wernicke concluded that the patient's lesion was in the posterior portion of the left superior temporal gyrus, now known as Wernicke's area, and that this region was the locus of the "storehouse of auditory word forms." Wernicke argued that, in speaking, word sounds were conveyed from Wernicke's area to Broca's area, where the motor programs for speech were developed. This connection gave this type of model its name.

Lichtheim (1885) deveoped a more general model of this type. Lichtheim recognized seven syndromes, listed in Table 1. Lichtheim argued that these syndromes followed lesions in the regions of the brain depicted in Figure 1. These syndromes were criticized on neuro-anatomical grounds (Marie, 1906; Moutier, 1908), dismissed as simplifications of reality that were of help only to schoolboys (Head, 1926), and ignored in favor of different approaches to language (Jackson, 1878; Goldstein, 1948). Nonetheless, they endured. Benson and Geschwind (1971) reviewed the major approaches to aphasia as they saw them and concluded that all researchers recognized the same basic patterns of aphasic impairments, despite using different nomenclature. Three more syndromes have been added by theorists such as Benson (1979), and Lichtheim's model has been rounded out with specific hypotheses about the neuro-anatomical bases for several functions that he could only guess at.

Additional neuroanatomical foundation was first suggested in a very influential paper by Geschwind (1965). Geschwind argued that the inferior parietal lobe was a tertiary association cortical area that received projections from the association cortex immediately adjacent to the primary visual, auditory, and somesthetic cortices in the occipital, temporal, and parietal lobes. Because of these anatomical connections, the inferior parietal lobe served as a cross-modal association region, associating word sounds with the sensory qualities of objects. This underlay word meaning, in Geschwind's view. Damasio and Tranel (1993) extended this model to

Table 1. Aphasic Syndromes Described by Lichtheim (1885)

Syndrome	Clinical Manifestations	Hypothetical Deficit	Classical Lesion Location
Broca's aphasia	Major disturbance in speech production with sparse, halting speech, often misarticulated, frequently missing function words and bound morphemes	Disturbances in the speech planning and production mechanisms	Posterior aspects of the 3rd frontal convolution (Broca's area)
Wernicke's aphasia	Major disturbance in auditory comprehension; fluent speech with disturbances of the sounds and structures of words (phonemic, morphological, and semantic paraphasias); poor repetition and naming	Disturbances in the permanent representations of the sound structures of words	Posterior half of the first temporal gyrus and possibly adjacent cortex (Wernicke's area)
Pure motor speech disorder	Disturbance of articulation; apraxia of speech, dysarthria, anarthria, aphemia	Disturbance of articulatory mechanisms	Outflow tracts from motor cortex
Pure word deafness	Disturbance of spoken word comprehension, repetition often impaired	Failure to access spoken words	Input tracts from auditory system to Wernicke's area
Transcortical motor aphasia	Disturbance of spontaneous speech similar to Broca's aphasia with relatively preserved repetition; comprehension relatively preserved	Disconnection between conceptual representations of words and sentences and the motor speech production system	White matter tracts deep to Broca's area connecting it to parietal lobe
Transcortical sensory aphasia	Disturbance in single-word comprehension with relatively intact repetition	Disturbance in activation of word meanings despite normal recognition of auditorily presented words	White matter tracts connecting parietal lobe to temporal lobe or portions of inferior parietal lobe
Conduction aphasia	Disturbance of repetition and spontaneous speech (phonemic paraphasias)	Disconnection between the sound patterns of words and the speech production mechanism	Lesion in the arcuate fasciculus and/or cortico-cortical connections between Wernicke's and Broca's areas

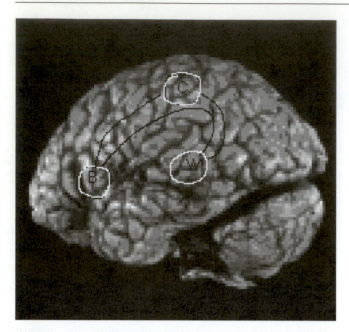

Figure 1. The classical connectionist model (modified from Lichtheim, 1885). W indicates Wernicke's area, the site of long-term storage of word sounds. B indicates Broca's area, the site for speech planning. C represents the concept center, which Wernicke thought was diffusely located in parietal lobe. Information flows along the pathways indicated by lines. The presence of these pathways ("connections") gives this type of model its name.

actions, arguing that associations between word sounds and memories of actions were created in the association cortex in the inferior frontal lobe. Geschwind (1965) and Damasio and Damasio (1980) also argued that the anatomical link between Wernicke's area and Broca's area (in which a lesion caused conduction aphasia) was the white matter tract known as the arcuate fasciculus.

The three and a half decades that have passed since publication of Geschwind's paper have brought new evidence for these syndromes and their relationships to brain lesions. Aphasic syndromes have been related to the brain using a series of neuroimaging techniques, first radionuclide scintigraphy with technetium[99], then computed tomography, magnetic resonance imaging, and positron emission tomography. All have confirmed the relationship of the major syndromes to lesion locations. These aphasic syndromes and their relationships to the brain figure prominently in recent reviews of aphasia in leading medical journals (e.g., Damasio, 1992).

Despite this revival, the connectionist approach to aphasic syndromes is under renewed attack.

A major limitation of the classical syndromes is that they stay at arm's length from the linguistic details of language impairments. The classical aphasic syndromes basically reflect the relative ability of patients to perform entire language tasks (speaking, comprehension, etc.), not the integrity of specific operations within the language processing system. Linguistic descriptions in these syndromes are incomplete and unsystematic. For instance, the speech production problem seen in Broca's aphasia can consist of one or more of a large number of impairments: dysprosodic speech, poorly articulated speech, agrammatism, an unusual number of short phrases. If all we know about a patient is that she or he has Broca's aphasia, we cannot tell which of these problems (or other) that person has.

A second problem is that identical deficits occur in different syndromes. For instance, certain types of naming problems can occur in any aphasic syndrome (Benson, 1979). Because of this, most applications of the clinical taxonomy result in widespread disagreements as to a patient's classification (Holland, Fromm, and Swindell, 1986) and to a large number of "mixed" or "unclassifiable" cases (Lecours, Lhermitte, and Bryans, 1983). The criteria for inclusion in a syndrome are often somewhat arbitrary: How bad does a patient's comprehension have to be for the patient to be identified as having Wernicke's aphasia instead of conduction aphasia, or global aphasia instead of Broca's aphasia? There have been many efforts to answer this question (see, e.g., Goodglass and Kaplan, 1972, 1982; Kertesz, 1979), but none is satisfactory.

A third problem with the classical aphasic syndromes is that they are not as well correlated with lesion sites as the theory claims they should be. These syndromes are related to lesion sites reasonably well only in cases of rapidly developing lesions, such as stroke. Even in these types of lesions, the syndromes are never applied to acute and subacute phases of the illness. Even in the chronic phase of diseases such as stroke, at least 15% of patients have lesions that are not predictable from their syndromes (Basso et al., 1985), and some researchers think this figure is much higher—as much as 40% or more, depending on what counts as an exception to the rule (de Bleser, 1988). We now know that the relationship between lesion location and syndrome is more complex than we had thought, even in cases in which the classical localization captures part of the picture. Broca's aphasia, for instance, does not usually occur in the chronic state after lesions restricted to Broca's area but requires much larger lesions (Mohr et al., 1978). Some theorists have argued that the localizing value of the classical syndromes reflects the co-occurrence of variable combinations of language processing deficits with motor impairments that affect the fluency of speech (Caplan, 1987; McNeil and Kent, 1991). From this point of view, the localizing value of the classical syndromes is due to the invariant location of the motor system.

Finally, the classical syndromes offer very limited help to the clinician planning therapy, because the syndromes give insufficient information about what is wrong with a patient. For example, knowing that a patient has Broca's aphasia does not tell the therapist what aspects of speech need remediation—articulation of sound segments, prosody, production of grammatical elements, formulation of syntactic structures, and so on. Nor does it guarantee that the patient does not need therapy for a comprehension problem; it only implies that any comprehension problem is mild relative to the problems of other aphasics or to the patient's speech problem. Finally, it does not guarantee that the patient does not have other problems, such as anomia, difficulty reading, and the like. In practice, most clinicians do not believe that they have adequately described a patient's language problems when they have identified that patient as having one of the classic aphasic syndromes. Rather, they specify the nature of the disturbance found in the patient within each language-related task; for example, they indicate that a patient with Broca's aphasia is agrammatic, has a mild anomia, and so on. Detailed psycholinguistic and linguistic descriptions of aphasic impairments are slowly replacing the disconnection approach to syndromes.

It is a feature of the history of science, and some think a tenet of the philosophy of science, that people do not abandon a theory because it has inadequacies. Some philosophers of science think that no theory is ever proven wrong. According to this view, theories are abandoned because people get tired of them, and people get tired of theories because they have others that they think are better. This perspective on science applies to the connectionist approach to aphasic syndromes. The classic syndromes have not been abandoned, but their acceptance is waning, and there are new developments that address some of their inadequacies.

Acknowledgment

Work was supported in part by a grant from NIDCD (DC00942).

—*David Caplan*

References

Basso, A., Lecours, A. R., et al. (1985). Anatomoclinical correlations of the aphasias as defined through computerized tomography: Exceptions. *Brain and Language, 26*, 201–229.

Benson, D. F. (1979). *Aphasia, alexia and agraphia*. London, Churchill Livingstone.

Benson, D. F., and Geschwind, N. (1971). Aphasia and related cortical disturbances. In A. B. Baker and L. H. Baker (Eds.), *Clinical neurology*. New York: Harper and Row.

Broca, P. (1861). Remarques sur le siege de la faculte de la parole articulee, suives d'une observation d'aphemie (perte de parole). *Bulletin de la Societe d'Anatomie, 36*, 330–357.

Caplan, D. (1987). Discrimination of normal and aphasic subjects on a test of syntactic comprehension. *Neuropsychologia, 25*, 173–184.

Damasio, A. R. (1992). Aphasia. *New England Journal of Medicine, 326*, 531–539.

Damasio, A., and Tranel, D. (1993). Nouns and verbs are retrieved with differently distributed neural systems. *Proceedings of the National Academy of Science of the United States of America, 90*, 4957–4960.

Damasio, H., and Damasio, A. R. (1980). The anatomical basis of conduction aphasia. *Brain, 103*, 337–350.

de Bleser, R. (1988). Localization of aphasia: Science or fiction? In D. Denes, C. Semenza, and P. Bisiacchi (Eds.), *Perspectives on cognitive neurology*. Hove, U.K.: Erlbaum.

Geschwind, N. (1965). Disconnection syndromes in animals and man. *Brain, 88*, 237–294, 585–644.

Goldstein, K. (1948). *Language and language disturbances*. New York: Grune and Stratton.

Goodglass, H., and Kaplan, E. (1972). *The assessment of aphasia and related disorders*. Philadelphia: Lea and Febiger.

Goodglass, H., and Kaplan, E. (1982). *The assessment of aphasia and related disorders* (2nd ed.). Philadelphia: Lea and Febiger.

Head, H. (1926). *Aphasia and kindred disorders of speech*. New York: Macmillan.

Holland, A. L., Fromm, D., and Swindell, C. S. (1986). The labeling problem in aphasia: An illustrative case. *Journal of Speech and Hearing Disorders, 51*, 176–180.

Jackson, H. H. (1878). On affections of speech from disease of the brain. Reprinted in J. Taylor (Ed.), *Selected writings of John Hughlings Jackson*. New York: Basic Books, 1958.

Kertesz, A. (1979). *Aphasia and associated disorders: Taxonomy, localization and recovery*. New York: Grune and Stratton.

Lecours, A. R., Lhermitte, F., and Bryans, B. (1983). *Aphasiology*. Paris: Baillard.

Lichtheim, L. (1885). On aphasia. *Brain, 7*, 433–484.

Marie, P. (1906). Revision de la question de l'aphasie: La troisieme circonvolution frontale gauche ne joue aucun role special dans la fonction du langage. *Semaine Medicale, 26*, 241–247.

McNeil, M. R., and Kent, R. D. (1991). Motoric characteristics of adult aphasic and apraxic speakers. In G. R. Hammond (Ed.), *Advances in psychology: Cerebral control of speech and limb movements* (pp. 317–354). New York: Elsevier/North Holland.

Mohr, J. P., Pessin, M. S., Finkelstein, S., Funkenstein, H., Duncan, G. W., and Davis, K. R. (1978). Broca aphasia: Pathologic and clinical. *Neurology, 28*, 311–324.

Moutier, F. (1908). *L'Aphasie de Broca*. Paris: Steinheil.

Wernicke, C. (1874). *Der Aphasische Symptomenkomplex*. Breslau: Cohn and Weigart. Reprinted in translation in *Boston Studies in Philosophy of Science, 4*, 34–97.

Aphasiology, Comparative

Comparative aphasiology is the systematic comparison of aphasia symptoms across languages, including the comparison of acquired reading problems across languages and writing systems. The goal of study is to ensure that theories that claim to account for the various constellations of aphasic symptoms can handle the similarities and differences seen in aphasic speakers of languages of different types (see Menn, 2001, for a discussion of language typology in the context of comparative aphasiology). Serious experimental and clinical comparative work began in the 1980s; however, researchers long before that time understood that comparative data are essential. Otherwise, general theories of aphasia would depend on data from the few, closely related languages of the countries in Europe and North America where research in neurolinguistics was being undertaken: English, French, German, and, for a time, Russian.

The clearest example of such a premature class of theories was the "least pronunciation effort" approach to agrammatism. This approach focused on the prevalence of bare-stem forms in agrammatic output in English, French, and German and suggested that such forms were used to avoid extra articulatory effort. A more phonologically sophisticated theory (Kean, 1979), relying on the same small database, proposed that agrammatic speakers were constrained to produce only the minimum phonological word. However, the languages then available for study have bare-stem forms that are not only short but also grammatically unmarked (mostly first- or third-person singular present tense of verbs and the singular of nouns) and very frequent. Therefore, the data could also support a markedness-based or a frequency-based account. Or the underlying problem could be morphological or morphosyntactic instead of articulatory or phonological.

A reason to think that the problem is actually morphological (problems with retrieving inflections) or morphosyntactic (problems with computing which inflections the syntax demands) is that endings of participles and infinitive forms are better preserved than other verb forms in English, Italian, French, and German. Is this because they have no tense marking or no person marking? Or is there another reason?

To test the hypothesis that a problem with inflections is a specific type of problem with morphosyntax, we look for languages where inflections are controlled in different ways. For example, if problems with verbs are blamed on difficulty with person or number agreement, we should see whether verb problems also exist in languages without agreement, such as Japanese. Or the problem may be deeper than morphosyntax: the verb problem could be due to a semantic difference between nominal and verbal types of elements, as suggested by experimental work on Chinese, which has no agreement or inflection (Bates, Chen, et al., 1991; Chen and Bates, 1998). Or perhaps multiple factors interact—a more difficult claim to test.

Another type of problem that demands a comparative approach is the question of why there are so few adjectives in aphasic language. From, say, a German-centered point of view, we might ask, Is this a conceptual problem, an agreement problem (nonexistent in English, so that could not be the sole problem), or a problem in inserting elements between article and noun (in which case, Romance languages, where most NPs have article-noun-adjective order, should not show the effect)?

Issue after issue requiring a comparative approach can be listed in the same way. Would relative clauses that do not require movement (as in Chinese or Japanese) be deployed better than ones that do? Is the observed problem with the passive voice in English to be explained in terms of movement rules and traces, in terms of its morphological complexity, in terms of its low frequency, or in terms of its pragmatic unnaturalness in a single-sentence test paradigm? Are irregular verbs preserved better than regular ones because of their generally greater frequency or because, as some theorists claim, they are stored in different places in the brain or deployed using different mechanisms? (Jaeger et al., 1996; Pinker, 1999).

Recent History

By 1980, comparative language acquisition studies (e.g., the work published in Slobin, 1985–1995) were well established and provided both intellectual and logistical models for comparative aphasiology. Bellugi's team at the Salk Institute began to compare aphasic syndromes in hearing/speaking and deaf/signing individuals (Bellugi, Poizner, and Klima, 1989), and an international group coordinated by Bates at the University of California–San Diego began using psycholinguistic techniques to do cross-linguistic studies of English and Italian, eventually expanding to Chinese, Russian, Spanish, and other languages. At the Aphasia Research Center of the Boston University School of Medicine, a team focused on morphosyntax in agrammatic narratives (Cross Language Aphasia Study I, Menn and Obler, 1988, 1990a) created a standard elicitation protocol and began to collect data from speakers with agrammatic aphasia and matched controls. Data were collected on 14 languages: the non-Indo-European languages Mandarin Chinese, Finnish, Hebrew, and Japanese and the Indo-European languages Dutch, English, French, German, Hindi, Icelandic, Polish, Serbo-Croatian, and Swedish. Many of these languages (plus Hungarian and Turkish) are also represented in special issues of *Brain and Language* (1991, 41:2) and *Aphasiology* (1996, 10:6). Michel Paradis has led international work on bilingual aphasia, including the development of the extensive set of Bilingual Aphasia Tests; Paradis (2001), which was also published as a special issue of *Journal of Neurolinguistics* (14:2–4), includes contributions on non-Indo-European Basque and Hungarian and Indo-European Afrikaans, Catalan, Czech, Farsi (Persian), Friulian, Greek, and Spanish, as well as material on African-American English and more data on Finnish, Polish, Hebrew, and Swedish.

Methods of Study

Comparative studies raise special methodological issues because of the need to ensure that all materials pose comparable levels of difficulty across languages and cultures. Drawings acceptable in one country may be anomalous in another; words that are (apparently) translation equivalents may not be comparably frequent, and so on (Menn et al., 1996). Several chapters in Paradis (2001) point out the importance of allowing for the effects of bilingualism and multiple dialect use, which are present in most of the world's population. The presentation of comparative production data requires an elaborated interlinear translation format, so that any reader, familiar with the language or not, can see what the subject actually said, what he or she should have said, and what the errors were. A widely used version is derived from the interlinear morphemic translation style codified by Lehmann (1982). The example below is taken from Farsi data (Nilipour, 2000).

1.   sar[-am]
2. *man [be] dast [va]   sar   xombâre [xor-d]*
3. I   [to] hand [and] head[-my] shrapnel [hit:PAST:3SG]
4. I hand, head shrapnel [hit].
5. pro [postposition] Noun [conjunction] Noun [possessive clitic] Noun [Verb]

Line 2 is the original as spoken, but edited to remove hesitations and phonetic or phonemic errors. Omitted words are supplied in square brackets if they can be reconstructed from the context. Line 1 gives the target forms for each substitution error, placed on the first line directly above the incorrect form. The third line is a morph-by-morph translation into the language of publication, with standard abbreviations indicating case, tense, aspect, and so on, with abbreviations for affixes. Line 4 contains a "smooth" translation into the language of the publication. Lines 1 and 4 are as similar as possible in their degree and types of errors—i.e., equally agrammatic, equally paraphasic. Line 5, not used in all publications, identifies part of speech, and codes for functor (all lowercase) versus content word (first letter uppercase), making it easier to count members of these categories. This is done because so much psycholinguistic theorizing hinges on form class and on the content/functor distinction.

Comprehension Studies and Recent Findings

Bates's group (e.g., Bates, Friederici, and Wulfeck, 1987a) has used a task in which hearers are presented with a string of two nouns and a transitive verb (e.g., "The cow the pencils kick") and must decide which of two nouns (or noun phrases) is the agent. The string is presented in all orders, whether grammatical or not in the language in question, and often with conflicting cues from word order, animacy, and number agreement. Their key finding has been that people with aphasia show the same language-specific preferences for interpreting these strings—the same tendency to place more reliance on word order, animacy, or agreement in making their interpretations—as do speakers without neurological impairment. Thus, agrammatic aphasia, in particular, cannot be an eradication of grammar. Further confirmation of this claim comes from Serbo-Croatian: Lukatela, Shankweiler, and Crain (1995) used a slightly more natural picture-choice comprehension task to show that people with agrammatic aphasia were able to distinguish between subject-gap sentences ("The lady is kissing the man who is holding an umbrella") and object-gap sentences ("The lady is kissing the man that the umbrella is covering"), even when these sentences were constructed with the same word order, so that the hearers had to rely only on case markers and agreement markers (subject-verb agreement, modifier-noun agreement, agreement between pronouns and their referents,

etc.). (Stimuli that convey this complex syntactic structure without varying the word order cannot be constructed in most European languages.)

While these results showed that agrammatic aphasics could use morphological information, Bates's group has shown that morphological cues are also the ones most likely to be underutilized by speakers with all forms of aphasia, as well as by control subjects who are loaded with competing experimental task demands (Blackwell and Bates, 1995).

Note that not all comparative studies make direct contrasts across two or more languages. A study is also comparative if it selects a language to work in specifically because that language enables us to tease apart variables of interest. The elaborate morphology and free word order of Serbo-Croatian allowed Lukatela and colleagues to examine comprehension of morphology with word order held constant. Similarly, gender agreement in French was used by Jakubowicz and Goldblum (1995, p. 242) to construct an experiment contrasting the preservation of grammatical morphemes in nonfluent aphasia. They found that "local" (within noun phrase) markings were better preserved than ones requiring computation across major syntactic boundaries. Luzzatti and De Bleser (1996) reported a similar result for production.

Production Studies and Findings

A variety of production studies have supported the following general claims. (1) The greater the semantic importance of a morpheme, the more likely that it will be produced. For example, although grammatical morphemes are in general prone to errors, and free grammatical morphemes tend to be omitted by speakers with nonfluent aphasias, negation is almost never omitted (Menn and Obler, 1990b; see also Friederici, Weissenborn, and Kail, 1991). (2) The larger the paradigm of choices for a given form, the more likely that errors will be made (Bates, Wulfeck, and MacWhinney, 1991; Paradis, 2001b). Aphasic production errors in morphosyntax tend to be only one semantic feature away from the target (gender or number or case or tense); the direction of errors is probabilistic, but more frequent forms are more likely to be produced correctly (Dressler, 1991). However, an individual may have a preferred "default" form not shared by other aphasic speakers of the same language (Magnúsdóttir and Thráinsson, 1991). (3) In paradigms with multiple stem forms, errors tend to keep the same stem as the target (Mimouni and Jarema, 1997). Semantically appropriate case forms may be chosen even when the verb or preposition that would control that case is not produced. Most errors, especially those of nonfluent aphasics, are misselections from existing paradigms, but a few, notably some instances in Basque, involve the creation of nonexistent forms from existing morphemes (Laka and Erriondo Korostola, 2001) or the production of nonexistent stem forms (Swedish: Månsson and Ahlsén, 2001).

(4) Classifier languages show classifier errors (Tzeng et al., 1991), with nonfluent aphasic speakers tending to omit them or to fall back on a "neutral" classifier; speakers with fluent aphasia tend to commit more substitution errors, as is characteristic of their production patterns across morpheme categories and languages.

Of course, widening the database also broadens the questions: Why are utterance-final particles preserved in Japanese aphasia but not so well in Chinese (Paradis, 2001b)? Why does canonical word order make comprehension and elicited production easier across languages, even those that have "free" word order, and why is some noncanonical order occasionally used as a production default? Cross-linguistic psycholinguistic and computational-linguistic approaches seem to be the most promising avenues to further understanding of aphasia, and, more generally, to the question of how language is represented in the human brain.

Note. Given the state of the art and the extent of individual variation within aphasia syndromes, I use the terminology of various authors cited, without attempting to differentiate between the overlapping diagnostic categories of Broca's aphasia and agrammatic aphasia (agrammatism); "non-fluent" aphasia includes both of these categories, plus several others from the traditional clinical categories. "Fluent" aphasia includes anomic aphasia (anomia) and Wernicke's aphasia. Textbook anomic aphasia has fluent articulation, disfluencies due only to word-finding difficulties, and no comprehension problems; textbook Wernicke's aphasia has word-finding problems, comprehension problems, fluent articulation, and possible use of empty speech or nonsense "words" to compensate for impaired lexical retrieval.

—*Lise Menn*

References

Bates, E., Chen, S., Tzeng, O., Li, P., and Opie, M. (1991). The noun-verb problem in Chinese aphasia. *Brain and Language, 41*, 203–233.

Bates, E., Friederici, A., and Wulfeck, B. (1987a). Comprehension in aphasia: A cross-linguistic study. *Brain and Language, 32*, 19–67.

Bates, E., Wulfeck, B., and MacWhinney, B. (1991). Cross-linguistic studies of aphasia: An overview. *Brain and Language, 41*, 123–148. [Special issue]

Bellugi, U., Poizner, H., and Klima, E. S. (1989). Language, modality, and the brain. *Trends in Neurosciences, 10*, 380–388.

Blackwell, A., and Bates, E. (1995). Inducing agrammatic profiles in normals: Evidence for the selective vulnerability of morphology under cognitive resource limitation. *Journal of Cognitive Neuroscience, 7*, 228–257.

Chen, S., and Bates, E. (1998). The dissociation between nouns and verbs in Broca's and Wernicke's aphasia: Findings from Chinese. *Aphasiology, 12*, 5–36.

Dressler, W. U. (1991). The sociolinguistic and patholinguistic attrition of Breton phonology, morphology, and morphonology. In H. W. Seliger and R. M. Vago (Eds.), *First language attrition* (pp. 99–112). Cambridge, U.K.: Cambridge University Press.

Friederici, A., Weissenborn, J., and Kail, M. (1991). Pronoun comprehension in aphasia: A comparison of three languages. *Brain and Language, 41*, 289–310.

Jaeger, J. J., Lockwood, A. H., Kemmerer, D. L., Van Valin, R. D., Murphy, B. W., and Khalak, H. G. (1996). A positron emission tomography study of regular and irregular verb morphology in English. *Language, 72*, 451–497.

Jakubowicz, C., and Goldblum, M.-C. (1995). Processing of number and gender inflections by French-speaking aphasics. *Brain and Language, 51*, 242–268.

Kean, M.-L. (1979). Agrammatism: A phonological deficit? *Cognition, 7*, 69–83.

Laka, I., and Erriondo Korostola, L. (2001). Aphasia manifestations in Basque. In M. Paradis (Ed.), *Manifestations of aphasia symptoms in different languages* (pp. 49–73). Amsterdam: Pergamon.

Lehmann, C. (1982). Directions for interlinear morphemic translations. *Folia Linguistica, 16*, 199–224.

Lukatela, K., Shankweiler, D., and Crain, S. (1995). Syntactic processing in agrammatic aphasia by speakers of a Slavic language. *Brain and Language, 49*, 50–76.

Luzzatti, C., and De Bleser, R. (1996). Morphological processing in Italian agrammatic speakers: Eight experiments in lexical morphology. *Brain and Language, 54*, 26–74.

Magnúsdóttir, S., and Thráinsson, H. (1991). Subject-verb agreement in aphasia. In H. A. Sigurdsson, T. G. Indridason, and E. Rögnvaldson (Eds.), *Papers from the 12th Scandinavian Conference on Linguistics* (pp. 256–266). Reykjavík, Iceland: Linguistic Institute, University of Iceland.

Månsson, A.-C., and Ahlsén, E. (2001). Grammatical features of aphasia in Swedish. In M. Paradis (Ed.), *Manifestations of aphasia symptoms in different languages* (pp. 281–296). Amsterdam: Pergamon.

Menn, L. (2001). Comparative aphasiology. In F. Boller and J. Grafman (Eds.), *Handbook of neuropsychology* (2nd ed.), vol. 3: *Language and aphasia* (R. S. Berndt, vol. ed., pp. 51–68). Amsterdam: Elsevier.

Menn, L., Niemi, J., and Ahlsén, E. (1996). Cross-linguistic studies of aphasia: Why and how. *Aphasiology, 10*, 523–532.

Menn, L., and Obler, L. K. (1988). Findings of the Cross-Language Aphasia Study: Phase I. Agrammatic narrative. *Aphasiology, 2*, 347–350.

Menn, L., and Obler, L. K. (1990a). *Agrammatic aphasia: A cross-language narrative sourcebook*. Amsterdam: John Benjamins.

Menn, L., and Obler, L. K. (1990b). Conclusion: Cross-language data and theories of agrammatism. In L. Menn and L. K. Obler (Eds.), *Agrammatic aphasia* (vol. II, pp. 1369–1389). Amsterdam: John Benjamins.

Mimouni, Z., and Jarema, G. (1997). Agrammatic aphasia in Arabic. *Aphasiology, 11*, 125–144, 1997.

Nilipour, R. (2000). Agrammatic language: Two cases from Farsi. *Aphasiology, 14*, 1205–1242.

Paradis, M. (Ed.). (2001a). *Manifestations of aphasia symptoms in different languages*. Amsterdam: Pergamon.

Paradis, M. (2001b). By way of a preface: The need for awareness of aphasia syndromes in different languages. In M. Paradis (Ed.), *Manifestations of aphasia symptoms in different languages*. Amsterdam: Pergamon.

Pinker, S. (1999). *Words and rules*. New York: Basic Books.

Slobin, D. (Ed.). (1985–1995). *The cross-linguistic study of language acquisition* (vols. 1–5). Hillsdale, NJ: Erlbaum.

Tzeng, O. J. L., Chen, S., and Hung, D. L. (1991). The classifier problem in Chinese aphasia. *Brain and Language, 41*, 184–202.

Further Readings

Ahlsén, E., Nespoulous, J.-L., Dordain, M., Stark, J., Jarema, G., Kadzielawa, D., et al. (1996). Noun-phrase production by agrammatic patients: A cross-linguistic approach. *Aphasiology, 10,* 543–560.

Bastiaanse, R., Edwards, S., and Kiss, K. (1996). Fluent aphasia in three languages: Aspects of spontaneous speech. *Aphasiology, 10,* 561–576.

Bastiaanse, R., and van Zonneveld, R. (1998). On the relation between verb inflection and verb position in Dutch agrammatic aphasics. *Brain and Language, 64,* 165–181.

Bates, E., Friederici, A., and Wulfeck, B. (1987b). Grammatical morphology in aphasia: Evidence from three languages. *Cortex, 23,* 545–574.

Bates, E., and Wulfeck, B. (1989). Comparative aphasiology: A cross-linguistic approach to language breakdown. *Aphasiology, 3,* 111–142.

Eng, N., Obler, L. K., Harris, K. S., and Abramson, A. S. (1996). Tone perception deficits in Chinese-speaking Broca's aphasics. *Aphasiology, 10,* 649–656.

Grodzinsky, Y. (1984). The syntactic characterization of agrammatism. *Cognition, 16,* 99–120.

Grodzinsky, Y. (1990). *Theoretical perspectives on language deficits.* Cambridge, MA: MIT Press.

Halliwell, J. F. (2000). Korean agrammatic production. *Aphasiology, 14,* 1187–1204.

Hickok, G., Wilson, M., Clark, L., Klima, E. S., Kritchevsky, M., and Bellugi, U. (1999). Discourse deficits following right hemisphere damage in deaf signers. *Brain and Language, 66,* 233–248.

Jarema, G. (1998). The breakdown of morphology in aphasia: A cross-linguistic perspective. In B. Stemmer and W. Whitaker (Eds.), *Handbook of neurolinguistics* (pp. 221–234). Orlando, FL: Academic Press.

Jarema, G., and Kehayia, E. (1992). Impairment of inflectional morphology and lexical storage. *Brain and Language, 43,* 541–564.

Kegl, J., and Poizner, H. (1997). Cross-linguistic/cross-modal syntactic consequences of left-hemisphere damage: Evidence from an aphasic signer and his identical twin. *Aphasiology, 11,* 1–38.

MacWhinney, B., and Osmán-Sági, J. (1991). Inflectional marking in Hungarian aphasics. *Brain and Language, 41,* 165–183.

Menn, L. (1989). Comparing approaches to comparative aphasiology. *Aphasiology, 3,* 143–150.

Menn, L., O'Connor, M. P., Obler, L. K., and Holland, A. L. (1995). *Non-fluent aphasia in a multi-lingual world.* Amsterdam: John Benjamins.

Menn, L., Reilly, K. F., Hayashi, M., Kamio, A., Fujita, I., and Sasanuma, S. (1998). The interaction of preserved pragmatics and impaired syntax in Japanese and English aphasic speech. *Brain and Language, 61,* 183–225.

Miceli, G., Mazzucchi, A., Menn, L., and Goodglass, H. (1983). Contrasting cases of Italian agrammatic aphasia without comprehension disorder. *Brain and Language, 19,* 65–97.

Miceli, G., Silveri, M. C., Villa, G., and Caramazza, A. (1984). On the basis of agrammatics' difficulty in producing main verbs. *Brain and Language, 36,* 447–492.

Nicol, J. L., Jakubowicz, C., and Goldblum, M. C. (1996). Sensitivity to grammatical marking in English-speaking and French-speaking non-fluent aphasics. *Aphasiology, 10,* 593–622.

Niemi, J., and Laine, M. (1997). Syntax and inflectional morphology in aphasia: Quantitative aspects of Wernicke speakers' narratives. *Journal of Quantitative Linguistics, 4,* 181–189.

Sasanuma, S., and Fujimura, O. (1971). Selective impairment of phonetic and nonphonetic transcription of words in Japanese aphasic patients: Kana vs. kanji in visual recognition and writing. *Cortex, 7,* 1–18.

Slobin, D. (1991). Aphasia in Turkish: Speech production in Broca's and Wernicke's patients. *Brain and Language, 41,* 149–164.

Tzeng, O. J. L. (1992). Reading and lateralization. In W. Bright (Ed.), *International Encyclopedia of Linguistics* (vol. 3). New York: Oxford University Press.

Vakareliyska, C. (1993). Implications from aphasia for the syntax of null-subject sentences: Underlying subject slot in Bulgarian. *Cortex, 29,* 409–430.

Wulfeck, B., Bates, E., and Capasso, R. (1991). A cross-linguistic study of grammaticality judgments in Broca's aphasia. *Brain and Language, 41,* 311–336.

Yiu, E., and Worrall, L. E. (1996). Agrammatic production: A cross-linguistic comparison of English and Cantonese. *Aphasiology, 10,* 623–648.

Argument Structure: Representation and Processing

In a Principles and Parameters syntax framework, sentences are derived by two operations, merger and movement. Merger takes two categories as input (e.g., V and NP) and merges them into a single, higher-order category (e.g., VP). There are, however, constraints on the categories that can be merged successfully. Consider the following pairs:

1a.   [NP The girl] sneezed
1b.   *[NP The girl] sneezed [NP the boy]

2a.   [NP The girl] defeated [NP the boy]
2b.   *[NP The girl] defeated

3a.   [NP The girl] gave [NP the prize] [PP to [NP the boy]]
3b.   *[NP The girl] gave [NP the prize]

The (a) examples above are well-formed sentences; the (b) versions, containing the same verbs but different structures following the verbs, are ill-formed. Thus, not all verbs can fit into all sentence structures. How, then, does a theory of syntax account for these facts? Borrowing from logic, we can say that sentences are composed of a verb (i.e., predicate) and a set of *arguments*. A verb denotes an activity or event and an argument denotes a *participant* in the activity or event. So, in the grammatical (a) versions above, the sentences contain the appropriate number of arguments the verb entails; in the ungrammatical (b) versions there is either an extra argument (as in (1b)) or a required argument is missing (as in (2b) and (3b)), hence violating the *argument structure* of the verb.

Not all the phrases in a sentence function as arguments of a verb. Consider:

4. [The girl] defeated [the boy] *on the beach/this after-noon/with great finesse.*

The bracketed NPs are clearly participants in the event denoted by *defeated*, and thus are arguments of the verb. However, the italicized phrases do not represent participants in the event. Instead, they carry additional information (i.e., where the event took place, when, and the manner in which it took place). These expressions are considered to be *adjuncts*; that is, they are adjunctive or in addition to the information specified by the verb. Simplifying a bit, adjuncts are typically optional while arguments are often required.

Thematic Roles.   The NPs that are participants/arguments of the verb in (4) play different *semantic* roles in relation to the verb *defeated*. A more comprehensive account of argument structure, then, needs to consider a description of these roles. For example, in (4) the NP *the boy* is the Agent of *defeat*, while *the girl* is the affected object and hence the Patient (or Theme). Some common thematic roles, then, are Agent, Experiencer, Theme/Patient, Goal, and Location.

A verb (that is, a lexical category) assigns its thematic roles to its arguments through *theta marking*. For example, the verb *defeat* is said to theta-mark the subject argument with the Agent role and the object argument with the Theme (Patient) role:

5. <u>defeat</u>   V

  (Agent Theme)

[NP The girl] defeated [NP the boy]   *The girl defeated

Thus, each lexical category (e.g., verb) has a set of argument structure features that must be satisfied in the sentence in which the word appears. If those features are not satisfied, the sentence will be ungrammatical.

Verbs can also have clauses as arguments; these too need to be theta-marked:

6. <u>know</u>   V

  (Experiencer Proposition)

[NP The coach] knew [CP that the girl defeated the boy]

The verb *know* assigns Experiencer to the subject NP argument and Proposition to the CP argument.

Processing.   Canonical linking rules have been hypothesized to play a key role in the acquisition (van der Lely, 1994) and the processing of such verb-argument structures (see, e.g., McRae, Spivey-Knowlton, and Tanenhaus, 1998). This linking or mapping refers to the regular, most frequent relation found between thematic roles and syntactic functions (Pesetsky, 1995). For example, if an individual knows that a verb involves an Agent, Patient/Theme, and Goal, she can infer that

those arguments can serve the role of subject, object, and oblique object, respectively. The verb *donate*, for example, requires three arguments—a subject NP, a direct object NP, and an indirect (oblique) object NP—as in:

7. [The girl/AGENT] donated [the present/THEME] to [the boy/GOAL].

Unlike (7), where the properties of the verb *donate* entail canonical linking, there are verbs with properties that entail noncanonical linking. Consider, for example, *receive*, which entails a reversal of the canonical assignment of Agent and Goal arguments:

8. [The boy/GOAL] received [the present/THEME] from [the girl/AGENT].

Sentences (7) and (8) reflect a well-known bias that suggests the "sender" seems more volitional and is a more plausible candidate for the Agent role than a "receiver" (Dowty, 1991). Importantly, there are no *positional* or *configurational* distinctions between the arguments to signal the difference in thematic order in the above examples; that is, the underlying syntax between the constructions appears to be the same. Thus, the distinction is based on the *inherent* properties of the verb.

Unlike the sentences above, where thematic roles can be directly assigned from inherent lexical information and linking relationships, sentences with so-called displaced arguments require *indirect* thematic role assignment. For example, consider the following noncanonical cleft-object sentence: "It was *the boy* who the girl kissed _____ yesterday." The direct object NP *the boy* has been displaced from its canonical, post-verb argument position in the sentence, leaving a *gap*. Such constructions are often referred to as *filler-gaps*. Verb-argument structure properties influence such constructions rather directly; for example, in the cleft-object case, a verb must license a direct object argument position in order to form a filler-gap dependency.

Given its syntactic and semantic importance, then, argument structure (in various forms) has played a privileged role in accounts of language processing. One of the earliest attempts to show that such lexically based information has repercussions for normal adult sentence processing was that of Fodor, Garrett, and Bever (1968). They inserted verbs differing in grammatical complexity (defined, in current terms, by the types of arguments each allowed) into matched sentences and found that off-line performance on those sentences decreased when verbs were more complex. Similar effects were later found on-line (e.g., Shapiro, Zurif, and Grimshaw, 1987).

What is important here is not just the fact that there are observed "effects" of argument structure, but what those effects suggest about the architecture of the sentence processing system. Briefly, most current accounts claim that when a verb (or any theta-assigning head of a phrase, including prepositions) is encountered in a sentence, its various argument structure configurations are momentarily activated (see, e.g., Pritchett, 1992; Mac-

Donald, Pearlmutter, and Seidenberg, 1994). On some accounts this information is ordered in terms of "preference," which then helps determine which of a set of parses the system initially attempts (Shapiro, Nagel, and Levine, 1993; Trueswell, Tanenhaus, and Kello, 1993). Such preference effects suggest that argument structure information may be used immediately to help analyze sentence input. Indeed, an influential set of theories (e.g., MacDonald, Pearlmutter, and Seidenberg, 1994) suggests just that.

However, there remains an equally influential alternative which suggests that there are (at least) two passes through a sentence (Frazier and Clifton, 1996). The first pass considers only categorical information (e.g., DET, N, NP, V, VP, etc.) and perhaps the number of arguments a verb entails, and essentially builds a skeletal phrase structure representation of the input; the second pass considers lexical-semantic and contextual information. In some of these accounts, detailed thematic information is explicitly claimed to be part of the second-pass analysis (Friederici, Hahne, and Mecklinger, 1996).

Finally, the representation and processing of argument structure has important implications for language disorders underlying aphasia. Briefly, the "mapping deficit" account (e.g., Schwartz et al., 1987) has suggested that the sentence comprehension patterns evinced by some agrammatic Broca's aphasic individuals may be explained by their inability to "map" thematic roles onto grammatical (i.e., subject, object) positions, particularly in sentences that have noncanonical mapping. A more detailed and circumscribed account of the deficit is offered by the TRACE DELETION HYPOTHESIS (e.g., Grodzinsky, 2000). Here, the claim is that knowledge of argument structure is intact for these individuals (for on-line evidence of this fact, see Shapiro et al., 1993). However, traces of moved referential NPs or arguments are deleted, and hence indirect thematic role assignment is blocked. Instead, these individuals appear to use an "agent-first" strategy for arguments that cannot receive a grammatically computed thematic role, explaining performance on a wide range of sentence types.

Unlike Broca's aphasic individuals, those individuals most likely characterized as Wernicke's syndrome type appear to be insensitive to the argument structure properties of verbs, even where on-line comprehension is at issue (Shapiro et al., 1993; Russo, Peach, and Shapiro, 1998). Yet, their deficit does not seem to affect on-line comprehension of sentences with moved arguments (Zurif et al., 1993). These patterns therefore suggest a double dissociation between the activation of argument structures and the syntactic parsing routines underlying the comprehension of sentences with moved arguments.

—Lewis P. Shapiro

References

Dowty, D. (1991). Thematic proto-roles and argument selection. *Language*, 3, 547–619.

Fodor, J. A., Garrett, M., and Bever, T. G. (1968). Some syntactic determinants of sentential complexity: II. Verb structure. *Perception and Psychophysics*, 6, 453–461.

Frazier, L., and Clifton, C. (1996). *Construal*. Cambridge, MA: MIT Press.

Friederici, A. D., Hahne, A., and Mecklinger, A. (1966). Temporal structure of syntactic parsing: Early and late event-related brain potential effects. *Journal of Experimental Psychology: Learning, Memory, and Cognition*, 22, 1219–1248.

Grodzinsky, Y. (2000). The neurology of syntax: Language use without Broca's area. *Behavioral and Brain Sciences*, 23, 47–117.

MacDonald, M. C., Pearlmutter, N. J., and Seidenberg, M. S. (1994). Lexical nature of syntactic ambiguity resolution. *Psychological Review*, 101, 676–703.

McRae, K., Spivey-Knowlton, M. J., and Tanenhaus, M. K. (1998). Modeling the influence of thematic fit (and other constraints) in on-line sentence comprehension. *Journal of Memory and Language*, 38, 283–312.

Pesetsky, D. (1995). *Zero syntax*. Cambridge, MA: MIT Press.

Pritchett, B. (1992). *Grammatical competence and parsing performance*. Chicago: University of Chicago Press.

Russo, K. D., Peach, R. K., and Shapiro, L. P. (1998). Verb preference effects in the sentence comprehension of fluent aphasic individuals. *Aphasiology*, 12, 537–545.

Schwartz, M. F., Linebarger, M. C., Saffran, E. M., and Pate, D. C. (1987). Syntactic transparency and sentence interpretation in aphasia. *Language and Cognitive Processes*, 2, 55–113.

Shapiro, L. P., Gordon, B., Hack, N., and Killackey, J. (1993). Verb-argument structure processing in complex sentences in Broca's and Wernicke's aphasia. *Brain and Language*, 45, 423–447.

Shapiro, L. P., Nagel, N., and Levine, B. A. (1993). Preferences for a verb's complements and their use in sentence processing. *Journal of Memory and Language*, 32, 96–114.

Shapiro, L. P., Zurif, E., and Grimshaw, J. (1987). Sentence processing and the mental representation of verbs. *Cognition*, 27, 219–246.

Trueswell, J. C., Tanenhaus, M. K., and Kello, C. (1993). Verb-specific constraints in sentence processing: Separating effects of lexical preference from garden-paths. *Journal of Experimental Psychology: Learning, Memory, and Cognition*, 19, 528–553.

van der Lely, H. K. J. (1994). Canonical linking rules: Forward versus reverse linking in normally developing and specifically language-impaired children. *Cognition*, 51, 29–72.

Zurif, E. B., Swinney, D., Prather, P., Solomon, J., and Bushell, C. (1993). An on-line analysis of syntactic processing in Broca's and Wernicke's aphasia. *Brain and Language*, 45, 448–464.

Further Readings

Canseco-Gonzalez, E., Shapiro, L. P., Zurif, E. B., and Baker, E. (1990). Predicate-argument structure as a link between linguistic and nonlinguistic representations. *Brain and Language*, 39, 391–404.

Friederici, A. D., and Frisch, S. (2000). Verb argument structure processing: The role of verb-specific and argument-specific information. *Journal of Memory and Language*, 43, 476–507.

Grodzinsky, Y., Shapiro, L. P., and Swinney, D. A. (Eds.). (2000). *Language and the brain: Representation and processing*. San Diego, CA: Academic Press.

Kemmerer, D. (2000). Grammatically relevant and grammatically irrelevant features of verb meaning can be independently impaired. *Aphasiology*, 14, 997–1020.

McRae, K., Ferretti, T. R., and Amyote, L. (1997). Thematic roles as verb-specific concepts. *Language and cognitive processes: Special issue on lexical representations in sentence processing.*

Rayner, K., Carlson, M., and Frazier, L. (1983). The interaction of syntax and semantics during sentence processing. *Journal of Verbal Learning and Verbal Behavior, 22,* 358–374.

Shapiro, L. P., and Levine, B. A. (1990). Verb processing during sentence comprehension in aphasia. *Brain and Language, 38,* 21–47.

Shapiro, L. P., Zurif, E., and Grimshaw, J. (1989). Verb representation and sentence processing: contextual impenetrability. *Journal of Psycholinguistic Research, 18,* 223–243.

Tanenhaus, M. K., Boland, J. E., Mauner, G. A., and Carlson, G. N. (1993). More on combinatory lexical information: Thematic structure in parsing and interpretation. In G. T. M. Altmann and R. Shillcock (Eds.), *Cognitive models of speech processing: The Second Sperlonga Meeting* (pp. 297–319). Hove, U.K.: LEA.

Attention and Language

The construct of attention has a long and occasionally tortuous history. Though regarded as central to psychology and as fundamental to human experience by James (1890), Wundt (1973), and other founders of psychology, its inability to be characterized unitarily has led many to regard it as theoretically incoherent (Cohen, 1993). Fischler (2001) has discussed the multicomponential nature of attention and the information-processing, factor-analytic, and brain systems contexts in which these processes are studied. The processes or components of attention are frequently characterized as (1) overall *arousal*, (2) *orienting* to novel stimuli, (3) *selectivity* to endogenous or exogenous stimuli, (4) *division* among concurrent tasks, (5) *executive control* of attention (resource allocation), and (6) *vigilance* or sustained attention. Though conceptualized as independent processes or components, the demonstration of this modularity has been difficult to instantiate, and studies designed to do so often remain confounded. For example, selective focus of one's conceptual and perceptual systems to external stimuli requires a mechanism for inhibiting some stimuli while allowing passage and activation of the intended stimuli. This notion invokes the distinctions between top-down and bottom-up processing, resource- versus data-driven processing, and controlled versus automatic processing. It also invokes the notions of selective versus divided attention, as well as an executive system that is capable of directing or allocating mental effort toward specific stimuli or actions. These attentional processes accomplish this in finitely timed intervals and in controlled amounts. Indeed, the models of attention are complex, and the study of attention is untidy. However, the struggle has produced a large and continuous flow of theoretical and experimental evidence supporting its validity as a field of study. The importance of attention in theories of consciousness, cognition, and brain dysfunction justifies the pursuit.

In his important treatise on attention and effort, Kahneman (1973) specified some defining attributes of attention. Among his attributes, he suggested that attention is a *limited capacity* commodity (whether viewed as a single or multiple pool system). Attention is *mobile* and can be shifted either through mechanisms of orienting, enduring dispositions, or through the executive control system. The distributor of processing resources allots attention according to a policy that (1) is biased toward novel stimuli, (2) has the ability to allocate attention to a particular domain or message, and (3) operates as a function of externally generated arousal levels. That attention is limited in capacity has been a central organizing principle for much of the research in attention and has given rise to the "dual task" paradigm, a widely used research method for investigating attention. The dual task is an experimental procedure whereby two tasks are performed concurrently and some aspect of each task is manipulated independently. The tasks are frequently manipulated by having the subject voluntarily allocate different percentages of attention or effort to each task (e.g., 50%/50%, 25%/75%, 75%/25%, 100%/0%, 0%/100%). If attention is shared between the two tasks, a trading of performance levels is expected and is typically expressed as a performance operating curve (POC). While the validity of the voluntary allocation part of the design has been challenged (Gopher, Brickner, and Navon, 1982), an alternative method is frequently used in which the inherent difficulty of the two tasks is manipulated parametrically. Again, a trading of performance levels is expected if the two tasks share a common pool or source of attention, and a POC is plotted and measured in order to test this hypothesis. The dual task paradigm, however, is not the only or even the most widely used approach to study attention. Without doubt, the Stroop test (Stroop, 1935) is the most widely researched attention task. In this task, unwanted intrusion of information is assessed through the rapid identification of colors or words of stimuli that are either congruent (e.g., written word "red" in red print) or incongruent (e.g., written word "red" in blue print). In this task, the subject is required to identify either the word or the color, and accuracy and response times are measured. Naming the color of a written word in the incongruent condition produces poorer accuracy and longer response times than in congruent conditions, indicating a competition for activation and inhibition of linguistic and nonlinguistic intentions and stimuli. N400 evoked potentials (Kutas and Hillyard, 1980; Bentin, 1987; Holcomb, 1988) and functional imaging (e.g., Just et al., 1996) are also common methods used to assess the role of attention in language processing.

Experimental paradigms are not the only source of evidence that attention is a construct worthy of study. Introspection also has provided a motivation for entertaining the notion of attention and its relationship to language. Indeed, most adults have had the experience of having read several pages of written material only to discover that nothing of what was read was remembered because the mind had wandered and focused on reviewing yesterday's particularly puzzling diagnostic or a previous argument with a colleague or the dean, or had focused on planning an upcoming holiday, course lecture, or treatment plan. Likewise, most have discovered the need to turn the radio off when encountering a difficult driving condition or courteously requesting the children to refrain from their backseat banter while formulating a response to the patrolman approaching the car following an apparent traffic violation. Although it is quite intuitive that attention to both internal and external stimuli plays an important role in many (perhaps all) language tasks, major syntheses and analyses of the general attention literature (e.g., Lang, Simons, and Balaban, 1997; Pashler, 1998) and the neuropsychological deficits of attention (e.g., Cohen, 1993; van Zomeren and Brouwer, 1994) have failed to address the role of attention in language processing. Indeed, not one of these major texts devoted to attention have addressed the role of attention in developmental disorders of language such as specific language impairment (SLI), or in acquired disorders affecting language processing, such as those of aphasia or traumatic brain injury. Only very recently has this subject received space in edited books on language and aphasia (e.g., Nadeau, Rothi, and Crosson, 2001) and only relatively recently have theoretical formulations (McNeil, Odell, and Tseng, 1991) of how attention might account for language impairments, and summary reviews (Murray, 2000; Crosson, 2001a; Fischler, 2001) offered explanations or hypotheses of how attention might interact with language impairments.

Language knowledge is characterized by the information that is represented in the brain along with the rules that govern it. Linguistic theory attempts to account for the structure of the information (rules and representations) that is stored in memory. Psycholinguistic theory attempts to account for conditions under which the rules and representations are stored or accessed and the various ways in which the different components are combined to produce or comprehend sounds, morphophonemes, words, phrases, sentences, and discourse. Informing and directing the linguistic system requires each individual language user to engage in a finitely tuned interplay between internally generated intentions, linguistic knowledge, and a massive amount of sensory information that is continuously available, in addition to the selection (planning), programming, and execution of appropriate responses. This temporally demanding interplay creates an astonishing array of factors that have to be sorted and managed at all instances in time and on a continuous basis. It is the domain and role of attention and resource allocation to account for the gating (inhibition) and activation of endogenous intentions and exogenous stimuli involved in the formulation, comprehension, and production of language. Indeed, the role of attention in normal language processing has a long history, and evidence supports the conclusion that all levels of language processing require and compete for attentional resources with other language processes and with the processing of nonlinguistic information. For example, the attentional demands placed on language processing have been illustrated for lexical/semantic processing through priming paradigms (Neely, 1977), through evoked potentials (Kutas and Hillyard, 1980), and through dual-task studies (Arvedson and McNeil, 1987; Murray, 2000). Attentional demands for language have also been demonstrated in dual-task studies for syntactic processing by Blackwell and Bates (1995), for phonemic processing by Tseng, McNeil, and Milenkovic (1993), for auditory prosody processing by Slansky and McNeil (1997), and between language and nonlinguistic tasks by LaPointe and Erickson (1991).

Disorders of language are common and account for a sizable proportion of all communication disorders. Within the various classification systems for language disorders, it is widely recognized that there are multiple causes. Most systems acknowledge deficits at the representational level, including the rules used to govern these representations. Deficits at this level are often referred to as deficits of linguistic competence. A variety of performance factors are also recognized that can cause an otherwise competent or intact linguistic system to malfunction. Examples of performance deficits include disorders of linguistic-specific memory processes (Baddeley, 1993; Crosson, 2001b) and slowed perceptual or cognitive mechanisms (Tallal, Stark, and Mellits, 1985). Disorders of various aspects of the attentional system include orienting of attention (Robin and Rizzo, 1989), selective attention (Petry et al., 1994; Murray, Holland, and Beeson, 1998), inability to engage or disengage attention (Posner, Snyder, and Davidson, 1980), and resource allocation (McNeil, Odell, and Tseng, 1991). The construct of attentional deficits underlying language deficits is neither new (e.g., Kreindler and Fradis, 1968) nor restricted to aphasia. Campbell and McNeil (1985), for example, illustrated attentional deficits in an acquired pediatric language disorder population, and Barkley (1996) has applied the construct to attention deficit-hyperactivity disorder. However, restricting the discussion to the language impairment in aphasia, the past decade has seen a renewed interest in various aspects of attention, but primarily in the allocation of processing resources.

While skepticism remains apparent in some circles, it is widely recognized that explanations of language and other domains of cognition (e.g., memory, learning, executive function) that fail to account for attentional phenomena will remain incomplete. This is especially true for those areas of cognitive dysfunction resulting from brain damage (congenital or acquired, regardless of the time or cause of the injury) and developmental disabilities.

—*Malcolm R. McNeil*

References

Arvedson, J. C., and McNeil, M. R. (1987). Accuracy and response times for semantic judgments and lexical decisions with left and right hemisphere lesions. *Clinical Aphasiology*, *17*, 188–201.

Baddeley, A. D. (1993). Working memory or working attention? In A. D. Baddeley and L. Weiskrantz (Eds.), *Attention: Selection, awareness and control. A tribute to Donald Broadbent* (pp. 152–170). Oxford: Oxford University Press.

Barkley, R. A. (1996). Critical issues in research on attention. In G. R. Lyon and N. A. Krasnegor (Eds.), *Attention, memory, and executive function* (pp. 450–456). Baltimore: Paul H. Brookes.

Bentin, S. (1987). Event-related potentials, semantic processes, and expectancy factors in word recognition. *Brain and Language*, *31*, 308–327.

Blackwell, A., and Bates, E. (1995). Inducing agrammatic profiles in normals: Evidence for the selective vulnerability of morphology under cognitive resource limitation. *Journal of Cognitive Neuroscience*, *7*, 228–257.

Campbell, T. F., and McNeil, M. R. (1985). Effects of presentation rate and divided attention on auditory comprehension in children with an acquired language disorder. *Journal of Speech and Hearing Research*, *28*, 513–520.

Cohen, R. A. (1993). *The neuropsychology of attention*. New York: Plenum Press.

Crosson, B. (2001a). Systems that support language processes: Attention. In S. E. Nadeau, L. J. Gonzalez Rothi, and B. Crosson (Eds.), *Aphasia and language: Theory to practice* (pp. 372–398). New York: Guilford Press.

Crosson, B. (2001b). Systems that support language processes: Verbal working memory. In S. E. Nadeau, L. J. Gonzalez Rothi, and B. Crosson (Eds.), *Aphasia and language: Theory to practice* (pp. 399–418). New York: Guilford Press.

Fischler, I. (2001). Attention, resource allocation, and language. In S. E. Nadeau, L. J. Gonzalez Rothi, and B. Crosson (Eds.), *Aphasia and language: Theory to practice* (pp. 348–371). New York: Guilford Press.

Gopher, D., Brickner, M., and Navon, D. (1982). Different difficulty manipulations interact differently with task emphasis: Evidence for multiple resources. *Journal of Experimental Psychology: Human Perception and Performance*, *8*, 146–158.

Holcomb, P. J. (1988). Automatic and attentional processing: An event-related brain potential analysis of semantic priming. *Brain and Language*, *35*, 371–395.

James, H. (1890). *The principles of psychology* (2 vols.). New York: Holt.

Just, M. A., Carpenter, P. A., Keller, T. A., Eddy, W. F., and Thulborn, K. R. (1996). Brain activation modulated by sentence comprehension. *Science*, *274*, 114–116.

Kahneman, D. (1973). *Attention and effort*. Englewood Cliffs, NJ: Prentice Hall.

Kreindler, A., and Fradis, A. (1968). *Performances in aphasia: A neurodynamical diagnostic and psychological study*. Paris: Gauthier-Villars.

Kutas, M., and Hillyard, S. A. (1980). Reading senseless sentences: Brain potentials reflect semantic incongruity. *Science*, *207*, 203–205.

Lang, P. J., Simons, R. F., and Balaban, M. T. (1997). *Attention and orienting: Sensory and motivational processes*. Mahwah, NJ: Erlbaum.

LaPointe, L. L., and Erickson, R. J. (1991). Auditory vigilance during divided task attention in aphasic individuals. *Aphasiology*, *5*, 511–520.

McNeil, M. R., Odell, K. H., and Tseng, C.-H. (1991). Toward the integration of resource allocation into a general theory of aphasia. *Clinical Aphasiology*, *20*, 21–39.

Murray, L. L. (2000). The effects of varying attentional demands on the word retrieval skills of adults with aphasia, right hemisphere brain damage, or no brain damage. *Brain and Language*, *72*, 40–72.

Murray, L. L., Holland, A. L., and Beeson, P. M. (1998). Spoken language of individuals with mild fluent aphasia under focused and divided-attention conditions. *Journal of Speech, Language, and Hearing Research*, *41*, 213–227.

Nadeau, S. E., Gonzalez Rothi, L. J., and Crosson, B. (Eds.). (2001). *Aphasia and language: Theory to practice*. New York: Guilford Press.

Neely, J. H. (1977). Semantic priming and retrieval and lexical memory: Roles of inhibitionless spreading activation and limited-capacity attention. *Journal of Experimental Psychology: General*, *106*, 226–254.

Pashler, H. E. (1998). *The psychology of attention*. Cambridge, MA: MIT Press.

Petry, M., Crosson, B., Rothi, L. J., Bauer, R. M., and Schauer, C. A. (1994). Selective attention and aphasia in adults: Preliminary findings. *Neuropsychologia*, *32*, 1397–1408.

Posner, M. I., Snyder, C. R. R., and Davidson, B. J. (1980). Attention and the detection of signals. *Journal of Experimental Psychology: General*, *109*, 160–174.

Robin, D. A., and Rizzo, M. (1989). The effects of focal cerebral lesions on intramodal and cross-modal orienting of attention. *Clinical Aphasiology*, *18*, 61–74.

Slansky, B. L., and McNeil, M. R. (1997). Resource allocation in auditory processing of emphatically stressed stimuli in aphasia. *Aphasiology*, *4–5*, 461–472.

Stroop, J. R. (1935). Studies of interference in serial verbal reactions. *Journal of Experimental Psychology*, *18*, 643–662.

Tallal, P., Stark, R. E., and Mellits, D. (1985). The relationship between auditory temporal analysis and receptive language development: Evidence from studies of developmental language disorder. *Neuropsychologia*, *4*, 527–534.

Tseng, C.-H., McNeil, M. R., and Milenkovic, P. (1993). An investigation of attention allocation deficits in aphasia. *Brain and Language*, *45*, 276–296.

van Zomeren, A. H., and Brouwer, W. H. (1994). *Clinical neuropsychology of attention*. New York: Oxford University Press.

Wundt, W. M. (1973). *An introduction to psychology*. New York: Arno.

Further Readings

Ballesteros, S., Manga, D., and Coello, T. (1989). Attentional resources in dual-task performance. *Bulletin of the Psychonomic Society*, *27*, 425–428.

Erickson, R. J., Goldinger, S. D., and LaPointe, L. L. (1996). Auditory vigilance in aphasic individuals: Detecting non-linguistic stimuli with full or divided attention. *Brain and Cognition*, *30*, 244–253.

Friedman, A., Polson, M. C., and Dafoe, C. G. (1988). Dividing attention between the hands and the head: Performance trade-offs between rapid finger tapping and verbal memory. *Journal of Experimental Psychology: Human Perception and Performance*, *14*, 60–68.

Gopher, D., and Sanders, A. F. (1984). S-Oh-R: Oh stages! Oh resources. In W. Prinz and A. F. Sanders (Eds.), *Cognition and motor processes*. Berlin: Springer-Verlag.

Hirst, W., and Kalmar, D. (1987). Characterizing attentional resources. *Journal of Experimental Psychology: General*, *116*, 68–81.

Maxfield, L. (1997). Attention and semantic priming: A review of prime task effects. *Consciousness and Cognition: An International Journal*, *6*, 204–218.

Murray, L. L. (1999). Attention and aphasia: Theory, research and clinical implications. *Aphasiology*, *13*, 91–112.

Murray, L. L., Holland, A. L., and Beeson, P. M. (1997a). Auditory processing in individuals with mild aphasia: A study of resource allocation. *Journal of Speech, Language, and Hearing Research*, *40*, 792–808.

Murray, L. L., Holland, A. L., and Beeson, P. M. (1997b). Grammaticality judgments of mildly aphasic individuals under dual-task conditions. *Aphasiology*, *11*, 993–1016.

Navon, D. (1984). Resources: A theoretical soup stone? *Psychological Review*, *91*, 2216–2234.

Navon, D., and Gopher, D. (1979). On the economy of the human processing system. *Psychological Review*, *86*, 214–255.

Navon, D., and Gopher, D. (1979). Task difficulty, resources and dual-task performance. *Attention and Performance*, *15*, 297–315.

Norman, D., and Bobrow, D. (1975). On data limited and resource limited processing. *Journal of Cognitive Psychology*, *7*, 44–60.

Schneider, W., and Shiffrin, R. M. (1977). Controlled and automatic human information processing: I. Detection, search, and attention. *Psychological Review*, *84*, 1–66.

Shiffrin, R. M., and Schneider, W. (1977). Controlled and automatic human information processing: II. Perceptual learning, automatic attending and general theory. *Psychological Review*, *84*, 127–190.

Strum, W., and Willmes, K. (1991). Efficacy of a reaction training on various attentional and cognitive functions in stroke patients. *Neuropsychological Rehabilitation*, *1*, 259–280.

Auditory-Motor Interaction in Speech and Language

Carl Wernicke argued that cortical areas involved in the sensory representation of speech played an important role in speech production (Wernicke, 1874/1969). His argument was based on the clinical observation that the speech output of aphasic patients with posterior lesions in the left hemisphere was fluent but error prone. Modern evidence from both lesion and neuroimaging studies strongly supports Wernicke's claim, and recent work has made progress in identifying an auditory-motor interface circuit for speech.

Developmental considerations make a strong case for the existence of an auditory-motor integration network for speech (Doupe and Kuhl, 1999). In learning to articulate the speech sounds in the local linguistic environment, there must be a mechanism by which (1) sensory representations of speech uttered by others can be stored, (2) articulatory attempts can be compared against these stored representations, and (3) the degree of mismatch revealed by this comparison can be used to shape future articulatory attempts. This auditory-motor integration network is still functional in adults, as revealed by the fact that it is possible to repeat pseudo-

words accurately and by the effects of late-onset deafness on speech output (Waldstein, 1989).

Clinical evidence supports the view that "sensory" cortex participates in speech production. The classical fluent aphasias—Wernicke's aphasia, conduction aphasia, transcortical sensory aphasia, and anomic aphasia—are all associated with left posterior cerebral lesions, that is, with regions that are commonly thought to be sensory in nature. Yet each of these fluent aphasias has prominent speech output symptoms: semantic and/or phonemic paraphasias (speech errors), paragrammatism (inappropriate use of grammatical markers), and anomia (naming difficulties) (Damasio, 1992). This observation demonstrates the general point that posterior "sensory" systems play an important role in speech production.

Evidence relevant to the more specific issue of auditory-motor integration comes from conduction aphasia (Hickok, 2001). A hallmark of conduction aphasia is the predominance of phonemic paraphasias, which can be evident across a large range of production tasks, including spontaneous speech, naming, reading aloud, and repetition (Goodglass, 1992). The preponderance of phonemic errors has led some authors to characterize conduction aphasia as a selective impairment in phonological encoding for production (Wilshire and McCarthy, 1996). Although the classical model holds that conduction aphasia is a disconnection syndrome involving damage to the arcuate fasciculus (Geschwind, 1965), recent evidence has shown that the syndrome can be caused by damage to, or electrical stimulation of, auditory-related cortical fields in the left superior temporal gyrus (Damasio and Damasio, 1980; Anderson et al., 1999). This region has been strongly implicated in speech perception, based on neuroimaging data (Zatorre et al., 1996; Norris and Wise, 2000), suggesting some degree of overlap in the systems supporting sensory and motor aspects of speech. This argument raises an apparent paradox, namely, that damage to systems strongly implicated in speech perception (i.e., left superior temporal gyrus) leads to a syndrome, conduction aphasia, characterized predominantly by a production deficit. This paradox can be resolved, however, on the assumption that speech perception is largely bilaterally organized, and that residual abilities of right hemisphere auditory systems function sufficiently well to support auditory comprehension (Hickok, 2000; Hickok and Poeppel, 2000).

Recent neuroimaging studies have supported and extended findings from the clinical literature. The left superior temporal gyrus has been shown to activate during a variety of speech production tasks (where speech is produced covertly, so that there is no external auditory input) including picture naming (Levelt et al., 1998; Hickok et al., 2000), repetition (Buchsbaum, Hickok, and Humphries, 2001), and word generation (Wise et al., 1991). Importantly, evidence from an MEG study of picture naming (Levelt et al., 1998) has shown that this left superior temporal activation occurs during a time frame prior to articulatory processes, suggesting that this region is involved in phonological code retrieval in preparation for speaking and is not merely a form of motor-to-sensory feedback mechanism, although the latter mechanism may also exist.

Two studies have looked explicitly for overlap in activation associated with speech perception and speech production. The first used positron emission tomography to map areas of overlap when participants listened to stories versus performed a verb generation task (Papathanassiou et al., 2000). A region of overlap was found in the superior temporal gyrus, predominantly on the left, as expected, based on results reviewed earlier. Additional areas of overlap included inferior temporal regions and portions of the left inferior frontal gyrus. The second study (Buchsbaum et al., 2001) used functional magnetic resonance imaging to map activated regions when subjects first listened to and then covertly rehearsed a set of three multisyllabic pseudo-words. Two left posterior sites responded both to the auditory and motor phases of the trial: a site in the sylvian fissure at the parietal-temporal boundary (area Spt) and a more ventral site in the superior temporal sulcus. Brodmann's area 44 (posterior Broca's area) and a more dorsal premotor site also responded to both the auditory and motor phases of the trial. The activation time course of area Spt and of area 44 in that study were particularly strongly correlated, suggesting a tight functional relation. A viable hypothesis is that the STS site supports auditory representations of speech and that the Spt site serves as an interface system translating between auditory and motor representations of speech. This hypothesis is consistent with recent work in vision demonstrating the existence of visuomotor systems in the dorsal parietal lobe that compute coordinate transformations, such as transformations of retinocentric to head- and body-centered coordinates, which allows visual information to interface with various motor-effector systems that act on that visual input (Andersen, 1997; Rizzolatti, Fogassi, and Gallese, 1997).

Sensorimotor interaction is pervasive across many hierarchical levels in the central nervous system. The empirical record supports conceptual arguments for sensorimotor interaction in speech and language and has begun to elucidate sensorimotor cortical circuits for speech. This work helps bridge the gap between functional anatomical models of speech and language and models of the functional organization of cortex more generally (Hickok and Poeppel, 2000).

—*Gregory Hickok*

References

Anderson, J. M., Gilmore, R., Roper, S., Crosson, B., Bauer, R. M., Nadeau, S., et al. (1999). Conduction aphasia and the arcuate fasciculus: A reexamination of the Wernicke-Geschwind model. *Brain and Language, 70,* 1–12.

Andersen, R. (1997). Multimodal integration for the representation of space in the posterior parietal cortex. *Philosophical Transactions of the Royal Society of London. Series B. Biological Sciences, 352,* 1421–1428.

Buchsbaum, B., Hickok, G., and Humphries, C. (2001). Role of left posterior superior temporal gyrus in phonological processing for speech perception and production. *Cognitive Science, 25,* 663–678.

Damasio, A. R. (1992). Aphasia. *New England Journal of Medicine, 326,* 531–539.

Damasio, H., and Damasio, A. R. (1980). The anatomical basis of conduction aphasia. *Brain, 103,* 337–350.

Doupe, A. J., and Kuhl, P. K. (1999). Birdsong and human speech: Common themes and mechanisms. *Annual Review of Neuroscience, 22,* 567–631.

Geschwind, N. (1965). Disconnexion syndromes in animals and man. *Brain, 88,* 237–294, 585–644.

Goodglass, H. (1992). Diagnosis of conduction aphasia. In S. E. Kohn (Ed.), *Conduction aphasia* (pp. 39–49). Hillsdale, NJ: Erlbaum.

Hickok, G. (2000). Speech perception, conduction aphasia, and the functional neuroanatomy of language. In Y. Grodzinsky, L. Shapiro, and D. Swinney (Eds.), *Language and the brain* (pp. 87–104). San Diego, CA: Academic Press.

Hickok, G. (2001). Functional anatomy of speech perception and speech production: Psycholinguistic implications. *Journal of Psycholinguistic Research, 30,* 225–234.

Hickok, G., Erhard, P., Kassubek, J., Helms-Tillery, A. K., Naeve-Velguth, S., Strupp, J. P., et al. (2000). A functional magnetic resonance imaging study of the role of left posterior superior temporal gyrus in speech production: Implications for the explanation of conduction aphasia. *Neuroscience Letters, 287,* 156–160.

Hickok, G., and Poeppel, D. (2000). Towards a functional neuroanatomy of speech perception. *Trends in Cognitive Sciences, 4,* 131–138.

Levelt, W. J. M., Praamstra, P., Meyer, A. S., Helenius, P., and Salmelin, R. (1998). An MEG study of picture naming. *Journal of Cognitive Neuroscience, 10,* 553–567.

Norris, D., and Wise, R. (2000). The study of prelexical and lexical processes in comprehension: Psycholinguistics and functional neuroimaging. In M. S. Gazzaniga (Ed.), *The new cognitive neurosciences* (pp. 867–880). Cambridge, MA: MIT Press.

Papathanassiou, D., Etard, O., Mellet, E., Zago, L., Mazoyer, B., and Tzourio-Mazoyer, N. (2000). A common language network for comprehension and production: A contribution to the definition of language epicenters with PET. *Neuroimage, 11,* 347–357.

Rizzolatti, G., Fogassi, L., and Gallese, V. (1997). Parietal cortex: From sight to action. *Current Opinion in Neurobiology, 7,* 562–567.

Waldstein, R. S. (1989). Effects of postlingual deafness on speech production: Implications for the role of auditory feedback. *Journal of the Acoustical Society of America, 88,* 2099–2144.

Wernicke, C. (1874/1969). The symptom complex of aphasia: A psychological study on an anatomical basis. In R. S. Cohen and M. W. Wartofsky (Eds.), *Boston studies in the philosophy of science* (pp. 34–97). Dordrecht: Reidel.

Wilshire, C. E., and McCarthy, R. A. (1996). Experimental investigations of an impairment in phonological encoding. *Cognitive Neuropsychology, 13,* 1059–1098.

Wise, R., Chollet, F., Hadar, U., Friston, K., Hoffner, E., and Frackowiak, R. (1991). Distribution of cortical neural networks involved in word comprehension and word retrieval. *Brain, 114*(Pt. 4), 1803–1817.

Zatorre, R. J., Meyer, E., Gjedde, A., and Evans, A. C. (1996). PET studies of phonetic processing of speech: Review, replication, and reanalysis. *Cerebral Cortex, 6,* 21–30.

Further Readings

Indefrey, P., and Levelt, W. J. M. (2000). The neural correlates of language production. In M. S. Gazzaniga (Ed.), *The new cognitive neurosciences* (pp. 845–865). Cambridge, MA: MIT Press.

Liberman, A. M., and Mattingly, I. G. (1985). The motor theory of speech perception revised. *Cognition, 21*, 1–36.

MacKay, D. G. (1987). *The organization of perception and action: A theory for language and other cognitive skills.* New York: Springer-Verlag.

Milner, A. D., and Goodale, M. A. (1995). *The visual brain in action.* Oxford: Oxford University Press.

Poeppel, D. (2001). Pure word deafness and the bilateral processing of the speech code. *Cognitive Science, 21*, 679–693.

Augmentative and Alternative Communication: General Issues

It is estimated that from 8 to 12 out of every 1000 individuals have a communication disorder severe enough to require the use of augmentative and alternative communication (AAC) intervention (Beukelman and Ansel, 1995). A large percentage of these individuals are children with spoken language disorders and a range of etiologies. Manual signs, communication boards, and computers with voice output have been developed to provide a means by which children with severe spoken language disorders can acquire language and communication skills. AAC is a language intervention approach.

The American Speech-Language-Hearing Association defines AAC as an area of research, clinical, and educational practice that attempts to compensate, either permanently or temporarily, for the impairment and disability patterns of individuals with severe expressive and receptive communication disorders that affect spoken, gestural, and/or written modes of communication. AAC is comprised of a system of four integrated components: symbols, aids, techniques, and strategies. The first component, symbols, are visual, auditory, and/or tactile, used to represent vocabulary and described as either aided or unaided. An aided AAC symbol employs the use of an external medium (e.g., photographs, pictures, line drawings, objects, Braille, or written words), while an unaided AAC symbol utilizes the AAC user's body (e.g., sign language, eye pointing, vocalizations). Aids are the second component; an aid is an object used to transmit or receive messages and includes, for example, communication boards, speech-generating devices, or computers. A technique, the third component, is the approach or method used for generating or selecting messages as well as the types of displays used to view messages. Messages may be generated or selected via direct selection or scanning. Direct selection permits a child to communicate messages from a large set of options using, for example, manual signing or pointing with a finger or headstick to a symbol. Scanning is used when message choices are presented to the child in a sequence and the child makes his or her selection by linear scanning, row-column scanning, or encoding. Displays may be either fixed (i.e., the symbol remains the same before and after activation) or dynamic (i.e., the symbol visually changes with its selection). Finally, strategies, the fourth component, are the specific intervention approaches in which AAC symbols, aids, and techniques are used to facilitate or develop language and communication skills via AAC (see ASHA, 1991; ASHA, in preparation, for complete definitions).

The role an AAC system plays in a particular child's life will vary depending on the type and severity of the child's language disorder. Children who use AAC include those individuals who present with congenital disorders as well as those individuals with an acquired language disorder. Children with congenital language disorders include children with cerebral palsy, dual sensory impairments, developmental apraxia of speech, language learning disabilities, mental retardation, autism, and pervasive developmental disorders. Acquired language disorders may include traumatic brain injury (TBI) and a range of other etiologies (e.g., sickle cell anemia) that affect language skills.

Children with language disorders who can employ AAC systems may range in age from toddlers to adolescents (Romski, Sevcik, and Forrest, 2001). The role AAC plays in language intervention depends on the child's individual communication needs. It is not restricted to use with children who do not speak at all and may benefit children with limited or unintelligible speech as well as those young children who may be at significant risk for failure to develop spoken communication. There are no exclusionary criteria or prerequisites for learning to use an AAC system (National Joint Committee, in preparation). Every child can communicate! Communication is defined in the broadest sense as "any act by which one person gives to or receives from another person information about that person's needs, desires, perceptions, knowledge, or affective states" (National Joint Committee, 1992). The modes by which children can communicate range along a representational continuum from symbolic (e.g., spoken words, manual signs, arbitrary visual-graphic symbols, printed words) to iconic (e.g., actual objects, photographs, line drawings, pictographic visual-graphic symbols) to nonsymbolic (e.g., signals such as crying or physical movement) (Sevcik, Romski, and Wilkinson, 1991). AAC interventions incorporate a child's full communication abilities, including vocalizations, gestures, manual signs, communication boards, and speech-generating devices. Even if a child uses some vocalizations and gestures, AAC systems can augment communication with familiar and unfamiliar partners across multiple environments. Some children with severe spoken language disorders who have no conventional way to communicate may express their communicative wants and needs in socially unacceptable ways, such as through aggressive or destructive, self-stimulatory, and/or perseverative means. AAC systems can replace these unacceptable means with conventional communication (Mirenda, 1997). AAC is truly multimodal, permitting a child to use every mode possible to communicate messages and ideas.

While AAC is an intervention approach, a team assessment is needed to describe, within a functional context, the child's language and communicative strengths and weaknesses and to determine what type of AAC system will permit the child to develop language and communication skills in order to participate in daily activities. AAC assessment is an ongoing process and includes a characterization of the child's current communication development (i.e., speech comprehension skills, communication modes), an inventory of the child's environments including partners and opportunities for communication, and a description of the child's physical abilities to access communication, including vision, hearing, and fine and gross motor skills. Fine and gross motor access includes physical access to an AAC system and in some cases seating and positioning options for optimal communication. A collaborative team approach to AAC service delivery incorporates families and a range of professional disciplines including, though not limited to, speech-language pathologists, general and special educators, and physical and occupational therapists. AAC abilities may change over time, although sometimes very slowly, and thus the AAC system selected for the present may need to be modified as a child grows and develops.

Not surprisingly, standardized psychological and speech and language assessment batteries are often difficult to employ with children with severe spoken language disorders because of the severity of their oral communication impairments. These assessments may not reveal an accurate picture of a child's abilities since many of these assessments are language-based and may be biased against a child who cannot speak. Often, the children are unable to obtain basal scores on such tests or their scores are so far below those of their chronological age peers that converting a raw score into a standard score is not possible. Systematic behavioral observation within everyday environments and informal measures that inventory and describe communication demands in these settings are employed to measure the communication skills of children who will employ AAC systems rather than standardized tests within isolated settings.

For most children who use AAC systems, language and communication development is the most important goal. Like all language and communication interventions, the long-term goal is to facilitate meaningful communication interactions during daily activities and routines. Goals should not only focus on the technological means of access the child uses, but on the development of language and effective communication skills. Depending on the child's current language and communication skills, goals may range from developing a basic vocabulary of single symbols or signs to express basic wants and needs to using sentences of symbols and signs to convey complex communicative messages (Reichle, York, and Sigafoss, 1991; Romski and Sevcik, 1996). It is essential that AAC system use take place in inclusive environments. The literature strongly suggests that AAC

systems can be embedded effectively within ongoing events of everyday life (Beukelman and Mirenda, 1998). Using AAC systems in inclusive settings requires that the team work together to ensure that the child has access to his or her AAC device throughout the day and that all adults and children who may interact with the child serve to support the child's communications as needed.

One frequently asked question is whether the use of AAC systems hinders speech development. Developing natural speech and literacy abilities are extremely important goals of AAC intervention. The empirical evidence suggests that AAC system use may result in increases in vocalizations and in some cases the development of intelligible speech (Beukelman and Mirenda, 1998). There is no evidence to suggest that AAC hinders or halts speech development. The use of AAC systems may also facilitate the development of early literacy skills and later reading.

In summary, for children with severe spoken communication disabilities, the AAC assessment is an ongoing process that includes information about the child's communication development, the child's environments, and the child's physical abilities. Children with severe language disorders who use AAC systems can demonstrate communication achievements far beyond traditional expectations. Recommended assessment and intervention practices are continuing to develop. The use of appropriate AAC systems enables the child to communicate effectively at home, school, play, and work. In addition to the development of communication skills, AAC increases social interactions with family and friends and participation in life activities.

See also AUGMENTATIVE AND ALTERNATIVE COMMUNICATION APPROACHES IN CHILDREN.

—*Mary Ann Romski, Rose A. Sevcik, and Melissa Cheslock*

References

American Speech-Language-Hearing Association. (1991). Report: Augmentative and alternative communication. *ASHA, 33*(Suppl. 5), 9–12.

American Speech-Language-Hearing Association. (in preparation). Service delivery by speech-language pathologists to individuals using augmentative and alternative communication: Knowledge and skillls.

Beukelman, D. R., and Ansel, B. (1995). Research priorities in augmentative and alternative communication. *Augmentative and Alternative Communication, 11*, 131–134.

Beukelman, D., and Mirenda, P. (1998). *Augmentative and alternative communication: Management of severe communication impairments* (2nd ed.). Baltimore: Paul H. Brookes.

Mirenda, P. (1997). Supporting individuals with challenging behavior through functional communication training and AAC: Research review. *Augmentative and Alternative Communication, 13*, 207–225.

National Joint Committee for the Communicative Needs of Persons with Severe Disabilities. (1992). Guidelines for meeting the communication needs of persons with severe disabilities. *ASHA, 34*(Suppl. 7), 1–8.

National Joint Committee for the Communicative Needs of Persons with Severe Disabilities. (in preparation). Position statement and report on the eligibility of persons with severe disabilities to benefit from communication services and supports.

Reichle, J., York, J., and Sigafoos, J. (1991). *Implementing augmentative and alternative communication: Strategies for learners with severe disabilities*. Baltimore: Paul H. Brookes.

Romski, M. A., and Sevcik, R. A. (1996). *Breaking the speech barrier: Language development through augmented means*. Baltimore: Paul H. Brookes.

Romski, M. A., Sevcik, R. A., and Forrest, S. (2001). Assistive technology and augmentative communication in inclusive early childhood programs. In M. J. Guralnick (Ed.), *Early childhood inclusion: Focus on change* (pp. 465–479). Baltimore: Paul H. Brookes.

Sevcik, R. A., Romski, M. A., and Wilkinson, K. (1991). Roles of graphic symbols in the language acquisition process for persons with severe cognitive disabilities. *Augmentative and Alternative Communication*, 7, 161–170.

Further Readings

American Speech-Language-Hearing Association. http://www .asha.org/.

Communication Aids Manufacturer's Association. http://www .aacproducts.org/

Glennen, S., and DeCoste, D. (1997). *The handbook of augmentative and alternative communication*. San Diego, CA: Singular Publishing Group.

International Society for Augmentative and Alternative Communication. http://www.isaac.org/

Lloyd, L., Fuller, D., and Arvidson, H. (1997). *Augmentative and alternative communication: A handbook of principles and practices*. Needham Heights, MA: Allyn and Bacon.

McEwen, I., and Lloyd, L. (1990). Positioning children with cerebral palsy to use augmentative and alternative communication. *Language, Speech, and Hearing Services in Schools*, 21, 15–21.

Reichle, R., Beukelman, D., and Light, J. (2002). *Implementing an augmentative communication system: Exemplary strategies for beginning communicators*. Baltimore: Paul H. Brookes.

Bilingualism and Language Impairment

This article is concerned with children who grow up learning two languages simultaneously. These are children who are exposed to two languages on a regular and consistent basis beginning within the first year of birth. (Children who begin learning a second language after 1 year of age are not considered because their pattern of development may be quite different from that of simultaneous bilinguals.) Understanding the nature of and developing appropriate treatment for impairment in simultaneous bilingual acquisition (i.e., bilingual impairment) is of the utmost importance because of the large number of such children worldwide. This article discusses key features of normal bilingual acquisition and factors that can influence bilingual acquisition that do not implicate impairment. It is imperative to understand normal bilingual development if valid diagnosis and

treatment of bilingual impairment is to occur. Research on impaired bilingual acquisition and its treatment are then discussed.

What Do We Know About Normal Bilingual Development?

Contrary to the widespread view that simultaneous acquisition of two languages is beyond a child's normal capacity, research on prenatal and newborn infants indicates that there are no neurocognitive limitations on infants' innate capacity to acquire two languages simultaneously (Genesee, 2001). Indeed, a growing body of research on children acquiring two languages simultaneously indicates that key milestones in phonological, lexical, syntactic, and pragmatic development occur within the same age range for bilingual children as for monolingual children (Paradis, 2000; Deuchar and Quay, 2000; Comeau and Genesee, 2001; Genesee, 2002a). Of course, there is considerable individual variation in the rate and pattern of normal language development among bilingual children as among monolingual children, and this should be taken into account when identifying possible cases of bilingual impairment. Delay in the emergence of key milestones and variations in pattern of development are not necessarily symptomatic of underlying impairment, although they might warrant careful monitoring.

Phonology.   Preverbal bilingual children progress from a stage in which there appears to be no system in either language to distinct phonological patterns in each (Deuchar and Quay, 2000; Paradis, 2000). En route to acquiring the target system, young bilingual children may demonstrate phonological patterns that deviate from those exhibited by monolingual children. The deviations that occur are not necessarily symptomatic of impairment but may simply reflect the bilingual child's transitional mastery of the complex dual phonological input that the child is exposed to. In the long run, most children exposed to two languages simultaneously and consistently exhibit no phonological difficulties as they mature, as demonstrated by young children's remarkable ability to acquire native-like accents, in comparison to the notorious phonological disadvantage of older second-language learners.

Vocabulary.   Bilingual children generally utter their first words around the same time as monolingual children, and the lexical repertoire of bilingual children is generally of the same magnitude and scope as that of same-age monolingual children when both languages are combined (Genesee and Nicoladis, 1995). When their vocabulary in each language is considered separately, it may be smaller and more restricted in scope than that of same-age monolingual children. Such differences are most likely attributable to the distinct environments in which they acquire each language and usually disappear with age as the child's experiences in each language expand. It is not uncommon for domain-specific differences in lexical proficiency to persist into adulthood, however, if the bilingual individual's contexts for acquiring and using both languages are distinct.

Many bilingual children exhibit "dominance" in one language; this can be reflected in syntactic and pragmatic as well as lexical domains. Dominance can express itself as differential proficiency, preference, or accuracy of use in one language in comparison to the other. In the case of vocabulary, for example, this can result in the child overusing words from the dominant language even in contexts where the nondominant language is appropriate. Dominance is a normal feature of bilingual acquisition and can continue into adulthood, often as a result of greater exposure to one language. Such imbalances do not usually imply impairment. Dominance should be considered carefully when understanding bilingual children's language development since it can explain their reliance on or more advanced proficiency in one language in comparison to the other.

Syntax. Contrary to earlier views (Volterra and Taeschner, 1978, for example), it is now clear that bilingual children develop separate grammatical systems for each language (Genesee, 2000; Meisel, 2001). This is evident as soon as they begin producing language that is clearly organized according to grammatical principles (in English, from the two-word stage onward). For the most part, bilingual children demonstrate the same stages and patterns of syntactic development in each language as children who acquire the same languages monolingually (e.g., Deuchar and Quay, 2000; Juan-Garau and Pérez-Vidal, 2000). Some bilingual children may show transfer (or so-called interference) effects such that a grammatical pattern (rule) from one language appears inappropriately when the child uses the other language (Döpke, 2000; Yip and Matthews, 2000). Such transfer effects are usually limited in scope and generally reflect grammatical overlap in the two languages. When transfer occurs, it is often, although not always, associated with much greater proficiency in or exposure to one of the languages. Transfer effects are usually short-term, provided the child continues to receive consistent and rich exposure to both languages. Some bilingual children also exhibit more advanced levels of syntactic development in one language than the other (Paradis and Genesee, 1996). This can be due to greater exposure to that language, inherent differences in the acquisition of specific syntactic patterns in the two languages, or simply a preference for one language. These patterns are normal and are not due to impairment.

Pragmatics. There is an extensive body of research on the development of pragmatic (or conversational) skills in bilingual children. Bilingual children are able to use their two languages differentially and appropriately with others, even strangers with whom they have had no or limited contact; this is evident even in children in the one and early two-word stage (Genesee, Nicoladis, and Paradis, 1995; Lanza, 1997; Comeau and Genesee, 2001; Genesee, 2002b). Bilingual children's pragmatic abilities can be limited by their proficiency. In particular, they

may not stick to the language of their conversational partner if their vocabulary, syntactic, or pragmatic skills in that language are not well-developed. In such situations, the child may call up the resources of the other language and code mix. Code mixing is the use of sounds, words, syntax, or pragmatic patterns from both languages in the same utterance or stretch of conversation. Some bilingual children may even prefer to code mix because they are accustomed to using and hearing others use two languages in the same conversation. Indeed, some bilingual children may never have encountered a monolingual person and thus are not used to communicating with adults whose skills are limited to one language. Indeed, code mixing is a normal part of interpersonal communication among fully proficient bilingual adults, and thus young bilingual people are often exposed to proficient adult bilinguals who mix.

Contrary to earlier views, it is now clear that bilingual code mixing is not a sign of linguistic confusion or incompetence (Genesee, Nicoladis, and Paradis, 1995; Meisel, 1989, 2001). To the contrary, child bilingual code mixing, like adult code mixing, is not random but is constrained according to the grammars of the two participating languages (Allen et al., 1999; Paradis, Nicoladis, and Genesee, 2000). In other words, children do not usually violate the grammatical rules of either language when they code mix. Bilingual code mixing in children is also situationally constrained, and bilingual children can adjust their rates of code mixing according to the rates of mixing of their interlocutors (Comeau, Genesee, and Lapagarette, in press). In short, code mixing is a communicative resource that bilingual children use to extend their communicative competence.

Bilingual children's language usage, including their code mixing, is shaped by the sociocultural context in which they acquire their languages, leading in some cases to patterns that could be misinterpreted. For example, a bilingual child may speak a language variety with phonological, lexical, or grammatical features that would be considered deviant from the point of view of the standard language but are normal in the child's variety (Crago, 1992). They may exhibit conversational patterns, such as silence, that could be interpreted as lack of pragmatic competence or even language disability from the perspective of mainstream norms but are normal and appropriate in the child's cultural community (see Crago, 1992, for an example among the Inuit). It is important to consider sociocultural factors as possible explanations of patterns of bilingual usage that might otherwise be attributed to impairment.

What Do We Know About Impairment in Bilingual Acquisition?

It is often thought that children exposed to two languages early in development will experience a higher incidence of impairment than monolingual children and that their impairment is likely to be unique and more severe than that of monolingual children. These expectations are based on the assumption, noted earlier, that acquisition of two languages simultaneously (or consecutively) during the preschool years exceeds the child's innate endowment to learn language. In effect, it is thought that bilingualism causes the impairment. However, such an assumption is misguided. While we currently lack adequate normative studies of the incidence of impairment in bilingual children, the extant evidence provides no reason to believe that exposure to two languages causes more delayed or impaired development than one would find in a monolingual population. Moreover, given the overwhelming evidence that bilingual children demonstrate the same milestones and patterns of development as monolingual children, there is no reason to expect unique patterns of impairment among bilingual children. Indeed, Paradis et al. (2003) found that the pattern and severity of impairment in a group of French-English children with a clinical diagnosis of impairment did not differ from that of age- and language-matched monolingual and bilingual controls also with impairment. In contrast, Crutchley and her colleagues found that bilingual children referred to special language units for children with language impairment in Britain exhibited more severe and unique patterns of difficulty on a variety of standardized measures in comparison to their monolingual counterparts (Crutchley, Conti-Ramsden, and Botting, 1997). However, these findings must be interpreted with caution, since, as noted by the authors, there may have been a bias toward inclusion of more severely impaired bilingual children in this sample. As well, the use of norm-referenced tests standardized on monolingual children may bias interpretation toward impairment, since normal bilingual-specific patterns of development were not taken into account. In support of the acquisition results, treatment studies with impaired bilingual children (both simultaneous and consecutive) have demonstrated that outcomes following bilingual treatment are just as positive or even more positive than those following monolingual treatment (Gutierrez-Clellen, 1999; Perozzi and Sanchez, 1992; Thordardottir, Weismer, and Smith, 1997). In sum, and contrary to the bilingualism-as-risk notion, there is no evidence that bilingual impairment is more severe than or different in kind from monolingual impairment, and there is no evidence to support monolingual treatment over bilingual treatment.

On the basis of this evidence, it is recommended that impairment in children acquiring two languages simultaneously be assessed in the same manner as in monolingual children, taking into account what we know about normal bilingual acquisition and the factors that can influence it: exposure, dominance, and sociocultural context. In addition to current best practices in assessment of monolingual children, the following principles should be observed when assessing bilingual children in order to ensure a valid diagnosis of impairment. (1) Evidence for impairment should be attested in both languages. (2) The pattern of impairment in each language should resemble that of monolingual children with impairment acquiring the same languages. (3) Standardized language tests that are normed on monolingual children should not be used normatively, nor should they be the sole basis for the diagnosis of impairment in bilingual children, since the latter may demonstrate normal patterns of performance that could be construed as impaired when compared with monolingual norms (Dodd, So, and Wei, 1996). Standardized tests that are normed exclusively on monolingual children are not likely to make allowances for the sociocultural and exposure differences that bilingual children experience learning two languages, and as a result, they are likely to misrepresent performance differences that bilingual children present as underlying impairment. Decision criteria that recognize alternative paths to normal language development must be used in the diagnosis of impairment in children acquiring two (or more) languages simultaneously.

There is no evidence that language impairment is due to or exacerbated by the simultaneous acquisition of two languages. It is likely that impairment is due to a fundamental problem in the child's innate capacity to acquire language that manifests itself in whatever language or languages the child is learning. Thus, children in the process of acquiring two languages who are suspected of impairment should not be limited to one language on the assumption that this will benefit their language development. Nor should treatment be restricted to one language only. To the contrary, children who have been exposed to two languages from birth may experience significant personal trauma and sociocultural disadvantages if they are deprived of the benefits of knowing two languages. Moreover, restricting children suspected of impairment to one language may entail significant long-term economic, professional, personal, and social disadvantages in the case of individuals living in bilingual communities. While we still have much to learn about typical and impaired bilingual acquisition, there is no evidence at present that would recommend or justify a decision that bilingual children with impairment learn only one language.

See also BILINGUALISM, SPEECH ISSUES IN.

Acknowledgments

I would like to thank Martha Crago and Elin Thordardottir for helpful suggestions on earlier versions of this chapter. I would also like to thank the Social Sciences and Humanities Research Council, Ottawa, Canada, for support of my research cited in this chapter.

—*Fred Genesee*

References

Allen, S., Genesee, F., Fish, S., and Crago, M. (1999, November). *Grammatical constraints on early bilingual code-mixing: Evidence from children learning Inuktitut and English*. Paper presented at the Boston University Conference on Language Development.

Comeau, L., and Genesee, F. (2001). Bilingual children's repair strategies during dyadic communication. In J. Cenoz and F. Genesee (Eds.), *Trends in bilingual acquisition* (pp. 231–256). Amsterdam: John Benjamins.

Comeau, L., Genesee, F., Lapagarette, L. (in press). The modeling hypothesis and child bilingual code-mixing. *International Journal of Bilingualism*.

Crago, M. (1992). Communicative interaction and second language acquisition: The Inuit example. *TESOL Quarterly*, 26, 487–505.

Crutchley, A., Conti-Ramsden, G., and Botting, N. (1997). Bilingual children with specific language impairment and standardized assessments: Preliminary findings from a study of children in language units. *International Journal of Bilingualism*, 1, 117–134.

Deuchar, M., and Quay, S. (2000). *Bilingual acquisition: Theoretical implications of a case study*. Oxford, U.K.: Oxford University Press.

Dodd, B. J., So, L. K. H., and Wei, L. (1996). Symptoms of disorder without impairment: The written and spoken errors of bilinguals. In B. Dodd, R. Campbell, and L. Worrall (Eds.), *Evaluating theories of language: Evidence from disordered communication* (pp. 119–136). San Diego, CA: Singular Publishing Group.

Döpke, S. (2000). Generation of and retraction from cross-linguistically motivated structures in bilingual first language acquisition. *Bilingualism: Language and Cognition*, 3, 209–226.

Genesee, F. (2001). Bilingual first language acquisition: Exploring the limits of the language faculty. In M. McGroarty (Ed.), *21st annual review of applied linguistics* (pp. 153–168). Cambridge, U.K.: Cambridge University Press.

Genesee, F. (2002a). Rethinking bilingual acquisition. In J. M. Dewaele (Ed.), *Bilingualism: Challenges and directions for future research* (pp. 158–182). Clevedon, U.K.: Multilingual Matters.

Genesee, F. (2002b). Portrait of the bilingual child. In V. Cook (Ed.), *Portraits of the second language user* (pp. 170–196). Clevedon, U.K.: Multilingual Matters.

Genesee, F., and Nicoladis, E. (1995). Language development in bilingual preschool children. In E. E. Garcia and B. McLaughlin (Eds.), *Meeting the challenge of linguistic and cultural diversity in early childhood education* (pp. 18–33). New York: Teachers College Press.

Genesee, F., Nicoladis, E., and Paradis, J. (1995). Language differentiation in early bilingual development. *Journal of Child Language*, 22, 611–631.

Gutierrez-Clellen, V. F. (1999). Language choice in intervention with bilingual children. *American Journal of Speech-Language Pathology*, 8, 291–302.

Juan-Garau, M., and Pérez-Vidal, C. (2000). Subject realization in the syntactic development of a bilingual child. *Bilingualism: Language and Cognition*, 3, 173–192.

Lanza, E. (1997). *Language mixing in infant bilingualism: A sociolinguistic perspective*. Oxford, U.K.: Clarendon Press.

Meisel, J. M. (1989). Early differentiation of languages in bilingual children. In K. Hyltenstam and L. Obler (Eds.), *Bilingualism across the lifespan: Aspects of acquisition, maturity and loss* (pp. 13–40). Cambridge, U.K.: Cambridge University Press.

Meisel, J. M. (2001). The simultaneous acquisition of two first languages: Early differentiation and subsequent development of grammars. In J. Cenoz and F. Genesee (Eds.), *Trends in bilingual acquisition research* (pp. 11–42). Amsterdam: John Benjamins.

Paradis, J. (2000). Beyond one system or two: Degrees of separation between the languages of French-English bilingual children. In S. Döpke (Ed.), *Cross-linguistic structures in simultaneous bilingualism* (pp. 175–200). Amsterdam: John Benjamins.

Paradis, J., Crago, M., Genesee, F., and Rice, M. (2003). Bilingual children with specific language impairment: How do they compare with their monolingual peers? *Journal of Speech, Language, and Hearing Research*, 46, 113–127.

Paradis, J., and Genesee, F. (1996). Syntactic acquisition in bilingual children: Autonomous or interdependent? *Studies in Second Language Acquisition*, 18, 1–25.

Paradis, J., Nicoladis, E., and Genesee, F. (2000). Early emergence of structural constraints on code-mixing: Evidence from French-English bilingual children. *Bilingualism: Language and Cognition*, 3, 245–261.

Perozzi, J. A., and Sanchez, M. L. C. (1992). The effect of instruction in L1 on receptive acquisition of L2 for bilingual children with language delay. *Language, Speech, and Hearing Services in Schools*, 23, 348–352.

Thordardottir, E. T., Weismer, S. E., and Smith, M. E. (1997). Vocabulary learning in bilingual and monolingual clinical intervention. *Child Language Teaching and Therapy*, 13, 215–227.

Volterra, V., and Taeschner, T. (1978). The acquisition and development of language by bilingual children. *Journal of Child Language*, 5, 311–326.

Yip, V., and Matthews, S. (2000). Syntactic transfer in a Cantonese-English bilingual child. *Bilingualism: Language and Cognition*, 3, 193–208.

Further Readings

Cummins, J. (1981). The role of primary language development in promoting educational success for language minority students. In *Schooling and language minority students: A theoretical framework* (pp. 3–49). Los Angeles: California State University, Evaluation, Dissemination and Assessment Center.

Doyle, A. B., Champagne, M., and Segalowitz, N. (1978). Some issues in the assessment of linguistic consequences of early bilingualism. In M. Paradis (Ed.), *Aspects of bilingualism* (pp. 13–20). Columbia, SC: Hornbeam Press.

Genesee, F. (1989). Early bilingual development: One language or two? *Journal of Child Language*, 16, 161–179.

Goodz, N. S. (1989). Parental language mixing in bilingual families. *Journal of Infant Mental Health*, 10, 25–44.

Grosjean, F. (1982). *Life with two languages: An introduction to bilingualism*. Cambridge, MA: Harvard University Press.

Hoffmann, C. (1991). *An introduction to bilingualism*. London: Longman.

Köppe, R., and Meisel, J. M. (1995). Code-switching in bilingual first language acquisition. In L. Milroy and P. Muysken (Eds.), *One speaker, two languages: Cross-disciplinary perspectives on code-switching* (pp. 276–301). Cambridge, MA: Cambridge University Press.

Meisel, J. M. (1990). *Two first languages: Early grammatical development in bilingual children*. Dordrecht: Foris.

Pearson, B. Z., Fernández, S. C., and Oller, D. K. (1993). Lexical development in bilingual infants and toddlers: Comparison to monolingual norms. *Language Learning*, 43, 93–120.

Pearson, B. Z., Fernández, S., and Oller, D. K. (1995). Cross-language synonyms in the lexicons of bilingual infants: One language or two? *Journal of Child Language*, 22, 345–368.

Petitto, L. A., Katerelos, M., Levy, B. G., Gauna, K., Tetreault, K., and Ferraro, V. (2001). Bilingual signed and spoken language acquisition from birth: Implications for the mechanism underlying early bilingual language acquisition. *Journal of Child Language*, 28, 453–496.

Communication Disorders in Adults: Functional Approaches to Aphasia

Functional communication has been a clinical theme since Martha Taylor Sarno first used the term as a label for her Functional Communication Profile (1968). Since then, the concept of functional communication has broadened in scope, with the result that there are now within this field two pertinent connotations for the word functional. Both are applicable to functional approaches to assessment and treatment of communication disorders in adults. Elman and Bernstein-Ellis (1995) suggest that the first connotation invokes a sense of the basics: for example, having the language necessary for signaling survival needs or rudimentary wants, for getting help, or for using "yes" and "no" reliably and accurately. Functional in the second sense connotes smooth running, getting through the worst of one's communication problem, or learning satisfactory compensatory skills that permit individuals only occasionally to have to remind themselves that they still have residual problems in communicating.

The term *communication* as used in the assessment and treatment of adult language disorders also has two connotations. For some clinicians, communication is almost synonymous with language, and their work emphasizes recovery or restitution of language skills. But clinicians whose interest is on functional communication utilize a more comprehensive definition. For them, communication typically encompasses not only language, but also other behaviors that permit individuals to exchange information and socialize even when they speak different languages. Most pertinent to adult language disorders are gesturing, drawing, and other ways of getting messages across, or learning how to guide others to provide the support and scaffolding that facilitates interpersonal interchange.

These expanded definitions are crucial to understanding the differences between functional and more traditional approaches to assessment and treatment of the language disorders that are acquired in adulthood, typically the result of insults to the brain and occurring to individuals who previously had normal language and communication. For such individuals, understanding the way that language functions in communication remains relatively spared, in contrast to their deficits of impaired lexicon, grammar, and phonology. As a result, functional approaches tend to stress communication strengths rather than linguistic deficits.

Because they emphasize everyday language and communication use, functional approaches rely heavily on the context in which such activities occur. They focus on authentic interpersonal exchange and interaction across a variety of settings, as well as communicative activities that occur in everyday life. Functional approaches also include usual conversational partners and emphasize their new role in facilitating as normal communication as is possible. With this background in mind, the following summarizes functional approaches to assess-

ment and treatment of aphasia. Although functional approaches can be applied to disorders such as traumatic brain injury and dementia, the bulk of the literature concerns aphasia, and it will be featured here.

Functional Assessment

A recent report from the National Committee on Vital and Health Statistics (2001) foreshadows the emerging emphasis on the need to lay "the groundwork for greater use of functional status information in and beyond clinical care." This report also supports the World Heath Organization's revised International Classification of Functioning, Disability and Health (ICF, 1999). The ICF makes it clear that in addition to measuring impairment such as aphasia, assessment must also consider how that impairment limits an individual's ability to go about the activities of daily living. The ICF takes one more step: It also requires the assessment of the effects of activity limitations on the ability to resume one's previous level of participation in society. Measuring activities and limitations brought about by aphasia, as well as how one's participation is affected, is precisely the domain of functional assessment. Such assessment does not substitute for tests that inventory the nature and extent of aphasic impairment. However, it dictates that such procedures must be supplemented by other measures.

Functional communication assessment measures are far-ranging. They include observing aphasic persons' communicative interactions, interviewing aphasic individuals and their families about communication needs, and analyzing their discourse and conversation. A few formal tests, such as Communicative Activities of Daily Living (CADL-2; Holland, Frattali, and Fromm, 1999) and rating scales such as the ASHA FACS (Frattali et al., 1995), the Functional Communication Profile (FCP; Sarno, 1969), and the Communication Effectiveness Inventory (CETI; Lomas et al., 1989) are used to measure activities and activity limitations in ICF terms.

The natural alignment of functional and pragmatic approaches also extends to ICF's next level, addressing restrictions in societal participation. Being able to resume activities and to participate in society clearly relates to quality of life. There are many quality-of-life measures available, but few at present focus specifically on the effects of communication problems. Nonetheless, effective functional assessment at the level of participation should be considered through interview and observation until more formal measures are available. This is because the ultimate goal of good therapy (functionally oriented or not) is to improve the quality of an aphasic person's life in this broadest sense.

We now turn our attention to functional approaches to the treatment of adult communication disorders. Specific clinical techniques for functional treatment are methodologically similar to those that are used in more traditional, impairment-focused treatments. That is, principles of learning and counseling are also used in functional treatment approaches. However, there is a great difference in the tasks that comprise traditional and functional treatments. In the latter, both stimuli and treatment tasks are geared to everyday events and interactions, or to communication strategies that can be used when language skills break down.

An individual's own pattern, style, and opportunities for communication are emphasized. As a result, the process is less clinician-driven and more the result of collaboration between aphasic individuals, their families, and their clinicians than are most other approaches. Functional approaches encourage the participation of aphasic individuals as well as their families in choosing treatment goals that are almost always cast in everyday terms. The clinician's role in the goal-setting phase treatment is to guide and counsel about how realistic the goals are, or to propose modifications that might be acceptable. For example, instead of the clinician's unilateral decision to work on general impairments in word retrieval (which might target words chosen on the basis of their frequency of occurrence or imageability), a collaborative approach might result in work that features retrieving the names of family, friends, and pets. Thus, even if traditional wisdom suggests that treatment should begin with easy targets and proceed from them hierarchically, the functionally motivated clinician might conclude that personal relevance is more important. The Functional Communication Planner (Worrall, 1999) provides a systematic format for determining the focus of such treatment.

There are many variations to the functional treatment theme when it is directed specifically toward the aphasic person in individual treatment. Perhaps the best known functional approaches involve training aphasic individuals to use strategies that facilitate their speech or aid in improving their comprehension. Some examples include supplementing or even substituting speech attempts with drawing or writing, or, for auditory comprehension, teaching aphasic persons to request repetition of a message that he or she does not understand. Often these alternative strategies are practiced in activities that promote the exchange of unknown information in a manner that approximates the normal interchange of everyday communication (PACE treatment; Davis and Wilcox, 1985).

Other approaches involve developing and practicing scenarios and scripts that can be used to recount important aspects of the person's life, such as how an aphasic man met his wife. A related approach might be to work on specific situations of personal relevance. These situation-specific scripts can be as diverse as a script that aids an individual in getting help in an emergency to consulting with a travel agent to plan a trip or even telling a few jokes. Finally, group treatment focused on conversational skills is becoming increasingly more frequent, as illustrated by the rich examples provided in Elman's book (1999).

There are also a number of ways to train others in the aphasic person's environment to take a disproportionate share of the burden of communication. Supported conversation (Kagan, 1998) is one such approach. Others include conversational coaching (Holland, 1991), and less formal training, accomplished both through didactic means and by counseling. Partner-centered approaches have been successfully used with family members, volunteers and even clinicians. The approaches share the rationale that communication can be improved not only by improving communication skills in aphasic individuals, but also when others in the communicative environment learn how to listen more effectively, how to encourage multimodal communicative attempts, and how to ask questions of aphasic people more appropriately.

In summary, functional approaches rely on a real-world perspective. Clinicians typically ask, How will this affect this person's daily life, and that of his or her family? Finally, functions of language, such as being able to invite, deny, or request, are essential to daily social interactions, and therefore to functional approaches.

In the last 35 years, researchers and clinicians have refined their abilities to assess everyday communication and to measure the functional outcomes of treatment efforts. Treatment methods that focus on the functional have also been expanded, and data now support the observation that functional changes can be achieved as a result. Qualitative as well as quantitative research on functional approaches can be expected to expand our knowledge over the next corresponding time period.

—*Audrey L. Holland and Jacqueline J. Hinckley*

References

Davis, G. A., and Wilcox, M. J. (1985). *Adult aphasia rehabilitation: Applied pragmatics.* San Diego, CA: College-Hill Press.

Elman, R., and Bernstein-Ellis, E. (1995). What is functional? *American Journal of Speech-Language Pathology, 4,* 115–117.

Elman, R. J. (1999). *Group treatment for neurogenic communication disorders: The expert clinician's approach.* Woburn, MA: Butterworth-Heinemann.

Frattali, C., Thompson, C., Holland, A., Ferketic, M., and Wohl, C. (1995). *Functional Assessment of Communication Skills for Adults (ASHA FACS).* Rockville, MD: American Speech-Language-Hearing Association.

Holland, A. L. (1991). Pragmatic aspects of intervention in aphasia. *Journal of Neurolinguistics, 6,* 197–211.

Holland, A., Frattali, C., and Fromm, D. (1991). *Commmunicative Activities of Daily Living (CADL-2).* Austin, TX: Pro-Ed.

Kagan, A. (1998). Supported conversation for adults with aphasia: Methods and resources for training conversation partners. *Aphasiology, 12,* 816–831.

Lomas, J., Pickard, L., Bester, S., Elbard, H., Finlayson, A., and Zoghabib, C. (1989). The Communicative Effectiveness Index: Development and psychometric evaluation of a functional communication measure for adult aphasia. *Journal of Speech and Hearing Disorders, 54,* 113–124.

National Committee on Vital Health Statistics. (2001). *Report on the use of the ICF for recording functional status information.* Available: www.ncvhs.hhs.gov/010716rp.htm.

Sarno, M. T. (1969). *Functional Communication Profile: A manual of directions* (Rehabilitation Monograph No. 42). New York: NYU Medical Center.

World Health Organization. (1999). International Classification of Function and Disability (ICF). Available: www.who.int/inf-pr-1999/en/note99-19.html.

Worrall, L. (1999). Functional Communication Planner. Oxon, U.K.: Winslow.

Further Readings

Aten, J., Caliguiri, M., and Holland, A. (1982). The efficacy of functional communication therapy for chronic aphasic patients. *Journal of Speech and Hearing Disorders, 47,* 93–96.

Bates, E. (1976). *Language in context.* New York: Academic Press.

Brumfitt, S. (1993). Losing your sense of self: What aphasia can do. *Aphasiology, 7,* 569–574.

Burns, M., Dong, K., and Oehring, A. (1995). Family involvement in the treatment of aphasia. *Topics in Stroke Rehabilitation, 2,* 68–77.

Doyle, P. J., Goldstein, H., Bourgeois, M., and Nakles, K. (1989). Facilitating generalized requesting behavior in Broca's aphasia: An experimental analysis of a generalization training procedure. *Journal of Applied Behavior Analysis, 22,* 157–170.

Elman, R., and Bernstein-Ellis, E. (1999). The efficacy of group communication treatment in adults with chronic aphasia. *Journal of Speech, Language, and Hearing Research, 42,* 411–419.

Hirsch, F., and Holland, A. (1999). Assessing quality of life after aphasia. In L. Worrall and C. Frattali (Eds.), *Functional communication in aphasia.* New York: Thieme.

Holland, A. (1982). Observing functional communication of aphasic adults. *Journal of Speech and Hearing Disorders, 47,* 50–56.

Holland, A., and Hinckley, J. (2002). Assessment and treatment of pragmatic aspects on communication in apahasia. In A. Hillis (Ed.), *Handbook of adult language disorders: Integrating cognitive neuropsychology, neurology and rehabilitation.* New York: Psychology Press.

Hopper, T., and Holland, A. (1998). Situation-specific treatment for aphasia. *Aphasiology, 12,* 933–944.

Jordan, L., and Kaiser, W. (1996). *Aphasia: A Social Approach.* London: Chapman and Hall.

LaPointe, L. (2002). Functional and pragmatic directions in aphasia treatment. In R. de Bleser and I. Papathanasiou (Eds.), *The sciences of aphasia, Vol. 1, From theory to therapy.* Oxford: Elsevier.

Lyon, J. G., Cariski, D., Keisler, L., Rosenbek, J., Levine, R., Kumpula, J., et al. (1997). Communication partners: Enhancing participation in life and communication for adults with aphasia in natural settings. *Aphasiology, 11,* 693–708.

Marshall, R. C. (1993). Problem-focused group treatment for clients with mild aphasia. *American Journal of Speech-Language Pathology, 2,* 31–37.

Newhoff, M., and Apel, K. (1990). Impairments in pragmatics. In L. L. LaPointe (Ed.), *Aphasia and related neurogenic language disorders.* New York: Thieme.

Oelschlaeger, M., and Damico, J. (1999). Participation of a conversation partner in the word searches of a person with aphasia. *American Journal of Speech-Language Pathology, 8,* 62–71.

Parr, S. (1992). Everyday reading and writing practices of normal adults: Implications for aphasia assessment. *Aphasiology, 6,* 273–283.

Parr, S. (1995). Everyday reading and writing in aphasia: Role change and the influence of pre-morbid literacy practice. *Aphasiology, 9,* 223–238.

Penn, C. (1998). The profiling of syntax and pragmatics in aphasia. *Clinical Linguistics and Phonetics, 2,* 179–208.

Penn, C. (1999). Pragmatic assessment and therapy for persons with bain damage: What have clinicians gleaned in two decades? *Brain and Language, 68,* 535–552.

Pound, C., Parr, S., Lindsay, J., and Woolf, C. (2000). *Beyond aphasia: Therapies for living with communication disability.* Oxon, U.K.: Winslow.

Prutting, C. A., and Kirchner, D. (1983). Applied pragmatics. In T. Gallagher and C. A. Prutting (Eds.), *Pragmatic assessment and intervention issues in language.* San Diego, CA: College-Hill Press.

Sarno, M. T. (1993). Aphasia rehabilitation: Psychosocial and ethical considerations. *Aphasiology, 7,* 321–324.

Simmons-Mackie, N., and Damico, J. (1996a). The contribution of discourse markers to communicative competence in aphasia. *American Journal of Speech-Language Pathology, 5,* 37–43.

Simmons-Mackie, N., and Damico, J. (1996b). Accounting for handicaps in aphasia: Assessment from an authentic social perspective. *Disability and Rehabilitation, 18,* 540–549.

Wilcox, M., Davis, G., and Leonard, L. (1978). Aphasics' comprehension of contextually conveyed meaning. *Brain and Language, 6,* 362–377.

Worrall, L., and Frattali, C. (2000). *Functional communication in aphasia.* New York: Thieme.

Communication Disorders in Infants and Toddlers

Prior to 1986, many speech-language pathologists serving infants and toddlers with communication disorders used an expert service delivery model. In the expert model, the speech-language pathologist is viewed as the professional who provides solutions by way of direct intervention to a child. Service delivery is often direct, and families have little control over the focus of and method of intervention. However, with passage of Public Law 99-457, a shift in service delivery philosophies occurred, with a new emphasis on a family-centered model (Donahue-Kilburg, 1992).

PL 99-457, Part H, mandated comprehensive, coordinated, community-based and family-centered services for infants and toddlers exhibiting disabilities in physical, cognitive, communication, social or emotional, and/or adaptive development. A range of services, including speech-language services and audiology, are available at no cost to the parents except where federal or state law provides for a system of payment by families. Reauthorization of IDEA in 1997 led to a change in name (now referred to as Part C). The reauthorization emphasizes services to children in natural environments (i.e., locations where the child would be served if he or she did not have a disability), using family-directed service delivery to identify family needs, and affirms families as members of the evaluation team.

Interagency coordinating councils (ICCs) exist at the federal, state, and local levels. Eligibility criteria for early intervention services under Part C is decided by each state's lead ICC, and as a result, varies from state to state. Eligibility is often determined by the presence of a developmental delay in physical, cognitive, speech and language, social or emotional, and adaptive (i.e., self-help) skills; or eligibility may be based on the degree of risk that the child has for developing a delay. There are three types of risks: established risk, biological risk, and environmental risk. In the case of established risk, a child displays a diagnosed medical condition, such as Down syndrome, fragile X syndrome, or Turner's syndrome, that is known to influence development negatively. Children with an established risk qualify for early intervention services. In contrast, a child who is biologically at risk exhibits characteristics (e.g., very low birth weight, otitis media, prematurity) that may result in developmental difficulties. A child with an environmental risk is exposed to conditions that may interfere with normal development, such as poor nutrition, poor environmental stimulation, or caregivers with substance abuse problems. Children with biological or environmental risks are considered to be at risk rather than to have an established risk. Some states include children who are at risk in their eligibility criteria for services; others do not.

One group of toddlers seen by speech-language pathologists who have been studied extensively display slow expressive language development (SELD). SELD is characterized by an expressive vocabulary of less than 50 words at 24 months of age and no word combinations, with no known hearing, cognitive, emotional/behavioral, gross neurological, oral-motor, or environmental deprivation (Rescorla, 1989; Paul, 1993). Paul (1996) concluded that children with SELD should not be regarded as having a disorder; rather, they should be considered at risk for further language impairment. Her longitudinal study of children identified as having SELD indicated that approximately 74% of the children identified with SELD as toddlers were no longer classified as having an expressive language delay by kindergarten age. Paul recommended a "watch-and-see" policy for children with SELD who do not display other risk factors. The watch-and-see policy would monitor children on a regular basis for their linguistic progress. However, other researchers have opposed such a policy, for a variety of reasons (van Kleeck, Gillam, and Davis, 1997). Children with specific language impairment (SLI), which can include receptive and expressive language skills, may also be seen for early intervention services. Risk factors for SLI include heredity, long periods of untreated otitis media, and parental characteristics such as low socioeconomic status, directive interaction style, and extreme parental concern (Olswang, Rodriquez, and Timler, 1998).

The family plays a vital role in providing services to infants and toddlers with communication disorders. They are part of the team from the referral stage through assessment, intervention, and dismissal. It is critical to consider the cultural variables that contribute to each family's unique system of functioning when working with families of infants and toddlers with communication disorders. The speech-language pathologist should understand each family's cultural belief system as it applies to views about disabilities, communication behaviors, and childrearing. Adopting a family-guided approach to early intervention requires a nonjudgmental respect for the family's views. The first step to understanding and respecting family and cultural views is to understand one's own family and culture. This places the speech-language pathologist in a position to understand differences of opinion and reduce potential misunderstandings. The next step is to learn about the family's belief system by observing, listening, and sharing information. Skills in interviewing and counseling are crucial for obtaining and clarifying information in a nonthreatening and respectful manner.

Unlike the expert model, which focuses only on the client's needs, the family-guided model focuses on both the family and the child. Child assessment and family assessment may both take place. A family assessment is voluntary and often conducted through interviews and surveys designed to collect information about the family's resources, priorities, and concerns. Child assessments must be multidisciplinary and comprehensive, conducted by trained personnel, and include both strengths and weaknesses of the child. The assessment should also be nondiscriminatory and confidential. Informed consent must be obtained. Professionals have 45 days from screening to complete the evaluation process that may determine the presence of a disorder and determine eligibility.

Assessment of infants and toddlers includes a variety of tasks and a range of informational questions asked of family members. Areas assessed include infant state behaviors, respiration, oral-motor skills (including sucking and swallowing evaluations), nonverbal communication behaviors, play behaviors, caregiver-child interaction, receptive and expressive vocabulary skills, phonological skills, word combinations, syntactic development, functions for language use, and cognitive skills (Donahue-Kilburg, 1992; Dickson, Linder, and Hudson, 1993; Paul, 2001). Assessment in the neonatal intensive care unit may involve working with nurses and parents and revolves around making the environment as positive as possible for the infant (Ziev, 1999). Assessment includes formal, standardized tests, informal methods such as play-based assessment and temptation tasks, and parental report.

Often assessment is conducted in an arena format, where one member of the team serves as the primary facilitator. Other team members observe and make notes about the child's behavior in their specialty area. In a transdisciplinary arena assessment, the primary facilitator will adopt the roles of the other professionals. Families can be involved in assessment by providing information, observing and collecting information, and interacting with their child. The level of involvement is the family's choice. It is important to remember that families are dynamic systems and that roles and functions of family members can change. A family initially reluctant to participate may want to participate in the next session. Frequent communication is necessary to ensure that services remain family-guided and family-friendly.

Families also assist the speech-language pathologist in determining outcomes rather than goals. These outcomes can be child-oriented, family-oriented, or both. The outcomes are written in family-friendly language, often in the family's own words. These outcomes are written in the form of an Individual Family Service Plan (IFSP). Importantly, the IFSP is a process as well as document. The process begins at referral and involves getting to know the family and child. It is an informal transferal of information that builds the foundation of trust and respect underlying future interactions. The written IFSP will contain information about the person who serves as the family service coordinator, the child's status in the areas of physical, cognitive, communication, social-emotional, and adaptive development, a plan that indicates the frequency and length of services, who will pay for services, the method of providing services, and how service will be provided in natural environments. The family service provider is selected by the family and is the main coordinator of services. The IFSP also includes a transition plan for children leaving Part C services and entering preschool (or Part B) services. It is optional on the part of the family whether or not they want the IFSP to contain information on the family's resources, concerns, and priorities. IFSPs can be used for children ages 0–6 years. Thus, on transitioning to Part B services, families may choose an IFSP instead of an Individual Education Plan.

Once outcomes have been selected, the type of intervention approach is determined. It is important to understand the family's view of speech and language development and the role they believe they play in their child's development of speech and language. Family members may choose to play an integral role in the intervention; others may prefer to have the intervention conducted by the speech-language pathologist. Intervention studies thus far have provided evidence that early intervention with infants and toddlers can facilitate prelinguistic behaviors, expressive vocabulary, phonology, social skills, and early word combinations (Girolametto et al., 1996, 1997, 1999; Robertson and Ellis Weismer, 1999; Yoder and Warren, 1998; Loeb and Armstrong, 2001). Some child-oriented techniques include parallel talk, recasting, and expansions. Some interventions focus modeling language effectively in everyday routines and scripts. The ultimate goal of this early intervention for children with established risk and those who are at risk is to reduce the likelihood that they will require future intervention and special education services and will gain the skills needed to participate socially and academically as they grow.

See also SPEECH DISORDERS IN CHILDREN: BIRTH-RELATED RISK FACTORS.

—*Diane Frome Loeb*

References

Dickson, K., Linder, T. W., and Hudson, P. (1993). Observation of communication and language development. In T. Linder (Ed.), *Transdisciplinary play-based assessment* (pp. 163–215). Baltimore: Paul H. Brookes.

Donahue-Kilburg, G. (1992). *Family-centered early intervention for communication disorders: Prevention and treatment.* Gaithersburg, MD: Aspen.

Girolametto, L., Pearce, P. S., and Weitzman, E. (1996). Interactive focused stimulation for toddlers with expressive language delays. *Journal of Speech, Language, and Hearing Research, 39,* 1274–1283.

Girolametto, L., Pearce, P. S., and Weitzman, E. (1997). Effects of lexical intervention on the phonology of late talkers. *Journal of Speech, Language, and Hearing Research, 40,* 338–348.

Girolametto, L., Weizman, E., Wiigs, M., and Pearce, P. S. (1999). The relationship between maternal language measures and language development in toddlers with expressive vocabulary delays. *American Journal of Speech-Language Pathology, 8,* 364–374.

Loeb, D. F., and Armstrong, N. (2001). Case studies on the efficacy of expansions and subject-verb-object models in early language intervention. *Child Language Teaching and Therapy, 17,* 35–54.

Olswang, L., Rodriquez, B., and Timler, G. (1998). Recommending intervention for toddlers with specific language learning difficulties: We may not have all the answers, but we know a lot. *American Journal of Speech-Language Pathology, 7,* 23–32.

Paul, R. (1993). Patterns of development in late talkers: Preschool years. *Journal of Childhood Communication Disorders, 15,* 7–14.

Paul, R. (1996). Clinical implications of the natural history of slow expressive language development. *American Journal of Speech-Language Pathology, 5,* 5–20.

Paul, R. (2001). *Language disorders from infancy through adolescence* (2nd ed.). St. Louis: Mosby.

Rescorla, L. (1989). The Language Development Survey: A screening tool for delayed language in toddlers. *Journal of Speech and Hearing Disorders, 54,* 587–599.

Robertson, S. B., and Ellis Weismer, S. (1999). Effects of treatment on linguistic and social skills in toddlers with delayed language development. *Journal of Speech, Language, and Hearing Research, 42,* 1234–1248.

van Kleeck, A., Gillam, R. B., and Davis, B. (1997). When is "Watch and see" warranted? A response to Paul's 1996 articles, "Clinical implications of the natural history of slow expressive language development." *American Journal of Speech-Language Pathology, 6,* 34–39.

Yoder, P., and Warren, S. (1998). Maternal responsivity predicts the prelinguistic communication intervention that facilitates generalized intentional communication. *Journal of Speech, Language, and Hearing Research, 41,* 1207–1219.

Ziev, M. S. R. (1999). Earliest intervention: Speech-language pathology services in the neonatal intensive care unit. *ASHA,* May/June, 32–36.

Further Readings

American Speech-Language-Hearing Association. (1989). Communication-based services for infants, toddlers, and their families, *ASHA, 31,* 32–34.

Billeaud, F. P. (2000). *Communication disorders in infants and toddlers* (2nd ed.). Needham Heights, MA: Allyn and Bacon.

Bliele, K. M. (1997). Language intervention with infants and toddlers. In L. McCormick, D. F. Loeb, and R. L. Schiefelbusch (Eds.), *Supporting children with communication difficulties in inclusive settings* (pp. 307–333). Needham Heights, MA: Allyn and Bacon.

Calandrella, A. M., and Wilcox, J. M. (2000). Predicting language outcomes for young prelinguistic children with developmental delay. *Journal of Speech, Language, and Hearing Research, 43*, 1061–1071.

Gallagher, T. M., and Watkin, K. L. (1998). Prematurity and language developmental risk: Too young or too small? *Topics in Language Disorders, 3*, 15–25.

Guralnick, M. J. (2001). *Early childhood inclusion*. Baltimore: Paul H. Brookes.

Hammer, C. H., and Weiss, A. L. (2000). African American mothers' views of their infants' language development and language-learning environment. *American Journal of Speech-Language Pathology, 9*, 126–140.

Ore, G. (1997). A silver lining. *Infant-Toddler Intervention, 7*, 79–92.

Rescorla, L., and Alley, A. (2001). Validation of the Language Development Survey (LDS): A parent report tool for identifying language delay in toddlers. *Journal of Speech, Language, and Hearing Research, 44*, 556–566.

Rescorla, L., Roberts, J., and Dahlsgaard, K. (1997). Late talkers at 2: Outcome at age 3. *Journal of Speech, Language, and Hearing Research, 44*, 434–445.

Rescorla, L., and Schwartz, E. (1990). Outcome of toddlers with specific expressive language delay. *Applied Psycholinguistics, 11*, 393–407.

Scherer, T. (1999). The speech and language status of toddlers with cleft lip and/or palate following early vocabulary intervention. *American Journal of Speech-Language Pathology, 8*, 81–93.

Tannock, R., and Girolametto, L. (1992). Reassessing parent-focused language intervention programs. In S. Warren and J. Reichle (Eds.), *Causes and effects in communication and language intervention* (pp. 49–79). Baltimore: Paul H. Brookes.

Thal, D. (2001). *Language and gesture in early identified late-talkers*. Paper presented at the Symposium for Research on Child Language Disorders, Madison, WI.

Tomblin, J. B. (1996). Genetic and environmental contributions to the risk for specific language impairment. In M. Rice (Ed.), *Toward a genetics of language*. Mahwah, NJ: Erlbaum.

Wetherby, A., Warren, S., and Reichle, J. (1998). *Transitions in prelinguistic communication*. Baltimore: Paul H. Brookes.

Yoder, P. J., and Warren, S. F. (2001). Relative treatment effects of two prelinguistic communication interventions on language development in toddlers with developmental delays vary by maternal characteristics. *Journal of Speech, Language, and Hearing Research, 44*, 224–237.

Ziev, M. S. R. (1999). Earliest intervention: Speech-language pathology services in the neonatal intensive care unit. *ASHA*, May/June, 32–36.

Communication Skills of People with Down Syndrome

Down syndrome is the most common genetic disorder in children. The genotype involves an extra copy of the short arm of chromosome 21, either as trisomy (95% of cases), a translocation, or expressed mosaicly. This condition is not inherited and occurs on average in about 1 in 800 live births in the United States. Incidence increases as maternal and paternal age increase. Down syndrome affects almost every system in the body. For example, brain size is smaller in adults though the same size at birth, 50% of these children have significant heart defects requiring surgery, neuronal density in the brain is significantly reduced, middle ear infection persists into adulthood, hypotonia ranges from mild to severe, and cognitive performance ranges from normal performance to severe mental retardation. The remainder of this article will summarize the specific speech, language and communication features associated with this syndrome.

The unique features of speech, language, and hearing ability of children with Down syndrome have been detailed by Miller, Leddy, and Leavitt (1999). First is the frequent hearing loss in infants and children, with more than 75% of young children found to have at least a mild hearing problem at sometime in childhood. These hearing problems can fluctuate, but about one-third of children have recurring problems throughout early childhood that can lead to greater language and speech delay. These results suggest particular attention be directed to monitoring responsiveness to everyday speech and frequent hearing testing through childhood. Second, there are unique verbal language characteristics of persons with Down syndrome. Children experience slower development of language relative to other cognitive skills. Communication performance is characterized by better language comprehension than production. Vocabulary use is better than the mastery of the grammar of the language. Progress in speech and language performance is linked to several related factors, including hearing status, speech-motor function status, and advancing cognitive skills associated with a stimulating verbal and nonverbal environment. Progress in speech, language, and communication should be expected beyond early childhood through adolescents (Chapman, Hesketh, and Kistler, 2002). A third unique feature is a protracted period of unintelligible speech. Speech intelligibility is a persistent problem of persons with Down syndrome through late childhood. Most family members have some difficulty understanding the speech of their children in everyday communication. Treatment protocols can improve speech intelligibility, leading to improved communication of children and adults. Finally, the development of writing and literacy skills in persons with Down syndrome should be expected. Children participating in early reading and writing experiences experience better communication and academic skills than their peers with less literacy experience.

Early reading programs have been successful at teaching sight word vocabulary to children as young as 3 years of age.

Assessment Principles

The following principles have evolved from our research over the past 10 years. Children with Down syndrome are very challenging to evaluate. The first and perhaps the only principle is to not make any assumptions about perceptual, motor, and cognitive skills or the child's experience with oral and written language. We suggest the following as guidelines for developing an assessment protocol. Access *all* information sources about current communication abilities across contexts—school, home, day care, and community. Review all data available on motor and cognitive development as well as perceptual (hearing and vision) status to direct the assessment decision-making process. Use flexible communication assessment protocols that can meet the specific attention shifts and motivational challenges of people with Down syndrome. Make sure the context of the assessment matches the child's performance level (i.e., play-based, observation, and standardized measures). Contrast measures conducted within familiar contexts, child- or family-centered approaches to assessment, with those taken in the absence of relevant context, i.e., standardized tests. Assess the child's communication environments as well as the child's independence in activities of daily living. Keep in mind that many persons with Down syndrome have a history of failing tests, "escaping" boring formal assessment procedures. Cover all bases evaluating cognition performance, hearing, verbal and printed language comprehension and production, oral nonspeech function, and speech behaviors. Remember that a child's performance in the office or clinic may represent a very thin slice of the full range of his or her capability.

Limitations of Standardized Tests Relevant for Children with Down Syndrome

Coggins (1998) identifies a number of limitations of standardized measures when testing children with developmental disabilities. Most tests are examiner directed, limiting the child's initiations and spontaneous language to single words or phrases. It is often difficult to translate test results into clinically useful outcomes. Rigid test administration guidelines make it difficult to use most measures with atypical children. Parents are typically excluded from active participation in the assessment process.

Challenges for Accurate Assessment

Consistency of Responding. One of the most frustrating characteristics of these children is the lack of consistency of responding in assessment tasks. This variability is associated with two things in our experience. The first is rapid shifts in *attention* and the second is *motivation*.

Clearly, these constructs are interrelated and it would be impossible to determine which is causal for any specific behavior. We have found that motivation is central to maintaining consistent response patterns. If we can provide a task that is sufficiently motivating, attention is maintained and responses are more consistent. Our work suggests that successful assessments can be conducted by careful preparation and understanding the interests of each child, what activities they like, what holds their attention at home and school, and then selecting assessment materials that can be imbedded into these activities.

Memory. The work of Michael Marcell (Marcell and Weeks, 1988) documents verbal short-term memory deficits. This has significant implications for assessment of language comprehension and production, particularly when using standardized procedures that require processing specific stimuli and remembering it long enough to provide to appropriate response. Clearly, memory deficits may also be contributing to behaviors that may be labeled as inattention or that result in inconsistent response patterns. In our experience, providing visual support enhances performance when verbal abilities are tested. This may involve pictures, graphic material, or printed words.

Motor Limitations. It has been widely reported that children with Down syndrome have motor deficits. Hypotonia is frequently cited as a cause, but there are little data to support this claim. Motor deficits are quite variable, with some children performing at age level and others show significant motor limitations delaying the onset of ambulation and other motor milestones. Testing protocols must take into consideration the motor demands on the child relative to the child's motor abilities. Make sure that the assessment tasks require motor responses within the child's capabilities.

Vision. France (1992) provides a detailed account of the visual deficits of children with Down syndrome. He followed a group of 90 children and reported that 49% had visual acuity deficits, with myopia being the most common. He also documented oculomotor imbalance in over 40% of the children, convergent strabismus accounting for the majority of these cases. In the majority of these cases only glasses were required to achieve normal vision. The message here is to make sure the children can see the stimuli during testing.

Hearing. Hearing remains an issue for children with Down syndrome because of frequent episodes of otitis media. Monitoring hearing should be done every 6 months for the first 10 years of life. In our work we have found that 33% of our children always had a hearing loss, 33% had a loss sometimes, and only 33% never had a loss. This was after screening out all of those children with significant hearing loss due to other causes. When oral language is tested, it is important to know the child's hearing status on the day of testing.

Summary. Designing a testing protocol requires attention to the skills and abilities the child is expected to bring to the task. These include attention and motivation differences, memory deficits, hearing and visual deficits, and motor limitations. Each of these can compromise the outcome of the assessment if accommodations are not made. It is also clear that in order to optimize the consistency of responding, alternative testing formats will have to be implemented. These testing formats will need to be less rigid, be context-based, and be child-centered rather than examiner-centered. A skilled clinician will have to follow the child's lead to implement functional, criterion reference, play-based assessments. Observational methods will also provide important information.

Who Is Responsible for the Development of Communication Skills?

The answer is that everyone is responsible—parents, teachers, and speech-language pathologists—but parents have the most pervasive role in the process. A recent book by Betty Hart and Todd Risley documents the contribution parents make to their children's language development in the first 3 years of life (Hart and Risley, 1995). Their results support what we have known for some time about language development: (1) parents are the first teachers of speech, language, and communication skills; (2) children will follow their parent's model of communication action and style; and (3) social relations are central for the development of communication skills.

Promoting Family Communication Supporting Language Development

The language and cognitive development of typical children can be improved by simply talking to them, by producing more and longer utterances with more complex vocabulary. This strategy can be used if we keep in mind children's ability to comprehend the language addressed to them and how parents adjust their own language to optimize the child's chances of understanding the message. Parents automatically adjust their language to children on almost every linguistic dimension, phonological, syntactic, and semantic, including slowing their rate of speech. The advice to talk more to children must be understood to mean talk more while adjusting language input to meet the child's level of language comprehension. This will facilitate processing the message. Communication is the product of this game. More talk in the absence of the rest of the features necessary for successful communication cannot improve language development. If this were not true, children's language would improve as a function of the amount of time they spend listening to the radio or watching television.

Families that are successful communicators perhaps talk more to their children, but the increased talking is in the context of *exchanging* messages. Families are generally encouraging as a communication style, urging their children to try new experiences, discussing their activities, and providing new challenging opportunities. As we consider increasing the frequency of communication with children with Down syndrome, we find that family styles are similar to those of typical children. Parents adjust their language and encourage their child's performance through attention and support for task completion. Increasing the frequency of talk should be encouraged in the context of family communication about the child's daily activities.

Guidelines for developing optimal environments for talking with children (Miller, 1981) include six rules: (1) Be enthusiastic. No one wants to talk with someone who does not appear to be interested in what they are saying. (2) Be patient. Allow children time and space to perform. Don't be afraid of pauses. Don't overpower the child with requests or directions. (3) Listen and follow the child's lead. Help maintain the child's focus (topic and meaning) with your responses, comments, and questions. (4) Value the child. Recognize the child's comments as important and worth your individual attention. (5) Don't play the fool. A valued conversational partner has something to say worth listening to, so pay attention. (6) Learn to think like a child. Consider that the child's perspective of the world is different at different levels of cognitive development.

Research on language learning in children with Down syndrome has documented that language learning is occurring and continues through adolescence (Chapman et al., 2002). The recent research on family communication style and frequency of communication may account for why some children with Down syndrome learn language more rapidly than other children. In our experience, families with children making good progress with their language and communication skills share common features. They select language levels relative to their child's ability to *understand* the message and not at their ability to produce messages. They have *realistic* communication goals. These families expect that their child will *learn to read*. They focus on understanding the *content* of their child's message and are not as concerned with the form of message. They make sure hearing testing is scheduled every six months through the developmental period. And they plan *frequent outings* to provide their children with varied experiences outside the home.

Who Is Running the Show, Parents Versus Professionals?

Diane Crutcher (1993) has powerfully presented the key issues underlying tensions between parents and professionals in speech and language. She articulates three issues parents perceive as limitations of speech-language intervention. The first is the lack of professional time, awareness, or unwillingness to explore intervention techniques specifically for their individual child. Second is the failure to modify intervention techniques into strategies that fit a family's natural lifestyle. The time constraints that most clinicians work under promote a "one size fits all" mentality. A lack of sensitivity to individual family styles and needs renders many family intervention programs ineffective, with families judged as uninterested when in fact it is the therapists that have failed. The third limitation is the failure of speech-language professionals to realize that families have other aspects of their lives that need attention, i.e., the activities of daily living, financial challenges, health concerns, other educational issues, and other family members. She also points out that most school and clinic settings allow limited time for family interaction, perhaps once-a-year visits. While most of these limitations can be attributed to job settings, we must ensure that the family context not be overlooked when designing effective intervention sequences for children with Down syndrome.

See also MENTAL RETARDATION.

—*Jon F. Miller*

References

Chapman, R. S., Hesketh, L. J., and Kistler, D. (2002). Predicting longitudinal change in language production and comprehension in individuals with Down syndrome: Hierarchical linear modeling. *Journal of Speech, Language, and Hearing Research, 45*, 902–915.

Coggins, T. (1998). Clinical assessment of emerging language: How to gather evidence and make informed decisions. In A. Wetherby, S. Warren, and J. Reichle (Eds.), *Transitions in Prelinguistic Communication.* Baltimore: Paul H. Brookes.

Crutcher, D. (1993). Parent perspectives: Best practice and recommendations for research. In A. Kaiser and D. Gray (Eds.), *Enhancing children's communication: Research foundations for intervention.* Baltimore: Paul H. Brookes.

France, T. (1992). Ocular disorders in Down syndrome. In I. Lott and E. McCoy (Eds.), *Down syndrome: Advances in medical care* (pp. 147–156). New York: Wiley-Liss.

Hart, B., and Risley, T. (1995). *Meaningful differences.* Baltimore: Paul H. Brookes.

Marcell, M., and Weeks, S. (1988). Short-term memory difficulties and Down syndrome. *Journal of Mental Deficiency Research, 32*, 153–162.

Miller, J. (1981). *Assessing language production in children.* Boston: Allyn and Bacon.

Miller, J., Leddy, M., and Leavitt, L. (1999). *Improving the communication of people with Down syndrome.* Baltimore: Paul H. Brookes.

Further Readings

Chapman, R. (1997). Language development in children and adolescents with Down syndrome. *Mental Retardation and Developmental Disabilities Research Reviews, 3*, 307–312.

Cole, K., Dale, P., and Thal, D. (Eds.). (1996). *Assessment of communication and language.* Baltimore: Paul H. Brookes.

Miller, J., and Paul, R. (1995). *The clinical assessment of language comprehension.* Baltimore: Paul H. Brookes.

Paul, R. (1995). *Language disorders from infancy through adolescence.* New York: Mosby.

Warren, S., and Yoder, P. (1997). Communication, language and mental retardation. In W. E. MacLean (Ed.), *Ellis' handbook of mental deficiency, psychological theory and research* (3rd ed., pp. 379–403). Mahwah, NJ: Erlbaum.

Wetherby, A., Warren, S., and Reichle, J. (1998). *Transitions in prelinguistic communication.* Baltimore: Paul H. Brookes.

Dementia

Dementia is a syndrome characterized by deficits in multiple cognitive domains, including short- and long-term memory and at least one of the following: aphasia, apraxia, agnosia, and impaired executive function (American Psychiatric Association, 1994). The deficits must be sufficiently potent to affect social and occupational functioning and apparent in the absence of delirium. Dementia is associated with many disorders, but most commonly with Alzheimer's disease (AD) and Lewy body disease (LBD). Other common dementia-producing diseases are vascular disease and Parkinson's disease (PD).

Because communicative functioning is a manifestation of cognition, it is necessarily affected when an individual experiences the multiple cognitive deficits that define the syndrome of dementia. However, differences in the nature and distribution of neuropathology in the common dementia-associated diseases produce unique patterns of communication deficits.

Effect of Alzheimer's Neuropathology on Communicative Function

The neurochemical alterations, neurofibrillary tangles, and neuritic plaques that characterize AD begin in the entorhinal cortex, perforant pathway, and hippocampal formation. Gradually, cells throughout the neocortex are affected, especially those in temporoparietal cortex. The formation of tangles and plaques eventuates in cell death and interferes with intercellular transmission. Subcortical structures and the motor strip are relatively free of neuropathology throughout much of the disease, which accounts for the fact that the speech of individuals with AD is spared.

Because AD begins in the hippocampal complex, an area important for the formation of recent or episodic memory, the typical initial manifestation is loss of memory for recent events. With disease progression to frontal cortex and temporoparietal association areas, other declarative memory systems are affected, specifically semantic and lexical memory. Because the basal ganglia and motor cortex are spared throughout most of the disease course, procedural memory also is spared.

In the early stages of AD, communicative functions dependent on recent memory, such as holding a conversation, are affected. Affected individuals forget what they have just heard, seen, or said. Many sentences are left unfinished, with forgotten communicative intentions, and repetitiousness is common. Comprehension of written materials, particularly long passages, diminishes because of memory impairment. The mechanics of reading are spared, however, and individuals with mild AD can still write, though they make frequent spelling errors.

The expression of grammar and syntax is remarkably intact, although occasional errors may be made. Individuals with mild AD can usually follow three-stage commands, answer comparative questions, name familiar items on confrontation, generate exemplars in a category, define familiar words, and describe pictures, although their descriptions do not contain as much factual information as those of age-matched healthy elders (Bayles and Tomoeda, 1993; Hopper, Bayles, and Kim, 2001).

By the middle stages of AD, when affected individuals have become disoriented for time and place and memory problems are more florid, communication is more disrupted (Bayles and Tomoeda, 1995). Meaningful verbal output diminishes because individuals have increasing trouble generating a series of meaningful ideas. Writing words to dictation may remain, but writing letters or pieces of any length is problematic. The ability to read is retained, although affected individuals rapidly forget what they have read. Grammar and syntax continue to resist prominent disease effects.

Persons with mid-stage AD can greet, name, and express many needs. Most can participate in short conversations, especially if those conversations involve only two people; however, they frequently have trouble retrieving desired names. They can answer questions and understand common gestures. Two-stage commands are comprehensible by most persons with mid-stage AD, and some can follow three-stage commands. Reading comprehension for single words remains good. Most individuals with mid-stage disease can still name on confrontation and produce exemplars in a category, but not as efficiently or accurately as normal elders. Verbal output continues to diminish in terms of meaningfulness, and sentence fragments are more common.

By the end stage of the disease, memory loss is extensive, disorientation may extend to self as well as time and place, and problem-solving skills are minimal. Urinary and then fecal incontinence develop, and ultimately ambulatory ability is severely compromised or lost. Nonetheless, a few linguistic skills are intact (Bayles et al., 2000). Most individuals retain some functional vocabulary, although a small percentage are mute. Much of the language produced by those who still speak is nonsensical. Nonetheless, many patients can follow a one-stage command demonstrating comprehension of language. The majority can read a simple word. Many retain common social phrases such as "I don't care" and "I don't know," and can contribute to a conversation.

Effects of Lewy Body Pathology on Communicative Function

Lewy bodies are spherical, intracytoplasmic neuronal inclusions that have a dense hyaline core and a halo of radiating filaments composed of proteins containing ubiquitin and associated enzymes (McKeith and O'Brien, 1999). They were first described in the literature by the German neuropathologist Friederich Lewy in 1912. Lewy bodies are classically associated with Parkinson's disease, particularly in the basal ganglia, brainstem, and diencephalic nuclei. They may also be widespread in the cerebral cortex. Diffuse distribution of Lewy bodies is associated with dementia, and 10%–15%

of cases of dementia (Cummings and Benson, 1992; McKeith et al., 1992) have this cause. Patients with LBD often have concomitant Alzheimer's pathology, and some have proposed that LBD is a variant of AD. However, there are cases of pure LBD, which argues for the theory that LBD is neuropathologically distinct (see Cercy and Bylsma, 1997, for a review).

Symptoms of LBD include fluctuating cognition in 80%–90% of patients (Byrne et al., 1989; McKeith et al., 1992), visual or auditory hallucinations, paranoid delusions, extrapyramidal features, and confusion (McKeith and O'Brien, 1999). Intellectual deterioration is more rapid than that observed in AD patients and disease duration is shorter.

Like the dementia of AD, LB dementia has an insidious onset and progressive course (Hansen, Salmon, and Galasko, 1990), producing the temporoparietal features of aphasia, apraxia, and agnosia (Byrne et al., 1989). Because the extrapyramidal features may be later occurring, LBD in its early stages may be misdiagnosed as AD. Prominent memory deficits may not be the presenting feature but may appear as the disease progresses.

The literature on the effects of LBD on language and communicative functioning is scant. However, it is reasonable to expect that the associated confusion, memory and attentional deficits will disrupt communication in much the same way that they do in AD. Because fluctuating cognitive status is a prominent feature of LBD, clinicians can expect wide fluctuation in communication skills.

Heyman and colleagues (1999) compared the neuropsychological test performance of individuals with AD with that of individuals with AD plus LBD. Both groups of patients were severely impaired on measures of mental status, verbal fluency, confrontation naming, concentration, visuospatial/constructional abilities, constructional praxis, and word list learning and recognition. The sole significant difference between the two groups appeared on the delayed recall of a word list, with AD-only patients being more impaired.

Vascular Dementia

Dementia can be produced by disease of the brain's vascular system, and the distribution of disease defines the nature of the neuropsychological deficits. However, the many possible variations in the nature and distribution of vascular disease make it impossible to specify a typical profile of neuropsychological deficits. For example, individuals with an infarct in the territory of the left posterior cerebral artery involving the temporo-occipital region might exhibit amnesia, whereas an individual with an infarcts in the left anterior cerebral artery involving the medial frontal region may have prominent executive dysfunction, with both nonetheless meeting the criteria for dementia. Similarly, individuals with cortical infarct differ from those with subcortical infarcts.

Individuals at greatest risk for developing vascular dementia are those who have experienced one or more clinically evident ischemic strokes (Desmond et al.,

1999). In fact, one-fourth to one-third develop dementia within 3 months (Pohjasvaara et al., 1998; Tatemichi et al., 1992). Examination of neuropsychological abilities has revealed inconsistent patterns of strengths and weaknesses (Reichman et al., 1991), but executive functions often are disproportionately impaired, as are motor aspects of language production (Powell et al., 1988).

Parkinson's Dementia

Parkinson's disease is associated with a loss of striatal dopaminergic neurons, particularly in the pars compacta region of the substantia nigra. Tremor is the best recognized symptom and is present in approximately half of individuals with PD (Martin et al., 1983). Often tremor begins unilaterally, increasing with stress and disappearing in sleep. Other early symptoms include aching, paresthesias, and numbness and tingling on one side of the body that ultimately spread to the other side. Other classic motor symptoms are rigidity, slowness of movement, and alterations in posture.

Not all individuals with PD develop dementia, and prevalence estimates vary. Marttila and Rinne (1976), in one of the most comprehensive studies of prevalence, reported it to be 29%. Other investigators have reported similar estimates of dementia prevalence (Rajput and Rozdilsky, 1975; Mindham, Ahmed, and Clough, 1982; Huber, Shuttleworth, and Christy, 1989). Widely debated is the cause of the dementia, with some attributing it to cortical degeneration and others to subcortical damage that impairs neurological control of attention (Brown and Marsden, 1988). Rinne and colleagues (2000) argue that reduced fluorodopa uptake in the caudate nucleus and frontal cortex produces impaired performance on neuropsychological tests that require executive function.

Individuals with PD, regardless of whether they develop dementia, have speech motor deficits because the disease damages the basal ganglia and striatal-cortical circuitry, which are involved in motor function. Those who develop dementia have problems communicating for other reasons, namely deficits in memory, attention, and executive functions. However, considerable evidence exists that language knowledge generally is preserved (Pirozzolo et al., 1982; Bayles and Tomoeda, 1983; Huber et al., 1986). Bayles (1997) argued that impaired performance on tests that manipulate language, such as confrontation naming and sentence comprehension, result more from nonlinguistic cognitive deficits than a loss of linguistic knowledge.

See also ALZHEIMER'S DISEASE.

—*Kathryn A. Bayles*

References

American Psychiatric Association. (1994). *Diagnostic and statistical manual of mental disorders—Fourth edition*. Washington, DC: Author.

Bayles, K. A. (1997). The effect of Parkinson's disease on language. *Journal of Medical Speech-Language Pathology, 5*, 157–166.

Bayles, K. A., and Tomoeda, C. K. (1983). Confrontation naming impairment in dementia. *Brain and Cognition, 19*, 98–114.

Bayles, K. A., and Tomoeda, C. K. (1993). *The Arizona Battery for Communication Disorders of Dementia*. Austin, TX: Pro-Ed.

Bayles, K. A., and Tomoeda, C. K. (1994). *The Functional Linguistic Communication Inventory*. Austin, TX: Pro-Ed.

Bayles, K. A., and Tomoeda, C. K. (1995). *The ABC's of dementia*. Austin, TX: Pro-Ed.

Bayles, K. A., Tomoeda, C. K., Cruz, R. F., and Mahendra, N. (2000). Communication abilities of individuals with late-stage Alzheimer disease. *Alzheimer Disease and Associated Disorders, 14*, 176–181.

Brown, R. G., and Marsden, C. D. (1988). Internal versus external cues and the control of attention in Parkinson's disease. *Brain, 111*, 323–345.

Byrne, E. J., Lennox, G., Lowe, J., and Godwin-Austen, R. B. (1989). Diffuse Lewy body disease: Clinical features in 15 cases. *Journal of Neurology, Neurosurgery, and Psychiatry, 52*, 709–717.

Cercy, S. P., and Bylsma, F. W. (1997). Lewy bodies and progressive dementia: A critical review and meta-analysis. *Journal of the International Neuropsychological Society, 3*, 179–194.

Cummings, J. L., and Benson, D. F. (1992). Dementia: Definition, prevalence, classification and approach to diagnosis. In J. L. Cummings and D. F. Benson (Eds.), *Dementia: A clinical approach*. Boston: Butterworth-Heinemann.

Desmond, D. W., Erkinjuntti, T., Sano, M., Cummings, J. L., Bowler, J. V., Pasquier, F., et al. (1999). The cognitive syndrome of vascular dementia: Implications for clinical trials. *Alzheimer Disease and Associated Disorders, 13*, S21–S29.

Hansen, L., Salmon, D., and Galasko, D. (1990). The Lewy body variant of Alzheimer's disease: A clinical and pathologic entity. *Neurology, 40*, 1–8.

Heyman, A., Fillenbaum, G. G., Gearing, M., Mirra, S. S., Welsh-Bohmer, K. A., Peterson, B., et al. (1999). Comparison of Lewy body variant of Alzheimer's disease with pure Alzheimer's disease. *Neurology, 52*, 1839–1844.

Hopper, T., Bayles, K. A., and Kim, E. (2001). Retained neuropsychological abilities of individuals with Alzheimer's disease. *Seminars in Speech and Language, 22*, 261–273.

Huber, S. J., Shuttleworth, E. C., and Christy, J. A. (1989). Magnetic resonance imaging in dementia of Parkinson's disease. *Journal of Neurology, Neurosurgery, and Psychiatry, 52*, 1221–1227.

Huber, S. J., Shuttleworth, E. C., Paulson, G. W., et al. (1986). Cortical vs subcortical dementia: Neuropathological differences. *Archives of Neurolology, 30*, 1326–1330.

Lewy, F. H. (1912). Paralysis agitans: I. Pathologische Anatomie. In Lewandowsky (Ed.), *Handbuch der Neurologie*. New York: Springer.

Martin, W. E., Loewenson, R. B., Resch, J. A., and Baker, A. B. (1983). Parkinson's disease: A clinical analysis of 100 patients. *Neurology, 23*, 783–390.

Marttila, R. J., and Rinne, U. K. (1976). Dementia in Parkinson's disease. *Acta Neurologica Scandinavica, 54*, 431–441.

McKeith, I. G., and O'Brien, J. (1999). Dementia with Lewy bodies. *Australian and New Zealand Journal of Psychiatry, 33*, 800–808.

McKeith, I. G., Perry, R. H., Fairbairn, A. F., Jabeen, S., and Perry, E. K. (1992). Operational criteria for senile dementia of Lewy body type (SDLT). *Psychological Medicine, 22*, 911–922.

Mindham, R. H. S., Ahmed, S. W., and Clough, C. G. (1982). A controlled study of dementia in Parkinson's disease. *Journal of Neurology, Neurosurgery, and Psychiatry, 45,* 969–974.

Pirozzolo, F. J., Hansch, E. C., Mortimer, J. A., et al. (1982). Dementia in Parkinson's disease: A neuropsychological analysis. *Brain and Cognition, 1,* 71–83.

Pohjasvaara, T., Erkinjuntti, T., Ylikoski, R., Hietanen, M., Vataja, R., and Kaste, M. (1998). Clinical determinants of poststroke dementia. *Stroke, 29,* 75–81.

Powell, A. L., Cummings, J. L., Hill, M. A., and Benson, D. F. (1988). Speech and language alterations in multi-infarct dementia. *Neurology, 38,* 717–719.

Rajput, A. H., and Rozdilsky, B. (1975). Parkinsonism and dementia: Effects of L-dopa. *Lancet, 1,* 1084.

Reichman, W., Cummings, J., McDanniel, K., Flynn, F., and Gornbein, J. (1991). Visuoconstructional impairment in dementia syndromes. *Behavioral Neurology, 4,* 153–162.

Rinne, J. O., Portin, R., Ruottinen, H., Nurmi, E., Bergman, J., Haaparanta, M., et al. (2000). Cognitive impairment and the brain dopaminergic system in Parkinson disease. *Archives of Neurology, 57,* 470–475.

Tatemichi, T. K., Desmond, D. W., Mayeux, R., et al. (1992). Dementia after stroke: Baseline frequency, risks, and clinical features in a hospitalized cohort. *Neurology, 42,* 1185–1193.

Further Readings

Azuma, T., and Bayles, K. A. (1997). Memory impairments underlying language difficulties in dementia. *Topics in Language Disorders, 18,* 58–71.

Azuma, T., Cruz, R., Bayles, K. A., Tomoeda, C. K., Wood, J. A., and Montgomery, E. B. (2000). Incidental learning and verbal memory in individuals with Parkinson's disease. *Journal of Medical Speech-Language Pathology, 3,* 163–174.

Bayles, K. A. (1991). Age at onset of Alzheimer's disease. *Archives of Neurology, 48,* 155–159.

Bayles, K. A. (1993). Pathology of language behavior in dementia. In G. Blanken, J. Dittman, H. Grimm, J. C. Marshall, and C. W. Wallesch (Eds.), *Linguistic disorders and pathologies: An international handbook* (pp. 388–409). Berlin: Walter de Gruyter.

Bayles, K. A., Azuma, T., Cruz, R. F., Tomoeda, C. K., Wood, J. A., and Montgomery, E. B. (1999). Gender differences in language of Alzheimer disease patients revisited. *Alzheimer Disease and Associated Disorders, 13,* 138–146.

Bayles, K. A., and Kaszniak, A. W., with Tomoeda, C. K. (1987). *Communication and cognition in normal aging and dementia.* Austin, TX: Pro-Ed.

Bayles, K. A., and Tomoeda, C. K. (1995). *The ABCs of dementia* (2nd ed.). Austin, TX: Pro-Ed.

Bayles, K. A., Tomoeda, C. K., Kaszniak, A. W., and Trosset, M. W. (1991). Alzheimer's disease effects on semantic memory: Loss of structure or impaired processing? *Journal of Cognitive Neuroscience, 3,* 166–182.

Bayles, K. A., Tomoeda, C. K., and Trosset, M. W. (1993). Alzheimer's disease: Effects on language. *Developmental Neuropsychology, 9,* 131–160.

Bayles, K. A., Tomoeda, C. K., Wood, J. A., Cruz, R., and McGeagh, A. (1996). Comparison of sensitivity to Alzheimer's dementia of the ABCD and other measures. *Journal of Medical Speech Language Pathology, 4,* 183–194.

Bayles, K. A., Tomoeda, C. K., Wood, J. A., Montgomery, E. B., Cruz, R. F., McGeagh, A., et al. (1996). Change

in cognitive function in idiopathic Parkinson's disease. *Archives of Neurology, 53,* 1140–1146.

Cheri, H. C. (1989). Dementia. *Archives of Neurology, 46,* 806–814.

Ehrlich, J. S., Oler, L. K., and Clark, L. (1997). Ideational and semantic contributions to narrative production in adults with dementia of the Alzheimer's type. *Journal of Communication Disorders, 30,* 79–99.

Grossman, M., D'Esposito, M., Hughes, E., Onishi, K., Biassou, N., White-Devine, T., et al. (1996). Language comprehension profiles in Alzheimer's disease, multi-infarct dementia, and frontotemporal degeneration. *Neurology, 47,* 183–189.

Nebes, R. (1992). Semantic memory dysfunction in Alzheimer's disease: Disruption of semantic knowledge or information processing limitation. In L. R. Squire and N. Butters (Eds.), *Neuropsychology of memory* (2nd ed., pp. 233–240). New York: Guilford Press.

Orange, J. B., and Purves, B. (1996). Conversational discourse and cognitive impairment: Implications for Alzheimer's disease. *Journal of Speech-Language Pathology and Audiology, 20,* 139–150.

Sabat, S. R. (1994). Language function in Alzheimer's disease: A critical review of selected literature. *Language and Communication, 14,* 331–351.

Snowdon, D. A., Kemper, S. J., Mortimer, J. A., Greiner, L. H., Wekstein, D. R., and Markesbery, W. R. (1996). Linguistic ability in early life and cognitive function and Alzheimer's disease in late life. *Journal of the American Medical Association, 275,* 528–532.

Tomoeda, C. K., and Bayles, K. A. (1993). Longitudinal effects of Alzheimer disease on discourse production. *Alzheimer Disease and Associated Disorders, 7,* 223–236.

Dialect Speakers

A dialect refers to any variety of language that is shared by a group of speakers. It is not possible to speak a language without also speaking a dialect (Wolfram and Schilling-Estes, 1998). Although all dialects of a language are equally systematic and complex, on a social level, dialects are often described as falling on a continuum of standardness. The most standard dialect of a language generally reflects an idealized prestige form that is rarely spoken by anyone in practice. Rules for producing this standard, however, can be found in formal grammar guides and dictionaries. Versions of the standard can also be found in formal texts that have been written by established writers. Next in standardness are a number of formal and informal oral dialects. These dialects reflect the language patterns of actual speakers. Norms of acceptability for these dialects vary as a function of the regional and social characteristics of different communities and of different speakers within these communities. Nonstandard dialects represent the other end of the continuum. These dialects also reflect spoken language, but they include socially stigmatized linguistic structures. Other terms used to describe nonstandard dialects are nonmainstream and vernacular.

At the linguistic level, scholars repeatedly highlight the arbitrary nature of a dialect's social acceptability (i.e., standardness). In fact, Milroy and Milroy (2000) argue that contradictory and changing attitudes to the same linguistic phenomenon can emerge at different times in the history of a language. For example, as these authors note, before World War II, absence of postvocalic /r/ in words such as *car* and *park* was not stigmatized in New York City. By 1966, however, r-lessness had become a stigmatized marker of casual style and lower social class. English dialects containing r-lessness continue to be stigmatized in the United States, but in England, English dialects with this same linguistic pattern have high status.

Most linguistic patterns that occur in the standard dialects of a language also occur in those that are nonstandard. Seymour, Bland-Stewart, and Green (1998) refer to these language patterns as *noncontrastive*, because all dialects of a language are thought to share these forms. Despite the similarity that exists among dialects, nonstandard versions are typically described by listing only those language patterns that do not appear in the standard varieties. Seymour, Bland-Stewart, and Green refer to these patterns as the *contrastive* features. Descriptions of nonstandard dialects become even narrower when they are generated by the media and general public, because these descriptions tend to highlight only the contrastive patterns that are highly stigmatized (Rickford and Rickford, 2000). Zero marking of the copula *be* (i.e., *he walking*) is an example of a pattern that is frequently showcased for African-American English (AAE) (Rickford, 1999). Other stereotypic patterns include the use of *ya'll* and *fixing to* to describe versions of Southern White English (SWE), *a- prefixing* (e.g., *he was a-walking ...*) to characterize Appalachian English, and pronouncing *think* and *that* as *tink* and *dat* to depict Cajun English.

Although it is relatively easy to identify the language forms that differentiate a nonstandard dialect from one that is viewed as standard, it is much more difficult to identify patterns that distinguish one nonstandard dialect of a language from another. One reason for this is that many nonstandard dialects of a language share the same contrastive patterns. Unique contrastive patterns for different nonstandard dialects are particularly rare when the dialects being compared are produced in the same community and by speakers of the same social class. Oetting and McDonald (2001, 2002) illustrated this finding by comparing the contrastive patterns of two nonstandard dialects spoken in southeastern Louisiana. The data for this comparison were language samples of children who lived in the same rural community and attended the same schools. Forty of the children were African American and spoke a southern rural version of AAE, and 53 were white and spoke a rural version of SWE. The AAE and SWE dialects spoken by the children were deemed distinct through the use of a listener judgment task and a discriminant function analysis of 35 different nonstandard (i.e., contrastive) language patterns found in the transcripts. Nevertheless, of the 35 contrastive patterns examined, 31 of them were found in the conversational speech of both the AAE and SWE child speakers.

Besides contrastive forms, there are three other ways in which dialects differ from one another. One way is in the frequency with which particular language forms are produced. Wolfram's (1986) analysis of consonant cluster reduction in 11 different English dialects is useful for illustrating this finding. His data showed cluster reduction occurring 3% of the time for standard English and northern white working-class English, 4% for northern African-American working-class English, 10% for southern white working-class English, 36% for southern African-American working-class English, 5% for Appalachian working-class English, 10% for Italian-American working-class English, 22%–23% for Chicano working-class and Puerto Rican working-class (New York City) English, 60% for Vietnamese English, and 81% for Native American Puebloan English. For each dialect listed, the percentage reflects the degree to which consonant clusters were reduced in regular past tense contexts that were followed by a nonconsonant (e.g., "Tom live in"). As can be seen, all 11 of the dialects showed cluster reduction, but the frequency with which this pattern occurred in each dialect greatly varied.

A second way in which dialects differ from one another has to do with the linguistic environments in which particular language forms occur. The effects of linguistic context on language use are often described as *linguistic constraints* or *linguistic conditions* (Chambers, 1995). Studies of linguistic constraints typically occur with language forms that show systematic variability in their surface structure. An example of a *variable form* is one that can be overtly expressed (i.e., present in the surface grammar; *he is walking*) in some contexts but is zero-marked (i.e., absent from the surface grammar; *he walking*) in others.

One of the most widely studied variable forms is the copula *be*, and research on this structure has typically involved nonstandard versions of AAE. At least six different linguistic constraints have been found to influence AAE speakers' use of the copula *be*. These constraints include the type of preceding noun phrase (noun phrase versus personal pronoun versus other pronoun), the phonological characteristics of the preceding environment (vowel versus consonant; voiced versus unvoiced consonant), the person, number, and tense of the verb context (first, second, third; present versus past), the grammatical function of the *be* form (copula versus auxiliary), the nature of the following predicate clause (locative versus adjective versus noun), and the phonological characteristics of the following environment (vowel versus consonant) (Rickford, 1999). The person, number, and tense of the verb context, the grammatical function of the *be* form, and the nature of the following predicate clause also have been shown to affect copula *be* marking in various nonstandard SWE dialects (Wolfram, 1974; Wynn, Eyles, and Oetting, 2000). Other morphosyntactic structures of English that have been found to be influenced by linguistic constraints include, but are not limited to, negation, do support, verb agreement, relative pronouns, plural marking, and question inversion (Poplack, 2000).

A third way in which dialects differ from one another is in the semantic meanings or grammatical entailments of some forms (Labov, 1998). These particular cases involve language patterns that occur in most dialects of a language, but their meanings or use in the grammar are unique to a particular dialect. These patterns are often described as *camouflaged forms* because, on the surface, the contrastive nature of these forms can be difficult to notice (Wolfram and Schilling-Estes, 1998). Use of *had + Ved* is an example of a camouflaged pattern. In most dialects of English, this structure carries past perfect meaning (e.g., "I already *had eaten* the ice cream when she offered the pie"). In some English dialects such as AAE, however, *had + Ved* also can express preterite (i.e., simple past) meaning (Rickford and Rafal, 1996). Ross, Oetting, and Stapleton (in press) provide the following sample from a 6-year-old AAE speaker to illustrate the preterite meaning of this form: "Then my mama said, 'It's your mama. Let me talk to your daddy.' Then she *had told* my daddy to come with us and bring a big rope so they could pull the car home."

Dialect use is affected by factors that are both internal and external to a speaker (Milroy, 1987; Chambers, 1995; Wolfram and Schilling-Estes, 1998). Internal factors that have been shown to influence the type and density of one's dialect include age, sex, race, region of the country, socioeconomic status, type of community, and type of social network. Interestingly, regardless of race, region, community, and network, members of lower social classes produce a greater frequency of contrastive dialect forms than members of higher classes. Greater frequencies of contrastive patterns also have been found for younger adults than for older adults, and for males than for females. Exceptions to these generalities do exist, however. For example, Dubois and Horvath (1998) documented a V-shaped age pattern rather than a linear one in their study of Cajun English. They also found that the type and degree of the age pattern (V-shaped versus linear) depended on the speaker's sex and type of social network. In particular, the V-shaped pattern was more pronounced for men than for women, and only women from closed social networks showed the V-shaped pattern. Women in open networks showed a linear pattern. Interestingly, though, the linear trend reflected higher frequencies of nonstandard dialect use by the older women than younger women. This finding contrasts with what is typically reported in other nonstandard dialect work, namely, that older adults present fewer instances of nonstandard forms than younger adults.

Some of the external factors that have been shown to affect dialect use include the type of speaking style (casual versus formal; interview versus conversation), speaking partner (familiar versus unfamiliar; with authority versus without), modality of expression (speaking versus writing versus reading), genre (persuasive versus informative versus imaginative), and type of speech act (comment versus request for information) (for data, see Farr-Whitman, 1981; Labov, 1982; Smitherman, 1992; Lucas and Borders, 1994). Influences of these external factors on dialect use interact in complex ways with those that are internal to a speaker. The dynamic interactions that occur between and among these variables help explain why dialect use is often described as fluid, flexible, and constantly changing.

The challenge for scientists in communication disorders is to learn how a speech or language disorder affects a person's use of language, regardless of the dialect spoken. Thus far, most descriptions of childhood language impairment have been made within the context of standard dialect varieties only. Extending the study of childhood language impairment to different nonstandard dialects is a topic of current scholarly work and debate (see DIALECT VERSUS DISORDER).

—Janna B. Oetting

References

Chambers, J. (1995). *Sociolinguistic Theory*. Malden, MA: Blackwell.

Christian, D. (2000). Reflections of language heritage: Choice and chance in vernacular English dialects. In J. Peyton, P. Griffin, W. Wolfram, and R. Fasold (Eds.), *Language in action* (pp. 213–229). Cresskill, NJ: Hampton Press.

Dubois, S., and Horvath, B. (1998). Let's tink about dat: Interdental fricatives in Cajun English. *Language Variation and Change, 10*, 245–261.

Farr-Whitman, M. (1981). Dialect influence in writing. In M. Farr-Whiteman (Ed.), *Writing: The nature, development, and teaching of written communication* (pp. 153–166). Hillsdale, NJ: Erlbaum.

Labov, W. (1982). *The social stratification of English in New York City*. Washington, DC: Center for Applied Linguistics.

Labov, W. (1998). Co-existent systems in African-American vernacular English. In S. Mufwene, J. Rickford, G. Bailey, and J. Baugh (Eds.), *African-American English* (pp. 110–153). New York: Routledge.

Lucas, C., and Borders, D. (1994). *Language diversity and classroom discourse*. Norwood, NJ: Ablex.

Milroy, J., and Milroy, L. (2000). *Authority in language: Investigating standard English* (3rd ed.). New York: Routledge.

Milroy, L. (1987). *Language and social networks* (2nd ed.). New York: Basil Blackwell.

Oetting, J., and McDonald, J. (2001). Nonmainstream dialect use and specific language impairment. *Journal of Speech, Language, and Hearing Research, 44*, 207–223.

Oetting, J., and McDonald, J. (2002). Methods for characterizing study participants' nonmainstream dialect use in studies of specific language impairment. *Journal of Speech, Language, and Hearing Research, 45*, 505–518.

Poplack, S. (Ed.). (2000). *The English history of African American English*. Maldon, MA: Blackwell.

Rickford, J. (1999). *African American vernacular English*. Malden, MA: Blackwell.

Rickford, J., and Rafal, C. (1996). Preterite had + V-ed in the narratives of African American preadolescents. *American Speech, 71*, 227–254.

Rickford, J., and Rickford, R. (2000). *Spoken souls*. New York: Wiley.

Ross, S., Oetting, J., and Stapleton, B. (in press). Preterite had-Ved: A narrative discourse structure of AAE. *American Speech*.

Seymour, H., Bland-Stewart, L., and Green, L. (1998). Difference versus deficit in child African American English. *Language, Speech, and Hearing Services in Schools, 29*, 96–108.

Smitherman, G. (1992). Black English, diverging or converging? The view from the national assessment of educational progress. *Language and Education, 6*, 47–64.

Wolfram, W. (1974). The relationship of white southern speech to Vernacular Black English. *Language, 50*, 498–527.

Wolfram, W. (1986). Language variation in the United States. In O. Taylor (Ed.), *Nature of communication disorders in culturally and linguistically diverse populations* (pp. 73–115). San Diego, CA: College-Hill Press.

Wolfram, W., and Schilling-Estes, N. (1998). *American English*. Malden, MA: Blackwell.

Wynn, C., Eyles, L., and Oetting, J. (2000). *Nonmainstream dialect use and copula be: Analysis of linguistic constraints.* Paper presented at the annual convention of the American Speech, Language, Hearing Association, Washington, DC.

Further Readings

Bernstein, C., Nunnally, T., and Sabino, R. (Eds.). (1997). *Language variety in the South revisited.* Tuscaloosa: University of Alabama Press.

Feagin, C. (1979). *Variation and change in Alabama English: A sociolinguistic study of the white community.* Washington, DC: Georgetown University Press.

Labov, W. (1994). *Principles of linguistic change: Internal factors.* Maldon, MA: Blackwell.

Labov, W. (2001). *Principles of linguistic change: Social factors.* Maldon, MA: Blackwell.

Montgomery, M., and Bailey, G. (Eds.). (1986). *Language variety in the South.* Tuscaloosa: University of Alabama Press.

Mufwene, J., Rickford, J., Bailey, G., and Baugh, J. (Eds.). (1998). *African-American English* (pp. 85–109). New York: Routledge.

Peyton, J., Griffin, P., Wolfram, W., and Fasold, R. (Eds.). (2001). *Language in action: New studies of language in society essays in honor of Roger W. Shuy* (pp. 213–229). Cresskill, NJ: Hampton Press.

Washington, J., and Craig, H. (1994). Dialectal forms during discourse of poor, urban, African American preschoolers. *Journal of Speech and Hearing Research, 37*, 816–823.

Washington, J., and Craig, H. (1998). Socioeconomic status and gender influences on children's dialectal variations. *Journal of Speech and Hearing Research, 41*, 618–626.

Wyatt, T. (1991). *Linguistic constraints on copula be production in Black English child speech.* Doctoral dissertation, University of Massachusetts, Amherst.

Dialect Versus Disorder

In 1983, the American Speech-Language-Hearing Association (ASHA) published a position statement on the topic of social dialects. A major point of the publication was to formally recognize the difference between language variation that is caused by normal linguistic processes (i.e., dialects) and variation that is caused by an atypical or disordered language system (i.e., language impairment). Through the position statement, ASHA also formally rebuked the practice of diagnosing and treating any dialect of a language as an impairment. The data used to support this stance were sociolinguistic findings regarding the systematic and complex nature of all dialects, including those that are socially stigmatized (see DIALECT SPEAKERS).

ASHA's position statement remains relevant today. Research on children's acquisition and use of different dialects is still a relatively new area of scientific endeavor, but small strides have been made. For example, there now exist numerous articles describing different dialects of English, and current publications about childhood language development, assessment, and treatment now routinely include discussions of dialect diversity. The different types of testing biases that may surface when the language tester and testee come from different linguistic or cultural backgrounds have also been described (Fagundes et al., 1998; Wilson, Wilson, and Coleman, 2000). A few traditional speech and language tests have added alternative scoring procedures for some nonstandard dialects (Garn-Nunn and Perkins, 1999; Ryner, Kelly, and Krueger, 1999). Alternative or new dialect scoring methods also have been created for the analysis of children's conversational language samples (Nelson, 1991; Stockman, 1996; McGregor et al., 1997; Seymour, Bland-Stewart, and Green, 1998).

Most of the advances listed started with methods and materials that were designed for speakers of standard English. Two different types of changes were then made to these methods. One change involved broadening the range of language forms that are considered normal by including the contrastive patterns of different dialects. The other type of change was to restrict the analysis to only the noncontrastive patterns. Contrastive patterns are those that show variation in surface structure across different dialects of a language (Seymour, Bland-Stewart, and Green, 1998). In English, one contrastive pattern is the copula/auxiliary *be*. In standard dialects of English, overt marking of *be* is obligatory in utterances such as "you are walking." In other dialects, such as African-American English (AAE) and Southern White English (SWE), overt marking of *be* in this context is optional. As a result, "you walking" and "you are walking" are both felicitous in these dialects. The use of contrast analysis when working with language sample data is an example of an alternative assessment method that treats the contrastive patterns of different dialects as normal (McGregor et al., 1997). With this method, the only language patterns that can be viewed as errors are those that cannot occur in the child's dialect.

Noncontrastive patterns are those that do not show surface variation across different dialects of a language (Seymour, Bland-Stewart, and Green, 1998). One noncontrastive pattern of English is S-V-O word order (Martin and Wolfram, 1998). This pattern is thought to be noncontrastive because all dialects of English thus far have been shown to present this word order. Other patterns thought to be noncontrastive in English include various forms of complex syntax that make sentential coordination and subordination possible. An example of a language assessment method that restricts the analysis to the noncontrastive patterns of dialects is Stockman's (1996) Minimal Competency Core (MCC) analysis. The goal of MCC analysis is to identify and then evaluate a common core of language that can be found in multiple dialects of a language. As a criterion-referenced procedure, MCC specifies a minimum level of competency for each language pattern and each age level examined. One of the language items included in MCC is a child's mean length of utterance (MLU). For English-speaking 3-year-olds, Stockman (1996) sets the minimum MLU at 3.27 morphemes. She also lists 15 consonants in the initial position and a set of semantic expressions and pragmatic functions that all 3-year-olds should be able to demonstrate, regardless of the English dialect they use. Another example of a relatively new assessment tool that targets the noncontrastive features of dialects is that formulated by Craig, Washington, and Thompson-Porter (1998b), which uses Wh- questions and passive probes.

All of these advances treat the contrastive patterns of dialects as problematic for diagnostic purposes. The problem, as articulated by Seymour, Bland-Stewart, and Green (1998), is that some contrastive patterns of some nonstandard English dialects can look very similar to those that are produced by standard English-speaking children who have a language impairment. Some of the surface patterns that are generated by both language learning conditions include zero marking of be (e.g., "you walking"), zero marking of past tense (e.g., "yesterday she fall"), and zero marking of third person (e.g., "today he walk"). Seymour, Bland-Stewart, and Green refer to these patterns and other contrastive forms as presenting a diagnostic conundrum because interpretations of their use as markers of either a normal dialect or a grammatical impairment are difficult. These authors also state that the exclusion of the contrastive patterns within assessment is necessary only until more is known about children's acquisition and use of these patterns. As more research is completed, new methods that include the contrastive patterns should be made possible.

Recently, research has begun to focus on children's acquisition and use of the contrastive patterns of dialects. Findings from some of these studies suggest that these particular language forms may not be as problematic as they first seemed. For example, at least four studies have examined the effect of these patterns on standard calculations of children's average utterance length and utterance complexity. Each of these studies has shown children's use of the contrastive patterns to play a minimal role within these calculations. For three of the studies, the focus has been on the contrastive patterns of AAE (Craig, Washington, and Thompson-Porter, 1998a; Jackson and Roberts, 2001; Smith, Lee, and McDade, 2001). The participants in these studies have ranged in age from 3 to 9 years. Measures of length have been calculated on utterances, C-units, and T-units, and measures of complexity have involved counts of complex syntax. In every case, children's use of the con-

trastive patterns of AAE has been shown to be relatively unrelated to the length and complexity indices. For example, Jackson and Roberts (2001) report correlations between children's use of contrastive AAE patterns and their utterance length and complexity scores to be at or below −.11.

Oetting, Cantrell, and Horohov (1999) also examined the effect of contrastive dialect forms on standard calculations of utterance length and utterance complexity. The participants in their study were children who spoke a rural Louisiana version of SWE, and they ranged in age from 4 to 6 years. Approximately one-third of the children were classified as specifically language impaired (SLI); the others were classified as normal. Three language indices, MLU, developmental sentence score (DSS), and Index of Productive Syntax (IPSyn), were evaluated. To examine the effect of the contrastive forms, scores for MLU, DSS, and IPSyn were calculated twice for each child, once using samples that contained utterances with contrastive forms and once using the same samples with the contrastive utterances removed. Results indicated that the diagnostic classification of each child as either normal or SLI was the same, regardless of whether utterances with the contrastive forms were included or excluded.

Recent studies also suggest that grammatical weaknesses of children with SLI can be identified within the contrastive forms. In addition to evaluating indices of utterance length and complexity, Oetting, Cantrell, and Horohov (1999) examined the grammatical profile of SLI within the context of nine contrastive forms of SWE. For five of the forms (i.e., third person regular, contractible copula, contractible auxiliary, uncontractible auxiliary, and auxiliary does), the children with SLI were found to present rates of overt marking that were lower than those of their SWE-speaking age-matched and language-matched peers. In a second study, Oetting and McDonald (2001) examined the grammatical weaknesses of SLI in the context of two nonstandard dialects, SWE and a rural Louisiana version of AAE. In this study, 35 different contrastive patterns were coded. Differences between the normal children and those with SLI were identified for 14 of the contrastive patterns. A full model discriminant function that involved counts of all 35 patterns resulted in 90% of the children being correctly classified as either normal or impaired. Stepwise analyses yielded slightly different discriminant functions for identifying children with SLI in the SWE dialect as compared to the AAE dialect, but both models included language forms needed to formulate questions and mark tense. The finding that both dialect groups with SLI were shown to have trouble with these two areas of grammar is consistent with SLI studies that have been completed with standard English speakers, nonstandard English speakers, and speakers of languages other than English (e.g., Rice, Wexler, and Hershberger, 1998; Seymour, Bland-Stewart, and Green, 1998; Craig and Washington, 2000; Paradis and Crago, 2000).

A few recent studies also have examined the developmental tragectories of particular contrastive patterns in isolation (Wyatt, 1996; Henry et al., 1997; Jackson, 1998; Burns et al., 1999; Wynn, Eyles, and Oetting, 2000; Ross, Oetting, and Stapleton, in press). The contrastive patterns examined in these studies have included aspectual *be* and preterite *had + Ved* in AAE, copula *be* in AAE and SWE, and negative concord in Bristol English and Belfast English. Each of these studies has shown normally developing children to be remarkably capable of learning the distributional properties of their native dialect. This finding occurs even when children who speak different dialects of a language live in the same community and attend the same schools (Wynn, Eyles, and Oetting, 2000; Ross, Oetting, and Stapleton, in press). Of the studies listed that also included children with SLI, some group differences (normal versus impaired) have been identified, but the nature of these differences warrants further study.

Understanding the ways in which a childhood language impairment manifests within the contrastive and noncontrastive forms of different dialects is a topic of ongoing study. Additional work also is needed to extend the study of childhood language impairment to other language-learning situations. Two such situations are bilingual language acquisition and second language learning. Until this research is completed, our tools for identifying children with language weaknesses and our understanding of language impairment as a construct will remain limited.

—*Janna B. Oetting*

References

ASHA Committee on the Status of Racial Minorities. (1983). Position paper: Social dialects and implications of the position on social dialects. *ASHA, 25,* 23–27.

Burns, F., Paulk, C., Johnson, V., and Seymour, H. (1999). *Constraint analysis of typical and impaired African American English-speaking children.* Paper presented at the annual convention of the American Speech, Language, and Hearing Association, San Francisco.

Craig, H., and Washington, J. (2000). An assessment battery for identifying language impairments in African American children. *Journal of Speech, Language, and Hearing Research, 43,* 366–379.

Craig, H., Washington, J., and Thompson-Porter, C. (1998a). Average C-unit lengths in the discourse of African American children from low-income, urban homes. *Journal of Speech, Language, and Hearing Research, 41,* 433–444.

Craig, H., Washington, J., and Thompson-Porter, C. (1998b). Performances of young African American children on two comprehension tasks. *Journal of Speech, Language, and Hearing Research, 41,* 445–457.

Fagundes, D., Haynes, W., Haak, N., and Moran, M. (1998). Task variability effects of the language test performance of southern lower socioeconomic class African American and caucasian five-year-olds. *Language, Speech, and Hearing Services in Schools, 29,* 148–157.

Garn-Nunn, P., and Perkins, L. (1999). Appalachian English and standardized language testing: Rational and recommendations for test adaption. *Contemporary Issues in Communication Sciences and Disorders, 26,* 150–159.

Henry, A., Maclaren, R., Wilson, J., and Finlay, C. (1997). The acquisition of negative concord in non-standard English. In E. Hughes, M. Hughes, and A. Greenhill (Eds.), *Proceedings of the 21st Annual Boston University Conference on Language Development* (pp. 269–280). Sommerville, MA: Cascadilla Press.

Jackson, J. (1998). *Linguistic aspect in African-American English speaking children: An investigation of aspectual 'be.'* Doctoral dissertation, University of Massachusetts, Amherst.

Jackson, S., and Roberts, J. (2001). Complex syntax production of African American preschoolers. *Journal of Speech, Language, and Hearing Research, 44,* 1083–1096.

Martin, S., and Wolfram, W. (1998). The sentence in African American Vernacular English. In S. Salikoko, J. Rickford, G. Bailey, and J. Baugh (Eds.), *African American Vernacular English: Structure, history, and use* (pp. 11–37). New York: Routledge.

McGregor, K., Williams, D., Hearst, S., and Johnson, A. (1997). The use of contrastive analysis in distinguishing difference from disorder: A tutorial. *American Journal of Speech Language Pathology, 6,* 45–56.

Nelson, N. (1991). *Black English sentence scoring.* Unpublished manuscript, Western Michigan University, Kalamazoo.

Oetting, J., Cantrell, J., and Horohov, J. (1999). A study of specific language impairment (SLI) in the context of nonstandard dialect. *Clinical Linguistics and Phonetics, 13,* 25–44.

Oetting, J., and McDonald, J. (2001). Nonmainstream dialect use and specific language impairment. *Journal of Speech, Language, and Hearing Research, 44,* 207–223.

Paradis, J., and Crago, M. (2000). Tense and temporality: A comparison between children learning a second language and children with SLI. *Journal of Speech, Language, and Hearing Research, 43,* 834–848.

Rice, M., Wexler, K., and Hershberger, S. (1998). Tense over time: The longitudinal course of tense acquisition in children with specific language impairment. *Journal of Speech, Language, and Hearing Research, 41,* 1412–1431.

Ross, S., Oetting, J., and Stapleton, B. (in press). Preterite had-Ved: A narrative discourse structure of AAE. *American Speech.*

Ryner, P., Kelly, D., and Krueger, D. (1999). Screening low-income African American children using the BLT-2S and the SPELT-P. *American Journal of Speech Language Pathology, 8,* 44–52.

Seymour, H., Bland-Stewart, L., and Green, L. (1998). Difference versus deficit in child African American English. *Language, Speech, and Hearing Services in Schools, 29,* 96–108.

Smith, T., Lee, E., and McDade, H. (2001). An investigation of T-units in African American English-speaking and standard American English-speaking fourth-grade children. *Communication Disorders Quarterly, 22,* 148–157.

Stockman, I. (1996). The promises and pitfalls of language sample analysis as an assessment tool for linguistic minority children. *Language, Speech, and Hearing Services in Schools, 27,* 355–366.

Wilson, W., Wilson, J., and Coleman, T. (2000). Culturally appropriate assessment: Issues and strategies. In T. Coleman (Ed.), *Clinical management of communication disorders in culturally diverse children* (pp. 101–127). Boston: Allyn and Bacon.

Wyatt, T. (1996). The acquisition of the African American English copula. In A. Kamhi, K. Pollock, and J. Harris (Eds.), *Communication development and disorders in African American children* (pp. 95–116). Baltimore: Paul H. Brooks.

Wynn, C., Eyles, L., and Oetting, J. (2000). *Nonmainstream dialect use and copula be: Analysis of linguistic constraints.* Paper presented at the annual convention of the American Speech, Language, and Hearing Association, Washington, DC.

Further Reading

Wolfram, W., Adger, C., and Christian, D. (1999). *Dialects in schools and communities.* Mahwah, NJ: Erlbaum.

Discourse

The term *discourse* is applied to language considerations beyond the boundaries of isolated sentences, although a discourse in its simplest form may be manifested as a single utterance in context, such as "Children at play." Discourse studies emerge from a variety of disciplines, with major contributions from linguistics and psychology. Linguists have been motivated primarily by the desire to explain phenomena that cannot be accounted for at the word and sentence levels, such as reference or given/new information, while psychologists have emphasized strategic processes and the role of cognitive factors, such as memory, in the production and comprehension of discourse. This entry focuses on seminal linguistic research areas that have had a strong influence on the field.

A construct that defines the nature of discourse study, regardless of discipline or perspective, is *coherence*. A discourse is coherent when it "hangs together," or makes sense. This notion of coherence pervades the approaches of a variety of discourse analysts. With some, it is used as a technical term in its own right. With others, it forms an underlying attribute of other constructs. Despite differences in terminology or focus, discourse approaches are similar in their analysis of an organization that supersedes any single sentence or utterance. Thus, the main goal of discourse analysis is to differentiate discourse from random sequences of sentences or utterances.

Discourse models generally assume that discourse coherence is realized through the integration of a variety of resources: the information contained in the text, shared knowledge, and the relevant features of the situation in which the text is embedded. Thus, linguistic form and meaning alone are insufficient for discourse comprehension and production. For that reason, discourse paradigms represent a dramatic shift from more traditional linguistic pursuits that focus exclusively on linguistic forms in isolation.

The knowledge structures that contribute to the formation of coherence are thought to be varied, conventional, and differentiated from each other by the kind of information they contain. For instance, *story schema* (Mandler, 1984) or *superstructure* (van Dijk and Kintsch, 1983) represent knowledge of the way in which events unfold in a story (narrative), and how a story typically begins and ends. *Script knowledge* (Schank and Abelson, 1977) specifies the sequence of steps in common everyday routines, such as going to a restaurant or making a sandwich. Knowledge structures also include knowledge of common patterns of conversational exchange, such as question-answer sequences (Schegloff, 1980).

Discourse analyses differ primarily in the degree to which they focus on the relative contributions of text, shared knowledge, and context. One influential model (van Dijk and Kintsch, 1983) is quite detailed in its account of the transformation of semantic content into cognitive information content. It represents the semantics of a text as a set of propositions. These propositions display coherence through inference at a local level, as *microstructures*, and at a global level, as *macrostructures* that represent the topic or gist of the text. The micro- and macrostructures constitute the *text base*, which is integrated with shared knowledge. The product of that integration is a representation of the events depicted in the text, conceptualized as the *situation model*. Thus, this is a model of discourse as a process involving transformation of information.

Linguists have also contributed greatly to our understanding of the various means by which discourse is coherently organized above the level of the sentence, and how the surface features of a text contribute to these higher levels of organization (Halliday, 1985). The research has centered largely on narrative, in part because of its universality as a genre and the fundamental nature of the temporal organization on which it is based. The extensive research on narrative has historical roots in Propp's (1928/1968) analysis of folk tales (from the field of rhetoric) and Bartlett's (1932) study of narrative remembering (from the field of psychology).

In linguistics, an early and influential framework for analyzing narrative structure was provided by Labov and Waletzky (1967) and extended in Labov's later work (1972). The model is organized around the role of sentential grammar in discourse-level structure. In this framework, the verbal sequence of clauses is matched to the sequence of events that occurred, as the means by which past experience is recapitulated in the narrative. The overall structure of the narrative progresses from orientation to complicating action to resolution. An additional component of the overall structure is evaluation, which is expressed through a wide range of lexico-grammatical devices. Thus, this work established a fundamental approach to analyzing how an event sequence is realized in linguistic form. Contemporary adaptations of this seminal approach to narrative analysis are numerous (Bamberg, 1997).

Work on textual *cohesion* (Halliday and Hasan, 1976) provides another view of the relationship between discourse organization and its component linguistic units. Halliday and Hasan define cohesion as "the set of possibilities that exist in the language for making text hang together [as a larger unit]" (p. 18). *Cohesive ties*, which are surface features of text, provide the relevant semantic relation between pieces of the text. These ties can be lexical or grammatical and include devices such as reference, conjunction, and ellipsis. Thus, cohesion is similar to coherence in that it is a relational concept; text is cohesive when it is coherent with respect to itself. The notion of cohesion has been widely applied, especially in the area of reference.

Linguistic accounts of discourse genre are another means of analyzing how discourse can be coherent. Although narrative has been the most extensively studied genre, Longacre (1996) provides a typology of various discourse genres (e.g., procedural, expository, narrative) in terms of both underlying knowledge structure and their linguistic realization. In his framework, discourse is classified by the nature of the relationship between the events and doings in the discourse, the nature of reference to agents in the discourse, and whether the events happened in the past or are not yet realized. As is typical of linguistic approaches, Longacre further specifies the surface linguistic characteristics of each discourse type, such as the types of tense and aspect markings on the verb, the typical forms of personal reference, and the nature of the linkage between sentences for each discourse genre. For instance, he specifies how the setting of narrative usually contains stative verbs, while the complicating action contains action verbs. He further analyzes how the peak or climax of the story can be marked through devices such as shifts in tense or changes in length and syntactic complexity (Longacre, 1981).

An especially detailed account of how thinking is transformed into language is found in cognitive-linguistic work using narratives (Chafe, 1980). Chafe's framework addresses ways in which the flow of thought is matched to units of language during the process of verbalization. Not only does he address lexicosyntactic contributions to discourse formation, he also considers the way in which syntax and intonation interact in discourse production.

Several of the discourse theorists explore the commonality and variability of narrative features across languages and cultures. These pursuits reflect an interest in universality that is pervasive in the field of linguistics in general. Contributions in this area include studies of cross-linguistic differences in expression of the basic features of narrative, such as verbs or the marking of reference (Longacre, 1996); ethnic linguistic devices used in the various narrative components, such as evaluation (Labov, 1972); variations in linguistic expression both within individuals and across individuals from different cultures (Chafe, 1980); and cultural presuppositions reflected in the content of narratives (Polanyi, 1989).

Conversational discourse represents a discourse type very different from the other discourse genres. Research on conversational discourse emphasizes the role of context and social interaction (e.g., Schiffrin, 1994). A basic unit of analysis for this genre is the *speech act*, a construct derived from early work in the philosophy of language (Austin, 1965; Searle, 1969). Speech acts are utterances defined by their pragmatic functions, such as making statements, asking questions, making promises, and giving orders. The sequence of speech acts can display a coherence that extends beyond any one speech act. On this basis, van Dijk (1981) proposes his notion of a *macro-speech act*, which consists of sequences of speech acts that function socially as one unit. The use of these speech acts during turn-taking in conversation is also rule-governed (Sacks, Schegloff, and Jefferson, 1974; Schegloff, 1982). Another important pragmatic framework that guides the overall coherence of information exchange is that of a *cooperative principle* (Grice, 1975). It subsumes the maxims of *quantity*, *quality*, *relation*, and *manner*, which guide the amount, clarity, and relevance of information required in conversations between interlocutors. Finally, some of the most recent and socially relevant work in conversational discourse extends the notion of context by focusing strongly on context in a variety of social settings. In this research, context is specified broadly to include participants and their relative roles in particular societal settings in a given culture (e.g., Tannen, 1994).

The advantage of discourse analysis lies in its potential to address both linguistic and cognitive factors underlying a range of normal and disordered communication performance.

See also DISCOURSE IMPAIRMENTS.

—*Hanna K. Ulatowska and Gloria Streit Olness*

References

Austin, J. L. (1965). *How to do things with words*. New York: Oxford University Press.

Bamberg, M. G. W. (Ed.). (1997). *Oral versions of personal experience: Three decades of narrative analysis. Journal of Narrative and Life History*, 7. [Special issue]

Bartlett, F. (1932). *Remembering*. Cambridge, U.K.: Cambridge University Press.

Chafe, W. L. (1980). The deployment of consciousness in the production of a narrative. In *Advances in discourse processes: Vol. 4. The Pear stories: Cognitive, cultural, and linguistic aspects of narrative production* (pp. 9–50) (R. O. Freedle, series ed., and W. L. Chafe, vol. ed.). Norwood, NJ: Ablex.

Grice, H. P. (1975). Logic and conversation. In P. Cole and J. Morgan (Eds.), *Syntax and semantics: Vol. 3. Speech acts* (pp. 41–58). New York: Academic Press.

Halliday, M. A. K. (1985). *An introduction to functional grammar*. London: Edward Arnold.

Halliday, M. A. K., and Hasan, R. (1976). *Cohesion in English*. London: Longman.

Labov, W. (1972). *Language in the inner city: Studies in the Black English Vernacular*. Philadelphia: University of Pennsylvania Press.

Labov, W., and Waletzky, J. (1967). Narrative analysis: Oral versions of personal experience. In J. Helm (Ed.), *Essays of the verbal and visual arts: Proceedings of the 1996 Annual Spring Meeting of the American Ethnological Society* (pp. 12–44). Seattle: University of Washington Press.

Longacre, R. E. (1981). A spectrum and profile approach to discourse analysis. *Text, 1*, 337–359.

Longacre, R. E. (1996). *The grammar of discourse* (2nd ed.). New York: Plenum Press.

Mandler, J. M. (1984). *Stories, scripts and scenes: Aspects of schema theory*. Hillsdale, NJ: Erlbaum.

Polanyi, L. (1989). *Telling the American story*. Cambridge, MA: MIT Press.

Propp, V. (1968/1928). *Morphology of the folktale* (L. Scott, trans.). Austin: University of Texas Press.

Sacks, H., Schegloff, E. A., and Jefferson, G. (1974). A simplest systematics for the organization of turn-taking in conversation. *Language, 50,* 696–735.

Schank, R. C., and Abelson, R. P. (1977). *Scripts, plans, goals, and understanding.* Hillsdale, NJ: Erlbaum.

Schegloff, E. A. (1980). Preliminaries to preliminaries: "Can I ask you a question?" *Sociological Inquiry, 50,* 104–152.

Schegloff, E. A. (1982). Discourse as an interactional achievement: Some uses of "uh huh" and other things that come between sentences. In D. Tannen (Ed.), *Georgetown University Round Table on Languages and Linguistics. Analyzing discourse: Text and talk* (pp. 71–93). Washington, DC: Georgetown University Press.

Schiffrin, D. (1994). *Approaches to discourse.* Cambridge, MA: Blackwell.

Searle, J. (1969). *Speech acts.* Cambridge, U.K.: Cambridge University Press.

Tannen, D. (1994). *Gender and discourse.* New York: Oxford University Press.

van Dijk, T. A. (1981). *Studies in the pragmatics of discourse.* The Hague: Mouton.

van Dijk, T. A., and Kintsch, W. (1983). *Strategies of discourse comprehension.* New York: Academic Press.

Further Readings

Brown, G., and Yule, G. (1983). *Discourse analysis.* Cambridge, U.K.: Cambridge University Press.

Bruner, J. (1991). The narrative construction of reality. *Critical Inquiry, 18,* 1–21.

Chafe, W. L. (1979). The flow of thought and the flow of language. In T. Givón (Ed.), *Syntax and semantics: Vol. 12. Discourse and syntax* (pp. 159–182). New York: Academic Press.

Clark, H., and Haviland, J. (1977). Comprehension and the given-new contract. In R. O. Freedle (Ed.), *Discourse processes: Advances in research and theory. Vol. 1. Discourse production and comprehension* (pp. 1–40). Norwood, NJ: Ablex.

Gee, J. P. (1986). Units in the production of narrative discourse. *Discourse Processes, 9,* 391–422.

Gee, J. P. (1991). A linguistic approach to narrative. *Journal of Narrative and Life History, 1,* 15–39.

Grice, H. P. (1957). Meaning. *Philosophical Review, 67,* 377–388.

Grimes, J. E. (1975). *The thread of discourse.* The Hague: Mouton.

Gumperz, J. (1982). *Discourse strategies.* Cambridge, U.K.: Cambridge University Press.

Kintsch, W. (1988). The role of knowledge in discourse comprehension: A constructive-integration model. *Psychological Review, 85,* 363–394.

Linde, C. (1993). *Life stories: The creation of coherence.* Oxford, U.K.: Oxford University Press.

Martin, J. R. (1992). *English text: System and structure.* Amsterdam: Benjamins.

Ochs, E. (1979). Planned and unplanned discourse. In T. Givón (Ed.), *Syntax and semantics: Vol. 12. Discourse and syntax* (pp. 51–80). New York: Academic Press.

Ochs, E. (1997). Narrative. In T. A. van Dijk (Ed.), *Discourse studies: A multidisciplinary introduction. Vol. 1. Discourse as structure and process* (pp. 185–207). Thousand Oaks, CA: Sage.

Sacks, H. (1992). *Lectures on conversation.* Cambridge, MA: Blackwell.

Schegloff, E. A. (1990). On the organization of sequences as a source of "coherence" in talk-in-interaction. In B. Dorval (Ed.), *Conversational organization and its development* (pp. 51–77). Norwood, NJ: Ablex.

Schiffrin, D. (1994). *Approaches to discourse.* Oxford, U.K.: Blackwell.

Tannen, D. (Ed.). (1984). *Coherence in spoken and written discourse.* Norwood, NJ: Ablex.

Tannen, D. (1984). *Conversational style.* Norwood, NJ: Ablex.

van Dijk, T. A. (1972). *Some aspects of text grammars.* The Hague: Mouton.

van Dijk, T. A. (1977). *Text and context: Explorations in the semantics and pragmatics of discourse.* New York: Longman.

van Dijk, T. A. (1980). *Macrostructures.* The Hague: Mouton.

van Dijk, T. A. (1981). *Studies in the pragmatics of discourse.* The Hague: Mouton.

van Dijk, T. A. (Ed.). (1997). *Discourse as structure and process.* Thousand Oaks, CA: Sage.

Wierzbicka, A. (1985). Different cultures, different languages, different speech acts. *Journal of Pragmatics, 9,* 145–163.

Discourse Impairments

The history of aphasiology dates back more than a century, but impairments of discourse abilities have only recently been described. Whereas changes in discourse abilities have always been part of the qualitative description of language following a brain lesion, the conceptual frameworks needed to identify impaired components of discourse in brain-damaged individuals have been available only since the late 1970s (Joanette and Brownell, 1990). Initial descriptions of discourse impairments essentially referred to traditional linguistic indicators, such as the noun-verb ratio or the percentage of subordinate clauses (e.g., Berko-Gleason et al., 1980; Obler and Albert, 1984). With increasing knowledge about the organization of the meaning conveyed in discourse, more specific descriptors have been introduced, such as coherence (e.g., Irigaray, 1973) or T-units (e.g., Ulatowska et al., 1983). However, those concepts and descriptors were not connected with a broader conceptual framework of discourse. Only recently have general integrative discourse models made it possible to link these various discourse components and to capture the different levels of cognitive processing needed in order to convey or understand verbal communication. This article summarizes discourse impairments associated with different pathological conditions with reference to these integrated frameworks.

Levels of Discourse Processing

Discourse is a set of utterances aimed at conveying a message among interlocutors. It can take many forms, such as narrative, argument, or conversation. Because it combines language components in a communicative context, discourse may be the most elaborate linguistic activity. The complexity of this activity can be captured through multilevel models, such as that proposed by

Carl Frederiksen (Frederiksen et al., 1990), in which each level of processing can be analyzed separately. Selective impairments of these levels, leading to distinct discourse patterns, may be used to differentiate among various adult populations with neurological disorders.

Seminal work by Kintsch and van Dijk (1978) largely inspired current integrated discourse models (for a review, see Mross, 1990). According to these models, discourse processing—production or comprehension—results from a number of cognitive operations that take place on four levels of representation:

- *Surface level*—Traditional linguistic units such as phonemes or graphemes, morphemes, words, and their combination into sentences constitute the surface level. Impairments at this level are described elsewhere in this book.
- *Semantic level*—Concepts expressed in discourse, along with the links between them, constitute the semantic level of processing. The smallest semantic unit is the microproposition, which is made up of a predicate (typically expressed by verbs or prepositions) and one or more arguments (typically expressed by nouns). Discourse meaning can thus be represented as a semantic network made up of a list of hierarchically related micropropositions. The main ideas of a discourse can be represented by macropropositions. On the receptive side, these macropropositions are constructed by applying rules in order to condense, eliminate, or generalize micropropositions. The latter are related through logical, inferential, or pragmatic links to the world depicted by the discourse. Mirror processing stages allow one to go from the main ideas of communicative intent to micropropositional discourse. The semantic level of discourse largely depends on the individual's semantic memory (general knowledge) and is independent of the linguistic (surface) level.
- *Situational level*—The processing of micropropositions and the relations among them leads to the construction of a situation model based on the subject's world knowledge. The situational level corresponds to the representation of the situation or events depicted in the discourse constructed by the interlocutor.
- *Structural level*—Finally, the structural level corresponds to the sequential and temporal organization of meaning units in a discourse. This level is known as the structure of a discourse and is identified as the discourse *schema*, *script*, or *frame*. It is at this level that distinctions among narrative, argumentative, procedural, or conversational discourse can be made.

Impairments of Discourse by Level of Processing

Surface-level impairments constitute the essence of aphasia as traditionally defined: phoneme, morpheme, word, and sentence impairments. The presence of impairments at this level usually makes it difficult to appreciate other levels of discourse. This explains why discourse impairments are most likely to be noticed in individuals without surface-level deficits, such as those with right hemisphere damage, traumatic brain injury, or early-stage Alzheimer's disease.

Few studies have looked for impairments at the microstructural level. In one such study, Joanette et al. (1986) showed that both patients with right hemisphere damage and normal controls produced discourse with similar microstructure. Stemmer and Joanette (1998) confirmed this observation but found that individuals with left hemisphere damage tended to produce more fragmented micropropositions, lacking in arguments. This resulted in a disruption of the connective structure of discourse, which requires predicates and arguments to be connected in order to form a semantic network of propositions. Numerous other studies have looked at cohesion, which can be considered representative of the microstructural level. *Cohesion* refers to the quality of local relationships between the elements of discourse and is frequently expressed through linguistic markers such as pronouns and conjunctions. Patients with traumatic brain injury, dementia, and in some cases right hemisphere damage have been reported to produce incohesive discourse typically characterized by the use of vague words or pronouns without clear referents. The lack of cohesion prevents the interlocutor from knowing what the speaker is talking about. In an incohesive discourse, micropropositions are also incomplete, since arguments are neither present nor identifiable, thus leading to a break in local coherence. Because local coherence is not established, discourse with cohesive problems can be viewed as a disconnected or incomplete semantic network.

The relationships among the elements of discourse form the macrostructure of a discourse. At this level, a logical progression of ideas ensures the global coherence of the discourse. Several authors have reported impairments at this level in the narrative discourse of patients with right brain damage, dementia, and traumatic brain injury (Nicholas et al., 1985; Glosser, 1993; Coelho, Liles, and Duffy, 1994; Ehrlich, 1994). Frequently the problem lies in the absence of principal ideas. Such discourse is incomplete and difficult to interpret. Another problem occurs when discourse contains unexpected information, in which case it is referred to as tangential. In such cases the links among ideas are not explicit and do not seem logical; this may happen with right-hemisphere-damaged individuals. Often, individuals who produce tangential discourse do not stay with the topic and jump from one subject to another. Such behavior may be attributed to some pragmatic inability to take the interlocutor's point of view into account and establish a common reference (Chantraine, Joanette, and Ska, 1998).

Discourse processing also requires the elaboration of a situation model. The presence of such a model testifies to the fact that the individual is able to make inferences by bridging several pieces of information. This ability is frequently impaired in patients with diffuse lesions (traumatic brain injury and dementia) or right brain damage. In some cases, patients' understanding is partial and remains at a superficial level. If such patients perceive contradictions, they often try to resolve them by invoking a plausible explanation from their own experience rather than from the information included or presupposed in the discourse. The difficulty in integrating information into a situation model has been proposed as an explanation for the inability to understand jokes, metaphors, or indirect requests that has been reported in patients with right brain damage and traumatic brain injury. In the case of dementia, it is thought to result from degradation of the semantic system itself.

The structural level of discourse is the level at which information is organized with respect to a given script, such as a narrative, which has to contain minimally a setting, a complication, and a resolution. Preservation of the text structure can guide the production or comprehension of discourse. Although text structure is considered to be robust, patients with traumatic brain injury and dementia have shown impairments at this level. For example, individuals with Alzheimer's disease may omit some components of the narrative schema, even when pictures are provided to support their production (Ska and Guénard, 1993). Script deficits in discourse are thought to result from impairments similar to those affecting routine activities of daily life through planning, organizing, selecting, and inhibiting information (Grafman, 1989). Patients with frontal lesions, for example, may exhibit difficulties in the sequential ordering of and hierarchical relations among actions belonging to a given script (Sirigu et al., 1995a, 1995b).

Discourse abilities and their impairments constitute a privileged component of communication and language that researchers can study in order to appreciate the interaction between so-called linguistic and other components of cognition. Although long addressed in purely descriptive terms, discourse impairments can now be understood with reference to comprehensive models of normal discourse processing. A description of discourse according to these models allows researchers to identify the levels characteristically impaired in individuals with particular brain lesions. The relationship between the various levels of discourse impairment and the different brain diseases or lesions is gradually becoming clearer. The availability of such specific descriptions will lead to a better understanding of the communicative disability affecting individuals with discourse impairments and should help clinicians develop strategies in order to help affected individuals overcome this disability.

See also DISCOURSE.

—*Bernadette Ska, Anh Duong, and Yves Joanette*

References

Berko-Gleason, G., Goodglass, H., Obler, L., Green, E., Hyde, M., and Weintraub, S. (1980). Narrative strategies of aphasic and normal speaking subjects. *Journal of Speech and Hearing Research, 23*, 370–382.

Chantraine, Y., Joanette, Y., and Ska, B. (1998). Conversational abilities in patients with right hemisphere damage. *Journal of Neurolinguistics, 11*, 21–32.

Coelho, C. A., Liles, B. Z., and Duffy, R. J. (1994). Cognitive framework: A description of discourse abilities in traumatically brain-injured adults. In R. L. Bloom, L. K. Obler, S. De Santi, and J. S. Ehrlich (Eds.), *Discourse analysis and applications: Studies in adult clinical populations* (pp. 81–94). Hillsdale, NJ: Erlbaum.

Ehrlich, J. S. (1994). Studies of discourse production in adults with Alzheimer's disease. In R. L. Bloom, L. K. Obler, S. De Santi, and J. S. Ehrlich (Eds.), *Discourse analysis and applications: Studies in adult clinical populations* (pp. 149–160). Hillsdale, NJ: Erlbaum.

Frederiksen, C. H., Bracewell, R. J., Breuleux, A., and Renaud, A. (1990). The cognitive representation and processing of discourse function and dysfunction. In Y. Joanette and H. H. Brownell (Eds.), *Discourse ability and brain damage: Theoretical and empirical perspectives* (pp. 69–110). New York: Springer-Verlag.

Glosser, G. (1993). Discourse production patterns in neurologically impaired and aged population. In H. H. Brownell and Y. Joanette (Eds.), *Narrative discourse in neurologically impaired and normal aging adults* (pp. 191–212). San Diego, CA: Singular Publishing Group.

Grafman, J. (1989). Plans, actions and mental sets: Managerial knowledge units in the frontal lobes. In E. Perecman (Ed.), *Integrating theory and practice in clinical neuropsychology* (pp. 93–138). Hillsdale, NJ: Erlbaum.

Irigaray, L. (1973). *Le langage des déments.* The Hague: Mouton.

Joanette, Y., and Brownell, H. H. (Eds.). (1990). *Discourse ability and brain damage: Theoretical and empirical perspectives.* New York: Springer-Verlag.

Joanette, Y., Goulet, P., Ska, B., and Nespoulous, J. L. (1986). Informative content of narrative discourse in right brain-damaged right-handers. *Brain and Language, 29*, 81–105.

Kintsch, W., and van Dijk, T. A. (1978). Toward a model of text comprehension and production. *Psychological Review, 85*, 363–394.

Mross, E. F. (1990). Text-analysis: Macro- and microstructural aspects of discourse processing. In Y. Joanette and H. H. Brownell (Eds.), *Discourse ability and brain damage: Theoretical and empirical perspectives* (pp. 50–68). New York: Springer-Verlag.

Nicholas, M., Obler, L. K., Albert, M. L., and Helm-Estabrooks, N. (1985). Empty speech in Alzheimer's disease and fluent aphasia. *Journal of Speech and Hearing Research, 28*, 405–410.

Obler, L. K., and Albert, M. L. (1984). Language in aging. In M. L. Albert (Ed.), *Neurology of aging* (pp. 245–253). New York: Oxford University Press.

Sirigu, A., Zalla, T., Pillon, B., Grafman, J., Agid, Y., and Dubois, B. (1995a). Selective impairments in managerial knowledge following pre-frontal cortex damage. *Cortex, 31*, 301–316.

Sirigu, A., Zalla, T., Pillon, B., Grafman, J., Agid, Y., and Dubois, B. (1995b). Encoding of sequence and boundaries of script following prefrontal lesions. *Cortex, 32*, 297–310.

Ska, B., and Guénard, D. (1993). Narrative schema in dementia of the Alzheimer's type. In H. H. Brownell and Y. Joanette (Eds.), *Narrative discourse in neurologically impaired and normal aging adults* (pp. 299–316). San Diego, CA: Singular Publishing Group.

Stemmer, B., and Joanette, Y. (1998). The interpretation of narrative discourse of brain-damaged individuals within the framework of a multilevel discourse model. In M. Beeman and C. Chiarello (Eds.), *Right hemisphere language comprehension: Perspectives from cognitive neuroscience* (pp. 329–348). Mahwah, NJ: Erlbaum.

Ulatowska, H. K., Freedman-Stern, R., Weiss Doyal, A., and Maccaluso-Haynes, S. (1983). Production of narrative discourse in aphasia. *Brain and Language, 19*, 317–334.

Functional Brain Imaging

Several techniques are now available to study the functional anatomy of speech and language processing by measuring neurophysiological activity noninvasively. This entry reviews the four dominant methods, electroencephalography (EEG) and magnetoencephalography (MEG), which measure the extracranial electromagnetic field, and positron emission tomography (PET) and functional magnetic resonance imaging (fMRI), which measure local changes in blood flow associated with active neurons. Each of these techniques has inherent strengths and weaknesses that must be taken into account when designing and interpreting experiments.

EEG and MEG respectively measure the electrical and magnetic field generated by large populations of synchronously active neurons with millisecond temporal resolution (Hamalainen et al., 1993; Nunez, 1995). Asynchronous activity cannot be easily detected because the signals produced by individual cells tend to cancel each other out rather than summing to produce a measurable signal at sensors or electrodes outside the head. The bulk of EEG and MEG signals appear to be generated not by action potentials but by postsynaptic potentials in the dendritic trees of pyramidal cells.

Although EEG has excellent temporal resolution, on the order of milliseconds, it is limited by poor spatial resolution because of the smearing of the potentials by the skull (Nunez, 1981). As a consequence, it is very difficult to identify the source of a signal from the distribution of electric potentials on the scalp. For any given surface distribution, there are many possible source distributions that might have produced the surface pattern—thus, *the inverse problem has no unique solution*. This complication is particularly significant where there are multiple generators, as is often the case in speech and language studies. The signals from different neural generators are mixed together in the potentials recorded at scalp electrodes.

EEG measures the electrical field produced by synchronous neural activity; MEG measures the magnetic fields associated with these electric current sources. There are important differences, however, between MEG and EEG signals. First, magnetic fields are unaffected by the tissue they pass through, so there is far less distortion of the signal between the source and the sensor in comparison to EEG (Hamalainen et al., 1993). Second, because most MEG is a measure of only the radial component of the magnetic field, MEG is effectively blind to activity that occurs in cortical areas that are oriented roughly parallel to the sensor (i.e., mostly gyral convexities). Conveniently for speech scientists, most of human auditory cortex is buried inside the sylvian fissure, making MEG ideal for recording auditory or speech-evoked fields. MEG has a temporal resolution comparable to that of EEG. Theoretically, MEG has somewhat better spatial resolution than EEG because magnetic fields pass unaffected through the tissues of the head, but this benefit is partly cancelled by the greater distance imposed between MEG sensors and the brain. Source localization in MEG is still limited by the non-uniqueness of the inverse problem, which becomes increasingly troublesome as the number of signal generators increases.

Most EEG and MEG studies in speech and language use an event-related potential (ERP) design. In such a design, the onset of EEG recording is time-locked to the onset of an event—say, the presentation of a stimulus—and the resulting EEG response is recorded. Because the ERP signal is a small component of the overall EEG signal, the event of interest must be repeated several times (up to 100), and the responses averaged. Another increasingly popular use of electromagnetic responses involves mapping regional correlations (synchrony) in oscillatory activity during cognitive and perceptual processes (Singer, 1999), which has been suggested to reflect cross-region binding.

Unlike the electromagnetic recording techniques, hemodynamic techniques such as PET and fMRI measure neural activity only indirectly (Villringer, 2000). The basic phenomenon underlying these methods is that an increase in neural activity leads to an increase in metabolic demand for glucose and oxygen, which in turn appears to be fed by a localized increase in cerebral blood flow (CBF) to the active region. It is these hemodynamic reflections of the underlying neural activity that PET and fMRI measure, although in different ways.

PET measures regional CBF (rCBF) in a fairly straightforward manner (Cherry and Phelps, 1996): water (typically) is labeled with a radioactive tracer, oxygen 15; the radiolabeled material is introduced into the bloodstream, typically intravenously; metabolically active regions in the brain have an increased rate of blood delivery, and therefore receive a greater concentration of the radioactive tracer; the regional concentrations of the tracer in the brain can then be measured using a PET scanner, which detects the decay of the radioactive tracer. As the tracer material decays, positrons are emitted from the radioactive nucleus and collide with electrons. Such a collision results in annihilation of the positron and electron and the generation of two gamma rays that travel away from the site of the collision in opposite directions and exit the head. The PET scanner, which is composed of a ring of gamma ray sensors, detects the simultaneous arrival of two gamma rays on opposite sides of the sensor array, and from this information the location of the collision site can be determined. PET also measures other aspects of local energy metabolism using different labeled compounds, based on the same principle, namely, that the amount of the agent taken up is proportional to the local metabolic rate. Oxygen metabolism is measured with oxygen labeled with oxygen 15, and glucose metabolism is measured with a molecule similar to glucose called deoxyglucose labeled with fluorine 18. The spatial resolution of PET is ultimately limited by the average distance a positron travels before it collides with an electron, which is in the range of a few millimeters. In practice, however, a typical PET study has a spatial resolution of about 1 cm.

The temporal resolution of PET is poor, ranging from approximately 1 minute for oxygen-based experiments to 30 minutes for glucose-based studies.

Typical PET experiments contrast rCBF maps generated in two or more experimental conditions. For example, one might contrast the rCBF map produced by listening to speech sounds with that produced in a resting baseline scan with no auditory input. Subtracting the resting baseline map from the speech-sound activation map would yield a different map highlighting just those brain regions that show a relative increase in metabolic activity during speech perception. Many studies attempt to isolate subcomponents of a complex process by using a variety of clever control conditions rather than a resting baseline. Whereas this general approach has yielded important insights, it must be used cautiously because it makes several assumptions that may not hold true. One of these, the "pure insertion" assumption, is that cognitive operations are built largely of noninteracting stages, such that manipulating one stage will not affect processes occurring at another stage. This assumption has been seriously questioned, however (Sartori and Umilta, 2000). Another assumption of the subtraction method is that the component processes of interest have neural correlates that are to some extent modularly organized, and further that the modules are sufficiently spatially distinct to be detected using current methods. In some cases this assumption may be valid, but in others it may not be, so again, caution is warranted in interpreting results of subtraction-based designs. These issues arise in fMRI designs as well.

Experimental designs that do not rely on subtraction logic are becoming increasingly popular. Correlational studies, for example, typically scan the participants under several parametrically varied levels of a variable and look for rCBF patterns across scans that correlate with the manipulated variable. For example, one might look for brain regions that show systematic increases in rCBF as a function of increasing memory load or of increasing rate of stimulus presentation. Alternatively, it is possible in a between-subject design to look for correlations between rCBF and performance on a behavioral measure.

In order to increase signal-to-noise ratios in PET studies, data from several participants are averaged. To account for individual differences in brain anatomy, each participant's PET scans are normalized to a standard stereotaxic space and spatially smoothed prior to averaging (Evans, Collins, and Holmes, 1996). Group averaged CBF maps are then overlaid onto normalized anatomical MR images for spatial localization. Group averaging does improve the signal-to-noise ratio, but it also has drawbacks. First, there is some loss of spatial resolution. This is important, not just in terms of localizing the precise site of an activation, but also in terms of the ability to detect activations in the first place: spatially smaller activations are less likely to be detected than larger ones, even if they are equally robust, simply because there is a reduced likelihood of small activations overlapping precisely in spatial location across subjects.

A related drawback is that it is often hard to distinguish between a difference in activation level and a difference in spatial distribution.

fMRI also is sensitive to hemodynamic changes, but not in the same way as PET. fMRI is based on a rather surprising physiological fact: when a region of brain is activated, both CBF and the metabolic rate of oxygen increase, but the CBF increase is much larger. This means that the local venous blood is more oxygenated during activation, even though the metabolic rate of oxygen has increased. The physiological significance of this is still not understood, but one possibility is that the increased level of tissue oxygen is necessary to drive a higher oxygen flux into the mitochondria. The most commonly used fMRI technique is sensitive to these changes in the oxygen concentration of blood; this is the BOLD, or blood oxygenation level dependent, signal (Chen and Ogawa, 2000). The BOLD signal is intrinsic to the blood response, and so, unlike in PET, no radioactive tracers are needed. A typical fMRI experiment involves imaging the brain repeatedly, collecting a volume of images every few seconds for a period of several minutes, during which time the participant is presented with alternating blocks of two (or more) stimulus or task conditions. Brain areas that are differentially active in one condition versus another will show a modulation of the MR image intensity over time that correlates with the stimulus (task) cycles. Under ideal conditions the spatial resolution of fMRI comes close to the size of a cortical column, although in most applications the resolution is closer to 3–6 mm (Kim et al., 2000). The temporal resolution of fMRI is limited by the variability of the hemodynamic response. Under ideal conditions, fMRI appears to be capable of resolving stimulus onset asynchronies in the range of a few hundreds of milliseconds, and there is some indication that even better temporal resolution (tens of milliseconds) is possible (Bandettini, 2000). However, in most applications the temporal resolution ranges from about 1 s to tens of seconds, depending on the design.

Because fMRI measures intrinsic signals, it is possible to present the stimulus (task) conditions in short alternating blocks, or even as a series of individual events, within a single scan, unlike a PET study (Aguirre, 2000). Typical block design experiments present four to eight cycles of alternating blocks of different stimulus (task) conditions per scan. Event-related fMRI designs, which are modeled on ERP experiments, present stimuli individually rather than in blocks. This affords greater flexibility in experimental design: items consisting of different conditions can be randomly intermixed to decrease predictability of the upcoming items, and the blood responses to items can be sorted and averaged in a variety of ways, for example by accuracy or reaction time of simultaneously collected behavioral responses. The disadvantages of event-related designs include decreased amplitude of the response due to shorter stimulus durations, and increased sensitivity to regional differences in response onset, which can provide better information in the temporal domain but also can make it difficult to model the hemodynamic response equally well across all activated brain regions.

fMRI is more sensitive than PET, allowing the detection of reliable signals in individual subjects. Despite this distinct advantage, most fMRI analyses are modeled on PET procedures, with spatial normalization of individual data sets, group averaging, and overlaying of activation maps onto normalized anatomical images. Also, as in PET experiments, most fMRI experiments utilize subtraction-based designs or correlational methods. Although fMRI has several advantages over PET, it also has several drawbacks related primarily to artifacts introduced into the signal from head motion, physiological noise (respiration, cardiac pulsations), and inhomogeneities in the magnetic field coming from a variety of sources. Another drawback, particularly relevant for speech/language studies, is the greater than 100 dB noise generated by the magnet during image acquisition. A potentially promising solution to this latter problem involves presenting auditory stimuli during silent periods between image acquisition (Hall et al., 1999).

—*Gregory Hickok*

References

Aguirre, G. K. (2000). Experimental design for brain fMRI. In C. T. W. Moonen and P. A. Bandettini (Eds.), *Functional MRI* (pp. 369–380). New York: Springer.

Bandettini, P. A. (2000). The temporal resolution of functional MRI. In C. T. W. Moonen and P. A. Bandettini (Eds.), *Functional MRI* (pp. 205–220). New York: Springer.

Chen, W., and Ogawa, S. (2000). Principles of BOLD functional MRI. In C. T. W. Moonen and P. A. Bandettini (Eds.), *Functional MRI* (pp. 103–113). New York: Springer.

Cherry, S. R., and Phelps, M. E. (1996). Imaging brain function with positron emission tomography. In A. W. Toga and J. C. Mazziotta (Eds.), *Brain mapping: The methods* (pp. 191–221). San Diego, CA: Academic Press.

Evans, A. C., Collins, D. L., and Holmes, C. J. (1996). Computational approaches to quantifying human neuroanatomical variability. In A. W. Toga and J. C. Mazziotta (Eds.), *Brain mapping: The methods* (pp. 343–361). San Diego, CA: Academic Press.

Hall, D. A., Haggard, M. P., Akeroyd, M. A., Palmer, A. R., Summerfield, A. Q., Elliott, M. R., et al. (1999). "Sparse" temporal sampling in auditory fMRI. *Human Brain Mapping*, 7, 213–223.

Hamalainen, M., Hari, R., Ilmonieli, R., Knuutila, J., and Lounasmaa, O. V. (1993). Magnetoencephalography: Theory, instrumentation, and applications to noninvasive studies of the working human brain. *Reviews of Modern Physics*, 65, 413–497.

Kim, S.-G., Lee, S. P., Goodyear, B., and Silva, A. C. (2000). Spatial resolution of BOLD and other fMRI techniques. In C. T. W. Moonen and P. A. Bandettini (Eds.), *Functional MRI* (pp. 195–203). New York: Springer.

Nunez, P. L. (1981). *Electric fields of the brain: The neurophysics of EEG*. New York: Oxford University Press.

Nunez, P. L. (1995). *Neocortical dynamics and human EEG rhythms*. New York: Oxford University Press.

Sartori, G., and Umilta, C. (2000). How to avoid the fallacies of cognitive subtraction in brain imaging. *Brain and Language*, 74, 191–212.

Singer, W. (1999). Neurobiology: Striving for coherence. *Nature*, 397, 391–393.

Villringer, A. (2000). Physiological changes during brain activation. In C. T. W. Moonen and P. A. Bandettini (Eds.), *Functional MRI* (pp. 3–13). New York: Springer.

Inclusion Models for Children with Developmental Disabilities

During 1998–99, 5,541,166 students with disabilities, or 8.75% of the school-age population ages 6–21 years, received special education and related services under Part B of the federal Individuals with Disabilities Education Act (IDEA) (U.S. Department of Education, 2000). IDEA specifies 13 disability categories based on etiological groupings. The largest single category of disability served is specific learning disabilities (50.8%), with speech and language impairments the second largest category (19.4%). Children with mental retardation account for 11.0%, while children with autism, considered a low incidence disability, constitute 1% of those receiving special education and related services. Since the original passage in 1975 of IDEA's forerunner, the Education for All Handicapped Children Act, the categorical model has served as the basis for determining who qualifies for special education in accord with two premises. First, each disability category represents a separate and distinct condition that may co-occur with others but is not identical (Lyon, 1996), and second, dissimilar disability conditions, or deficits, require educational programs that differ from regular education programs.

The concept of inclusive schooling emerged during the 1980s and gained momentum in the 1990s in response to the two categorical premises of IDEA and its predecessor. Special education was viewed as a form of de facto segregation for children with disabilities. Furthermore, special education had assumed the mantle of a placement setting rather than seeing its primary function under federal regulations as the source of specially designed instruction and support services intended to meet children's unique learning needs (Giangreco, 2001). Because of these reasons, major educational reforms were necessary to transform schools and instruction (Skrtic, 1992). Educational equity and excellence for all students required "a restructured system of education, one that eliminates categorical special needs programs by eliminating the historical distinction between general and special education" (Skrtic, Sailor, and Gee, 1996, p. 146). Inclusive schooling became the democratic mechanism proposed to accomplish this restructuring. From the perspectives of curriculum and instruction, inclusive practices in a single system of education should foster engaged learning. All classrooms should be learner-centered, children should be supported to become active and self-regulated learners, and instructional practices should be grounded to theme-based units, cooperative learning, team teaching, and student-teacher dialogue that scaffolds critical inquiry in both intellectual and social realms (National Research Council, 1999, 2000).

IDEA specifies that children with disabilities must be educated in the least restrictive environment. This means that, to the greatest possible extent, a child should be educated with children who do not have disabilities and an explanation must be provided in the Individualized Educational Plan (IEP) of the degree, if any, to which a child will not participate in regular class activities (Office of Special Education and Rehabilitation Services [OSERS], 2000). In the practical implementation of this requirement in the past 10 years, the terms *least restrictive environment*, *mainstreaming*, and *inclusion* often have become confused (Osborne, 2002). *Least restrictive environment* is a *legal requirement*. It specifies that children can be removed from the regular education classroom for special education placement only if the nature and severity of the child's disability are such that education in regular classes with the use of supplementary aids and services cannot be satisfactorily achieved (OSERS, 2000). In other words, maintenance in the regular education classroom means that children receive special education and related services for less than 21% of the school day. *Mainstreaming* is an *educational practice* that refers to the placement of students in regular education for part of the school day, such as physical education or science classes.

Inclusion is neither specified in law nor regulations as a placement. Similar to resource rooms and self-contained classrooms as optional placement settings, inclusion is also an option along the educational continuum of the least restrictive environment. In its broadest sense, inclusion is an *educational philosophy* about schooling. Inclusive schools are communities of learners "where everyone belongs, is accepted, supports, and is supported by his or her peers and other members of the school community while his or her educational needs are met" (Stainback, Stainback, and Jackson, 1992, p. 5). Full inclusion is the complete integration of the regular and special education systems where all children with disabilities receive their education, including special education and related services, as an integral part of the regular education curriculum. A major criticism of full inclusion models has been that placement decisions begin to take precedence over decisions about children's individual educational needs (Bateman, 1995). In contrast, partial inclusion, which is more typical of current inclusive schooling, pertains to those situations in which one or more classrooms within a school or school district are inclusive. Most advocates of full inclusion would consider partial inclusion as inconsistent with the philosophy of inclusive schooling. Moreover, judicial tests of inclusion have primarily involved students with moderate to severe cognitive disabilities. In general, in case law situations, courts have ruled that "inclusionary placement" should be the placement of choice, with a segregated placement occurring only when the evidence is overwhelming, despite the school district's best efforts, that inclusion is not feasible (Osborne, 2002).

Depending on state education laws, speech-language pathologists may provide either special education (instructional) services or, in conjunction with special education, related (support) services. The provision of related services must meet standards of educational necessity and educational relevance (Giangreco, 2001). In full and partial inclusion, special education and related services, as specified in an IEP, may be delivered through multiple models, all of which are premised on collaboration. In this sense, collaboration means that team participants have particular beliefs and possess certain skills (Silliman et al., 1999; Giangreco, 2000). These include (1) a shared belief in the philosophy of inclusion, (2) empowerment as decision makers combined with respect for varying decision-making values, (3) flexibility in problem solving about how best to meet the language and literacy needs of individual students, (4) the shared expertise made possible through coteaching strategies, and (5) high expectations for all students, regardless of their educational and disability status.

Based on the collaboration concept, the American Speech-Language-Hearing Association (ASHA, 1996) supported "inclusive practices" as an option for optimally meeting the educational needs of children and youth. A flexible array of service delivery models for implementing inclusive practices was also specified in accord with children's needs at different points in time. These four general models are not viewed as mutually exclusive or exhaustive. One model is *direct service delivery* in the form of "pull-out" services, considered appropriate only when there is a short-term objective for a child to achieve, such as acquisition of a new communication skill through direct teaching. A second model is *classroom-based service delivery*, in which the speech-language pathologist and teachers collaborate, for example through team teaching, to incorporate children's IEP goals across the curriculum. The composition of team teaching models varies, but the teams may include a regular education teacher, a teacher of specific learning disabilities, and a speech-language pathologist who works full-time in the classroom (e.g., Silliman et al., 1999). A third model is *community-based service delivery*, in which communication goals are specifically addressed in community settings, such as a vocational education program that is a focus of a transition service plan. This plan is designed to bridge between the secondary education curriculum and adulthood and must be included in an IEP for students beginning at age 14 years (OSERS, 2000). The *consultative model of service delivery* is a fourth model; its main characteristic is indirect assistance. This model may be most appropriate when a child's communication needs are so specific that they do not apply to other children in the classroom (ASHA, 1996).

For any inclusion model to be effective in meeting children's diverse needs, two foundations must be functional. One concerns the change process that serves to translate conceptually sound research into everyday instructional practices. The process of changing beliefs and practices must be explicitly understood, supported, and crafted to the particular educational situation (Skrtic, 1992; Gersten and Brengelman, 1996). The second fundamental support involves the building and sustaining of educational partnerships. A team's capacity to sustain innovative and educationally relevant practices requires the successful integration of collaborative principles and practices (Giangreco et al., 2000).

Few studies have evaluated the outcomes of inclusion programs for students with language impairments. At least three predicaments have contributed to this situation. The first is the co-occurring disabilities dilemma. Few inclusion programs have been reported in the literature that specifically focus on children classified as having language impairment as the primary condition. The absence of data can be attributed in part to the categorical model, which fails to account adequately for co-occurring disabilities, much less the existence of category overlap. For example, the U.S. Department of Education (2000) continues to report that, for identification and assessment purposes, "learning disabilities and language disorders may be particularly hard to distinguish … because these two disabilities present in similar ways" (p. II-32). Procedural requirements contribute one part of this dilemma. State education agencies typically report unduplicated counts of children with disabilities. Only the primary disability category is provided. For example, specific learning disability, mental retardation, or autism is often reported as the primary condition, with language impairment classified as the secondary condition. However, when duplicated counts are available, such as the count of all disabilities for each child that the Florida Department of Education provides (U.S. Department of Education, 2000), language impairment emerges as the most frequent disability associated with another disability.

Second is the broad variations in research purposes and methods. Most outcome studies have primarily addressed the social benefits of inclusion for children with severe development disabilities, such as autism or Down syndrome. The results are complicated to evaluate because of significant disparities among studies in their definitions of inclusion, sample characteristics, such as ages, grades, gender, and type of disabilities, and the instructional or intervention focus (McGregor and Vogelsberg, 1999; Murawski and Swanson, 2001).

Two major issues confront the design of future research on the efficacy of inclusive practices (ASHA, 1996). First, in studying the cognitive and social complexities of teaching and learning, multiple research methodologies pursued in a systematic manner are necessary for exploring, developing, and testing hypotheses (Friel-Patti, Loeb, and Gillam, 2001) about the efficacy of the four inclusion models. Second, in moving past the social outcome focus, research strategies should examine individual differences in the ability to benefit academically and linguistically from inclusive education as a product of variations in instructional practices, expanding the scope of investigation beyond children's performance on standardized measures of language and academic performance.

A third predicament is the broad variation in instructional practices in inclusive classrooms. The fact that disruptions in language and communication development are implicated in a wide range of disabilities but not acknowledged as central to children's literacy learning (Catts et al., 1999) also has significant ramifications for research on academic outcomes of inclusion. For example, the effects of inclusion on emerging reading skill have been reported in a limited manner, primarily for children classified with learning (severe reading) disabilities (Klingner et al., 1998), less so for children with language impairment (Silliman et al., 2000). In general, the reading instruction for these children remained undifferentiated from the reading practices used with other students in the classroom, resulting in minimal gains. Thus, shifting a child to inclusion from a special education placement, or even maintaining a child in the regular education classroom, may mean that little has changed for that child in reality.

One implication for instructional practices is that educational team members, including speech-language pathologists, should be skilled in designing multilevel instruction that takes into account the individual child's needs for the integration of oral language dimensions with evidence-based practices for learning to read, write, and spell (National Institute of Child Health and Human Development, 2000). A second implication, supported by ASHA (2001), is that speech-language pathologists are critical stakeholders in children's literacy learning. They have the professional responsibility to bring their knowledge of language to the planning and implementation of prevention, identification, assessment, and intervention programs in order to facilitate children's literacy development.

—*Elaine R. Silliman*

References

American Speech-Language-Hearing Association. (1996, Spring). Inclusive practices for children and youth with communication disorders: Position statement and technical report. *ASHA, 38*(Suppl. 16), 35–44.

American Speech-Language-Hearing Association. (2001). Roles and responsibilities of speech-language pathologists with respect to reading and writing in children and adolescents (position statement, executive summary of guidelines, technical report). *ASHA, Suppl. 21*, 17–27.

Bateman, B. D. (1995). Who, how, and where: Special education's issues in perpetuity. In J. M. Kaufman and D. P. Hallahan (Eds.), *The illusion of full inclusion: A comprehensive critique of a current special education bandwagon* (pp. 75–90). Austin, TX: Pro-Ed.

Catts, H. W., Fey, M. E., Zhang, X., and Tomblin, J. B. (1999). Language basis of reading and reading disabilities: Evidence from a longitudinal investigation. *Scientific Studies of Reading, 3*, 331–361.

Friel-Patti, S., Loeb, D. F., and Gillam, R. B. (2001). Looking ahead: An introduction to five exploratory studies of Fast ForWord. *American Journal of Speech-Language Pathology, 10*(3), 195–202.

Gersten, R., and Brengelman, S. U. (1996). The quest to translate research into classroom practice. *Remedial and Special Education, 17*, 67–74.

Giangreco, M. F. (2000). Related services research for students with low-incidence disabilities: Implications for speech-language pathologists in inclusive classrooms. *Language, Speech, and Hearing Services in Schools, 31,* 230–239.

Giangreco, M. F. (2001). *Guidelines for making decisions about IEP services.* Montpelier, VT: Vermont Department of Education [on-line]. Available: http://www.state.vt.us/educ/Cses/sped/main.htm.

Giangreco, M. F., Prelock, P. A., Reid, R. R., Dennis, R. E., and Edelman, S. W. (2000). Roles of related service personnel in inclusive schools. In R. A. Villa and J. S. Thousand (Eds.), *Restructuring for caring and effective education: Piecing the puzzle together* (pp. 360–388). Baltimore: Paul H. Brookes.

Klingner, J. K., Vaughn, S., Hughes, M. T., Schumm, J. S. S., and Elbaum, B. (1998). Outcomes for students with and without learning disabilities in inclusive classrooms. *Learning Disabilities: Research and Practice, 13,* 153–161.

Lyon, G. R. (1996, Spring). Learning disabilities. *The Future of Children, 6*(1), 54–76.

McGregor, G., and Vogelsberg, T. T. (1999). *Inclusive schooling practices and research foundations: A synthesis of the literature that informs best practices about inclusive schooling.* Baltimore: Paul H. Brookes.

Murawski, W. W., and Swanson, H. L. (2001). A meta-analysis of co-teaching research: Where are the data? *Remedial and Special Education, 22,* 258–267.

National Institute of Child Health and Human Development. (2000). *Report of the National Reading Panel. Teaching children to read: An evidence-based assessment of the scientific research literature on reading and its implications for reading instruction: Reports of the subgroups* (NIH Publication No. 00-4754). Washington, DC: U.S. Government Printing Office.

National Research Council. (1999). *How people learn: Bridging research and practice.* Washington, DC: National Academy Press.

National Research Council. (2000). *How people learn: Brain, mind, experience, and school* (expanded ed.). Washington, DC: National Academy Press.

Osborne, A. G., Jr. (2002). Legal, administrative and policy issues in special education. In K. G. Butler and E. R. Silliman (Eds.), *Speaking, reading, and writing in children with language learning disabilities: New paradigms for research and practice* (pp. 297–314). Mahwah, NJ: Erlbaum.

Office of Special Education and Rehabilitation Services, U.S. Department of Education. (2000, July). *A guide to the individualized education program* [on-line]. Available: http://www.ed.gov/offices/OSERS.

Silliman, E. R., Bahr, R., Beasman, J., and Wilkinson, L. C. (2000). Scaffolds for learning to read in an inclusion classroom. *Language, Speech, and Hearing Services in Schools, 31,* 265–279.

Silliman, E. R., Ford, C. S., Beasman, J., and Evans, D. (1999). An inclusion model for children with language learning disabilities: Building classroom partnerships. *Topics in Language Disorders, 19*(3), 1–18.

Skrtic, T. M. (1992). The special education paradox: Equity as the way to excellence. In T. Hehir and T. Latus (Eds.), *Special education at the century's end: Evolution of theory and practice since 1970* (pp. 203–272). Cambridge, MA: Harvard University Press.

Skrtic, T. M., Sailor, W., and Gee, K. (1996). Voice, collaboration, and inclusion: Democratic themes in educational and social reform initiatives. *Remedial and Special Education, 17,* 142–157.

Stainback, S., Stainback, W., and Jackson, H. J. (1992). Toward inclusive classrooms. In S. Stainback and W. Stainback (Eds.), *Curriculum considerations in inclusive classrooms: Facilitating learning for all students* (pp. 3–17). Baltimore: Paul H. Brookes.

U.S. Department of Education, Office of Special Education Programs. (2000). 22nd Annual Report to Congress on the Implementation of the Individuals with Disabilities Act [on-line]. Available: http://www.ed.gov/offices/OSERS/.

Further Readings

Catts, H. W., and Kamhi, A. G. (1999). Causes of reading disabilities. In H. W. Catts and A. G. Kamhi (Eds.), *Language and reading disabilities* (pp. 95–127). Boston, MA: Allyn and Bacon.

Ehren, B. J. (2000). Maintaining a therapeutic focus and sharing responsibility for student success: Keys to in-classroom speech-language services. *Language, Speech, and Hearing Services in Schools, 31,* 219–229.

Farber, J., and Klein, E. (1999). Classroom-based assessment of a collaborative intervention program with kindergarten and first grade children. *Language, Speech, and Hearing Services in Schools, 30,* 83–91.

Hadley, P. A., Simmerman, A., Long, M., and Luna, M. (2000). Facilitating language development for inner-city children: Experimental evaluation of a collaborative classroom-based intervention. *Language, Speech, and Hearing Services in Schools, 31,* 280–295.

Idol, L. (1997). Key questions related to building collaborative and inclusive schools. *Journal of Learning Disabilities, 30,* 384–394.

National Research Council. (2000). *From neurons to neighborhoods: The science of early childhood development.* Washington, DC: National Academy Press.

Prelock, P. A. (2000a). Prologue: Multiple perspectives for determining the roles of speech-language pathologists in inclusionary classrooms. *Language, Speech, and Hearing Services in Schools, 31,* 213–218.

Prelock, P. A. (2000b). Epilogue: An intervention focus for inclusionary practice. *Language, Speech, and Hearing Services in Schools, 31,* 296–298.

Prelock, P. A., Beatson. J., Contompasis, S. H., and Bishop, K. K. (1999). A model for family-centered interdisciplinary practice in the community. *Topics in Language Disorders, 19*(3), 36–51.

Pressley, M., and El-Dinary, P. B. (1997). What we know about translating comprehension-strategies instruction research into practice. *Journal of Learning Disabilities, 30,* 486–488.

Rankin-Erickson, J. L., and Pressley, M. (2000). A survey of instructional practices of special education teachers nominated as effective teachers of literacy. *Learning Disabilities: Research and Practice, 15,* 206–225.

Salisbury, C. L., and Dunst, C. J. (1997). Home, school, and community partnerships: Building inclusive teams. In B. Rainforth and J. York-Barr (Eds.), *Collaborative teams for students with severe disabilities: Integrating therapy and educational services* (pp. 57–87). Baltimore: Paul H. Brookes.

Snow, C. E., Burns, M. S., and Griffin, P. (1998). *Preventing reading difficulties in young children.* Washington, DC: National Academy Press.

Speece, D. L., MacDonald, V., Kilsheimer, L., and Krist, J. (1997). Research to practice: Preservice teachers reflect on reciprocal teaching. *Learning Disabilities: Research and Practice, 12,* 177–187.

Stone, C. A. (1998). The metaphor of scaffolding: Its utility for the field of learning disabilities. *Journal of Learning Disabilities*, *31*, 344–364.

Tabors, P. O., and Snow, C. E. (2001). Young bilingual children and early literacy development. In S. B. Neuman and D. K. Dickinson (Eds.), *Handbook of early literacy research* (pp. 159–178). New York: Guilford Press.

Tager-Flusberg, H. (Ed.). (1999). *Neurodevelopmental disorders*. Cambridge, MA: MIT Press.

Thousand, J., Diaz-Greenberg, R., Nevin, A., Cardelle-Elawar, M., Beckett, C., and Reese, R. (1999). Perspective: Perspectives on a Freirean dialectic to promote inclusive education. *Remedial and Special Education*, *20*, 323–328.

Westby, C. E. (1994). The vision of full inclusion: Don't exclude kids by including them. *Journal of Childhood Communication Disorders*, *16*, 13–22.

Zigmond, N. (1995). An exploration of the meaning and practice of the context of full inclusion of students with learning disabilities. *Journal of Special Education*, *29*, 109–115.

Language Development in Children with Focal Lesions

Many lines of evidence support the concept that the left hemisphere plays an essential and specialized role in language processing in adults. Studies of adults with focal brain injury find that approximately 95% of cases of aphasia are associated with left hemisphere damage (Goodglass, 1993). In the traditional view, damage to the third frontal convolution, Broca's area, is associated with problems in language production, whereas damage to the first temporal convolution, Wernicke's area, is associated with problems in language comprehension. However, the picture is more complex. The ability to predict the location of injury from the aphasic syndrome (or vice versa) is limited, and the right hemisphere remains involved in aspects of language processing, such as interpretation of prosody and metaphor and comprehension of complex syntax (Just et al., 1996). Nonetheless, the left hemisphere contribution to language seems to be necessary.

How, when, and why does the left hemisphere become specialized for language functions? The study of children who sustain focal left hemisphere damage prior to or during language development provides one experimental approach to address these issues. Rarely, children who have not yet learned to speak or who are still developing language skills sustain brain injury to areas of the left hemisphere that typically serve language function in adults. These children afford a naturalistic experimental opportunity to address the theoretical questions about the neural substrate of language learning.

If children with left hemisphere damage prior to language learning subsequently demonstrate serious delays in language development, the implication is that the mechanisms for language development reside within the damaged regions of the left hemisphere, a position called *early specialization*. Such findings would suggest that the neural architecture for language is determined by innate and probably genetic mechanisms. If, by contrast, children with left hemisphere damage successfully master language skills, the implication is that, at least under extreme circumstances, alternative organizations can be established. Such findings would suggest that the neural architecture of language is an outcome of language learning. In its strongest formulation, this second position asserts *equipotentiality*, that is, that either hemisphere can serve language functions as long as the neural commitment occurs before language learning forces left hemisphere specialization (Lenneberg, 1967). If children with left hemisphere damage show only minor delays, the implication is that alternative neural organizations are less favorable to language development or processing than the classical language areas (Satz, Strauss, and Whitaker, 1990), an intermediate position called *constrained plasticity* or *ontogenetic specialization*. This last position would suggest that some aspects of brain structure may be determined by early and possibly genetic factors, but that the full development of left hemisphere specialization emerges through development.

Challenges in the study of children with early focal brain injury complicate obtaining and interpreting findings. Before modern neural imaging modalities became available, the localization of damage was often uncertain; this review considers empirical studies that used computed tomography or magnetic resonance imaging for lesion location. Because early focal brain injuries are rare, published studies usually consist of small, heterogeneous samples. Age at onset, extent of lesion, time since injury, and associated problems vary within and across these groups, making meta-analyses impossible. The language capabilities of the infants, had they not sustained injury, remain uncertain. Other variables, including presence of seizure disorder or use of anticonvulsant medications, mediate outcomes (Vargha-Khadem et al., 1992). Given all the sources of potential variability, the use of group means to describe brain-injured populations may combine disparate groups and mask important distinctions. A preferable approach is individual profiling in the setting of a contrastive group of age- and developmentally matched children (Bishop, 1983).

An initial question to be addressed in considering the language development of children with focal lesions is their overall intelligence and cognitive profiles. If these children have severe intellectual impairments, then any language deficits should be evaluated in relation to cognitive measures such as intelligence quotient (IQ) tests. Most studies concur that children with focal injury to either hemisphere, even those with total surgical removal of a hemisphere, score at or near the population mean (Bates, Vicari, and Trauner, 1999). In children, unlike in adults, differential hemispheric mediation of verbal and performance or nonverbal functions is not typically found (Vargha-Khadem et al., 1992; Vargha-Khadem, Isaacs, and Muter, 1994; Bates, Vicari, and Trauner, 1999). The near-normal intellectual performance of children with focal damage is a testament to the plasticity of the human brain.

Development of Functional Communication Skills

Children with left hemisphere damage to the classical speech areas are not aphasic. Individual differences occur in fluency, intelligibility, frequency of initiation, and volume of output. However, in light of the chronic sensory and motor deficits that follow injury in these children and the severe disruption of language that follows similar injuries in adults, it is remarkable that their conversational language is normal or near normal (Bates et al., 1997).

Despite the favorable prognosis, children with focal injury to either hemisphere may experience developmental delays in the onset of babbling and communicative gestures (Marchman, Miller, and Bates, 1991), vocabulary development, and use of word combinations in parent-child conversations (Thal et al., 1991; Feldman et al., 1992). Once these children begin to acquire functional skills, they are comparable in their rate of developmental progress to each other and to children developing typically (Feldman et al., 1992). By age 4, children with focal left hemisphere damage can master even the complex morphosyntactic structures of Hebrew, at least using a criterion that multiple complex structures are present in the spoken output (Levy, Amir, and Shalev, 1994).

Location of injury is not related to rate of development in the manner predicted from studies of adults with brain injury. Children with right hemisphere damage initially show greater delays in initial word comprehension and production than children with left hemisphere damage, and children with posterior left hemisphere damage, presumably including Wernicke's area, develop more slowly than children with damage to other areas of the left hemisphere, including Broca's area (Thal et al., 1991; Bates et al., 1997). These findings implicate the centrality of pattern recognition and subsequently of language comprehension in the development of language production.

Children with focal damage achieve high-level language skills. By school age, they can produce narrative discourse. Their productions are shorter and syntactically less sophisticated than those of age-matched peers, but narrative skills are comparable in children with left hemisphere and right hemisphere damage (Reilly, Bates, and Marchman, 1998). Most children with early focal damage also learn to read, write, and spell, although the strategies they use may vary as a function of the side of the lesion (Dennis, Lovett, and Wiegel-Crump, 1981).

These findings suggest that a wide neural network involving both cerebral hemispheres is necessary to launch language development, so that damage to a neural substrate in either hemisphere may delay language development. Once language skills begin to develop and an initial neural network is beginning to be established, neural organization progresses at a similar rate as in an intact system. The system is capable of high-level skills, such as narrative discourse and reading, but damage anywhere in the system may reduce the levels of functioning in these areas, presumably because these skills, even in maturity, require an extensive neural network.

Performance on Specific and Formal Measures

Despite adequacy of conversational language, children with left hemisphere damage show subtle to moderate impairments in selective aspects of language. In children with injuries acquired during childhood, expressive and receptive complex syntax is particularly vulnerable (Aram, Ekelman, and Whitaker, 1986, 1987; Aram and Ekelman, 1987). At school age, an on-line sentence comprehension task suggested that their strategies for interpreting syntactic structures were developmentally delayed compared with those of normal learners (Feldman, MacWhinney, and Sacco, 2002). However, children with right hemisphere damage also showed developmental delays on this task. An alternative explanation to the interpretation that syntax skills may be particularly vulnerable to left hemisphere injuries is that subjects with left hemisphere damage have greatest difficulty with the most developmentally advanced areas on an experimental assessment (Bishop, 1983). In this regard, children who sustain left hemisphere damage in the perinatal period have also been shown to have more difficulties in lexical retrieval (Aram, Ekelman, and Whitaker, 1987), comprehension of difficult verbal material, and formulating sentences than children with right hemisphere injury (MacWhinney et al., 2000). They also show relatively more difficulties with reading, writing, and spelling than children with right hemisphere damage (Woods and Carey, 1978). The procedures that demonstrate the selective weaknesses of children with left hemisphere damage require precise and constrained performance, as opposed to the relatively free form of conversation.

On-line reaction time methodology has been used in school-age children with focal lesions to determine whether particular information processing abilities are selectively compromised in children with left hemisphere damage (MacWhinney et al., 2000). Children with both left and right hemisphere damage had slower reaction times than age-matched normal peers on all of the auditory and visual reaction time tasks studied. The two tasks that best distinguished children with left hemisphere damage from children with other lesions and normal children were verbally repeating numbers presented in the auditory mode and naming numbers presented in the visual mode, both tasks that require rapid verbal output.

Age at Injury

In most studies, the younger the child at the time of focal injury, the higher is the subsequent level of functioning in IQ and language. In children who sustain injuries after age 5, verbal IQ is more likely to be affected with left hemisphere damage and performance IQ with right hemisphere damage. Children who undergo total hemispherectomy for intractable seizures have better language if the operation is done before 1 year of age than after 1 (Dennis and Whitaker, 1976). Nonetheless, Vargha-Khadem and colleagues (1997) reported the case of a previously nonverbal child who began to speak at age 9 years, after he had undergone a hemispherectomy of the left hemisphere for seizures and a reduction in anticonvulsant medications. The ability to develop language appears to be preserved under some circumstances into middle childhood.

Brain Reorganization After Early Injury

Language functioning can be relocated to the right hemisphere after early damage to the left hemisphere. Previously, the method used to determine the eloquent hemisphere was a sodium amytal carotid infusion, used in the presurgical evaluation of individuals with intractable seizures. If this anesthetic disrupts language when infused into the carotid artery on one side but not the other, then that side is considered the "eloquent" hemisphere. Rasmussen and Milner (1977) found evidence that individuals with early left hemisphere injury were far more likely to have language in the right hemisphere than individuals with no previous left hemisphere injury, although some individuals with early left hemisphere injury retained language functioning in the left hemisphere.

Functional imaging offers a noninvasive method to reexplore this issue. The methods are appropriate for normal individuals as well as clinical populations and can be used to determine the areas of activation for many different tasks. In adults, functional magnetic resonance imaging (fMRI) has shown that a wide network of areas is involved in sentence interpretation (Just et al., 1996); activation was more likely to include right hemisphere locations as the sentence difficulty increased. Booth and colleagues (2000) used a similar fMRI paradigm to compare six children with perinatal injuries, four with damage to left hemisphere areas, to normal adults and normal children. In adults and normal children, a sentence comprehension task produced more activation in the left hemisphere than in the right hemisphere; greatest activation in the superior temporal, middle temporal, inferior frontal, and prefrontal areas; and right hemisphere recruitment for difficult sentences, particularly in the adults. The children with left hemisphere damage performed less accurately than normal children on the task. These children activated primarily a right hemisphere network and did not show an increase in activation as a function of sentence difficulty. The children with left hemisphere damage also had very poor performance on a mental rotation task that typically activates right hemisphere areas. This finding suggests that reorganization of language to the right hemisphere may compromise skills typically served by the right hemisphere.

A variety of basic science methods show that cortical tissue can take on a variety of functions, suggesting that the cortex is pluripotential, if not equipotential. Synaptic connections seem to be formed and preserved on the basis of experience. Experience-dependent commitment of neural substrate may explain some of the variability in the neural organization of basic functions seen across individuals. Many studies also demonstrate experience-dependent progressive specialization of neural tissue. In language development, studies of normal infants and toddlers using event-related potentials have shown that in the initial development of a language skill, such as word learning or recognition of syntactic markers, a bilateral network becomes activated. As skill level increases, the function lateralizes to the left hemisphere (Mills, Coffey-Corina, and Neville, 1993, 1997).

The language of children with focal injuries leads to similar views on the neural basis of language learning. The development of language initially seems to use a wide bilateral neural network, such that damage to either hemisphere delays the onset. For reasons that remain unclear, a slight advantage to the left hemisphere for language function results in progressive specialization of the left hemisphere as learning proceeds. If the left hemisphere is damaged, then the other cortical areas specialize to serve language function.

Language functions may be preserved in adjacent regions of the left hemisphere or in homologous regions of the right hemisphere, depending on multiple factors. Given the pluripotential nature of cortex, children with left hemisphere damage perform well in conversational language. However, they have selective difficulties when tasks require syntactic skills and other rapid, precise, or constrained linguistic processing. However, children with right hemisphere injury may also have subtle to moderate language disturbances. The plasticity of the brain for language function may come about at the expense of other neuropsychological functions, including visual-spatial processing. Functional imaging holds enormous promise for investigating the organization of language and other skills in intact individuals developing typically as well as in children with focal injuries.

—Heidi M. Feldman

References

Aram, D. M., and Ekelman, B. L. (1987). Unilateral brain lesions in childhood: Performance on the Revised Token Test. *Brain and Language, 32,* 137–158.

Aram, D. M., Ekelman, B. L., and Whitaker, H. A. (1986). Spoken syntax in children with acquired unilateral hemisphere lesions. *Brain and Language, 27,* 75–100.

Aram, D. M., Ekelman, B. L., and Whitaker, H. A. (1987). Lexical retrieval in left and right brain-lesioned chidlren. *Brain and Language, 38,* 105–121.

Bates, E., Thal, D., Trauner, D., Fenson, J., Aram, D., Eisele, J., and Nass, R. (1997). From first words to grammar in children with focal brain injury. *Developmental Neuropsychology, 13,* 447–476.

Bates, E., Vicari, S., and Trauner, D. (1999). Neural mediation of language development: Perspectives from lesion studies of infants and children. In H. Tager-Flusberg (Ed.), *Neurodevelopmental disorders* (pp. 533–581). Cambridge, MA: MIT Press.

Bishop, D. (1983). Linguistic impairment after left hemi-decortication for infantile hemiplegia? A reappraisal. *Quarterly Journal of Experimental Psychology, 35*(A), 199–207.

Booth, J. R., MacWhinney, B., Thulborn, K. R., Sacco, K., Voyvodic, J., and Feldman, H. M. (2000). Patterns of brain activation in children with strokes engaged in three cognitive tasks. *Developmental Neuropsychology, 18*, 139–169.

Dennis, M., Lovett, M., and Wiegel-Crump, C. A. (1981). Written language acquisition after left or right hemidecortication in infancy. *Brain and Language, 12*, 54–91.

Dennis, M., and Whitaker, H. A. (1976). Language acquisition following hemidecortication: Linguistic superiority of the left over the right hemisphere. *Brain and Language, 3*, 404–433.

Feldman, H. M., Holland, A. L., Kemp, S. S., and Janosky, J. E. (1992). Language development after unilateral brain injury. *Brain and Language, 42*, 89–102.

Feldman, H. M., MacWhinney, B., and Sacco, K. (2002). Sentence processing in children with early left hemisphere brain injury. *Brain and Language, 83*, 335–352.

Goodglass, D. (1993). *Understanding aphasia.* San Diego, CA: Academic Press.

Just, M., Carpenter, P., Keller, T., Eddy, W., and Thulborn, K. (1996). Brain activation modulated by sentence comprehension. *Science, 274*, 114–116.

Lenneberg, E. H. (1967). *Biological foundations of language.* New York: Wiley.

Levy, Y., Amir, N., and Shalev, R. (1994). Morphology in a child with a congenital, left-hemisphere brain lesion: Implications for normal acquisition. In *Constraints on language acquisition: Studies of atypical children.* Hillsdale, NJ: Erlbaum.

MacWhinney, B., Feldman, H., Sacco, K., and Valdes-Perez, R. (2000). Online measures of basic language skills in children with early focal brain lesions. *Brain and Language, 71*, 400–431.

Marchman, V. A., Miller, R., and Bates, E. (1991). Babble and first words in children with focal brain injury. *Applied Psycholinguistics, 12*, 1–22.

Mills, D. L., Coffey-Corina, S. A., and Neville, H. J. (1993). Language acquisition and cerebral specialization in 20-month-old infants. *Journal of Cognitive Neuroscience, 53*, 317–334.

Mills, D. L., Coffey-Corina, S. A., and Neville, H. J. (1997). Language comprehension and cerebral specialization from 13 to 20 months. *Developmental Neuropsychology, 13*, 397–445.

Rasmussen, T., and Milner, B. (1977). The role of early left brain injury in determining implications for models of language development. *Annals of the New York Academy of Sciences, 299*, 355–369.

Reilly, J. S., Bates, E. A., and Marchman, V. A. (1998). Narrative discourse in children with early focal brain injury. *Brain and Language, 61*, 335–375.

Satz, P., Strauss, E., and Whitaker, H. (1990). The ontogeny of hemispheric specialization: Some old hypotheses revisted. *Brain and Language, 38*, 596–614.

Thal, D., Marchman, V., Stiles, J., Aram, D., Trauner, D., Nass, R., and Bates, E. (1991). Early lexical development in children with focal brain injury. *Brain and Language, 40*(4), 491–527.

Vargha-Khadem, F., Carr, L. J., Isaacs, E., Brett, E., Adams, C., and Mishkin, M. (1997). Onset of speech after left hemispherectomy in a nine-year-old boy. *Brain, 120*(Pt. 1), 159–182.

Vargha-Khadem, F., Isaacs, E., and Muter, V. (1994). A review of cognitive outcome after unilateral lesions sustained during childhood. *Journal of Child Neurology, 9*(Suppl. 2), 67–73.

Vargha-Khadem, F., Isaacs, E., van der Werf, S., Robb, S., and Wilson, J. (1992). Development of intelligence and memory in children with hemiplegic cerebral palsy: The deleterious consequences of early seizures. *Brain, 115*(Pt. 1), 315–329.

Woods, B., and Carey, S. (1978). Language deficits after apparent clinical recovery from aphasia. *Annals of Neurology, 6*, 405–409.

Further Readings

Bates, E. (1999). Language and the infant brain. *Journal of Communication Disorders, 32*, 195–205.

Bishop, D. V. (1997). Cognitive neuropsychology and developmental disorders: Uncomfortable bedfellows. *Quarterly Journal of Experimental Psychology. A. Human Experimental Psychology, 50*, 899–923.

Dennis, M., Spiegler, B. J., and Hetherington, R. (2000). New survivors for the new millennium: Cognitive risk and reserve in adults with childhood brain insults. *Brain and Cognition, 42*, 102–105.

Eisele, J. A., and Aram, D. M. (1995). Lexical and grammatical development in children with early hemisphere damage: A cross-sectional view from birth to adolescence. In P. Fletcher and B. MacWhinney (Eds.), *Handbook of child language* (pp. 664–689). Oxford, U.K.: Blackwell.

Rivkin, M. J. (2000). Developmental neuroimaging of children using magnetic resonance techniques. *Mental Retardation and Developmental Disabilities Research Reviews, 6*, 68–80.

Semrud-Clikeman, M. (1997). Evidence from imaging on the relationship between brain structure and developmental language disorders. *Seminars in Pediatric Neurology, 4*, 117–124.

Vargha-Khadem, F. (2001). Generalized versus selective cognitive impairments resulting from brain damage sustained in childhood. *Epilepsia, 42*(Suppl. 1), 37–40.

Vargha-Khadem, F., Isaacs, E., Watkins, K., and Mishkin, M. (2000). Ontogenetic specialization of hemispheric function. In C. E. Polkey and M. Duchowney (Eds.), *Intractable focal epilepsy: Medical and surgical treatment* (pp. 405–418). London: Harcourt.

Volpe, J. J. (2001). Perinatal brain injury: From pathogenesis to neuroprotection. *Mental Retardation and Developmental Disabilities Research Reviews, 7*, 56–64.

Language Disorders in Adults: Subcortical Involvement

The first suggestion of a link between subcortical structures and language was made by Broadbent (1872), who proposed that words were generated as motor acts in the basal ganglia. Despite this suggestion, according to the classical anatomo-functional models of language organization proposed by Wernicke (1874) and Lichtheim (1885), subcortical brain lesions could only produce language deficits if they disrupted the white matter fibers that connect the various cortical language centres. Consequently, aphasia has traditionally been regarded as a language disorder resulting from damage to the language areas of the dominant cerebral cortex. Since the late 1970s, however, this traditional view has been challenged by the findings of an increasing number of cliniconeuroradiological correlation studies that have documented the occurrence of adult language disorders in association with apparently subcortical vascular lesions. In particular, the introduction in recent decades of new neuroradiological methods for lesion localization *in vivo*, including computed tomography in the 1970s and more recently magnetic resonance imaging, has led to an increasing number of reports in the literature of aphasia following apparently purely subcortical lesions. (For reviews of *in vivo* correlation studies, see Alexander, 1989; Cappa and Vallar, 1992, and Murdoch, 1996.) Therefore, although the concept of subcortical aphasia remains controversial, recent years have seen a growing acceptance of a role for subcortical structures in language. Despite an abundance of theoretical models, however, the precise nature of that role remains elusive.

Subcortical structures most commonly purported to have a linguistic role include the basal ganglia, the thalamus, and the subcortical white matter pathways. Some evidence for a role for the cerebellum in language has also been reported (Leiner, Leiner, and Dow, 1993). The basal ganglia comprise the corpus striatum (including the caudate nucleus and the putamen and internal capsule), the globus pallidus, the subthalamic nucleus, and the substantia nigra. Although these nuclei are primarily involved in motor functions, the corpus striatum and globus pallidus have frequently been included in models of subcortical participation in language. In addition, several thalamic nuclei have also been implicated in language, in particular the ventral anterior nucleus, which has direct connections to the premotor cortex and indirect connections to the temporoparietal cortex via the pulvinar. The basal ganglia and the thalamus are linked to the cerebral cortex by way of a series of circuits referred to as the cortico-striato-pallido-thalamo-cortical loops. The majority of contemporary theories specify these loops as the neuroanatomical basis of subcortical participation in language.

Although there is general agreement that critical white matter pathways and the thalamus are involved in language, controversy and uncertainty surround the possible linguistic role of striatocapsular structures. Although in vivo correlation studies have documented beyond reasonable doubt that language impairments can occur in association with lesions confined to the striatocapsular region of the dominant hemisphere, considerable variability has been reported in the nature and degree of these language impairments, with no unitary striatocapuslar aphasia being identified (Kennedy and Murdoch, 1993; Nadeau and Crosson, 1997). Varied impairments have been noted in spontaneous speech, confrontation naming, repetition, auditory comprehension, and reading comprehension. A number of authors have suggested that a difference exists between the type of aphasia associated with anterior striatocapsular

lesions compared to posterior striatocapsular lesions. For example, Naeser et al. (1982) noted that patients with capsular-putaminal lesions extending into the anterior-superior white matter typically had good comprehension and slow but grammatical speech. In contrast, those with capsular-putaminal lesions including posterior white matter extension showed poor comprehension and fluent Wernicke's-type speech, while those with anterior-superior and posterior white matter involvement were globally aphasic. Further support for this anterior-posterior distinction was provided by Cappa et al. (1983) and Murdoch et al. (1986). Despite this apparent consensus, several other studies have questionned the accuracy and utility of the anterior-posterior dichotomy by describing a number of cases in which the patterns of language impairment could not be accounted for in terms of this anatomical distinction (Kennedy and Murdoch, 1993; Wallesch, 1985).

In contrast to the striatocapsular lesions, language disturbances following thalamic lesions present a more uniform clinical picture, and it is generally accepted that a typical thalamic aphasia can be characterized by the clinical presentation. Most commonly the aphasia resulting from thalamic injury is of a mixed transcortical presentation, sharing some features with both transcortical motor and transcortical sensory aphasia (Cappa and Vignolo, 1979; Murdoch, 1996). The features of thalamic aphasia most commonly reported include preserved repetition, variable but often relatively good auditory comprehension, a reduction in spontaneous speech output, a predominance of semantic paraphasic errors, and anomia. Lesions of the dominant anterolateral thalamus (including the ventral anterior, ventral lateral, and anterior nuclei) have been highlighted as the loci of aphasic deficits, given that infarctions in this region more consistently lead to aphasic disturbances than lesions involving the posterior parts of the thalamus (Cappa et al., 1986).

Attempts to explain the clinical manifestations of subcortical aphasia have culminated in the formulation of several theories of subcortical participation in language. These theories, largely developed on the basis of speech and language data collected from subjects who have sustained cerebrovascular accidents involving the thalamus or striatocapsular region, have been expressed as neuroanatomically based models. Two models of subcortical participation in language have been quite influential. The first of these, the response/release/semantic feedback model (Crosson, 1985), proposes a role for subcortical structures in regulating the release of preformulated language segments from the cerebral cortex. According to this model, the conceptual, word-finding, and syntactic processes that fall under the rubric of language formulation occur in the anterior cerebral cortex. The monitoring of anteriorly formulated language segments, as well as the semantic and phonological decoding of incoming language, occurs in the posterior temporoparietal cortex. Language segments are conveyed from the anterior language formulation center to the posterior language center via the thalamus prior to release for motor programming. This operation allows the posterior semantic decoding centers to monitor the language segment for semantic accuracy. If an inaccuracy is detected, then the information required for correction is conveyed via the thalamus back to the anterior cortex. If the language segment is found to be accurate during monitoring, then it is released from a buffer in the anterior cortex for subsequent motor programming. In addition to subcortical structures participating in the preverbal semantic monitoring process, the model also specifies that the striatocapsular structures are involved in the release of the formulated language segment for motor programming. Specifically, it is suggested that this release occurs through the cortico-striato-pallido-thalamo-cortical loop in the following way. Once the language segments have been verified for semantic accuracy, the temporoparietal cortex releases the caudate nucleus from inhibition. The caudate nucleus then serves to weaken inhibitory pallidal regulation of thalamic excitatory outputs in the anterior language center, which in turn arouses the cortex to enable the generation of motor programs for semantically verified language segments. According to this model, Crosson (1985) hypothesized that subcortical lesions within the cortico-striato-pallido-thalamo-cortical loop would produce language deficits confined to the lexical-semantic level.

Crosson's (1985) original conception of the response-release mechanism has since been revised and elaborated in terms of the neural substrates involved (Crosson, 1992a, 1992b). Although the actual response-release mechanism in the modified version resembles that in the original conception, the route for this release is altered. The formulation of a language segment causes frontal excitation of the caudate, which increases inhibition of specific fields within the globus pallidus; however, this level of inhibition alone is not sufficient to alter pallidal output to the thalamus. An increase in posterior language cortex excitation to the caudate, which occurs once a language segment has been semantically verified posteriorly, provides a boost to the inhibition of the pallidum. The pallidal summation of this anterior and posterior inhibitory input allows the release of the ventral anterior thalamus from inhibition by the globus pallidus, causing the thalamic excitation of the frontal language cortex required to trigger the release of the language segment for motor programming. Overall, the revised model provides an integrated account of how subcortical structures might influence language output through a neuroregulatory mechanism that is consistent with knowledge of cortical-subcortical neurotransmitter systems and structural features.

A second model of subcortical participation in language was proposed by Wallesch and Papagno (1988). This model, referred to as the lexical selection model, also proposes that subcortical structures participate in language processes via a cortico-striato-pallido-thalamo-cortical loop. Wallesch and Papagno (1988) postulated that the subcortical components of the loop constitute a frontal lobe system comprised of parallel modules with integrative and decision-making capabilities rather than the simple neuroregulatory function proposed in Crosson's (1985) model. Specifically, the basal ganglia system and thalamus were hypothesized to process situational as well as goal-directed constraints and lexical information from the frontal cortex and posterior language area, and to subsequently participate in the process of determining the appropriate lexical item, from a range of cortically generated lexical alternatives, for verbal production. The most appropriate lexical alternative is then released by the thalamus for processing by the frontal cortex and programming for speech. Cortical processing of selected lexical alternatives is made possible by inhibitory influences of the globus pallidus on a thalamic gating mechanism. This most appropriate lexical alternative has an inhibitory effect on the thalamus, promoting closure of the thalamic gate, resulting in activation of the cerebral cortex and production of the desired response. Cortical processing of subordinate alternatives is suppressed as a consequence of pallidal disinhibition of the thalamus, and the inhibition of cortical activity.

Despite the apparent differences in the two models, they both ascribe an important role to the subcortical nuclei in language processing, especially at the lexical level of language organization. It is equally apparent that each of these models has a number of limitations and that no one model has achieved uniform acceptance. A major limitation of these models is that neither explains the considerable variability in clinical presentation of subcortical aphasia. According to Cappa (1997), a further problem is that the models suggest such extensive and widely distributed systems subserving lexical processing that specific predictions appear to be difficult to disprove on the basis of pathological evidence. Put more simply, these models do not lend themselves readily to empirical testing. Yet another limitation arises from the nature of the research on which these models are based. The available models of subcortical participation in language are largely based on the observation that certain contrasting deficits of language production arise in subjects with particular subcortical vascular lesions when tested on traditional tests of language function. These language measures were typically designed for taxonomic purposes regarding traditional cortical-based aphasia syndromes and may be inadequate for developing models of brain functioning (Caramazza, 1984). It has also been argued that language deficits associated with subcortical vascular lesions may actually be related to concomitant cortical dysfunction via various pathophysiological mechanisms. For instance, cortical infarction may not have been detected by neuroimaging. Also, subcortical lesions may result in diaschisis or the functional deactivation of distant related cortical structures (Metter et al., 1983). Further, language dysfunction following subcortical lesions may be related to decreases in cortical perfusion, causing widespread cortical damage that may or may not be detected by neuroimaging (Nadeau and Crosson, 1997). As yet, however, the relationship between the structural site and etiology of subcortical lesions, the extent of cortical hypometabolism and hypoperfusion, and associated language function remains to be fully elucidated.

Further clarification of the role of subcortical structures in language is likely to come through the use of functional imaging techniques and neurophysiological methods such as electrical and magnetic evoked responses, as well as from the study of the language abilities of patients with circumscribed neurosurgical lesions involving subcortical structures (e.g., thalamotomy and pallidotomy). Functional imaging techniques such as positron emission tomography (PET) and functional magnetic resonance imaging (fMRI) enable brain images to be collected while the subject is performing various language production tasks (e.g., picture naming, generating nouns) or during language comprehension (e.g., listening to stories). These techniques therefore enable visualization of the brain regions involved in a language task, with a spatial resolution as low as a few millimeters. The use of fMRI in the future is therefore likely to further inform the debate as to the role of subcortical structures in language. A review of the extensive literature on PET studies indicates that some studies published since 1994 have demonstrated activation of the thalamus and basal ganglia during completion of language tasks such as picture naming (Price, Moore, et al., 1996) and word repetition (Price, Wise, et al., 1996).

In summary, although a role for the thalamus in language is generally accepted, some controversy still exists as to whether the structures of the striatocapsular region participate directly in language processing or play a role as supporting structures for language. Contemporary theories suggest that the role of subcortical structures in language is essentially neuroregulatory, relying on quantitative neuronal activity. Although these theories have a number of limitations, for the present they do serve as frameworks for generating experimental hypotheses which can then be tested in order to advance our understanding of subcortical brain mechanisms in language.

—*Bruce E. Murdoch*

References

Alexander, M. P. (1989). Clinico-anatomical correlations of aphasia following predominantly subcortical lesions. In F. Boller and J. Grafman (Eds.), *Handbook of neuropsychology* (pp. 47–66). Amsterdam: Elsevier.

Broadbent, G. (1872). *On the cerebral mechanism of speech and thought.* London.

Cappa, S. F. (1997). Subcortical aphasia: Still a useful concept? *Brain and Language, 58,* 424–426.

Cappa, S. F., Cavallotti, G., Guidotti, M., Papagno, C., and Vignolo, L. A. (1983). Subcortical aphasia: Two clinical-CT scan correlation studies. *Cortex, 19,* 227–241.

Cappa, S. F., Papagno, C., Vallar, G., and Vignolo, L. A. (1986). Aphasia does not always follow left thalamic hemorrhage: A study of five negative cases. *Cortex, 22,* 639–647.

Cappa, S. F., and Vallar, G. (1992). Neuropsychological disorder after subcortical lesions: Implications for neural models of language and spatial attention. In G. Vallar, S. F. Cappa, and C. W. Wallesch (Eds.), *Neuropsychological dis-orders associated with subcortical lesions* (pp. 7–41). New York: Oxford University Press.

Cappa, S. F., and Vignolo, L. A. (1979). Transcortical features of aphasia following left thalamic hemorrhage. *Cortex, 15,* 121–130.

Caramazza, A. (1984). The logic of neuropsychological research and the problem of patient classification in aphasia. *Brain and Language, 21,* 9–20.

Crosson, B. (1985). Subcortical functions in language: A working model. *Brain and Language, 25,* 257–292.

Crosson, B. (1992a). *Subcortical functions in language and memory.* New York: Guilford Press.

Crosson, B. (1992b). Is the striatum involved in language? In G. Vallar, S. F. Cappa, and C. W. Wallesch (Eds.), *Neuropsychological disorders associated with subcortical lesions* (pp. 268–293). Oxford: Oxford University Press.

Kennedy, M., and Murdoch, B. E. (1993). Chronic aphasia subsequent to striatocapsular and thalamic lesions in the left hemisphere. *Brain and Language, 44,* 284–295.

Leiner, H. C., Leiner, A. L., and Dow, R. S. (1993). Cognitive language functions of the human cerebellum. *Trends in Neurosciences, 16,* 444–447.

Lichtheim, L. (1885). On aphasia. *Brain, 7,* 433–484.

Metter, E. J., Riege, W. H., Hanson, W. R., Kuhl, D. E., Phelps, M. E., Squire, L. R., et al. (1983). Comparison of metabolic rates, language and memory in subcortical aphasias. *Brain and Language, 19,* 33–47.

Murdoch, B. E. (1996). The role of subcortical structures in language: Illuminations from clinico-neuroradiological studies of brain damaged subjects. In B. Dodd, R. Campbell, and L. Worrall (Eds.), *Evaluating theories of language: Evidence from disordered communication* (pp. 137–160). London: Whurr.

Murdoch, B. E., Thompson, D., Fraser, S., and Harrison, L. (1986). Aphasia following non-haemorrhagic lesions in the left striatocapsular region. *Australian Journal of Human Communication Disorders, 14,* 5–21.

Nadeau, S. E., and Crosson, B. (1997). Subcortical aphasia. *Brain and Language, 58,* 355–402.

Naeser, M. A., Alexander, M. P., Estabrooks, N., Levine, H. L., Laughlin, S. A., and Geschwind, N. (1982). Aphasia with predominantly subcortical lesion sites: Description of three capsular/putaminal aphasia syndromes. *Archives of Neurology, 39,* 2–14.

Price, C. J., Moore, C., Humphreys, G. W., Frackowiak, R. S., and Friston, K. J. (1996). The neural signs sustaining object recognition and naming. *Proceedings of the Royal Society of London, B, 263,* 1501–1507.

Price, C. J., Wise, R. J., Warburton, E. A., Moore, C. J., Howard, D., Patterson, K., et al. (1996). Hearing and saying: The functional neuroanatomy of auditory word processing. *Brain, 119,* 919–931.

Wallesch, C. W. (1985). Two syndromes of aphasia occurring with ischemic lesions involving the left basal ganglia. *Brain and Language, 25,* 357–361.

Wallesch, C. W., and Papagno, C. (1988). Subcortical aphasia. In F. C. Rose, R. Whurr, and M. A. Wyke (Eds.), *Aphasia* (pp. 256–287). London: Whurr.

Wernicke, C. (1874). *Der aphasische Symtomencomplex.* Breslau: Cohn and Weigert.

Further Readings

Alexander, M. P., Naeser, M. A., and Palumbo, C. L. (1987). Correlations of subcortical CT lesion sites and aphasia profiles. *Brain, 110,* 961–991.

Basso, A., Della-Sala, S., and Farabola, M. (1987). Aphasia arising from purely deep lesions. *Cortex, 23,* 29–44.

Crosson, B. (1999). Subcortical mechanisms in language: Lexical-semantic mechanisms and the thalamus. *Brain and Cognition, 40,* 414–438.

Crosson, B., Zawacki, T., Brinson, G., Lu, L., and Sadek, J. R. (1997). Models of subcortical functions in language: Current status. *Journal of Neurolinguistics, 10,* 277–300.

Fabbro, F., Clarici, A., and Bava, A. (1996). Effects of left basal ganglia lesions on language production. *Perceptual and Motor Skills, 82,* 1291–1298.

Friederici, A. D., von Cramon, Y., and Kotz, S. (1999). Language related brain potentials in patients with cortical and subcortical left hemisphere lesions. *Brain, 122,* 1033–1047.

Kennedy, M., and Murdoch, B. E. (1991). Patterns of speech and language recovery following left striatocapsular haemorrhage. *Aphasiology, 5,* 489–510.

Kirk, A., and Kertesz, A. (1994). Cortical and subcortical aphasias compared. *Aphasiology, 8,* 65–82.

Metter, E. J. (1992). Role of subcortical structures in aphasia: Evidence from studies of resting cerebral glucose metabolism. In G. Vallar, S. F. Cappa, and C. W. Wallesch (Eds.), *Neuropsychological disorders associated with subcortical lesions* (pp. 478–500). Oxford: Oxford University Press.

Parent, A., and Hazrati, L. N. (1995). Functional anatomy of the basal ganglia: 1. The cortico-basal ganglia-thalamo-cortical loop. *Brain Research Reviews, 20,* 91–127.

Vignolo, L. A., Macario, M., and Cappa, S. F. (1992). Clinical-CT scan correlations in a prospective series of patients with acute left-hemispheric subcortical stroke. In G. Vallar, S. F. Cappa, and C. W. Wallesch (Eds.), *Neuropsychological disorders associated with subcortical lesions* (pp. 335–343). Oxford: Oxford University Press.

Wallesch, C. W. (1997). Symptomatology of subcortical aphasia. *Journal of Neurolinguistics, 10,* 267–275.

Wallesch, C. W., Johannsen-Harbach, H., Bartels, C., and Herrmann, M. (1997). Mechanisms of and misconceptions about subcortical aphasia. *Brain and Language, 58,* 403–409.

Language Disorders in African-American Children

Interest in language disorders among African-American children arises from the recognition that a significant number of these children speak a form of English variously referred to as Black English, African-American English, African-American Vernacular English and Ebonics (see DIALECT SPEAKERS). African-American English (AAE), the term preferred here, differs sufficiently from Standard American English (SAE) to adversely affect the educational and clinical treatment of African-American children. In addressing this issue, the American Speech, Language, and Hearing Association (ASHA) has taken the official position that children should not be viewed as having a speech and language problem because they speak AAE (ASHA, 1983). ASHA's position is consistent with that of the Linguistic Society of America (LSA), which asserts AAE to be legitimate, systematic, and rule-governed (LSA, 1997). Despite proclamations of this kind, child speakers of

AAE are overrepresented in special education classes, in part because of their linguistic background (Kuelen, Weddington, and Debose, 1998).

An important factor contributing to this overrepresentation is clinicians' failure to differentiate legitimate patterns of AAE from symptoms of a language disorder. This failure results from an assessment process that relies heavily on identifying deviations from SAE as signs of impairment. Moreover, when these deviations are the sole symptoms and no confirming evidence exists of concomitant disorders such as hearing impairment, cognitive-intellectual deficits, neurological impairment, or psycho-emotional problems, the reliance on deviant SAE patterns for diagnosis is even greater.

A case in point is specific language impairment (SLI), a disorder presumably restricted to aberrant language symptoms without a known cause (Watkins and Rice, 1994). Because the language symptoms of SLI can appear similar to legitimate language patterns of AAE (Seymour, Bland-Stewart, and Green, 1998), African-American children are at risk for SLI misdiagnosis. This kind of misdiagnosis epitomizes linguistic and cultural bias in assessment, which has been a major issue of concern to clinical professionals committed to equity and fairness in testing. Although far from resolved, linguistic bias in testing has been addressed by focusing on three related areas: language acquisition milestones for AAE, reduction of bias in assessment methods, and reduction of bias in intervention strategies.

Language Acquisition Milestones for AAE. Much of what is known about language acquisition in SAE undoubtedly also applies to the AAE-speaking child. However, it is not altogether clear whether speakers of AAE and SAE follow parallel tracks in mastering their respective adult systems. Acquisition data on AAE suggest that the two are quite similar until approximately the age of 3, at which point they diverge (Cole, 1980). This claim rests largely on evidence that young children from both language groups produce similar kinds of developmental "errors." However, these similarities may not occur for the same reasons, since several early developmental patterns also appear to match the adult AAE system. For example, absent morphological inflections are common in the emerging language of AAE and SAE as well as in adult AAE.

Whether these early patterns are a function of development or are manifestations of the AAE system is an important question. It may be that AAE development and maturation are uniquely influenced by adult AAE in ways unlikely for SAE. Some preliminary evidence to support this position comes from the work of Wyatt (1995), who showed that African-American preschoolers followed the same adult AAE constraint conditions in their optional use of zero copulas. No comparable analysis has been done on zero copulas at earlier periods or for developmental SAE patterns, however.

Evidence of differences in acquisition becomes clearer as children's language systems mature and AAE patterns become more evident (Washington and Craig, 1994).

Features that once appeared similar between AAE and SAE begin to disappear in SAE and may even increase in frequency in AAE, as with the zero copula after the age of 3 (Kovac, 1980). Between the preschool period and age 5, archetypical AAE features are observed in children across socioeconomic levels, but their density is greater among low socioeconomic classes and among males (Wyatt, 1995; Washington and Craig, 1998).

Although the descriptive accounts of early AAE have provided important information about the characteristics and pervasiveness of child AAE, still limited milestone data exist about age ranges at which language structures are mastered and the appropriate form those structures should take. In contrast, a rich source of acquisition data in SAE establishes when children of various ages acquire language milestones in ways consistent with their SAE peers. This disparity in milestone data between AAE and SAE requires a somewhat different assessment strategy in order to reduce bias.

Reduction of Bias in Assessment Methods. Of the several kinds of possible bias in language disorders (Taylor and Payne, 1983), perhaps the most intractable is linguistic and cultural bias associated with existing standardized tests. These tests are biased because they have not been specifically designed for and standardized on AAE. As a consequence, alternative and "nonstandardized" assessment methods have been recommended (Seymour and Miller-Jones, 1981; Leonard and Weiss, 1983; Stockman, 1996). These methods include language sampling analysis and criterion-referenced language probes, which are both common methods in the clinical process and typically complement norm-referenced testing. Their specific use with AAE-speaking children is important because they offer a less biased, richer, more dynamic and naturalistic source for analysis than is found in the more linguistically biased, relatively restrictive, and artificial context of standardized tests.

However, there are disadvantages with language sampling and language probes as well. They are time-intensive and possibly less reliable, and they too are limited by the inadequate normative descriptions of AAE. In an attempt to minimize the importance of specific AAE norms in the assessment process, several authors have proposed focusing alternative assessment methods on those language elements that are not specific to AAE features. Such a focus circumvents difficult questions about the status of patterns such as absent language elements. Stockman (1996) proposed the Minimal Competency Core (MCC), which is a criterion-referenced measure that represents the lowest end of a competency scale of obligatory language patterns that typically developing children should demonstrate, irrespective of their language backgrounds. Similarly, Craig and Washington (1994) advocated the avoidance of several AAE-specific features dominated by morphosyntax by focusing on complex sentence constructions common to both AAE and SAE. Also, Seymour, Bland-Stewart, and Green (1998) showed that language features that

did not contrast between AAE and SAE were better predictors of language disorders than those that were contrastive.

Each of the above recommendations can be useful in identifying possible language disorders. However, to determine the nature of the problem requires a more in-depth and complete analysis of the child's language, since language disorders are likely to extend beyond only language behaviors shared between AAE and SAE, or only in complex sentences. To ignore AAE features or any aspect of the child's language in determining the nature of a problem could yield an incomplete and distorted profile. Therefore, it is necessary to examine the child's productive capacity for a variety of targeted language structures that have been identified in a representative sample of language and that can be probed further under various linguistic and situational contexts (Seymour, 1986). With sufficient evidence about the nature of a child's language problems, the foundation then exists for intervention.

Reduction of Bias in Intervention Strategies. Decisions about intervention strategies depend directly on evidence obtained about the nature of the child's problem. For reasons stated earlier, this evidence can be more valid and less biased when alternative or no standardized testing methods are used. However, because these methods are time-consuming and require a multiple phase process, Seymour (1986) advocated a diagnostic-intervention model in which intervention is part of ongoing assessment. In this model, intervention is based on diagnostic hypotheses formulated from an initial and tentative diagnosis, and then tested by language probes. The process is one of repeatedly formulating hypotheses, testing them, and reformulating them, again and again, as needed.

The test-retest approach is recommended for AAE-speaking children largely because of the uncertainty about the nature of AAE. This uncertainty is less a factor in identifying a language disorder, since identification can be made without focusing on AAE features. However, when determining the nature of the child's problem and treating those problems, AAE features should not be avoided if a complete and accurate account of the child's language is the objective. Consider the kind of diagnostic information needed for an AAE-speaking child who fails to produce any copulas, unlike optional copula use by his AAE-speaking peers. At least two intervention strategies are possible: (1) to apply an SAE model by targeting copulas wherever they are obligatory in SAE, or (2) to follow an AAE model and target copulas in a manner consistent with optional use. Unfortunately, no matter how desirable the latter course of action might be, it is unlikely without greater knowledge of the linguistic conditions that determine optional use.

Consequently, a default to an SAE model in situations where clinical solutions for AAE are not readily apparent may be inevitable until AAE is more fully described and viewed as a complete grammar comprised of systems (Green, 1995), rather than as simply a list of structures defined by their contrast with SAE. A system's account requires answers to some complex linguistic and social questions about African-American children's development and use of language in a context characterized by linguistic duality.

—Harry N. Seymour

References

American Speech-Language-Hearing Association. (1983). Position paper on social dialects. *ASHA, 25*, 23–25.

Cole, L. (1980). A developmental analysis of social dialect features in the spontaneous language of preschool Black children. *Dissertation Abstracts International, 41*(06), 2132B (University Microfilms No. AAC8026783).

Craig, H. K., and Washington, J. A. (1994). The complex syntax skills of poor, urban, African American preschoolers at school entry. *Language, Speech, and Hearing Services in Schools, 25*, 181–190.

Green, L. (1995). Study of verb classes in African American English. *Linguistics and Education, 7*, 65–81.

Kovac, C. (1980). Children's acquisition of variable features. *Dissertation Abstracts International, 42*(02), 687A (University Microfilms No. AAC8116548).

Kuelen, J. E., Weddington, G. T., and Debose, C. E. (1998). *Speech, language, learning, and the African American child.* Boston: Allyn and Bacon.

Leonard, L. B., and Weiss, A. L. (1983). Application of nonstandardized assessment procedures to diverse linguistic populations. *Topics in Language Disorders, 3*, 35–45.

Linguistic Society of America. (1997). Resolution on the Oakland "Ebonics" issue. Adopted at the annual meeting, Chicago, IL.

Seymour, H. N. (1986). Clinical intervention for language disorders among nonstandard speakers of English. In O. L. Taylor (Ed.), *Communication disorders in culturally and linguistically diverse populations.* San Diego, CA: College-Hill Press.

Seymour, H. N., Bland-Stewart, L., and Green, L. J. (1998). Difference versus deficit in child African-American English. *Language, Speech, and Hearing Services in Schools, 29*, 96–108.

Seymour, H. N., and Miller-Jones, D. (1981). Language and cognitive assessment of Black children. In N. Lass (Ed.), *Speech and language: Advances in basic research and practice* (pp. 203–263). New York: Academic Press.

Stockman, I. (1996). The promise and pitfalls of language sample analysis as an assessment tool for linguistic minority children. *Language, Speech, and Hearing Services in Schools, 27*, 355–366.

Taylor, O., and Payne, K. (1983). Culturally valid testing: A proactive approach. *Topics in Language Disorders, 3*, 8–20.

Washington, J., and Craig, H. (1994). Dialectal forms during discourse of poor, urban, African American preschoolers. *Journal of Speech and Hearing Research, 37*, 816–823.

Washington, J. A., and Craig, H. K. (1998). Socioeconomic status and gender influences on children's dialectal variations. *Journal of Speech, Language, and Hearing Research, 41*, 618–626.

Watkins, R. V., and Rice, M. L. (1994). *Specific language impairments in children.* Baltimore: Paul H. Brookes.

Wyatt, T. (1995). Language development in African American English child speech. *Linguistics and Education, 7*, 7–22.

Further Readings

Adler, S., and Birdsong, S. (1983). Reliability and validity of standardized testing tools used with poor children. *Topics in Language Disorders, 3*, 76–87.

Battle, D. E. (Ed.). (1993). *Communication disorders in multicultural populations.* Boston: Andover.

Baugh, J. (1983). *Black street speech: Its history, structure and survival.* Austin: University of Texas Press.

Burling, R. (1973). *English in black and white.* New York: Holt, Rinehart and Winston.

Dillard, J. L. (1972). *Black English: It's history and usage in the United States.* New York: Random House.

Edwards, J. R. (1979). *Language and disadvantage.* Amsterdam: Elsevier.

Green, L. (2002). *African American English: A linguistic introduction.* New York: Cambridge University Press.

Kamhi, A. G., Pollock, K. E., and Harris, J. L. (1996). *Communication development and disorders in African American children: Research, assessment, and intervention.* Baltimore: Paul H. Brookes.

Labov, W. (1970). The logic of nonstandard English. In F. Williams (Ed.), *Language and poverty.* Chicago: Markham.

Labov, W. (1972). *Language in the inner city: Studies in the Black English Vernacular.* Philadelphia: University of Pennsylvania Press.

Leonard, L. (1998). *Children with specific language impairment.* Cambridge, MA: MIT Press.

Mufwene, S. S., Rickford, J. R., Bailey, G., and Baugh, J. (1998). *African-American English.* London: Rutledge.

Rickford, J. R. (1999). *African American Vernacular English.* Oxford: Blackwell.

Seymour, H. N., and Roeper, T. (1999). Grammatical acquisition of African American English. In O. Taylor and L. Leonard (Eds.), *Language acquisition across North America: Cross-cultural and cross-linguistic perspectives* (pp. 109–153). San Diego, CA: Singular Press Publishing Group.

Seymour, H. N., Abdulkarim, L., and Johnson, V. (1999). The Ebonics controversy: An educational and clinical dilemma. *Topics in Language Disorders, 19*, 66–77.

Smith, E. (1998). What is Black English? What is Ebonics? In L. Delpit and T. Perry (Eds.), *The real Ebonics debate: Power, language, and the education of African American children.* Boston: Beacon Press.

Smitherman, G. (1977). *Talkin' and testifyin': The language of Black America.* Boston: Houghton-Mifflin.

Stockman, I., and Vaughn-Cooke, F. (1982). Semantic categories in the language of working class black children. In C. E. Johnson and C. L. Thew (Eds.), *Proceedings of the Second International Child Language Conference, 1*, 312–327.

Stockman, I., and Vaughn-Cooke, F. (1989). Addressing new questions about black children's language. In R. Fasold and D. Shiffrin (Eds.), *Language change and variation* (pp. 274–300). Amsterdam: John Benjamins.

Taylor, O. (1986). *Treatment of communication disorders in culturally and linguistically diverse populations.* San Diego, CA: College-Hill Press.

Terrell, S., and Terrell, F. (1983). Distinguishing linguistic difference from disorders. *Topics in Language Disorders, 3*, 1–7.

Vaughn-Cooke, F. B. (1983). Improving language assessment in minority children. *ASHA, 25*, 29–34.

Williams, R. L. (Ed.). (1975). *Ebonics: The true language of Black folks.* St. Louis: Institute of Black Studies.

Wolfram, W., and Fasold, R. W. (1974). *The study of social dialects in American English.* Englewood Cliffs, NJ: Prentice Hall.

Wolfram, W. (1976). Levels of sociolinguistic bias in testing. In D. S. Harrison and T. Trabasso (Eds.), *Black English: A seminar*. Hillsdale, NJ: Erlbaum.

Language Disorders in Latino Children

The Latino population encompasses a diverse group of people who self-identify as descendants of individuals who came to the United States from a predominantly Spanish-speaking country. Over the past decade, the Latino population in the United States has increased four times faster than the general population (Guzmán, 2001). It is estimated that the size of the Latino population will represent one-quarter of the U.S. population, or approximately 81 million Latinos, by the year 2050. The large growth of the Latino population is largely attributable to its high fertility rate (National Center for Health Statistics, 1999); a large proportion of the population is in the childbearing years, and families tend to be larger. Children under the age of 15 account for 30.5% of the Latino population.

The Latino population is linguistically diverse with respect to dialects and languages spoken. The dialects spoken in the country of origin and subsequently brought to the United States evolved from the different regional dialects spoken by the original settlers, the languages spoken by the native peoples of the Americas, and the languages spoken by later immigrants. There are two major groups of Spanish dialects, radical and conservative (Guitart, 1996). The radical dialects are spoken primarily in the coastal areas of Spanish-speaking countries and the Caribbean, while the conservative dialects are spoken in the interior parts of the countries. The dialects vary in phonology, morphosyntax, semantics, and pragmatics, with the most drastic qualitative differences seen in phonology and lexicon. The differences in morphosyntax are more quantitative than qualitative. The specific dialects spoken by Latino children will be influenced by the dialects spoken in their community. Other factors influencing the dialect spoken include the degree of contact with Spanish and English speakers, whether the speaker is learning both languages simultaneously or sequentially, and the prestige attached to the various dialects with which the individual comes in contact (Poplack, 1978; Wolfram, Adger, and Christian, 1999).

Speaking Spanish is one of the major ties that bind the Latino population, and approximately 80% of the population reportedly speaks it. The vast majority of the Latino population consider themselves bilingual; a small percentage is monolingual in either English or Spanish. Twenty-eight percent of the Latino population report that they "do not speak English well" or speak it "not at all" (U.S. Census Bureau, 2000). The number of monolingual Spanish speakers and bilingual English-Spanish speakers reflects the fact that 35% of the Latino population is foreign born and that the majority of foreign-born Latinos entered the United States in the last three decades. Continuous immigration and growth of the Latino population, coupled with greater acceptability of linguistic diversity in the United States, might reverse the previous trend, in which immigrants lost their native language by the third generation (Veltman, 1988). The more likely trend is for a continuous growth of a Latino population that is bilingual.

Bilingualism is not a one-dimensional concept. Rather, bilingualism may be viewed as existing on several continua representing different language competencies in form, content, and use of the language (Valdes and Figueroa, 1994). Collectively, these individual competencies will dictate the child's linguistic proficiency in a language. The degree to which proficiency is exhibited in any one language at a particular point in time is influenced by the situation, the topic, individuals, and context (Romaine, 1995; Zentella, 1997). A shift in topic or a shift in participants may result in a switching of the code. This type of code switching is a verbal skill that requires a large degree of linguistic competence. Code switches are also made by less proficient speakers as a way to compensate for insufficient knowledge of one language.

Latino children exhibit varying degrees of proficiency in both English and Spanish. Given the pervasiveness of English language media, the use of Spanish by the majority of Latino families, and the communities in which Latinos are raised, it is doubtful that many Latino children reach school age as true monolingual Spanish speakers. Some of the children may be considered to be sequential bilinguals because their major exposure prior to entering school was to Spanish and their linguistic skills in English are minimal. These children's main exposure to English will come when they enter school. Impressionistically, many of these children are indistinguishable from monolingual Spanish speakers (e.g., Spanish-speaking children in Mexico). However, differences become apparent when their Spanish is compared with the language spoken by true monolingual Spanish speakers (Merino, 1992). Children who have been exposed to both languages at home and who tend to communicate in both languages, the so-called simultaneous bilinguals, show a wide range of linguistic skills in English and Spanish by the time they reach the school-age years. However, their exposure to and use of Spanish makes even the most English-fluent members of this group different from their monolingual peers. In environments that do not foster the development of the child's first language, language attrition occurs. Some language patterns attributable to language attrition are similar to patterns seen in children with language disorders (e.g., gender errors) (Restrepo, 1998; Anderson, 1999).

Given the large linguistic variability in the population, differentiating between a language difference (expected community variation) and a language disorder (communication that deviates significantly from the norms of the community; Taylor and Payne, 1994) is not simple. Our existing literature on language development in Latino children focuses primarily on a limited number of grammatical structures used by monolingual Spanish-speaking children (Gutierrez-Clellen, 1998; Goldstein,

2000; Bedore and Leonard, 2001). However, most Latino children are either bilingual or in the process of becoming bilingual, and therefore existing normative data on language acquisition by monolingual children (e.g., Miller and Leadholm, 1992; Sebastían and Slobin, 1994) do not accurately represent the language development of the majority of Latino children.

Assessments are further complicated by the fact that most of the available assessment protocols assume a high degree of homogeneity of exposure to the content of test items and to the sociolinguistic aspects of the testing situation. The cross-cultural child socialization literature suggests that Latino children's home routines are not always compatible with the content or the routines typically required in a language assessment (Iglesias and Quinn, 1997). Thus, poor performance on a particular assessment may reflect lack of experience rather than a child's inability to learn (Peña and Quinn, 1997).

The growing number of Latinos and their over-representation in statistical categories that place children at higher risk for disabilities or developmental delays (Arcia et al., 1993; Annie E. Casey Foundation, 2000; Iglesias, 2002) make it imperative that our assessment protocols not only accommodate linguistic differences across groups but also takes into account children's experiences. A variety of assessment protocols that take into consideration the languages and dialects spoken and the child's experiences have been suggested (Erickson and Iglesias, 1986; Peña, Iglesias, and Lidz, 2001; Wyatt, 2002). These protocols suggest the judicious use of standardized tests, taking into consideration norming samples and possible situational test biases, and consideration of alternative nonstandardized assessment procedures such as ethnographic analyses, criterion-referenced assessments, and dynamic assessments. Further, consistent with IDEA regulations (Individuals with Disabilities Act Amendments of 1997) and ASHA's position statement on the assessment of cultural-linguistic minority populations (American Speech-Language-Hearing Association, 1985), the assessments need to be provided and administered in the child's native language. In many cases this will require the examiner to be bilingual in Spanish and English or will require the use of qualified interpreters (Kayser, 1998).

The interpretation of the assessment results must take into consideration the growing literature on language development in Latino populations (Goldstein, 2000); with recognition that performance may differ from the expected norm because of a language difference rather than a language disorder. Although most children will show normal development in one or both languages, some will demonstrate weaker than expected performance in one or both languages. The data obtained must be carefully examined in the context of the languages and the dialects to which the child has been exposed and the experiences the child brings to the testing situation.

Intervention, if warranted, will require a culturally competent approach to services delivery in which the families' belief systems, including views on disability, are respected and intervention approaches are culturally and linguistically congruent with those of the children's families (Lynch and Hanson, 1992; Maestas and Erickson, 1992; van Kleeck, 1994; Iglesias and Quinn, 1997). The language of intervention should be based on the children's linguistic competencies, parents' preference, and functionality, not on the clinician's lack of proficiency in speaking the child's language. The bilingual literature on typical and atypical language learners strongly supports the notion that intervention should be conducted in the child's strongest and most environmentally functional language (Gutierrez-Clellen, 1999). In many cases, this will mean using Spanish as the language of intervention. The skills gained in the acquisition of the first language will facilitate acquisition of the second.

—*Aquiles Iglesias*

References

American Speech-Language-Hearing Association. (1985). Clinical management of communicatively handicapped minority language populations. *ASHA, 27,* 29–32.

Anderson, R. (1999). Loss of gender agreement in L1 attrition: Preliminary results. *Bilingual Research Journal, 23,* 389–407.

Annie E. Casey Foundation. (2000). *Kids count data book.* Baltimore: Author.

Arcia, E., Keyes, L., Galalgher, J. J., and Chabhar, M. (1993). *Status of young Mexican-American children: Implications for early intervention systems.* Chapel Hill, NC: Carolina Institute for Child and Family Policy.

Bedore, L., and Leonard, L. (2001). Grammatical morphology deficits in Spanish-speaking children with specific language impairment. *Journal of Speech and Hearing Research, 44,* 904–924.

Erickson, J., and Iglesias, A. (1986). Assessment of communication disorders in non-English proficient children. In O. Taylor (Ed.), *Nature of communication disorders in culturally and linguistically diverse populations* (pp. 181–217). San Diego, CA: College-Hill Press.

Goldstein, B. (2000). *Cultural and linguistic diversity resource guide for speech-language pathologists.* San Diego, CA: Singular Publishing Group.

Guitart, J. (1996). Spanish in contact with itself and the phonological characterization of conservative and radical styles. In J. Jensen (Ed.), *Spanish in contact: Issues in bilingualism* (pp. 151–157). Somerville, MA: Cascadilla Press.

Gutierrez-Clellen, V. F. (1998). Syntactic skills of Spanish-speaking children with low school achievement. *Language, Speech, and Hearing Services in Schools, 29,* 207–215.

Gutierrez-Clellen, V. F. (1999). Language choice in intervention with bilingual children. *American Journal of Speech-Language Pathology, 8,* 291–302.

Guzmán, B. (2001). *The Hispanic population, Census 2000 briefs.* Washington, DC: U.S. Census Bureau.

Iglesias, A. (2002). Latino culture. In D. Battle (Ed.), *Communication disorders in multicultural populations* (pp. 179–202). Woburn, MA: Butterworth-Heinemann.

Iglesias, A., and Quinn, R. (1997). Culture as a context for early intervention. In K. Thurman, J. Cornwell, and S. R. Gottwald (Eds.), *Contexts of early intervention: Systems and settings* (pp. 55–72). Baltimore: Paul H. Brookes.

Individuals with Disabilities Act Amendments of 1997, USC 1400 et seq. (1997).

Kayser, H. (1998). *Assessment and intervention resource for Hispanic children*. San Diego, CA: Singular Publishing Group.

Lynch, E., and Hanson, M. J. (1992). *Developing cross-cultural competence: A guide for working with young children and their families*. Baltimore: Paul H. Brookes.

Maestas, A. G., and Erickson, J. G. (1992). Mexican immigrant mothers' beliefs about disabilities. *American Journal of Speech-Language Pathology, 1,* 5–10.

Merino, B. (1992). Acquisition of syntactic and phonological features in Spanish. In H. W. Langdon and L. R. Cheng (Eds.), *Hispanic children and adults with communication disorders* (pp. 57–98). Gaithersburg, MD: Aspen.

Miller, J., and Leadholm, B. (1992). *Language sample analysis guide: The Wisconsin guide for the identification and description of language impairment in children*. Madison: Wisconsin Department of Education.

National Center for Health Statistics. (1999). *National vital statistics* (No. 47-18). Washington, DC: National Center for Health Statistics.

Peña, E., Iglesias, A., and Lidz, C. S. (2001). Reducing test bias through dynamic assessment of children's word learning ability. *American Journal of Speech-Language Pathology, 10,* 138–154.

Peña, E., and Quinn, R. (1997). Task familiarity: Effects on the test performance of Puerto Rican and African American children. *Language, Speech, and Hearing Services in Schools, 28,* 323–332.

Poplack, S. (1978). Dialect acquisition among Puerto Rican bilinguals. *Language in Society, 7,* 89–103.

Restrepo, M. A. (1998). Identifiers of predominantly Spanish-speaking children with language impairment. *Journal of Speech and Hearing Research, 41,* 1398–1411.

Romaine, S. (1995). *Bilingualism*. Cambridge, U.K.: Blackwell.

Sebastián, E., and Slobin, D. I. (1994). Development of linguistic forms: Spanish. In D. I. Slobin (Ed.), *Relating events in narrative. A crosslinguistic developmental study* (pp. 239–284). Hillsdale, NJ: Erlbaum.

Taylor, O., and Payne, K. (1994). Language and communication differences. In W. Secord (Ed.), *Human communication disorders: An introduction* (pp. 136–173). Upper Saddle River, NJ: Prentice Hall.

U.S. Census Bureau. (2000). Age by language spoken at home by ability to speak English for the population 5 years and over. Available: http://www.census.gov. [Accessed Aug. 6, 2001.]

Valdes, G., and Figueroa, R. A. (1994). *Bilingualism and testing: A special case of bias*. Norwood: Ablex.

van Kleeck, A. (1994). Potential bias in training parents as conversational partners with their children who have delays in language development. *American Journal of Speech-Language Pathology, 3,* 67–78.

Veltman, C. J. (1988). *The future of the Spanish language in the United States*. Washington, DC: Hispanic Policy Development Project.

Wolfram, W., Adger, C. T., and Christian, D. (1999). *Dialects in schools and communities*. Mahwah, NJ: Erlbaum.

Wyatt, T. A. (2002). Assessing the communicative abilities of clients from diverse cultural and language backgrounds. In D. Battle (Ed.), *Communication disorders in multicultural populations* (pp. 415–450). Boston: Butterworth-Heinemann.

Zentella, A. C. (1997). *Growing up bilingual*. Malden, MA: Blackwell.

Further Readings

Anderson, R. (1996). Assessing the grammar of Spanish-speaking children: A comparison of two procedures. *Language, Speech, and Hearing Services in the Schools, 27,* 333–344.

Bedore, L. (1999). The acquisition of Spanish. In O. Taylor and L. Leonard (Eds.), *Language acquisition in North America* (pp. 167–207). San Diego, CA: Singular Publishing Group.

Bedore, L. (2001). Assessing morphosyntax in Spanish-speaking children. *Seminars in Speech and Language, 22,* 65–77.

Goldstein, B., and Iglesias, A. (2002). Issues of cultural and linguistic diversity. In R. Paul (Ed.), *Introduction to clinical methods in communication disorders* (pp. 261–279). Baltimore: Paul H. Brookes.

Gutierrez-Clellen, V. F., and Heinrich-Ramos, L. (1993). Referential cohesion in the narratives of Spanish-speaking children: A developmental study. *Journal of Speech and Hearing Research, 36,* 559–568.

Gutierrez-Clellen, V. F., and Hoffstetter, R. (1994). Syntactic complexity in Spanish narratives: A developmental study. *Journal of Speech and Hearing Research, 35,* 363–372.

Gutierrez-Clellen, V. F., and Quinn, R. (1993). Assessing narratives of children from diverse cultural/linguistic groups. *Language, Speech, and Hearing Services in Schools, 24,* 2–9.

Gutierrez-Clellen, V. F., Restrepo, M. A., Bedore, L., Peña, E., and Anderson, R. (2000). Language sample analysis in Spanish-speaking children: Methodological considerations. *Language, Speech, and Hearing Services in Schools, 31,* 88–98.

Iglesias, A. (2001). What test should I use? *Seminars in Speech and Language, 22,* 3–15.

Jackson-Maldonado, D., Thal, D., Marchman, V., Bates, E., and Gutierrez-Clellen, V. (1993). Early lexical development of Spanish-speaking infants and toddlers. *Journal of Child Language, 20,* 523–549.

Kohnert, K. J., Bates, E., and Hernandez, A. E. (1999). Balancing bilinguals: Lexical-semantic production and cognitive processing in children learning Spanish and English. *Journal of Speech and Hearing Research, 41,* 1103–1114.

Kvaal, J. T., Shipstead-Cox, N., Nevitt, S. G., Hodson, B., and Launer, P. B. (1988). The acquisition of 10 Spanish morphemes by Spanish-speaking children. *Language, Speech, and Hearing Services in Schools, 19,* 384–394.

Langdon, H. W. (1994). Meeting the needs of the non-English-speaking parents of a communicatively disabled child. *Clinics in Communication Disorders, 4,* 227–236.

Oller, D. K., and Eilers, E. R. (2002). *Language and literacy in bilingual children*. Buffalo, NY: Multilingual Matters.

Ortiz, S. A. (2001). Assessment of cognitive abilities in Hispanic children. *Seminars in Speech and Language, 22,* 17–37.

Perez-Leroux, A. T., and Glass, W. R. (1997). *Contemporary perspectives on the acquisition of Spanish: Developing grammars*. Somerville, MA: Cascadilla Press.

Seliger, H. W., and Vago, R. M. (1991). *First language attrition*. New York: Cambridge University Press.

Silva-Corvalan, C. (1995). *Spanish in four continents*. Washington, DC: Georgetown University Press.

Language Disorders in School-Age Children: Aspects of Assessment

Approximately 7% of kindergarten children have a primary language disorder characterized by a significant delay in the comprehension or production of spoken language. Although these children have normal intelligence and hearing and are free of obvious neurological deficits such as cerebral palsy and severe emotional disturbances such as autism, their limitations in spoken language often persist throughout childhood, adolescence, and well into adulthood.

In addition, children with this disorder, often called specific language impairment, frequently demonstrate limitations in written language development during the school-age years, including problems in decoding print, comprehending text, spelling, and producing essays for school assignments. Problems in the social use of language, particularly during peer interactions, frequently affect these children as well.

Phonology

Most typically developing children have mastered the sound system of their native language by 7 or 8 years of age. In contrast, children with language disorders may demonstrate errors in the production of speech sounds during adolescence. Common errors include distortions of sibilants (s, z) and liquids (l, r), reduction of consonant clusters (kl, sp), imprecise articulation during rapid speech (Johnson et al., 1999), and difficulty articulating polysyllabic words (*thermometer*, *rhinoceros*; Catts, 1986). Phonological errors can impair intelligibility and make the child overly self-conscious. For these reasons, they should be addressed during language intervention. Standardized tests that can be used to identify phonological disorders include the Arizona Articulation Proficiency Scale and the Goldman-Fristoe Test of Articulation.

Phonological disorders in young children are sometimes predictive of later problems in learning to read, particularly when additional deficits in phonological awareness are present. Problems in phonological awareness—the ability to analyze and manipulate the sounds of the language—commonly occur in school-age children with language disorders and underlie their difficulties in learning to decode and to spell words (Catts, 1993; Lombardino et al., 1997). Unfortunately, difficulties in decoding text can seriously hamper a child's reading comprehension, just as difficulties in spelling can hamper the writing process. It is therefore very important that deficits in phonological awareness be addressed during language intervention.

Phonological awareness can be evaluated with a variety of tasks. For example, sound deletion requires the child to delete a particular sound or syllable in a word ("Say *tall* without the *t*," "Say *haircut* without the *hair*"), and sound segmenting requires that the number of sounds or syllables in a word be counted ("How many sounds do you hear in *crab*?" "How many syllables do you hear in *elephant*?"). Standardized tests of phonological awareness, such as the Comprehensive Test of Phonological Processing, can also be used to identify deficits in school-age children.

Syntax and Morphology

The conversational speech of school-age children with language disorders is often characterized by utterances that are shorter and simpler than those of their peers with typical language development. For example, by age 10 or 12 years, a typical child can produce discourse such as the following: "The other day, while I was waiting for bus 28, which goes to the mall, my friend Harry, who lives in Brighton, stopped by and wanted to play a game of checkers. Finally, after we had played about an hour, the bus arrived and we had to stop, but I was glad because he had already beaten me four games." These two sentences, containing 32 and 28 words, respectively, and six verbs each (both finite and nonfinite), would be well beyond the syntactic competence of school-age children with language disorders.

To express the same content, the child with a language disorder might need to employ a series of eight or ten shorter utterances. Although those utterances might be free of grammatical errors, it is unlikely that they would contain the advanced, low-frequency syntactic structures used by the typical child, such as the adverbial clause containing an adjective clause (*while I was waiting for bus 28, which goes to the mall*), the elaborated subject (*my friend Harry, who lives in Brighton*), the perfect aspect (*had played, had beaten*), or the adverbial conjunct *finally* to link ideas across sentences. In addition, the child with a language disorder might exhibit numerous false starts, hesitations, and revisions—"maze behavior" (Loban, 1976)—and may struggle to call up the details of the situation, producing a laborious and confusing message.

Similar problems can be observed in written language when children are asked to produce narrative, persuasive, or expository texts for school assignments. School-age children with language disorders characteristically produce shorter texts with fewer details, poorer organization, and a greater number of grammatical and spelling errors than their age-matched peers (e.g., Gillam and Johnston, 1992; Snowling, Bishop, and Stothard, 2000). They may also show evidence of morphological difficulties in writing. For example, they may omit the plural and past tense markers ("*They use their skate yesterday*"), or they may fail to use past irregular verbs correctly in obligatory contexts ("*He teached them to read*") even as late as 12 years of age (Windsor, Scott, and Street, 2000). Problems in the use of derivational morphemes—prefixes and suffixes such as *non-*, *-tion*, and *-ment*—also occur in the speech and writing of children with language disorders (Moats and Smith, 1992).

The best way to evaluate a child's syntax and morphology is to analyze spoken and written language samples with the aid of computer programs such as Systematic Analysis of Language Transcripts (Miller and Chapman, 2000). Standardized language tests can also be administered, such as the Clinical Evaluation of Language Fundamentals–3, the Oral and Written Language Scales, the Test of Language Development–Primary, and the Test of Language Development–Intermediate.

Semantics

Compared to their age-matched peers, school-age children with language disorders frequently demonstrate limitations in lexical knowledge, particularly in relation to words that express abstract (*pride, courage*), polysemous (*deep, absorbing*), or technical (*equation, parabola*) meanings (Wiig and Secord, 1998). Figurative expressions such as metaphors (*The lawyer was a bulldozer questioning the witness*), idioms (*throw in the towel, read between the lines*), and proverbs (*Every cloud has a silver lining*) also pose comprehension difficulties, along with slang expressions (*grandma lane*), sarcasm ("*Your room is SO clean now!*"), and humor (Q: "Which sport is the quietest?" A: "Bowling. You can hear a pin drop") (Nippold and Fey, 1983; Lutzer, 1988; Spector, 1990; Milosky, 1994). Word retrieval, the ability to call up words with speed and accuracy, is often impaired as well, particularly in relation to low-frequency (*tambourine*) or abstract (*religions*) words (German, 1994).

Deficiencies in semantic development can seriously limit a child's spoken and written communication, affecting social development and academic progress. For example, difficulties in word retrieval and humor comprehension can prevent a child from freely engaging in telling jokes and riddles, a popular pastime among school-age children. Because teachers' classroom talk and the textbooks used in schools frequently contain difficult words and expressions, children with semantic deficits often fail to understand much of what they hear and read. These effects are cyclical, because listening and reading themselves are major sources of language-learning input during the school-age years. As a result, children who are deficient in listening and reading will continue to fall farther behind their peers in language development as they grow older.

Semantic development in school-age children can be evaluated through the use of standardized tests such as the Peabody Picture Vocabulary Test–III, the Test of Word Knowledge, and the Test of Word Finding–2. Informal observation of a child's use of words, phrases, and expressions in social and academic contexts can also be informative. Deficiencies in listening and reading comprehension can be identified using standardized tests such as the Clinical Evaluation of Language Fundamentals–3 and the Woodcock Reading Mastery Tests–Revised, and by inspecting the child's scores on academic achievement tests.

Pragmatics

Problems in pragmatics—the social use of language—commonly occur in school-age children with language disorders. Because of their phonological, syntactic, morphological, and semantic deficits, children with language disorders may receive social penalties from their typically developing peers in the form of teasing, hurtful comments, and personal rejection. This type of negative feedback can cause a child to avoid social situations and the opportunities they present for language development. For example, through regular interactions with peers, children are able to observe others using complex language and can themselves practice using appropriate phonological patterns, syntactic structures, morphemes, words, and figurative expressions in varied contexts such as greeting others, having conversations, exchanging information, agreeing and disagreeing, and persuading others to do things. A variety of pragmatic difficulties have been reported in school-age children with language disorders. In relation to peer interactions, these difficulties include limitations in the ability to access ongoing play groups; to collaborate, persuade, and negotiate; to engage in extended conversations; and to deliver bad news tactfully (Bliss, 1992; Brinton et al., 1997; Brinton, Fujiki, and Higbee, 1998; Brinton, Fujiki, and McKee, 1998; Fujiki et al., 2001).

Pragmatic development can be evaluated through role-playing tasks and social skills rating scales. Although the specific sources of pragmatic deficits are often unclear, in some cases they stem from limitations in the child's social cognition—knowledge of the thoughts, feelings, and beliefs of others—and from deficits in the ability to use words, morphemes, and syntactic structures that mark politeness and empathy (e.g., "*I don't know why you weren't chosen for the play, but I'm sure you'll get the lead next time*") (Bliss, 1992). These problems, which can limit a child's ability to maintain friendships, should be addressed in concert with other language goals.

See also LANGUAGE DISORDERS IN SCHOOL-AGE CHILDREN: OVERVIEW.

—*Marilyn A. Nippold*

References

Bliss, L. S. (1992). A comparison of tactful messages by children with and without language impairment. *Language, Speech, and Hearing Services in Schools, 23,* 343–347.

Brinton, B., Fujiki, M., and Higbee, L. M. (1998). Participation in cooperative learning activities by children with specific language impairment. *Journal of Speech, Language, and Hearing Research, 41,* 1193–1206.

Brinton, B., Fujiki, M., and McKee, L. (1998). Negotiation skills of children with specific language impairment. *Journal of Speech, Language, and Hearing Research, 41,* 927–940.

Brinton, B., Fujiki, M., Spencer, J. C., and Robinson, L. A. (1997). The ability of children with specific language impairment to access and participate in an ongoing interaction. *Journal of Speech, Language, and Hearing Research, 40,* 1011–1025.

Catts, H. W. (1986). Speech production/phonological deficits in reading-disordered children. *Journal of Learning Disabilities, 19,* 504–508.

Catts, H. W. (1993). The relationship between speech-language impairments and reading disabilities. *Journal of Speech, Language, and Hearing Research, 36,* 948–958.

Fujiki, M., Brinton, B., Isaacson, T., and Summers, C. (2001). Social behaviors of children with language impairment on the playground: A pilot study. *Language, Speech, and Hearing Services in Schools, 32*, 101–113.

German, D. J. (1994). Word finding difficulties in children and adolescents. In G. P. Wallach and K. G. Butler (Eds.), *Language learning disabilities in school-age children and adolescents: Some principles and applications* (pp. 323–347). New York: Macmillan.

Gillam, R. B., and Johnston, J. R. (1992). Spoken and written language relationships in language/learning-impaired and normally achieving school-age children. *Journal of Speech and Hearing Research, 35*, 1303–1315.

Johnson, C. J., Beitchman, J. H., Young, A., Escobar, M., Atkinson, L., Wilson, B., et al. (1999). Fourteen-year follow-up of children with and without speech/language impairments: Speech/language stability and outcomes. *Journal of Speech, Language, and Hearing Research, 42*, 744–760.

Loban, W. (1976). *Language development: Kindergarten through grade twelve.* Urbana, IL: National Council of Teachers of English.

Lombardino, L. J., Riccio, C. A., Hynd, G. W., and Pinheiro, S. B. (1997). Linguistic deficits in children with reading disabilities. *American Journal of Speech-Language Pathology, 6*, 71–78.

Lutzer, V. D. (1988). Comprehension of proverbs by average children and children with learning disorders. *Journal of Learning Disabilities, 21*, 104–108.

Miller, J., and Chapman, R. (2000). *SALT: Systematic Analysis of Language Transcripts* [Computer program to analyze language samples]. Madison, WI: Language Analysis Laboratory, Waisman Research Center, University of Wisconsin–Madison.

Milosky, L. M. (1994). Nonliteral language abilities: Seeing the forest for the trees. In G. P. Wallach and K. G. Butler (Eds.), *Language learning disabilities in school-age children and adolescents: Some principles and applications* (pp. 275–303). New York: Macmillan.

Moats, L. C., and Smith, C. (1992). Derivational morphology: Why it should be included in language assessment and instruction. *Language, Speech, and Hearing Services in Schools, 23*, 312–319.

Nippold, M. A., and Fey, S. H. (1983). Metaphoric understanding in preadolescents having a history of language acquisition difficulties. *Language, Speech, and Hearing Services in Schools, 14*, 171–180.

Snowling, M., Bishop, D. V. M., and Stothard, S. E. (2000). Is preschool language impairment a risk factor for dyslexia in adolescence? *Journal of Child Psychology and Psychiatry, 41*, 587–600.

Spector, C. C. (1990). Linguistic humor comprehension of normal and language-impaired adolescents. *Journal of Speech and Hearing Disorders, 55*, 533–541.

Wiig, E., and Secord, W. (1998). Language disabilities in school-age children and youth. In G. Shames, E. Wiig, and W. Secord (Eds.), *Human communication disorders: An introduction* (pp. 185–226). Boston: Allyn and Bacon.

Windsor, J., Scott, C. M., and Street, C. K. (2000). Verb and noun morphology in the spoken and written language of children with language learning disabilities. *Journal of Speech, Language, and Hearing Research, 43*, 1322–1336.

Further Readings

Catts, H., and Kamhi, A. (1999). *Language and reading disabilities.* Boston: Allyn and Bacon.

Fey, M. E., Windsor, J., and Warren, S. E. (Eds.). (1995). *Language intervention: Preschool through the elementary years.* Baltimore: Paul H. Brookes.

Moats, L. C. (2000). *Speech to print: Language essentials for teachers.* Baltimore: Paul H. Brookes.

Nippold, M. A. (1998). *Later language development: The school-age and adolescent years.* Austin, TX: Pro-Ed.

Paul, R. (2001). *Language disorders from infancy through adolescence: Assessment and intervention* (2nd ed.). St. Louis: Mosby.

Wallach, G. P., and Butler, K. G. (Eds.). (1994). *Language learning disabilities in school-age children and adolescents: Some principles and applications.* New York: Macmillan.

Language Disorders in School-Age Children: Overview

Even though the symptoms and severity of a child's language disorder may change over time, language disorders tend to be chronic. Preschoolers who are identified with language disorders are at substantial risk for experiencing language disorders during the school years and are also at risk for the academic, social, and vocational difficulties often associated with language disorders. Like younger children with language disorders, school-age children with language disorders are characterized by their heterogeneity. This heterogeneity manifests itself in the severity of the disorder, with some children showing mild grammatical difficulties, others showing no syntactic knowledge, and still others having no expressive language. For children with severe language disorders, spoken language may present inordinate difficulties. In these instances, children may use augmentative forms of communication, such as graphic systems, manual signs, and electronic speech output devices, to facilitate language development or to serve as alternate forms of communication.

The heterogeneity of language disorders in school-age children is also evident in the particular aspects of language that are disordered, with some children, for example, showing word-finding deficits, others having difficulty understanding complex directions, and yet others exhibiting global language deficits. Conventionally, a distinction is drawn between language disorders that affect only the production of language (expressive language disorders) and those that affect language comprehension in addition to production (mixed receptive-expressive language disorders). Children with either expressive or mixed language disorders may have a concomitant speech disorder, reflecting difficulty with speech sound representation and/or production. Disorders of reading and writing also may accompany language disorders (see LANGUAGE IMPAIRMENT AND READING DISABILITY).

For some children, language is the only developmental area in which they experience obvious difficulty; these children are often identified as having specific language impairment (SLI) (see SPECIFIC LANGUAGE IMPAIRMENT IN

CHILDREN). Omission of grammatical markers may be the most salient language characteristic in SLI, but it is not the only language deficit that may hinder a child's academic performance. In other children the language disorder is secondary to other cognitive, motor, or sensory disorders.

Several populations of school-age children are at risk for language disorders. These populations include children with developmental disabilities, such as children with MENTAL RETARDATION, AUTISM, or a pervasive developmental disorder, and also children in whom only subtle cognitive deficits are implicated. Among the latter are children with learning disabilities or disorders as well as children with attention deficit disorder, characterized by frequent instances of inattention and impulsiveness, and children with disruptive behavior disorder, marked by aggressive behavior or the violation of social norms. Children with hearing impairments are also at risk for language disorders. Although most school-age language disorders are developmental, children may have acquired language disorders resulting from closed head injuries, seizure disorders, or focal lesions such as stroke or tumors. Taken together, children with language disorders constitute a large group of students for whom language poses substantial difficulties.

About 5% of students in the United States show a learning disorder (American Psychiatric Association, 1994). Learning disorders are identified as disorders of reading, written expression, and mathematics. However, many children with learning disorders appear to have an associated difficulty with spoken language that substantially affects their ability to meet classroom language demands. The comorbidity of language disorders, learning disorders, and also attention deficit and disruptive behavior disorders is well-established. The overlap between disorders is at some level intuitive. For instance, children with attention deficit disorder often show deficits in executive functions, such as difficulties in goal setting, monitoring behavior, and self-awareness (Ylvisaker and DeBonis, 2000). These characteristics may have deleterious effects on the child's ability to deal with the complex language tasks encountered in the classroom.

Traditionally, a distinction was made between language delay and language deviance. For example, children with mental retardation were considered to show a delayed profile of language development, consistent with delay in other cognitive abilities. Children with autism were considered to show deviant language characterized by patterns not found for typically achieving children. Current research suggests that this global distinction does not fully capture the language profiles of children with language disorders. Contrary to the idea of simple delay, for example, children and adolescents with Down syndrome show greater deficits in expressive than in receptive language (Chapman et al., 1998). And contrary to the notion of overall language deviance, children and adolescents with autism have been found to produce narratives similar to those of children with mental retardation (Tager-Flusberg and Sullivan, 1995).

Across populations of children, difficulties in all domains of language, semantic, syntactic, and pragmatic, have been found. Current thinking in speech-language pathology, however, is not to address individual skills in isolation but to focus on broader aspects of the child's language and the learning environment that will best promote the child's current and future communicative success (Fey, Catts, and Larrivee, 1995). This includes recognizing the link between language, especially phonological awareness (awareness of the sound structure of words), and literacy skills (Catts and Kamhi, 1999). Oral narrative production is another area that has received attention, in part because the ability to tell a cohesive story rests on other language and cognitive skills and in part because good narrative skills seem to be associated with good academic performance (Hughes, McGillivray, and Schmidek, 1997). Also, children with language disorders are at risk for fewer and less effective social interactions than other children of the same age. Thus, the language foundations for social interaction, particularly conversational skills, constitute a major area to be addressed.

The school years cover a broad developmental range, and language disorders during adolescence are as important to identify as disorders occurring at earlier ages. However, language development is more gradual and individual in adolescence than it is in younger children, and identification of a disorder may be particularly challenging. Later language developments, such as the acquisition of figurative language (e.g., metaphors and idioms), advanced lexical and syntactic skills (e.g., defining abstract words, using complex sentences), analogical reasoning, and effective conversational skills, such as negotiation and persuasion, each develop over an extended period. At the same time, competence with these language skills is fundamental for dealing effectively with the academic and social curricula of high school. Adolescents with language disorders are at risk for dropping out of school or in other ways not making a successful transition to employment or university after high school. Thus, emphasizing adolescents' functional competence in social communication has been increasingly advocated.

Both standardized and nonstandardized measures are used to assess school-age language disorders in children and adolescents. Although below-average performance on standardized tests compared with chronological or developmental norms remains the primary way of identifying the presence of a language disorder, criterion-referenced assessments provide a more direct guide to intervention. In criterion-referenced assessments, the emphasis is on how well the child reaches certain levels of achievement rather than on how the child's language performance compares with that of other children of the same age. For instance, criterion-referenced assessments can be used to determine how well a child understands vocabulary used in classroom textbooks or how effectively a child initiates conversations with other children. (Paul, 2001, describes many standardized and criterion-referenced language assessments.)

Another form of nonstandardized assessment focuses on the underlying cognitive processing skills that potentially are linked to some language disorders. This evaluation includes tasks assessing verbal working memory (e.g., recalling an increasing number of real words), phonological working memory (e.g., imitating nonsense words), and auditory perception (e.g., discriminating speech and nonspeech sounds). School-age children with language disorders have been distinguished from their age peers by lower accuracy on verbal working memory and nonword repetition tasks (Ellis Weismer, Evans, and Hesketh, 1999; Ellis Weismer et al., 2000). Dynamic assessment also has been advocated as an effective nonstandardized assessment strategy (Olswang, Bain, and Johnson, 1992). In dynamic assessment, aspects of a language task are altered systematically to examine the conditions under which a child can achieve optimal success. Thus, dynamic assessment can be used to determine a child's potential for benefiting from intervention, and also what guidance or structure will be most helpful in intervention. Criterion-referenced, processing-dependent, and dynamic assessments may be especially important for children from culturally and linguistically diverse backgrounds, for whom many current standardized language tests may be inadequate or inappropriate (Restrepo, 1998; Craig and Washington, 2000).

See also SPEECH DISORDERS IN CHILDREN: SPEECH-LANGUAGE APPROACHES; SPECIFIC LANGUAGE IMPAIRMENT IN CHILDREN.

—*Jennifer Windsor*

References

American Psychiatric Association. (1994). *Diagnostic and statistical manual of mental disorders—Fourth edition.* Washington, DC: American Psychiatric Press.

Catts, H. W., and Kamhi, A. (Eds.). (1999). *Language and reading disabilities.* Boston: Allyn and Bacon.

Chapman, R. S., Seung, H., Schwartz, S., and Kay-Raining Bird, E. (1998). Language skills of children and adolescents with Down syndrome: II. Production deficits. *Journal of Speech, Language, and Hearing Research, 41,* 861–873.

Craig, H., and Washington, J. (2000). An assessment battery for identifying language impairments in African American children. *Journal of Speech, Language, and Hearing Research, 43,* 366–379.

Ellis Weismer, S., Evans, J., and Hesketh, L. (1999). An examination of verbal working memory capacity in children with specific language impairment. *Journal of Speech, Language, and Hearing Research, 42,* 1249–1260.

Ellis Weismer, S., Tomblin, B., Zhang, X., Buckwalter, P., Chynoweth, J., and Jones, M. (2000). Nonword repetition performance in school-age children with and without language impairment. *Journal of Speech, Language, and Hearing Research, 43,* 865–878.

Fey, M. E., Catts, H., and Larrivee, L. (1995). Preparing preschoolers for the academic and social challenges of school. In M. E. Fey, J. Windsor, and S. Warren (Eds.), *Language intervention: Preschool through the elementary years* (pp. 3–37). Baltimore: Paul H. Brookes.

Hughes, D., McGillivray, L., and Schmidek, M. (1997). *Guide to narrative language: Procedures for assessment.* Eau Claire, WI: Thinking Publications.

Olswang, L. B., Bain, B., and Johnson, G. (1992). Using dynamic assessment with children with language disorders. In S. F. Warren and J. Reichle (Eds.), *Causes and effects in communication and language intervention* (pp. 187–215). Baltimore: Paul H. Brookes.

Paul, R. (2001). *Language Disorders from Infancy through Adolescence: Assessment and Intervention* (2nd ed). St. Louis: Mosby.

Restrepo, M. A. (1998). Identifiers of predominantly Spanish-speaking children with language impairment. *Journal of Speech, Language, and Hearing Research, 41,* 1398–1411.

Tager-Flusberg, H., and Sullivan, K. (1995). Attributing mental states to story characters: A comparison of narratives produced by autistic and mentally retarded individuals. *Applied Psycholinguistics, 16,* 241–256.

Ylvisaker, M., and DeBonis, D. (2000). Executive function impairment in adolescence: TBI and ADHD. *Topics in Language Disorders, 20,* 29–57.

Further Readings

Bishop, D. V. M. (1994). Grammatical errors in specific language impairment: Competence or performance limitations? *Applied Psycholinguistics, 15,* 507–550.

Bishop, D. V. M., Bishop, S., Bright, P., James, C., Delaney, T., and Tallal, P. (1999). Different origin of auditory and phonological processing problems in children with language impairment: Evidence from a twin study. *Journal of Speech, Language, and Hearing Research, 42,* 155–168.

Boudreau, D., and Chapman, R. (2000). The relationship between event representation and linguistic skill in narratives of children and adolescents with Down syndrome. *Journal of Speech, Language, and Hearing Research, 43,* 1146–1159.

Campbell, T., Dollaghan, C., Needleman, H., and Janosky, J. (1997). Reducing bias in language assessment: Processing-dependent measures. *Journal of Speech, Language, and Hearing Research, 40,* 519–525.

Chapman, S. B., Watkins, R., Gustafson, C., Moore, S., Levin, H., and Kufera, J. (1997). Narrative discourse in children with closed head injury, children with language impairment, and typically developing children. *American Journal of Speech-Language Pathology, 6,* 66–75.

Fey, M. E., Windsor, J., and Warren, S. (Eds.). (1995). *Language intervention: Preschool through the elementary years.* Baltimore: Paul H. Brookes.

Gallagher, T. M. (1999). Interrelationships among children's language, behavior, and emotional problems. *Topics in Language Disorders, 19,* 1–15.

Gillam, R., and Johnston, J. (1992). Spoken and written language relationships in language/learning-impaired and normally achieving school-age children. *Journal of Speech and Hearing Research, 35,* 1303–1315.

Kay-Raining Bird, E., Cleave, P., and McConnell, L. (2000). Reading and phonological awareness in children with Down syndrome: A longitudinal study. *American Journal of Speech-Language Pathology, 9,* 319–330.

Leadholm, B. J., and Miller, J. (1992). *Language Sample Analysis: The Wisconsin guide.* Madison: Wisconsin Department of Public Instruction.

Leonard, L. B. (1998). *Children with specific language impairment.* Cambridge, MA: MIT Press.

Marchman, V. A., Wulfeck, B., and Ellis Weismer, S. (1999). Morphological productivity in children with normal language and SLI: A study of the English past tense. *Journal of Speech, Language, and Hearing Research, 42,* 206–219.

McCauley, R. J. (1996). Familiar strangers: Criterion-referenced measures in communication disorders. *Language, Speech, and Hearing Services in Schools, 27, 122–131.

McCormick, L., Frome Loeb, D., and Schiefelbusch, R. (1997). Supporting children with communication difficulties in inclusive settings: School-based language intervention. Boston: Allyn and Bacon.

Nippold, M. A. (2000). Language development during the adolescent years: Aspects of pragmatics, syntax, and semantics. Topics in Language Disorders, 20, 15–28.

Scott, C. M., and Stokes, S. (1995). Measures of syntax in school-age children and adolescents. Language, Speech, and Hearing Services in Schools, 26, 309–319.

Rice, M. L. (1993). "Don't talk to him; he's weird." A social consequences account of language and social interaction. In A. P. Kaiser and D. Gray (Eds.), Enhancing Children's Communication: Research Foundations for Intervention (pp. 139–158). Baltimore: Paul H. Brookes.

Romski, M. A., and Sevcik, R. (1992). Developing augmented language in children with severe mental retardation. In S. F. Warren and J. Reichle (Eds.), Causes and effects in communication and language intervention (pp. 113–130). Baltimore: Paul H. Brookes.

Scott, C. M., and Windsor, J. (2000). General language performance measures in spoken and written discourse produced by school-age children with and without language learning disabilities. Journal of Speech, Language, and Hearing Research, 43, 324–339.

Wallach, G. P., and Butler, K. (1994). Language learning disabilities in school-age children and adolescents: Some principles and applications. New York: Merrill.

Windsor, J., Doyle, S., and Siegel, G. (1994). Language acquisition after mutism: A longitudinal case study of autism. Journal of Speech and Hearing Research, 37, 96–105.

Language Impairment and Reading Disability

Reading is a language-based activity. As such, there is frequently an overlap between developmental language impairments and reading disabilities. Evidence of a relationship between these developmental disabilities has come from two perspectives. One has been the study of the language development of children with reading disabilities, and the other has been the investigation of the reading outcomes of children with spoken language impairments.

Language Problems in Children with Reading Disabilities

Numerous studies have documented that children with reading disabilities have problems in language development. Most investigations have involved concurrent examination of language problems in children with existing reading disabilities (Vogel, 1974; Bradley and Bryant, 1983; McArthur et al., 2000), while a few have studied the early language abilities of children who later became reading disabled (Scarborough, 1990; Catts et al., 1999). The latter approach is critical to determining the direction of causality.

Children who become poor readers often have language problems, or at least a history of these problems.

Poor readers may have difficulties in vocabulary, grammar, or text-level processing (Vogel, 1974; Catts et al., 1999; McArthur et al., 2000). In at least some cases, these deficits are severe enough for children to have been identified as language impaired (Catts et al., 1999; McArthur et al., 2000).

In addition to these language deficits, children with reading disabilities have difficulties in other areas of language processing, specifically phonological processing (Bradley and Bryant, 1983; Fletcher et al., 1994; Catts et al., 1999). The most noteworthy of these deficits are problems in phonological awareness. Phonological awareness is the explicit awareness of, or sensitivity, to the sounds of speech. It is one's ability to attend to, reflect on, or manipulate phonemes. Children with reading disabilities are consistently more impaired in phonological awareness than in any other single ability (Torgesen, 1996). Poor readers often have difficulties making judgments about the sounds in words or in their ability to segment or blend phonemes. Such problems make it difficult for children to learn how the alphabet represents speech and how this knowledge can be used to decode printed words.

Children with reading disabilities have also been reported to have other deficits in phonological processing (Wagner and Torgesen, 1987). Poor readers have problems in phonological retrieval (i.e., rapid naming), phonological memory, and phonological production (reviewed in Catts and Kamhi, 1999). Although these difficulties in phonological processing often co-occur with those in phonological awareness, there are notable exceptions. For example, one current theory proposes that phonological awareness and rapid naming are somewhat independent, so that poor readers may have deficits in either area alone or in combination (Wolf and Bowers, 1999). However, it is proposed that children with deficits in both areas, or what is termed a double deficit, are at greatest risk for reading difficulties.

Although most children with reading disabilities have a history of language problems, the overlap between language and reading disabilities is not complete. In each group of poor readers who have been studied, at least some participants do not appear to have a history of language problems. When language problems are defined on the basis of difficulties in vocabulary, grammar, or text-level processing, about half of poor readers show no evidence of a language impairment (Mattis, 1978; Catts et al., 1999; McArthur et al., 2000). However, when phonological processing deficits are also included, the percentage of unaffected poor readers is about 25%–30% (Catts et al., 1999). These results are due, at least in part, to the fact that other nonlinguistic factors likely contribute to reading disabilities. Current theories include visual deficits and speed of processing problems as alternative or additional causes of reading problems (Eden et al., 1995; Nicholson and Fawcett, 1999). However, the lack of an apparent association between reading disabilities and language impairments may also be the result of discontinuities in the growth of various aspects of language and reading abilities. These discontinuities may obscure the relationship between language and reading disabilities at certain points in time and highlight the association at others (Scarborough, 2001).

Reading Outcomes in Children with Language Impairments

The overlap between language impairments and reading disabilities has also been established by studies of the reading outcomes of children with language impairments. In the earliest of these studies, children with a clinical history of language impairments were located later in childhood or adulthood and their academic achievement was compared with their earlier speech-language abilities (Aram and Nation, 1980; Hall and Tomblin, 1978). More recently, studies have identified children with language impairment in preschool or kindergarten and followed them into the school grades (Bishop and Adams, 1990; Catts, 1993; Stothard et al., 1998; Rescorla, 2000; Catts et al., 2002). Both lines of research indicate that children with a history of language impairments are at high risk for reading problems. In almost every instance, the reading outcomes of children with language impairment have been found to differ significantly from those of children with typical language development. In addition, many children with a history of language impairments could be classified as reading disabled. Across studies, the percentage of children with language impairment who have been found to have subsequent reading problems has varied from approximately 40% to 90%, with a median value of about 50%.

Despite a strong tendency for children with language impairment to develop reading problems, not all of these children become poor readers. Research indicates that the type and severity of the language disorder are related to reading outcome. Children with more severe or broader-based language impairments are at greater risk for reading disabilities than those with less severe problems or problems confined to a single dimension of language (i.e., expressive language) (Rescorla, 2000; Catts et al., 2002). Also, children with language impairments who have concomitant nonverbal cognitive deficits (i.e., low nonverbal IQ) have poorer reading achievement than those with normal nonverbal cognitive abilities (Bishop and Adams, 1990; Catts et al., 2002). Phonological processing abilities are also related to reading outcome in children with language impairments. For example, Catts (1993) found that measures of phonological awareness and rapid naming were predictive of reading achievement, especially word recognition abilities, in children with language or articulation impairments.

The persistence of a language impairment may be an important predictor of reading outcome in many children. Some children with language impairment appear to resolve their language difficulties prior to school entry, while others continue to manifest language impairments into the school years. Those who continue to have significant language problems are at a much greater risk for reading disabilities in the early school grades than those with improved language abilities. Bishop and Adams (1990), for example, reported that children with language impairments at age 4 who were no longer language impaired at age 5½ had normal reading achievement at age 8. Catts et al. (2002) further found that children with language impairments in kindergarten who did not show language impairments in second grade had significantly better reading outcomes than those who continued to have language problems. Finally, the "persistence hypothesis" is also supported by evidence that change in language impairment status is related to severity of language difficulties, type of language impairment, and nonverbal IQ, each of which has been associated with reading outcome in children with language impairment (Bishop and Adams, 1990, Catts et al., 2002).

These conclusions, however, are compromised somewhat by long-term follow-up data. Specifically, Stothard et al. (1998) showed that the children studied by Bishop and Adams (1990) who had improved in language abilities by age 5½ and who did not have reading problems at age 8½ subsequently did have language and reading problems when tested at age 15. In fact, 52% were found to read significantly below grade level. These results are consistent with Scarborough's proposal of "illusory recovery" (Scarborough, 2001). According to this proposal, children who appear to have resolved their language problems early on, later show language impairments and demonstrate significant disabilities. Scarborough (2001) has argued that illusory recovery and apparent relapse may be the result of nonlinear growth in language development. She suggests that different aspects of language are characterized by spurts and plateaus in growth. Thus, individual differences in language development may be more apparent at some stages than others.

Nonlinear growth in different aspects of reading development may also influence the observation of a relationship between language and reading disabilities. For example, in the early stages, reading development is characterized by rapid improvement in word recognition skills, which rest heavily on phonological processing abilities. At later stages, individual differences become more related to language comprehension abilities (Hoover and Gough, 1990). Thus, children with deficits in phonological processing will most likely have problems in the early stages of learning to read, while those with vocabulary and grammar deficits will be especially at risk in the later stages of reading development.

In summary, the two lines of research reviewed here converge in support of a close relationship between language impairments and reading disabilities. However, this relationship is not complete and may be complicated by nonlinearities in both language and reading development.

—*Hugh W. Catts*

References

Aram, D., and Nation, J. (1980). Preschool language disorders and subsequent language and academic difficulties. *Journal of Communication Disorders, 13,* 159–179.

Bishop, D. V. M., and Adams, C. (1990). A prospective study of the relationship between specific language impairment, phonological disorders and reading retardation. *Journal Child Psychology and Psychiatry, 31*, 1027–1050.

Bradley, L., and Bryant, P. (1983). Categorizing sounds and learning to read: A causal connection. *Nature, 301*, 419–421.

Catts, H. (1993). The relationship between speech-language impairments and reading disabilities. *Journal of Speech and Hearing Research, 36*, 948–958.

Catts, H. W., Fey, M. E., Tomblin, J. B., and Zhang, X. (2002). A longitudinal investigation of reading outcomes of children with language impairments. *Journal of Speech, Language, and Hearing Research, 45*, 1142–1157.

Catts, H. W., Fey, M. E., Zhang, X., and Tomblin, J. B. (1999). Language basis of reading and reading disabilities: Evidence from a longitudinal investigation. *Scientific Studies in Reading, 3*, 331–361.

Catts, H. W., and Kamhi, A. G. (1999). *Language and reading disabilities*. Needham Heights, MA: Allyn and Bacon.

Eden, G. F., Stein, J. F., Wood, M. H., and Wood, F. B. (1995). Verbal and visual problems in reading disability. *Journal of Learning Disabilities, 28*, 272–290.

Fletcher, J. M., Shaywitz, S. E., Shankweiler, D. P., Katz, L., Liberman, I. Y., Stuebing, K. K., et al. (1994). Cognitive profiles of reading disability: Comparisons of discrepancy and low achievement definitions. *Journal of Educational Psychology, 86*, 6–23.

Hall, P., and Tomblin, J. B. (1978). A follow-up study of children with articulation and language disorders. *Journal of Speech and Hearing Disorders, 43*, 227–241.

Hoover, W. A., and Gough, P. B. (1990). The simple view of reading. *Reading and Writing: An Interdisciplinary Journal, 2*, 127–160.

Mattis, S. (1978). Dyslexia syndromes: A working hypothesis that works. In A. L. Benton and D. Pearl (Eds.), *Dyslexia: An appraisal of current knowledge* (pp. 45–58). New York: Oxford University Press.

McArthur, G. M., Hogben, J. H., Edwards, V. T., Heath, S. M., and Mengler, E. D. (2000). On the "specifics" of specific reading disability and specific language impairment. *Journal of Child Psychology and Psychiatry, 41*, 869–874.

Nicholson, R. I., and Fawcett, A. J. (1999). Developmental dyslexia: The role of the cerebellum. *Dyslexia, 5*, 155–177.

Rescorla, L. (2000). Do late-talkers turn out to have reading difficulties a decade later? *Annals of Dyslexia, 50*, 87–102.

Scarborough, H. S. (1990). Very early language deficits in dyslexic children. *Child Development, 61*, 1728–1743.

Scarborough, H. S. (2001). Connecting early language and literacy to later reading (dis)abilities: Evidence, theory, and practice. In S. Neuman and D. Dickison (Eds.), *Handbook for early literacy research*. New York: Guilford Press.

Stothard, S. E., Snowling, M. J., Bishop, D. V. M., Chipchase, B., and Kaplan, C. (1998). Language impaired preschoolers: A follow-up in adolescence. *Journal of Speech, Language, and Hearing Research, 41*, 407–418.

Torgesen, J. (1996). *Phonological awareness: A critical factor in dyslexia*. Baltimore: Orton Dyslexia Society.

Vogel, S. A. (1974). Syntactic abilities in normal and dyslexic children. *Journal of Learning Disabilities, 7*, 47–53.

Wagner, R. K., and Torgesen, J. K. (1987). The nature of phonological processing and its causal role in the acquisition of reading skills. *Psychological Bulletin, 101*, 1–21.

Wolf, M., and Bowers, P. G. (1999). The double-deficit hypothesis for the developmental dyslexias. *Journal of Learning Disabilities, 91*, 415–438.

Language Impairment in Children: Cross-Linguistic Studies

For many years the study of language impairment in children focused almost exclusively on children learning English. The past decade has seen a decided and salutary broadening of this exclusive focus as researchers from many nations have become interested in understanding the impaired language acquisition of children speaking diverse languages. The concern for understanding the cross-linguistic nature of developmental language impairment has followed in the path of investigations into the cross-linguistic nature of typical language development that were initiated by Slobin and his colleagues (e.g., Slobin, 1985).

Cross-linguistic studies of language impairment in children have both a theoretical and a practical impetus. Theoretically, the study of typical and impaired language development across a number of structurally different languages should reveal commonalities as well as differences in how children learn languages. Such studies should help researchers determine what is universal and what is variable in the ways that children learn languages. By sorting the variable from the universal, such research enhances knowledge about the properties of language development that are general to the process of language learning and those that are determined by the structure of the language that the child is exposed to. Practically, understanding what form impairment takes in various languages improves the possibilities for assessment and treatment in those languages. Understanding the contribution of input to the nature and timing of acquisition in a specific language has important consequences for developing intervention approaches. On the other hand, understanding the common properties of language learning helps to clarify in what ways impairment results from possible disruptions of basic human biological and cognitive mechanisms.

Most cross-linguistic studies of children with language impairment have been concerned with the morphological deficits experienced by children with specific language impairment (SLI) (see SPECIFIC LANGUAGE IMPAIRMENT IN CHILDREN). Some such grammatical deficits are found to occur in almost all languages that have been studied so far, regardless of their structure. Other deficits are particular to individual language families. One deficit that appears to exist in many languages has to do with the acquisition of verbal inflection. Finite verbal inflections and auxiliary verbs produced by children with SLI are optionally missing or substituted for in the following languages: German (Clahsen, Bartke, and Gollner, 1997; Rice, Ruff Noll, and Grimm, 1997), Dutch (de Jong, 1999), Swedish (Hansson, 1997), Norwegian (Meyer Bjerkan, 1999), English (Rice and Wexler, 1996), French (Jakubowicz and Nash, 2001; Paradis and Crago, 2001), Italian (Bottari, Cipriani, and Chilosi, 1996; Bortolini, Caselli, and Leonard, 1997; Bottari et al., 2001), Japanese (Fukuda and Fukuda, 2001), Greek (Clahsen and

Dalalakis, 1999), Inuktitut (Crago and Allen, 2001), and Arabic (Abdalla, 2002).

Various language families show interesting patterns that relate to the structure or typology of those particular groups of languages. For example, studies of Germanic languages such as Dutch, Swedish, and German have shown that there are word order consequences related to the omission of finite verb inflections and auxiliaries in the speech of children with SLI.

Studies of Romance languages such as Italian and French have demonstrated that children with SLI have greater trouble acquiring the past tense than the present tense, while English-speaking children with SLI have difficulty with both tenses. Impaired speakers of French and Italian also have difficulty with the production of object clitics. Surprisingly, however, Italian and French children with SLI differ in their acquisition of determiners. Italian-speaking children have more difficulty with this aspect of their grammar than the French-speaking children. It is unfortunate that in the family of Romance languages, there are no comparable acquisition studies of children with SLI learning Spanish, either in the Americas or in Europe.

Speakers of non-Indo-European languages such as Inuktitut and Arabic have different patterns of impairment than other groups. For instance, Arabic speakers replace incorrect verbal inflections with a default form that is typically tense-bearing in the adult language. This is different from the Germanic and Romance languages, where tense-bearing morphemes, such as verbal inflections or auxiliary verbs, tend to be dropped, resulting in a nonfinite verb form such as an infinitive, a participle, or the verb stem appearing as the main verb in the sentence. Specific language impairment in Inuktitut has been shown to present yet another dimension. Here, the trouble a child with impairment had with verbal inflection did not resemble younger normally developing children. This is a different pattern than has been found in many other languages where children with SLI show a pattern of optional verbal inflection that resembles that of younger normally developing children.

Cross-linguistic studies can also play a particularly useful role in verifying hypotheses about the nature of the deficits experienced by children with SLI. They allow researchers to check out explanations based on particular languages with results from typologically different languages. For instance, Leonard, one of the pioneers of cross-linguistic studies of child language impairment, hypothesized from his study of English-speaking children that a plausible explanation for the grammatical deficit in SLI was that these children had difficulty establishing a learning paradigm for morphology in languages where the morphemes had low phonological saliency. He and his colleagues sought systematic cross-linguistic verification for this explanation by studying children with SLI who were learning languages with more salient morphology, such as Italian (Leonard et al., 1992) or Hebrew (Dromi, Leonard, and Shteiman, 1993; Dromi et al., 1999). Indeed, such children appeared to have less difficulty with the acquisition of their verbal

morphology. However, succeeding studies of other languages with very phonologically salient verbal inflections, such as Inuktitut and Japanese, have shown that children with SLI did, in fact, have difficulty with the acquisition of verbal inflections. This demonstrates how a series of cross-linguistic studies can be useful in establishing whether a certain theoretical explanation of SLI is meaningful across languages.

Even though the number of languages that are being studied is expanding, there are only a few studies that can be considered truly cross-linguistic in design. These few genuine cross-linguistic studies involve either a format that compares in one study two groups of subjects who speak two different languages or a specific language in which the grammatical variables tested are as identical as possible to a previously studied language. In addition, studies in which investigators have examined the grammatical properties of children speaking a single specific language also display some methodological shortcomings impeding well-founded conclusions. They have varied in the age and criteria of selection of the children being studied. They have also varied in the particular properties of the children's grammar that were assessed. Regrettably, such design issues have made the kinds of comparisons that are essential to establishing the universal and variable properties of acquisition and impairment often inconclusive.

In summary, despite certain limitations, the expansion of studies of language impairment in children to include a wider variety of languages has enlivened theoretical debate, led to new, linguistically based understandings, and enriched perspectives on this communicative disorder. It is important that studies of language impairment in childhood continue to encompass more and different languages. In fact, languages spoken by the vast majority of children in the world's population remain virtually unexplored. It is equally important that more studies be designed to be truly cross-linguistic in nature, with variables and criteria for impairment established as uniformly as possible. The study of bilingual children with impairment provides a unique opportunity for the cross-linguistic observation of language impairment. These children are perfectly matched to themselves as the learners of two languages (see BILINGUALISM AND LANGUAGE IMPAIRMENT). Finally, just as important as understanding how children with language impairment learn different languages is recognizing that they are also members of different cultures. Language and culture are inextricably linked and as such they influence each other as well as the manifestations of and beliefs about childhood language impairment.

— *Martha Crago and Johanne Paradis*

References

Abdalla, F. (2002). *Specific language impairment in Arabic-speaking children: Deficits in morphosyntax.* Unpublished dissertation, McGill University, Montreal.

Bortolini, U., Caselli, M. C., and Leonard, L. (1997). Grammatical deficits in Italian-speaking children with specific language impairment. *Journal of Speech, Language, and Hearing Research*, 40, 809–820.

Bottari, P., Cipriani, P., and Chilosi, A. (1996). Root infinitives in Italian SLI children. In A. Stringfellow, D. Cahana-Amitay, E. Hughes, and A. Zukowski (Eds.), *BUCLD 20* (pp. 75–86). Somerville, MA: Cascadilla Press.

Bottari, P., Cipriani, P., Chilosi, A., and Pfanner, L. (2001). The Italian determiner system in normal acquisition, specific language impairment, and childhood aphasia. *Brain and Language*, 77, 283–293.

Clahsen, H., Bartke, S., and Göllner, S. (1997). Formal features in impaired grammars: A comparison of English and German SLI children. *Journal of Neurolinguistics*, 10, 151–171.

Clahsen, H., and Dalalakis, J. (1999). Tense and agreement in Greek SLI: A case study. *Essex Research Reports in Linguistics*, 1–25.

Crago, M., and Allen, S. (2001). Early finiteness in Inuktitut: The role of language structure and input. *Language Acquisition*, 9(1), 59–111.

de Jong, J. (1999). *Specific language impairment in Dutch: Inflectional morphology and argument structure*. Enschede, The Netherlands: Print Partners Ipskamp.

Dromi, E., Leonard, L., Adam, G., and Zadunaisky-Ehrlich, S. (1999). Verb agreement morphology in Hebrew-speaking children with specific language impairment. *Journal of Speech, Language, and Hearing Research*, 42, 1414–1431.

Dromi, E., Leonard, L., and Shteiman, M. (1993). The grammatical morphology of Hebrew-speaking children with specific language impairment: Some competing hypotheses. *Journal of Speech and Hearing Research*, 36, 760–771.

Fukuda, S., and Fukuda, S. (2001). The acquisition of complex predicates in Japanese specifically language-impaired and normally developing children. *Brain and Language*, 77, 305–320.

Hansson, K. (1997). Patterns of verb usage in Swedish children with SLI: An application of recent theories. *First Language*, 17, 195–217.

Jakubowicz, C., and Nash, L. (2001). Functional categories and syntactic operations in (ab)normal language acquisition. *Brain and Language*, 77, 321–339.

Leonard, L., Bortolini, U., Caselli, M., McGregor, K., and Sabbadini, L. (1992). Morphological deficits in children with specific language impairment: The status of features in the underlying grammar. *Language Acquisition*, 2, 151–179.

Meyer Bjerkan, K. (1999). *Do SLI children have an optional infinitive stage?* San Sebastian, Spain: International Association for the Study of Child Language.

Paradis, J., and Crago, M. (2001). The morphosyntax of specific language impairment in French: An extended optional default account. *Language Acquisition*, 9(4), 269–300.

Rice, M., Ruff Noll, K., and Grimm, H. (1997). An extended optional infinitive stage in German-speaking children with specific language impairment. *Language Acquisition*, 6, 255–296.

Rice, M., and Wexler, K. (1996). Toward tense as a clinical marker of specific language impairment. *Journal of Speech, Language, and Hearing Research*, 39, 1236–1257.

Slobin, D. (1985). *The cross-linguistic study of language acquisition*. Mahwah, NJ: Erlbaum.

Further Readings

Bastiaanse, R., and Bol, G. (2001). Verb inflection and verb diversity in three populations: Agrammatic speakers, normally developing children, and children with specific language impairment. *Brain and Language*, 77, 274–282.

Crago, M., and Paradis, J. (2003). Two of a kind: Commonalities and variation in across learners and languages. In Y. Levy and J. Schaeffer (Eds.), *Linguistic competence across populations: Towards a definition of Specific Language Impairment* (pp. 97–110). Mahwah, NJ: Erlbaum.

Hakansson, G. (1998). Language impairment and the realization of finiteness. In A. Greenhill, M. Hughes, H. Littlefield, and H. Walsh (Eds.), *BUCLD 22* (pp. 314–324). Somerville, MA: Cascadilla Press.

Jakubowicz, C., Nash, L., Rigaut, C., and Gérard, C. (1998). Determiners and clitic pronouns in French-speaking children with SLI. *Language Acquisition*, 7, 113–160.

Jakubowicz, C., Nash, L., and van der Velde, M. (1999). Inflection and past tense morphology in French SLI. In A. Greenhill, H. Littlefield, and C. Tano (Eds.), *BUCLD 23* (pp. 289–300). Somerville, MA: Cascadilla Press.

Paradis, J., and Crago, M. (2000). Tense and temporality: A comparison between children learning a second language and children with SLI. *Journal of Speech, Language, and Hearing Research*, 43, 834–847.

Paradis, J., Crago, M., Genesee, F., and Rice, M. (2000). *Dual language disorders: Extended optional infinitive in bilingual children with specific language impairment*. Paper presented at the Boston University Conference on Language Development, Boston.

Roberts, S., and Leonard, L. (1997). Grammatical deficits in German and English: A crosslinguistic study of children with specific language impairment. *First Language*, 17, 131–150.

Language in Children Who Stutter

A connection between language and stuttering in young children is intuitive. As noted by Yairi (1983) and others (e.g., Ratner, 1997), stuttering first appears in children between ages 2 and 4 years, during a time of rapid expansion in expressive and receptive language ability. Moreover, the repetitions and prolongations that characterize stuttering are observed as the child uses sounds to form words and words to form phrases and sentences. The apparent link between domains has given rise to theoretical accounts of stuttering that emphasize linguistic variables. For example, one working account of stuttering suggests that underlying difficulties with phonological encoding, difficulties that self-correct prior to actual language production but that slow language processing, yield disfluencies (Postma and Kolk, 1993). Linguistic factors are implicated in several other theoretical accounts of stuttering as well (Wingate, 1988; Perkins, Kent, and Curlee, 1991).

Despite the intuitive appeal of connections between language and stuttering, many of the most fundamental questions in this area of inquiry continue to be debated. The language abilities of young children who stutter have been the focus of research and controversy for many years (see Yairi et al., 2001, and Wingate, 2001, for examples of the ongoing dialogue on this topic). In addition to examinations of the language development status of young children who stutter, the connection between language and stuttering in young children has been studied in other ways, namely, through evaluation of linguistic variables that appear to exert an influence on stuttering behavior. Relevant linguistic variables include grammatical complexity and location of stuttering events in the language planning or production process. In both areas, the developmental status of children who stutter and the study of linguistic influences on stuttering, a growing body of knowledge speaks to the associations of language and stuttering in young children. This article highlights key research findings in these areas and summarizes what is known about the interface of language and stuttering in young children.

Language Ability and Stuttering in Young Children

The scholarly literature reveals a relatively longstanding view of the child who stutters as more likely to have language learning difficulties or impairments than typically developing peers. Through analysis of spontaneous language sample data, a group of scholars has empirically evaluated the expressive language abilities of a large cohort of young children who stutter (Watkins and Yairi, 1997; Watkins, Yairi, and Ambrose, 1999). The Illinois Stuttering Research Project has prospectively tracked a group of young children who stutter, beginning as near stuttering onset as possible and continuing longitudinally for a number of years to monitor persistence in versus recovery from stuttering. This work has focused on expressive language abilities, comparing the performance of young children who stutter with normative expectations on a range of language sample measures, such as mean length of utterance (MLU, a general index of grammatical ability), number of different words (NDW, a general measure of vocabulary skills), and Developmental Sentence Score (DSS, an index of grammatical skills). The researchers found that, as a group, children who stutter perform at or above normative expectations in their expressive language skills. More specifically, Watkins, Yairi, and Ambrose (1999) reported data based on analysis of 83 preschoolers who stuttered. Children who entered the study between the ages of 2 and 3 years (i.e., exhibited stuttering onset between ages 2 and 3 years) scored about 1 SD above normative expectations on several expressive language measures calculated from spontaneous samples. Children who entered the study between the ages of 3 and 4 years or 4 and 5 years performed at or near normative expectations. Interestingly, the children whose stuttering would ultimately persist (roughly 25% of the total sample) did not differ in expressive language skills from the children who would later recover from stuttering, when their language skills were compared near the time of stuttering onset. Figure 1 provides a sample of the findings of Watkins, Yairi, and Ambrose (1999), showing the MLU for children who entered the longitudinal study at three different age groupings relative to normative expectations.

The findings of several other investigators lend support to these results regarding expressive language skills

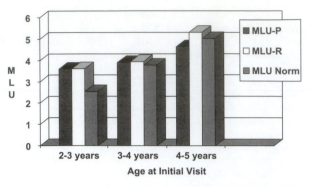

Figure 1. Mean length of utterance, compared with normative expectations, for children whose stuttering persists or recovers. (From Watkins, R. V., Yairi, E., and Ambrose, N. G. [1999]. Early childhood stuttering: III. Initial status of expressive language abilities. *Journal of Speech, Language, and Hearing Research*, *42*, 1125–1135. Reproduced with permission.)

in young children who stutter. More than a decade ago, Nippold (1990) reported that there was no compelling evidence that children who stuttered had a higher rate of language learning difficulties than the general population. In 2001, Miles and Ratner reported the performance of a group of young children who stuttered on a range of expressive and receptive language measures; the children in their sample scored at or slightly above the average level of performance on every reported measure (i.e., the group scored at or above a percentile rank of 50 or at or above a standard score of 100 on the measures used). Rommel and colleagues (1999) in Germany reported that preschool-age participants who stuttered had language skills at or above age expectations. Anderson and Conture (2000) also reported language scores at or above average for a group of children who stuttered.

In light of these findings, there is little empirical support for the hypothesis that language development and stuttering are linked to a common, underlying communication difficulty, at least in any significant number of young children. On closer examination of the research literature, methodological issues appear that may account for the view that children who stutter frequently have concomitant language difficulties. Several early studies of language ability in young children who stuttered did not consider socioeconomic status, potentially comparing young children who stuttered and were from lower or middle-income backgrounds with typically developing youngsters from university-based families (see Ratner, 1997). Furthermore, several past studies of language ability in young children who stuttered did not evaluate the children's skills in light of normative expectations. Other studies reported higher than expected rates of concomitant language disabilities in young children who stuttered but evaluated children long after stuttering onset, or included children of very different ages. When relations between language ability and stuttering are examined long after stuttering onset, children may well have learned to adapt their expressive language in various ways in order to limit or reduce stuttering events. Such studies may be interesting, but they ask very different questions from those addressed by investigations of language skills near the onset of stuttering. Any or all of these methodological choices could have considerable impact on findings pertaining to patterns and pathways of language acquisition in youngsters who stutter, and all could be in the direction that predict a less favorable performance for children who stutter in comparison with typically developing children.

In general, there is a growing consensus that language development is not particularly vulnerable in young children who stutter. Continued study of language strengths or challenges in conjunction with stuttering may reveal developmental asynchronies (e.g., perhaps early precocious language skill is a particular risk factor for stuttering, or perhaps accelerated language development in one domain, such as syntax or semantics, creates difficulties with fluency when proficiencies in other domains, such as motoric abilities, are less sophisticated). These possibilities await empirical study and will require detailed linguistic analyses to evaluate.

Linguistic Influences on Stuttering

There is ample evidence that stuttering events are influenced by linguistic variables. Brown (1945) was perhaps the first researcher to suggest linguistic influences on stuttering events with his groundbreaking report of apparent influences of a word's grammatical form class (i.e., content versus function word) on stuttering loci in adults who stuttered. In brief, Brown reported that adults who stuttered were significantly more likely to be disfluent on content words (e.g., nouns and verbs) than on function words (e.g., prepositions and pronouns).

Since Brown's seminal work, researchers have continually refined analyses in the study of linguistic influences on stuttering. We now know, for example, that young children are generally more likely to stutter on sentences of greater grammatical complexity than on sentences of less grammatical complexity (Logan and Conture, 1995; Yaruss, 1999). Furthermore, the content-function variable appears not to be the most relevant influence on stuttering loci; instead, stuttering events are significantly more likely on either a content word or on a phrase-initial function word that precedes a content word than in other phrasal locations (Au-Yeung, Howell, and Pilgrim, 1998). The underlying influence here is thought to be the planning unit in language formulation, such that disfluencies are significantly more likely to occur at the beginning of a language planning unit, when remaining components of the unit continue to be refined for production.

These findings reveal that aspects of language planning, formulation, and production exert an influence on stuttering for children and adults. These findings support the view that linguistic variables are relevant in characterizing stuttering events. It is noteworthy, however, that linguistic factors appear to influence disfluencies in the same way for stutterers and nonstutterers alike. That is, linguistic variables such as grammatical complexity and the loci of stuttering tend to influence individuals whose disfluencies occur at typical rates in language production as well as individuals whose disfluencies are frequent enough to yield identification as a "stutterer."

The domain of language is relevant in the study of early childhood stuttering. The majority of young children who stutter display expressive language abilities at or above normative expectations. In addition, a number of linguistic variables, such as the grammatical complexity of an utterance, exert an influence on the likelihood of a stuttering event. It may be informative for future investigation in this area of inquiry to move toward detailed and specific analyses of profiles of language strength and evaluation of synchrony versus asynchrony within and across developmental domains.

See also SPEECH DISFLUENCY AND STUTTERING IN CHILDREN.

—*Ruth V. Watkins*

References

Anderson, J., and Conture, E. (2000). Language abilities of children who stutter: A preliminary study. *Journal of Fluency Disorders, 25,* 283–304.

Au-Yeung, J., Howell, P., and Pilgrim, L. (1998). Phonological words and stuttering on function words. *Journal of Speech, Language, and Hearing Research, 41,* 1019–1030.

Brown, S. F. (1945). The loci of stutterings in the speech sequence. *Journal of Speech Disorders, 10,* 181–192.

Logan, K. J., and Conture, E. G. (1995). Length, grammatical complexity, and rate differences in stuttered and fluent conversational utterances of children who stutter. *Journal of Fluency Disorders, 20,* 35–61.

Miles, S., and Ratner, N. B. (2001). Parental language input to children at stuttering onset. *Journal of Speech, Language, and Hearing Research, 44,* 1116–1130.

Nippold, M. (1990). Concomitant speech and language disorders in stuttering children: A critique of the literature. *Journal of Speech and Hearing Disorders, 55,* 51–60.

Perkins, W. H., Kent, R. D., and Curlee, R. F. (1991). A theory of neuropsycholinguistic function in stuttering. *Journal of Speech and Hearing Research, 34,* 734–752.

Postma, A., and Kolk, H. (1993). The covert repair hypothesis: Prearticulatory repair processes in normal and stuttered disfluencies. *Journal of Speech and Hearing Research, 36,* 472–487.

Ratner, N. B. (1997). Stuttering: A psycholinguistic perspective. In R. Curlee and G. Siegel (Eds.), *Nature and treatment of stuttering: New directions* (2nd ed., pp. 99–127). Boston: Allyn and Bacon.

Rommel, D., Hage, A., Kalehne, P., and Johannsen, H. S. (1999). Developmental, maintenance, and recovery of childhood stuttering: Prospective longitudinal data 3 years after first contact. In K. Baker, L. Rustin, and K. Baker (Eds.), *Proceedings of the Fifth Oxford Disfluency Conference.* Berkshire, U.K.: Chappel Gardner.

Watkins, R. V., and Yairi, E. (1997). Language production abilities of children whose stuttering persisted or recovered. *Journal of Speech and Hearing Research, 40,* 385–399.

Watkins, R. V., Yairi, E., and Ambrose, N. G. (1999). Early childhood stuttering: III. Initial status of expressive language abilities. *Journal of Speech, Language, and Hearing Research, 42*, 1125–1135.

Wingate, M. (1988). *The structure of stuttering: A psycholinguistic perspective*. New York: Springer-Verlag.

Wingate, M. (2001). SLD is not stuttering. *Journal of Speech, Language, and Hearing Research, 44*, 381–383.

Yairi, E. (1983). The onset of stuttering in two- and three-year-old children. *Journal of Speech and Hearing Disorders, 48*, 171–177.

Yairi, E., Watkins, R. V., Ambrose, N. G., and Paden, E. (2001). What is stuttering? *Journal of Speech, Language, and Hearing Research, 44*, 384–390.

Yaruss, S. (1999). Utterance length, syntactic complexity, and childhood stuttering. *Journal of Speech, Language, and Hearing Research, 42*, 329–344.

Language of the Deaf: Acquisition of English

Effective English language skills are essential for the education of deaf children and for the integration of deaf individuals into the wider, hearing society. However, the average deaf student's English language competence over the course of his or her schooling is limited. Although periodic reviews of nationwide achievement testing reveal some improvement in the average reading levels of deaf students over the past 30 years, the increase is small, and in English literacy skills most deaf students fall farther and farther behind their hearing peers over the course of their schooling. The average reading comprehension scores for deaf students in the United States rises from the second-grade level at age 9 to around the fourth-grade level at age 17 (de Villiers, 1992). Among white deaf high school graduates, only about 15% read above the sixth-grade level, and the percentage is only about 5% for those who are from African-American or Hispanic backgrounds (Allen, 1994).

The hearing child and the typical deaf child are in very different stages of language development when they reach the point of formal schooling and reading instruction. Normally hearing 5- or 6-year-old children have a speaking vocabulary of several thousand words and have mastered most of the complex syntax of English. Thus, for hearing children, the acquisition of reading is primarily learning to map printed English onto an existing knowledge of spoken English (Adams, 1990).

For the deaf child, the situation is quite different. Impairment of hearing has a negative effect on the acquisition of a spoken language from early in the child's life, and all of the major milestones in normal language acquisition are considerably delayed. For example, around 6 months of age, normal-hearing infants begin producing the first approximations to consonant-vowel combinations, or syllables, over quite a wide range of speech-like sounds (so-called "marginal" babbling). A few months later "canonical" babbling emerges, in which the child produces a more restricted set of phonetic units in repetitive, rhythmic syllabic organization, and there is an abrupt decline in non-speech-like vocalizations. Canonical babbling increasingly uses the phonemes found in the adult input language, yet it makes no reference to any real-world objects or actions. However, the parents of these hearing infants treat their infants' babbles as if they were meaningful, engaging in reciprocal "dialogues" and commenting on the infants' utterances. For deaf infants, early vocalization and marginal babbling is not delayed, and they produce a similar range of speech-like sounds, which suggests that this stage is biologically driven. But canonical babbling is considerably delayed and appears to be deviant in both vocal quantity and quality (Mogford, 1993). So, hearing parents of deaf infants do not respond to their infant's vocalizations as proto-communications, being more likely to ignore or talk through them. Thus, most deaf infants are already at a disadvantage toward the end of the first year of life, both in their ability to extract the phonemes of their spoken language from the input and reproduce them, and in the initial structuring of conversational dialogues in parent-infant interaction (Paul, 2001).

Phonology

Speech intelligibility is a persistent problem for deaf children with moderate to profound hearing loss (>60 dB·loss in the better ear), particularly if the major hearing loss is in the higher frequencies of sound (>1500 Hz). Studies report from 50% to 80% of moderate to profoundly deaf children having either "very hard to understand" or "totally unintelligible" speech (Carney, 1986). Omission or distortion of consonant sounds is common and has a major impact on intelligibility (Osberger and McGarr, 1982). Many of the speech errors of deaf children reflect the phonological processes and constraints operating in normal speech development in young hearing children (e.g., consonant cluster reduction, fronting of place of articulation, voicing errors, or deletion of final consonants), but they persist in the speech of deaf children well into later childhood (Murphy and Dodd, 1995). Control of voice quality and intonation is also difficult for children with substantial hearing loss. Consequently, instances of consistently high or low pitch, nasalized speech, and rhythmical errors such as unusual breath groups and either misplaced syllabic stress or added syllables are common and produce a characteristic set of deaf "accents" in spoken English (Osberger and McGarr, 1982; Paterson, 1994; Murphy and Dodd, 1995).

Vocabulary

As measured by parental reports on the MacArthur Communicative Development Inventory (CDI), the average hearing child progresses rapidly from an expressive vocabulary of approximately 100 words at 18 months to 300 words at 2 years and 550 words at 3 years (Fenson et al., 1993). In contrast, the average deaf toddler with hearing parents produces about 30 words at 2 years and 200 words at 3 years, whether those words are spoken or signed (Mayne, Yoshinago-Itano, Sedey, and Carey, 2000). Deaf children whose hearing loss was identified by 6 months of age and who have above-average cognitive skills fare best, showing a vocabulary spurt in the third year of life similar to that found in hearing children, though about 6 months later (Mayne et al., 2000). However, even these successful deaf children fall below the 25th percentile for hearing children on norms for the CDI at 30–36 months of age (see also Mayne, Yoshinago-Itano, and Sedey, 2000). Thus, the average 5- to 6-year-old deaf child is some 2 years behind hearing peers in vocabulary size when the child begins the task of learning to read.

Syntax

The English of deaf children also exhibits characteristic syntactic problems. For example, tense markers on the verb and many other grammatical morphemes and function words (e.g., articles "a" and "the," or copula and auxiliary verbs) are inconsistently provided or missing from most deaf children's spoken or signed English when they reach the early grades of formal schooling. These aspects of English grammar continue to provide great difficulty for deaf children during the school years (Quigley and King, 1980; de Villiers, 1988). In the terms of generative grammar (Radford, 1990; Leonard, 1995), the functional categories Inflectional Phrase (IP) and Determiner Phrase (DP), which host the marking of tense for verbs and specification for nouns, may be incompletely specified in the grammar of deaf children. If so, one might expect problems also with a final functional category that structures the embedding of clauses, the Complementizer Phrase (CP) (de Villiers, de Villiers, and Hoban, 1994). Hearing children at the age of 5 or 6 have mastered a variety of multiclause embedded sentence forms—especially temporal and causal adverbial clauses, complement structures, and relative clauses— that are essential for creating cohesion in narrative discourse and other extended conversation (de Villiers, 1988, 1991; Engen, 1994). However, in deaf children, clauses and sentences tend to be strung together with "and" or "then," and complex embedded structures are usually missing or malformed in their English production and also are poorly comprehended (Engen and Engen, 1983; de Villiers, de Villiers, and Hoban, 1994; Engen, 1994; Berent, 1996). Thus the spoken, signed, or written English narratives of deaf students can often be characterized as a list of sentences each describing an event, but with little cohesion or coherence because the characters and events are not linguistically linked together by referential, causal, and temporal cohesion markers (de Villiers, 1991; Engen, 1994).

In summary, when deaf children reach the point of acquiring English literacy skills, they usually have a severely limited vocabulary and lack knowledge of the complex syntax of English that is critical for combining sentences together into cohesive text. Indeed, much of the deaf child's English language learning comes from printed English, and the task of learning to read becomes one of both cracking the print code *and* learning the

language at the same time. The better the child's English language skills are before formal schooling, the easier the task of reading acquisition becomes.

New Developments

This pattern of delay and difficulty with language and literacy in deaf youngsters is mitigated by two technological advances that are transforming language intervention with deaf toddlers. The first is the implementation of universal newborn hearing screening programs, with the potential for identifying almost all infants with a significant degree of hearing loss within the first few months of life. By 2000, some two dozen states in the United States had mandated universal screening of hearing for infants prior to hospital discharge. Researchers in the state of Colorado demonstrated that identification of hearing loss prior to 6 months of age followed by effective ongoing intervention services and parent training programs was a major contributor to successful language outcomes for deaf children (Yoshinaga-Itano and Appuzzo, 1998a, 1998b; Yoshinago-Itano, Sedey, et al., 1998).

The second important advance is the development of multichannel cochlear implant technology. Electrodes implanted into the cochlear now bypass the hair cells and stimulate the auditory nerve directly. An external receiver and processor analyzes the incoming speech according to a predetermined strategy and transforms the complex pattern of sound frequencies and amplitudes into a corresponding pattern of electrical stimulation across a number of electrodes in the cochlear. Over the past 15 years, major developments in the complexity of the analysis that can be carried out in the externally worn speech processor (increasingly miniaturized by developing computer technology) first led to remarkable improvements in speech perception in postlingually deafened adults with implants. Now younger and younger profoundly deaf children who lost their hearing at or soon after birth and who would not benefit much from conventional hearing aids are receiving cochlear implants, some as young as 18 months of age (Niparko et al., 2000). Children who receive an implant early in life, followed by intensive auditory and speech training, can achieve speech intelligibility and conversational fluency that exceed the levels typically observed in profoundly deaf children who use hearing aids (Fryauf-Bertschy et al., 1997; Spencer, Tye-Murray, and Tomblin, 1998; Tomblin et al., 1999; Svirsky et al., 2000). However, there remains substantial individual variation in the degree of success of these implants with prelingually deaf toddlers (Pisoni et al., 2000). Although some children exhibit dramatic improvement in their speech perception and production, and may even acquire grammatical and vocabulary skills at a rate matching that of hearing children, others show only limited spoken language gains even after 3 or 4 years of implant use. The sources of this variability are still rather poorly understood but may include such factors as age at implantation, preimplant residual hearing, type of speech processor used, and success at tuning or "mapping" the implant, as well as the educational and family environment (Fryauf-Bertschy et al., 1997; Niparko et al., 2000; Osberger and Fisher, 2000; Pisoni et al., 2000).

Conclusion

In summary, most children who are born with a moderate to profound hearing loss or who become deaf in the first few years of life suffer a pervasive disruption in their acquisition of all aspects of spoken English (and its signed forms). This leads to major difficulties in the children's acquisition of literacy skills. Early identification of hearing loss and the immediate implementation of intervention strategies involving the best available technologies for amplification, and parental training in early language intervention in a rich interactional context, seem to offer the best outcome for these children in their acquisition of English.

—*Peter A. de Villiers*

References

Adams, M. (1990). *Beginning to read: Thinking and learning about print*. Cambridge, MA: MIT Press.

Allen, T. (1994). *Who are the deaf and hard-of-hearing students leaving high school and entering postsecondary education?* Washington, DC: Gallaudet University.

Berent, G. (1996). The acquisition of English syntax by deaf learners. In W. Ritchie and T. Bhatia (Eds.), *Handbook of second language acquisition*. San Diego, CA: Academic Press.

Carney, A. (1986). Understanding speech intelligibility in the hearing impaired. In K. Butler (Ed.), *Hearing impairment and language disorders: Assessment and intervention*. Gaithersburg, MD: Aspen.

de Villiers, J. G., de Villiers, P. A., and Hoban, E. (1994). The central problem of functional categories in the English syntax of deaf children. In H. Tager-Flusberg (Ed.), *Constraints on language acquisition: Studies of atypical children*. Hillsdale, NJ: Erlbaum.

de Villiers, P. A. (1988). Assessing English syntax in hearing-impaired children: Elicited production in pragmatically motivated situations. In R. Kretschmer and L. Kretschmer (Eds.), *Communication assessment of hearing-impaired children: From conversation to classroom*. *Journal of the Academy of Rehabilitative Audiology: Monograph Supplement, 21,* 41–71.

de Villiers, P. A. (1991). English literacy development in deaf children: Directions for research and intervention. In J. Miller (Ed.), *Research on child language disorders: A decade of progress*. Austin, TX: Pro-Ed.

de Villiers, P. A. (1992). Educational implications of deafness: Language and literacy. In R. Eavey and J. Klein (Eds.), *Hearing loss in childhood: A primer*. Columbus, OH: Ross Laboratories.

Engen, E. (1994). English language acquisition in deaf children in programs using manually-coded English. In A. Vonen, K. Arnesen, R. Enerstvedt, and A. Nafstad (Eds.), *Bilingualism and literacy: Proceedings of an international workshop*. Oslo, Norway: Skadalan Publications.

Engen, E., and Engen, T. (1983). *Rhode Island Test of Language Structure*. Austin, TX: Pro-Ed.

Fenson, L., Dale, P., Reznick, D., Thal, E., Bates, E., Hartung, J., et al. (1993). *MacArthur Communication Developmental Inventories*. San Diego, CA: Singular Publishing Group.

Fryauf-Bertschy, H., Tyler, R., Kelsay, D., Gantz, B., and Woodworth, G. (1997). Cochlear implant use by prelingually deafened children: The influences of age at implant and length of device use. *Journal of Speech, Language, and Hearing Research, 40,* 183–199.

Leonard, L. (1995). Functional categories in the grammars of children with specific language impairment. *Journal of Speech and Hearing Research, 38,* 1270–1283.

Mayne, A., Yoshinago-Itano, C., and Sedey, A. (2000). Receptive vocabulary development of infants and toddlers who are deaf and hard of hearing. *Volta Review, 100,* 29–52.

Mayne, A., Yoshinago-Itano, C., Sedey, A., and Carey, A. (2000). Expressive vocabulary development of infants and toddlers who are deaf and hard of hearing. *Volta Review, 100,* 1–28.

Mogford, K. (1993). Oral language acquisition in the prelinguistically deaf. In D. Bishop and K. Mogford (Eds.), *Language development in exceptional circumstances*. Hillsdale, NJ: Erlbaum.

Murphy, J., and Dodd, B. (1995). Hearing impairment. In B. Dodd (Ed.), *Differential diagnosis and treatment of children with speech disorder*. San Diego, CA: Singular Publishing Group.

Niparko, J., Kirk, K., Mellon, N., Robbins, L., Tucci, D., and Wilson, B. (Eds.). (2000). *Cochlear implants: Principles and practices*. Philadelphia: Lippincott, Williams, and Wilkins.

Osberger, M., and Fisher, L. (2000). Preoperative predictors of postoperative implant performance in children. *Annals of Otology, Rhinology and Laryngology, 109*(Suppl. 185), 44–46.

Osberger, M., and McGarr, N. (1982). Speech production characteristics of the hearing-impaired. In N. Lass (Ed.), *Speech and language: Advances in basic research and practice*. New York: Academic Press.

Paterson, M. (1994). Articulation and phonological disorders in hearing-impaired school aged children with severe and profound sensorineural hearing losses. In J. Bernthal and N. Bankson (Eds.), *Child phonology: Characteristics, assessments and intervention with special populations*. New York: Thieme.

Paul, P. (2001). *Language and deafness* (3rd ed.). San Diego, CA: Singular Publishing Group.

Pisoni, D., Cleary, M., Geers, A., and Tobey, E. (2000). Individual differences in effectiveness of cochlear implants in children who are prelingually deaf: New process measures of performance. *Volta Review, 100,* 111–164.

Quigley, S., and King, C. (1981). An invited article: Syntactic performance of hearing-impaired and normal individuals. *Applied Psycholinguistics, 1,* 329–356.

Radford, A. (1990). *Syntactic theory and the acquisition of English syntax*. Oxford, U.K.: Blackwell.

Spencer, L., Tye-Murray, N., and Tomblin, J. (1998). The production of English inflectional morphology, speech production and listening performance in children with cochlear implants. *Ear and Hearing, 19,* 310–318.

Svirsky, M., Robbins, A., Kirk, K., Pisoni, D., and Miyamoto, R. (2000). Language development in profoundly deaf children with cochlear implants. *Psychological Science, 11,* 153–158.

Tomblin, J. B., Spencer, L., Flock, S., Tyler, R., and Gantz, B. (1999). A comparison of language achievement in children with cochlear implants and children using hearing aids. *Journal of Speech, Language, and Hearing Research, 42,* 497–511.

Yoshinaga-Itano, C., and Appuzzo, M. (1998a). Identification of hearing loss after age 18 months is not early enough. *American Annals of the Deaf, 143,* 380–387.

Yoshinaga-Itano, C., and Appuzzo, M. (1998b). The development of deaf and hard-of-hearing children identified early through the high risk registry. *American Annals of the Deaf, 143,* 416–424.

Yoshinago-Itano, C., Sedey, A., Coulter, D., and Mehl, A. (1998). Language of early- and late-identified children with hearing loss. *Pediatrics, 102,* 1161–1171.

Further Readings

Annals of Otology, Rhinology, and Laryngology. (2000). *Supplement 185, 109*(12). [Special issue]

Bench, R. (1992). *Communication skills in hearing impaired children.* London, U.K.: Whurr.

Geers, A., and Moog, J. (1989). Factors predictive of the development of literacy in profoundly hearing-impaired adolescents. *Volta Review, 91,* 69–86.

Geers, A., and Moog, J. (Eds.). (1994). *Effectiveness of cochlear implants and tactile aids for deaf children. Volta Review, 96*(5). [Special issue]

Jeanes, R., Nienhuys, T., and Rickards, F. (2000). The pragmatic skills of profoundly deaf children. *Journal of Deaf Studies and Deaf Education, 5,* 237–247.

Lederberg, A., and Spencer, P. (2001). Vocabulary development of deaf and hard of hearing children. In M. D. Clark, M. Marschark, and M. Karchmer (Eds.), *Context, cognition, and deafness.* Washington, DC: Gallaudet University Press.

Levitt, H., McGarr, N., and Geffner, D. (1987). *Development of language and communication skills in hearing-impaired children* (ASHA Monograph No. 26). Rockville, MD: American Speech-Hearing-Language Association.

Novelli-Olmstead, T., and Ling, D. (1984). Speech production and speech discrimination by hearing-impaired children. *Volta Review, 86,* 72–80.

Osberger, M. (Ed.). (1986). *Language and learning skills of hearing-impaired students* (ASHA Monograph No. 23). Rockville, MD: American Speech-Language-Hearing Association.

Schirmer, B. (1994). *Language and literacy development in children who are deaf.* New York: Maxwell Macmillan International.

Stoker, R., and Ling, D. (Eds.). (1992). Speech production in hearing-impaired children and youth: Theory and practice. *Volta Review, 94*(5). [Special issue]

Wood, D., Wood, H., Griffiths, A., and Howarth, I. (1986). *Teaching and talking with deaf children.* London, U.K.: Wiley.

Yoshinago-Itano, C., and Sedey, A. (Eds.). (2000). Language, speech, and social-emotional development of children who are deaf or hard of hearing: The early years. *Volta Review, 100*(5). [Special issue]

Language of the Deaf: Sign Language

Hearing loss limits deaf children's access to spoken languages, but deaf communities around the world acquire natural sign languages that create complete communication systems with the same subtlety and level of syntactic and semantic complexity as any spoken language. At the core of these communities are the 8%–10% of deaf children with deaf parents who are exposed to sign language from birth. But some deaf children with hearing parents are also exposed to a natural sign language through contact with native-signing deaf children and adults in educational settings. Thus, deaf children may be speech-delayed, but they are not necessarily language-delayed or disordered in any sense.

Characteristics of American Sign Language and Other Natural Sign Languages

This entry focuses on American Sign Language (ASL) because it is the natural sign language used in the United States and it has been the most extensively studied. However, many of the issues raised here about the unique properties of natural sign languages and the normal pattern of acquisition of those languages by deaf children exposed to complete and early input apply to all natural sign languages.

ASL and other natural sign languages are formally structured at different levels and follow the same universal constraints and organizational principles of all natural languages. Like the distinctive features of spoken phonology, a limited set of handshapes, movements, and places of articulation on the face and body distinguish different lexical signs. For example, in ASL the signs for SUMMER, UGLY, and DRY are produced with the same handshape and movement, but in different locations on the face (Bellugi et al., 1993). Just as in spoken languages, the syntactic rules of ASL operate on underlying abstract categories defined by their linguistic function, such as subjects and objects, or noun phrases and verb phrases. Furthermore, grammatical processes are recursive, embedding one phrase or clause within another (Liddell, 1980).

On the other hand, the visual-spatial modality of natural sign languages leads to several distinctive properties. Spoken languages are mostly sequential, in that the order of speech elements determines meaning. For example, temporal or adverbial modulations in meaning are expressed in spoken English by inflectional suffixes and prefixes that are added to the verb root. In contrast, multiple features of meaning are communicated simultaneously in sign languages: the place, direction, and manner in which signs are produced frequently add to or modulate the meaning of a sign. For example, ASL has evolved a system of simultaneous inflectional morphology on the verb that indicates person, number, distributional aspect, and such temporal aspects as the repetition, habituality, and duration of the action. The single sign GIVE, for example, can be inflected to communicate the meanings "give to me," "give regularly," "give to them," "give to a number of people at different times," "give over time," "give to each," and "give to each over time" (Bellugi et al., 1993).

Second, sign languages use space as a grammatical and semantic device. For example, in ASL the noun referring to a particular person or object can be assigned (or *indexed*) to a location in space, typically to one or other side of the signer. Referring back to that place

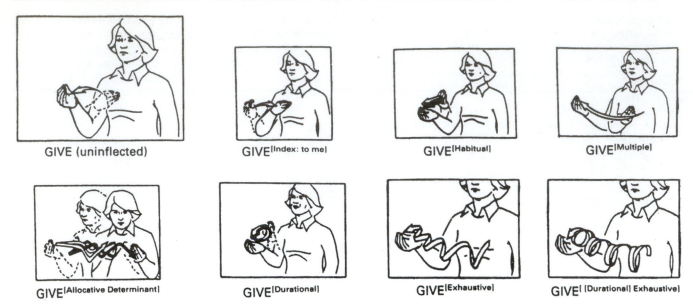

Figure 1. (From Bellugi, U., et al. [1993]. The acquisition of syntax and space in young deaf signers. In D. Bishop and K. Mogford [Eds.], *Language development in exceptional circumstances*. Hillsdale, NJ: Erlbaum. Reproduced with permission.)

in space by pointing to it then acts as an anaphoric pronoun. Similarly, for verbs such as GO, GIVE, INFORM, or TEACH that involve directionality or movement in their meaning, the starting and end points of the sign and its direction of movement between points in space are used as an agreement marker on the verb to indicate the subject and recipient of the action (Wilbur, 1987; Bellugi et al., 1993).

Third, ASL makes extensive use of simultaneous nonmanual facial expressions and body movements as adverbial, grammatical, and semantic devices. Some of the facial expressions accompanying signed sentences seem to be expressions of intensity or attitude, such as pursing the lips or puffing out the cheeks, but others have obligatory syntactic roles. Raising the eyebrows and tilting the head forward slightly changes a declarative sentence into a yes/no question. Topicalized clauses such as relative clauses specifying information about a referent are marked by raised eyebrows and the head tilted back (Liddell, 1980). Finally, ASL has several ways to negate an utterance, and a nonmanual marker—a headshake with the eyebrows squeezed together—is used with or without the negative signs for NO and NOT to negate a clause (Humphries, Padden, and O'Rourke, 1980; Wilbur, 1987).

In reporting speech or action, the person whose perspective is to be taken is assigned to a location in space (Emmory and Reilly, 1995). Then the signer turns his body as if signing from the perspective of that location and signs what the person did or said. This "role shift" is analogous to direct speech in spoken languages. It is accompanied by a break in eye gaze away from the conversational partner and the use of "first-person" pronouns in the role of the character involved. Reporting action also uses a role shift of the signer's body in

space, but it employs different pronoun usage and facial markers to indicate that the actor's perspective is being taken (Emmory and Reilly, 1995).

Finally, like some spoken languages, ASL incorporates classifiers, linguistic markers that identify such features as the size, shape, animacy, and function of objects. In ASL different handshapes encode these properties of the objects and are incorporated into movement verbs (Wilbur, 1987; Schick, 1990). The most iconic of the classifier handshapes are those that reflect the size and shape of the object referred to. So, a single handshape depicts all medium-sized cylindrical objects, such as a cup, a small tube, and a vase. Other classifiers are more abstract, representing classes of objects that do not resemble each other (or the classifier sign) in size or shape. Thus, one classifier is used to represent all vehicles, including boats and bicycles. Some classifier signs can serve as pronouns in sentences (Humphries, Padden, and O'Rourke, 1980).

Acquisition of ASL by Native-Signing Children

Deaf children exposed at an early age to a sufficiently rich input acquire a full natural sign language as effortlessly and rapidly as hearing children acquire their native spoken language. Deaf babies "babble" in sign at about the same age as their hearing peers babble in speech, repeating the handshape or movement components of signs in a rhythmic fashion (Pettito and Marentette, 1991). Just as in canonical babbling the child's phonetic repertoire comes to be restricted to that of the child's native language, so too the sign-babbling deaf child shifts to incorporating only the restricted set of handshapes and movements found in the input sign language. Notably, the phonetic units found in "canonical" manual babbling are the same ones later used in the first meaningful signs (Pettito, 2000).

Although there is considerable variation among children, the first signs with a clear reference may emerge a month or two earlier in deaf children than the first spoken words of hearing children. Motor control over the hands and arms sufficient to produce recognizable signs develops a little ahead of control over the vocal articulators (Bonvillian, 1999). Early vocabularies in sign or speech refer to the same categories of objects and actions: the significant people, animals, objects, and actions in the common environment of most toddlers, hearing or deaf. Some signs in ASL are iconic in that they resemble the referent. For example, the sign for CAT is made by stroking the side of the upper lip to indicate whiskers. However, while iconicity may facilitate the comprehension of some signs, semantic domain and phonological complexity seem to be stronger determinants of early sign productions (Bonvillian, 1999).

The phonological properties of early signs are affected by motor control and perceptual salience, as well as by linguistic constraints (Conlin et al., 2000; Marentette and Mayberry, 2000). For example, sign location seems to be the most accurately produced feature of early signs because the place of articulation is perceptually more salient than the handshape and manner of movement and requires less fine motor control. Signing children produce a pattern of regular substitutions of phonetic elements in their early signs, just like the phonological substitutions in hearing toddlers' early spoken words (Bellugi et al., 1993).

By around 2 years of age, children begin to master the pronoun system, in ASL a system of pointing gestures to the self ("me"), to one's conversational partner ("you"), or to indexed referential spaces ("he," "she," "it"). Despite the iconic transparency of first- and second-person pronouns, signing children follow the same developmental timeline and exhibit the same problems as speaking children do in learning pronouns that shift reference, depending on who is the speaker and addressee. They even tend to make the same reversal error in early acquisition of "I/me" and "you," using a point facing outward toward their conversational partner when referring to themselves, and pointing to themselves when referring to "you" (Pettito, 1987). More abstract pronouns that involve pointing to an indexed referent assigned to a location in signing space are the last acquired, around age 5 (Hoffmeister and Wilbur, 1980).

In two- and three-word signed utterances, semantic relationships between sentence elements emerge in a reliable order of acquisition that seems to be determined by the conceptual development of the child: reference to the existence or disappearance of objects, then action relationships, and finally state relationships (properties, possession, or location of objects), just as in early spoken language acquisition (Brown, 1973; Newport and Ashbrook, 1977).

Although much of the syntax of ASL is conveyed through spatial morphology rather than word order, young signing children begin by producing uninflected root forms of these verbs and use more fixed word orders in their early sentences to express grammatical and semantic relationships, typically the most frequent sign order seen in the adult input (Newport and Meier, 1985). The use of agreement morphology on these verbs emerges over the period between age 2 and 5 years, being mastered first for referents that are present in the discourse context and only later for absent referents indexed in space (Newport and Meier, 1985). The pattern of development and the errors are predicted not by iconicity, the fact that the path of the action is clearly traced in space, but by a linguistic model of morphological complexity observed in spoken languages (Newport and Meier, 1985; Slobin, 1985). Just as speaking children overgeneralize inflectional rules like the regular -ed past tense (e.g., "holded" for "held") or use noncausative verbs in a causative sense (e.g., "He falled me down"), signing deaf children overgeneralize spatial agreement marking to verb signs in ASL that cannot be used in that way. So, verbs like SAY or LIKE, which cannot be directionally marked, are sometimes extended toward the object, and verbs like DRINK and EAT may be signed as if coming from an indexed referent in space, not in their required location on the signer (Bellugi et al., 1993).

Classifiers first emerge at around age 3 but are mastered over a long period of time, with some forms still giving children trouble at age 6 or 7. Size and shape classifier handshapes resemble their referents more closely and are acquired first (Schick, 1990). Mastery of the more abstract classifiers depends not only on mastery of the syntax and semantics of ASL, but also on the child's conceptual development in classifying such objects as cars, boats, and bicycles all together as a functional class.

Despite our natural attention to affective markers in facial expressions, nonmanual syntactic and semantic markers can be difficult for both first and second language learners of ASL to acquire (Reilly, 2000). The marker itself may appear early, but its full linguistic use can take several years to master. Thus the negative headshake is first used by native-signing deaf children in the second year to negate signs, but young children experience difficulty in timing this nonmanual marker to coincide with the correct manual signs, and they may ungrammatically extend the headshake across more than one clause or sentence (Anderson and Reilly, 1997).

Thus the same developmental processes and constraints apply to the natural acquisition of ASL and other sign languages as to the normal development of any spoken language. The pattern of acquisition is primarily dictated by the linguistic and cognitive complexity of forms, not by their iconicity in the visual mode of the language.

Natural Sign Language Versus Artificial Signed Versions of Spoken Language

In several countries, signed versions of the native spoken language have been created by educators. Unlike natural sign languages, they are typically signed simultaneously with the spoken language as a form of sign-supported speech. In the United States there are several versions of manually coded English (MCE). The most widely used of these are Signed English, Signed Exact English, and Seeing Essential English. These all use lexical signs from ASL and English word order, but they vary in the degree to which created signs encode all of the function words or derivational and inflectional morphology of English.

The educational value of these MCE systems over ASL and oral or written English is hotly disputed. They have two primary drawbacks. First, because signs take longer to produce than words, signing a sentence in a linear sequence following that of English takes much longer than speaking the same sentence in English. The simultaneous speaker-signer either has to slow down her speech to an unnatural extent or has to leave out aspects of the signed portion of the message. Thus, deaf children receive either an incomplete and ungrammatical language input or a simplified one, so that their exposure to complex English syntax is artificially reduced.

Second, several universal features of natural sign languages that have evolved to allow effective and rapid communication of meaning in a visual-spatial mode are not incorporated into MCE systems. These features include the use of space as a grammatical and semantic device, simultaneous morphology, and nonmanual linguistic markers. Indeed, in several respects MCE systems directly violate these universal principles and so can be very confusing for deaf children who have been exposed to ASL (Johnson, Liddell, and Erting, 1989). Deaf children may then naturalize MCE so that it more closely conforms to ASL's use of space and simultaneity (Suppala, 1991).

Going Beyond the Input

Many deaf children are exposed to incomplete versions of ASL, from deaf parents who are not native signers or hearing parents still learning ASL. In this input morphological rules in particular may be inconsistently used. However, children systematize their sign language to make consistent rules out of what are only statistical regularities in their parents' signing (Newport, 1999; Newport and Aslin, 2000). For example, spatial agreement markers on verbs of motion that were correct only about two-thirds of the time in the parental input were used correctly more than 90% of the time by their children at age 7. The children create a more regular rule out of inconsistently used morphology, thus going beyond the input to acquire a more complete form of ASL.

Even with no conventional signed input, deaf children of hearing parents in oral environments create rich gestural systems, although these are not complete languages (Goldin-Meadow, 2001). Over a longer period of time and several generations of deaf signers, a more complete sign language may emerge. This phenomenon is seen in the creation of a new Nicaraguan Sign Language out of many home gestural systems by deaf children brought together from isolated villages into a centralized school for the deaf in Nicaragua in the early 1980s. Motivated by the pressure to communicate among themselves, the deaf students evolved a more and more complex sign language, with each generation of students inheriting a more complex form of the language and then elaborating it. Several researchers have identified the emergence of many of the apparently universal features of natural sign languages in the evolution of Nicaraguan Sign Language over the past 20 years, among them componentiality of lexical signs, simultaneity of meaning expression, nonmanual syntactic markers, and the use of space for grammatical purposes (Kegl, Senghas, and Coppola, 1999; Senghas, 2000).

A Critical Period for Sign Language Acquisition

There seems to be a sensitive or even critical period in early childhood in which exposure to a relatively complete sign language must take place. Deaf individuals exposed to ASL for the first time in late childhood or adolescence are less proficient ASL users in adulthood than those who learn ASL in the first few years of life, even though they may have been using ASL as their primary means of communication for decades (Fischer, 1998; Mayberry and Eichen, 1991; Newport, 1991).

ASL and Finger Spelling

There are some influences on ASL from the surrounding dominant English language culture, for example the importation of loan words from English that are finger-spelled using the manual alphabet to represent English letters. Finger-spelled vocabulary is highly selective, almost always nouns and rarely verbs. In everyday conversations these finger-spelled words are frequently the names of people and places, but in educational settings finger spelling is used to represent technical words and concepts for which there is not a natural sign in ASL. Padden (1998) has argued that this is similar to the way in which most if not all spoken languages import foreign vocabulary words. Indeed, deaf children of deaf parents who cannot yet read or write English begin to produce finger-spelled words as "signs" before they learn to connect them to English orthography.

Padden and Ramsey (1998) suggest that finger spelling may interact with ASL skills in providing deaf children with better access to English literacy learning. They find that deaf teachers using ASL in the classroom actually finger-spell more words than hearing teachers. Most important, these deaf teachers effectively chain together the different expressive modes of communication, switching from finger spelling to printed text to finger spelling, or from ASL sign to finger spelling to text, in order to facilitate the connection between text and meaning and to develop better print decoding skills. In Padden and Ramsey's study, the deaf students with better ASL and finger-spelling skills developed better English-reading skills.

ASL and English Literacy

The extent to which the development of phonological decoding from print to spoken phonemes is necessary for fluent reading in deaf students is still in dispute. However, skill in ASL does not interfere with learning to read printed English. Rather, it is a strong independent contributor to reading comprehension levels for deaf children in educational settings using sign language, even when controlling for having deaf or hearing parents (Hoffmeister et al., 1997; Strong and Prinz, 1997). Having a fluent sign language can facilitate learning to read in several ways: by increasing the children's comprehension of the instructional process (if the teacher is also fluent in ASL), increasing the number of semantic concepts the child understands, developing extended discourse skills that are critical to early reading, and fostering metacognitive skills such as communication monitoring and planning (Nelson, 1998).

Conclusion

The visual-spatial nature of sign languages—the fact that they are articulated with the hands and perceived through the eyes—does not relegate them to the realm of pantomime and gesture. Natural sign languages are as subtle and complex as any spoken language and are structured according to universal linguistic principles. Deaf children exposed to a complete and consistent natural sign language early in childhood acquire the language normally, following the same stages and learning processes as are observed in hearing children acquiring their native spoken language.

—*Peter A. de Villiers and Jennie Pyers*

References

Anderson, D., and Reilly, J. (1997). The puzzle of negation: How children move from communicative to grammatical negation in ASL. *Applied Psycholinguistics, 18*, 411–429.

Bellugi, U., vanHoek, K., Lillo-Martin, D., and O'Grady, L. (1993). The acquisition of syntax and space in young deaf signers. In D. Bishop and K. Mogford (Eds.), *Language development in exceptional circumstances*. Hillsdale, NJ: Erlbaum.

Bonvillian, J. (1999). Sign language development. In M. Barrett (Ed.), *The development of language*. Hove, U.K.: Psychology Press.

Brown, R. (1973). *A first language*. Cambridge, MA: Harvard University Press.

Conlin, K., Mirus, G., Mauk, C., and Meier, R. (2000). The acquisition of first signs: Place, handshape and movement. In C. Chamberlain, J. Morford, and R. Mayberry (Eds.), *Language acquisition by eye*. Mahwah, NJ: Erlbaum.

Emmory, K., and Reilly, J. (1995). *Sign, gesture, and space*. Hillsdale, NJ: Erlbaum.

Fischer, S. (1998). Critical periods for language acquisition: consequences for deaf education. In A. Weisel (Ed.), *Issues unresolved: New perspectives on language and deaf education*. Washington, DC: Gallaudet University Press.

Goldin-Meadow, S. (2001). *The resilience of language*. Philadelphia: Psychology Press.

Gustason, G. (1990). Signing exact English. In H. Bornstein (Ed.), *Manual communication: Implications for education*. Washington, DC: Gallaudet University Press.

Hoffmeister, R., de Villiers, P. A., Engen, E., and Topol, D. (1997). English reading achievement and ASL skills in deaf students. In E. Hughes, M. Hughes, and A. Greenhill (Eds.), *Proceedings of the 21st Annual Boston University Conference on Language Development*. Somerville, MA: Cascadilla Press.

Hoffmeister, R., and Wilbur, R. (1980). The acquisition of sign language. In H. Lane and F. Grosjean (Eds.), *Recent perspectives on American Sign Language*. Hillsdale, NJ: Erlbaum.

Humphries, T., Padden, C., and O'Rourke, T. (1980). *A basic course in American Sign Language*. Silver Springs, MD: T.J. Publishers.

Johnson, R., Liddell, S., and Erting, C. (1989). *Unlocking the curriculum: Principles for achieving success in deaf education* (Working Paper 89-3). Washington, DC: Gallaudet Research Institute, Gallaudet University.

Kegl, J., Senghas, A., and Coppola, M. (1999). Creation through contact: Sign language emergence and sign language change in Nicaragua. In M. DeGraff (Ed.), *Language creation and language change: Creolization, diachrony, and development*. Cambridge, MA: MIT Press.

Liddell, S. (1980). *American Sign Language syntax*. The Hague, Netherlands: Mouton.

Marentette, P., and Mayberry, R. (2000). Principles for an emerging phonological system: A case study of early ASL acquisition. In C. Chamberlain, J. Morford, and R. Mayberry (Eds.), *Language acquisition by eye*. Mahwah, NJ: Erlbaum.

Mayberry, R., and Eichen, E. (1991). The long-lasting advantage of learning sign language in childhood: Another look at the critical period for language acquisition. *Journal of Memory and Language, 30*, 486–512.

Nelson, K. (1998). Toward a differentiated account of facilitators of literacy development and ASL in deaf children. *Topics in Language Disorders, 18*, 73–88.

Newport, E. (1991). Contrasting concepts of the critical period for language. In S. Carey and R. Gelman (Eds.), *The epigenesis of mind: Essays on biology and cognition*. Hillsdale, NJ: Erlbaum.

Newport, E. (1999). Reduced input in the study of signed languages: Contributions to the study of creolization. In M. DeGraff (Ed.), *Language creation and language change: Creolization, synchrony, and development*. Cambridge, MA: MIT Press.

Newport, E., and Ashbrook, E. (1977). The emergence of semantic relations in American Sign Language. *Papers and Reports on Child Language Development, 13*, 16–21.

Newport, E., and Aslin, R. (2000). Innately constrained learning: Blending of old and new approaches to language acquisition. In S. C. Howell, S. Fish, and T. Keith-Lucas (Eds.), *Proceedings of the 24th Annual Boston University Conference on Language Development*. Somerville, MA: Cascadilla Press.

Newport, E., and Meier, R. (1985). The acquisition of American Sign Language. In D. Slobin (Ed.), *The cross-linguistic study of language acquisition. Vol. 1. The data*. Hillsdale, NJ: Erlbaum.

Padden, C. (1998). Early bilingual lives of deaf children. In I. Parasnis (Ed.), *Cultural and language diversity and the deaf experience*. New York: Cambridge University Press.

Padden, C., and Ramsey, C. (1998). Reading ability in signing deaf children. *Topics in Language Disorders, 18*, 40–46.

Pettito, L. (1987). On the autonomy of language and gesture: Evidence from the acquisition of personal pronouns in American Sign Language. *Cognition, 27*, 1–52.

Petitto, L. (2000). The acquisition of natural signed languages: Lessons in the nature of human language and its biological functions. In C. Chamberlain, J. Morford, and R. Mayberry (Eds.), *Language acquisition by eye.* Mahwah, NJ: Erlbaum.

Pettito, L., and Marentette, P. (1991). Babbling in the manual mode: Evidence for the ontogeny of language. *Science, 251*, 1493–1496.

Reilly, J. (2000). Bringing affective expression into the service of language: Acquiring perspective marking in narratives. In K. Emmory and H. Lane (Eds.), *The Signs of Language revisited: An anthology to honor Ursula Bellugi and Edward Klima.* Mahwah, NJ: Erlbaum.

Schick, B. (1990). The effects of morphosyntactic structure on the acquisition of classifier predicates in ASL. In C. Lucas (Ed.), *Sign language research: Theoretical issues.* Washington, DC: Gallaudet University Press.

Senghas, A. (2000). The development of early spatial morphology in Nicaraguan Sign Language. In S. C. Howell, S. Fish, and T. Keith-Lucas (Eds.), *Proceedings of the 24th Annual Boston University Conference on Language Development.* Somerville, MA: Cascadilla Press.

Slobin, D. (1985). Crosslinguistic evidence for the language-making capacity. In D. Slobin (Ed.), *The crosslinguistic study of language acquisition. Vol. 2. Theoretical issues.* Hillsdale, NJ: Erlbaum.

Strong, M., and Prinz, P. (1997). A study of the relationship between American Sign Language and English literacy. *Journal of Deaf Studies and Deaf Education, 2*, 37–46.

Supalla, S. (1991). Manually coded English: The modality question in signed language development. In P. Siple and S. Fischer (Eds.), *Theoretical issues in sign language research. Vol. 2. Psychology.* Chicago: University of Chicago Press.

Wilbur, R. (1987). *American Sign Language: Linguistics and applied dimensions* (2nd ed.). Columbus, OH: Merrill.

Further Readings

Akamatsu, C. T., and Stewart, D. (1998). Constructing simultaneous communication: The contributions of natural sign language. *Journal of Deaf Studies and Deaf Education, 3*, 302–319.

Chamberlain, C., Morford, J., and Mayberry, R. (Eds.). (2000). *Language acquisition by eye.* Mahwah, NJ: Erlbaum.

Emmorey, K., and Reilly, J. (1998). The development of quotation and reported action: Conveying perspective in ASL. In E. Clark (Ed.), *Proceedings of the Twenty-Ninth Annual Child Language Research Forum.* Chicago: Center for the Study of Language and Information.

Hoffmeister, R. (1990). American Sign Language and education of the deaf. In H. Bornstein (Ed.), *Manual communication: Implications for education.* Washington, DC: Gallaudet University Press.

Klima, E., and Bellugi, U. (1979). *The signs of language.* Cambridge, MA: Harvard University Press.

Lane, H., Hoffmeister, R., and Bahan, B. (1996). *A journey into the DEAF-WORLD.* San Diego, CA: Dawn Sign Press.

Marschark, M. (1993). *Psychological development of deaf children.* New York: Oxford University Press.

Mayberry, R. (1993). First-language acquisition after childhood differs from second-language acquisition: The case of American Sign Language. *Journal of Speech and Hearing Research, 36*, 1258–1270.

Mayer, C., and Akamatsu, C. (1999). Bilingual-bicultural models of literacy education for deaf students: Considering the claims. *Journal of Deaf Studies and Deaf Education, 4*, 1–8.

Meier, R., and Newport, E. (1990). Out of the hands of babes: On a possible sign advantage in language acquisition. *Language, 66*, 1–23.

Padden, C., and Humphries, T. (1988). *Deaf in America: Voices from a culture.* Cambridge, MA: Harvard University Press.

Parasnis, I. (Ed.). (1998). *Cultural and language diversity and the deaf experience.* New York: Cambridge University Press.

Schein, J., and Stewart, D. (1995). *Language in motion: Exploring the nature of sign.* Washington, DC: Gallaudet University Press.

Linguistic Aspects of Child Language Impairment—Prosody

In linguistics, "prosody" refers to sound patterns in language involving more than a single segment or phoneme. Since the early 1980s, the study of prosody has blossomed, both in linguistics and in the allied areas of computer speech analysis and synthesis, adult sentence processing, infant speech perception, and language production. The study of prosody has provided insight into the word and sentence productions of young children with normally developing language and language disorders. In particular, prosody has proven a useful tool for examining children's "deviant" utterances; that is, utterances that deviate from what we would expect from an adult speaker with normal speech and language. For example, a child's production of "blue" as "bu" will be considered a deviant utterance for purposes of this discussion.

The article begins with a brief overview of two aspects of prosody, syllable shape and meter, that have been the focus of many studies of child language production. It then provides examples of some recent studies that demonstrate effects of syllable shape and meter on deviant productions of children with normal and disordered language. To foreshadow the general finding across the studies presented here, we state that syllable shapes and metrical patterns that are frequent across the world's languages or in the language the child is learning are most resistant to deviations.

Beginning with *syllable shape*, it has been noted that all languages of the world have syllables comprising a consonant plus a vowel (CV). Only some languages allow additional syllable shapes, such as V, VC, CVC, CCVC, and so on. In linguistic terms, the CV syllable shape is said to be "unmarked." Even when languages allow syllable shapes other than CV, the shapes are often restricted. For example, Japanese allows only CVC syllables ending in /n/.

Furthermore, in languages like English that allow consonant clusters (syllables of the shape CCVC, CVCC, etc.), these clusters generally conform to a sonority sequencing principle (e.g., Hooper, 1976). Briefly, sonority may be conceptualized as the openness of the vocal tract for a particular segment. Vowels are the most sonorous; glides are less sonorous, followed by liquids, nasals, fricatives, and stops. Clements (1990) argues that an ideal syllable structure is one in which a sequence of segments increases from the onset to the vowel with no or a minimal decline from the vowel to the coda. English word-initial consonant clusters such as /pr/ and /kw/, which comprise a stop plus liquid or glide, are consistent with this principle, as are English word-final clusters such as /rp/ and /nt/.

The foregoing discussion of syllable shapes concerns what is allowed in words of a language. It is also important to note that even languages that allow a variety of syllable shapes nevertheless have strong statistical tendencies toward particular shapes. For example, English CVC words are very likely to end in /t/ and very unlikely to end in /dʒ/. These statistical tendencies are the subject of a growing interest in researchers studying prosody and its role in child language production.

Let us now turn to *meter*. In many languages, multisyllabic words exhibit a characteristic stress pattern. For example, the majority of words in English have the pattern found in "apple" and "yellow," that is, a stressed or strong syllable followed by an unstressed or weak syllable. Stressed syllables are louder, longer, and higher in pitch than unstressed syllables. The frequency of the strong-weak word pattern is consistent with the observation that the basic unit of stress in English is a trochaic (strong-weak) foot, with a foot defined as a grouping of a single strong syllable plus adjacent weak syllables.

Feet not only explain the dominant stress pattern of words in a language, they also help us to understand how lexical words like nouns and verbs combine with grammatical words like determiners and auxiliary verbs in phrases. For example, when we say phrases like "drink of water" and "pick a card," we tend to combine the grammatical words (in this case "of" and "a") with the preceding strong syllable, even though these words belong syntactically with the following word (in a prepositional phrase and noun phrase, respectively). That is, English speakers tend to create trochaic feet whenever they can, giving the language a characteristic metrical pattern.

The discussion up to this point has revealed that languages of the world and particular languages are biased toward specific syllable shapes (e.g., CV) and meters (e.g., trochaic). Beginning with syllable shape, let us now consider how these prosodic biases affect the productions of children with normally developing and disordered language. Two of the most frequent syllable shape deviations from a standard target produced by children are final consonant or coda deletion and consonant cluster reduction. With respect to coda deletion, this phenomenon has been viewed as one in which the speaker is resorting to the most common syllable shape, CV. However, recent studies indicate that there are significant differences in the rate at which children omit different codas in different prosodic environments. Zamuner and Gerken (1998) reported that normally developing 2-year-olds produced more codas and more coda types on nonsense words when the coda occurred in a stressed syllable (either on a monosyllabic item or an item with a weak-strong stress pattern, e.g., /məbɪb/). Zamuner (2001) discovered that children from the same population produced obstruent codas, which are more frequent in English, sooner than sonorant codas on CVC nonsense words. She also found that the same coda was produced less frequently when it occurred in nonsense names exhibiting less frequent biphones (e.g., CV, VC) than more frequent biphones.

With respect to consonant cluster reduction, several studies have shown a role for syllable shape, and in particular sonority sequencing, in this phenomenon (e.g., Barlow and Dinnsen, 1998; Ohala, 1999). These studies have revealed that children with normal language and language disorders were more likely to produce the least sonorous consonant of an initial cluster and the least sonorous consonant of a final cluster. That is, they produced CV sequences that were closer to the ideal syllable shape suggested by Clements (1990).

Turning now to the role of meter in language production, several researchers have noted that children are more likely to omit weak syllables from the beginning of words like "giraffe" and "banana" and, more generally weak syllables that do not belong to a trochaic foot (e.g., Wijnen, Krikhaar, and Den Os, 1994). The bias to produce trochaic feet has also been observed at the level of sentence production, where the determiner "the" is more likely to be preserved in a sentence like "He pats the zebra" ("pats the" forms a trochaic foot) than "He brushes the bear" (the syllabic verb inflection makes the formation of a trochaic foot containing "the" impossible; Gerken, 1996). Thus, the effects of prosody are not restricted to what have traditionally been considered phonological deviations but extend to morphosyntactic deviations as well. It is interesting to note that not all languages show as strong a bias toward trochaic feet as English does. For example, Spanish has many words like "banana," which exhibit a weak-strong-weak pattern. Spanish-learning children have been shown to produce determiners at an earlier age than their English-learning counterparts, again suggesting a role for prosody in children's morphosyntactic development (Lleó and Demuth, 1999).

At least some of children's weak syllable omissions appear to occur during late stages of language production rather than during utterance planning, as evidenced by work by Carter (1999). Normally developing 2-year-olds and older children with language impairment produced sentences like "He kissed Cassandra" and "He kissed Sandy." Note that the former sentence type was frequently produced with the first syllable of the name omitted (Cassandra → Sandra). Acoustic measurements revealed that, even though the two types of sentences contained the same number of overtly produced syllables (four), children produced the first sentence type with a longer duration, suggesting that they reserved a timing slot for the syllable they eventually omitted. One possible source of weak syllable omissions is a lack of complete control over the motor sequences involved in producing trochaic vs. weak-strong feet (Goffman, 1999).

Finally, several studies have revealed joint effects of syllable shape and meter on deviant utterances. In the Zamuner and Gerken study discussed above, children showed different rates of coda preservation for strong and weak syllables. Ohala (1998) found that young children with normal language were less likely to reduce word-medial consonant clusters in words with a strong-strong stress pattern. In a study of weak syllable omission in young children with normal language, Kehoe and Stoel-Gammon (1997) noted more omissions of the middle syllable of words like "elephant," which exhibit a strong-weak-weak pattern, if the syllable began with a sonorant consonant. Carter (1999) found that adults with a variety of types of aphasia were more likely to omit word-initial weak syllables with V and VC syllable shapes than CV shapes. It seems likely that such results would be found in children with normal and disordered language as well.

In summary, linguistic studies of canonical syllable shapes and metrical patterns across languages and within particular languages provide the tools for fine-grained analyses of deviant forms produced by children with normal and disordered language. The results of these analyses feeds a growing consensus that those forms that are very frequent in languages of the world or in the child's target language are generally more robust and less susceptible to deviations from the accepted standard. Further research is needed to reveal the mechanism underlying prosody's clear effect on language production (see also PROSODIC DEFICITS).

—*LouAnn Gerken*

References

Barlow, J., and Dinnsen, D. (1998). Asymmetrical cluster reduction in a disordered system. *Language Acquisition, 7*, 1–49.

Carter, A. (1999). An integrated acoustic and phonological investigation of weak syllable omissions. Unpublished doctoral dissertation, University of Arizona.

Clements, G. (1990). The role of the sonority cycle in core syllabification. In J. Kingston and M. Beckman (Eds.), *Papers in laboratory phonology* (pp. 283–333). New York: Cambridge University Press.

Gerken, L. A. (1996). Prosodic structure in young children's language production. *Language, 72*, 683–712.

Goffman, L. (1999). Prosodic influences on speech production in children with specific language impairment and speech deficits: Kinematic, acoustic, and transcription evidence. *Journal of Speech, Language, and Hearing Research, 42*, 1499–1517.

Hooper, J. (1976). *An introduction to generative phonology*. New York: Academic Press.

Kehoe, M., and Stoel-Gammon, C. (1997). Truncation patterns in English-speaking children's word productions. *Journal of Speech and Hearing Research, 40*, 526–541.

Lleó, C., and Demuth, K. (1999). Prosodic constraints on the emergence of grammatical morphemes: Crosslinguistic evidence from Germanic and Romance languages. In A. Greenhill, H. Littlefield, and C. Tano (Eds.), *Proceedings of the 23rd Annual Boston University Conference on Language Development* (pp. 407–418). Somerville, MA: Cascadilla Press.

Ohala, D. (1998). Medial cluster reduction in early child speech. In E. Clark (Ed.), *Proceedings of the Twenty-ninth Annual Child Language Research Forum* (pp. 128–135). Palo Alto, CA: Stanford University Press.

Ohala, D. (1999). The influence of sonority on children's cluster reductions. *Journal of Communication Disorders, 32*, 397–422.

Wijnen, F., Krikhaar, E., and Den Os, E. (1994). The (non)-realization of unstressed elements in children's utterances: Evidence for a rhythmic constraint. *Journal of Child Language, 21*, 59–83.

Zamuner, T. (2001). Input-based phonological acquisition: Codas, frequency and universal grammar. Unpublished doctoral dissertation, University of Arizona.

Zamuner, T., and Gerken, L. A. (1998). Young children's production of coda consonants in different prosodic environments. In E. Clark (Ed.), *Proceedings of the Twenty-ninth Annual Child Language Research Forum* (pp. 121–128). Palo Alto, CA: Stanford University Press.

Further Readings

Allen, G., and Hawkins, S. (1980). Phonological rhythm: Definition and development. In G. Yeni-Komshian, J. Kavanagh, and G. Ferguson (Eds.), *Child phonology. Vol. I. Production*. New York: Academic Press.

Barlow, J., and Gierut, J. (1999). Optimality theory in phonological acquisition. *Journal of Speech, Language, and Hearing Research, 42*, 1482–1498.

Bortolini, U., and Leonard, L. (1996). Phonology and grammatical morphology in specific language impairment: Accounting for individual variation in English and Italian. *Applied Psycholinguistics, 17*, 85–104.

Chiat, S., and Hirson, A. (1987). From conceptual intention to utterance: A study of impaired language output in a child with developmental dysphasia. *British Journal of Disorders of Communication, 22*, 37–64.

Demuth, K. (1996). The prosodic structure of early words. In J. Morgan and K. Demuth (Eds.), *Signal to syntax*. Mahwah, NJ: Erlbaum.

Echols, C. (1993). A perceptually-based model of children's earliest productions. *Cognition, 46*, 245–296.

Ellis Weismer, S. (1997). The role of stress in language processing and intervention. *Topics in Language Disorders, 17*, 41–52.

Fee, E. J. (1997). The prosodic framework for language learning. *Topics in Language Disorders, 17*, 53–62.

Fikkert, P. (1994). *On the acquisition of prosodic structure*. Dordrecht: Holland Institute of Generative Linguistics.

Gerken, L. A. (1994). A metrical template account of children's weak syllable omissions. *Journal of Child Language, 21*, 565–584.

Gerken, L. A., and McGregor, K. (1998). An overview of prosody and its role in normal and disordered child language. *American Journal of Speech Language Pathology, 7*, 38–48.

Hammond, M. (1999). *The phonology of English: A prosodic optimality-theoretic approach*. London: Oxford University Press.

Hogg, R., and McCully, C. B. (1987). *Metrical phonology*. Cambridge, UK: Cambridge University Press.

Klein, H. B. (1981). Production strategies for the pronunciation of early polysyllabic lexical items. *Journal of Speech and Hearing Research, 24*, 535–551.

McGregor, K. (1994). Article use in the spontaneous samples of children with specific language impairment: The importance of considering syntactic contexts. *Clinical Linguistics and Phonetics, 8*, 153–160.

Nespor, M., and Vogel, I. (1986). *Prosodic phonology*. Dordrecht, Holland: Foris.

Panagos, J. M., and Prelock, P. A. (1997). Prosodic analysis of child speech. *Topics in Language Disorders, 17*, 1–10.

Selkirk, E. (1984). *Phonology and syntax*. Cambridge, MA: MIT Press.

Selkirk, E. (1996). The prosodic structure of function words. In J. Morgan and K. Demuth (Eds.), *Signal to syntax*. Mahwah, NJ: Erlbaum.

Shattuck-Hufnagel, S., and Turk, A. (1996). A prosody tutorial for investigators of auditory sentence processing. *Journal of Psycholinguistic Research, 25*, 193–247.

Melodic Intonation Therapy

Among the many published approaches for the treatment of aphasia, melodic intonation therapy (MIT) is one of the few techniques whose clinical effectiveness has been established by peer review (American Academy of Neurology, 1994). The effectiveness of the program is based on the specific guidelines for patient candidacy, its formalized protocol, and a variety of reports testifying to improved communication competence following MIT. After evaluating the available evidence, the American Academy of Neurology considers the program to be promising when administered by a qualified speech-language pathologist.

The guiding principles and procedures associated with MIT were set forth in the early works of Albert, Sparks, and Helm (1973), Sparks, Helm, and Albert (1974), and Sparks and Holland (1976). More recent descriptions of the program can be found in Helm-Estabrooks and Albert (1991) and Sparks (2001). Generally, three principles form the conceptual foundation for MIT. First, in most of the population, the right cerebral hemisphere mediates music and speech prosody. Second, the right hemisphere is preserved in most individuals with aphasia, and as a result, singing abilities are generally preserved even in the most severe cases of aphasia. Third, the preserved musical and prosodic capabilities of the right hemisphere can be exploited to rehabilitate language production in patients with aphasia.

The goals of MIT are to facilitate some recovery of language production in severely nonfluent speakers with poorly articulated or severely restricted verbal output. Good candidates have poor repetition but at least moderately preserved to essentially normal language comprehension. Attempts at self-correction are evident. They are emotionally stable, if sometimes depressed, and highly motivated to improve their speech. A coexisting buccofacial apraxia is usually observed, as well as right hemiplegia that is greater in the arm than leg. The program therefore seems to be particularly suited for patients with Broca's or mixed nonfluent aphasia with accompanying apraxia of speech (Tonkovich and Peach, 1989; Square, Martin, and Bose, 2001). These characteristics also generally exclude patients with Wernicke's, transcortical, or global aphasia.

The initial computed tomographic profile for good candidates included a large lesion in Broca's area extending superiorly to the left premotor and sensorimotor cortex for the face and deep to the periventricular white matter, putamen, and internal capsule. The lesion also typically spared Wernicke's area and the temporal isthmus. No lesions of the right hemisphere were detected; this evidence was used to support the preservation of melodic functions in these patients (Naeser and Helm-Estabrooks, 1985). Naeser (1994) subsequently identified two important areas in the subcortical white matter that appeared to have an important role regarding recovery of spontaneous speech. Lesions of good responders involved no more than half of the total area, including the medial subcallosal fasciculus and the middle one-third of the periventricular white matter. The extent of lesion in cortical language areas, including Broca's area, could not be used to discriminate among individuals who responded well or poorly to MIT. Lesions may have involved Wernicke's area or the subcortical temporal isthmus, but when they did, they involved less than half of those areas.

During the beginning stages of an MIT program, emphasis is placed on the production of syntactically and phonologically simplified phrases and sentences that gradually increase in complexity throughout the course of the program. Ideally, language materials are thematically related and relevant to the patient's daily needs and background. A large corpus of materials is recommended to vary the stimuli from session to session and to decrease practice effects. It is debatable whether the use of supplementary pictures or written sentences is appropriate (Helm-Estabrooks and Albert, 1991; Sparks, 2001). Frequent treatment, perhaps twice daily, is essential, but when unattainable, family members might be used to assist with the program (Sparks, 2001).

MIT focuses on three elements represented in the spoken prosody of verbal utterances: the melodic line or variation in pitch in the spoken phrase or sentence, the tempo and rhythm of the utterance, and the points of stress for emphasis. The intoned pattern has a range of only three or four whole notes that is selected from several reasonable speech prosody patterns for the target sentence. Tempo is slowed by syllable lengthening; phrase accuracy appears to be best when syllable durations approximate 2.0 s per syllable. The effects of this tempo are most pronounced when patients are required to intone utterances independent of the clinician (Laughlin, Naeser, and Gordon, 1979). Rhythm and stress are exaggerated by elevating intoned notes and increasing loudness. Clinicians tap out and further reinforce the rhythm and stress of the utterances using the patient's hand. The emphasis on slow tempo, precise rhythm, and distinct stress appears to facilitate the processing of the structure and the articulation of the intoned utterances.

The MIT program consists of four levels. In level I, the clinician hums a melody pattern within the three- to four-note range and aids the patient in tapping the rhythm and stress of the stimulus melody to establish the process of intoning melody patterns with hand tapping. Level II requires the patient to tap and repeat the clinician's production of the intoned utterance and to respond to a probe question eliciting an intoned repetition of the intoned utterance. Hand tapping is not used in response to probe questions. The clinician provides assistance by intoning the utterance in unison with the patient and then fading his participation so that the patient subsequently intones the utterance on his own. In level III, unison intoning of the utterance is followed by immediate fading of the clinician's participation. The patient then produces the target utterance following an enforced delay after the clinician presents it. Finally, the patient gives an appropriate intoned response to an intoned probe question from the clinician. A backup procedure is introduced at this level to provide the patient an opportunity to correct errors. The backups consist of repeating the previous step and attempting the failed step again, and as such constitute an "indirect" approach to correcting errors. The goal of level IV is normal speech prosody. Latencies for delayed repetition are increased, and the training sentences become more complex. A technique called *Sprechgesang* (speech-song) is used in the transition to speech prosody. In this technique, the constant pitch of the intoned words is replaced by the variable pitch of speech while retaining the tempo, rhythm, and stress of the intoned sentence. Unison production of the target sentence in *Sprechgesang* is followed by fading, delayed spoken repetition using normal speech prosody, and production using normal prosody in response to a probe question with normal speech prosody.

MIT uses a scoring method where values of 2, 1, or 0 can be obtained. Full scores (i.e., 1 for items with no backups, 2 for items with backups) are assigned to successful responses, while partial scores (i.e., 1) are assigned to responses that require a backup where available. No score is assigned to unsuccessful responses following multiple attempts. The average score for three sessions must be higher than the average score of the three previous sessions for the participant to remain in the program. An overall score of 90% or better for five consecutive sessions is required to advance from one level of MIT to the next.

The neurophysiological model offered by the developers of MIT to account for its effectiveness has been controversial since it was first proposed. Berlin (1976) stated that the evidence linking the right hemisphere to the interpretation of nonverbal acoustic processes like music is insufficient to conclude that MIT activates the right hemisphere in some way to control motor speech gestures. Instead, he suggested that good candidates for MIT might have an intact left primary motor area that is deprived of input from the damaged left Broca's area. Improved speech production might then result from transcallosal input to left hemisphere speech motor centers arising from the MIT-activated right hemisphere homologue of Broca's area. An alternative explanation involved input from a disconnected intact left Broca's area to an intact left primary motor area via a transcallosal pathway involving the right hemisphere homologues to these areas.

Belin et al. (1996) used positron emission tomography to investigate recovery from nonfluent aphasia following treatment with MIT. Changes in cerebral blood flow were measured while the participant listened to and repeated simple words, and during repetition of intoned words. Abnormal activation of right hemisphere structures homotopic to those normally activated in the intact left hemisphere was observed during the simple word tasks performed without intoning, while word repetition with intoning reactivated essential motor language zones, including Broca's area and the adjacent left prefrontal cortex. Belin et al. concluded that MIT is more strongly associated with exaggerated speech prosody than with singing and therefore recruits language-related brain areas of the left hemisphere rather than right hemisphere areas.

Boucher et al. (2001) investigated whether the processing of melodic contours in music applies similarly to the processing of speech prosody. According to these authors, melody is associated with musical tone and rhythm. Tonal elements include pitch, timbre, and chord and correspond to intonation in speech. Musical rhythm refers to the timing distribution of tonal elements and is comparable to the stress points of speech. Although there is support for right hemisphere processing of intonation, Boucher et al. (2001) provide evidence that the left hemisphere is involved in the processing of rhythm, and consequently question whether melody-based interventions such as MIT facilitate speech production because of right hemisphere contributions. Following interventions in two speakers with nonfluent aphasia using stimuli emphasizing tone or rhythm in varying conditions, equal or greater success in responding was found for conditions emphasizing rhythm than for conditions emphasizing melodic intoning. Boucher et al. concluded that the right hemisphere explanation for the facilitating effects of MIT could not be supported strongly.

—*Richard K. Peach*

References

Albert, M., Sparks, R., and Helm, N. (1973). Melodic intonation therapy for aphasia. *Archives of Neurology, 29,* 130–131.

American Academy of Neurology. (1994). Assessment: Melodic intonation therapy. *Neurology, 44,* 566–568.

Belin, P., Van Eeckhout, P., Zilbovicius, M., Remy, P., Francois, C., Guillaume, S., et al. (1996). Recovery from nonfluent aphasia after melodic intonation therapy: A PET study. *Neurology, 47,* 1504–1511.

Berlin, C. I. (1976). On "Melodic Intonation Therapy for aphasia" by R. W. Sparks and A. L. Holland. *Journal of Speech and Hearing Disorders, 41*, 298–300.

Boucher, V., Garcia, L. J., Fleurant, J., and Paradis, J. (2001). Variable efficacy of rhythm and tone in melody-based interventions: Implications for the assumption of a right-hemisphere facilitation in non-fluent aphasia. *Aphasiology, 15*, 131–149.

Helm-Estabrooks, N., and Albert, M. L. (1991). *Manual of aphasia therapy*. Austin, TX: Pro-Ed.

Laughlin, S. A., Naeser, M. A., and Gordon, W. P. (1979). Effects of three syllable durations using the melodic intonation therapy technique. *Journal of Speech and Hearing Research, 22*, 311–320.

Naeser, M. A. (1994). Neuroimaging and recovery of auditory comprehension and spontaneous speech in aphasia with some implications for treatment in severe aphasia. In A. Kertesz (Ed.), *Localization and neuroimaging in neuropsychology* (pp. 245–295). San Diego, CA: Academic Press.

Naeser, M. A., and Helm-Estabrooks, N. (1985). CT scan lesion localization and response to melodic intonation therapy with nonfluent aphasia cases. *Cortex, 21*, 203–223.

Sparks, R., Helm, N., and Albert, M. (1974). Aphasia rehabilitation resulting from melodic intonation therapy. *Cortex, 10*, 303–316.

Sparks, R. W. (2001). Melodic intonation therapy. In R. Chapey (Ed.), *Language intervention strategies in aphasia and related neurogenic communication disorders* (4th ed., pp. 703–717). Philadelphia: Lippincott Williams and Wilkins.

Sparks, R. W., and Holland, A. L. (1976). Method: Melodic intonation therapy for aphasia. *Journal of Speech and Hearing Disorders, 41*, 287–297.

Square, P. A., Martin, R. E., and Bose, A. (2001). Nature and treatment of neuromotor speech disorders in aphasia. In R. Chapey (Ed.), *Language intervention strategies in aphasia and related neurogenic communication disorders* (4th ed., pp. 847–884). Philadelphia: Lippincott Williams and Wilkins.

Tonkovich, J. D., and Peach, R. K. (1989). What to treat: Apraxia of speech, aphasia, or both. In P. A. Square (Ed.), *Acquired apraxia of speech in aphasic adults* (pp. 115–144). London: Erlbaum.

Further Readings

Baum, S., and Pell, M. (1999). The neural bases of prosody: Insights from lesion studies and neuroimaging. *Aphasiology, 13*, 581–608.

Behrens, S. (1985). The perception of stress and lateralization of prosody. *Brain and Language, 26*, 332–348.

Blumstein, S., and Cooper, W. (1974). Hemispheric processing of intonation contours. *Cortex, 10*, 146–158.

Keith, R., and Aronson, A. (1975). Singing as a therapy for apraxia of speech and aphasia. *Brain and Language, 2*, 483–488.

Pell, M. (1999). Fundamental frequency encoding of linguistic and emotional prosody by right-hemisphere damaged speakers. *Brain and Language, 69*, 161–192.

Robinson, G., and Solomon, D. (1974). Rhythm is processed by the speech hemisphere. *Journal of Experimental Psychology, 102*, 508–511.

Van Lancker, D., and Sidtis, J. (1992). The identification of affective-prosodic stimuli by left- and right-hemisphere-damaged subjects: All errors are not created equal. *Journal of Speech and Hearing Research, 35*, 963–970.

Yamadori, A., Osumi, Y., Masuhara, G., and Okubo, M. (1977). Preservation of singing in Broca's aphasia. *Journal of Neurology, Neurosurgery, and Psychiatry, 40*, 221–224.

Memory and Processing Capacity

Research on the role of working memory in language disorders has stemmed mainly from the phonological loop model (e.g., Baddeley, 1986; Gathercole and Baddeley, 1993) or the capacity theory of comprehension (e.g., Just and Carpenter, 1992). These models differ in their conception of working memory and in the paradigms typically used to assess this construct (cf. Montgomery, 2000a); however, a central premise of both frameworks is that there is a limited pool of operational resources available to perform computations, such that processing and storage of linguistic information is degraded when demands exceed available resources. Numerous investigations based on these two approaches have demonstrated an association between working memory capacity and normal language functioning in children and adults. In young children, individual differences in phonological working memory predict vocabulary development and are related to differences in word repertoire, utterance length, and grammatical construction use (e.g., Gathercole and Baddelely, 1990b; Adams and Gathercole, 2000). School-age children's performance on working memory measures is significantly correlated with spoken language comprehension as well as with reading recognition and comprehension (e.g., Gaulin and Campbell, 1994; Swanson, 1996). Working memory capacity predicts a number of verbal abilities in adults, including reading comprehension levels, understanding of ambiguous passages and syntactically complex sentences, and the ability to make inferences (e.g., King and Just, 1991; Carpenter, Miyake, and Just, 1994).

Investigators have examined short-term or working memory abilities in children with varying profiles of language and cognitive deficits, including children with Down syndrome, Williams' syndrome, Landau-Kleffner syndrome, learning disabilities, and specific language impairment (SLI). Of special interest are children with SLI, who demonstrate significant language deficits in the absence of any clearly identifiable cause such as mental retardation or hearing loss. One theoretical camp views SLI in terms of limited processing capacity. There are various formulations of limited capacity accounts of SLI, including hypotheses about specific deficits in phonological working memory and hypotheses regarding more generalized difficulties in information processing and storage that affect performance across modalities (cf. Leonard, 1998). Difficulties discussed here are limited to poor nonword repetition, reduced listening span, and poor serial recall.

Children with SLI exhibit deficits in nonword repetition, a paradigm that has been used extensively by Baddeley and colleagues (and others as well) as a measure of phonological working memory (Gathercole and Baddeley, 1990a; Montgomery, 1995; Dollaghan and Campbell, 1998; Edwards and Lahey, 1998; Ellis Weismer et al., 2000; Briscoe, Bishop, and Norbury, 2001). Nonword repetition has proved to be useful clinically as a culturally nonbiased measure for distinguishing between children with and without language disorders. In one of the initial investigations of nonword repetition in SLI, Gathercole and Baddeley (1990a) concluded that children with SLI demonstrate significantly poorer phonological working memory than controls matched on nonverbal cognition or language level (however, see van der Lely and Howard, 1993; Howard and van der Lely, 1995). The findings of Gathercole and Baddeley (1990a) were replicated by Montgomery (1995), who similarly interpreted his results as indicating that children with SLI have reduced phonological memory capacity.

Other studies have sought to determine whether difficulties with nonword repetition reflect cognitive processes other than working memory deficits (Edwards and Lahey, 1998; Briscoe, Bishop, and Norbury, 2001). After a thorough investigation of possible explanations for nonword repetition deficits in SLI, Edwards and Lahey (1998) concluded that neither auditory discrimination nor response processes could account for the difficulties. Instead, they attributed the deficits to problems in the formation or storage of phonological representations in working memory. Children with SLI usually do not differ from normal language peers in their ability to repeat short, simple nonwords; rather, breakdowns on nonword repetition tasks typically occur on the most complex stimuli (Ellis Weismer et al., 2000; Briscoe, Bishop, and Norbury, 2001). When children with SLI were compared with children with mild to moderate hearing loss, both groups showed similar difficulty with longer nonwords, but children with SLI also displayed deficits on digit recall and were more negatively affected by phonological complexity (Briscoe, Bishop, and Norbury, 2001). These investigators concluded that auditory perceptual deficits are not sufficient to explain the range of language and literacy difficulties observed in children with SLI and suggested that some kind of processing capacity limitation underlay their language deficits.

Several genetic investigations of developmental language disorder have examined phonological memory as indexed by nonword repetition. Bishop, North, and Donlan (1996) administered a nonword repetition task to participants in a study of twins with language impairment. Children with persistent language impairment as well as those with resolved language impairment exhibited significant deficits in nonword repetition. Comparison of nonword repetition performance in monozygotic and dizygotic twin pairs revealed a significant heritability component. Based on these results, Bishop et al. suggested that deficits in nonword repetition provide a phenotypic marker of heritable forms of developmental language disorder. Bishop and colleagues (1999) replicated the earlier results and found that nonword repetition gave high estimates of group heritability. This measure was a better predictor of low language

scores than was a measure of auditory processing (Tallal's Auditory Repetition Test). Tomblin and colleagues (2002) recently investigated candidate genes associated with developmental language disorder, testing for associations between candidate loci in a sample of 476 children and their parents. A two-stage approach was used to search for loci associated with language disorder, as diagnosed by standardized tests of listening and speaking or by a measure of phonological memory (nonword repetition). Preliminary results were suggestive of an association of CFTR (a marker on chromosome 7) with both the phonological memory and spoken language phenotypes.

Another paradigm widely employed in research on the association between language and working memory abilities uses a listening/reading span task (e.g., Daneman and Carpenter, 1980). The person is required to perform two tasks concurrently (involving processing and storage), such as making true/false judgments about sentences and recalling the last word in each sentence following the presentation of all sentences in a set. The number of sentences within a set increases throughout the task in order to assess memory span. Ellis Weismer, Evans, and Hesketh (1999) found that children with SLI evidenced limitations in verbal working memory compared to age-matched controls, based on their performance on a listening span task developed by Gaulin and Campbell (1994). Findings primarily pointed to quantitative differences between the groups involving reduced capacity for the children with SLI; however, there were some indications of qualitative differences in terms of distinct patterns of word-recall errors and different patterns of associations between working memory and performance on language and nonverbal cognitive measures. Montgomery (2000a, 2000b) examined the relation between working memory and sentence processing in children with SLI. Using an adaptation of Daneman and Carpenter's listening span task, he demonstrated that children with SLI exhibit reduced capacity under dual-load conditions. Performance on the listening span measure was significantly correlated with performance on an off-line sentence comprehension task but not with on-line sentence processing. Montgomery concluded that the slower real-time sentence processing in children with SLI was primarily a function of inefficient lexical retrieval operations rather than limitations in working memory; however, he posited that their difficulties with off-line sentence comprehension tasks were related to difficulties coordinating the requisite processing and storage functions, revealing limitations in functional working memory capacity.

Serial memory deficits in children with SLI have been documented by Gillam and colleagues (Gillam, Cowan, and Day, 1995; Gillam, Cowan, and Marler, 1998). The initial study employed a suffix effect procedure in which a spoken list to be recalled was followed by a "suffix" (nonword item) that was not to be recalled. The suffix had a disproportionately negative effect on recency recall for the children with SLI when strict serial position criteria for scoring were imposed. The subsequent investigation by Gillam et al. sought to determine the nature of working memory deficiencies in children with SLI, using a modality effect paradigm in which input modality, rate of input, and response modality were manipulated. To control for differences in capacity across the groups, trials were administered at a level consistent with each child's working memory span. Children with SLI and controls demonstrated traditional primacy, recency, and modality effects and similar performance when audio-visual stimuli were paired with spoken responses. However, children with SLI exhibited reduced recency effects and poor recall when visually presented items were paired with pointing responses. The investigators concluded that neither output processes nor auditory temporal processing could account for the working memory deficits in children with SLI. They suggested instead that children with SLI have problems retaining or transforming phonological codes, particularly on tasks requiring multiple mental operations. They further speculated that these capacity limitations in working memory may be due to rapid decay of phonological representations or to performance limitations involving the use of less demanding coding and retrieval strategies.

In conclusion, there is considerable evidence that children with SLI have limitations in working memory, yet there are a number of unresolved issues. In light of the known heterogeneity of the SLI population, it seems unlikely that any single factor can account for the language difficulties of all children. Additional research is warranted to examine individual variation within this population and to explore whether limitations in working memory are differentially implicated in various subtypes of SLI. Another important issue pertains to whether deficits in working memory capacity are restricted to processing of verbal material or extend to nonverbal information as well. That is, it is important to determine whether the evidence supports a domain-specific model or a generalized capacity deficit model. Finally, future studies should determine whether memory limitations are actually a causal factor in SLI, an outgrowth of the language problems, or an independent area of difficulty for children with language disorder.

—*Susan Ellis Weismer*

References

Adams, A. M., and Gathercole, S. (2000). Limitations in working memory: Implication for language development. *International Journal of Language and Communication Disorder*, *35*, 95–116.

Baddeley, A. (1986). *Working memory*. Oxford, U.K.: Clarendon Press.

Bishop, D. V. M., North, T., and Donlan, C. (1996). Nonword repetition as a behavioral marker for inherited language impairment: Evidence from a twin study. *Journal of Child Psychology and Psychiatry*, *36*, 1–13.

Bishop, D. V. M., Bishop, S., Bright, P., James, C., Delaney, T., and Tallal, P. (1999). Different origin of auditory and phonological processing problems in children with language impairment: Evidence from a twin study. *Journal of Speech, Language, and Hearing Research*, *42*, 155–168.

Briscoe, J., Bishop, D. V. M., and Norbury, C. F. (2001). Phonological processing, language, and literacy: A comparison of children with mild-to-moderate sensorineural hearing loss and those with specific language impairment. *Journal of Child Psychology and Psychiatry*, *42*, 329–340.

Carpenter, P., Miyake, A., and Just, M. (1994). Working memory constraints in comprehension: Evidence from individual differences, aphasia, and aging. In M. A. Gernsbacher (Ed.), *Handbook of psycholinguistics* (pp. 1075–1122). San Diego, CA: Academic Press.

Daneman, M., and Carpenter, P. (1980). Individual differences in working memory and reading. *Journal of Verbal Learning and Verbal Behavior*, *19*, 450–466.

Dollaghan, C., and Campbell, T. (1998). Nonword repetition and child language impairment. *Journal of Speech, Language, and Hearing Research*, *41*, 1136–1146.

Edwards, J., and Lahey, M. (1998). Nonword repetitions of children with specific language impairment: Exploration of some explanations for their inaccuracies. *Applied Psycholinguistics*, *19*, 279–309.

Ellis Weismer, S., Evans, J., and Hesketh, L. J. (1999). An examination of verbal working memory capacity in children with specific language impairment. *Journal of Speech, Language, and Hearing Research*, *42*, 1249–1260.

Ellis Weismer, S., Tomblin, J. B., Zhang, X., Buckwalter, P., Chynoweth, J. G., and Jones, M. (2000). Nonword repetition performance in school-age children with and without language impairment. *Journal of Speech, Language, and Hearing Research*, *43*, 865–878.

Gathercole, S., and Baddeley, A. (1990a). Phonological memory deficits in language disordered children: Is there a causal connection? *Journal of Memory and Language*, *29*, 336–360.

Gathercole, S., and Baddeley, A. (1990b). The role of phonological memory in vocabulary acquisition: A study of young children learning new words. *British Journal of Psychology*, *81*, 439–454.

Gathercole, S., and Baddeley, A. (1993). *Working memory and language processing*. Hove, U.K.: Erlbaum.

Gaulin, C., and Campbell, T. (1994). Procedure for assessing verbal working memory in normal school-age children: Some preliminary data. *Perceptual and Motor Skills*, *79*, 55–64.

Gillam, R., Cowan, N., and Day, L. (1995). Sequential memory in children with and without language impairment. *Journal of Speech and Hearing Research*, *38*, 393–402.

Gillam, R., Cowan, N., and Marler, J. (1998). Information processing by school-age children with specific language impairment: Evidence from a modality effect paradigm. *Journal of Speech, Language, and Hearing Research*, *41*, 913–926.

Howard, D., and van der Lely, H. (1995). Specific language impairment in children is *not* due to a short-term memory deficit: Response to Gathercole and Baddeley. *Journal of Speech and Hearing Research*, *38*, 466–472.

Just, M., and Carpenter, P. (1992). A capacity theory of comprehension: Individual differences in working memory. *Psychological Review*, *99*, 122–149.

King, J., and Just, M. (1991). Individual differences in syntactic processing: The role of working memory. *Journal of Memory and Language*, *30*, 580–602.

Leonard, L. (1998). *Children with specific language impairment*. Cambridge, MA: MIT Press.

Montgomery, J. (1995). Sentence comprehension in children with specific language impairment: The role of phonological working memory. *Journal of Speech and Hearing Research*, *38*, 177–189.

Montgomery, J. (2000a). Relation of working memory to off-line and real-time sentence processing in children with specific language impairment. *Applied Psycholinguistics, 21,* 117–148.

Montgomery, J. (2000b). Verbal working memory and sentence comprehension in children with specific language impairment. *Journal of Speech, Language, and Hearing Research, 43,* 293–308.

Swanson, H. L. (1996). Individual and age-related differences in children's working memory. *Memory and Cognition, 24,* 70–82.

Tomblin, J. B., Murray, J. C., Nishimura, C., Zhang, X., Ellis Weismer, S., O'Brien, M., and Palmer, P. (2002). *Positive association and sibpair linkage results on children with impairments in spoken language and phonological memory.* Unpublished manuscript, Department of Speech Pathology and Audiology, University of Iowa, Iowa City.

van der Lely, H., and Howard, D. (1993). Children with specific language impairment: Linguistic impairment or short-term memory deficit? *Journal of Speech and Hearing Research, 36,* 1193–1207.

Further Readings

Chapman, R., and Hesketh, L. J. (2000). Behavioral phenotype of individuals with Down syndrome. *Mental Retardation and Developmental Disabilities Research Reviews, 6,* 84–95.

Cohen, N., Vallance, D., Barwick, M., Im, N., Menna, R., Horodezky, N., and Issacson, L. (2000). The interface between ADHD and language impairment: An examination of language, achievement, and cognitive processing. *Journal of Child Psychology and Psychiatry, 41,* 353–362.

Cowan, N. (1996). Short-term memory, working memory, and their importance in language processing. *Topics in Language Disorders, 17,* 1–18.

de Jong, P. F. (1998). Working memory deficits of reading disabled children. *Journal of Experimental Child Psychology, 70,* 75–96.

Donlan, C., and Masters, J. (2000). Correlates of social development in children with communication disorders: The concurrent predictive value of verbal short-term memory. *International Journal of Language and Communication Disorders, 35,* 211–226.

Ellis Weismer, S. (1996). Capacity limitations in working memory: The impact on lexical and morphological learning by children with language impairment. *Topics in Language Disorders, 17,* 33–44.

Evans, J., Alibali, M., and McNeil, N. (2001). Divergence of verbal expression and embodied knowledge: Evidence from speech and gesture in children with specific language impairment. *Language and Cognitive Processes, 16,* 309–331.

Farmer, M. (2000). Language and social cognition in children with specific language impairment. *Journal of Child Psychology and Psychiatry, 41,* 627–636.

Fazio, B. (1999). Arithmetic calculation, short-term memory, and language performance with specific language impairment: A 5-year follow-up. *Journal of Speech, Language, and Hearing Research, 42,* 420–431.

Gillam, R. (Ed.). (1998). *Memory and language impairments in children and adults.* Frederick, MD: Aspen.

Jarrold, C., and Baddeley, A. (1999). Genetically dissociated components of working memory: Evidence from Down's and Williams syndrome. *Neuropsychologia, 37,* 637–651.

Jarrold, C., Baddeley, A., and Hewes, A. (2000). Verbal short-term memory deficits in Down syndrome: A consequence of

problems in rehearsal? *Journal of Child Psychology and Psychiatry, 41,* 223–244.

Metz-Lutz, M. N., Seegmuller, C., Kleitz, C., de Saint-Martin, A., Hirsch, E., and Marescaux, C. (1999). Landau-Kleffner syndrome: A rare childhood epileptic aphasia. *Journal of Neurolinguistics, 12,* 167–179.

Nation, K., Adams, J., Bowyer-Crane, C., and Snowling, M. (1999). Working memory deficits in poor comprehenders reflect underlying language impairments. *Journal of Experimental Child Psychology, 73,* 139–158.

Oakhill, J., Cain, K., and Yuill, N. (1998). Individual differences in children's comprehension skill: Toward an integrated model. In C. Hulme and R. M. Joshi (Eds.), *Reading and spelling: Development and disorders* (pp. 343–367). Mahwah, NJ: Erlbaum.

Swanson, H. L. (1999). Reading comprehension and working memory in learning-disabled readers: Is the phonological loop more important than the executive system? *Journal of Experimental Child Psychology, 72,* 1–31.

Zera, D. A., and Lucian, D. (2001). Self-organization and learning disabilities: A theoretical perspective for the interpretation and understanding of dysfunction. *Learning Disability Quarterly, 24,* 107–118.

Mental Retardation

Mental retardation is characterized by "significantly subaverage intellectual functioning, existing concurrently with related limitations in two or more of the following adaptive skills areas: communication, self-care, home-living, social skills, community use, self-direction, health and safety, functional academics, leisure and work" (Luckerson et al., 1992, p. 5). Mental retardation thus applies to a broad range of children and adults, from those with mild deficits who function fairly well in society to those with extremely severe deficits who require a range of support in order to function. Regardless of the extent of mental retardation, the likelihood that communication development will be delayed is high. In fact, language delays or disorders are often an early outward signal of mental retardation.

Prior to the 1960s, a child who was diagnosed with mental retardation received little or no attention from investigators or practitioners in communication disorders because it was thought that the child could not learn and thus would make few gains in speech development. Following changes in policy and federal legislation, the 1960s saw the emergence of the modern scientific study of mental retardation. Since then, significant research findings about language and communication development have enhanced the speech, language, and communication outcomes for children and adults with mental retardation.

With respect to communication, children and adults with mental retardation can be broadly divided according to whether or not the individual speaks. Most children and adults with mental retardation or developmental disabilities do learn to communicate through speech, either spontaneously or with the aid of speech and language intervention during the developmental period (Rosenberg and Abbeduto, 1993). A substantial body of research has addressed the language and communication abilities of children and adults with mental retardation who speak. In particular, strong empirical findings about the communication abilities of children and adults with Down syndrome, fragile X syndrome, and Williams syndrome suggest a complex picture, with different relations between language comprehension and production and between language and cognition. The development of communicative and language intervention approaches for children with mental retardation who speak is an area of remarkable developments (Kaiser, 1993). Psycholinguistic research findings and behavioral instructional procedures have provided the foundation for language intervention protocols for teaching children with mental retardation specific speech and language skills. An early emphasis on direct instruction was followed by a shift away from the formal aspects of language and toward the teaching of lexical and pragmatic skills, measuring generalization, and the use of intervention approaches in a natural environment to promote the child's social competence. Techniques include milieu teaching, parent-implemented intervention, and peer-mediated approaches. These are each identifiable, distinct language interventions with supporting empirical evidence that they work. Perhaps the most important recent development is the extension of intervention approaches to infants and toddlers with developmental disabilities, a move reflecting examinations of interventions targeted to intentional communication and language comprehension (Bricker, 1993). Overall, the field has developed by expanding the content and focus of intervention programs and fine-tuning the procedures used to deliver the interventions. Greater sophistication in language intervention strategies now permits an examination of the relationship between the characteristics a child brings to the intervention and the attributes of the intervention itself.

Some children and adults with mental retardation, however, encounter significant difficulty developing oral communication skills. Such difficulty during childhood results in inability to express oneself, to maintain social contact with family, to develop friendships, and to function successfully in school. As the child moves through adolescence and into adulthood, inability to communicate continues to compromise his or her ability to participate in society, from accessing education and employment to engaging in leisure activities and personal relationships. For the most part, individuals who experience considerable difficulty communicating are those with the most significant degrees of mental retardation. They may also exhibit other disabilities, including seizure disorders, cerebral palsy, sensory impairments, or maladaptive behaviors. They range in age from very young children just beginning development to adults with a broad range of life experiences, including a history of institutionalization. These children and adults can and now do benefit from language and communication intervention focusing on the development and use of functional communication skills, although the areas of concentration vary with age and experience.

One intervention approach that has been developed for use with individuals with severe communication difficulties is augmentative and alternative communication (AAC). AAC encompasses all forms of communication, from simple gestures, manual signs and picture communication boards to American Sign Language and sophisticated computer-based devices that can speak in phrases and sentences for their users. Children with mental retardation who can benefit from AAC are usually identified based on communication profiles. The majority of children with mental retardation who use AAC have more severe forms of mental retardation. These children never develop any speech, or develop only a few words, or are echolalic. For them, AAC provides a means with which to develop receptive and expressive language skills (Romski and Sevcik, 1996).

See also COMMUNICATION SKILLS OF PEOPLE WITH DOWN SYNDROME; MENTAL RETARDATION AND SPEECH IN CHILDREN.

—*Mary Ann Romski and Rose A. Sevcik*

References

Bricker, D. (1993). Then, now, and the path between: A brief history of language intervention. In A. Kaiser and D. Gray (Eds.), *Enhancing children's communication: Research foundations for intervention* (pp. 11–31). Baltimore: Paul H. Brookes.

Kaiser, A. (1993). Parent-implemented language intervention: An environmental system perspective. In A. Kaiser and D. Gray (Eds.), *Enhancing children's communication: Research foundations for intervention* (pp. 63–84). Baltimore: Paul H. Brookes.

Luckasson, R., Coulter, D. L., Polloway, E. A., Reiss, S., Schalock, R. L., Snell, M. E., et al. (1992). *Mental retardation: Definition, classification, and systems of supports* (9th ed.). Washington, DC: AAMR.

Romski, M. A., and Sevcik, R. A. (1996). *Breaking the speech barrier: Language development through augmented means.* Baltimore: Paul H. Brookes.

Rosenberg, S., and Abbeduto, L. (1993). *Language and communication in mental retardation: Development, processes, and intervention.* Hillsdale, NJ: Erlbaum.

Further Readings

Chapman, R. (1997). Language development in children and adolescents with Down syndrome. *Mental Retardation and Developmental Disabilities Research Reviews, 3,* 307–312.

Miller, J. F., Leddy, M., and Leavitt, L. (1999). *Improving the communication of people with Down syndrome.* Baltimore: Paul H. Brookes.

National Joint Committee for the Communication Needs of Persons with Severe Disabilities. (2001). Access to communication services and supports: Concerns regarding the application of restrictive "eligibility" policies. Unpublished document. Washington, DC: Author.

Romski, M. A., and Sevcik, R. A. (1997). Augmentative and alternative communication for children with developmental disabilities. *Mental Retardation and Developmental Disabilities Research Reviews, 3,* 363–368.

Sevcik, R. A., and Romski, M. A. (1997). Comprehension and language acquisition: Evidence from youth with severe cognitive disabilities. In L. B. Adamson and M. A. Romski (Eds.), *Communication and language acquisition: Discoveries from atypical language development* (pp. 184–201). Baltimore: Paul H. Brookes.

Warren, S., and Yoder, P. (1997). Communication, language, and mental retardation. In W. McLean (Ed.), *Ellis' handbook of mental deficiency, psychological theory and research* (pp. 379–403). Mahwah, NJ: Erlbaum.

Morphosyntax and Syntax

This article discusses issues in the linguistic analysis of morphosyntax and syntax in children with language disorders. It presupposes familiarity with generative linguistic theory. The goal is to illustrate what kinds of grammatically based explanations are available to theories of disorders. The task of such explanations is to unify superficially diverse markers of a disorder into natural classes that linguistic theory motivates or to characterize observed errors. The discussion is divided, as suggested by recent generative theory, into issues concerning the lexicon versus issues concerning the computation of larger structures from lexical atoms.

The lexicon can be subdivided along various dimensions, any of which might be relevant in capturing dissociations found in nonnormal language development. A primary split divides content words, i.e., nouns, verbs, adjectives, and adverbs, from all other morphemes, i.e., functional or closed-class elements. (I ignore the challenging issue of where adpositions belong; they likely are heterogeneous, a dichotomy among them being evinced in adult disorders [Rizzi, 1985; Grodzinsky, 1990].) In Chomskyan syntax of the 1980s (cf. Emonds, 1985; Chomsky, 1986; Fukui, 1986) there was a seemingly arbitrary split between functional meanings that were treated as autonomous syntactic functional categories (e.g., Tense, Determiner, Agreement, Complementizer) and those that were not (e.g., number marking on nouns, participial affixes, infinitival suffixes on verbs). Some attempts were made to understand disorders of acquisition in terms of this heterogeneous system (cf. Leonard, 1998). However, the harder linguists have looked, the more functional heads for which they have found structural evidence. On parsimony grounds we now expect *all* functional meanings to be represented in syntactic positions separate from those of content words (cf. van Gelderen, 1993; Hoekstra, 2000; Jakubowicz and Nash, 2001).

Among functional elements (morphemes or features thereof) a further distinction is made, dubbed "interpretability" by Chomsky (1995). Some morphemes encode elements of meaning and contribute directly to the interpretation of a sentence; for example, the English noun plural suffix *-s* combines with a noun whose meaning describes a kind of entity, and adds information about number; for example, *dog + s* = caninehood + more-than-one. Plural *-s* is therefore an interpretable morpheme. This contrasts with the 3sg present indicative verbal suffix *-s*, which makes no semantic contribution, because what is semantically "one" or "more than one" is the subject of the sentence—a noun phrase. Numerosity (and person) are properties of noun meanings, not verb meanings. The inflection *-s* appears on the verb as a consequence of the number and person of the subject, that information having been copied onto the verb. Agreement is therefore an uninterpretable morpheme: it replicates a bit of meaning represented elsewhere, surfacing only because the morphosyntax of English requires it. It has no impact at Logical Form. Such morphemes are seen as a plausible locus for impairment (cf. Clahsen, Bartke, and Göllner, 1997).

A second common kind of uninterpretable morphology is case marking. Many case markings have nothing to do with meaning. For example, in *She saw me* and *I was seen by her*, the difference between accusative *me* and nominative *I* does not correspond to any change in the semantic role played by the speaker; rather, it reflects purely syntactic information. A third kind of uninterpretable morphology arises in concord. For instance, in Latin the forms of many words within a noun phrase reflect its case and number, as well as the gender of the head noun: for example, *ill-as vi-as angust-as* "those-acc.fem.pl streets-acc.fem.pl narrow-acc.fem.pl."

Among the uninterpretable features there may be a further distinction to be drawn, as follows. Person and number information is interpretable on noun phrases but not on verbs; in a sense, there is an asymmetry between the contentful versus the merely duplicated instantiation of those features (cf. Clahsen, 1989). Case is different: it is taken to be uninterpretable both on the recipient/checkee (noun phrase) and on the source/checker (verb, preposition, or Tense); it does not exist at Logical Form at all. Thus, symmetrically uninterpretable functional elements such as Case constitute another natural class. Grammatical gender is also an example of a morphosyntactic feature that has no semantic counterpart. There are two ways in which gender marking might be impaired, calling for different explanations: first, children might not be able to consistently recall the gender of particular nouns; second, children might not be able to consistently copy gender information from the noun, which is associated with gender in the lexicon, to other parts of a noun phrase (a problem with concord).

Turning now from the lexicon to the syntax, under Minimalism the transformational operations Merge and Move are restricted in a way that effectively builds some former filters into their definitions. Taking this seriously, certain ways of talking about language disorders in terms of missing or dysfunctional subcomponents of syntax no longer make much sense. For example, in the theory of Chomsky (1981), it was plausible to talk about, say, bounding theory (which encompasses the constraints on movement operations) being inoperative as a consequence of some disorder; this simply meant that certain structures that were always generable by Move α were no longer declared invalid after the fact by virtue of a movement that was too long. There is no natural translation of this idea into Minimalist machinery because locality is part of what defines an operation as a Move. A language disorder could in principle involve a change in this definition, but we cannot think of this as simply excising a piece of the grammar. Similarly, since movement in Minimalism is just a means to an end, it makes little sense to think of eliminating movement while leaving the rest of the theory intact; the system is now designed such that movement is the only way to satisfy a fundamental requirement that drives the computational system, namely, the need to create valid Logical Forms by eliminating uninterpretable features.

The syntactic accounts of language disorders that have been suggested often involve impoverished structure. One way to execute this is to posit that particular functional heads are either missing from syntactic structures or do not contain (all) the features that they would for adults (cf. Wexler, 1998). Another way is by reference to the position of the heads in the clausal structure rather than by reference to their content. Thus, it can be proposed that all structure above a particular point, say VP, is either missing (Radford, 1990) or optionally truncated (Rizzi, 1994). The extent to which particularly the tree pruning variant of this idea (Friedmann and Grodzinsky, 1997) can be characterized as simply lesioning one independently motivated piece of grammar is open to debate.

The division between stored representations and computational procedures is also relevant in (particularly inflectional) morphology, where the contrast between general rules and stored probabilistic associations has a long history (Pinker, 1999). Where precisely the line should be drawn differs, depending on one's theory of morphology. For instance, if there are any rules at all, then surely the process that adds (a predictable allomorph of) -d to form the past tense of a verb is a rule, and unless *all* morphology is seen as executed by rules, the relationship between *am* and *was* is stored in the lexicon as an idiosyncratic fact about the verb *be*, not encoded as a rule. But in between lie numerous subregularities that could be treated either way. For example, the alternation in *sing-sang*, *drink-drank*, and so on could be represented as a family of memorized associations or as a rule (with some memorized exceptions) triggered by the phonological shape of the stem ([ɪŋ]). Most psychologically oriented research has assumed that there is only one true rule for each inflectional feature such as [past tense] (supplying the default), while the generative phonology tradition has used numerous rules to capture subpatterns within a paradigm, only the most general of which corresponds to the default in having no explicit restriction on its domain. Thus, although a dissociation between rules and stored forms is expected under virtually any approach, precise predictions vary.

There are several ways in which (inflectional) morphology might be impaired. One of the two mechanisms might be entirely inoperative, in which case either every inflected form would have to be memorized by rote (no rules; cf. Gopnik, 1994) or every word would have to be treated as regular (no associations). The latter would be evinced by overregularizations. The former might yield overirregularizations if, in the absence of a rule, analogy-based associations were unchecked and overextended; alternatively, it might have a subtler symptomology whereby any verb could be correctly learned once its past tense was heard, but in a Wug-testing situation nonce forms could not be inflected. A more moderate impairment might entail that at least some irregular forms would be demonstrably learnable, but in production they would not always be retrieved reliably or quickly enough to block a general rule (Clahsen and Temple, 2002), apparently violating the Elsewhere Condition.

We turn now to the logic governing ways in which the most commonly produced error types from the child language disorder literature can be explained. Under the strong separation of computational combinatoric machinery versus lexical storage pursued in Minimalist syntax, it is possible for children with normal syntactic structures to sound very unlike adults, because in their lexicon certain morphemes either are missing or have incorrect features associated with them. For example, the fact that some children learning English might never produce -s in an obligatory 3sg context could be consistent with them having mastered the syntax of agreement, if their lexicon has a missing or incorrect entry for 3sg. Consequently, it is important to document the lexical inventory, that is, whether each child does at least sometimes produce the forms of interest or can in some way be shown to know them. Similarly, suppose that children learning a given language produce agreement mismatch errors of just one type, namely, that non-3sg subjects appear with 3sg verb forms. That is, suppose that in Spanish we find errors like *yo tiene* ("I has (3sg)") but no errors like *ella tengo* ("she have (1sg)"). One could postulate that 3sg forms (e.g., *tiene*) are unspecified for person and number features and are inserted whenever more specific finite forms (e.g., *tengo*) are unavailable, or that *tiene* has wrongly been learned as a 1sg form. In either case, again, the syntax might be fully intact.

Errors due to lexical gaps should pattern differently from errors due to syntactically absent heads. Consider the Tense head as an example. The meaning of tense itself (past versus present) can be expressed morphologically in the Tense head position, and in addition Tense is commonly thought to house the uninterpretable feature that requires the presence of an overt subject in non-null subject languages (the unhelpfully named EPP feature), and the uninterpretable feature that licenses nominative case on its specifier (the subject). If Tense were completely missing from the grammar of some children, this would predict not only that they would produce no tense morphemes, but also that they would not enforce the overt subject requirement and would not (syntactically) require nominative case on subjects. If, on the other hand, what is observed is not an absence of tense marking but rather an incorrect choice of how to express Tense morphophonologically (e.g., *singed*, instead of *sang*), this would not be compatible with absence of the Tense head and would not predict the other syntactic consequences mentioned. Only omission of an inflectional marking or perhaps supernumerary inflection (e.g., *Did he cried?*) could have a syntactic cause; incorrect allomorph selection could not.

If a feature such as Tense is expressed some of the time but not always, this could have two underlying causes that lead to different syntactic expectations. One possibility is that Tense is part of the syntactic representation in all cases and its inconsistent expression reflects some intermittent problem in its morphophonological spell-out (cf. Phillips, 1995; Marcus, 1995); in that case no syntactic consequences are predicted. The other possibility is that Tense is intermittently absent from syntactic representations. In just this scenario we expect that the syntactic properties controlled by the Tense head should be variable (e.g., subjects are sometimes nominative, sometimes not), and furthermore, utterance by utterance, syntax and morphology should correlate: the Tense morpheme should be missing if and only if nominative case is not assigned/checked and the overt subject requirement is not enforced.

It is crucial to understand such predicted contingencies as claims concerning the distribution of *contrasting* forms. It seems clear that some children go through a stage during which, for example, some of the English pronoun forms are not produced at all; this is particularly common for *she*. What behavior we should expect at this stage depends on assumptions about the architecture of the syntax-morphology interface. Taking an "early insertion" view, under which only complete words from the lexicon can be inserted in syntactic derivations, a child lacking a lexical entry for the features [pron, 3sg, fem, NOM] should be unable to generate a sentence requiring such an item. In contrast, on a "late insertion" nonblocking approach such as Distributed Morphology (Halle and Marantz, 1993), there is always some form (perhaps phonologically null) that can be used to realize the output of a syntactically valid derivation. The syntactic tree is built up using feature bundles such as [pron, 3sg, fem, NOM], without regard to which vocabulary item might fill such a position. The architecture dictates that if there is no vocabulary entry with exactly this set of features, then the item containing the greatest subset of these features will be inserted. Thus, a child who knows the word *her* and knows that it is a feminine singular pronoun could insert it in such a tree, producing *Her goes* from a fully adultlike finite clause structure.

We conclude with some methodological points. Generative grammar's conception of linguistic knowledge as a cognitive (hence also neural) representation in the mind of an individual at some particular time dictates that, in analyzing behavioral data collected over an extended period or from multiple children, pooled data cannot be directly interpreted at face value. For example, suppose we analyze transcripts of three children's spontaneous productions sampled over a period of 6 months and find that in obligatory contexts for some grammatical morpheme, say 3sg -*s*, the overall rate of use is 67%. Virtually nothing can be concluded from this datum. It could represent (among other possibilities) a scenario in which two children were producing -*s* at

100% (i.e., talking like adults in this regard) and the third child never produced -*s*. In this circumstance we would have no evidence of a developmental stage at which -*s* is optional, and the third child's productions would be consistent with her simply not knowing the form of the 3sg present tense verbal inflection in English. At another extreme, if each of the three children were producing -*s* in two-thirds of obligatory contexts, we would have to posit a grammar in which Tense or Agreement are optional (or else multiple concurrent grammars). The same logic applies in the temporal dimension: a period of 0% production followed by a period of 100% production calls for a different analysis from a period during which production is at 50% within single recording sessions. Therefore, data reporting needs to facilitate assessment of the extent to which samples being pooled represent qualitatively comparable grammars. In addition to measures of central tendency and variance, this calls for the kind of distributional information found in "box-and-whiskers" plots.

Furthermore, to say that a child "has acquired X" by a certain age, where X is some morpheme or class of morphemes, is not strictly meaningful from the linguistic perspective adopted here. We can speak of attaining levels of normal or adult performance, and we can speak of having established a lexical entry with the correct feature specifications, but there is nothing in grammar that could correspond to a claim such as the following: "A child is taken to have acquired X once her rate of production of X morphemes in obligatory contexts is greater than 90%" (cf. Brown, 1973). This begs the question of what the grammar was like when production of X was at 85%: If X was not at that time a part of her grammar, how did the child manage to create the illusion of using it correctly so much of the time? Also, rates of production in obligatory contexts must be complemented by correct usage rates; one is scarcely interpretable without the other. If X is always used correctly, then even very low production rates signal knowledge of the properties of X and the syntactic conditions on its distribution. But if X is also frequently used incorrectly, neither type of knowledge can be inferred.

—*Carson T. Schütze*

References

Brown, R. (1973). *A first language: The early stages.* Cambridge, MA: Harvard University Press.

Chomsky, N. (1981). *Lectures on government and binding.* Dordrecht: Foris.

Chomsky, N. (1986). *Knowledge of language: Its nature, origin, and use.* New York: Praeger.

Chomsky, N. (1995). *The Minimalist program.* Cambridge, MA: MIT Press.

Clahsen, H. (1989). The grammatical characterization of developmental dysphasia. *Linguistics, 27,* 897–920.

Clahsen, H., and Temple, C. (2003). Words and rules in children with Williams syndrome. In Y. Levy and J. Schaeffer (Eds.), *Language competence across populations: Toward a definition of Specific Language Impairment* (pp. 323–352). Hillsdale, NJ: Erlbaum.

Clahsen, H., Bartke, S., and Göllner, S. (1997). Formal features in impaired grammars: A comparison of English and German SLI children. *Journal of Neurolinguistics*, *10*, 151–171.

Emonds, J. E. (1985). *A unified theory of syntactic categories.* Dordrecht: Foris.

Friedmann, N., and Grodzinsky, Y. (1997). Tense and agreement in agrammatic production: Pruning the syntactic tree. *Brain and Language*, *56*, 397–425.

Fukui, N. (1986). A theory of category projection and its applications. Ph.D. dissertation, MIT, Cambridge, MA.

Gelderen, E. van (1993). *The rise of functional categories.* Amsterdam: John Benjamins.

Gopnik, M. (1994). Impairments of syntactic tense in a familial language disorder. *McGill Working Papers in Linguistics*, *10*, 67–80.

Grodzinsky, Y. (1990). *Theoretical perspectives on language deficits.* Cambridge, MA: MIT Press.

Halle, M., and Marantz, A. (1993). Distributed morphology and the pieces of inflection. In K. L. Hale and S. J. Keyser (Eds.), *The view from Building 20: Essays in linguistics in honor of Sylvain Bromberger* (pp. 111–167). Cambridge, MA: MIT Press.

Hoekstra, T. (2000). The function of functional categories. In L. Cheng and R. Sybesma (Eds.), *The first Glot International state-of-the-article book* (pp. 1–25) Berlin: Mouton de Gruyter.

Jakubowicz, C., and Nash, L. (2001). Functional categories and syntactic operations in (ab)normal language acquisition. *Brain and Language*, *77*, 321–339.

Leonard, L. B. (1998). *Children with specific language impairment.* Cambridge, MA: MIT Press.

Marcus, G. F. (1995). Children's overregularization of English plurals: A quantitative analysis. *Journal of Child Language*, *22*, 447–459.

Phillips, C. (1995). Syntax at age two: Cross-linguistic differences. In C. T. Schütze, J. Ganger, and K. Broihier (Eds.), *Papers on language processing and acquisition* (MIT Working Papers in Linguistics 26, pp. 325–382). Cambridge, MA: MIT Press.

Pinker, S. (1999). *Words and rules: The ingredients of language.* New York: Basic Books.

Radford, A. (1990). *Syntactic theory and the acquisition of English syntax: The nature of early child grammars of English.* Oxford: Blackwell.

Rizzi, L. (1985). Two notes on the linguistic interpretation of Broca's aphasia. In M.-L. Kean (Ed.), *Agrammatism* (pp. 153–164). Orlando, FL: Academic Press.

Rizzi, L. (1994). Some notes on linguistic theory and language development: The case of root infinitives. *Language Acquisition*, *3*, 371–393.

Wexler, K. (1998). Very early parameter setting and the unique checking constraint: A new explanation of the optional infinitive stage. *Lingua*, *106*, 23–79.

Further Readings

Avrutin, S., Haverkort, M., and van Hout, A. (Eds.). (2001). *Language acquisition and language breakdown. Brain and Language*, *77*(3). [Special issue]

Bishop, D. (Ed.). (2001). *Language and cognitive processes in developmental disorders. Language and Cognitive Processes*, *16*(2–3). [Special issue]

Capirci, O., Sabbadini, L., and Volterra, V. (1996). Language development in Williams syndrome: A case study. *Cognitive Neuropsychology*, *13*, 1017–1039.

Clahsen, H., and Almazan, M. (1998). Syntax and morphology in Williams syndrome. *Cognition*, *68*, 167–198.

Clahsen, H., and Almazan, M. (2001). Compounding and inflection in language impairment: Evidence from Williams syndrome (and SLI). *Lingua*, *111*, 729–757.

Curtiss, S., Katz, W., and Tallal, P. (1992). Delay versus deviance in the language acquisition of language-impaired children. *Journal of Speech and Hearing Research*, *35*, 373–383.

Curtiss, S., and Schaeffer, J. (1997). Syntactic development in children with hemispherectomy: The Infl-system. In E. Hughes, M. Hughes, and A. Greenhill (Eds.), *Proceedings of the 21st Annual Boston University Conference on Language Development* (pp. 103–114). Somerville, MA: Cascadilla Press.

Dalalakis, J. (1996). *Developmental language impairment: Evidence from Greek and its implications for morphological representation.* Ph.D. dissertation, McGill University, Montreal.

Fowler, A. E., Gelman, R., and Gleitman, L. R. (1994). The course of language learning in children with Down syndrome. In H. Tager-Flusberg (Ed.), *Constraints on language acquisition: Studies of atypical children* (pp. 91–140). Hillsdale, NJ: Erlbaum.

Gopnik, M., and Goad, H. (1997). What underlies inflectional error patterns in genetic dysphasia? *Neurolinguistics*, *10*, 109–137.

Harris, N. G. S., Bellugi, U., Bates, E., Jones, W., and Rossen, M. (1997). Contrasting profiles of language development in children with Williams and Down syndromes. *Developmental Neuropsychology*, *13*, 345–370.

Levy, Y., Amir, N., and Shalev, R. (1992). Linguistic development of a child with a congenital, localized LH lesion. *Cognitive Neuropsychology*, *9*, 1–32.

Levy, Y., and Kavé, G. (1999). Language breakdown and linguistic theory: A tutorial overview. *Lingua*, *107*, 95–143.

McGill Working Papers in Linguistics, *10*, 1994. [Special issue on the linguistic aspects of familial language impairment]

Oetting, J. B., and Horohov, J. E. (1997). Past tense marking by children with and without Specific Language Impairment. *Journal of Speech, Language, and Hearing Research*, *40*, 62–74.

Oetting, J. B., and Rice, M. (1993). Plural acquisition in children with Specific Language Impairment. *Journal of Speech and Hearing Research*, *36*, 1236–1248.

Rice, M. L. (Ed.). (1996). *Toward a genetics of language.* Mahwah, NJ: Erlbaum.

Rossen, M., Klima, E. S., Bellugi, U., Bihrle, A., and Jones, W. (1996). Interaction between language and cognition: Evidence from Williams syndrome. In J. H. Beitchman, N. J. Cohen, M. M. Konstantareas, and R. Tannock (Eds.), *Language, learning, and behavior disorders: Developmental, biological, and clinical perspectives* (pp. 367–382). New York: Cambridge University Press.

Stevens, T., and Karmiloff-Smith, A. (1997). Word learning in a special population: Do individuals with Williams syndrome obey lexical constraints? *Journal of Child Language*, *24*, 737–765.

Stromswold, K. (1998). Genetics of spoken language disorders. *Human Biology*, *70*, 297–324.

Tager-Flusberg, H. (Ed.). (1994). *Constraints on language acquisition: Studies of atypical children.* Hillsdale, NJ: Erlbaum.

Ullman, M. T., and Gopnik, M. (1999). Inflectional morphology in a family with inherited specific language impairment. *Applied Psycholinguistics*, *20*, 51–117.

van der Lely, H. K. J. (Ed.). (1998). *Language impairment in children. Language Acquisition,* 7(2–4). [Special issue]

van der Lely, H. K. J., and Christian, V. (2000). Lexical word formation in children with grammatical SLI: A grammar-specific versus an input-processing deficit? *Cognition,* 75, 33–63.

van der Lely, H. K. J., and Stollwerck, L. (1996). A grammatical specific language impairment in children: An autosomal dominant inheritance? *Brain and Language,* 52, 484–504.

Zukowski, A. (2001). *Uncovering grammatical competence in children with Williams syndrome.* Ph.D. dissertation, Boston University, Boston.

Otitis Media: Effects on Children's Language

Whether recurrent or persistent otitis media during the first few years of life increases a child's risk for later language and learning difficulties continues to be debated. Otitis media is the most frequent illness of early childhood, after the common cold. Otitis media with effusion (OME) denotes fluid in the middle ear accompanying the otitis media. OME generally causes mild to moderate fluctuating conductive hearing loss that persists until the fluid goes away. It has been proposed that a child who experiences repeated and persistent episodes of OME and associated hearing loss in early childhood will have later language and academic difficulties. Unlike the well-established relationship between moderate or severe permanent hearing loss and language development, a relationship between OME and later impairment in language development is not clear. This entry describes the possible effect of OME on language development in early childhood, research studies examining the OME–language learning linkage, and the implications of this literature for clinical practice. For information about the relationship of OME to children's speech development, see EARLY RECURRENT OTITIS MEDIA AND SPEECH DEVELOPMENT.

More than 80% of children have had at least one episode of otitis media before 3 years of age, and more than 40% have had three or more episodes (Teele, Klein, and Rosner, 1989). The middle ear transmits sounds from the outer ear to the inner ear, from which information is carried by the acoustic nerve to the brain. In OME, the middle ear is inflamed, the tympanic membrane between the outer and middle ear is thickened, and fluid is present in the middle ear cavity. The fluid can persist for several weeks or even months after the onset of an episode of otitis media. The fluid generally results in a mild to moderate conductive hearing loss. The hearing loss is typically around 26 dB HL, but it can range from no hearing loss to a moderate loss (around 50 dB HL), making it hard to hear conversational speech. It has been suggested that frequent and persistent hearing loss during the first few years of life, a time that is critical for language learning, causes later language difficulties.

The OME-associated hearing loss, which is often variable in degree, recurrent, and at times asymmetrical, has been hypothesized to disrupt the rapid rate of language-processing, causing a loss of language information. This disruption has been hypothesized to affect children's language acquisition in the areas of phonology, vocabulary, syntax, and discourse in several ways. First, the disruption and variability in auditory input due to OME may cause children to encode information incompletely and inaccurately into their phonological working memory. Consequently, children's lexical development may be hindered if they have inaccurate representations of words, which may then result in imprecise lexical recognition or production. Second, OME-associated hearing loss may result in difficulties acquiring inflectional morphology and grammar. Children may not hear or may inaccurately hear certain grammatical morphemes that are of low phonetic substance, such as inflections of short duration and low intensity (e.g., third person /s/, past tense /"ed"/) and unstressed function words ("is," "the"). Third, children's use of language may also be affected because they may miss subtle nuances of language (e.g., intonation marks, questions), which interferes with their ability to follow conversations. Children with prolonged or frequent OME may also learn to tune out, particularly in noisy situations, resulting in attention difficulties for auditory-based information. Difficulty maintaining sustained attention could compromise children's ability to sustain discourse (i.e., to follow and elaborate on the topic of the conversation) and to organize and produce coherent narratives (both requiring auditory memory and recall).

Recent models of a potential linkage between a history of OME and subsequent impaired language development hypothesize that not only factors inherent in the child but also the child's environment and the interaction between the child and the environment can affect this relationship (Roberts and Wallace, 1997; Vernon-Feagans, Emanual, and Blood, 1997; Roberts et al., 1998; Vernon-Feagans, 1999). These additional factors include both risk factors (e.g., the child has poor phonemic awareness skills, the mother has less than a high school education, the child care environment is noisy) and protective factors (e.g., the child has an excellent vocabulary, a literacy-rich home environment, and a responsive child care environment). Thus, it is proposed that the potential impact of OME on children's language development depends on the number and timing of OME episodes and associated hearing loss; the child's cognitive, linguistic, and perceptual abilities; the responsiveness and supportiveness of the child's environment; and interactions among these variables.

Over the past three decades, more than 90 original studies have examined whether children who had frequent episodes of OME in early childhood score lower on measures of language than children without such a history. Earlier studies examining an association between OME and later language were retrospective in design (the children's history of OME was documented by parents reporting the frequency with which children had OME or by a review of medical records collected by different medical providers) and were more likely to contain measurement errors. More recent studies of the OME–language linkage were prospective, with children's OME histories documented longitudinally from early infancy and repeated at specific sampling intervals. Prospective studies are more likely to have greater objectivity and accuracy over time, avoiding many of the methodological limitations of previous studies.

Several prospective studies have found a relationship between a history of otitis media in early childhood and later language skills during the preschool and early elementary school years. More specifically, in comparison with children who infrequently experienced otitis media, infants and preschoolers with a history of OME scored lower on standardized assessments of receptive and expressive language (Teele et al., 1984; Wallace et al., 1988; Friel-Patti and Finitzo-Hieber, 1990) and in specific language areas, including syntax (Teele et al., 1990), vocabulary (Teele et al., 1984), and narratives (Feagans et al., 1987). However, many studies failed to find associations between an early history of OME and later measures of overall receptive or expressive language, vocabulary, or syntax (Teele et al., 1990; Peters et al., 1994; Paradise et al., 2000; Roberts et al., 2000).

Several ongoing prospective studies are providing new and important information on whether a history of OME in early childhood causes later language difficulties. Three recent experimental studies (Maw et al., 1999; Rovers et al., 2000; Paradise et al., 2001) examined whether prompt insertion of tympanostomy tubes (to drain the fluid for children with frequent or persistent OME) improved children's language development, compared with delaying the insertion of tympanostomy tubes. Paradise and colleagues (2001) randomized 429 children (at mean age of 15 months) who had persistent or frequent OME to have tympanostomy tubes inserted either promptly or 6–9 months later and reported no language differences between the two treatment groups at age 3 years of age. Rovers and colleagues (2000) also did not find that prompt insertion of tympanostomy tubes improved children's language development. Maw and colleagues (1999) did find effects on language development 9 months after treatment; however, 18 months after treatment there were no longer differences between the groups.

Other prospective studies considered the impact of multiple factors such as the educational level of the mother and the extent of hearing loss a child experienced during early childhood on children's language development. The Pittsburgh group (Feldman et al., 1999; Paradise et al., 2000) reported weak but significant correlations between OME in the first 3 years of life and language development (accounting for 1%–3% of the variance in language skills), after controlling for many family background variables. Roberts and colleagues (1995, 1998, 2000) prospectively studied the relationship of both children's OME and hearing history to language development. They did not find a direct relationship between OME or hearing history and children's language

skills between 1 and 5 years of age (Roberts et al., 1995, 1998, 2000). They did find that the caregiving environment (responsiveness of the child's home and child care environments) mediated the relationship between children's history of OME and associated hearing loss and later communication development at 1 and 2 years of age (Roberts et al., 1995, 1998, 2000, 2002). That is, children with more OME and associated hearing loss tended to live in less responsive caregiving environments, and these environments were linked to lower performance on measures of receptive and expressive language skills. More recently, Roberts and colleagues reported that children with greater incidence of OME scored lower in expressive language upon entering school but caught up with their peers in expressive language by second grade. However, a child's home environment was much more strongly related to early expressive language skills than was OME. These and other ongoing prospective studies highlight the importance of examining the multiple factors that affect children's language development.

The potential impact of frequent and persistent hearing loss due to OME on later language skills may be particularly important to examine in children from special populations who are already at risk for language and learning difficulties. Children who have Down syndrome, fragile X syndrome, Turner's syndrome, Williams's syndrome, cleft palate, and other craniofacial differences often experience frequent and persistent OME in early childhood (Zeisel and Roberts, 2003; Casselbrant and Mandel, 1999). This increased risk for OME among special populations may be due to craniofacial structural abnormalities, hypotonia, or immune system deficiencies. A few retrospective studies have reported that a history of OME further delays the language development of children from special populations (Whiteman, Simpson, and Compton, 1986; Lonigan et al., 1992).

The question of whether recurrent OME affects the later acquisition of language is still unresolved, in part because of the conflicting findings of studies that have examined this issue. There is increasing support from prospective studies that for typically developing children, OME may not be a substantial risk factor for later language development. Although a few studies report a very mild association between OME and later impairment of receptive and expressive language skills during infancy and the preschool years, the effect is generally very small, accounting for only about 1%–4% of the variance. Furthermore, it is clear that the caregiving environment at home and in child care plays a much more important role than OME in children's later language development. Future research should examine if frequent hearing loss due to OME relates to children's language development. The impact of a history of OME and associated hearing loss on the language development of children from special populations should also be further studied. Some typically developing children as well as children from special populations may be at increased risk for later language and learning difficulties due to a history of OME and associated hearing loss. Until further research can resolve whether such a relationship between a chronic history of OME and later language skills exists and can determine what aspects of language are affected, hearing status and language skills need to be considered in the management of young children with histories of OME.

Several strategies have been recommended for young children who are experiencing chronic OME (Roberts and Medley, 1995; Roberts and Wallace, 1997; Vernon-Feagans, 1999; Roberts and Zeisel, 2000). First, a child's hearing, speech, and language should be tested after 3 months of bilateral OME, or after four to six episodes of otitis media in a 6-month period, or when families or caregivers are concerned about a child's development. Second, families and other caregivers (e.g., child care providers) of young children with recurrent or persistent OME need clear and accurate information in order to make decisions about the child's medical and educational management. Third, children who experience recurrent or persistent OME, similar to all children, will benefit from a highly responsive language- and literacy-enriched environment. Caregivers should respond to communication attempts, provide frequent opportunities for children to participate in conversations, and read often to their children. Fourth, children with chronic OME will benefit from an optimal listening environment in which the speech signal is easy to hear and background noise is kept to a minimum. Fifth, some children with a history of OME may exhibit language and other developmental difficulties, and benefit from early intervention. Finally, the results of ongoing research studies combined with previous studies should help determine whether a history of OME in early childhood places children at risk for later language difficulties, and if so, how to then target intervention strategies.

—*Joanne E. Roberts*

References

Casselbrant, M. L., and Mandel, E. M. (1999). Epidemiology. In R. M. Rosenfeld and C. D. Bluestone (Eds.), *Evidence-based otitis media* (pp. 117–136). St. Louis: B. C. Decker.

Feagans, L., Sanyal, M., Henderson, F., Collier, A., and Applebaum, M. (1987). Relationship of middle ear diseases in early childhood to later narrative and attentions skills. *Journal of Pediatric Psychology*, *12*, 581–594.

Feldman, H. M., Dollaghan, C. A., Campbell, T. F., Colborn, D. K., Kurs-Lasky, M., Jaosky, J. E., et al. (1999). Parent-reported language and communication skills of one and two years of age in relation to otitis media in the first two years of life. *Pediatrics*, *104*, 52.

Friel-Patti, S., and Finitzo-Hieber, T. (1990). Language learning in a prospective study of otitis media with effusion in the first two years of life. *Journal of Speech and Hearing Research*, *33*, 188–194.

Lonigan, C. J., Fischel, J. E., Whitehurst, G. J., Arnold, D. S., and Valdez-Menchaca, M. C. (1992). The role of otitis media in the development of expressive language disorder. *Developmental Psychology*, *28*, 430–440.

Maw, R., Wilks, J., Harvey, I., Peters, T. J., and Golding, J. (1999). Early surgery compared with watchful waiting for glue ear and effect on language development in preschool children: A randomised trial. *Lancet*, *353*, 960–963.

Paradise, J. L., Dollaghan, C. A., Campbell, T. F., Feldman, H. M., Bernard, B. S., Colborn, D. K., et al. (2000). Language, speech sound production, and cognition in three-year-old children in relation to otitis media in their first three years of life. *Pediatrics*, *105*, 1119–1130.

Paradise, J. L., Feldman, H. M., Campbell, T. F., et al. (2001). Effect of early or delayed insertion of tympanostomy tubes on developmental outcomes at the age of three years. *New England Journal of Medicine*, *344*, 1179–1187.

Peters, S. A. F., Grievink, E. H., van Bon, W. H. J., and Schilder, A. G. M. (1994). The effects of early bilateral otitis media with effusion on educational attainment: A prospective cohort study. *Journal of Learning Disabilities*, *27*, 111–121.

Roberts, J. E., Burchinal, M. R., Medley, L. P., Zeisel, S. A., Mundy, M., Roush, J., et al. (1995). Otitis media, hearing sensitivity, and maternal responsiveness in relation to language during infancy. *Journal of Pediatrics*, *126*, 481–489.

Roberts, J. E., Burchinal, M. R., Jackson, S. C., Hooper, S. R., Roush, J., Mundy, M., et al. (2000). Otitis media in early childhood in relation to preschool language and school readiness skills among African American children. *Pediatrics*, *106*, 1–11.

Roberts, J. E., Burchinal, M. R., and Zeisel, S. A. (2002). Otitis media in early childhood in relation to children's school-age language and academic skills. *Pediatrics*, *110*, 1–11.

Roberts, J. E., Burchinal, M. R., Zeisel, S. A., Neebe, E. C., Hooper, S. R., Roush, J., et al. (1998). Otitis media, the caregiving environment, and language and cognitive outcomes at two years. *Pediatrics*, *102*, 346–352.

Roberts, J. E., and Medley, L. (1995). Otitis media and speech-language sequelae in young children: Current issues in management. *American Journal of Speech-Language Pathology*, *4*, 15–24.

Roberts, J. E., and Wallace, I. F. (1997). Language and otitis media. In J. E. Roberts, I. F. Wallace, and F. Henderson (Eds.), *Otitis media in young children: Medical, developmental and educational considerations* (pp. 133–161). Baltimore: Paul H. Brookes.

Roberts, J. E., and Zeisel, S. A. (2000). *Ear infections and language development*. American Speech-Language-Hearing Association and the National Center for Early Development and Learning. Rockville, MD.

Rovers, M. M., Straatman, H. M., Ingels, K., van der Wilt, G., van den Broek, P., and Zielhuis, G. (2000). The effect of ventilation tubes on language development in infants with otitis media with effusion: A randomized trial. *Pediatrics*, *106*, e42.

Teele, D. W., Klein, J. O., Rosner, B. A., and the Greater Boston Otitis Media Study Group. (1984). Otitis media with effusion during the first three years of life and development of speech and language. *Pediatrics*, *74*, 282–287.

Teele, D. W., Klein, J. O., and Rosner, B. A. (1989). Epidemiology of otitis media during the first seven years of life in children in greater Boston. *Journal of Infectious Diseases*, *160*, 83–94.

Teele, D. W., Klein, J. O., Chase, C., Menyuk, P., Rosner, B. A., and the Greater Boston Otitis Media Study Group. (1990). Otitis media in infancy and intellectual ability, school achievement, speech, and language at age 7 years. *Journal of Infectious Diseases*, *162*, 685–694.

Vernon-Feagans, L. (1999). Impact of otitis media on speech, language, cognition, and behavior. In R. M. Rosenfeld and C. D. Bluestone (Eds.), *Evidence-based otitis media* (pp. 353–398). St. Louis: B. C. Decker.

Vernon-Feagans, L., Emanuel, D. C., and Blood, I. (1997). The effect of otitis media on the language and attention skills of daycare attending toddlers. *Developmental Psychology, 30,* 701–708.

Wallace, I. F., Gravel, J. S., McCarton, C. M., Stapelis, D. R., Bernstein, R. S., and Ruben, R. J. (1988). Otitis media, auditory sensitivity, and language outcomes at one year. *Laryngoscope, 98,* 64–70.

Whiteman, B. C., Simpson, G. B., and Compton, W. C. (1986). Relationship of otitis media and language impairment in adolescents with Down syndrome. *Mental Retardation, 24,* 353–356.

Zeisel, S. A., and Roberts, J. E. (2003). Otitis media in young children with disabilities. *Infants and Young Children: An Interdisciplinary Journal of Special Care Practices, 16,* 106–119.

Further Readings

Bluestone, C. D., and Klein, J. O. (2001). *Otitis media in infants and children.* Philadelphia: Saunders.

Casby, M. W. (2001). Otitis media and language development: A meta-analysis. *American Journal of Speech-Language Pathology, 10,* 65–80.

Gravel, J. S., and Wallace, I. F. (1992). Listening and language at 4 years of age: Effects of otitis media. *Journal of Speech and Hearing Research, 35,* 588–595.

Gravel, J. S., and Wallace, I. F. (2000). Effects of otitis media with effusion on hearing in the first three years of life. *Journal of Speech, Language, and Hearing Research, 43,* 631–644.

Kavanagh, J. F. (Ed.). (1986). *Otitis media and child development.* Parkton, MD: York Press.

National Institute of Child Health and Human Development Early Child Care Research Network. (2001). Child care and common communicable illnesses. *Archives of Pediatrics and Adolescent Medicine, 155,* 481–488.

Paradise, J. L., Feldman, H. M., Colborn, K., Campbell, T. F., Dollagahn, C. A., Rockette, H. E., et al. (1999). Parental stress and parent-rated child behavior in relation to otitis media in the first three years of life. *Pediatrics, 104,* 1264–1273.

Rach, G. H., Zielhuis, G. A., van Baarle, P. W., and van den Broek, P. (1991). The effect of treatment with ventilating tubes on language development in preschool children with otitis media with effusion. *Clinical Otolaryngology, 16,* 128–132.

Rach, G. H., Zielhuis, G. A., and van den Broek, P. (1988). The influence of chronic persistent otitis media with effusion on language development of 2- to 4-year-olds. *International Journal of Pediatric Otorhinolaryngology, 15,* 253–261.

Roberts, J. E., Wallace, I. F., and Henderson, F. (Eds.). (1997). *Otitis media in young children: Medical, developmental and educational considerations.* Baltimore: Paul H. Brookes.

Wallace, I. F., Gravel, J. S., Schwartz, R. G., and Ruben, R. J. (1996). Otitis media, communication style of primary caregivers, and language skills of 2 year olds: A preliminary report. *Journal of Developmental Behavioral Pediatrics, 17,* 27–35.

Perseveration

Perseveration, a term introduced by Neisser in 1895, refers to the inappropriate continuation or repetition of an earlier response after a change in task requirements. Although individuals without brain damage may display occasional perseverative behaviors (e.g., Ramage et al., 1999), as Allison (1966) pointed out, when perseveration is pronounced, "it is a reliable, if not a pathognomonic sign of disturbed brain function" (p. 1029). Indeed, perseveration has been described in association with a variety of neurological and psychiatric conditions, including stroke, head injury, dementia, Parkinson's disease, and schizophrenia.

Perseveration is such a notable and fascinating clinical phenomenon that for more than 100 years, various researchers have attempted to more precisely describe its characteristics, label its subtypes, and identify its neuropathological correlates and neuropsychological mechanisms. Good agreement has emerged from these studies as to the characteristics of various forms of perseveration, with rather little agreement as to labels for subtypes. And although most investigators agree that the frontal lobes and their associated white matter pathways play a prominent role in perseveration, other areas of the brain have been implicated. The neuropsychological mechanisms responsible for perseveration also are uncertain and probably vary according to subtypes. Among the mechanisms implicated are persistent memory traces, failure to inhibit prepotent responses, pathological inertia, and failure to disengage attention. For a review of some of this literature, see Hotz and Helm-Estabrooks (1995a).

It is important for professionals working with individuals having neurological conditions to be aware of perseveration and recognize its subtypes, because this behavior can contaminate experimental and clinical test results and reduce communicative effectiveness. Perseveration can occur in any behavioral output modality, including speech, writing, gesturing, drawing, and other forms of construction. Three primary forms of perseveration have been described, with one of these forms having four subtypes. The terms used here are derived from several sources (e.g., Santo-Pietro and Rigrodsky, 1986; Sandson and Albert, 1987; Lundgren et al., 1994; Hotz and Helm-Estabrooks, 1995b).

Stuck-in-set perseveration is the inappropriate maintenance of a category or framework of response after introduction of a new task. For example, as a part of a standardized test, an individual with traumatic brain injury without aphasia was asked to list as many animals as he could in 1 minute. He listed ten animals before he was given the following instructions: "Now I want you to name as many words as you can that start with the letter *m.* [He was shown a lowercase *m.*] Here are the rules. Do not name words that begin with a capital *M.* Do not say the same words with a different ending, like *mop,* then *mopped* or *mopping.* [The written letter *m* was removed.] Okay, you have 1 minute to name as many words you can think of that start with the letter *m*." In response, the man said "monkey," "mouse" in the first few seconds, then "man" after 15 seconds. He produced no further responses for the remaining time. Thus, although he understood the concept of listing *m* words, he could not disengage from the idea of listing animals, and his score for producing words according to a letter/sound category was contaminated by stuck-in-set perseveration.

Continuous perseveration is the inappropriate prolongation or continuation of a behavior without an intervening response or stimulus. For example, a woman with Alzheimer's disease was given the following spoken and written instructions: "Draw a clock. Put in all the numbers. Set the hands to 10 minutes after 11." She wrote numbers 1 through 18 in the circle provided before she ran out of space. She then drew a hand to the number 10, but continued to draw hands to each number. Thus, either she was unable to disengage from the idea of drawing clock hands or she was unable to inhibit that particular graphomotor activity.

Recurrent perseveration is the inappropriate recurrence of a previous response following presentation of a new stimulus or after giving a different intervening response. For example, a man with fluent aphasia was asked to write the days of the week. He wrote, "Monday, Tuesday, Wednesday, Tuesday, Friday, Saturday, Monday, Sunday."

Various subtypes of recurrent perseveration have been described and labeled. A primary distinction can be made between carryover of part of the phonemic structure of a previous word and repetition of an entire word.

An example of *phonemic carryover perseveration*, in which part of the phonemic makeup of a previous word is inappropriately repeated, is "comb" for *comb*, then "klower" for *flower*.

Within the category of *whole-word carryover*, three types of perseveration occur, semantic, lexical, and program-of-action perseveration.

Semantic perseverations are words that are semantically related to the target (e.g., repetition of the naming response *apple* when shown a lemon).

Lexical perseverations are words that have no obvious semantic relation to the target (e.g., repetition of the word *key* when asked to name scissors).

Program-of-action perseverations are repeated words that begin with the same initial sound as a previous response (e.g., repetition of the response *wristwatch* for subsequent objects, such as *wrench*, whose names begin with /r/).

Although, as mentioned earlier, perseveration occurs in association with many neurological and psychiatric conditions, perseverative behavior is especially notable in acquired aphasia. The results of their study of perseverative behaviors in aphasic individuals prompted Albert and Sandson (1986) to suggest that it "may even comprise an integral part of [the] specific language deficits in aphasia" (p. 105). This suggestion is supported by the work of other investigators (e.g., Santo-Pietro and

Rigrodsky, 1982; Emery and Helm-Estabrooks, 1989; Helm-Estabrooks et al., 1998). There is good evidence that perseverative behaviors are unrelated to time post onset of aphasia but are correlated significantly with aphasia severity. Thus, perseveration can be a persistent problem for individuals with aphasia and interfere with all modalities of communicative expression. As such, perseveration is an important treatment target for speech and language clinicians working with aphasic individuals, although few approaches have been described thus far. Exceptions are the program designed by Helm-Estabrooks, Emery, and Albert (1987) to reduce verbal recurrent perseveration, and the strategies described by Bryant, Emery, and Helm-Estabrooks (1994) to manage various forms of perseveration in severe aphasia. See Helm-Estabrooks and Albert (2003) for updated descriptions on these methods.

—*Nancy Helm-Estabrooks*

References

Albert, M. L., and Sandson, J. (1986). Perseveration in aphasia. *Cortex*, 22, 103–115.

Allison, R. S. (1966). Perseveration as a sign of diffuse and focal brain damage. I. *British Medical Journal*, 2, 1027–1032.

Bryant, S. L., Emery, P. A., and Helm-Estabrooks, N. (1994). Management of different forms of perseveration in severe aphasia. *Seminars in Speech and Language*, 15, 71–84.

Emery, P., and Helm-Estabrooks, N. (1989). The role of perseveration in aphasic confrontation naming performance. *Proceedings of Clinical Aphasiology Conference*, 18, 64–83.

Emery, P., and Helm-Estabrooks, N. (1995). Whole word perseverations: Where do they come from? *Brain and Language*, 51, 29–31.

Helm-Estabrooks, N., and Albert, M. L. (2003). *Manual of aphasia and aphasia therapy*. Austin, TX: Pro-Ed.

Helm-Estabrooks, N., Emery, P., and Albert, M. L. (1987). Treatment of aphasic perseveration (T.A.P.) program: A new approach to aphasia therapy. *Archives of Neurology*, 44, 1253–1255.

Helm-Estabrooks, N., Ramage, A., Bayles, K., and Cruz, R. (1998). Perseverative behavior in fluent and non-fluent aphasic adults. *Aphasiology*, 12, 689–698.

Hotz, G., and Helm-Estabrooks, N. (1995a). Perseveration: Part I. A review. *Brain Injury*, 9, 151–159.

Hotz, G., and Helm-Estabrooks, N. (1995b). Perseveration: Part II. A study of perseveration in closed-head injury. *Brain Injury*, 9, 161–172.

Lundgren, K., Helm-Estabrooks, N., Magnusdottir, S., and Emery, P. (1994). Exploring mechanisms underlying "recurrent" perseveration: An aphasic naming study. *Brain and Language*, 47, 370–373.

Neisser, A. (1895). Krankenvorstellung. *Allgemeine Zeitschrifte fur Psychitrie*, 51, 1016–1021.

Ramage, A., Bayles, K., Helm-Estabrooks, N., and Cruz, R. (1998). Frequency of perseveration in normal subjects. *Brain and Language*, 66, 329–340.

Sandson, J., and Albert, M. L. (1984). Varieties of perseveration. *Neuropsychologia*, 22, 715–732.

Santo-Pietro, M. J., and Rigrodsky, S. (1986). Patterns of oral-verbal perseveration in adult aphasics. *Brain and Language*, 29, 1–17.

Further Readings

Bayles, K. A., Tomoeda, C. K., Kaszniak, A. W., Sterns, L. Z., and Eagans, K. K. (1985). Verbal perseveration of dementia patients. *Brain and Language, 25,* 102–116.

Brown, J. W., and Chobor, K. L. (1989). Frontal lobes and the problem of perseveration. *Journal of Neurolinguistics, 4,* 65–85.

Helm-Estabrooks, N., Bayles, K., and Bryant, S. (1994). Four forms of perseveration in dementia and aphasia patients and normal elders. *Brain and Language, 47,* 457–460.

Freedman, T., and Gathercole, C. E. (1966). Perseveration: The clinical symptoms in chronic schizophrenia and organic dementia. *British Journal of Psychiatry, 112,* 27–32.

Fuld, P. A., Katzman, R., Davis, P., and Terry, R. D. (1982). Intrusions as a sign of Alzheimer's dementia: Chemical and pathological verification. *Annals of Neurology, 11,* 155–159.

Hudson, J. (1968). Perseveration. *Brain, 91,* 143–582.

Luria, A. R. (1965). Two kinds of motor perseveration in massive injury of the frontal lobes. *Brain, 88,* 1–9.

Shindler, A. G., Caplan, L. R., and Hier, D. B. (1984). Intrusions and perseverations. *Brain and Language, 23,* 148–158.

Yamadori, A. (1981). Verbal perseverations in aphasia. *Neuropsychologia, 19,* 591–594.

Phonological Analysis of Language Disorders in Aphasia

Various approaches have been utilized in the study of phonological disorders in aphasia, but each usually shares certain assumptions of the others. This overview presents these different orientations with the recognition that there is a good deal of overlap in each.

Neurolinguistic

Renee Beland (and several colleagues) have used "underspecification theory" to capture the types of phonological errors in fluent aphasics and the constraints on those errors (Beland, 1990; Beland, Caplan, and Nespoulous, 1990). The phonological model here has three levels: the minimally specified level, a lexical level, and a surface level. Feature markedness, phonotactic patterns, and syllable constituent slots (onset, rime, nucleus, coda) are then used to describe the nature and location of phonemic paraphasias and the constraints on those paraphasias.

As a student of Roman Jakobson, Sheila Blumstein (1973) is the intermediary between Prague School phonological studies of aphasic errors (e.g., Jakobson, 1968) and a host of neurolinguistic studies of paraphasia published since the early 1970s. Her contributions to the study of the neuropsychology and neurobiology of human language sound structure are herculean (see Blumstein, 1995, 1998, for discussion of much of her work). Her initial study of the typology of phonemic paraphasia set the stage for numerous ensuing studies.

Susan Kohn (1989, 1993) has provided a wealth of information on phonological breakdown in fluent aphasics, usually patients with conduction aphasia and Wernicke's aphasia. Her studies have focused on the difficulties these patients have with constructing phonemic strings once the full-form lexical representations have been accessed in their stored form. Through the mechanisms of models (Shattuck-Hufnagel, 1979; Garrett, 1984), Kohn has successfully characterized many paraphasic types, located the production process where the error occurs, and specified which type of error is diagnostic of distinct aphasic syndromes. She has incorporated syllable structure constraints, phonotactic patterns, and the principle of sonority. Furthermore, Kohn, Smith, and Alexander (1996) have charted the recovery patterns of Wernicke's patients who in the acute stages produced neologistic jargon. They observed that in certain of these patients the aphasia resolved to a chronic stage in which the patients were clearly getting closer to underlying lexical representations and producing less severe phonemic paraphasia, with lower number of random segments in those errors. In another set of patients the aphasia resolved to a chronic stage in which the patients maintained severe lexical access disruptions, producing less neology but more lexical blocks, circumlocutions, and other errors indicative of lingering anomia.

David Caplan (1987) and colleagues (Caplan and Waters, 1992) have published widely on phonological breakdown in aphasia. He, as well as Kohn, has analyzed the phonemic string construction difficulties of the syndrome of "reproduction" conduction aphasia. He localizes this disruption at the point where final sound production is called for from either a semantic input, an auditory/lexical input, or a written input. That is, the patient will produce phonemic errors in object naming, in repetition, or in reading aloud. Any one patient may produce paraphasias with all or certain ones of these inputs. Cognitive neuropsychological dissociations are numerous here.

Buckingham and Kertesz (1976) analyzed the neologistic jargon of several patients with fluent aphasia. Each patient revealed a good deal of phonemic errors, but many errors rendered underlying targets opaque. Other forms, however, were opaque and otherwise abstruse where there was no clear transparency of any certain underlying lexical target. All patients had severe anomia, which led to the suggestion that there could be two separate productive mechanisms or processes that might give rise to the production of these nonrecognizable word-form errors, but in that study the question was left unexplored. The issue was broached again in Buckingham (1977), but not until Butterworth (1979) was a specific idea put forth, that of a "random generator." Subsequently, Buckingham (1990a) attempted to mollify the critics of the random generator by showing that the idea was in a sense a metaphor for the use and appreciation of general phonological knowledge, which for all speakers underlies the ability to recognize "possible words" in a language and to produce "nonce" forms when necessary. The issue of a dual route for the neologism has reappeared recently. Gagnon and

Schwartz (1996) found no bimodal distribution in their corpus of phonemic paraphasias and neologisms, and thus argued for a single route for their productions. In contradistinction, Kohn, Smith, and Alexander (1996) observed patients who demonstrated both routes, one for phonemic paraphasia and another that involved some sort of a "backup mechanism for 'reconstructing' a phonological representation when either partial or no stored phonological information about a word is made available to the production system" (p. 132), which reduces to some kind of generating device.

In Buckingham (1990b), the principle of sonority (see Ohala, 1992, for some criticism of this principle) was invoked to provide an account of the structural constraints on phonemic paraphasia, and shortly thereafter Christman (1994) extended the utilization of sonority to capture the pattern constraints on a large corpus of neologisms, where she statistically demonstrated that neologisms abided by both sonority and phonotactic dictates. A major portion of her contribution was to show how sonority could go beyond mere phonotactics to characterize neologistic word production.

Slips, Paraphasia, and the Continuity Thesis

Slips-of-the-tongue have always played a role in the modeling, characterization, analysis, and explanation of paraphasia. There is a direct line from Hughlings-Jackson in the second half of the nineteenth century to modern psycholinguistic studies of the "lapsus linguae," all of which have assumed at least some degree of continuity between the functional errors in normality and the paraphasias in pathology (Buckingham, 1999).

Phonological Breakdown and Connectionist Modeling

Wheeler and Touretzky (1997) have combined a model of segmental "licensing" from phonological autosegmental theory with a connectionist simulation of phonological disruptions in fluent aphasia with no psycholinguistic mechanisms at all. In an impressive and surprising fashion, they were able to simulate most error types and conditions described in such work as Buckingham (1986).

Dell et al. (1997) have published one of the most in-depth investigations of a connectionist system (of the interactive activation type) that simulated normal naming and aphasic naming—and *only* naming. The three-level (semantic, lexical, segmental) system had upward and downward feedforward and feedback connections. The system was set up so that connection weight values and decay rate values could be varied globally throughout the system as a whole. Phonological errors (and other errors) that indicated level interaction were produced by lesioning only the decay rates: phonemic paraphasias that did not render targets opaque and formal verbal substitutions where error and target shared phonological features. Lesioning only connection weights, however, simulated phonological errors (and other errors) that did not indicate interaction between levels:

neologisms, where target words were not recognizable. Recovery patterns were then analyzed and simulated, where it appeared to the authors that although there was improvement in productions, the productions themselves remained either of the decay lesion type or of the connection lesion type. The only problem with phonological breakdown would be that those who had produced neologisms early on may resolve to a less severe phonemic paraphasia, where targets could be increasingly gleaned, thereby indicating level interaction. That scenario, of course, would mean that a connection weight lesion pattern would resolve to a decay rate lesion pattern. Most connectionist-oriented accounts do not provide for dual routes for neologisms (e.g., Gagnon and Schwartz, 1996; Gagnon et al., 1997; Goldman, Schwartz, and Wilshire, 2001; Nadeau, 2001), locating their production exclusively between the lexeme and the phoneme strata. For instance, the model of Hillis et al. (1999, p. 1820) accounts for phonemic paraphasias *and* neologisms with different degrees of connectionist weakenings between these two strata, where only a "few" nontarget subword units would be activated for phonemic paraphasias but "many" nontarget subword units would be activated for neologisms. It is not yet clear just how connectionist models will continue to eschew dual routes for neologisms.

Apraxia of Speech Meets Phonemic Paraphasia: Phonology or Phonetics?

Square, Roy, and Martin (1997) have recently discussed posterior lesion apraxia of speech patients, which accords with ideas suggested in Buckingham and Yule (1987). In addition, many presumed phonemic paraphasias in Broca's aphasia (e.g., Keller, 1978) could very plausibly stem from apraxic asynchronies (Buckingham and Yule, 1987). Speech perception disturbances have been observed in Broca's aphasics, and Wernicke's aphasics often present with articulatory abnormalities (Price, Indefrey, and van Turennout, 1999, p. 212). The perceptual function of the inferior frontal gyrus has also been observed by Hsieh et al. (2001). Galaburda has uncovered motor regions in layer III of the left temporal cortex in the plenum region (Galaburda, 1982), and Amaducci et al. (1981) have found asymmetrical concentrations of choline-acetyltransferase (ChAT) in this region from neurochemical assays at autopsy in human subjects. Recent reviews (e.g., Blumstein, 1995) have emphasized the highly distributed nature of the sound system throughout the left perisylvian cortex. Little wonder there is such a degree of indeterminacy with aphasic sound system disruptions in stroke. From purely linguistic reasoning, Ohala (1990) has challenged the claim that phonetics and phonology are separate systems; rather, they are totally integrated. Vocal tract embodiment is tightly linked to most so-called phonological properties (e.g., syllable constituency and phonotactics, sonority, feature markedness, coarticulatory processes), so that whatever element may be "phonologized" will remain forever linked to vocal tract dynamics (see

Christman, 1992; MacNeilage, 1998). It would seem that we are poised for major reevaluations in our understanding of how the human sound system breaks down in aphasia.

—Hugh W. Buckingham

References

Amaducci, L., Sorbi, S., Albanese, A., and Gianotti, G. (1981). Choline-acetyltransferase (ChAT) activity differs in right and left human temporal lobes. *Neurology, 31,* 799–805.

Beland, R. (1990). Vowel epenthesis in aphasia. In J.-L. Nespoulous and P. Villiard (Eds.), *Morphology, Phonology and Aphasia* (pp. 235–252). New York: Springer-Verlag.

Beland, R., Caplan, D., and Nespoulous, J.-L. (1990). The role of abstract phonological representations in word production: Evidence from phonemic paraphasias. *Journal of Neurolinguistics, 5,* 125–164.

Blumstein, S. (1973). *A phonological investigation of aphasic speech.* The Hague: Mouton.

Blumstein, S. (1995). The neurobiology of the sound structure of language. In M. S. Gazzaniga (Ed.), *The cognitive neurosciences* (pp. 915–929). Cambridge, MA: The MIT Press.

Blumstein, S. (1998). Phonological aspects of aphasia. In M. Sarno (Ed.), *Acquired aphasia* (pp. 157–185). San Diego, CA: Academic Press.

Buckingham, H. (1977). The conduction theory and neologistic jargon. *Language and Speech, 20,* 174–184.

Buckingham, H. (1986). The scan-copier mechanism and the positional level of language production: Evidence from aphasia. *Cognitive Science, 10,* 195–217.

Buckingham, H. (1990a). Abstruse neologisms, retrieval deficits and the random generator. *Journal of Neurolinguistics, 5,* 215–235.

Buckingham, H. (1990b). Principle of sonority, doublet creation, and the checkoff monitor. In J.-L. Nespoulous and P. Villiard (Eds.), *Morphology, phonology and aphasia* (pp. 193–205). New York: Springer-Verlag.

Buckingham, H. (1999). Freud's continuity thesis. *Brain and Language, 69,* 76–92.

Buckingham, H., and Kertesz, A. (1976). *Neologistic jargon aphasia.* Amsterdam: Swets and Zeitlinger.

Buckingham, H., and Yule, G. (1987). Phonemic false evaluation: Theoretical and clinical aspects. *Clinical Linguistics and Phonetics, 1,* 113–125.

Butterworth, B. (1979). Hesitation and the production of verbal paraphasias and neologisms in jargon aphasia. *Brain and Language, 18,* 133–161.

Caplan, D. (1987). *Neurolinguistics and linguistic aphasiology.* Cambridge, U.K.: Cambridge University Press.

Caplan, D., and Waters, G. (1992). Issues arising regarding the nature and consequences of reproduction conduction aphasia. In S. Kohn (Ed.), *Conduction aphasia* (pp. 117–149). Hillsdale, NJ: Erlbaum.

Christman, S. (1992). Abstruse neologism formation: Parallel processing revisited. *Clinical Linguistics and Phonetics, 6,* 65–76.

Christman, S. (1994). Target-related neologism formation in jargonaphasia. *Brain and Language, 46,* 109–128.

Dell, G., Schwartz, M., Martin, N., Saffran, E., and Gagnon, D. (1997). Lexical access in aphasic and nonaphasic speakers. *Psychological Review, 104,* 808–838.

Gagnon, D., and Schwartz, M. (1996). The origins of neologisms in picture naming by fluent aphasics. *Brain and Cognition, 32,* 118–120.

Galaburda, A. (1982). Histology, architectonics, and asymmetry of language areas. In M. Arbib, D. Caplan, and J. Marshall (Eds.), *Neural models of language processes* (pp. 435–445). New York: Academic Press.

Garrett, M. (1984). The organization of processing structure for language production: Applications to aphasic speech. In D. Caplan, A. Lecours, and A. Smith (Eds.), *Biological perspectives on language* (pp. 172–193). Cambridge, MA: MIT Press.

Goldmann, R. E., Schwartz, M. F., and Wilshire, C. E. (2001). The influence of phonological context on the sound errors of a speaker with Wernicke's aphasia. *Brain and Language, 78,* 279–307.

Hillis, A., Boatman, D., Hart, J., and Gordon, B. (1999). Making sense out of jargon: A neurolinguistic and computational account of jargon aphasia. *Neurology, 53,* 1813–1824.

Hsieh, L., Gandour, J., Wong, D., and Hutchins, G. (2001). Functional heterogeneity of inferior frontal gyrus is shaped by linguistic experience. *Brain and Language, 76,* 227–252.

Jakobson, R. (1968). *Child language, aphasia, and phonological universals* (A. R. Keiler, Trans.). The Hague: Mouton.

Keller, E. (1978). Parameters for vowel substitutions in Broca's aphasia. *Brain and Language, 5,* 265–285.

Kohn, S. (1989). The nature of the phonemic string deficit in conduction aphasia. *Aphasiology, 3,* 209–239.

Kohn, S. (1993). Segmental disorders in aphasia. In G. Blanken, J. Dittmann, H. Grimm, J. Marshall, and C.-W. Wallesch (Eds.), *Linguistic disorders and pathologies: An international handbook* (pp. 197–209). Berlin: Walter de Gruyter.

Kohn, S., Smith, K., and Alexander, M. (1996). Differential recovery from impairment to the phonological lexicon. *Brain and Language, 52,* 129–149.

MacNeilage, P. (1998). The frame/content theory of evolution of speech production. *Behavioral and Brain Sciences, 21,* 499–546.

Nadeau, S. E. (2001). Phonology: A review and proposals from a connectionist perspective. *Brain and Language, 79,* 511–579.

Ohala, J. (1990). There is no interface between phonology and phonetics: A personal view. *Journal of Phonetics, 18,* 153–171.

Ohala, J. (1992). Alternatives to the sonority hierarchy for explaining segmental sequential constraints. In M. Ziolkowski, M. Noske, and K. Deaton (Eds.), *Papers from the 26th Regional Meeting of the Chicago Linguistic Society. Vol. 2. The parasession on the syllable in phonetics and phonology* (pp. 319–338). Chicago: Chicago Linguistic Society.

Price, C., Indefrey, P., and van Turennout, M. (1999). The neural architecture underlying the processing of written and spoken word forms. In C. Brown and P. Hagoort (Eds.), *The neurocognition of language* (pp. 211–240). Oxford: Oxford University Press.

Shattuck-Hufnagel, S. (1979). Speech errors as evidence for a serial-ordering mechanism in sentence production. In W. Cooper and E. Walker (Eds.), *Sentence processing: Psycholinguistic studies presented to Merrill Garrett* (pp. 295–342). Hillsdale, NJ: Erlbaum.

Square, P., Roy, E., and Martin, R. (1997). Apraxia of speech: Another form of praxis disruption. In L. Rothi and K. Heilman (Eds.), *Apraxia: The neuropsychology of action* (pp. 173–206). East Sussex, U.K.: Psychology Press.

Wheeler, D., and Touretzky, D. (1997). A parallel licensing model of normal slips and phonemic paraphasias. *Brain and Language, 59,* 147–201.

Further Readings

Baum, S., and Slatkovsky, K. (1993). Phonemic false evaluation? Preliminary data from a conduction aphasia patient. *Clinical Linguistics and Phonetics, 7*, 207–218.

Beland, R., and Favreau, Y. (1991). On the special status of coronals in aphasia. In C. Paradis and J.-F. Prunet (Eds.), *Phonetics and phonology. Vol. 2. The special status of coronals* (pp. 201–221). San Diego, CA: Academic Press.

Blumstein, S. (1978). Segment structure and the syllable. In A. Bell and J. Hooper (Eds.), *Syllables and segments* (pp. 189–200). Amsterdam: North Holland.

Blumstein, S. (1990). Phonological deficits in aphasia. In A. Caramazza (Ed.), *Cognitive neuropsychology and neurolinguistics: Advances in models of cognitive function and impairment* (pp. 33–53). Hillsdale, NJ: Erlbaum.

Buckingham, H. (1980). On correlating aphasic errors with slips-of-the-tongue. *Applied Psycholinguistics, 1*, 199–220.

Buckingham, H. (1981). Where do neologisms come from? In J. Brown (Ed.), *Jargonaphasia* (pp. 39–62). New York: Academic Press.

Buckingham, H. (1987). Phonemic paraphasias and psycholinguistic production models for neologistic jargon. *Aphasiology, 1*, 381–400.

Buckingham, H. (1992). The mechanisms of phonemic paraphasia. *Clinical Linguistics and Phonetics, 6*, 41–63.

Buckingham, H. (1998). Explanations for the concept of apraxia of speech. In M. Sarno (Ed.), *Acquired aphasia* (pp. 269–307). San Diego, CA: Academic Press.

Butterworth, B. (1992). Disorders in phonological encoding. *Cognition, 42*, 261–286.

Caplan, D., and Waters, G. (1995). On the nature of the phonological output planning processes involved in verbal rehearsal: Evidence from aphasia. *Brain and Language, 48*, 191–220.

Caramazza, A. (2000). Aspects of lexical access: Evidence from aphasia. In Y. Grodzinsky, L. Shapiro, and D. Swinney (Eds.), *Language and the brain: Representation and processing* (pp. 203–228). San Diego: Academic Press.

Cutler, A. (Ed.). (1981). Slips-of-the-tongue and language production. *Linguistics, 19*, 561–847. [Special issue]

Demonet, J. F., Fiez, J. A., Paulesu, E., Petersen, S. E., and Zatorre, R. J. (1996). REPLY: PET studies of phonological processing: A critical reply to Peoppel. *Brain and Language, 55*, 352–379.

Ellis, A., Miller, D., and Sin, G. (1983). Wernicke's aphasia and normal language processing: A case study in cognitive neuropsychology. *Cognition, 15*, 111–144.

Gagnon, D., Schwartz, M., Martin, N., Dell, G., and Saffran, E. (1997). The origins of formal paraphasias in aphasics' picture naming. *Brain and Language, 59*, 450–472.

Garrett, M. (1982). Production of speech: Observations from normal and pathological language use. In A. Ellis (Ed.), *Normality and pathology in cognitive functions* (pp. 19–76). London: Academic Press.

Kohn, S. (1984). The nature of the phonological disorder in conduction aphasia. *Brain and Language, 23*, 97–115.

Kohn, S. (1988). Phonological production deficits in aphasia. In H. Whitaker (Ed.), *Phonological processes and brain mechanisms* (pp. 93–117). New York: Springer-Verlag.

Kohn, S., and Smith, K. (1994). Distinctions between two phonological output disorders. *Applied Psycholinguistics, 15*, 75–95.

Kohn, S., Melvold, J., and Shipper, V. (1998). The preservation of sonority in the context of impaired lexical-phonological output. *Aphasiology, 12*, 375–398.

Lecours, A. (1982). On neologisms. In J. Mehler, E. Walker, and M. Garrett (Eds.), *Perspectives on mental representation: Experimental and theoretical studies of cognitive processes and capacities* (pp. 217–247). Hillsdale, NJ: Erlbaum.

Lecours, A., and Lhermitte, F. (1969). Phonemic paraphasias: Linguistic structures and tentative hypotheses. *Cortex, 5*, 193–228.

Lecours, A., and Rouillon, F. (1976). Neurolinguistic analysis of jargonaphasia and jargonagraphia. In H. Whitaker and H. A. Whitaker (Eds.), *Studies in neurolinguistics. Vol. 2* (pp. 95–144). New York: Academic Press.

Martin, N., Dell, G., Saffran, E., and Schwartz, M. (1994). Origins of paraphasias in deep dysphasia: Testing the consequences of a decay impairment to an interactive activation model of lexical retrieval. *Brain and Language, 47*, 609–660.

Nickels, L. (1997). *Spoken word production and its breakdown in aphasia.* East Sussex, U.K.: Psychology Press.

Nickels, L., and Howard, D. (2000). When words won't come: Relating impairments and models of spoken word production. In L. Wheeldon (Ed.), *Aspects of language production* (pp. 115–142). East Sussex, U.K.: Psychology Press.

Poeppel, D. (1996). A critical review of PET studies of phonological processing. *Brain and Language, 55*, 317–351.

Poeppel, D. (1996). Some remaining questions about studying phonological processing with PET: Response to Demonet, Fiez, Paulesu, Petersen, and Zatorre (1996). *Brain and Language, 55*, 380–385.

Schwartz, M., Saffran, E., Block, D., and Dell, G. (1994). Disordered speech production in aphasic and normal speakers. *Brain and Language, 47*, 52–88.

Phonology and Adult Aphasia

The sound structure of language is the primary medium for language communication. As a result, deficits affecting phonology, defined as the sound structure of language, may have a critical impact on language communication in general, and specifically on the processes involved in both speaking and understanding.

Deficits in Speech Production

A number of stages of processing underlie speech production. The speaker must select a word candidate from the lexicon and access its phonological form. Once selected, the sound structure of the word or utterance must be planned—the phonological representation is encoded in terms of the phonological properties of the sound segments, their order and context, and the prosodic structure of the word as a whole. The next stage of processing is articulatory implementation, in which the more abstract phonological representation is converted into a set of motor commands or motor programs for the phonetic realization of the utterance.

There is some evidence to suggest that these stages of production may be dissociated in the aphasias (Nadeau, 2001). However, the patterns suggest that the dissociations are not complete, and hence the production system appears to be neurally distributed in the left perisylvian regions of the left hemisphere (Blumstein, 2000). In particular, patients with Broca's aphasia and other patients with anterior lesions appear to have predominantly articulatory implementation deficits and to a lesser extent phonological selection and planning impairments. In contrast, those with Wernicke's and conduction aphasia and patients with posterior lesions appear to have predominantly lexical selection and phonological planning deficits and to a minor degree articulatory implementation impairments.

The clearest evidence for a dissociation between the production stage of articulation implementation and the stages of phonological selection and planning comes from investigations of the acoustic patterns of speech productions. These studies show that persons with anterior aphasia, including those with Broca's aphasia, have a deficit in the articulatory implementation of speech. Articulatory timing and laryngeal control appear to be particularly affected. The timing disorder emerges in the production of those speech sounds requiring the coordination of two independent articulators, such as the production of voicing in stop consonants, as measured by voice-onset time (Blumstein et al., 1980), and the complex timing relation between syllables (Kent and McNeil, 1987; Gandour et al., 1993). Deficits in laryngeal control are evident in the production of sound segments as well as in the production of prosody. Individuals with these deficits show lower and more variable amplitudes of glottal excitation during the production of voicing in fricative consonants (Code and Ball, 1982) as well as changes in the spectral characteristics associated with the production of stop consonants (Shinn and Blumstein, 1983). Prosodic disturbances are characterized by a restricted fundamental frequency range (Danly and Shapiro, 1982). Additionally, the production of tone in languages such as Thai and Chinese is affected, although the global properties of tone, such as whether the tone is rising or falling, are maintained (Gandour et al., 1992).

Individuals with posterior aphasia, including those with Wernicke's and conduction aphasia, also appear to have a subtle articulatory implementation deficit that is different from that of individuals with anterior aphasia. Characteristics of this deficit include increased variability in a number of phonetic parameters, including vowel formant frequencies and vowel duration, and abnormal temporal patterns between syllables (Baum et al., 1990; Vijayan and Gandour, 1995).

Deficits in selection and planning emerge across a wide spectrum of aphasia, including left hemisphere anterior (Broca's) and posterior (conduction and Wernicke's) aphasia. Evidence in support of this is provided by similar patterns of phonological errors produced by these patients in spontaneous speech (Blumstein, 1973; Holloman and Drummond, 1991). Error types include phoneme substitution errors (e.g., "teams" → [kimz]), simplification errors (e.g., "brown" → [bawn]), addition errors (e.g., "bet" → [blɛt]), and environment errors (e.g., "degree" → [gədri] or "moon" → [mum]). These utterances deviate phonologically from the target word but are implemented correctly by the articulatory sys-

tem, reflecting an inability to correctly encode or activate the correct phonemic (i.e., phonetic feature) representation of the word. Evidence that the phonological representations are intact comes from the variability with which errors occur. An affected individual may make one or a series of phonological errors on a target word and also produce it correctly (Butterworth, 1992).

Despite these similarities, differences have emerged in the patterns of production in naming and repetition tasks, suggesting a difference in the locus of the underlying impairment. Persons with conduction aphasia produce many more phonological errors than persons with Wernicke's aphasia, and the patterns of production in individuals with conduction aphasia more nearly approximate the phonological representation of the target word than those of persons with Wernicke's aphasia. These results suggest that the basis of the deficit in Wernicke's aphasia more likely resides in the processes involved in lexical selection, whereas the basis of the deficit in conduction aphasia more likely lies in the processes involved in phonological planning (Kohn, 1993).

In sum, the evidence suggests that the neural system underlying speech production is a distributed neural network with functional subcomponents. Wernicke's area and the association cortices around it are implicated in the processes of lexical selection. The supramarginal gyrus and the white matter deep to it appear to be involved in phonological selection and planning. The motor areas including the frontal operculum, the premotor and motor regions posterior and superior to the frontal operculum, and the white matter below, including the basal ganglia and insula, appear to be involved in the articulatory implementation of speech (Dronkers, 1997; Damasio, 1998). Nonetheless, the evidence suggests that there is not a 1:1 relationship between these neurological landmarks and the stages of output, since all stages of speech production appear to be affected in all of the patients, although to varying degrees.

Deficits in Speech Perception

A number of stages of processing have been identified in auditory word reception. These stages include the extraction of generalized auditory patterns from the acoustic waveform, the conversion of this spectral representation to a more abstract phonetic feature/phonological representation, and the mapping of this phonological representation onto lexical form (i.e., a word in the lexicon) (Nadeau, 2001). Deficits at any one or all of these levels may potentially contribute to auditory comprehension impairments.

There is little evidence to suggest that aphasic patients have deficits at the stage of extracting generalized auditory patterns from the acoustic waveform (Polster and Rose, 1998). However, they show impairments in processing a number of auditory/phonetic parameters of speech, including temporal cues such as voice-onset time, a cue to the phonetic dimension of voicing, and spectral cues such as formant transitions, cues to the phonetic dimension of place of articulation (Blumstein et al.,

1984; Shewan, Leeper, and Booth, 1984). Increasing the duration of the formant transitions to allow more time to process the rapid spectral changes associated with the perception of place of articulation does not improve the performance of aphasic patients (Riedel and Studdert-Kennedy, 1985). In general, patients have great difficulty performing these tasks, particularly when the stimuli are synthetic speech stimuli as compared to natural speech stimuli and when the task requires labeling or naming the stimuli as compared to discriminating them. Nonetheless, the patterns of performance suggest that individuals with aphasia can map the spectral representations on to the phonetic features of language. Those who can perform the labeling and discrimination tasks typically show categorical perception similar to normal subjects. They perceive the stimuli as belonging to discrete phonetic categories, and they show peaks in discrimination at the phonetic boundaries between the phonetic categories. All of the deficits described above emerge across aphasic syndromes and do not correlate with the severity of auditory comprehension impairment (Basso, Casati, and Vignolo, 1977).

In contrast to the difficulty in perceiving acoustic dimensions associated with voicing and place of articulation, persons with aphasia are generally able to perceive those acoustic dimensions contributing to the perception of speech prosody, that is, intonation and stress. Even individuals with severe auditory comprehension impairments are able to use intonation cues to recognize whether an utterance is a command, a yes-no question, an information question, or a statement (Green and Boller, 1974). Nonetheless, some impairments have emerged in the perception of more local parameters of prosody, including word stress and tone (Gandour and Dardaranananda, 1983; Baum, 1998). However, no differences have emerged in the performance of persons with anterior and posterior aphasia.

Similar to studies of the acoustic-phonetic properties of speech, nearly all persons with aphasia show perceptual deficits in phonological processing (Blumstein, Baker, and Goodglass, 1977; Jauhiainen and Nuutila, 1977; Csepe et al., 2001). These deficits emerge in tasks requiring subjects to discriminate words or nonsense syllables contrasting by one or more phonetic features (e.g., "dime"—"time" or "da"—"ta") or to point to an auditorily presented target stimulus from a visual array of objects or written nonsense syllables that are phonologically similar. Individuals with aphasia have more difficulty on labeling and pointing tasks than on discrimination tasks. They also make more errors in the perception of nonsense syllables than in the perception of real words, although the patterns of performance are similar across these stimulus types. For all patients, the perception of consonants is worse than that of vowels; more errors occur when the stimuli contrast by a single phonetic feature; and more errors occur in the perception of place of articulation and voicing than in the perception of other phonetic feature contrasts.

The results of studies investigating the perception of speech challenge the view that the posterior left hemisphere, particularly Wernicke's area and associated temporal lobe structures, is selectively involved in speech receptive functions. Instead, the results are consistent with the view that phonetic/phonological processing has a distributed neural basis, one that involves the perisylvian regions of the left hemisphere (Hickok and Poeppel, 2000; Burton, 2001). Although persons with Wernicke's aphasia make a large number of errors on speech perception tasks, and although damage to the left supramarginal gyrus and the bordering parietal operculum is correlated with speech perception deficits (Gow and Caplan, 1996), some persons with anterior aphasia have shown poorer performance on these tasks than those with Wernicke's aphasia. Moreover, performance on speech perception tasks has failed to show a strong correlation with severity of auditory language comprehension. Thus, although phonetic and phonological processing deficits may contribute to the auditory comprehension impairments of aphasics, they do not appear to be the primary cause of such impairments.

See also PHONOLOGICAL ANALYSIS OF LANGUAGE DISORDERS IN APHASIA.

—*Sheila E. Blumstein*

References

Basso, A., Casati, G., and Vignolo, L. A. (1977). Phonemic identification defects in aphasia. *Cortex, 13*, 84–95.

Baum, S. (1998). The role of fundamental frequency and duration in the perception of linguistic stress by individuals with brain damage. *Journal of Speech and Hearing Research, 41*, 31–40.

Baum, S. R., Blumstein, S. E., Naeser, M. A., and Palumbo, C. L. (1990). Temporal dimensions of consonant and vowel production: An acoustic and CT scan analysis of aphasic speech. *Brain and Language, 39*, 33–56.

Blumstein, S. E. (1973). *A phonological investigation of aphasic speech.* The Hague: Mouton.

Blumstein, S. E. (2000). Deficits of speech production and speech perception in aphasia. In R. Berndt (Ed.), *Handbook of neuropsychology* (2nd ed., vol. 3, pp. 1–19). Amsterdam: Elsevier.

Blumstein, S. E., Baker, E., and Goodglass, H. (1977). Phonological factors in auditory comprehension in aphasia. *Neuropsychologia, 15*, 19–30.

Blumstein, S. E., Cooper, W. E., Goodglass, H., Statlender, S., and Gottlieb, J. (1980). Production deficits in aphasia: A voice-onset time analysis. *Brain and Language, 9*, 153–170.

Blumstein, S. E., Tartter, V. C., Nigro, G., and Statlender, S. (1984). Acoustic cues for the perception of place of articulation in aphasia. *Brain and Language, 22*, 128–149.

Burton, M. W. (2001). The role of the inferior frontal cortex in phonological processing. *Cognitive Science, 25*, 695–709.

Butterworth, B. (1992). Disorders of phonological encoding. *Cognition, 42*, 261–286.

Code, C., and Ball, M. (1982). Fricative production in Broca's aphasia: A spectrographic analysis. *Journal of Phonetics, 10*, 325–331.

Csepe, V., Osman-Sagi, J., Molnar, M., and Gosy, M. (2001). Impaired speech perception in aphasic patients: Event-related potential and neurophysiological assessment. *Neuropsychologia, 39*, 1194–1208.

Damasio, H. (1998). Neuroanatomical correlates of the aphasias. In M. T. Sarno (Ed.), *Acquired aphasia* (pp. 43–70). New York: Academic Press.

Danly, M., and Shapiro, B. (1982). Speech prosody in Broca's aphasia. *Brain and Language, 16,* 171–190.

Dronkers, N. F. (1997). A new brain region for coordinating speech articulation. *Nature, 384,* 159–161.

Gandour, J., and Dardarananda, R. (1983). Identification of tonal contrasts in Thai aphasic patients. *Brain and Language, 17,* 24–33.

Gandour, J., Dechongkit, S., Ponglorpisit, S., Khunadorn, F., and Boongird, P. (1993). Intraword timing relations in Thai after unilateral brain damage. *Brain and Language, 45,* 160–179.

Gandour, J., Ponglorpisit, S., Khunadorn, F., Dechongkit, S., Boongird, P., Boonklam, R., et al. (1992). Lexical tones in Thai after unilateral brain damage. *Brain and Language, 43,* 275–307.

Gow, D. W., Jr., and Caplan, D. (1996). An examination of impaired acoustic-phonetic processing in aphasia. *Brain and Language, 52,* 386–407.

Green, E., and Boller, F. (1974). Features of auditory comprehension in severely impaired aphasics. *Cortex, 10,* 133–145.

Hickok, G., and Poeppel, D. (2000). Towards a functional neuroanatomy of speech perception. *Trends in Cognitive Science, 4,* 131–138.

Holloman, A. L., and Drummond, S. S. (1991). Perceptual and acoustical analyses of phonemic paraphasias in nonfluent and fluent dysphasia. *Journal of Communication Disorders, 24,* 301–312.

Jauhiainen, T., and Nuutila, A. (1977). Auditory perception of speech and speech sounds in recent and recovered aphasia. *Brain and Language, 4,* 572–579.

Kent, R., and McNeil, M. (1987). Relative timing of sentence repetition in apraxia of speech and conduction aphasia. In J. Ryalls (Ed.), *Phonetic approaches to speech production in aphasia and related disorders* (pp. 181–220). Boston: College-Hill Press.

Kohn, S. E. (1993). Segmental disorders in aphasia. In G. Blanken, J. Dittman, H. Grimm, J. C. Marshall, and C. W. Wallesch (Eds.), *Linguistic disorders and pathologies: An international handbook* (pp. 197–209). New York: Walter de Gruyter.

Nadeau, S. E. (2001). Phonology: A review and proposals from a connectionist perspective. *Brain and Language, 79,* 511–579.

Polster, M. R., and Rose, S. B. (1998). Disorders of auditory processing: Evidence from modularity in audition. *Cortex, 34,* 47–65.

Riedel, K., and Studdert-Kennedy, M. (1985). Extending formant transitions may not improve aphasics' perception of stop consonant place of articulation. *Brain and Language, 24,* 223–232.

Shewan, C. M., Leeper, H., and Booth, J. (1984). An analysis of voice onset time (VOT) in aphasic and normal subjects. In J. Rosenbek, M. McNeill, and A. Aronson (Eds.), *Apraxia of speech* (pp. 197–220). San Diego, CA: College-Hill Press.

Shinn, P., and Blumstein, S. E. (1983). Phonetic disintegration in aphasia: Acoustic analysis of spectral characteristics for place of articulation. *Brain and Language, 20,* 90–114.

Vijayan, A., and Gandour, J. (1995). On the notion of a 'subtle phonetic deficit' in fluent/posterior aphasia. *Brain and Language, 48,* 106–119.

Further Readings

Baum, S. R. (1992). The influence of word length on syllable duration in aphasia: Acoustic analysis. *Aphasiology, 6,* 501–513.

Baum, S. R., Kelsch Daniloff, J., and Daniloff, R. (1982). Sentence comprehension by Broca's aphasics: Effects of some suprasegmental variables. *Brain and Language, 17,* 261–271.

Blumstein, S. E., Cooper, W. E., Zurif, E. B., and Caramazza, A. (1977). The perception and production of voice-onset time in aphasia. *Neuropsychologia, 15,* 371–383.

Boller, F. (1978). Comprehension disorders in aphasia: A historical overview. *Brain and Language, 5,* 149–165.

Buckingham, H. W., Jr. (1998). Explanations for the concept of apraxia of speech. In M. T. Sarno (Ed.), *Acquired aphasia* (pp. 269–308). New York: Academic Press.

Dronkers, N., Pinker, S., and Damasio, A. (2000). Language and the aphasias. In E. Kandel, J. Schwartz, and T. Jessell (Eds.), *Principles of neural science* (4th ed., pp. 1169–1187). New York: McGraw-Hill.

Gandour, J. (1998). Phonetics and phonology. In B. Stemmer and H. A. Whitaker (Eds.), *Handbook of neurolinguistics* (pp. 208–221). New York: Academic Press.

Gandour, J., Dechongkit, S., Ponglorpisit, S., and Khunadorn, F. (1994). Speech timing at the sentence level in Thai after unilateral brain damage. *Brain and Language, 46,* 419–438.

Hickok, G. (2000). Speech perception, conduction aphasia, and the functional neuroanatomy of language. In Y. Grodzinsky, L. Shapiro, and D. Swinney (Eds.), *Language and the brain* (pp. 87–104). New York: Academic Press.

Katz, W. (1988). Anticipatory coarticulation in aphasia: Acoustic and perceptual data. *Brain and Language, 35,* 340–368.

Katz, W., Machetanz, J., Orth, U., and Schonle, P. (1990). A kinematic analysis of anticipatory coarticulation in the speech of anterior aphasic subjects using electromagnetic articulography. *Brain and Language, 38,* 555–575.

Kent, R. D. (2000). Research on speech motor control and its disorders. *Journal of Communication Disorders, 33,* 391–428.

Kohn, S. E. (1989). The nature of the phonemic string deficit in conduction aphasia. *Aphasiology, 3,* 209–239.

Kohn, S. E. (Ed.). (1992). *Conduction aphasia.* Hillsdale, NJ: Erlbaum.

Lieberman, P. (2000). *Human language and our reptilian brain.* Cambridge, MA: Harvard University Press.

Miceli, G., Caltagirone, C., Gainotti, G., and Payer-Rigo, P. (1978). Discrimination of voice versus place contrasts in aphasia. *Brain and Language, 2,* 434–450.

Rosenbek, J. C., McNeil, M. R., and Aronson, A. E. (Eds.). (1984). *Apraxia of speech: Physiology, acoustics, linguistics, management.* San Diego, CA: College-Hill Press.

Ryalls, J. H. (Ed.). (1987). *Phonetic approaches to speech production in aphasia and related disorders.* Boston: College-Hill Press.

Poverty: Effects on Language

More than one in five children in the United States live in poverty, with pervasive consequences for their health and development. These consequences include effects on language. Children who live in poverty develop language at a slower pace than more advantaged children, and, after the age at which all children can be said to have acquired language, they differ from children from higher income backgrounds in their language skills and manner of language use. Children from low-income families are also overrepresented among children diagnosed as language-impaired.

These relations between poverty and language are robust, but they are complicated to describe and difficult to interpret. Poverty itself is not a homogeneous condition but occurs on a gradient and is usually associated with other variables that affect language, particularly education and ethnicity. Thus, the source of poverty effects is sometimes obscure. Further, the language children display is always a combined function of their language skill and language style. Thus, the nature of poverty effects is sometimes unclear. This article describes the observed associations between poverty and language development, and then considers why those associations occur. Much of the relevant literature does not use poverty per se as a variable but instead uses correlated variables such as education or a composite measure of socioeconomic status (SES). Thus, an important task in studying poverty effects is to identify the causal factors at work when poverty, low levels of parental education, and other associated factors are correlated with low levels of language achievement in children.

Language Differences Related to Income or SES. Before speech begins, infants who live in poverty produce speech sounds and babble in much the same way and on the same developmental timetable as all normally developing infants (Oller et al., 1995), and even at 3 years of age, SES is unrelated to the accuracy of children's articulation (Dollaghan et al., 1999). In contrast, virtually every other measure of language development reveals differences between children from low-income or low-SES families and children from higher income or higher SES families.

The clearest and largest SES-related difference is in the area of vocabulary. Recordings of spontaneous speech, maternal report measures, and standardized tests all show that children from low-income and low-SES families have smaller vocabularies than children from higher income and higher SES families (Rescorla, 1989; Hart and Risley, 1995; Dollaghan et al., 1999). By the age of 3 years, children from low-income families have productive vocabularies averaging around 500 words, while children from higher income families have productive vocabularies averaging more than 1000 words (Hart and Risley, 1995). Eighty percent of toddlers from low-income families score below the 50th percentile on the MacArthur Communicative Development Inventory (CDI) (Arriaga et al., 1998). Some findings suggest that low family income is more associated with measures of children's productive vocabulary than with measures of their receptive vocabulary (Snow, 1999). Two studies have reported SES-related differences in children's vocabulary, with lower SES children showing larger vocabularies. Both used the CDI, and both attributed their findings to lower SES mothers' tendencies to overestimate their children's abilities (Fenson et al., 1994; Feldman et al., 2000).

Grammatical development is also related to income or SES. Compared with higher SES children, children from lower social strata produce shorter responses to adult speech (McCarthy, 1930), score lower on standardized tests that include measures of grammatical development (Morrisset et al., 1990; Dollaghan et al., 1999), produce less complex utterances in spontaneous speech as toddlers (Arriaga et al., 1998) and at age 5 (Snow, 1999), and differ significantly on measures of productive and receptive syntax at age 6 (Huttenlocher et al., 2002). As an indicator of the magnitude of these effects on grammatical development, the low-income sample studied by Snow (1999) had an average MLU at age 3 years 9 months that would be typical of children more than a year younger, according to norms based on a middle-class sample. At age 5 years 6 months they had an average MLU typical of middle-class children age 3 years 1 month. On the other hand, the SES-related differences in productive syntax are not in whether children can or cannot use complex structures in their speech, but in the frequency with which they do so (Tough, 1982; Huttenlocher et al., in press). Studies of school-age children find SES-related differences in the communicative purposes to which language is put, such that children with less educated parents less frequently use language to analyze and reflect, to reason and justify, or to predict and consider alternative possibilities than children with more educated parents. The structural differences in children's language associated with SES may be a by-product of these functional differences (Tough, 1982).

SES-related differences in school-age children also appear in the ability to communicate meaning through language and to draw meaning from language, sometimes referred to as speaker and listener skills (Lloyd, Mann, and Peers, 1998). In the referential communication task, which requires children to describe one item in an array of objects so that a visually separated listener with the same array can identify that item, lower SES children are less able than higher SES children to produce sufficiently informative messages and to use information in messages addressed to them to make correct choices (Lloyd et al., 1998). Children from lower socioeconomic strata also perform less well than higher SES children in solving mathematics word problems. This poorer performance reflects a difference in language ability, not mathematical ability, because the same children show no difference in performance in math calculations (Jordan, Huttenlocher, and Levine, 1992).

The foregoing effects are effects of poverty or SES on variation within the normal range. On average, children from low-income families acquire language at a slower rate and demonstrate both differences in language use and poorer language skills than children from higher income families. Low SES is also a correlate of the diagnosis of specific language impairment (SLI) (Tomblin et al., 1997), although it is not clear what this means, given that SLI is defined in terms of delay relative to norms and that normative development is slower for lower SES children (Fazio, Naremore, and Connell, 1996). For this reason, there have been calls for sensitivity to SES effects on standardized measures in diagnosing SLI (Arriaga et al., 1998; Feldman et al., 2000), and efforts are underway to develop tests of language impairment that are direct tests of language learning ability rather than norm-referenced comparisons (Fazio, Naremore, and Connell, 1996; Campbell et al., 1997; Seymour, 2000).

Understanding the Relation Between Poverty and Language Development. Low family income cannot directly cause the depressed language skills associated with poverty but must operate via mediators that affect language. Potential mediators, or pathways, through which poverty operates may include factors with general effects on health and development, such as nutrition, exposure to environmental hazards, and quality of schools and child care, and may also include factors with specific effects on language, such as the opportunity for one-to-one contact with an adult (McCartney, 1984) and the language use of parents and classroom teachers (Huttenlocher et al., 2002).

A variety of evidence suggests that an important mediator of the relation between SES and language development in children is the nature of the language-learning environment provided by the family (Hoff, 2003) and that low levels of parental education, more than low income per se, affect the language-learning environment in the home. Two predictors of language development, the talk parents address to children and the exposure to books that parents provide, differ as a function of parental education. Compared with children of more educated parents, children of less educated parents hear less speech, hear less richly informative speech, receive less support for their own participation in conversation, and are read to less (Hart and Risley, 1995; Hoff-Ginsberg, 1998; U.S. Department of Education, 1998; Hoff, Laursen, and Tardif, 2002). When mediators of the relation between family SES and child language have been examined, properties of children's language-learning environments have been found to account for most of the variance attributable to SES both for syntax and for lexical development (Hoff, 2003; Huttenlocher et al., 2002). In fact, even variation within low-income samples is attributable to variation in language-learning environments. Among a group of 5-year-olds in Head Start programs (thus, children from low-income families), standard scores on a measure of comprehension vocabulary (the Peabody Picture Vocabulary Test) were significantly related to maternal use of sophisticated vocabulary (i.e., low-frequency words) and to the frequency of supportive mother-child interactions (Weizman and Snow, 2001). In a different sample of 4-year-olds in Head Start, variation in productive and comprehension vocabulary was accounted for by children's literacy experiences at home (Payne, Whitehurst, and Angell, 1994).

With respect to understanding the role of poverty in communication disorders, the literature presents a paradox. Poverty is associated with slow language development because poverty is associated with less supportive language-learning environments for children than more affluent situations. Poverty is also associated with the diagnosis of SLI, although most evidence suggests that the language environment is not the cause of SLI (Lederberg, 1980). In fact, studies of the heritability of language find a higher heritability for language impairment than for variation in language development within the normal range (Eley et al., 1999; Dale et al., 2000). If input is the mediator of poverty effects on language but input does not explain SLI, then why is poverty associated with SLI? The inescapable conclusion is that children can differ from the normative rate of development for two reasons: an impairment in the ability to learn language or an inadequate language-learning environment. Low percentile scores on measures of language development do not, by themselves, distinguish between these. While poverty does not cause language impairment or a communication disorder, the impoverished language-learning environment often associated with poverty can similarly impede language development.

See also SPECIFIC LANGUAGE IMPAIRMENT IN CHILDREN.

—*Erika Hoff*

References

Arriaga, R. J., Fenson, L., Cronan, T., and Pethick, S. J. (1998). Scores on the MacArthur Communicative Development Inventory of children from low- and middle-income families. *Applied Psycholinguistics, 19,* 209–223.

Campbell, T., Dollaghan, D., Needleman, H., and Janosky, J. (1997). Reducing bias in language assessment: Processing-dependent measures. *Journal of Speech, Language, and Hearing Research, 40,* 519–525.

Dale, P. S., Dionne, G., Eley, T. C., and Plomin, R. (2000). Lexical and grammatical development: A behavioral genetic perspective. *Journal of Child Language, 27,* 619–642.

Dollaghan, C. A., Campbell, T. F., Paradise, J. L., Feldman, H. M., Janosky, J. E., Pitcairn, D. N., et al. (1999). Maternal education and measures of early speech and language. *Journal of Speech, Language, and Hearing Research, 42,* 1432–1443.

Eley, T. C., Bishop, D. V. M., Dale, P. S., Oliver, B., Petrill, S. A., Price, T. S., et al. (1999). Genetic and environmental origins of verbal and performance components of cognitive delay in 2-year-olds. *Developmental Psychology, 35,* 1122–1131.

Fazio, B. B., Naremore, R. C., and Connell, P. J. (1996). Tracking children from poverty at risk for specific language impairment: A 3-year longitudinal study. *Journal of Speech and Hearing Research, 39,* 611–624.

Feldman, H. M., Dollaghan, C. A., Campbell, T. F., Kurs-Lasky, M., Janosky, J. E., and Paradise, J. L. (2000). Measurement properties of the MacArthur Communicative Development Inventory at ages one and two years. *Child Development, 71,* 310–322.

Fenson, L., Dale, P. A., Reznick, J. S., Bates, E., Thal, D. J., and Pethick, S. J. (1994). *Variability in early communicative development. Monographs of the Society for Research in Child Development, 59* (Serial No. 242).

Hart, B., and Risley, T. (1995). *Meaningful differences in the everyday experience of young American children.* Baltimore: Paul H. Brookes.

Hoff, E. (2003). Causes and consequences of SES-related differences in parent-to-child speech. In M. H. Bornstein (Ed.), *Socioeconomic status, parenting, and child development*. Mahwah, NJ: Erlbaum.

Hoff, E., Laursen, B., and Tardif, T. (2002). Socioeconomic status and parenting. In M. H. Bornstein (Ed.), *Handbook of parenting* (2nd ed.). Mahwah, NJ: Erlbaum.

Hoff-Ginsberg, E. (1998). The relation of birth order and socioeconomic status to children's language experience and language development. *Applied Psycholinguistics, 19*, 603–629.

Huttenlocher, J., Vasilyeva, M., Cymerman, E., and Levine, S. (2002). Language input at home and at school: Relation to child syntax. *Cognitive Psychology, 45*, 337–374.

Jordan, N., Huttenlocher, J., and Levine, S. (1992). Differential calculation abilities in young children from middle- and low-income families. *Developmental Psychology, 28*, 644–653.

Lederberg, A. (1980). The language environment of children with language delays. *Journal of Pediatric Psychology, 5*, 141–158.

Lloyd, P., Mann, S., and Peers, I. (1998). The growth of speaker and listener skills from five to eleven years. *First Language, 18*, 81–104.

McCarthy, D. (1930). *The language development of the preschool child*. Minneapolis: University of Minnesota Press.

McCartney, K. (1984). Effect of quality of day care environment on children's language development. *Developmental Psychology, 20*, 244–260.

Morrisset, C., Barnard, K., Greenberg, M., Booth, D., and Spieker, S. (1990). Environmental influences on early language development: The context of social risk. *Development and Psychopathology, 2*, 127–149.

Oller, D. K., Eilers, R. E., Basinger, D., Steffens, M. L., and Urbano, R. (1995). Extreme poverty and the development of precursors to the speech capacity. *First Language, 15*, 167–188.

Payne, A. C., Whitehurst, G. J., Angell, A. L. (1994). The role of home literacy environment in the development of language ability in preschool children from low-income families. *Early Childhood Research Quarterly, 9*, 427–440.

Rescorla, L. (1989). The Language Development Survey: A screening tool for delayed language in toddlers. *Journal of Speech and Hearing Disorders, 54*, 587–599.

Seymour, H. N. (2000). *The development of a dialect sensitive language test*. Paper presented at the Symposium on Research in Child Language Disorders, Madison, WI, June 3.

Snow, C. E. (1999). Social perspectives on the emergence of language. In B. MacWhinney (Ed.), *The emergence of language* (pp. 257–276). Mahwah, NJ: Erlbaum.

Tomblin, J. B., Records, N. L., Buckwalter, P., Zhang, X., Smith, E., and O'Brien, M. (1997). Prevalence of specific language impairment in kindergarten children. *Journal of Speech, Language, and Hearing Research, 40*, 1245–1260.

Tough, J. (1982). Language, poverty, and disadvantage in school. In L. Feagans and D. C. Farran (Eds.), *The language of children reared in poverty* (pp. 3–19). New York: Academic Press.

U.S. Department of Education, National Center for Education Statistics. (1998). Estimates of "read to every day" as published in Federal Interagency Forum on Child and Family Statistics, Table ED1. Washington, DC: Author.

Weizman, Z. O., and Snow, C. E. (2001). Lexical input as related to children's vocabulary acquisition: Effects of sophisticated exposure and support for meaning. *Developmental Psychology, 37*, 265–279.

Further Reading

Heath, S. B. (1983). *Ways with words*. Cambridge, U.K.: Cambridge University Press.

Pragmatics

Pragmatics may be defined as "the study of the rules governing the use of language in social contexts" (McTear and Conti-Ramsden, 1992, p. 19). Although there is some debate as to what should be included under the heading of pragmatics, traditionally it has been thought to incorporate behaviors such as communicative intent (speech acts), conversational management (turn taking, topic manipulation, etc.), presuppositional knowledge, and culturally determined rules for linguistic politeness. Some authors, working from a framework in which pragmatics is seen as the motivating force behind other components of language such as syntax and semantics, include an expanded list of behaviors within this domain. For example, from this latter perspective, behaviors such as those occurring in the interactive context of early language acquisition would be considered pragmatic. Despite difficulty in determining where the boundaries of pragmatics should be drawn, as one considers how language is used in real interactions with other people, it is impossible not to cross over into areas more typically seen as social or cultural rather than linguistic (Ninio and Snow, 1996).

Although the social implications of impaired communication skills have been considered for some time, the pragmatic aspects of language impairment did not become a serious topic of study until the mid-1970s, following the lead of researchers studying typical language acquisition (see Leonard, 1998). The innovations for language assessment and intervention that stemmed from this work motivated Duchan (1984) to characterize these efforts as "the pragmatics revolution." Gallagher (1991) summarized the contributions of pragmatics to assessment by noting that greater awareness of the pragmatic aspects of language resulted in a larger set of behaviors on which a diagnosis of language impairment could be made. It also highlighted the importance of contextual variables in spontaneous language production. Clinicians gained an understanding that controlling or standardizing these variables would fundamentally alter the nature of the interaction.

With respect to language intervention, goals were expanded to include a wide range of pragmatic behaviors. Further, providing intervention in more naturalistic contexts, thereby allowing communication to be motivated and reinforced by natural consequences, was highlighted. At the same time the value of using routines, scripts, and similar procedures to provide greater contextual support for language usage also gained favor among clinicians (Gallagher, 1991).

The study of pragmatics also brought insights into how communication might be linked to other aspects of behavior. A prime example, stemming from work with persons with pervasive developmental disabilities, was the insight that challenging behavior may have communicative intent. Further, providing the individual with a more appropriate means of communicating the same intent would often result in a notable decrease in the undesirable behavior (Carr and Durrand, 1985).

Additionally, much of the recent work focusing on the social skills and peer relationships of children with language impairment (e.g., Hadley and Rice, 1991; Craig and Washington, 1993; Brinton et al., 1997) is a natural extension of earlier work studying the interactional skills of these children. As Gallagher (1999) noted, "it was inevitable that the pragmatic language focus on communication would eventually lead to questions about the interpersonal and intrapersonal roles of language" (p. vi).

Despite the positive contributions to assessment and intervention procedures that have resulted from the study of pragmatics, a clear sense of the role of pragmatic behaviors in language impairment has been difficult to achieve. Research with some groups of children with language impairment has documented the presence of serious pragmatic problems. In other groups of children the nature of pragmatic difficulties has been more challenging to characterize. This variability can be seen by contrasting two groups for which language problems play a major role: children with autism spectrum disorders (ASD) and children with specific language impairment (SLI).

Children with ASD have communication deficits that may be grouped within two categories: (1) the capacity for joint attention to objects and events with other persons, and (2) the ability to understand the symbolic function of language (Wetherby, Prizant, and Schuler, 2000). Pragmatic deficits figure prominently within both categories. For example, with respect to joint attention, children with ASD produce a limited range of communicative intentions. They may communicate to direct the behavior of others but not for purposes requiring joint attention with another person, such as to share feelings or experiences. Children with ASD also have difficulty interpreting and responding to the emotional states of others. This may be reflected in a lack of responsiveness to positive affect as well as in behaviors such as the failure to appropriately coordinate eye gaze during interaction.

Problematic behaviors stemming from difficulty with symbol use include the often cited reliance on reenactment strategies (e.g., a preschool child who used the phrase "do ah" to mean that he was not feeling well, stemming from appropriate use in a prior context), as well as developing maladaptive ways of communicating to compensate for a lack of more conventional means (e.g., using head banging to communicate the desire to avoid an unpleasant task) (Wetherby, Prizant, and Schuler, 2000). Both of these examples of language use have important pragmatic implications.

Whereas it is accepted that pragmatic difficulties constitute a basic problem for children with ASD, the situation is less clear for children with SLI. It is well established that children in the latter group have difficulty with aspects of syntactic, morphological, and semantic development. Studies examining pragmatic behaviors have yielded more equivocal findings. For example, children with SLI have been found to be less capable of responding to stacked requests for clarification (Brinton, Fujiki, and Sonnenberg, 1988), less able to initiate utterances in conversation (Conti-Ramsden and Friel-Patti, 1983), and less adept at entering ongoing conversations (Craig and Washington, 1993) than typically developing peers at the same language level. Other researchers, however, have found that children with SLI performed similarly to typically developing peers on pragmatic variables when language level was controlled (e.g., Fey and Leonard, 1984; Leonard, 1986). In summarizing this work, it appears that many (but not all) children with SLI have difficulty with many (but not all) aspects of pragmatic language behavior. For some of these children, pragmatic deficits stem from problems with language form and content. For other children, pragmatic impairment is a central component of their language difficulty.

One way in which researchers have addressed the variability noted above has been to place children with SLI into subgroups more specifically characterizing the nature of their impairment. Several groups of researchers (e.g., Bishop and Rosenbloom, 1987; Conti-Ramsden, Crutchley, and Botting, 1997) have developed taxonomies identifying a group of children whose language impairments are pragmatic in nature. Labeled as "semantic pragmatic deficit syndrome," these children are described as having a variety of pragmatic problems in the face of relatively typical structural language skills. Areas of deficit include inappropriate topic manipulation, difficulty assessing shared information, an overly high level of verbosity, and a lack of responsiveness to questions. Word-finding problems and difficulty comprehending language are also associated with this subgroup. In work by Conti-Ramsden, Crutchley, and Botting (1997), semantic pragmatic deficit syndrome characterized approximately 10% of 242 participants with SLI. In follow-up work, Conti-Ramsden and Botting (1999) found that although the subcategories of impairment were stable over the course of a year, many individual children moved between subcategories.

It might be argued that children with pragmatic problems in the face of relatively good structural language (and who do not meet criteria for ASD) might form a separate category of impairment. Bishop (2000) argued that this is not an ideal solution because pragmatic impairment is not limited to children with good structural skills, nor is it always found in association with semantic difficulties. Rather, it may be more productive to view structurally based SLI and ASD as two ends of a continuum on which many combinations of pragmatic and structural language deficits may occur.

In summary, pragmatic impairment may be found in a wide range of children with language problems. In some cases, it may constitute a central component of the impairment. For other children, the problem may be secondary to other types of language problems. From a clinical standpoint, it is important to recognize that children with a variety of disabilities may have pragmatic problems. Given the close link between language and social behavior, it is perhaps as important to recognize that even language impairments that do not involve pragmatic behaviors are likely to have implications for social interaction. To be most productive, interventions should be structured not only to improve specific language skills but also to facilitate the use of language in interactions to improve relationships with peers and adults in the child's social world.

—*Martin Fujiki and Bonnie Brinton*

References

Bishop, D. V. M. (2000). Pragmatic language impairment: A correlate of SLI, a distinct subgroup, or part of the autistic continuum? In D. V. M. Bishop and L. B. Leonard (Eds.), *Speech and language impairments in children: Causes, characteristics, intervention and outcome* (pp. 99–113). Philadelphia: Taylor and Francis.

Bishop, D. V. M., and Rosenbloom, L. (1987). Classification of childhood language disorders. In W. Yule and M. Rutter (Eds.), *Language development and disorders: Clinics in developmental medicine*. London: MacKeith Press.

Brinton, B., Fujiki, M., and Sonnenberg, E. A. (1988). Responses to requests for clarification by linguistically normal and language-impaired children in conversation. *Journal of Speech and Hearing Disorders, 53,* 383–391.

Brinton, B., Fujiki, M., Spencer, J. C., and Robinson, L. A. (1997). The ability of children with specific language impairment to access and participate in an ongoing interaction. *Journal of Speech, Language, and Hearing Research, 40,* 1011–1025.

Carr, E. G., and Durrand, V. M. (1985). The social-communicative basis of severe behavior problems in children. In S. Reiss and R. R. Bootzin (Eds.), *Theoretical issues in behavior therapy* (pp. 219–254). New York: Academic Press.

Conti-Ramsden, G., and Botting, N. (1999). Classification of children with specific language impairment: Longitudinal considerations. *Journal of Speech, Language, and Hearing Research, 42,* 1195–1204.

Conti-Ramsden, G., Crutchley, A., and Botting, N. (1997). The extent to which psychometric tests differentiate subgroups of children with SLI. *Journal of Speech, Language, and Hearing Research, 40,* 765–777.

Conti-Ramsden, G., and Friel-Patti, S. (1983). Mothers' discourse adjustments to language-impaired and non-language-impaired children. *Journal of Speech and Hearing Disorders, 48,* 360–367.

Craig, H. K., and Washington, J. A. (1993). The access behaviors of children with specific language impairment. *Journal of Speech and Hearing Research, 36,* 322–336.

Duchan, J. (1984). Language assessment: The pragmatics revolution. In R. Naremore (Ed.), *Language science* (pp. 147–180). San Diego, CA: College-Hill Press.

Fey, M. E., and Leonard, L. (1984). Partner age as a variable in the conversational performance of specifically language-impaired and normal-language children. *Journal of Speech and Hearing Research, 27,* 413–423.

Gallagher, T. M. (1991). A retrospective look at clinical pragmatics. In T. M. Gallagher (Ed.), *Pragmatics of language: Clinical practice issues* (pp. 1–9). San Diego, CA: Singular Publishing Group.

Gallagher, T. M. (1999). Foreword (issue on children's language, behavior, and emotional problems). *Topics in Language Disorders, 19*(2), vi–vii.

Hadley, P. A., and Rice, M. L. (1991). Conversational responsiveness of speech- and language-impaired preschoolers. *Journal of Speech and Hearing Research, 34,* 1308–1317.

Leonard, L. B. (1986). Conversational replies of children with specific language impairment. *Journal of Speech and Hearing Research, 29,* 114–119.

Leonard, L. B. (1998). *Children with specific language impairment.* Cambridge, MA: MIT Press.

McTear, M., and Conti-Ramsden, G. (1992). *Pragmatic disability in children.* San Diego, CA: Singular Publishing Group.

Ninio, A., and Snow, C. E. (1996). *Pragmatic development.* Boulder, CO: Westview Press.

Wetherby, A. M., Prizant, B. M., and Schuler, A. L. (2000). Understanding the nature of communication and language impairments. In A. M. Wetherby and B. M. Prizant (Eds.), *Autism spectrum disorders: A transactional developmental perspective* (pp. 109–141). Baltimore: Paul H. Brookes.

Further Readings

Bishop, D. V. M., and Adams, C. (1989). Conversational characteristics of children with semantic-pragmatic disorder: II. What features lead to a judgement of inappropriacy? *British Journal of Disorders of Communication, 24,* 241–263.

Bishop, D. V. M., and Adams, C. (1992). Comprehension problems in children with specific language impairment: Literal and inferential meaning. *Journal of Speech and Hearing Research, 35,* 119–129.

Bishop, D. V. M., Chan, J., Hartley, J., Adams, C., and Weir, F. (2000). Conversational responsiveness in specific language impairment: Evidence of disproportionate pragmatic difficulties in a subset of children. *Development and Psychopathology, 12,* 177–199.

Blank, M., Gessner, M., and Esposito, A. (1979). Language without communication: A case study. *Journal of Child Language, 6,* 329–352.

Brinton, B., and Fujiki, M. (1982). A comparison of request-response sequences in the discourse of normal and language-disordered children. *Journal of Speech and Hearing Disorders, 47,* 57–62.

Brinton, B., and Fujiki, M. (1989). *Conversational management with language-impaired children.* Rockville, MD: Aspen.

Brinton, B., and Fujiki, M. (1994). Ways to teach conversation. In J. Duchan, L. Hewitt, and R. Sonnenmeier (Eds.), *Pragmatics: From theory to practice* (pp. 59–71). Englewood Cliffs, NJ: Prentice Hall.

Brinton, B., and Fujiki, M. (1995). Efficacy of conversational intervention with children with language impairment. In M. E. Fey, J. Windsor, and S. Warren (Eds.), *Communication intervention for school-age children* (pp. 183–212). Baltimore: Paul H. Brookes.

Brinton, B., Fujiki, M., and Powell, J. (1997). The ability of children with language impairment to manipulate topic in a structured task. *Language, Speech, and Hearing Services in Schools, 28,* 3–22.

Brinton, B., Fujiki, M., Winkler, E., and Loeb, D. (1986). Responses to requests for clarification in linguistically normal and language-impaired children. *Journal of Speech and Hearing Disorders*, 51, 370–378.

Conti-Ramsden, G., and Gunn, M. (1986). The development of conversational disability: A case study. *British Journal of Disorders of Communication*, 21, 339–351.

Craig, H. K. (1991). Pragmatic characteristics of the child with specific language impairment: An interactionist perspective. In T. M. Gallagher (Ed.), *Pragmatics of language: Clinical practice issues* (pp. 163–198). San Diego, CA: Singular Publishing Group.

Craig, H. K., and Evans, J. (1989). Turn exchange characteristics of SLI childrens' simultaneous and non-simultaneous speech. *Journal of Speech and Hearing Disorders*, 54, 334–347.

Craig, H. K., and Evans, J. L. (1993). Pragmatics and SLI: Within-group variations in discourse behaviors. *Journal of Speech and Hearing Research*, 36, 777–789.

Craig, H. K., and Gallagher, T. (1986). Interactive play: The frequency of related verbal responses. *Journal of Speech and Hearing Research*, 29, 375–383.

Duchan, J. F. (1995). *Supporting language learning in everyday life*. San Diego, CA: Singular Publishing Group.

Duchan, J. F., Hewitt, L. E., and Sonnenmeier, R. M. (Eds.). (1994). *Pragmatics: From theory to practice*. Englewood Cliffs, NJ: Prentice Hall.

Fujiki, M., and Brinton, B. (1991). The verbal noncommunicator: A case study. *Language, Speech and Hearing Services in Schools*, 22, 322–333.

Gallagher, T. M. (1991). *Pragmatics of language: Clinical practice issues*. San Diego, CA: Singular Publishing Group.

Gallagher, T. M. (1999). Interrelationships among children's language, behavior, and emotional problems. *Topics in Language Disorders*, 19(2), 1–15.

Gallagher, T. M., and Prutting, C. A. (1983). *Pragmatic assessment and intervention issues in language*. San Diego, CA: College-Hill Press.

McTear, M. F. (1985a). Pragmatic disorders: A case study of conversational disability. *British Journal of Disorders of Communication*, 20, 129–142.

McTear, M. F. (1985b). Pragmatic disorders: A question of direction. *British Journal of Disorders of Communication*, 20, 119–127.

Mentis, M. (1994). Topic management in discourse: Assessment and intervention. *Topics in Language Disorders*, 14(3), 29–54.

Nippold, M. A. (1994). Persuasive talk in social contexts: Development, assessment, and intervention. *Topics in Language Disorders*, 14(3), 1–12.

Prutting, C. A. (1982). Pragmatics as social competence. *Journal of Speech and Hearing Disorders*, 47, 123–134.

Prutting, C. A., and Kirchner, D. M. (1987). A clinical appraisal of the pragmatic aspects of language. *Journal of Speech and Hearing Disorders*, 52, 105–119.

Rapin, I. (1996). Developmental language disorders: A clinical update. *Journal of Child Psychology and Psychiatry and Allied Disciplines*, 37, 643–655.

Rapin, I., and Allen, D. (1983). Developmental language disorders: Nosologic considerations. In U. Kirk (Ed.), *Neuropsychology of language, reading and spelling* (pp. 155–184). New York: Academic Press.

Rollins, P. R., Pan, B. A., Conti-Ramsden, G., and Snow, C. E. (1994). Communicative skills in children with specific language impairments: A comparison with their language-matched siblings. *Journal of Communication Disorders*, 27, 189–206.

Westby, C. (1999). Assessment of pragmatic competence in children with psychiatric disorders. In D. Rogers-Adkinson and P. Griffith (Eds.), *Communication disorders and children with psychiatric and behavioral disorders* (pp. 177–258). San Diego, CA: Singular Publishing Group.

Windsor, J. (1995). Language impairment and social competence. In M. E. Fey, J. Windsor, and S. F. Warren (Eds.), *Language intervention: Preschool through the elementary years* (pp. 213–238). Baltimore: Paul H. Brookes.

Prelinguistic Communication Intervention for Children with Developmental Disabilities

The onset of intentional communication late in the first year of life marks an infant's active entry into his or her culture and ignites important changes in how others regard and respond to the infant. A significant delay in the onset of intentional communication is a strong indicator that the onset of productive language also will be delayed (McCathren, Warren, and Yoder, 1996; Calandrella and Wilcox, 2000). Such a delay may hold the infant in a kind of developmental limbo because the onset of intentional communication triggers a series of transactional processes that support the emergence of productive language just a few months later. In this article we discuss the research on the effects of prelinguistic communication interventions aimed at teaching infants and toddlers with developmental delays to be clear, frequent prelinguistic communicators.

The onset of coordinated attention occupies a "pivotal" juncture in prelinguistic communication development. Before the emergence of coordinated attention, an infant's intention is very difficult to discern (Bates, Benigni, Bretherton et al., 1979). Almost simultaneously with the emergence of coordinated attention, the child begins to move from preintentional to intentional communication. Requesting and commenting episodes provide the earliest contexts in which intentionality is demonstrated (Bates, O'Connell, and Shore, 1987). Both functions require the infant to shift his or her attention between his or her partner and an object. Requesting (also termed imperatives and protoimperatives in the literature) is commonly defined as behavior that clearly indicates that the child wants something. Commenting (also termed joint attention, indicating, declarative, and referencing in the literature) is the act of drawing another's attention to or showing a positive affect about an object or interest (Bates, Benigni, Bretherton et al., 1987). Although other communicative functions also emerge during this period (e.g., greeting, protesting), requesting and commenting are considered the fundamental pragmatic building blocks of both prelinguistic and linguistic communication (Bruner, Roy, and Ratner, 1980). They are also the two most frequent functions expressed during the prelinguistic period (Wetherby, Cain, Yonclas et al., 1988).

The Transactional Model of Development and Intervention

The effectiveness of prelinguistic intervention in enhancing later language development depends on the operation of a transactional model of social communication development (Sameroff and Chandler, 1975; McLean and Snyder-McLean, 1978). The model presumes that early social and communication development is facilitated by bidirectional, reciprocal interactions between children and their environment. For example, a change in the child such as the onset of intentional communication may trigger a change in the social environment, such as increased linguistic mapping (i.e., naming objects and actions that the child is attending to) by their caregivers. These changes then support further development in the child (e.g., increased vocabulary), and subsequently further changes by the caregivers (e.g., more complex language interaction with the child). In this way, both the child and the environment change over time and affect each other in reciprocal fashion as early achievements pave the way for subsequent development.

A transactional model may be particularly well suited to understanding social-communication development in young children because caregiver–child interaction can play such an important role in this process. The period of early development (age birth to 3 years) may represent a unique time during which transactional effects can have a substantial impact on development. Young children's relatively restricted repertoire during this early period can make changes in their behavior more salient and easily observable to caregivers. This in turn may allow adults to be more specifically contingent with their responses to developing skills of the child than is possible later in development, when children's behavioral repertoire is far more expansive and complex. During this natural window of opportunity, the transactional model may be employed by a clever practitioner to multiply the effects of relatively circumscribed interventions and perhaps alter the very course of the child's development in a significant way. But the actions of the practitioner may need to be swift and intense, or they may be muted by the child's steadily accumulating history.

The generation of strong transactional effects in which the growth of emotional, social, and communication skills is scaffolded by caregivers can have a multiplier effect in which a relatively small dose of early intervention may lead to long-term effects. These effects are necessary when we consider that a relatively "intensive" early intervention by a skilled clinician may represent only a few hours a week of a young child's potential learning time (e.g., 5 hours per week of intensive interaction would represent just 5 percent of the child's available social and communication skill learning time if we assume the child is awake and learning 100 hours per week). Thus, unless direct intervention accounts for a large portion of a child's waking hours, transactional effects are mandatory for early intervention efforts to achieve their potential.

Effects of Prelinguistic Communication Intervention

In their initial explorations of the effects of prelinguistic communication intervention, Yoder and Warren demonstrated that increases in the frequency and clarity of prelinguistic requesting by children with developmental delays as a result of the intervention covaried with substantial increases in linguistic mapping by teachers and parents who were naive as to the specific techniques and goals of the intervention (Warren, Yoder, Gazdag et al., 1993; Yoder, Warren, Kim et al., 1994). These studies also demonstrated strong generalization effects in that the intentional requesting function they taught was shown to generalize across people, setting, communication styles, and time. Based on the promising results of these initial studies, Yoder and Warren (1998, 1999a, 1999b, 2001a, 2001b) conducted a relatively large (N = 58) longitudinal experimental study of the effects of prelinguistic communication intervention on the communication and language development of children with general delays in development. This study represented an experimental analysis of the transactional model of early social communication development.

Fifty-eight children between the ages of 17 and 32 months (mean, 23; SD, 4) with developmental delays and their primary parent participated in this study. Fifty-two of these children had no productive words at the outset of the study; the remaining six children had between one and five productive words. All children scored below the l0th percentile on the expressive scale of the Communication Development Inventory (Fenson et al., 1991).

The children were randomly assigned to one of two treatment groups. Twenty-eight of the children received an intervention termed "prelinguistic milieu teaching" (PMT) for 20 minutes per day, 3 or 4 days per week, for 6 months. The other 30 children received an intervention termed "responsive small group" (RSG). PMT represented an adaptation of milieu language teaching (e.g., Warren and Bambara, 1989; Warren, 1992). RSG represented an adaptation of the responsive interaction approach (Wilcox, 1992; Wilcox and Shannon, 1998). These interventions are described in detail elsewhere (e.g., Warren and Yoder, 1998; Yoder and Warren, 1998). Caretakers were kept naive as to the specific methods, measures, records of child progress, and child goals throughout the study. This allowed Yoder and Warren to investigate how change in the children's behavior as a result of the interventions might affect the behavior of the primary caretaker, and how this in turn might affect the child's development later in time. Data were collected at five points in time for each dyad: at pretreatment, at post-treatment, and 6, 12, and 18 months after the completion of the intervention.

Both interventions had generalized effects on intentional communication development. However, the treatment that was most effective depended on the pretreatment maternal interaction style and the education level of the mother (Yoder and Warren, 1998, 2001b).

Specifically, Yoder and Warren found that for children of highly responsive, relatively well-educated mothers, PMT was effective in fostering intentional communication development. However, for children with relatively unresponsive mothers, RSG was relatively more successful in fostering generalized intentional communication development.

The two interventions differ along a few important dimensions that provide a plausible explanation for these effects. PMT uses a child-centered play context in which communication prompts for more advanced forms of communication are employed, as well as social consequences for target responses such as specific acknowledgment and compliance. RSG emphasizes following the child's attentional lead and being highly responsive to child initiation while avoiding the use of direct prompts for communication. Maternal interaction style may have influenced which intervention was most beneficial, because children may develop expectations concerning interactions with adults (including teachers and interventionists) based on their history of interaction with their primary caretaker(s). Thus, children with responsive parents may learn to persist in the face of communication breakdowns, such as might be occasioned by a direct prompt or time delay, because their history leads them to believe that their communication attempts will usually be successful. On the other hand, children without this history may cease communicating when their initial attempt fails. Thus, children of responsive mothers in the PMT group persisted when prompted and thus learned effectively in this context, while children with unresponsive parents did not. But when provided with a highly responsive adult who virtually never prompted them over a 6-month period, children of unresponsive mothers showed greater gains than children of responsive parents receiving the same treatment.

The effects of maternal responsivity as a mediator and moderator of intervention effects rippled throughout the longitudinal follow-up period. Yoder and Warren demonstrated that children in the PMT group with relatively responsive mothers received increased amounts of responsive input in direct response to their increased intentional communication (Yoder and Warren, 2001b). Furthermore, the effects of the intervention were found on both protoimperatives and protodeclaratives (Yoder and Warren, 1999a), became greater with time, and impacted expressive and receptive language development 6 and 12 months after intervention ceased (Yoder and Warren, 1999b, 2001a). It is important to consider this finding in light of the substantial number of early intervention studies in which the effects were reported to wash out over time (Farren, 2000). Finally, the finding that amount of responsive input by the primary caregiver was partly responsible for the association between intentional communication increases and later language development (Yoder and Warren, 1999a), coupled with the longitudinal relationship between maternal responsivity and expressive language development (Yoder and Warren, 2001a), supports the prediction of the transactional model that children's early intentional communi-

cation will elicit mother's linguistic mapping, which in turn will facilitate the child's vocabulary development.

Conclusion

Prelinguistic communication intervention represents a promising approach for young children with developmental delays. Research on this approach has been quite limited to date. However, it is clear that the effectiveness of specific interventions may be dependent to some extent on mediating effects of caretaker responsivity. Therefore, the combining specific child-centered techniques such as PMT with parent training aimed at enhancing caretaker responsivity may be the most efficacious approach.

See also COMMUNICATION DISORDERS IN INFANTS AND TODDLERS.

—*Steven F. Warren and Paul J. Yoder*

References

Bates, E., Benigni, L., Bretherton, I., Camaioni, L., and Volterra, V. (1979). *The emergence of symbols, cognition and communication in infancy*. New York: Academic Press.

Bates, E., O'Connell, B., and Shore, C. (1987). Language and communication in infancy. In J. Osofsky (Ed.), *Handbook of infant development* (pp. 149–203). New York: Wiley.

Bruner, J., Roy, C., and Ratner, R. (1980). The beginnings of request. In K. E. Nelson (Ed.), *Children's language* (Vol. 3, pp. 91–138). New York: Gardner Press.

Calandrella, A. M., and Wilcox, M. J. (2000). Predicting language outcome for young prelinguistic children with developmental delay. *Journal of Speech, Language, and Hearing Research, 43,* 1061–1071.

Farren, D. C. (2000). Another decade of intervention for children who are low income or disabled: What do we know now? In J. Shonkoff and S. Meisels (Eds.), *Handbook of early intervention* (2nd ed., pp. 510–548). Cambridge, U.K.: Cambridge University Press.

Fenson, L., Dale, P. S., Reznick, S., Thal, D., Bates, E., Hartung, J. P., Pethnick, S., and Reilly, J. S. (1991). *Technical manual for the MacArthur Communicative Development Inventories*. San Diego, CA: San Diego State University.

McCathren, R. B., Warren, S. F., and Yoder, P. J. (1996). Prelinguistic predictors of later language development. In K. N. Cole, P. S. Dale, and D. J. Thal (Eds.), *Communication and language intervention series: Vol. 6. Advances in assessment of communication and language* (pp. 57–76). Baltimore: Paul H. Brookes.

McLean, J., and Snyder-McLean, L. (1978). A transactional approach to early language training. Columbus, OH: Charles E. Merrill.

Sameroff, A. J., and Chandler, M. J. (1975). Reproductive risk and the continuum of care-taking casualty. In F. D. Horowitz, M. Hetherington, S. Scarr-Salapatck, and G. Siegel (Eds.), *Review of child development research* (Vol. 4, pp. 187–244). Chicago: University of Chicago Press.

Warren, S. F. (1992). Facilitating basic vocabulary acquisition with milieu teaching procedures. *Journal of Early Intervention, 16*(3), 235–251.

Warren, S. F., and Bambara, L. S. (1989). An experimental analysis of milieu language intervention: Teaching the action-object form. *Journal of Speech and Hearing Research, 54,* 448–461.

Warren, S. F., and Yoder, P. J. (1998). Facilitating the transition from preintentional to intentional communication. In A. Wetherby, S. Warren, and J. Reichle (Eds.), *Transitions in prelinguistic communication* (pp. 365–384). Baltimore: Paul H. Brookes.

Warren, S. F., Yoder, P. J., Gazdag, G. E., Kim, K., and Jones, H. A. (1993). Facilitating prelinguistic communication skills in young children with developmental delay. *Journal of Speech and Hearing Research, 36*, 83–97.

Wetherby, A. M., Cain, D. H., Yonclas, D. G., and Walker, V. G. (1988). Analysis of intentional communication of normal children from prelinguistic to the multiword stage. *Journal of Speech and Hearing Research, 31*, 240–252.

Wilcox, M. J. (1992). Enhancing initial communication skills in young children with developmental disabilities through partner programming. *Seminars in Speech and Language, 13*(3), 194–212.

Wilcox, M. J., and Shannon, J. S. (1998). Facilitating the transition from prelinguistic to linguistic communication. In A. Wetherby, S. Warren, and J. Reichle (Eds.), *Transitions in prelinguistic communication* (pp. 385–416). Baltimore: Paul H. Brookes.

Yoder, P. J., and Warren, S. F. (1998). Maternal responsivity predicts the extent to which prelinguistic intervention facilitates generalized intentional communication. *Journal of Speech, Language, and Hearing Research, 41*, 1207–1219.

Yoder, P. J., and Warren, S. F. (1999a). Maternal responsivity mediates the relationship between prelinguistic intentional communication and later language. *Journal of Early Intervention, 22*, 126–136.

Yoder, P. J., and Warren, S. F. (1999b). Self-initiated proto-declaratives and proto-imperatives can be facilitated in prelinguistic children with developmental disabilities. *Journal of Early Intervention, 22*, 337–354.

Yoder, P. J., and Warren, S. F. (2001a). Intentional communication elicits language-facilitating maternal responses in dyads with children who have developmental disabilities. *American Journal of Mental Retardation, 106*, 327–335.

Yoder, P. J., and Warren, S. F. (2001b). Relative treatment effects of two prelinguistic communication interventions on language development in toddlers with developmental delays vary by maternal characteristics. *Journal of Speech, Language, and Hearing Research, 44*, 224–237.

Yoder, P. J., Warren, S. F., Kim, K., and Gazdag, G. E. (1994). Facilitating prelinguistic communication skills in young children with developmental delay: II. Systematic replication and extension. *Journal of Speech and Hearing Research, 37*, 841–851.

Preschool Language Intervention

In 2000, the *British Medical Journal* published an important clinical trial of preschool speech and language services in 16 community clinics in Bristol, England (Glogowska et al., 2000). This study was the largest trial of its kind to address the communication problems of preschool children. Unfortunately, its findings were largely negative; after 12 months, the treatment group showed a significant advantage on only one of the five primary outcome variables, auditory comprehension, over a control group that had received only "watchful waiting" over the same time period. This lone treatment effect was small and, arguably, not clinically significant. Most children in both groups were still eligible for preschool speech and language services at the end of the 12-month study period.

As disappointing as these results are, it is important to note that the study was designed to study the *effectiveness* of early communication services as typically provided in one community in the United Kingdom (Law and Conti-Ramsden, 2000). Effectiveness studies evaluate treatment effects under relatively typical clinical conditions. As such, the investigators learned that, on average, the children in the treatment group received only 6.2 hours of intervention, or 30 minutes per month. In fact, the most intervention provided to any child was only 15 hours over a 12-month period! This study demonstrates most clearly that small, insignificant doses of early language intervention are not effective in eliminating or reducing the broad range of problems associated with preschool language impairment (see SPECIFIC LANGUAGE IMPAIRMENT IN CHILDREN; SOCIAL DEVELOPMENT AND LANGUAGE IMPAIRMENT; PRESCHOOL LANGUAGE INTERVENTION).

Unlike studies of effectiveness, which monitor client change under typical clinical conditions, *efficacy* studies are designed to determine, under more idealized, laboratory conditions, whether an intervention is directly responsible for positive outcomes. There is ample evidence that when preschool language interventions are applied regularly with reasonable intensity, they are efficacious, leading to clinically significant improvement in the children's language and early literacy skills. There are many varieties of preschool interventions, however, and clinicians must carefully consider the options available to them.

The principal differences between different preschool intervention approaches are best captured by determining where the interventions fall on a continuum of intrusiveness. Approaches that are highly intrusive use direct teaching methods in clinical settings, usually with the clinician as the intervention agent, to address predetermined treatment objectives, such as specific words or grammatical structures. In contrast to the prescriptive character of highly intrusive approaches, minimally intrusive approaches have goals that are stated more broadly, with less focus on specific targets. Example targets include the use of longer and more complex sentences, personal reports, and stories, with the child using an increasingly varied vocabulary. This gives the child latitude to learn from the rich set of linguistic options available in intervention contexts. In general, the clinician exerts limited control over the child's agenda. Descriptions and examples of approaches at each end of the intrusiveness continuum follow.

In protocols that are maximally intrusive, the child may examine a picture, object, or event presented by a clinician, who then presents a linguistic model and a request for the child to imitate. If the child imitates correctly, the clinician provides social or other reinforcement and then presents another stimulus set. If the child imitates incorrectly, the stimulus is repeated or simplified, and the child is prompted to imitate again. This procedure originally stems from stimulus-response psychology, but in contemporary versions, goals may be attacked in ways that are based on linguistic principles to encourage generalization to targets not directly trained (Connell, 1986).

These types of intrusive approaches were popular in the 1960s, 1970s, and 1980s, and experimental evidence indicates that they can be used to teach productive use of words, grammatical forms, and even conversational behaviors to preschool children with language impairments (Cole and Dale, 1986; Yoder, Kaiser, and Alpert, 1991). In contrast to the interventions studied by Glogowska et al. (2001), however, in these successful programs, intervention is provided intensively, often for 10 minutes to 2 hours daily, with outcomes measured after periods of several months of intervention.

Maximally intrusive intervention options have fallen out of favor because of evidence that language forms learned in this manner in the clinic do not transfer well to typical communicative contexts. Furthermore, because teaching focuses on discrete language acts, and there are no planned opportunities for the child to learn language incidentally, success depends to a large extent on the clinician's ability to identify the most appropriate communication targets for each child.

The minimally intrusive approach described by Norris and Hoffman (1990) is based on whole-language principles and differs dramatically from maximally intrusive methods. There are three general steps to this approach. The first involves selection of a theme around which the therapy room or preschool classroom is organized. This theme typically is repeated across sessions, as the children engage in dramatic play, shared book reading, art projects, and other theme-oriented activities. This thematic repetition provides greater familiarity, thus enabling children to become active participants in the activities, with reduced guidance from adults. It also provides for a natural repetition of language forms, such as words, grammatical structures, and story structures, making it easier for children to learn and use them. Second, the clinician follows the child's lead, waiting for the child to communicate rather than guiding the child's attention. Third, the clinician evaluates the child's communicative efforts and provides appropriate consequences. If the child's efforts are unclear, the clinician may ask for clarification (e.g., "You want what?" "Do you want a cookie or a pencil?"), use the *cloze* procedure by providing a model utterance for the child to complete (e.g., "Tell Sandy you want a ____"), or otherwise help the child to repair the communicative attempt. If the child communicates adequately, the child's message is affirmed with an appropriate verbal or nonverbal act. In addition, after the child's attempt (e.g., "Me eat cookie"), the clinician can *recast* the child's utterance by correcting its form (e.g., "Oh, you ate your cookie") or by altering its form in some way ("Can I have a cookie now?"). In interventions such as this, it is easy and appropriate to focus on early literacy skills, such as letter knowledge, rhyming, and phonological awareness. In keeping with the limited clinician intrusiveness, however, the clinician does not directly teach specific words, language structures, story structure, or early literacy targets, nor are efforts made to get the child to imitate or to produce language out of context.

As appealing as these child-oriented approaches are, there is only limited empirical evidence that they are efficacious in facilitating language use among children with language impairments. Furthermore, it has not been adequately demonstrated that focusing broadly on the communication of meaning leads to gains in the specific areas of grammatical, phonological, and discourse weakness exhibited by preschoolers with language impairment. Techniques such as following the child's lead, recasting the child's utterances, and following the child's utterances with open-ended questions can be efficiently taught to parents or paraprofessionals, and this is an important feature. For example, Dale et al. (1996) taught parents to use these procedures during shared book reading with their children over two relatively brief sessions. Parents made more changes as a result of the intervention than the children did, but outcomes were measured after only 2 months. A longer intervention period may have resulted in greater effects on the children's performance.

Contemporary language interventions typically are hybrids that fall somewhere between the extremes in intrusiveness. For example, so-called milieu interventions blend the identification of discrete intervention targets and direct teaching using imitation and other prompts (i.e., more intrusive components) with the principles of creating natural contexts for communication, following the child's lead, and recasting the child's utterances (i.e., less intrusive components). These approaches appear to be especially efficacious for children at the single-word or early multiword stages (Yoder, Kaiser, and Alpert, 1991). Gibbard (1994) demonstrated that parents can be taught to use milieu procedures in as few as 11 sessions over a 6-month period, yielding effects commensurate with those of clinician-administered treatment. When they are applied with moderate intensity, milieu approaches increase not only the length and complexity of children's utterances, but also the children's conversational assertiveness and responsiveness (Warren, McQuarter, and Rogers-Warren, 1984).

Another popular hybrid intervention is called focused stimulation. Most focused stimulation approaches create contexts within which the interventionist produces frequent models of the child's social and linguistic targets and creates numerous opportunities for the child to produce them. Interventionists follow the child's lead, recasting the child's utterances and using the child's language targets, but they do not prompt the child to imitate. Fey et al. (1993) used this type of approach over a 5-month period to facilitate the grammatical abilities of a group of 4- to 6-year-old children with impairments of grammatical production. They also trained parents to use these techniques over a 12-session parent intervention. The children who received intervention exclusively from their parents made gains that were, on average, equivalent to the gains of the children who received 3 hours of weekly individual and group intervention from a clinician. Observed gains in the parent group were not as consistent across children as were the gains of the children in the clinician group, however.

In sum, preschool language intervention of several different types can be efficacious. Although individual clinicians have their strong personal preferences, there are few experimental indications that any one approach is dramatically superior to the others. To achieve clinically meaningful effects, however, these interventions must be presented rigorously over periods of at least several months. Furthermore, it remains unclear whether existing approaches are sufficient to minimize the risks for later social, behavioral, and academic problems preschoolers with language impairments typically experience once they reach school. To this end, promising hybrid preschool classroom interventions have been developed that aim to enhance not only the children's spoken language, but their problems in social adaptation and early literacy as well (Rice and Wilcox, 1995; van Kleeck, Gillam, and McFadden, 1998).

—Marc E. Fey

References

Cole, K., and Dale, P. (1986). Direct language instruction and interactive language instruction with language-delayed preschool children: A comparison study. *Journal of Speech and Hearing Disorders, 29,* 209–217.

Connell, P. (1986). Teaching subjecthood to language-disordered children. *Journal of Speech and Hearing Disorders, 29,* 481–492.

Dale, P. S., Crain-Thoreson, C., Notari-Syverson, A., and Cole, K. (1996). Parent-child book reading as an intervention technique for young children with language delays. *Topics in Early Childhood Special Education, 16,* 213–235.

Fey, M. E., Cleave, P. L., Long, S. H., and Hughes, D. L. (1993). Two approaches to the facilitation of grammar in language-impaired children: An experimental evaluation. *Journal of Speech and Hearing Research, 36,* 141–157.

Gibbard, D. (1994). Parental-based intervention with preschool language-delayed children. *European Journal of Disorders of Communication, 29,* 131–150.

Glogowska, M., Roulstone, S., Enderby, P., and Peters, T. (2000). Randomised controlled trial of community based speech and language therapy in preschool children. *British Medical Journal, 321,* 1–5.

Law, J., and Conti-Ramsden, G. (2000). Treating children with speech and language impairments: Six hours of therapy is not enough. *British Medical Journal, 321,* 908–909.

Norris, J. A., and Hoffman, P. R. (1990). Language intervention within naturalistic environments. *Language, Speech, and Hearing Services in Schools, 21,* 72–84.

Rice, M. L., and Wilcox, K. A. (1995). *Building a language-focused curriculum for the preschool classroom. Vol. 1, A foundation for lifelong communication.* Baltimore: Paul H. Brookes.

Van Kleeck, A., Gillam, R. B., and McFadden, T. U. (1998). A study of classroom-based phonological awareness training for preschoolers with speech and/or language disorders. *American Journal of Speech-Language Pathology, 7,* 65–76.

Warren, S. F., McQuarter, R. T., and Rogers-Warren, A. K. (1984). The effects of mands and models on the speech of unresponsive language-delayed preschool children. *Journal of Speech and Hearing Disorders, 49,* 43–52.

Yoder, P., Kaiser, A., and Alpert, C. (1991). An exploratory study of the interaction between language teaching methods and child characteristics. *Journal of Speech and Hearing Research, 34,* 155–167.

Further Readings

Camarata, S. M., and Nelson, K. E. (1992). Treatment efficiency as a function of target selection in the remediation of child language disorders. *Clinical Linguistics and Phonetics, 6,* 167–178.

Camarata, S. M., Nelson, K. E., and Camarata, M. (1994). Comparison of conversational-recasting and imitative procedures for training grammatical structures in children with specific language impairment. *Journal of Speech and Hearing Research, 37,* 1414–1423.

Cleave, P. L., and Fey, M. E. (1997). Two approaches to the facilitation of grammar in children with language impairments: Rationale and description. *American Journal of Speech-Language Pathology, 6,* 22–32.

Culatta, B., and Horn, D. (1982). A program for achieving generalization of grammatical rules to spontaneous discourse. *Journal of Speech and Hearing Disorders, 47,* 174–180.

Fey, M. E. (1986). *Language intervention with young children.* Boston: Allyn and Bacon.

Fey, M. E., Catts, H. W., and Larrivee, L. (1995). Preparing preschoolers with language impairment for the academic and social challenges of school. In M. E. Fey, J. Windsor, and S. F. Warren (Eds.), *Language intervention: Preschool through the elementary years* (pp. 3–37). Baltimore: Paul H. Brookes.

Fey, M. E., Cleave, P. L., and Long, S. H. (1997). Two approaches to grammar facilitation in children with language impairments: Phase 2. *Journal of Speech and Hearing Research, 40,* 5–19.

Fey, M. E., Cleave, P. L., Ravida, A. I., Dejmal, A. R., Easton, D., and Long, S. H. (1994). Effects of grammar facilitation on the phonological performance of children with speech and language impairments. *Journal of Speech and Hearing Research, 37,* 594–607.

Fey, M. E., Krulik, T., Loeb, D. F., and Proctor-Williams, K. (1999). Sentence recast use by parents of children with typical language and children with specific language impairment. *American Journal of Speech-Language Pathology, 8,* 273–286.

Fey, M. E., and Proctor-Williams, K. (2000). Recasting, elicited imitation, and modeling in grammar intervention for children with specific language impairments. In D. V. M. Bishop and L. B. Leonard (Eds.), *Speech and language impairments in children: Cause, characteristics, intervention, and outcome* (pp. 177–194). London: Psychology Press.

Hayward, D., and Schneider, P. (2000). Effectiveness of teaching story grammar knowledge to pre-school children with language impairment: An exploratory study. *Child Language Teaching and Therapy, 16,* 255–284.

Kaiser, A. P., Yoder, P. J., and Keetz, A. (1992). Evaluating milieu teaching. In S. F. Warren and J. Reichle (Eds.), *Causes and effects in communication and language intervention* (pp. 9–47). Baltimore: Paul H. Brookes.

Law, J., Boyle, J., Harris, F., Harkness, A., and Nye, C. (1998). Screening for speech and language delay: A systematic review of the literature. *Health Technology Assessment*, *2*, 858–865.

Leonard, L. B. (1975). Modeling as a clinical procedure in language training. *Language, Speech, and Hearing Services in Schools, 6*, 72–85.

Leonard, L. B. (1998). The nature and efficacy of treatment. In L. B. Leonard (Ed.), *Children with specific language impairment* (pp. 193–210). Cambridge, MA: MIT Press.

Nelson, K. E., Camarata, S. M., Welsh, J., Butkovsky, L., and Camarata, M. (1996). Effects of imitative and conversational recasting treatment on the acquisition of grammar in children with specific language impairment and younger language-normal children. *Journal of Speech and Hearing Research, 39*, 850–859.

Notari-Syverson, A., O'Connor, R. E., and Vadasy, P. F. (1998). *Ladders to literacy: A preschool activity book.* Baltimore: Paul H. Brookes.

Nye, C., Foster, S., and Seaman, D. (1987). Effectiveness of language intervention with the language/learning disabled. *Journal of Speech and Hearing Disorders, 52*, 348–357.

Olswang, L. B., Bain, B. A., and Johnson, G. A. (1992). Using dynamic assessment with children with language disorders. In S. F. Warren and J. Reichle (Eds.), *Causes and effects in communication and language intervention* (pp. 187–215). Baltimore: Paul H. Brookes.

Paul, R. (2001). *Language disorders from infancy through adolescence: Assessment and Intervention* (2nd ed.). St. Louis: Mosby.

Proctor-Williams, K., Fey, M. E., and Loeb, D. F. (2001). Parental recasts and production of copulas and articles by children with specific language impairment and typical language. *American Journal of Speech-Language Pathology, 10*, 155–168.

Rice, M. L., and Hadley, P. A. (1995). Language outcomes of the language-focused curriculum. In M. L. Rice and K. A. Wilcox (Eds.), *Building a language-focused curriculum for the preschool classroom. Vol. 1. A foundation for lifelong communication* (pp. 155–169). Baltimore: Paul H. Brookes.

Robertson, S. B., and Ellis Weismer, S. (1997). The influence of peer models on the play scripts of children with specific language impairment. *Journal of Speech, Language, and Hearing Research, 40*, 49–61.

Schuele, C. M., Rice, M. L., and Wilcox, K. A. (1995). Redirects: A strategy to increase peer initiations. *Journal of Speech and Hearing Research, 38*, 1319–1333.

Weiss, A. L. (2001). *Preschool language disorders resource guide.* San Diego, CA: Singular Publishing Group.

Wilcox, M. J., Kouri, T. A., and Caswell, S. B. (1991). Early language intervention: A comparison of classroom and individual treatment. *American Journal of Speech-Language Pathology, 1*, 49–62.

Prosodic Deficits

Among the sequelae of certain types of brain damage are impairments in the production and perception of speech prosody. Prosody serves numerous functions in language, including signaling lexical differences when used phonemically in tone languages, providing cues to stress, sentence type or modality, and syntactic boundaries, and conveying a speaker's emotions. Any or all of these functions of prosody may be impaired subsequent to brain damage. The hemispheric lateralization of the brain lesion seems to play an important role in the nature of the ensuing deficits; however, the neural substrates for prosody are still far from clear (see Baum and Pell, 1999, for a review). Historically, clinical impressions led to the contention that subsequent to right hemisphere damage (RHD), patients would present with flat affect and monotonous speech, whereas patients with left hemisphere damage (LHD) would maintain normal speech prosody. As research progressed, several alternative theories concerning the control of speech prosody were posited. Among these are the hypothesis that affective or emotional prosody is controlled within the right hemisphere, and thus RHD would yield emotional prosodic deficits, whereas linguistic prosody is controlled within the left hemisphere, yielding linguistic prosodic deficits when damage is confined to the left hemisphere (e.g., Van Lancker, 1980; Ross, 1981). A second hypothesis proposes that prosody is principally controlled in subcortical regions and via cortical-subcortical connections (e.g., Cancelliere and Kertesz, 1990); evidence of prosodic deficits in individuals with Parkinson's disease supports this view. A third alternative contends that the individual acoustic cues to prosody (i.e., duration, amplitude, and fundamental frequency) are differentially lateralized to the right and left hemispheres, with temporal properties processed by the left hemisphere and spectral properties by the right hemisphere (e.g., Van Lancker and Sidtis, 1992). Whereas several recent investigations have utilized functional neuroimaging techniques in normal individuals to address these hypotheses (e.g., Gandour et al., 2000), by far the most data have been gathered in studies of individuals who have suffered brain damage. These investigations allow us to characterize the nature of prosodic deficits that may emerge in neurologically impaired populations. The discussion is divided into affective and linguistic prosodic impairments.

Beginning with deficits in the production and perception of affective prosody, one of the salient speech characteristics of individuals who have suffered RHD is a flat affect. That is, in conjunction with a reduction in emotional expression as reflected in facial expressions, clinical impressions suggest that individuals with RHD tend to produce speech that is reduced, if not devoid, of affect. In fact, based on clinical judgments of the speech of RHD patients with varying sites of lesion, Ross (1981) proposed a classification system for affective impairments, or aprosodias, that paralleled the popular aphasia syndrome classification system of Goodglass and Kaplan (1983). Ross's 1981 classification scheme sparked a good deal of research on affective prosodic deficits that ultimately resulted in its abandonment by the majority of investigators. However, the investigations it catalyzed contributed significantly to our understanding of prosodic impairments; much of the work inspired by Ross's proposal took advantage of increasingly reliable methods such as acoustic analysis of speech. When studying RHD patients in an acute stage, results seemed to support impairments in patients' ability to accurately signal emotions such as happiness, sadness, and anger.

However, the majority of investigations of patients who had reached a more chronic stage (i.e., at least 3 months post onset) reported few differences between RHD patients and normal controls in signaling various emotions, as reflected in acoustic measures as well as perceptual judgments. Occasionally, studies have reported affective prosodic impairments in speech production subsequent to LHD (e.g., Cancelliere and Kertesz, 1990), although such findings are far less frequent.

With respect to the perception of affective prosody, early studies again suggested deficits in the processing of emotions cued by vocal signals subsequent to RHD (see Baum and Pell, 1999). Additional investigations have also indicated that LHD patients may exhibit deficits in the perception of affective prosody, particularly when the processing load is heavy (e.g., Tompkins and Flowers, 1985). The finding that both LHD and RHD may yield impairments in prosodic processing led to the proposal that the individual acoustic properties that serve as prosodic cues (i.e., duration, F0, and amplitude) may be processed independently in the two cerebral hemispheres and that patients with RHD and LHD may rely to different degrees on multiple cues (e.g., Van Lancker and Sidtis, 1992).

With regard to linguistic prosody, in keeping with the hypothesized functional lateralization of prosody described earlier (Van Lancker, 1980), numerous investigations have demonstrated that individuals with LHD exhibit impairments in the production of linguistic prosody, particularly at the phonemic level (i.e., in tone languages such as Mandarin, Norwegian, or Thai; e.g., Gandour et al., 1992). Deficits in the ability to signal emphatic stress contrasts, declarative versus interrogative sentence types, and syntactic clause boundaries have also been shown subsequent to LHD (e.g., Danly and Shapiro, 1982), but some studies have shown similar impairments in RHD patients (e.g., Pell, 1999) or have demonstrated that the production of only certain acoustic cues, primarily temporal parameters, is affected in LHD patients (e.g., Baum et al., 1997). The clearest evidence for the role of the left hemisphere in the production of linguistic prosody comes from studies of the phonemic use of tone; while this is arguably the "most linguistic" of the functions of prosody, it is also the smallest unit (i.e., a single syllable) in which prosodic cues may be manifest. It has therefore been suggested that the size or domain of the production unit may play a role in the brain regions implicated in prosodic processing. As an obvious corollary, patients with LHD and RHD may display impairments limited to different domains of prosodic processing.

Impairments in the perception or comprehension of linguistic prosody have also been found in both LHD and RHD patient groups, with varying results depending on the nature of the stimuli or the task. Investigations focusing on the perception of stress cues have mainly reported reduced performance relative to normal by individuals with LHD. For instance, several studies have shown that LHD patients are impaired in the ability to identify phonemic (lexical) and emphatic stress (e.g., Emmorey, 1987). With regard to the perception of lin-

guistic prosodic cues at the phrase or sentence level, both individuals with RHD and LHD have difficulty identifying declarative, interrogative, and imperative sentence types on the basis of prosodic cues alone. LHD but not RHD patients tend to be relatively more impaired in linguistic than affective prosodic perception when direct comparisons are made within a single study (Heilman et al., 1984). Baum and colleagues (1997) have also noted impairments in the perception of phrase boundaries by both LHD and RHD patients. Investigations of individuals with basal ganglia disease due to Parkinson's or Huntington's disease have also reported deficits in the comprehension of prosody (e.g., Blonder, Gur, and Gur, 1989), suggesting that subcortical structures or cortical-subcortical connections are important in prosodic processing. Due to its multiple functions in language, understanding prosodic deficits and the neural substrates implicated in the processing of prosody is clearly a complex task.

Although this article has considered affective and linguistic prosody separately, this represents a somewhat artificial distinction, as they are integrated in natural speech production and perception. A handful of recent investigations have begun to address this integration, with mixed results appearing even in normal individuals (e.g., Pell, 1999). Exploring the integration of affective and linguistic prosody in individuals who have suffered brain damage only compounds the problem and the inconsistencies.

In summary, impairments in the production and perception of speech prosody may emerge subsequent to focal brain damage to numerous cortical and subcortical regions. The precise nature of the deficit may depend in part on the site of the lesion, but it seems to vary along the dimensions of the prosodic functional load (from affective to linguistic), the size or domain of the production or processing unit, and the specific acoustic parameters contributing to the prosodic signal. Prosodic deficits clearly interact with other communicative impairments, including disorders of linguistic and pragmatic processing, contributing to the symptom complexes associated with the aphasias, motor speech disorders, and right hemisphere communication deficits.

See also RIGHT HEMISPHERE LANGUAGE AND COMMUNICATION FUNCTIONS IN ADULTS; RIGHT HEMISPHERE LANGUAGE DISORDERS.

—*Shari R. Baum*

References

Baum, S., and Pell, M. (1999). The neural bases of prosody: Insights from lesion studies and neuroimaging. *Aphasiology*, 13, 581–608.
Baum, S., Pell, M., Leonard, C., and Gordon, J. (1997). The ability of right- and left-hemisphere-damaged individuals to produce and interpret prosodic cues marking phrasal boundaries. *Language and Speech*, 40, 313–330.
Blonder, L. X., Gur, R. E., and Gur, R. C. (1989). The effects of right and left hemiparkinsonism on prosody. *Brain and Language*, 36, 193–207.

Cancelliere, A., and Kertesz, A. (1990). Lesion localization in acquired deficits of emotional expression and comprehension. *Brain and Cognition, 13*, 133–147.

Danly, M., and Shapiro, B. E. (1982). Speech prosody in Broca's aphasia. *Brain and Language, 16*, 171–190.

Emmorey, K. (1987). The neurological substrates for prosodic aspects of speech. *Brain and Language, 30*(2), 305–320.

Gandour, J., Ponglorpisit, S., Khunadorn, F., Dechongkit, S., Boongird, P., Boonklam, R., et al. (1992). Lexical tones in Thai after unilateral brain damage. *Brain and Language, 43*, 275–307.

Gandour, J., Wong, D., Hsieh, L., Weinzapfel, B., Van Lancker, D., and Hutchins, G. (2000). A crosslinguistic PET study of tone perception. *Journal of Cognitive Neuroscience, 12*, 207–222.

Goodglass, H., and Kaplan, E. (1983). *The assessment of aphasia and related disorders*. Philadelphia: Lea and Febiger.

Heilman, K., Bowers, D., Speedie, L., and Coslett, H. (1984). Comprehension of affective and nonaffective prosody. *Neurology, 34*, 917–920.

Pell, M. (1999). Fundamental frequency encoding of linguistic and emotional prosody by right hemisphere damaged speakers. *Brain and Language, 69*, 161–192.

Ross, E. (1981). The aprosodias: Functional-anatomic organization of the affective components of language in the right hemisphere. *Archives of Neurology, 38*, 561–569.

Tompkins, C. A., and Flowers, C. R. (1985). Perception of emotional intonation by brain-damaged adults: The influence of task processing levels. *Journal of Speech and Hearing Research, 28*, 527–538.

Van Lancker, D. (1980). Cerebral lateralization of pitch cues in the linguistic signal. *International Journal of Human Communication, 13*(2), 227–277.

Van Lancker, D., and Sidtis, J. J. (1992). The identification of affective-prosodic stimuli by left- and right-hemisphere-damaged subjects: All errors are not created equal. *Journal of Speech and Hearing Research, 35*, 963–970.

Further Readings

Baum, S. (1998). The role of fundamental frequency and duration in the perception of linguistic stress by individuals with brain damage. *Journal of Speech, Language, and Hearing Research, 41*, 31–40.

Blonder, L. X., Pickering, J. E., Heath, R. L., Smith, C. D., and Butler, S. M. (1995). Prosodic characteristics of speech pre- and post-right hemisphere stroke. *Brain and Language, 51*, 318–335.

Borod, J. (1993). Cerebral mechanisms underlying facial, prosodic, and lexical emotional expression: A review of neuropsychological studies and methodological issues. *Neuropsychology, 7*(4), 445–463.

Gandour, J., Larsen, J., Dechongkit, S., Ponglorpisit, S., and Khunadorn, F. (1995). Speech prosody in affective contexts in Thai patients with right hemisphere lesions. *Brain and Language, 51*, 422–443.

Gandour, J., Wong, D., Hsieh, L., Weinzapfel, B., Van Lancker, D., and Hutchins, G. (2000). A crosslinguistic PET study of tone perception. *Journal of Cognitive Neuroscience, 12*, 207–222.

Gandour, J., Wong, D., and Hutchins, G. (1998). Pitch processing in the human brain is influenced by language experience. *NeuroReport, 9*, 2115–2119.

Ivry, R., and Robertson, L. (1998). *The two sides of perception*. Cambridge, MA: MIT Press.

Pell, M. (1996). On the receptive prosodic loss in Parkinson's disease. *Cortex, 32*, 693–704.

Pell, M. (1999). The temporal organization of affective and non-affective speech in patients with right-hemisphere infarcts. *Cortex, 35*, 455–477.

Pell, M., and Baum, S. (1997a). The ability to perceive and comprehend intonation in linguistic and affective contexts by brain damaged adults. *Brain and Language, 57*, 80–99.

Pell, M., and Baum, S. (1997b). Unilateral brain damage, prosodic comprehension deficits, and the acoustic cues to prosody. *Brain and Language, 57*, 195–214.

Ross, E., Thompson, R., and Yenkosky, J. (1997). Lateralization of affective prosody in brain and the callosal integration of hemispheric language functions. *Brain and Language, 56*, 27–54.

Zatorre, R. (1988). Pitch perception of complex tones and human temporal-lobe function. *Journal of the Acoustical Society of America, 84*, 566–572.

Zatorre, R., Evans, A., and Meyer, E. (1994). Neural mechanisms underlying melodic perception and memory for pitch. *Journal of Neuroscience, 14*, 1908–1919.

Zatorre, R., Evans, A., Meyer, E., and Gjedde, A. (1992). Lateralization of phonetic and pitch discrimination in speech processing. *Science, 256*, 846–849.

Reversibility/Mapping Disorders

Impaired comprehension of reversible sentences is widely observed in aphasia. Reversible sentences (e.g., *The cat chased the dog*) cannot be interpreted accurately without attention to word order and other syntactic devices, whereas the sole plausible interpretation of nonreversible sentences (e.g., *The cat drank the milk*) can be derived from content words via semantic or pragmatic inferencing. Impaired comprehension of reversible sentences, along with relatively intact comprehension of single words and nonreversible sentences, most frequently co-occurs with Broca's aphasia but is also observed in other forms of aphasia (Caramazza and Zurif, 1976; Martin and Blossom-Stach, 1986; Caramazza and Micelli, 1991). This comprehension pattern, termed asyntactic comprehension, has been studied intensively as evidence about the syntactic abilities of aphasic listeners.

Accounts of asyntactic comprehension differ in two dimensions. The first is *competence versus performance*: Does the failure to interpret reversible sentences correctly derive from a loss of linguistic knowledge or language-processing ability, or does this failure stem from performance factors such as resource limitations? The second dimension is *parsing versus mapping*: Does asyntactic comprehension derive from a failure to parse or from a failure to map an accurate parse onto a semantic representation?

Competence Versus Performance

Early competence-based interpretations of asyntactic comprehension pointed to loss of linguistic knowledge or damage to the human parser as a common underlying source for this comprehension impairment and for AGRAMMATISM, a speech production pattern found in some Broca's aphasics. *Agrammatism* is characterized by omission or misselection of grammatical morphemes and/or simplified, fragmentary grammatical structure. This hypothesis of a central syntactic disorder (Caramazza and Zurif, 1976; Berndt and Caramazza, 1980) was motivated by the observation that asyntactic comprehension and agrammatism of speech both suggest a limited exploitation of syntactic devices. However, double dissociations between asyntactic comprehension and agrammatic production (Goodglass and Menn, 1985) argue against a central account. Competence-based explanations—using the term "competence" broadly to apply to the absolute inability to perform specific linguistic operations as a result of either loss of knowledge or damage to the psychological mechanisms responsible for computing linguistic representations—are undermined by the findings that (1) asyntactic comprehension can be induced in normal subjects under resource-demanding conditions (Miyake, Carpenter, and Just, 1994; Blackwell and Bates, 1995); (2) aphasic performance varies greatly from session to session (Kolk and van Grunsven, 1985) and from task to task (Cupples and Inglis, 1993); and (3) asyntactic comprehenders frequently perform close to normally on grammaticality judgment tasks (Linebarger, Schwartz, and Saffran, 1983), detecting grammatical ill-formedness in the same structures that they do not reliably comprehend. These findings are more compatible with a performance account than with an account that implicates loss of the ability to perform the relevant language-processing operations even under optimal conditions.

Performance accounts differ regarding the nature of the hypothesized resource limitation. Some point to a global resource deficit (Blackwell and Bates, 1995); others invoke more specific limitations (Miyake et al., 1994; Caplan and Waters, 1995). Performance accounts also differ regarding the linguistic operations disrupted by the hypothesized resource limitation: some implicate parsing (Kolk, 1995); others point to subsequent interpretative processes.

Asyntactic Comprehension as Parsing Failure

This class of performance-based explanations posits a failure to retrieve the syntactic structure of the input sentence, a failure that may occur only when task demands are high (Frazier and Friederici, 1991; but see Linebarger, 1995). On the basis of patterns of performance on comprehension tasks, some investigators have attempted to pinpoint the grammatical locus of this failure, implicating, for example, the processing of closed-class elements (Bradley, Garrett, and Zurif, 1980), syntactically moved elements (Grodzinsky, 1990), or referential dependencies (Mauner, Fromkin, and Cornell, 1993). One difficulty for these more fine-grained hypotheses (see also Linebarger, 1995) is the variability observed in aphasic performance across different syntactic structures (Berndt, Mitchum, and Haendiges, 1996). For example, these accounts predict good performance on simple active sentences, and hence fail to account for the difficulties posed for some patients by such sentences (Schwartz, Saffran, and Marin, 1980). And even those aphasic patients who normally perform well on simple active reversible sentences may fail when the lexical content is manipulated so that the syntactically correct interpretation is the opposite of the interpretation supported by lexicosemantic heuristics, as in, for example, a semantic/pragmatic anomaly task requiring the subject to detect the anomaly of *The cheese ate the mouse* (Saffran, Schwartz, and Linebarger, 1998).

An additional point to note is that while the linguistically fine-grained accounts appeal to heuristics to explain observed patterns of comprehension, they invoke these heuristics only as a response to parsing failure. The Saffran et al. (1998) data, in contrast, suggest that heuristics may occur in parallel with, and sometimes in competition with, syntactic analysis. Such a view accords with studies of sentence processing in normals, where the influence of extragrammatical heuristics in normal sentence comprehension is well documented (Slobin, 1966; Bever, 1970; Trueswell, Tanenhaus, and Garnsey, 1994).

Asyntactic Comprehension as Mapping Failure

This explanation for asyntactic comprehension implicates the mapping between syntactic structure and semantic interpretation (Linebarger, Schwartz, and Saffran, 1983). On this account, asyntactic listeners do construct an adequate representation of the structure of the input sentence but fail to exploit this syntactic information for the recovery of meaning, specifically of thematic roles such as agent and theme. The frequently observed difficulty posed by passive and object-gapped sentences follows, on this account, from the fact that the order of content words in these structures conflicts with extragrammatical order-based heuristics (Caplan, Baker, and Dehaut, 1985). If such heuristics occur in parallel with grammatically based processing, as suggested by the literature on normals, then conflict between grammatical structure and extragrammatical heuristics would be predicted to lead to more errorful performance.

Evidence to choose between these two hypotheses is sparse. The grammaticality judgment data do not undermine the performance (as opposed to the competence) version of the parsing hypothesis, on the assumption that the grammaticality judgment task is less resource-demanding than the sentence-picture matching task or other paradigms that require not only syntactic analysis but also semantic interpretation. Parsing, on this account, is performed in optimal circumstances, but not when other task demands are high.

The grammaticality judgment data do not contradict the mapping account, either. This explanation for asyntactic comprehension posits a normal syntactic parse that is not adequately mapped onto an interpretation. In fact, patterns of performance observed within the grammaticality judgment task may be seen as supporting the mapping hypothesis. Errors related to constituent structure, verb subcategorization, and the legitimacy of syntactic gaps were detected more reliably by agrammatic patients than errors involving coindexation of pronouns and other referential elements (Linebarger, 1990); such patterns suggest an initial "first-pass" recovery of constituent structure that is not fully interpreted, a pattern which falls naturally from the mapping hypothesis.

The mapping hypothesis also receives support from a study in which aphasic subjects judged the plausibility of simple reversible sentences and, in addition, of "padded" versions of these sentences (Schwartz et al., 1987; see also Kolk and Weijts, 1995). In the padded versions, the basic SVO (subject-verb-object) structure was elaborated with extraneous material. For example, subjects were presented with *The bird swallowed the worm*, its padded counterpart, *As the sun rose, the bird in the cool wet grass swallowed the worm quickly and went away*, and with the role-reversed versions of these sentences. In addition, these same predicate argument structures were embedded in noncanonical structures such as passives, object gaps, and other deviations from the simple SVO structure that typically cause difficulties for asyntactic comprehenders. The agrammatic and conduction aphasic subjects in this study performed well above chance on both the simple and padded sentences; their performance declined to chance or near chance only on the noncanonical structures. The good performance on padded sentences supports the view that asyntactic comprehenders are able to construct an adequate representation of constituent structure, because the extraction of the elements critical to the plausibility judgment (*bird*, *swallow*, and *worm*) requires an analysis of the structure of the sentence. A nonsyntactic "nearest NP" strategy, for example, would lead subjects to reject the padded sentence above, since *grass* immediately precedes *swallowed*.

The literature on mapping therapy, an approach to remediation based on this hypothesis, contains reports (Jones, 1986; Byng, 1988) of striking gains resulting from a training protocol focusing on the relationship between grammatical functions such as subject/object and thematic roles such as agent/theme. While subsequent studies have reported a variety of outcomes for this approach to therapy, the reported successes suggest that for at least a subset of patients, the breakdown in processing may occur in the assignment of thematic roles on the basis of grammatical function.

Asyntactic Comprehension as Evidence About Language Processing

It can be argued that the fragility of linguistic processing in aphasia, whatever its cause, results in a disproportionate influence of extralinguistic processing based on lexical content and word order rather than grammatical structure. Therefore the patterns of misinterpretation observed in aphasic subjects may not directly reflect their linguistic impairments, but rather a complex interaction between inefficient or inaccurate linguistic analysis and extragrammatical interpretative processes. Furthermore, the heterogeneous patterns of interpretive errors even within specific subgroups such as agrammatics suggest that there may be no unitary explanation for the impaired comprehension of reversible sentences in aphasia.

See also ATTENTION AND LANGUAGE; MEMORY AND PROCESSING CAPACITY; TRACE DELETION HYPOTHESIS.

—*Marcia C. Linebarger*

References

Berndt, R. S., and Caramazza, A. (1980). A redefinition of the syndrome of Broca's aphasia: Implications for a neuropsychological model of language. *Applied Psycholinguistics*, *1*, 225–278.

Berndt, R. S., Mitchum, C. C., and Haendiges, A. N. (1996). Comprehension of reversible sentences in "agrammatism": A meta-analysis. *Cognition*, *58*, 289–308.

Bever, T. G. (1970). The cognitive basis for linguistic structures. In R. Hayes (Ed.), *Cognition and language development*. New York: Wiley.

Blackwell, A., and Bates, E. (1995). Inducing agrammatic profiles in normals: Evidence for the selective vulnerability of morphology under cognitive resource limitation. *Journal of Cognitive Neuroscience*, *7*, 228–257.

Bradley, D. C., Garrett, M. F., and Zurif, E. B. (1980). Syntactic deficits in Broca's aphasia. In D. Caplan (Ed.), *Biological studies of mental processes*. Cambridge, MA: MIT Press.

Byng, S. (1988). Sentence processing deficits: Theory and therapy. *Cognitive Neuropsychology*, *5*, 629–676.

Caplan, D., Baker, C., and Dehaut, F. (1985). Syntactic determinants of sentence comprehension in aphasia. *Cognition*, *21*, 117–175.

Caplan, D., and Waters, G. S. (1995). Aphasic disorders of syntactic comprehension and working memory capacity. *Cognitive Neuropsychology*, *12*, 637–649.

Caramazza, A., and Micelli, G. (1991). Selective impairment of thematic role assignment in sentence processing. *Brain and Language*, *41*, 402–436.

Caramazza, A., and Zurif, E. B. (1976). Dissociation of algorithmic and heuristic processes in language comprehension: Evidence from aphasia. *Brain and Language*, *3*, 572–582.

Cupples, L., and Inglis, A. L. (1993). When task demands induce "asyntactic" comprehension: A study of sentence interpretation in aphasia. *Cognitive Neuropsychology*, *10*, 201–234.

Frazier, L., and Friederici, A. (1991). On deriving the properties of agrammatic comprehension. *Brain and Language*, *40*, 51–66.

Goodglass, H., and Menn, L. (1985). Is agrammatism a unitary phenomenon? In M.-L. Kean (Ed.), *Agrammatism* (pp. 1–26). New York: Academic Press.

Grodzinsky, Y. (1990). *Theoretical perspectives on language deficits*. Cambridge, MA: MIT Press.

Jones, E. V. (1986). Building the foundations for sentence production in a non-fluent aphasic. *British Journal of Disorders of Communication*, *21*, 63–82.

Kolk, H. H. J. (1995). A time-based approach to agrammatic comprehension. *Brain and Language*, *50*, 282–303.

Kolk, H. H. J., and van Grunsven, M. F. (1985). Agrammatism as a variable phenomenon. *Cognitive Neuropsychology*, *2*, 347–384.

Kolk, H. H. J., and Weijts, M. (1995). Judgements of semantic anomaly in agrammatic patients: Argument movement, syntactic complexity, and the use of heuristics. *Brain and Language*, *54*, 86–135.

Linebarger, M. C. (1990). Neuropsychology of sentence parsing. In A. Caramazza (Ed.), *Cognitive neuropsychology and neurolinguistics: Advances in models of cognitive function* (pp. 55–122). Hillsdale, NJ: Erlbaum.

Linebarger, M. C. (1995). Agrammatism as evidence about grammar. *Brain and Language, 50*, 52–91.

Linebarger, M. C., Schwartz, M. F., and Saffran, E. M. (1983). Sensitivity to grammatical structure in so-called agrammatic aphasics. *Cognition, 13*, 361–392.

Martin, R. C., and Blossom-Stach, C. (1986). Evidence of syntactic deficits in a fluent aphasic. *Brain and Language, 28*, 196–234.

Mauner, G., Fromkin, V. A., and Cornell, T. L. (1993). Comprehension and acceptability judgments in agrammatism: Disruption in the syntax of referential dependency. *Brain and Language, 45*, 340–370.

Miyake, A., Carpenter, P., and Just, M. A. (1994). A capacity approach to asyntactic comprehension: Making normal adults perform like aphasic patients. *Cognitive Neuropsychology, 11*, 671–717.

Saffran, E. M., Schwartz, M., and Linebarger, M. C. (1998). Semantic influences on thematic role assignment: Evidence from normals and aphasics. *Brain and Language, 62*, 255–297.

Schwartz, M., Linebarger, M. C., Saffran, E. M., and Pate, D. S. (1987). Syntactic transparency and sentence interpretation in aphasia. *Language and Cognitive Processes, 2*, 85–113.

Schwartz, M. F., Saffran, E. M., and Marin, O. S. M. (1980). The word order problem in agrammatism: I. Comprehension. *Brain and Language, 10*, 249–262.

Slobin, D. I. (1966). Grammatical transformations and sentence comprehension in childhood and adulthood. *Journal of Verbal Learning and Verbal Behavior, 2*, 219–227.

Trueswell, J. C., Tanenhaus, M., and Garnsey, S. M. (1994). Semantic influences on parsing: Use of thematic role information in syntactic disambiguation. *Journal of Memory and Language, 33*, 285–318.

Right Hemisphere Language and Communication Functions in Adults

The role of the right cerebral hemisphere in language and communication represents a relatively young area of research that has grown rapidly since the late 1970s. Recent interest in the role of the right hemisphere reflects an emphasis on language as a tool for communication in natural contexts, and an awareness that normal language use is the product of many regions of the two hemispheres working in concert. Left hemisphere structures are routinely linked to the nuts and bolts of what might be termed basic language: phonology, lexical semantics, and syntax. In contrast, right hemisphere structures have been implicated in less tightly constrained domains, including some uses of prosody (the "melody" of speech), metaphor, discourse such as conversations, stories, indirect requests, and other forms of nonliteral language, and even the social-cognitive basis for discourse. These domains most closely associated with the right hemisphere are especially sensitive to context and are ideally suited to expressing nuance. This article will first present some general issues pertaining to research in these areas and then describe, in turn, representative findings relating to prosody, lexical processing and metaphor, and discourse.

Claims related to right hemisphere contributions to language and communication can be stated in a strong form: that a specific function is housed in some region of the right hemisphere that is necessary and sufficient to support that function. However, most claims are more general and also weaker: that normal task performance draws on intact right as well as left hemisphere structures. For example, understanding the point of an ironic comment rests on a listener's appreciation of phonology, word meaning, and grammatical relations, as well as a speaker's tone of voice, preceding context, and the speaker's mood. In simplistic terms, the right hemisphere's contributions to language and communication are typically layered on top of the foundation provided by the left hemisphere. Even weak claims for the right hemisphere's role are extremely important clinically because injury to the right hemisphere often results in impairments that significantly reduce a patient's ability to communicate effectively in natural settings.

Another general point concerns localization of function. Often, a group of patients with right hemisphere lesions is compared with a group of non-brain-injured controls. Although this type of comparison does not allow localization of a particular function to the right hemisphere, it still supports the weaker interpretation mentioned earlier. In addition, some studies provide strong support for right hemisphere localization by (1) directly comparing the effects of unilateral lesions of the right and left hemispheres, (2) using lateralized presentation to intact left or right hemispheres, or (3) using functional imaging (PET, fMRI) to examine "on-line" brain activation in non-brain-injured adults. There is growing support for the right hemisphere's unique contribution to language and communication.

Prosody.   Prosody refers to variation in frequency, amplitude, duration, timbre, and rhythm. Prosodic contour can be used to convey linguistic distinctions, such as distinguishing between meanings of words or phrases ("yellow jacket" meaning a kind of bee or a brightly colored piece of clothing) and between speech acts (a question versus statement signaled by a rising pitch toward the end of an utterance). Research with right hemisphere-injured patients suggests that both expressive and receptive deficits can occur, although there is disagreement across studies. In terms of production, there is some loss of control, sometimes manifested as an increased variability in pitch (specifically, fundamental frequency) after temporal and rolandic area lesions (e.g., Colsher, Cooper, and Graff-Radford, 1987). Patients with right hemisphere lesions are also impaired on a variety of discrimination and production tasks (Behrens, 1989; Weintraub, Mesulam, and Kramer, 1981).

Prosody can also be used to convey a range of emotions, such as anger or sadness. Ross (1981) has proposed a taxonomy of aprosodias to mirror the classical taxonomy of aphasias: a motor aprosodia associated with right frontal lesions, a receptive aprosodia associated with right temporal lesions, and a global aprosodia associated with extensive frontal-temporal-parietal lesions. Other research has confirmed the separation of an affective deficit from a linguistic prosody comprehension deficit based on direct comparison between the effects of left- and right-sided lesions (Heilman et al., 1984; Pell, 1998).

Lexical and Phrasal Metaphor. Several studies have used a sentence-picture matching task. Patients with right hemisphere lesions, more so than aphasic patients with left-sided lesions, tend to be overly literal, thereby missing the conventional meaning of phrasal metaphors such as "he has a heavy heart" or idioms such as "turning over a new leaf" (Van Lancker and Kempler, 1987). The characteristic literalness has been extended to single-word stimuli such as "warm," "cold," "deep," and "shallow" in a semantic similarity judgment task presented to left- and right-lesioned patient groups (Brownell et al., 1984). Functional imaging in normal adults confirms that regions in the right hemisphere (including the dorsolateral prefrontal cortex, middle temporal gyrus, and the precuneus in the medial parietal lobe) are differentially activated during metaphor processing compared to literal sentence processing (Bottini et al., 1994).

Studies of lexical semantic processing by the left and right hemispheres of normal adults, together with work on discourse, have been used to support a comprehensive model. Beeman (1998), as well as others, suggests that the left hemisphere is designed for focused processing of the closest (literal) associations to a word demanded by preceding context and for actively dampening activation of alternative meanings. The right hemisphere, in contrast, is sensitive to looser, more remote associations and allows them to persist over time. Extrapolating Beeman's model, one can imagine what happens when a potential metaphor is presented: "Microsoft Corporation is the tiger of the software industry." The right hemisphere maintains the various associations emanating from "Microsoft," the topic of the metaphor, and "tiger," the vehicle; the overlapping or shared associations between "Microsoft" and "tiger" provide the ground for the metaphor.

Discourse. Discourse processing requires that a listener integrate meaning across sentences and from non- or paralinguistic sources to achieve an understanding of an entire story, joke, or conversation. Several studies have documented that right hemisphere lesions more than left hemisphere lesions result in decreased humor appreciation (Shammi and Stuss, 1999). While patients with right-sided lesions have no trouble appreciating that short story jokes require an incongruous punch line, they are deficient in apprehending exactly how a punch line fits with the body of a joke on a deeper level, and they have analogous problems with other types of discourse for which comprehension requires a reinterpretation (Brownell et al., 2000). Patients with right hemisphere injuries have trouble extracting gist from extended narrative even in the absence of an obvious need for reinterpretation (Hough, 1990), although there are highly constrained situations in which they are able to perform inferences that span sentence boundaries (Leonard,

Waters, and Caplan, 1997). Another realm of impairment centers on nonliteral language. Several studies of sarcasm and irony comprehension suggest a problem using context (mood, sentence prosody) as a guide to uncovering a speaker's intended meaning (Tompkins and Flowers, 1985). Similarly, a host of studies show that right-sided lesions alter patient's production and comprehension of indirect requests, which also require consideration of the preceding context (Stemmer, Giroux, and Joanette, 1994).

An overlapping body of work examines whether an underlying social cognitive impairment affects discourse performance. The ability to explain behavior in terms of other people's mental states, referred to as theory of mind, has been examined in several populations, including people with autism and stroke patients. Comprehension of stories and cartoons that rely on theory of mind are relatively difficult for patients with right-sided lesions, but not for aphasic patients with left hemisphere lesions (Happé, Brownell, and Winner, 1999). Also, functional imaging studies in normal adults suggest greater activation linked to theory of mind in a variety of regions, including the right middle frontal gyrus and precuneus (Gallagher et al., 2000).

There are, of course, unresolved issues. The range of language and communication skills associated with right hemisphere injury is extensive. These skills seem to represent several domains that will need to be examined separately, even though powerful unifying constructs have been explored, such as coherence (Benowitz, Moya, and Levine, 1990) and working memory (Tompkins et al., 1994). Finally, our understanding of localization of function involving the right hemisphere is poorly developed. Functions often associated with the right hemisphere may be as appropriately tied to prefrontal regions in either hemisphere (McDonald, 1993; Stuss, Gallup, and Alexander, 2001).

See also DISCOURSE; DISCOURSE IMPAIRMENTS.

—*Hiram Brownell*

References

Beeman, M. (1998). Coarse semantic coding and discourse comprehension. In M. Beeman and C. Chiarello (Eds.), *Right hemisphere language comprehension: Perspectives from cognitive neuroscience* (pp. 255–284). Mahwah, NJ: Erlbaum.

Behrens, S. J. (1989). Characterizing sentence intonation in a right hemisphere–damaged population. *Brain and Language, 37,* 181–200.

Benowitz, L. I., Moya, K. L., and Levine, D. N. (1990). Impaired verbal reasoning and constructional apraxia in subjects with right hemisphere damage. *Neuropsychologia, 28,* 231–241.

Bottini, G., Corcoran, R., Sterzi, R., Paulesu, E., Schenone, P., Scarpa, P., et al. (1994). The role of the right hemisphere in the interpretation of figurative aspects of language: A positron emission tomography activation study. *Brain, 117,* 1241–1253.

Brownell, H., Griffin, R., Winner, E., Friedman, O., and Happé, F. (2000). Cerebral lateralization and theory of mind. In S. Baron-Cohen, H. Tager-Flusberg, and D. J. Cohen (Eds.), *Understanding other minds: Perspectives from autism and developmental cognitive neuroscience* (2nd ed., pp. 311–338). Oxford: Oxford University Press.

Brownell, H. H., Potter, H. H., Michelow, D., and Gardner, H. (1984). Sensitivity to lexical denotation and connotation in brain-damaged patients: A double dissociation? *Brain and Language, 22,* 253–265.

Colsher, P. L., Cooper, W. E., and Graff-Radford, N. (1987). Intonation variability in the speech of right-hemisphere damaged patients. *Brain and Language, 32,* 379–383.

Gallagher, H. L., Happé, F., Brunswick, N., Fletcher, P. C., Frith, U., and Frith, C. D. (2000). Reading the mind in cartoons and stories: An fMRI study of "theory of mind" in verbal and nonverbal tasks. *Neuropsychologia, 38,* 11–21.

Happé, F., Brownell, H., and Winner, E. (1999). Acquired theory of mind impairments following right hemisphere stroke. *Cognition, 70,* 211–240.

Heilman, K. M., Bowers, D., Speedie, L., and Coslett, H. B. (1984). Comprehension of affective and nonaffective prosody. *Neurology, 34,* 917–921.

Hough, M. S. (1990). Narrative comprehension in adults with right and left hemisphere brain-damage: Theme organization. *Brain and Language, 38,* 253–277.

Leonard, C. L., Waters, G. S., and Caplan, D. (1997). The use of contextual information by right brain-damaged individuals in the resolution of ambiguous pronouns. *Brain and Language, 57,* 309–342.

McDonald, S. (1993). Viewing the brain sideways? Frontal versus right hemisphere explanations of non-aphasic language disorders. *Aphasiology, 7,* 535–549.

Pell, M. (1998). Recognition of prosody following unilateral brain lesion: Influence of functional and structural attributes of prosodic contours. *Neuropsychologia, 36,* 701–715.

Ross, E. D. (1981). The aprosodias. *Archives of Neurology, 38,* 561–569.

Shammi, P., and Stuss, D. T. (1999). Humour appreciation: A role of the right frontal lobe. *Brain, 122,* 657–666.

Stemmer, B., Giroux, F., and Joanette, Y. (1994). Production and evaluation of requests by right hemisphere brain-damaged individuals. *Brain and Language, 47,* 1–31.

Stuss, D. T., Gallup, G. G., and Alexander, M. P. (2001). The frontal lobes are necessary for "theory of mind." *Brain, 124,* 279–286.

Tompkins, C. A., Bloise, C. G. R., Timko, M. L., and Baumgaertner, A. (1994). Working memory and inference revision in brain-damaged and normally aging adults. *Journal of Speech and Hearing Research, 37,* 896–912.

Tompkins, C. A., and Flowers, C. (1985). Perception of emotional intonation by brain-damaged adults: The influence of task processing levels. *Journal of Speech and Hearing Research, 28,* 527–538.

Van Lancker, D. R., and Kempler, D. (1987). Comprehension of familiar phrases by left but not by right hemisphere damaged patients. *Brain and Language, 32,* 265–277.

Weintraub, S., Mesulam, M.-M., and Kramer, L. (1981). Disturbances in prosody: A right hemisphere contribution to language. *Archives of Neurology, 38,* 742–744.

Further Readings

Baron-Cohen, S., Tager-Flusberg, H., and Cohen, D. J. (Eds.). (2000). *Understanding other minds: Perspectives from autism and developmental cognitive neuroscience* (2nd ed.). Oxford: Oxford University Press.

Beeman, M., and Chiarello, C. (Eds.). (1998). *Right hemisphere language comprehension: Perspectives from cognitive neuroscience.* Mahwah, NJ: Erlbaum.

Brownell, H. (2000). Right hemisphere contributions to understanding lexical connotation and metaphor. In Y. Grodzinsky, L. Shapiro, and D. Swinney (Eds.), *Language and the brain* (pp. 185–201). San Diego, CA: Academic Press.

Brownell, H., and Friedman, O. (2001). Discourse ability in patients with unilateral left and right hemisphere brain damage. In R. S. Berndt (Ed.), *Handbook of neuropsychology* (2nd ed., vol. 3, pp. 189–203). Amsterdam: Elsevier.

Deacon, T. W. (1997). *The symbolic species: The co-evolution of language and the brain.* New York: Norton.

Joanette, Y., Goulet, P., and Hannequin, D. (1990). *Right hemisphere and verbal communication.* New York: Springer-Verlag.

Myers, P. S. (1999). *Right hemisphere damage: Disorders of communication and cognition.* San Diego, CA: Singular Publishing Group.

Tompkins, C. A. (1995). *Right hemisphere communication disorders.* San Diego, CA: Singular Publishing Group.

Right Hemisphere Language Disorders

For nearly 150 years, the language-dominant left cerebral hemisphere has dominated research and clinical concern about language disorders that accompany brain damage in adults. However, it is now well established that unilateral right hemisphere brain damage can substantially impair language and communication. The language deficits associated with right hemisphere damage, while often quite socially handicapping (Tompkins et al., 1998), are little understood. This article focuses on disorders characterized by damage restricted to the right cerebral hemisphere in adults. Such individuals may have difficulties with some basic language tasks but are not generally considered to have aphasia, because phonology, morphology, syntax, and many aspects of semantics are largely intact. About 50% of adults with right hemisphere damage have a verbal communication disorder (Joanette et al., 1990). In one study, 93% of 123 adults with right hemisphere damage in a rehabilitation center had at least one cognitive deficit with the potential to disrupt communication and social interaction (Blake et al., 2002).

Heterogeneity typifies the population of adults with right hemisphere damage: not all will have all characteristic communicative problems, and some will have no discernible problems. This heterogeneity often is unaccounted for in sample selection or data analysis, and its potential effects are compounded by the small samples in most studies of language in patients with right hemisphere damage. A related difficulty involves control group composition in research on language deficits associated with right hemisphere damage. Non-brain-damaged samples typically comprise individuals who do not have complications associated with being a patient. Individuals with left brain damage often are excluded because they cannot perform the more complex tasks that are most revealing of language functioning after right hemisphere damage, and because differences in impairment profiles make it difficult to equate groups for severity. Consequently, it is impossible to determine whether observed deficits are specific to right hemisphere damage. Another major issue is the lack of consensus on how to define or even what to call language deficits associated with right hemisphere damage (cf. Myers, 1999), either in totality or as individual components of an aggregate syndrome. Conceptual and terminological imprecision, and apparent overlap, are common in referring to targets of inquiry such as nonliteral language processing, inferencing, integration, and reasoning from a theory of mind (Blake et al., 2002). Conclusions about language deficits after right hemisphere damage also are complicated by intraindividual performance variability, whether due to factors such as differential task processing requirements (e.g., Tompkins and Lehman, 1998), or to time following onset of injury (Colsher et al., 1987). Finally, many language difficulties ostensibly related to right hemisphere damage stem from or are exacerbated by other perceptual and cognitive impairments, some of which are as yet unidentified but others of which have not been evaluated consistently. Chief among these complications are hemispatial neglect, other attentional difficulties, and impairments of working memory and related processing resources.

Overview and Potential Accounts of Symptoms in Characteristic Deficit Domains

Prosody. Prosody is not uniquely a right hemisphere function (Baum and Pell, 1999). However, many adults with right hemisphere damage have difficulty producing and comprehending prosody, whether it serves linguistic functions or conveys nuance and affect (Joanette, Goulet, and Hannequin, 1990; Baum and Pell, 1999). Evidence is mixed on the occurrence and nature of prosodic problems in right hemisphere damage. Speech prosody is most commonly described as flat, but by contrast may be characterized by an abnormally high fundamental frequency and variability (Colsher, Cooper, and Graff-Radford, 1987). Dysarthrias often may be a source of spoken prosodic impairment (Wertz et al., 1998). Prosodic interpretation difficulties largely may be due to perceptual deficits, apart from the linguistic or emotional characteristics of a message (Tompkins and Flowers, 1985; Joanette, Goulet, and Hannequin, 1990). Some prosodic production and comprehension difficulties also may stem from more general emotional processing deficits (Van Lancker and Pachana, 1998).

Prosodic expression and comprehension deficits can be dissociated, and Ross (1981) proposed a taxonomy for prosodic impairments, relating them to right hemisphere lesion site. However, the proposed functional-anatomical correlations have not been substantiated in other research (e.g., Wertz et al., 1998), and the neurological correlates of prosodic disruption are more complex than Ross's framework suggests (Baum and Pell, 1999; Joanette, Goulet, and Hannequin, 1990).

Related Emotional and Nonverbal Processing Deficits. Emotional processing deficits also are a hallmark of right hemisphere damage (Van Lancker and Pachana, 1998), potentially contributing to difficulties with social exchange. Adults with right frontal lesions may be emotionally disinhibited, while those with more posterior damage may minimize and rationalize their deficits. Many adults with right hemisphere damage demonstrate reduced nonverbal animation and coverbal behaviors (Blonder et al., 1993). Some exhibit emotional interpretation deficits across modalities (pictures, body language, facial and vocal expressions, and complex discourse). Hypoarousal can occur in the presence of emotional stimuli, though not necessarily with impaired emotional recognition (Zoccolotti, Scabini, and Violani, 1982). Some work suggests problems in the way adults with right hemisphere damage apply a relatively intact appreciation of emotional material. For example, individuals with right hemisphere damage may do well inferring the affect conveyed by sentences that describe emotional situations (Tompkins and Flowers, 1985) but falter when required to match emotional inferences with specific stimulus representations or settings (Cicone, Wapner, and Gardner, 1980). Emotional misinterpretation also may reflect problems appreciating the visuospatial and acoustic/prosodic stimuli in which emotional messages are embedded.

Lexical-Semantic Processing. Right hemisphere damage is not usually considered to impair lexical structure, but it has been shown to diminish performance on tasks that involve lexical-semantic processing, such as picture naming, word-picture matching, word generation, and semantic judgment. These findings have been taken to indicate a general, subtle, but specific deficit in lexical-semantic processing (e.g., Gainotti et al., 1983). However, visual-perceptual problems could account for difficulties in many such tasks. Additionally, semantic priming studies indicate no lexical-semantic processing deficit after right hemisphere damage, under either automatic or controlled activation (Joanette and Goulet, 1998; Tompkins, Fassbinder, et al., 2002). This suggests that right hemisphere damage does not affect representation and initial activation processes in the lexical-semantic system (although currently it is not possible to rule out slowed initial processing). Because clear difficulties are evident only on metalinguistic tasks that obscure lexical-semantic operations per se, the "lexical-semantic deficits" of right hemisphere damage could reflect difficulties with other specific task requirements or more general attentional or working memory limitations (Joanette and Goulet, 1998; Tompkins, Fassbinder, et al., 2002).

Adults with right hemisphere damage also can have difficulty making semantic judgments about words with metaphorical or emotional content. Thus, some investigators have suggested that right hemisphere damage impairs specific semantic domains. A prominent account of difficulties with metaphorical meanings was derived from studies of hemispheric differences in non-brain-damaged individuals. This work suggests that as words are processed for comprehension, the right hemisphere is solely responsible for maintaining activation of a rather diffuse network of peripheral or secondary interpretations and remote associates of those words. This broad-based lexical-semantic activation is proposed to underpin figurative language interpretation, among other comprehension abilities (e.g., Beeman, 1998). By extrapolation, right hemisphere damage is assumed to impair the maintenance of weak associates and secondary meanings, making, for example, metaphorical interpretations unavailable. Contrary to this proposal, however, adults with right hemisphere lesions evince both initial, automatic priming and prolonged priming of metaphorical meanings of words (i.e., 1000 ms after hearing the word; Tompkins, 1990). Again, difficulties do not occur on implicit tasks with minimal strategic processing demands; thus, factors related to processing capacity and processing load cannot be excluded as the source of domain-specific deficits for metaphorical words in adults with right hemisphere damage (Joanette and Goulet, 1998; Tompkins, Fassbinder, et al., 2002). The processing of emotional words has not been investigated with implicit methods, so the influences of processing demands cannot be evaluated at present.

Discourse and Conversation. A growing literature suggests possible impairments of building, extracting, applying, or manipulating the mental structures that guide discourse processing after right hemisphere damage (Beeman, 1998; Tompkins, Fassbinder, et al., 2002). Again, contrasting findings abound (Tompkins, 1995). For example, although the output of adults with right hemisphere damage most often is described as verbose, digressive, and lacking in informative content, some produce a paucity of spoken discourse (Myers, 1999). Deficits in organizing and integrating elements of discourse structure may be evident as well. As with the lexical-semantic investigations, confounds introduced by typically metalinguistic assessment tasks (Tompkins and Baumgaertner, 1998) create difficulties for interpreting much of the literature on discourse in adults with right hemisphere lesions.

Discourse production often is investigated in terms of conversational pragmatics. In the few available studies, heterogeneity again is the rule, with some participants with right hemisphere damage displaying no deficits. Adults with right hemisphere damage most often are reported to have difficulties with eye contact and some, but not all, turn-taking parameters (Prutting and Kirchner, 1987; Kennedy et al., 1994). Idiosyncratic and ambiguous reference, poor re-use of common referents, and excessive attention to peripheral details also may occur (Chantraine, Joanette, and Ska, 1998).

Discourse comprehension problems are especially evident when adults with right hemisphere damage must reconcile multiple, seemingly incongruent inferences. They have particular problems with messages that induce conflicting interpretations, such those that contain ambiguities or violate canonical expectations. As summarized by Tompkins, Fassbinder, et al. (2002), inference generation per se is not a primary interpretive roadblock. Rather, difficulties appear to involve integration processes that are needed to revise or repair erroneous interpretations that were activated by such messages. Relatedly, adults with right hemisphere damage can have difficulty synthesizing their mental representations of stimulus elements and stimulus contexts in order to determine nonliteral intent, as expressed in jokes, idioms, indirect requests, connotative meanings of words, and conversational irony. Again, right hemisphere damage does not clearly affect the representation or activation of such nonliteral meanings, and adults with right-sided lesions can represent relevant elements of stimulus contexts in nonliteral processing tasks (see Tompkins, Fassbinder, et al., 2002). Finally, adults with right hemisphere damage may perform poorly on tasks that require reasoning from a "theory of mind," which involves an understanding of the ways in which knowledge, beliefs, and motivations guide behavior. Once again, these difficulties cannot be attributed to a failure to understand or represent individual elements of comprehension scenarios (Winner et al., 1998). Overall, for these deficit areas, impaired performance by adults with right-sided lesions is evident in conditions of relatively high processing demand.

There are several emerging accounts of difficulties experienced by adults with right hemisphere damage in constructing coherent, integrated mental structures that support discourse production and comprehension. Brownell and Martino (1998) implicate problems with "self-directed inference" (p. 325), which refers to comprehenders' efforts to discover and elaborate an interpretive framework when overlearned interpretive routines are inadequate. Reasoning from a theory of mind also is gaining popularity as an explanatory construct (Brownell and Martino, 1998). Another prominent hypothesis derives from characterization of the normal right hemisphere's "coarse semantic coding" properties (Beeman, 1998, p. 255), or the broad-based activation of diffuse, peripheral, and secondary meanings of words. Damage to the right hemisphere presumably creates difficulty in activating and/or maintaining the distant associates and subordinate meanings on which connotative interpretations, various inferences, and some discourse integration processes rely. However, Tompkins and colleagues (2000, 2001) demonstrated that adults with right hemisphere damage activate multiple meanings of lexical and inferential ambiguities, and that abnormally prolonged activation of contextually incompatible interpretations predicts aspects of discourse comprehension after right hemisphere lesions. These authors propose that right hemisphere damage may impair a comprehension mechanism by which contextually incompatible interpretations are suppressed, and they argue that this "suppression deficit" account accommodates a variety of other existing data. The suppression deficit and maintenance deficit views may be reconcilable by considering within-hemisphere site of lesion, a possibility currently under investigation (Tompkins, 2002). More generally, Stemmer and Joanette (1998) suggest that discourse deficits in individuals with right-sided lesions reflect difficulty with constructing and integrating new conceptual models. In a different vein, Brownell and Martino (1998) maintain that many impairments associated with right hemisphere damage stem from a social disconnection or diminished interest in people. Finally, because the expression of deficits in various domains seems to be moderated by processing abilities and demands, factors related to processing capacity and processing load need to be considered in a full account of impairments and skills in individuals with right hemisphere damage (Tompkins, Blake, et al., 2002; Tompkins, Fassbinder, et al., 2002).

Impact and Management

The cognitive and behavioral problems of adults with right hemisphere lesions can interfere with judgment and social skills, family relationships, functional living activities, and the potential to return to productive work (Klonoff et al., 1990; Tompkins et al., 1998). Clinical management typically is symptom driven, although various authors emphasize the value of a theoretically oriented approach (Tompkins, 1995; Myers, 1999). Treatment that focuses on the remediation of deficits may miss the bigger picture, in which therapeutic benefit is assessed in terms of its effects on daily life activities and psychosocial functioning (Tompkins et al., 1998; Tompkins, Fassbinder, et al., 2002). Treatment research is urgently needed for this population.

See also DISCOURSE IMPAIRMENTS; PROSIDIC DEFICITS.

—Connie A. Tompkins and Wiltrud Fassbinder

References

Baum, S. R., and Pell, M. D. (1999). The neural bases of prosody: Insights from lesion studies and neuroimaging. Aphasiology, 13, 581–608.

Beeman, M. (1998). Coarse semantic coding and discourse comprehension. In M. Beeman and C. Chiarello (Eds.), Right hemisphere language comprehension: Perspectives from cognitive neuroscience (pp. 255–284). Mahwah, NJ: Erlbaum.

Blake, M., Duffy, J. R., Myers, P. S., and Tompkins, C. A. (2002). Prevalence and patterns of right hemisphere cognitive/communicative deficits: Retrospective data from an inpatient rehabilitation unit. Aphasiology, 16, 537–547.

Blonder, L. X., Burns, A. F., Bowers, D., Moore, R. W., and Heilman, K. M. (1993). Right hemisphere facial expressivity during natural conversation. Brain and Cognition, 21, 44–56.

Brownell, H., and Martino, G. (1998). Deficits in inference and social cognition: The effects of right hemisphere brain damage on discourse. In M. Beeman and C. Chiarello (Eds.), Right hemisphere language comprehension: Perspectives from cognitive neuroscience (pp. 309–328). Mahwah, NJ: Erlbaum.

Chantraine, Y., Joanette, Y., and Ska, B. (1998). Conversational abilities in patients with right hemisphere damage. Journal of Neurolinguistics, 11, 21–32.

Cicone, M., Wapner, W., and Gardner, H. (1980). Sensitivity to emotional expressions and situations in organic patients. Cortex, 16, 145–158.

Colsher, P. L., Cooper, W. E., and Graff-Radford, N. (1987). Intonational variability in the speech of right-hemisphere damaged patients. Brain and Language, 32, 379–383.

Gainotti, G., Caltagirone, C., Miceli, G., and Masullo, C. (1983). Selective impairment of semantic-lexical discrimination in right-brain-damaged patients. In E. Perecman (Ed.), Cognitive processing in the right hemisphere (pp. 149–167). New York: Academic Press.

Joanette, Y., and Goulet, P. (1998). Right hemisphere and the semantic processing of words: Is the contribution specific or not? In E. G. Visch-Brink and R. Batiaanse (Eds.), Linguistic levels in aphasiology (pp. 19–34). San Diego, CA: Singular Publishing Group.

Joanette, Y., Goulet, P., and Hannequin, D. (1990). Right hemisphere and verbal communication. New York: Springer-Verlag.

Kennedy, M., Strand, E., Burton, W., and Peterson, C. (1994). Analysis of first-encounter conversations of right-hemisphere-damaged adults. Clinical Aphasiology, 22, 67–80.

Klonoff, P. S., Sheperd, J. C., O'Brien, K. P., Chiapello, D. A., and Hodak, J. A. (1990). Rehabilitation and outcome of right-hemisphere stroke patients: Challenges to traditional diagnostic and treatment methods. Neuropsychology, 4, 147–163.

Myers, P. S. (1999). Right hemisphere damage: Disorders of communication and cognition. San Diego, CA: Singular Publishing Group.

Prutting, C. A., and Kirchner, D. M. (1987). A clinical appraisal of the pragmatic aspects of language. Journal of Speech and Hearing Disorders, 52, 105–119.

Ross, E. D. (1981). The aprosodias: Functional-anatomic organization of the affective components of language in the right hemisphere. Archives of Neurology, 38, 561–569.

Stemmer, B., and Joanette, Y. (1998). The interpretation of narrative discourse of brain-damaged individuals within the framework of a multilevel discourse model. In M. Beeman and C. Chiarello (Eds.), Right hemisphere language comprehension: Perspectives from cognitive neuroscience (pp. 329–348). Mahwah, NJ: Erlbaum.

Tompkins, C. A. (1990). Knowledge and strategies for processing lexical metaphor after right or left hemisphere brain damage. Journal of Speech and Hearing Research, 33, 307–316.

Tompkins, C. A. (1995). Right hemisphere communication disorders: Theory and management. San Diego, CA: Singular Publishing Group.

Tompkins, C. A. (2002). Comprehension impairment and right brain damage. Grant funded by the National Institutes of Health: National Institute on Deafness and Other Communicative Disorders (DC01820).

Tompkins, C. A., and Baumgaertner, A. (1998). Clinical value of online measures for adults with right hemisphere brain damage. American Journal of Speech-Language Pathology, 7, 68–74.

Tompkins, C. A., Baumgaertner, A., Lehman, M. T., and Fassbinder, W. (2000). Mechanisms of discourse comprehension impairment after right hemisphere brain damage: Suppression in lexical ambiguity resolution. Journal of Speech, Language, and Hearing Research, 43, 62–78.

Tompkins, C. A., Blake, M. L., Baumgaertner, A., and Fassbinder, W. (2002). Characterizing comprehension difficulties after right brain damage: Attentional demands of suppression function. Aphasiology, 16, 559–572.

Tompkins, C. A., Fassbinder, W., Lehman-Blake, M. T., and Baumgaertner, A. (2002). The nature and implications of right hemisphere language disorders: Issues in search of answers. In A. Hillis (Ed.), *Handbook of adult language disorders: Integrating cognitive neuropsychology, neurology, and rehabilitation* (pp. 429–448). Philadelphia: Psychology Press.

Tompkins, C. A., and Flowers, C. R. (1985). Perception of emotional intonation by brain-damaged adults: The influence of task processing levels. *Journal of Speech and Hearing Research, 28,* 527–538.

Tompkins, C. A., and Lehman, M. T. (1998). Interpreting intended meanings after right hemisphere brain damage: An analysis of evidence, potential accounts, and clinical implications. *Topics in Stroke Rehabilitation, 5,* 29–47.

Tompkins, C. A., Lehman-Blake, M. T., Baumgaertner, A., and Fassbinder, W. (2001). Mechanisms of discourse comprehension impairment after right hemisphere brain damage: Suppression in inferential ambiguity resolution. *Journal of Speech, Language, and Hearing Research, 44,* 400–415.

Tompkins, C. A., Lehman, M. T., Wyatt, A., and Schulz, R. (1998). Functional outcome assessment of adults with right hemisphere brain damage. *Seminars in Speech and Language, 19,* 303–321.

Van Lancker, D., and Pachana, N. A. (1998). The influence of emotion on language and communication disorders. In B. Stemmer and H. A. Whitaker (Eds.), *Handbook of neurolinguistics* (pp. 301–311). San Diego, CA: Academic Press.

Wertz, R. T., Henschel, C. R., Auther, L. L., Ashford, J. R., and Kirshner, H. S. (1998). Affective prosodic disturbance subsequent to right hemisphere stroke: A clinical application. *Journal of Neurolinguistics, 11,* 89–102.

Winner, E., Brownell, H. H., Happe, F., Blum, A., and Pincus, D. (1998). Distinguishing lies from jokes: Theory of mind deficits and discourse interpretation in right hemisphere brain-damaged patients. *Brain and Language, 62,* 89–106.

Zoccolotti, P., Scabini, D., and Violani, C. (1982). Electrodermal responses in patients with unilateral brain damage. *Journal of Clinical Neuropsychology, 4,* 143–150.

Further Readings

Ardila, A., and Rosselli, M. (1993). Spatial agraphia. *Brain and Cognition, 22,* 137–147.

Beeman, M., and Chiarello, C. (1998). *Right hemisphere language comprehension: Perspectives from cognitive neuroscience.* Mahwah, NJ: Erlbaum.

Bihrle, A., Brownell, H. H., and Gardner, H. (1988). Humor and the right hemisphere: A narrative perspective. In H. A. Whitaker (Ed.), *Contemporary reviews in neuropsychology* (pp. 109–126). New York: Springer-Verlag.

Blonder, L. X., Bowers, D., and Heilman, K. M. (1991). The role of the right hemisphere in emotional communication. *Brain, 114,* 1115–1127.

Borod, J. C., Cicero, B. A., Obler, L. K., Welkowitz, J., Ehran, H. M., Santschi, C., et al. (1998). Right hemisphere emotional perception: Evidence across multiple channels. *Neuropsychology, 12,* 446–458.

Chiarello, C. (1998). On codes of meaning and the meaning of codes: Semantic access and retrieval within and between hemispheres. In M. Beeman and C. Chiarello (Eds.), *Right hemisphere language comprehension: Perspectives from cognitive neuroscience* (pp. 141–160). Mahwah, NJ: Erlbaum.

Cooper, W. E., and Klouda, G. V. (1987). Intonation in aphasic and right-hemisphere-damaged patients. In J. H. Ryalls (Ed.), *Phonetic approaches to speech production in*

aphasia and related disorders (pp. 59–77). Boston: Little, Brown.

Duffy, J. R., and Myers, P. S. (1991). Group comparisons across neurologic communication disorders: Some methodological issues. In T. E. Prescott (Ed.), *Clinical aphasiology* (pp. 1–14). Austin, TX: Pro-Ed.

Joanette, Y., and Ansaldo, A. I. (1999). Clinical note: Acquired pragmatic impairments and aphasia. *Brain and Language, 68,* 529–534.

Joanette, Y., and Goulet, P. (1990). Narrative discourse in right-brain-damaged right-handers. In Y. Joanette and H. H. Brownell (Eds.), *Discourse ability and brain-damage: Theoretical and empirical perspectives* (pp. 131–153). New York: Springer-Verlag.

Joanette, Y., and Goulet, P. (1994). Right hemisphere and verbal communication: Conceptual, methodological, and clinical issues. In M. Lemme (Ed.), *Clinical aphasiology* (pp. 1–24). Austin, TX: Pro-Ed.

Kennedy, M. R. T. (2000). Topic scenes in conversations with adults with right-hemisphere brain damage. *American Journal of Speech-Language Pathology, 9,* 72–86.

Kent, R. D., and Rosenbek, J. C. (1982). Prosodic disturbance and neurological lesion. *Brain and Language, 15,* 259–291.

Lehman-Blake, M. T., and Tompkins, C. A. (2001). Predictive inferencing in adults with right hemisphere brain damage. *Journal of Speech, Language, and Hearing Research, 44,* 639–654.

Lojek-Osiejuk, E. (1996). Knowledge of scripts reflected in discourse of aphasics and right-brain-damaged patients. *Brain and Language, 29,* 68–80.

Myers, P. S. (2001). Toward a definition of RHD syndrome. *Aphasiology, 15,* 913–918.

Myers, P. S., and Brookshire, R. H. (1996). Effect of visual and inferential variables on scene descriptions by right-hemisphere-damaged and non-brain-damaged adults. *Journal of Speech and Hearing Research, 39,* 870–880.

Stemmer, B., Giroux, F., and Joanette, Y. (1994). Production and evaluation of requests by right-hemisphere brain-damaged individuals. *Brain and Language, 47,* 1–31.

Tompkins, C. A., Bloise, C. G. R., Timko, M. L., and Baumgaertner, A. (1994). Working memory and inference revision in brain-damaged and normally aging adults. *Journal of Speech and Hearing Research, 37,* 896–912.

Tompkins, C. A., Boada, R., and McGarry, K. (1992). The access and processing of familiar idioms by brain-damaged and normally aging adults. *Journal of Speech and Hearing Research, 35,* 626–637.

Trupe, E. H., and Hillis, A. (1985). Paucity vs. verbosity: Another analysis of right hemisphere communication deficits. In R. H. Brookshire (Ed.), *Clinical aphasiology* (pp. 83–96). Minneapolis: BRK.

Segmentation of Spoken Language by Normal Adult Listeners

Listening to spoken language usually seems effortless, but the processes involved are complex. A continuous acoustic signal must be translated into meaning so that the listener can understand the speaker's intent. The mapping of sound to meaning proceeds via the lexicon—our store of known words. Any utterance we hear may be novel to us, but the words it contains are familiar, and to understand the utterance we must therefore identify the words of which it is composed.

We know a great many words; an educated adult's vocabulary has been estimated at around 150,000 words. Entries in the mental lexicon may include, besides stand-alone words, grammatical morphemes such as prefixes and suffixes and multiword phrases such as idioms and cliches. Languages also differ widely in how they construct word forms, and this too will affect what is stored in the lexicon. But in any language, listening involves mapping the acoustic signal onto stored meanings.

The continuity of utterances means that boundaries between individual words in speech are not overtly marked. Speakers do not pause between words but run them into one another. The problem of segmenting a speech signal into words is compounded by the fact that words themselves are not highly distinctive. All the words we know are constructed of just a handful of different sounds; on average, the phonetic repertoire of a language contains 30–40 contrasting sounds (Maddieson, 1984). As a consequence, words inevitably resemble other words, and may have other words embedded within them (thus *strange* contains *stray, strain, train, rain*, and *range*). Word recognition therefore involves identifying the correct form among a large number of similar forms, in a stream in which they abut one another without a break (*strange act* contains *jack* and *jacked*).

The only segmentation that is logically required is to find the words in speech. Whether listening also involves some intermediate level of coding is an issue of contention among speech researchers. Do listeners extract whole syllables from the speech stream and use this syllabic representation to contact the lexicon? Do they extract phonemes from the input, so that listening involves an intermediate stage in which heard utterances are represented as strings of phonemes? Or does listening involve matching speech input against holistic stored forms? The available evidence does not yet allow us to distinguish among these positions (and other variants).

There is agreement, however, on other aspects of the spoken-word recognition process. First, information in the signal is evaluated continuously and the results are passed to the lexicon. Coarticulatory effects that cause cues to adjacent phonemes to overlap in time are efficiently used. Thus *robe, rope, wrote, road*, and *rogue* all begin with *ro-*, but the vowel will in each case include anticipatory information about the place of articulation of the following consonant, and listeners can exploit this (e.g., to narrow the field of candidates to only *rope* and *robe*, eliminating *rogue, road*, and *wrote*).

Evidence for continuous evaluation comes from experiments in which listeners perform lexical decision (judging whether a spoken string is indeed a real word) on speech that has been cross-spliced so that the coarticulatory effects are no longer reliable. Thus, when listeners hear *troot* they should respond "no"—*troot* is not a word. If *troot* is cross-spliced so that a final *-t* is appended to a *troo-* from either *trook* or *troop* (which give coarticulatory cues to an upcoming velar or bilabial

consonant, respectively), then responses are slower than if the cues match. This shows that listeners are sensitive to the coarticulatory mismatch and must have processed the consonant place cues in the vowel. However, the responses are still slower when the mismatching *troo-* comes from *troop* than when it comes from *trook*. This suggests that the processing of consonant cues in the vowel has caused activation of the existing compatible real-word *troop* (Marslen-Wilson and Warren, 1994; McQueen, Norris, and Cutler, 1999).

Second, multiple candidate words are simultaneously activated during the listening process, including words that are merely accidentally present in a speech signal. Thus, hearing *strange-acting* may activate *stray, train, range, jack*, and so on, as well as the intended words.

Evidence for multiple activation comes from cross-modal priming experiments in which a word-initial fragment facilitates recognition of different words that it might become. Thus, lexical decision responses for visually presented "captain" or "captive" are both facilitated when listeners have just heard the fragment *capt-* (compared with some other control fragment). Moreover, both are facilitated even if only one of them matches the context (Zwitserlood, 1989).

Third, there is active competition between alternative candidate words. The more active a candidate word is, the more it may suppress its rivals, and the more competitors a word has, the more suppression it may undergo. Evidence for competition between simultaneously activated candidate words comes from experiments in which listeners must spot any real words occurring in spoken nonsense strings. If the rest of the string partially activates a competitor word, then spotting the real embedded word is slowed. For instance, listeners spot *mess* less rapidly in *domess* (which partially activates *domestic*, a competitor for the same portion of the signal that supports *mess*) than in *nemess* (which supports no other word; McQueen, Norris, and Cutler, 1994; see also Norris, McQueen, and Cutler, 1995; Vroomen and de Gelder, 1995; Soto-Faraco, Sebastián-Gallés, and Cutler, 2001).

Because activated and competing words need not be aligned with one another, the competition process offers a potential means of segmenting the utterance. Thus, although recognition of *strange-acting* may involve competition from *stray, range, jack*, and so on, this will eventually yield to joint inhibition from the two intended words, which receive greater support from the signal.

Adult listeners can also use information which their linguistic experience suggests to be correlated with the presence of a word boundary. For instance, in English the phoneme sequence [mg] never occurs word-internally, so the occurrence of this sequence must imply a word boundary (*some go, tame goose*); sequences such as [pf] or [ml] or [zw] never occur syllable-internally, so this sequence implies at least a syllable boundary (*cupful, seemly, beeswax*). Listeners more rapidly spot embedded words whose edges are aligned with such a boundary-correlated sequence (e.g., *rock* is spotted more easily in *foomrock* than in *foogrock*; McQueen, 1998). Also, words that begin with a common phoneme sequence are easier to extract from a preceding context than words that begin with an infrequent sequence (e.g., in *golnook* versus *golnag*, it will be easier to spot *nag*, which shares its beginning with *natural, navigate, narrow, nap*, and many other words; van der Lugt, 2001; see also Cairns et al., 1997).

These latter sources of information are, of course, necessarily language-specific. It is a characteristic of a particular vocabulary that more words begin with the *na-* of *nag* than with the *noo-* of *nook*; likewise, it is vocabulary-specific that sequences such as [pf] or [zw] or [ml] cannot occur within a syllable. Each of these three sequences is in fact legitimately syllable-internal in some language ([pf], for instance, in German: *Pferd, Kopf*).

Other language-specific information is also used in segmentation, notably rhythmic structure. In languages such as English and Dutch, most words begin with stressed syllables, and listeners find it easier to segment speech at the onset of stressed syllables (Cutler and Norris, 1988; Vroomen, van Zon, and de Gelder, 1996). This can be clearly seen in segmentation errors, as when a pop song line *She's a must to avoid* is widely misperceived as *She's a muscular boy*—the strong syllable *void* is taken to be the onset of a new word, while the weak syllables *to* and *a-* are taken to be noninitial (Cutler and Butterfield, 1992).

The stress rhythm of English and Dutch is not universal; many other languages have different rhythmic structures. Indeed, syllabically based rhythm in French is accompanied by syllabic segmentation in French listening experiments (Mehler et al., 1981; Cutler et al., 1986; Kolinsky, Morais, and Cluytens, 1995), while moraic rhythm in Japanese likewise accompanies moraic segmentation by Japanese listeners (Otake et al., 1993; Cutler and Otake, 1994).

Thus, although the type of rhythm is language-specific, its use in speech segmentation seems universal. Other universal constraints on segmentation exist, for example, to limit activation of spurious embedded competitors. It is harder to spot a word if the residual context contains only consonants (thus, *apple* is harder to find in *fapple* than in *vuffapple*; Norris et al., 1997), an effect explained as a primitive filter selecting for possible words—*vuff* is not a word, but it might have been one, while *f* could never be a word. This constraint would operate to rule out many spuriously present words in speech (such as *tray* and *ray* in *stray*). It is not affected by what may be a word in a particular language (Norris et al., 2001; Cutler, Demuth, and McQueen, 2002) and thus appears to be universal.

The ability to extract words from continuous speech starts early in life, as shown by experiments in which infants listen longer to passages containing words that they had previously heard in isolation than to wholly new passages (Jusczyk and Aslin, 1995); none of the passages can be comprehended by these young listeners, but they can recognize familiar strings embedded in the fluent speech. One-year-olds also detect familiar strings less easily if they are embedded in a context without a vowel (e.g., *rest* is found less easily in *crest* than in

caressed; Johnson et al., 2003); that is, they are already sensitive to the apparently universal constraint on possible words.

Finally, segmentation of second languages in later life is not aided by the efficiency with which listeners exploit language-specific structure in recognizing speech. Segmentation procedures suitable for the native language can be inappropriately applied to non-native input (Cutler et al., 1986; Otake et al., 1993; Cutler and Otake, 1994; Weber, 2001). This is one effect making listening to a second language paradoxically harder than, for instance, reading the same language.

See also PHONOLOGY AND ADULT APHASIA.

—Anne Cutler

References

Cairns, P., Shillcock, R., Chater, N., and Levy, J. (1997). Bootstrapping word boundaries: A bottom-up corpus-based approach to speech segmentation. *Cognitive Psychology, 33*, 111–153.

Cutler, A., and Butterfield, S. (1992). Rhythmic cues to speech segmentation: Evidence from juncture misperception. *Journal of Memory and Language, 31*, 218–236.

Cutler, A., Demuth, K., and McQueen, J. M. (2002). Universality versus language-specificity in listening to running speech. *Psychological Science, 13*, 258–262.

Cutler, A., Mehler, J., Norris, D., and Seguí, J. (1986). The syllable's differing role in the segmentation of French and English. *Journal of Memory and Language, 25*, 385–400.

Cutler, A., and Norris, D. (1988). The role of strong syllables in segmentation for lexical access. *Journal of Experimental Psychology: Human Perception and Performance, 14*, 113–121.

Cutler, A., and Otake, T. (1994). Mora or phoneme? Further evidence for language-specific listening. *Journal of Memory and Language, 33*, 824–844.

Johnson, E. K., Jusczyk, P. W., Cutler, A., and Norris, D. (2003). Lexical viability constraints on speech segmentation by infants without a lexicon. *Cognitive Psychology, 46*, 65–97.

Jusczyk, P. W., and Aslin, R. N. (1995). Infants' detection of sound patterns of words in fluent speech. *Cognitive Psychology, 29*, 1–23.

Kolinksy, R., Morais, J., and Cluytens, M. (1995). Intermediate representations in spoken word recognition: Evidence from word illusions. *Journal of Memory and Language, 34*, 19–40.

Maddieson, I. (1984). *Patterns of sounds*. Cambridge, U.K.: Cambridge University Press.

Marslen-Wilson, W. D., and Warren, P. (1994). Levels of perceptual representation and process in lexical access: Words, phonemes, and features. *Psychological Review, 101*, 653–675.

McQueen, J. (1998). Segmentation of continuous speech using phonotactics. *Journal of Memory and Language, 39*, 21–46.

McQueen, J. M., Norris, D., and Cutler, A. (1994). Competition in spoken word recognition: Spotting words in other words. *Journal of Experimental Psychology: Learning, Memory and Cognition, 20*, 621–638.

McQueen, J. M., Norris, D., and Cutler, A. (1999). Lexical influence in phonetic decision making: Evidence from subcategorical mismatches. *Journal of Experimental Psychology: Human Perception and Performance, 25*, 1363–1389.

Mehler, J., Dommergues, J.-Y., Frauenfelder, U. H., and Seguí, J. (1981). The syllable's role in speech segmentation. *Journal of Verbal Learning and Verbal Behavior, 20,* 298–305.

Norris, D., McQueen, J. M., and Cutler, A. (1995). Competition and segmentation in spoken word recognition. *Journal of Experimental Psychology: Learning, Memory and Cognition, 21,* 1209–1228.

Norris, D., McQueen, J. M., Cutler, A., and Butterfield, S. (1997). The possible-word constraint in the segmentation of continuous speech. *Cognitive Psychology, 34,* 191–243.

Norris, D., McQueen, J. M., Cutler, A., Butterfield, S., and Kearns, R. (2001). Language-universal constraints on speech segmentation. *Language and Cognitive Processes, 16,* 637–660.

Otake, T., Hatano, G., Cutler, A., and Mehler, J. (1993). Mora or syllable? Speech segmentation in Japanese. *Journal of Memory and Language, 32,* 258–278.

Soto-Faraco, S., Sebastián-Gallés, N., and Cutler, A. (2001). Segmental and suprasegmental mismatch in lexical access. *Journal of Memory and Language, 45,* 412–432.

van der Lugt, A. (2001). The use of sequential probabilities in the segmentation of speech. *Perception and Psychophysics, 63,* 811–823.

Vroomen, J., and de Gelder, B. (1995). Metrical segmentation and lexical inhibition in spoken word recognition. *Journal of Experimental Psychology: Human Perception and Performance, 21,* 98–108.

Vroomen, J., van Zon, M., and de Gelder, B. (1996). Cues to speech segmentation: Evidence from juncture misperceptions and word spotting. *Memory and Cognition, 24,* 744–755.

Weber, A. (2001). *Language-specific listening: The case of phonetic sequences.* Doctoral dissertation, University of Nijmegen, The Netherlands.

Zwitserlood, P. (1989). The locus of the effects of sentential-semantic context in spoken-word processing. *Cognition, 32,* 25–64.

Further Readings

Cutler, A., and Clifton, C. E. (1999). Comprehending spoken language: A blueprint of the listener. In C. Brown and P. Hagoort (Eds.), *Neurocognition of language* (pp. 123–166). Oxford: Oxford University Press.

Frauenfelder, U. H., and Floccia, C. (1998). The recognition of spoken words. In A. Friederici (Ed.), *Language comprehension, a biological perspective* (pp. 1–40). Heidelberg: Springer-Verlag.

Grosjean, F., and Frauenfelder, U. H. (Eds.). (1997). *Spoken word recognition paradigms.* Hove, U.K.: Psychology Press.

Jusczyk, P. W. (1997). *The discovery of spoken language.* Cambridge, MA: MIT Press.

McQueen, J. M., and Cutler, A. (Eds.). (2001). *Spoken word access processes.* Hove, U.K.: Psychology Press.

Semantics

The term *semantics* refers to linguistic meaning. Semantic development involves mapping linguistic forms onto our mental models of the world and organizing these maps into networks of related information. Semantic processing involves the comprehension and production of meaning as conveyed by linguistic forms, their combinations, and the nonlinguistic contexts in which they occur.

In this article, semantic development in selected populations of children with language disorders is described via intralinguistic referencing. Included are summaries of deficits in semantic processing that characterize each population as a whole, at early and later points in development.

Early Semantic Development in Children with Developmental Language Disorders

Children with autism or other pervasive developmental disorders (PDDs) typically demonstrate semantic systems that are weak relative to the formal systems of syntax, morphology, and phonology. This weakness is manifested as use of words without regard to conventional meaning, context-bound extensions of word meaning, and confusion regarding the mapping of personal pronouns onto their referents. Social and cognitive deficits are thought to contribute to this weakness. Whereas normally developing children readily make inferences about word meanings by reading social and contextual cues, such as the speaker's eye gaze and intentions, children with autism do not (Baron-Cohen, Baldwin, and Crowson, 1997). This failure is often viewed as part of a broader deficit in theory of mind. The theory of mind deficit is further reflected in a particular limitation of children with autism in the acquisition of words for cognitive states (Tager-Flusberg, 1992).

In SPECIFIC LANGUAGE IMPAIRMENT (SLI), semantics is generally a strength relative to the formal domains of MORPHOSYNTAX AND SYNTAX. However, children with SLI do demonstrate some semantic delay relative to their normal age-mates. For example, the appearance of first meaningful words is delayed an average of 11 months (Trauner et al., 1995). This delay is maintained throughout the early preschool years and is measurable with receptive vocabulary tests and experimental word-learning paradigms, which show that children with SLI are poor at fast mapping and long-term retention of words (Rice et al., 1994). Even when these children succeed at word mapping, the semantic elaboration of those words in the lexicon is sparser than age expectations would predict. This sparseness is associated with greater numbers of naming errors during picture naming (McGregor et al., 2002). In their spontaneous speech, these children exhibit less lexical diversity, especially verb diversity, than their normal age-mates (Watkins et al., 1995). Finally, for children with SLI, processing the subtle meanings carried by grammatical morphemes, derivational morphemes, and word order is particularly problematic (Bishop, 1997).

Short-term (working) memory deficits likely contribute to the delayed semantic development of children with SLI (Gathercole and Baddely, 1990). These deficits are associated with slower word learning, presumably because features of new words or their referents are not sufficiently represented in short-term memory to be committed to the long-term lexical store. Another possible contributor to weak lexical semantics is the limited ability of children with SLI to benefit from syntactic bootstrapping. On tasks requiring the acting out of unfamiliar verbs, children with SLI do not infer meanings from syntactic bootstrapping as well as their younger language-matched controls (van der Lely, 1994), or they require a great deal of processing effort to do so (O'Hara and Johnston, 1997).

Down syndrome is another condition in which intralinguistic referencing reveals semantics as a relative strength. In the Down syndrome population, receptive single-word vocabulary is unaffected in early childhood and may exceed nonverbal cognitive ability by adolescence (Chapman, 1995). However, children with Down syndrome demonstrate semantic delays relative to their normal (mental-age-matched) peers. Soon after the onset of first words, expressive vocabulary development begins to lag (Cardoso-Martins, Mervis, and Mervis, 1985). As children with Down syndrome learn to combine words into sentences, their expressive delays in lexical semantics relative to their MLU-matched peers are manifested as a lower rate of verb use per sentence (Hesketh and Chapman, 1998). As in SLI, children with Down syndrome have difficulty expressing meanings with grammatical morphemes and noncanonical word order (Kumin, Councill, and Goodman, 1998). Limited diversity of vocabulary is characteristic of their discourse (Chapman, 1995). Also, similar to children with autism, these children have difficulty expressing internal states; use of words to express volition, ability, or cognition is particularly compromised (Beeghly and Cicchetti, 1997).

The semantic delays of children with Down syndrome are multidetermined. Degree of mental retardation limits development of the semantic-conceptual system. Fluctuating mild to moderate hearing loss, which is highly prevalent in this population, also has some effect (see OTITIS MEDIA: EFFECTS ON CHILDREN'S LANGUAGE). Finally, as in SLI, limited short-term memory is thought to play a role (Chapman, 1995).

Early Semantic Development in Children with Acquired Language Disorders

In children who have acquired language disorders subsequent to unilateral focal lesions, intralinguistic profiles often vary according to location of the lesion in the brain. Children with right hemisphere lesions tend to have more pronounced deficits in semantics than in formal aspects of language; children with left hemisphere lesions demonstrate the reverse pattern (Eisele and Aram, 1994). This generalization is gross, and semantic involvement will vary across individuals. Overall, compared to their normal age-mates, children with unilateral lesions present with late onset of first words in both comprehension and production, with right-lesioned children having more significant comprehension deficits than left-lesioned children (Thal et al., 1991). In experimental word-learning studies, unilateral brain-lesioned children require more teaching trials than their normal peers to demonstrate comprehension (Keefe, Feldman,

and Holland, 1989). Also, these children have difficulty building semantic networks. For example, when asked to select two antonyms, synonyms, or class coordinates from lists of four words, both right- and left-lesioned schoolchildren made significantly more errors than their normal age-mates (Eisele and Aram, 1995). In spontaneous speech, their semantic deficits are manifested as low numbers and diversity of words (Feldman et al., 1992).

Type and extent of insult, as well as age at onset, influence semantic processing in children with acquired language disorders. In general, cognitive disorganization and poor long-term memory exacerbate semantic deficits in this population (Levin et al., 1982).

Later Semantic Development

Semantic weaknesses in older children and adolescents extend to the discourse level. In order to process discourse, children must integrate meanings across sentences (linguistic context) with regard to shared information, communicative goals, and the physical setting (nonlinguistic context). Not surprisingly, most individuals with language disorders, no matter their diagnostic category, have significant difficulties with semantics at the discourse level. Children with acquired language disorders have trouble recalling meaningful propositions from stories and, when producing stories, they have difficulty conjoining meaning across sentences via referential and lexical ties (Ewing-Cobbs et al., 1998). Children with developmental language disorders present with similar problems (Bishop and Adams, 1992). Processing the implicit meanings, abstract meanings, and nonliteral meanings characteristic of sophisticated discourse is also problematic for many children with either acquired or developmental language disorders. Some argue that a subgroup of children with developmental language disorders, who share certain characteristics of both SLI and PDD syndromes, have semantic-pragmatic disorders as their primary area of deficit. Such children are particularly deficient in all higher level semantic attainments (Rapin and Allen, 1983).

Semantic Development and Reading

Children with language impairments of both developmental and acquired types have a higher incidence of reading impairment than the general population (see LANGUAGE IMPAIRMENT AND READING DISABILITY). For example, roughly half of a group identified as having SLI at 5 years were reading-impaired at 15 years (Stothard et al., 1998). Part of this reading difficulty relates to weaknesses in semantics (poor phonological and grammatical processing also plays a role). These children may not have sufficient semantic representations on which to map orthography. Furthermore, they are less able to use semantic bootstrapping to infer the meaning of words in context (Snowling, 2000).

The developmental relation between lexical semantics and reading is reciprocal. Poor knowledge in the semantic domain contributes to poor reading, and poor reading exacerbates lags in semantic development. Children who have poor reading skills read fewer words over the course of a year and are less able to learn the words they do read than those who have good reading skills (Nagy and Anderson, 1984).

Children with hyperlexia, often viewed as a subgroup of the PDD spectrum, demonstrate a preoccupation with decoding written words to the exclusion of meaning. Word recognition skills in these children are reported to be as much as 7 years in advance of grade-level expectations, whereas reading comprehension is at or below grade level (Whitehouse and Harris, 1984). Such children demonstrate that form and meaning can be sharply divorced in developmental disorders.

Future Trends

Recent years brought improved methods for identifying lexical semantic deficits in children. Newly developed parent-report inventories provide valid estimates of the size of receptive lexicons in children functioning below the 16-month level and expressive lexicons in children functioning below the 30-month level (Fenson et al., 1993). For more skilled children, new ways of quantifying lexical-semantic abilities from discourse samples provide valid diagnostic indicators (Miller, 1996).

The near future promises a burgeoning interest in semantic development in children with language disorders. Increasingly, investigators, motivated by social interactionist and dynamical systems theories, are demonstrating that semantic ability is not a static collection of knowledge but a system that emerges from interactions among and between knowledge, context, and processing demands in real time. Aiding investigation of real-time semantic processing are new technologies and methods such as semantic priming, eye tracking, and event-related potentials. Aiding identification of semantic deficits is the inclusion of dynamic word-learning tasks in diagnostic batteries. When these sophisticated methods are widely employed, both the quality and the quantity of semantic representations in children affected by language impairments will receive increased attention.

—*Karla M. McGregor*

References

Baron-Cohen, S., Baldwin, D. A., and Crowson, M. (1997). Do children with autism use the speaker's direction of gaze strategy to crack the code of language? *Child Development*, *68*, 48–57.

Beeghly, M., and Cicchetti, D. (1997). Talking about self and other: Emergence of an internal state lexicon in young children with Down syndrome. *Development and Psychopathology*, *9*, 729–748.

Bishop, D. V. M. (1997). *Uncommon understanding: Development and disorders of language comprehension in children.* East Sussex, U.K.: Psychology Press.

Bishop, D. V. M., and Adams, C. (1992). Comprehension problems in children with specific language impairment: Literal and inferential meaning. *Journal of Speech and Hearing Research*, *35*, 119–129.

Cardoso-Martins, C., Mervis, C. B., and Mervis, C. A. (1985). Early vocabulary acquisition by children with Down syndrome. *American Journal of Mental Deficiency*, *90*, 177–184.

Chapman, R. S. (1995). Language development in children and adolescents with Down syndrome. In P. Fletcher and B. MacWhinney (Eds.), *Handbook of child language.* Oxford: Blackwell.

Eisele, J. A., and Aram, D. M. (1994). Differential effects of early hemisphere damage on lexical comprehension and production. *Aphasiology*, *7*, 513–523.

Ewing-Cobbs, L., Brookshire, B., Scott, M. A., and Fletcher, J. M. (1998). Children's narratives following traumatic brain injury: Linguistic structure, cohesion, and thematic recall. *Brain and Language*, *61*, 395–419.

Feldman, J. M., Holland, L., Kemp, S. S., and Janosky, J. E. (1992). Language development after unilateral brain injury. *Brain and Language*, *42*, 89–102.

Fenson, L., Dale, P., Reznick, S., Thal, D., Bates, E., Hartung, J., et al. (1993). *The Macarthur Communicative Development Inventories.* San Diego, CA: Singular Publishing Group.

Gathercole, S. E., and Baddeley, A. D. (1990). Phonological memory deficits in language disordered children: Is there a causal connection? *Journal of Memory and Language*, *29*, 336–360.

Hesketh, L. J., and Chapman, R. S. (1998). Verb use by individuals with Down syndrome. *American Journal on Mental Retardation*, *103*, 288–304.

Keefe, K. A., Feldman, H. M., and Holland, A. L. (1989). Lexical learning and language abilities in preschoolers with prenatal brain damage. *Journal of Speech and Hearing Disorders*, *54*, 395–402.

Kumin, L., Councill, C., and Goodman, M. (1998). Expressive vocabulary development in children with Down syndrome. *Down Syndrome Quarterly*, *3*, 1–7.

Levin, H., Eisenberg, H. M., Wigg, N. R., and Kobayashi, K. (1982). Memory and intellectual ability after head injury in children and adolescents. *Neurosurgery*, *11*, 668–673.

McGregor, K., Newman, R., Reilly, R., and Capone, N. (2002). Semantic representation and naming in children with specific language impairment. *Journal of Speech, Language, and Hearing Research*, *45*, 998–1014.

Miller, J. F. (1996). The search for the phenotype of disordered language performance. In M. L. Rice (Ed.), *Toward a genetics of language* (pp. 297–314). Mahwah, NJ: Erlbaum.

Nagy, W. E., and Anderson, R. C. (1984). How many words are there in printed school English? *Reading Research Quarterly*, *19*, 304–330.

O'Hara, M., and Johnston, J. (1997). Syntactic bootstrapping in children with specific language impairment. *European Journal of Disorders of Communication*, *32*, 147–164.

Rapin, I., and Allen, D. (1983). Developmental language disorders: Nosological considerations. In U. Kirk (Ed.), *Neuropsychology of language, reading, and spelling* (pp. 155–184). New York: Academic Press.

Rice, M., Oetting, J., Marquis, J., Bode, J., and Pae, S. (1994). Frequency of input effects on word comprehension of children with specific language impairment. *Journal of Speech and Hearing Research*, *37*, 106–122.

Snowling, M. J. (2000). Language and literacy skills: Who is at risk and why? In D. V. M. Bishop and L. B. Leonard (Eds.), *Speech and language impairments in children: Causes, characteristics, intervention and outcome* (pp. 245–259). Philadelphia: Psychology Press.

Stothard, S. E., Snowling, M. J., Bishop, D. V. M., Chipchase, B. B., and Kaplan, C. A. (1998). Language-impaired preschoolers: A follow-up into adolescence. *Journal of Speech, Language, and Hearing Research, 41,* 407–418.

Tager-Flusberg, H. (1992). Autistic children's talk about psychological states: Deficits in the early acquisition of a theory of mind. *Child Development, 63,* 161–172.

Thal, D. J., Marchman, V., Stiles, J., Aram, D., Trauner, D., Nass, R., et al. (1991). Early lexical development in children with focal brain injury. *Brain and Language, 40,* 491–527.

Trauner, D., Wulfeck, B., Tallal, P., and Hesselink, J. (1995). *Neurologic and MRI profiles of language impaired children* (Technical Report, Publication No. CND-9513). San Diego, CA: Center for Research in Language, UCSD.

Van der Lely, H. (1994). Canonical linking rules: Forward versus reverse linking in normally developing and specifically language-impaired children. *Cognition, 51,* 29–72.

Watkins, R. V., Kelly, D. J., Harbers, H. M., and Hollis, W. (1995). Measuring children's lexical diversity: Differentiating typical and impaired language learners. *Journal of Speech and Hearing Research, 38,* 1349–1355.

Whitehouse, D., and Harris, J. C. (1984). Hyperlexia in infantile autism. *Journal of Autism and Developmental Disorders, 14,* 281–289.

Further Readings

Bishop, D. V. M., and Adams, C. (1989). Conversational characteristics of children with semantic-pragmatic disorder: II. What features lead to a judgement of inappropriacy? *British Journal of Disorders of Communication, 24,* 241–263.

Bloom, P. (2000). *How children learn the meanings of words.* Cambridge, MA: MIT Press.

Chapman, R. S., Seung, J. K., Schwartz, S. E., and Kay-Raining Bird, E. (2000). Predicting language production in children and adolescents with Down syndrome: The role of comprehension. *Journal of Speech, Language, and Hearing Research, 43,* 340–350.

Dorman, C., and Katzir, B. (1994). *Cognitive effects of early brain injury.* Baltimore: Johns Hopkins University Press.

Dunn, M., Gomes, J., and Sebastian, M. J. (1996). Prototypicality of responses of autistic, language disordered, and normal children in a word fluency task. *Child Neuropsychology, 2,* 99–108.

Fletcher, P., and Peters, J. (1984). Characterizing language impairment in children: An exploratory study. *Language Testing, 1,* 33–49.

Frith, U. (1989). *Autism: Explaining the enigma.* Oxford: Blackwell.

Gathercole, S. E., and Baddeley, A. D. (1993). *Working memory and language.* Hillsdale, NJ: Erlbaum.

Hollich, G. J., Hirsh-Pasek, K., and Golinkoff, R. M. (2000). Breaking the language barrier: An emergentist coalition model for the origins of word learning. *Monographs of the Society for Research in Child Development, 65.*

Jordan, F. M. (1990). Speech and language disorders following childhood closed head injury. In B. E. Murdoch (Ed.), *Acquired neurological speech/language disorders in childhood* (pp. 124–147). London: Taylor and Francis.

Kail, R., and Leonard, L. B. (1986). Word-finding abilities in language-impaired children. *ASHA Monographs, 25.*

Kiernan, B., and Gray, S. (1998). Word learning in a supported-learning context by preschool children with specific language impairment. *Journal of Speech, Language, and Hearing Research, 41,* 161–171.

Lahey, M., and Edwards, J. (1999). Naming errors of children with specific language impairment. *Journal of Speech, Language, and Hearing Research, 42,* 195–205.

Leonard, L. B. (1998). *Children with specific language impairment.* Cambridge, MA: MIT Press.

McGregor, K. K., Friedman, R., Reilly, R., and Newman, R. (2002). Semantic representation and naming in young children. *Journal of Speech, Language, and Hearing Research, 45,* 332–346.

McGregor, K. K., and Waxman, S. R. (1998). Object naming at multiple hierarchical levels: A comparison of preschoolers with and without word-finding deficits. *Journal of Child Language, 25,* 419–430.

Mervis, C. B., and Bertrand, J. (1995). Acquisition of the novel name-nameless category (N3C) principle by young children who have Down syndrome. *American Journal of Mental Retardation, 100,* 231–243.

Nation, K., and Snowling, M. J. (1999). Developmental differences in sensitivity to semantic relations among good and poor comprehenders: Evidence from semantic priming. *Cognition, 70,* B1–B13.

Nippold, M. A. (1988). *Later language development* (2nd ed.). Austin, TX: Pro-Ed.

Oetting, J. B., Rice, M. L., and Swank, L. K. (1995). Quick incidental learning (QUIL) of words by school-age children with and without specific language impairment. *Journal of Speech and Hearing Research, 38,* 434–445.

Rescorla, L. (1989). The Language Development Survey: A screening tool for delayed language in toddlers. *Journal of Speech and Hearing Disorders, 54,* 587–599.

Secord, W. A., and Wiig, E. H. (1993). Interpreting figurative language expressions. *Folia Phoniatrica, 45,* 1–9.

Stanovich, K. E. (1986). Matthew effects in reading: Some consequences of individual differences in the acquisition of literacy. *Reading Research Quarterly, 21,* 360–406.

Social Development and Language Impairment

Social skills determine to a large extent the success we enjoy vocationally and avocationally and the amount of satisfaction we derive from our personal relationships. Social skill deficits in childhood have long been associated with a variety of negative outcomes, including criminality, underemployment, and psychopathology (cf. Gilbert and Connolly, 1991). The potential impact of developmental language impairments on social development is one of the most important issues facing families, educators, and speech-language pathologists. Unfortunately, there is little agreement on the definition of social skills as a psychological construct, making service planning in this area challenging. In their review, Merrell and Gimpel (1998) presented no less than 16 different definitions that enjoy wide currency and reflect the interests of a variety of disciplines, including psychology, psychiatry, special education, and social work. However, commonalities across these different perspectives can be extracted. In a meta-analysis of 21 multivariate studies that classified children's social skills (total N = 22,000), Caldarella and Merrell (1997) identified five core dimensions: peer relations, self-management, academics, compliance, and assertion.

What are the interrelationships between language impairments and these important areas of social development? Language impairments occur with a large variety of developmental disorders, and some, such as mental retardation, AUTISM, and pervasive developmental delay, include social skill deficits as a primary diagnostic feature. In order to address the question of how language impairment uniquely affects social development, however, we need to examine the social skills of children with specific language impairment (SLI) (see SPECIFIC LANGUAGE IMPAIRMENT IN CHILDREN). SLI refers to a language deficiency that occurs in the absence of other conditions commonly associated with language disorders in children. Children with SLI show normal hearing, age-appropriate scores on nonverbal tests of intelligence, and no obvious signs of neurological or socioemotional impairment. Children with SLI represent a heterogeneous group, and significant individual differences exist among children diagnosed with this disorder. However, a common profile in young, English-speaking children with SLI is a mild to moderate deficit in a range of language areas and a more significant deficit in the use of grammatical morphology.

According to Caldarella and Merrell (1997), a large number of social skills contribute to the dimension *peer relations*. These skills include specific discourse/pragmatic behaviors such as complimenting others and inviting others to play, as well as more general social attributes such as peer acceptance. Several studies have examined the peer interactions of preschool and school-age children with SLI and have documented the detrimental effect that language impairments can have on this area of social development. For example, children with SLI are likely to be ignored by their typically developing peers, respond less often when their peers make initiations, and rely more on adults to mediate their interactions (Craig and Evans, 1989; Hadley and Rice, 1991; Rice, Sell, and Hadley, 1991; Craig and Washington, 1993; Brinton, Fujiki, and Higbee, 1998; Brinton, Fujiki, and McKee, 1998). Sociometric analyses confirm further the impression that children with SLI experience limited peer acceptance (Gertner, Rice, and Hadley, 1994; Fujiki, Brinton, Hart, et al., 1999). Some studies suggest that problems in peer group acceptance may extend to difficulties establishing adequate friendships (Fujiki, Brinton, Morgan, et al., 1999), whereas others have reported no differences between children with SLI and typically developing children in the number and quality of close friendships (Redmond and Rice, 1998).

Although peer relations represent the sine qua non of social development, there are other important social skills. *Self-management* refers to the ability to control one's temper, follow rules and limits, and compromise with others (Caldarella and Merrell, 1997). A few studies have assessed this dimension in children with SLI. Stevens and Bliss (1995) examined conflict resolution abilities in 30 children with SLI in grades 3 through 7 and found no significant differences between this group and

a group of grade-matched typically developing controls during a role-enactment activity. Children with SLI produced fewer strategies during a more verbally demanding hypothetical problem-solving activity. Brinton, Fujiki, and McKee (1998) examined the negotiation skills of six children with SLI (8 to 12 years old) during conversational interactions with typically developing peers and found that children with SLI contributed fewer and less mature negotiation strategies. The strategies used by children in the SLI group resembled those produced by a younger group of children of equivalent language levels.

The third cluster of social skills identified by Caldarella and Merrell's (1997) meta-analysis was the *academics* dimension. This dimension captures behaviors regarded by teachers as important to school adjustment and is represented by such skills as completing tasks independently, following teachers' directions, and producing quality work. Indirect evidence for problems in this dimension comes from studies of SLI that have used rating scales to evaluate children's socioemotional characteristics. For example, Redmond and Rice (1998) compared standardized parent and teacher ratings of 17 children with SLI collected at kindergarten and first grade to ratings collected on typically developing children. The particular rating scales used included several items that relate to important academic skills (e.g., *has difficulty following directions; fails to carry out tasks; messy work*). These investigators found significant differences between groups on the teacher ratings of these problems but not on the parent ratings, suggesting that the social performance of children with SLI varies significantly across situations, depending on the verbal demands placed on them and the expectations of others. Levels of academic success may also influence academic social behaviors. In an epidemiological study of 164 second-grade children with language impairments, Tomblin et al. (2000) found that levels of classroom behavior problems were higher among children with SLI who also had reading disabilities than among children with SLI alone (see LANGUAGE DISORDERS AND READING DISABILITIES).

Prosocial behaviors such as cooperation and sharing are captured by Caldarella and Merrell's *compliance* dimension. Information on the consequences of SLI in this area of social skill development is limited. Farmer (2000) compared the performances of 16 10-year-old children with SLI with that of a group of typically developing children on a standardized teacher rating scale of prosocial behaviors and found no significant differences.

The final social skills dimension in Caldarella and Merrell's taxonomy is *assertion*. Several studies suggest children with SLI experience particular difficulty in this area. Craig and Washington (1993) examined the conversational skills of five 7-year-old children with SLI as they attempted to access ongoing peer interactions and found that three of the five children had considerable difficulty asserting themselves in this situation. Brinton et al. (1997) replicated these results with older children

(8–12 years old). Children with SLI have also been consistently characterized as shy, passive, and withdrawn by parents and teachers (Tallal, Dukette, and Curtiss, 1989; Fujiki, Brinton, and Todd, 1996; Redmond and Rice, 1998; Beitchman et al., 2001). Results from a recent 14-year longitudinal study of 77 children with speech and language impairments suggest that characterizations of low assertiveness may be longstanding and continue at least into young adulthood for some children with SLI (Beitchman et al., 2001).

In sum, a small but growing body of research suggests that language impairments place children at risk for negative social consequences, specifically in the areas of assertion and peer relations. Problems in these areas may be particularly detrimental for children with SLI because they can contribute to what Rice (1993) has described as a "negative social spiral." Rice suggested that in response to repeated instances of communicative failure, children with SLI may withdraw from peer interactions or rely more on adults to mediate peer interactions. However, these behavioral adjustments may turn out to be counterproductive for both social and linguistic development because they limit children's access to important socialization experiences and opportunities to improve their limited language skills.

Studies of children with SLI have consistently reported high levels of variability in social skill performance, a finding that has important clinical and research implications. Social skill deficits do not appear to be an inevitable consequence of developmental language impairments, nor can social skill differences between children be inferred from differences in either the type or severity of language deficits (e.g., Brinton and Fujiki, 1999; Fujiki et al., 1999; Donlan and Masters, 2000). Given the heterogeneity of children with developmental language disorders, it is important that treatment teams supplement the assessment of language impairment with a separate assessment of social skills in the areas of peer relations, self-management, academics, compliance, and assertion across different situational contexts (home, classroom, playground).

Future investigations may reveal that variability in children with language impairments is better accounted for by uncontrolled confounding factors. For example, although many studies suggest that SLI and attention-deficit/hyperactivity disorder commonly co-occur (cf. Cohen et al., 2000) the potential influence of this comorbidity on social skill development has not yet been considered. Likewise, a small portion of children diagnosed with SLI demonstrate limitations in social cognition commonly associated with autism and pervasive developmental delay. There has been a longstanding controversy over the diagnostic boundaries between SLI and autism spectrum disorders (cf. Bishop, 2000), and social skill outcomes may be an important distinguishing characteristic of children who fall outside preconceived categories. Large-scale investigations comparing the social skills of children with SLI only with those of children with SLI and other comorbid disorders are needed to delineate which language skills are associated with

specific areas of social skill development. The results of this line of research will inform important areas of clinical practice, such as diagnosis, prognosis, and treatment.

See also PSYCHOSOCIAL PROBLEMS ASSOCIATED WITH COMMUNICATIVE DISORDERS.

—*Sean M. Redmond*

References

Beitchman, J. H., Wilson, B., Johnson, C. J., Atkinson, L., Young, A., Adlaf, E., et al. (2001). Fourteen-year follow-up of speech/language impaired and control children: Psychiatric outcome. *Journal of the American Academy of Child and Adolescent Psychiatry, 40*, 75–82.

Bishop, D. V. M. (2000). Pragmatic language impairment: A correlate of SLI, a distinct subgroup, or part of the autistic continuum? In D. V. M. Bishop and L. B. Leonard (Eds.), *Speech and language impairments in children: Causes, characteristics, intervention and outcome* (pp. 99–114). Philadelphia: Taylor and Francis.

Brinton, B., and Fujiki, M. (1999). Social interactional behaviors of children with specific language impairment. *Topics in Language Disorders, 19*, 34–48.

Brinton, B., Fujiki, M., and Higbee, L. (1998). Participation in cooperative learning activities by children with specific language impairment. *Journal of Speech, Language, and Hearing Research, 41*, 1193–1206.

Brinton, B., Fujiki, M., and McKee, L. (1998). The negotiation skills of children with specific language impairment. *Journal of Speech, Language, and Hearing Research, 41*, 927–940.

Brinton, B., Fujiki, M., Spencer, J. C., and Robinson, L. A. (1997). The ability of children with specific language impairment to access and participate in an ongoing interaction. *Journal of Speech, Language, and Hearing Research, 40*, 1011–1025.

Caldarella, P., and Merrell, K. W. (1997). Common dimensions of social skills of children and adolescents: A taxonomy of positive behaviors. *School Psychology Review, 26*, 264–278.

Cohen, N. J., Vallance, D. D., Barwick, M., Im, N., Menna, R., Horodezky, N. B., et al. (2000). The interface between ADHD and language impairment: An examination of language, achievement, and cognitive processing. *Journal of Child Psychology and Psychiatry, 41*, 353–362.

Craig, H. K., and Evans, J. (1989). Turn exchange characteristics of SLI children's simultaneous and nonsimultaneous speech. *Journal of Speech and Hearing Disorders, 54*, 334–347.

Craig, H. K., and Washington, J. A. (1993). The access behaviors of children with specific language impairment. *Journal of Speech and Hearing Research, 36*, 322–336.

Donlan, C., and Masters, J. (2000). Correlates of social development in children with communicative disorders: The concurrent predictive value of verbal short-term memory span. *International Journal of Communication Disorders, 35*, 211–226.

Farmer, M. (2000). Language and social cognition in children with specific language impairment. *Journal of Child Psychology and Psychiatry and Allied Disciplines, 41*, 627–636.

Fujiki, M., Brinton, B., Hart, C. H., and Fitzgerald, A. (1999). Peer acceptance and friendship in children with specific language impairment. *Language, Speech, and Hearing Services in Schools, 30*, 183–195.

Fujiki, M., Brinton, B., Morgan, M., and Hart, C. H. (1999). Withdrawn and sociable behavior of children with language impairments. *Language, Speech, and Hearing Services in Schools, 30,* 183–195.

Fujiki, M., Brinton, B., and Todd, C. M. (1996). Social skills of children with specific language impairment. *Language, Speech, and Hearing Services in Schools, 27,* 195–202.

Gertner, B. L., Rice, M. L., and Hadley, P. A. (1994). Influence of communicative competence on peer preferences in a preschool classroom. *Journal of Speech and Hearing Research, 37,* 913–923.

Gilbert, D. G., and Connolly, J. J. (Eds.). (1991). *Personality, social skills, and psychopathology: An individual difference approach.* New York: Plenum Press.

Hadley, P. A., and Rice, M. L. (1991). Conversational responsiveness of speech- and language-impaired preschoolers. *Journal of Speech and Hearing Research, 34,* 1308–1317.

Merrell, K. W., and Gimpel, G. A. (1998). *Social skills of children and adolescents: Conceptualization, assessment, treatment.* Mahwah, NJ: Erlbaum.

Redmond, S. M., and Rice, M. L. (1998). The socioemotional behaviors of children with SLI: Social adaptation or social deviance? *Journal of Speech, Language, and Hearing Research, 41,* 688–700.

Rice, M. L. (1993). "Don't talk to him: He's weird": A social consequences account of language and social interactions. In A. P. Kaiser and D. B. Gray (Eds.), *Enhancing children's communication: Research foundations for intervention* (pp. 139–158). Baltimore: Paul H. Brookes.

Rice, M. L., Sell, M. A., and Hadley, P. A. (1991). Social interactions of speech- and language-impaired children. *Journal of Speech and Hearing Research, 34,* 1299–1307.

Stevens, L. J., and Bliss, L. S. (1995). Conflict resolution abilities of children with specific language impairment and children with normal language. *Journal of Speech and Hearing Research, 38,* 599–611.

Tallal, P., Dukette, D., and Curtiss, S. (1989). Behavior/emotional profiles of preschool language-impaired children. *Development and Psychopathology, 1,* 51–67.

Tomblin, J. B., Zhang, X., Buckwalter, P., and Catts, H. (2000). The association of reading disability, behavioral disorders, and language impairments among second-grade children. *Journal of Child Psychology and Psychiatry and Allied Disciplines, 41,* 473–482.

Further Readings

Beitchman, J. H., Cohen, N. J., Konstantareas, M. M., and Tannock, R. (Eds.). (1996). *Language, learning, and behavior disorders: Developmental, biological, and clinical perspectives.* New York: Cambridge University Press.

Bishop, D. V. M. (1997). *Uncommon understanding: Development and disorders of language comprehension in children.* East Sussex, U.K.: Psychology Press.

Botting, N., and Conti-Ramsden, G. (2000). Social and behavioral difficulties in children with language impairment. *Child Language Teaching and Therapy, 16,* 105–120.

Brinton, B., and Fujiki, M. (1989). *Conversational management with language-impaired children: Pragmatic assessment and intervention.* Rockville, MD: Aspen.

Brinton, B., Fujiki, M., Montague, E., and Hanton, J. L. (2000). Children with language impairments in cooperative work groups: A pilot study. *Language, Speech, and Hearing Services in Schools, 31,* 252–264.

Cantwell, D. P., and Baker, L. (1991). *Psychiatric and developmental disorders in children with communication disorder.* Washington, DC: American Psychiatric Press.

Craig, H. K. (1991). Pragmatic characteristics of the child with specific language impairment: An interactionist perspective. In T. M. Gallagher (Ed.), *Pragmatics of language: Clinical practice issues* (pp. 163–198). San Diego, CA: Singular Publishing Group.

Craig, H. K. (1993). Social skills of children with specific language impairment: Peer relationships. *Language, Speech, and Hearing Services in Schools, 24,* 206–215.

Craig, H. K. (1995). Pragmatic impairments. In P. Fletcher and B. MacWhinney (Eds.), *The handbook of child language* (pp. 623–640). Cambridge, MA: Blackwell.

DeThorne, L. S., and Watkins, R. V. (2001). Listeners' perceptions of language use in children. *Language, Speech, and Hearing Services in Schools, 32,* 142–148.

Donahue, M. L., Hartas, D., and Cole, D. (1999). Research on interactions among oral language and emotional/behavioral disorders. In D. Rogers-Adkinson and P. Griffith (Eds.), *Communication disorders and children with psychiatric and behavioral disorders* (pp. 69–98). San Diego, CA: Singular Publishing Group.

Elliot, S. N., and Gresham, F. M. (1991). *Social skills intervention guide: Practical strategies for social skills training.* Circle Pines, MN: American Guidance.

Farmer, M. (1997). Exploring the links between communication skills and social competence. *Educational and Child Psychology, 14,* 38–44.

Fey, M. E., and Leonard, L. B. (1983). Pragmatic skills of children with specific language impairment. In T. M. Gallagher and C. A. Prutting (Eds.), *Pragmatic assessment and intervention issues in language* (pp. 65–82). San Diego, CA: College-Hill Press.

Gallagher, T. M. (1991). Language and social skills: Implications for clinical assessment and intervention with school-age children. In T. M. Gallagher (Ed.), *Pragmatics of language: Clinical practice issues* (pp. 11–42). San Diego, CA: Singular Publishing Group.

Goldstein, H., and Gallagher, T. M. (1992). Strategies for promoting the social communicative competence of children with specific language impairment. In S. L. Odom, S. R. McConnell and M. A. McEvoy (Eds.), *Social competence of young children with disabilities* (pp. 189–213). Baltimore: Paul H. Brookes.

Goodyer, I. M. (2000). Language difficulties and psychopathology. In D. V. M. Bishop and L. B. Leonard (Eds.), *Speech and language impairments in children: Causes, characteristics, intervention and outcome* (pp. 227–244). Philadelphia: Taylor and Francis.

Gresham, F. M., and MacMillan, D. L. (1997). Social competence and affective characteristics of students with mild disabilities. *Review of Educational Research, 67,* 377–415.

Hummel, L. J., and Prizant, B. (1993). A socioemotional perspective for understanding social difficulties of school-age children with language disorders. *Language, Speech, and Hearing Services in Schools, 31,* 216–224.

Miller, C. A. (2001). False belief understanding in children with specific language impairment. *Journal of Communication Disorders, 34,* 73–86.

Merrell, K. W. (1999). *Behavioral, social, and emotional assessment of children and adolescents.* Mahwah, NJ: Erlbaum.

Prizant, B., Audet, L., Burke, G., Hummel, L., Maher, S., and Theadore, G. (1990). Communication disorders and emotional/behavioral disorders in children and adolescents. *Journal of Speech and Hearing Research, 55,* 179–192.

Redmond, S. M., and Rice, M. L. (2002). Stability of behavioral ratings of children with SLI. *Journal of Speech, Language, and Hearing Research, 45,* 190–200.

Rice, M. L., Hadley, P. A., and Alexander, A. L. (1993). Social biases toward children with speech and language impairments: A correlative causal model of language limitations. *Applied Psycholinguistics, 14,* 445–471.

Rutter, M., Mawhood, L., and Howlin, P. (1992). Language delay and social development. In P. Feltcher and D. Hall (Eds.), *Specific Speech and Language Disorders in Children* (pp. 63–78). San Diego, CA: Singular Publishing Group.

Windsor, J. (1995). Language impairment and social consequence. In M. E. Fey, J. Windsor, and S. F. Warren (Eds.), *Language intervention: Preschool through the elementary years* (pp. 213–240). Baltimore: Paul H. Brookes.

Specific Language Impairment in Children

Specific language impairment (SLI) is a term that is applied to children who show a significant deficit in their spoken language ability with no obvious accompanying problems such as hearing impairment, mental retardation, or neurological damage. This type of language disorder is regarded as developmental in nature because affected children exhibit language learning problems from the outset.

Although SLI is receiving increased attention in the research and clinical literature, it is not a newly discovered disorder. Children meeting the basic definition of SLI have been described in the literature since the 1800s, but have been given a wide range of clinical labels. More recent clinical labels used for children with SLI include developmental aphasia, developmental dysphasia, and developmental language disorder. The last continues to be used in the *DSM-IV* classification system, with the subtypes of "expressive" and "receptive and expressive" (American Psychiatric Association, 1994). These subtypes acknowledge that some children with SLI may have significant limitations primarily in the area of language production, whereas others may have major limitations in both the comprehension and production of language.

The prevalence of SLI is estimated to be approximately 7% among 5-year-olds, based on epidemiological data (Tomblin et al., 1997). Males outnumber females; the most recent evidence suggests a ratio of approximately 1.5 : 1.

Children with SLI are two to three times more likely than typically developing children to have parents or siblings with a history of language problems (Tallal, Ross, and Curtiss, 1989; Tomblin, 1989; Tallal et al., 2001). For children with family histories of language problems, there is reason to suspect a genetic basis rather than a primary environmental basis. Concordance rates for SLI are considerably higher for monozygotic twins than for same-sex dizygotic twins (Bishop, North, and Donlan, 1995). Rapid progress is being made in the genetic study of SLI. For a well-studied three-generational family that includes a high proportion of members with SLI, the evidence implicates a region on the long arm of chromosome 7 (Fisher et al., 1998). The same region was identified in a group of children with SLI who participated in an epidemiological study (Tomblin, 1999). However, other recent studies of clinically referred cases of SLI have revealed prominent areas of linkage on chromosomes 16 and 19, but not on chromosome 7 (SLI Consortium, 2002). Clearly, further refinement is needed before the genetic basis for SLI is fully understood (see Bishop, 2002).

In recent years, neuroanatomical evidence of differences between individuals with SLI and typically developing individuals has appeared in the literature (see Ahmed, Lombardino, and Leonard, 2000, for a recent review). The specific differences observed have varied across studies. For example, symmetry of the right and left perisylvian areas seems to be more likely in children with SLI than in controls. Interestingly, this pattern can also be seen in parents or siblings of children with SLI even when they do not exhibit a language disorder. Other studies have revealed a higher likelihood of atypical neuroanatomical patterns in children with SLI than in controls, but differences among the children with SLI in the particular pattern seen (e.g., ventricular enlargement, central volume loss).

Although a diagnosis of SLI is not given to children unless they meet the criteria noted above, many children with SLI nevertheless show subtle weaknesses in other areas. For example, as a group, these children are slower and less accurate on nonlinguistic cognitive tasks such as mental rotation (e.g., Miller et al., 2001), and less coordinated than their typically developing same-age peers (Powell and Bishop, 1992; Hill, 2001). These findings have led to proposals about the possible causes of SLI, but the presence of children with SLI who show none of these accompanying weaknesses raises the possibility that SLI and subtle cognitive and motor weakness are comorbid. That is, the conditions that cause SLI frequently co-occur with conditions that cause these other problems, but the latter are not responsible for SLI.

For children with SLI whose language problems are still present at 5 years of age, difficulties with language may continue into adolescence and even adulthood (Bishop and Adams, 1990; Beitchman et al., 1996). Comparisons of young adults with a history of SLI and same-age adults with no such history reveal differences favoring the latter on a range of spoken production and comprehension tasks (Tomblin, Freese, and Records, 1992).

Children with SLI are at greater risk for reading deficits than children with typical language development. This observation can be explained in part by the fact that children with SLI and those with developmental dyslexia are overlapping populations (McArthur et al., 2000). For example, prospective study of children from homes with a positive history of dyslexia reveals significantly more difficulties with spoken language than children with no such family history (Scarborough, 1990).

The language difficulties experienced by children with SLI cover most or all areas of language, including vocabulary, morphosyntax, phonology, and pragmatics. However, these areas of language are rarely affected to the same degree. In English, vocabulary and pragmatic skills are often relative strengths, whereas phonology and especially morphosyntax are relative weaknesses. This profile is not seen in all English-speaking children meeting the criteria for SLI. For example, some children with SLI show notable word-finding problems. There have been several attempts at determining whether the differences seen among children with SLI constitute distinct subtypes or instead represent different points on a continuum. Resolution of this issue will be important, as identification of the correct phenotype of SLI will be necessary for further progress in the genetic study of this disorder.

The heterogeneity of SLI notwithstanding, certain symptoms may have the potential to serve as "clinical markers" of SLI. For English-speaking children, two measures seem especially promising. One is a measure of the children's use of grammatical morphemes pertaining to grammatical tense and agreement, such as regular past -ed, third person singular -s, and copula and auxiliary forms of be (Rice and Wexler, 1996). The second is a measure of children's ability to repeat nonsense words containing several syllables (e.g., Dollaghan and Campbell, 1998). Both of these measures are quite accurate in distinguishing children with SLI from their normally developing age mates.

The linguistic profile of relative strengths and weaknesses in SLI seems to be shaped to a significant degree by the language being acquired. For example, children with SLI acquiring inflectionally rich languages such as Italian and Hebrew are not as severely impaired as their English-speaking counterparts in their use of grammatical inflections pertaining to tense and agreement. On the other hand, Swedish-speaking children with SLI show more serious problems in using appropriate word order than do children with SLI acquiring English (see Leonard, 1998, for a recent review).

Evidence for the efficacy of intervention is abundant in the literature. For example, for preschool-age children with SLI, approaches such as recasting have been relatively successful (Camarata and Nelson, 1992; Fey, Cleave, and Long, 1997). However, although the gains made in intervention usually go well beyond those that can be expected by maturation alone, no intervention approach has led to dramatic and rapid language gains by these children on a consistent basis. This is especially true when gains are defined in terms of use in spontaneous speech.

Attempts to explain the nature of SLI vary considerably. Most of these accounts focus on the extraordinary grammatical deficits often seen in children with SLI. It is possible to classify these alternative accounts according to their principal assumptions. Some accounts assume that children with SLI lack particular types of grammatical knowledge. For example, the "extended optional infinitive" account assumes that children with SLI go through a protracted period during which they assume that tense and agreement are optional rather than obligatory in main clauses (Rice and Wexler, 1996). The "representational deficit for dependent relationships" account assumes that children with SLI fail to grasp that movement or checking of grammatical features is obligatory (van der Lely, 1998).

Other types of accounts assume that children with SLI might have the potential to acquire normal grammar but have limitations in processing that slow their identification and interpretation of the relevant input and their ability to retrieve this information for production. In some cases the processing limitation is assumed to be quite general (Johnston, 1994; Ellis Weismer, 1996). In other cases the limitation is assumed to be specific to particular operations, such as phonological processing (Chiat, 2001) or the processing of brief or rapidly presented auditory information (e.g., Tallal et al., 1996).

Future research on SLI will make two types of contributions. Most obviously, greater understanding of this disorder should lead to more effective methods of assessment, treatment, and prevention. In addition, because the language disorder seen in SLI may in many cases occur in the absence of accompanying impairments, it constitutes a challenge for theories of language learning to explain.

See also LANGUAGE DISORDERS IN SCHOOL-AGE CHILDREN: OVERVIEW; SPEECH DISORDERS IN CHILDREN: A PSYCHOLINGUISTIC PERSPECTIVE.

—*Laurence B. Leonard*

References

Ahmed, S., Lombardino, L., and Leonard, C. (2001). Specific language impairment: Definitions, causal mechanisms, and neurobiological factors. *Journal of Medical Speech-Language Pathology, 9,* 1–15.

American Psychiatric Association. (1994). *Diagnostic and statistical manual of mental disorders—Fourth edition.* Washington, DC: Author.

Beitchman, J., Wilson, B., Brownlee, E., Walters, H., and Lancee, W. (1996). Long-term consistency in speech/language profiles: I. Developmental and academic outcomes. *Journal of the American Academy of Child and Adolescent Psychiatry, 35,* 804–814.

Bishop, D. (2002). Putting language genes in perspective. *Trends in Genetics, 18,* 57–59.

Bishop, D., and Adams, C. (1990). A prospective study of the relationship between specific language impairment, phonological disorders and reading retardation. *Journal of Child Psychology and Psychiatry, 31,* 1027–1050.

Bishop, D., North, T., and Donlan, C. (1995). Genetic basis of specific language impairment: Evidence from a twin study. *Developmental Medicine and Child Neurology, 37,* 56–71.

Camarata, S., and Nelson, K. E. (1992). Treatment efficiency as a function of target selection in the remediation of child language disorders. *Clinical Linguistics and Phonetics, 6,* 167–178.

Chiat, S. (2001). Mapping theories of developmental language impairment: Premises, predictions and evidence. *Language and Cognitive Processes, 16,* 113–142.

Dollaghan, C., and Campbell, T. (1998). Nonword repetition and child language impairment. *Journal of Speech, Language, and Hearing Research, 41,* 1136–1146.

Ellis Weismer, S. (1996). Capacity limitations in working memory: The impact on lexical and morphological learning by children with language impairment. *Topics in Language Disorders, 17*, 33–44.

Fey, M., Cleave, P., and Long, S. (1997). Two models of grammar facilitation in children with language impairments: Phase 2. *Journal of Speech, Language, and Hearing Research, 40*, 5–19.

Fisher, S., Vargha-Khadem, F., Watkins, K., Monaco, A., and Pembrey, M. (1998). Localisation of a gene implicated in a severe speech and language disorder. *Nature Genetics, 18*, 168–170.

Hill, E. (2001). Non-specific nature of specific language impairment: A review of the literature with regard to concomitant motor impairment. *International Journal of Language and Communication Disorders, 36*, 149–171.

Johnston, J. (1994). Cognitive abilities of children with language impairment. In R. Watkins and M. Rice (Eds.), *Specific language impairments in children* (pp. 107–121). Baltimore: Paul H. Brookes.

Leonard, L. (1998). *Children with specific language impairment.* Cambridge, MA: MIT Press.

McArthur, G., Hogben, J., Edwards, V., Heath, S., and Mengler, E. (2000). On the "specifics" of specific reading disability and specific language impairment. *Journal of Child Psychology and Psychiatry, 41*, 869–874.

Miller, C., Kail, R., Leonard, L., and Tomblin, J. B. (2001). Speed of processing in children with specific language impairment. *Journal of Speech, Language, and Hearing Research, 44*, 416–433.

Powell, R., and Bishop, D. (1992). Clumsiness and perceptual problems in children with specific language impairment. *Developmental Medicine and Child Neurology, 41*, 159–165.

Rice, M., and Wexler, K. (1996). Toward tense as a clinical marker of specific language impairment in English-speaking children. *Journal of Speech and Hearing Research, 39*, 1239–1257.

Scarborough, H. (1990). Very early language deficits in dyslexic children. *Child Development, 61*, 1728–1743.

SLI Consortium. (2002). A genomewide scan identifies two novel loci in specific language impairment. *American Journal of Human Genetics, 70*, 384–398.

Tallal, P., Hirsch, L., Realpe-Bonilla, T., Miller, S., Brzustowicz, L., Bartlett, C., et al. (2001). Familial aggregation in specific language impairment. *Journal of Speech, Language, and Hearing Research, 44*, 1172–1182.

Tallal, P., Miller, S., Bedi, G., Byma, G., Wang, X., Nagarajan, S., et al. (1996). Language comprehension in language-learning impaired children improved with acoustically modified speech. *Science, 271*, 81–84.

Tallal, P., Ross, R., and Curtiss, S. (1989). Familial aggregation in specific language impairment. *Journal of Speech and Hearing Disorders, 54*, 167–173.

Tomblin, J. B. (1989). Familial concentration of developmental language impairment. *Journal of Speech and Hearing Disorders, 54*, 287–295.

Tomblin, J. B. (1999). *Epidemiology and familial transmission of specific language impairment.* Paper presented at the annual meeting of the American Association for the Advancement of Science, Anaheim, CA.

Tomblin, J. B., Freese, P., and Records, N. (1992). Diagnosing specific language impairment in adults for the purpose of pedigree analysis. *Journal of Speech and Hearing Research, 35*, 832–843.

Tomblin, J. B., Records, N., Buckwalter, P., Zhang, X., Smith, E., and O'Brien, M. (1997). The prevalence of specific language impairment in kindergarten children. *Journal of Speech, Language, and Hearing Research, 40*, 1245–1260.

van der Lely, H. (1998). SLI in children: Movement, economy, and deficits in the computational-syntactic system. *Language Acquisition, 7*, 161–192.

Further Readings

Bishop, D. (1997). *Uncommon understanding: Development and disorders of comprehension in children.* Hove, U.K.: Psychology Press.

Catts, H., Fey, M., Zhang, X., and Tomblin, J. B. (2001). Estimating the risk of future reading difficulties in kindergarten children: A research-based model and its classroom implementation. *Language, Speech, and Hearing Services in Schools, 32*, 38–50.

Clahsen, H., Bartke, S., and Göllner, S. (1997). Formal features in impaired grammars: A comparison of English and German SLI children. *Journal of Neurolinguistics, 10*, 151–172.

Conti-Ramsden, G., Botting, N., and Faragher, B. (2001). Psycholinguistic markers for specific language impairment (SLI). *Journal of Child Psychology and Psychiatry, 42*, 741–748.

Conti-Ramsden, G., Botting, N., Simkin, Z., and Knox, E. (2001). Follow-up of children attending infant language units: Outcomes at 11 years of age. *International Journal of Language and Communication Disorders, 36*, 207–219.

Dromi, E., Leonard, L., Adam, G., and Zadunaisky-Ehrlich, S. (1999). Verb agreement morphology in Hebrew-speaking children with specific language impairment. *Journal of Speech, Language, and Hearing Research, 42*, 1414–1431.

Gillam, R. (Ed.). (1998). *Memory and language impairment in children and adults.* Gaithersburg, MD: Aspen.

Gopnik, M., and Crago, M. (1991). Familial aggregation of a developmental language disorder. *Cognition, 39*, 1–50.

Hansson, K., Nettelbladt, U., and Leonard, L. (2000). Specific language impairment in Swedish: The status of verb morphology and word order. *Journal of Speech, Language, and Hearing Research, 43*, 848–864.

Jakubowicz, C., and Nash, L. (2001). Functional categories and syntactic operations in (ab)normal language acquisition. *Brain and Language, 77*, 321–339.

Leonard, L. (2000). Specific language impairment across languages. In D. Bishop and L. Leonard (Eds.), *Speech and language impairments in children* (pp. 115–129). Hove, U.K.: Psychology Press.

Leonard, L., Eyer, J., Bedore, L., and Grela, B. (1997). Three accounts of the grammatical morpheme difficulties of English-speaking children with specific language impairment. *Journal of Speech, Language, and Hearing Research, 40*, 741–753.

McGregor, K. (1997). The nature of word-finding errors in preschoolers with and without word-finding deficits. *Journal of Speech, Language, and Hearing Research, 40*, 1232–1244.

Paradis, J., and Crago, M. (2000). Tense and temporality: A comparison between children learning a second language and children with SLI. *Journal of Speech, Language, and Hearing Research, 43*, 834–847.

Paul, R. (2000). Predicting outcomes of early expressive language delay: Ethical implications. In D. Bishop and L. Leonard (Eds.), *Speech and language impairments in children* (pp. 195–209). Hove, U.K.: Psychology Press.

Plante, E. (1996). Phenotypic variability in brain-behavior studies of specific language impairment. In M. Rice (Ed.), *Toward a genetics of language* (pp. 317–335). Baltimore: Paul H. Brookes.

Rice, M., Wexler, K., and Hershberger, S. (1998). Tense over time: The longitudinal course of tense acquisition in children with specific language impairment. *Journal of Speech, Language, and Hearing Research, 41,* 1412–1431.

Thal, D., and Katich, J. (1997). Issues in early identification of language impairment: Does the early bird always catch the worm? In K. Cole, P. Dale, and D. Thal (Eds.), *Assessment of communication and language* (pp. 1–28). Baltimore: Paul H. Brookes.

Syntactic Tree Pruning

AGRAMMATISM is a syntactic deficit following damage to the left hemisphere, usually in Broca's area and its vicinity (Zurif, 1995). The traditional view concerning speech production in agrammatism was that syntactic ability is completely lost, and agrammatic aphasics rely on nonlinguistic strategies to concatenate words into sentences (Goodglass, 1976; Berndt and Caramazza, 1980; Caplan, 1985), or that all functional elements are impaired in agrammatic speech production (Grodzinsky, 1990; Ouhalla, 1993). However, in recent years empirical evidence has accumulated to suggest that the deficit is actually finer-grained.

Speech production in agrammatism shows an intricate and intriguing pattern of deficit. Individuals with agrammatism correctly inflect verbs for agreement but substitute tense inflection; they produce well-formed yes/no questions (in some languages), but not Wh questions; they can produce untensed embedding but not full relative sentences, and coordination markers but not subordination markers. The *tree pruning hypothesis* (TPH) was suggested by Friedmann (1994, 2001) and

Friedmann and Grodzinsky (1997) to account for these seemingly unrelated deficits and for the dissociations between spared and impaired abilities within and across languages. The TPH is a linguistic generalization, formulated within the generative grammar framework, and was suggested to account for production only. (For a syntactic account of agrammatic comprehension, see TRACE DELETION HYPOTHESIS; Grodzinsky, 2000.) According to the TPH, individuals with agrammatic aphasia are unable to project the syntactic tree up to its highest node, and their syntactic tree is "pruned." As a result, syntactic structures and elements that require the high nodes of the tree are impaired, but structures and elements that involve only low nodes are preserved (Fig. 1).

According to syntactic theories within the generative tradition (e.g., Chomsky, 1995), sentences can be represented as phrase markers or syntactic trees. In these syntactic trees, content and function words are represented in different nodes (head nodes and phrasal nodes) (Fig. 1). Functional nodes include, among others, inflectional nodes: an agreement phrase (Agr$_s$P), which represents agreement between the subject and the verb in person, gender, and number, and a tense phrase (TP), representing tense inflection of the verb. Finite verbs move from V^0, their base-generated position within the VP, to Agr^0 and then to T^0 in order to check (or collect) their inflection. Thus, the ability to correctly inflect verbs for agreement and tense crucially depends on the AgrP and TP nodes.

The highest phrasal node in the tree is the complementizer phrase (CP), which hosts complementizers such as "that" and Wh morphemes such as "who" and "what" that moved from the base-generated position within the VP. Thus, the construction of embedded

Figure 1. A syntactic tree (Pollock, 1989). The arch represents a possible impairment site according to the tree pruning hypothesis. Nodes below the arch are intact and nodes above it are impaired.

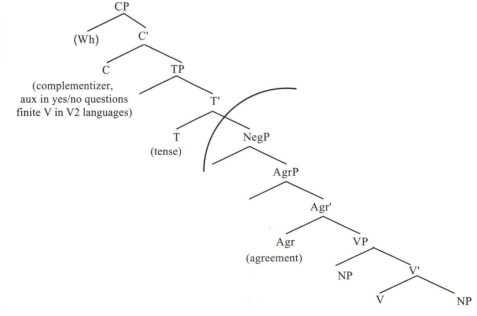

sentences and Wh questions depends on the CP node being intact and accessible.

Crucially, the nodes are hierarchically ordered in the syntactic tree: the lowest node is the verb phrase, the nodes above it are the agreement phrase and the tense phrase (in this order according to Pollock, 1989), and the complementizer phrase is placed at the highest point of the syntactic tree.

The TPH uses this hierarchical order and suggests that in agrammatism, the syntactic tree is pruned from a certain node and up. Persons with agrammatic aphasia who cannot project the syntactic tree up to the TP node are not able to produce structures that require TP or the node above it, CP. Persons with agrammatic aphasia whose tree is pruned at a higher point, CP, are unable to produce structures that involve the CP. Importantly, nodes below the pruning site are intact, and therefore structures that require only low nodes, such as AgrP and VP, are well-formed in agrammatic production.

How does tree pruning account for the intricate pattern of loss and sparing in agrammatic production? The implications of tree pruning for three syntactic domains—verb inflection, embedding, and question production—are examined here.

Inflections are impaired in agrammatic production, but in a selective way. In Hebrew and in Palestinian Arabic, tense inflection was found to be severely impaired, whereas agreement inflection was almost intact in a set of constrained tasks such as sentence completion, elicitation, and repetition (Friedmann, 1994, 2001; Friedmann and Grodzinsky, 1997). Subsequent studies reported a similar dissociation between tense and agreement in Spanish, Dutch, German, and English. If tense and agreement reside in different nodes in the syntactic tree, and if TP is higher than AgrP, this dissociation is explained by tree pruning: the TP is inaccessible, and therefore tense inflection is impaired, whereas the AgrP node, which is below the pruning site, remains intact, and subsequently agreement inflection is intact. This can also account for the findings from German and Dutch, according to which individuals with agrammatic aphasia frequently use nonfinite verbs in sentence-final position, instead of the required fully inflected main verbs in second position (Kolk and Heeschen, 1992; Bastiaanse and van Zonneveld, 1998). The lack of TP and CP prevents persons with agrammatic aphasia from moving the verbs to T to collect the required inflection, and to C to second position, and therefore they produce the verbs in a nonfinite form, which does not require verb movement to high nodes. Verbs that do not move to high nodes stay in their base-generated position within VP, which is the sentence-final position (see Friedmann, 2000).

Individuals with agrammatic aphasia are also known to use only simple sentences and to avoid *embedded sentences*. When they do try to produce an embedded sentence, either a relative clause (such as "I saw the girl that the grandmother drew") or a sentential complement of a verb ("The girl said that the grandmother drew her"), they fail, and stop before the complementizer (the embedding marker "that," for example), omit the

complementizer, use direct instead of indirect speech, or produce an ungrammatical sentence (Menn and Obler, 1990; Hagiwara, 1995; Friedmann, 1998, 2001). The difficulty posed by embedded constructions is explained by tree pruning, as full relative clauses and sentential embeddings require the CP, and when the CP is unavailable, these structures are impaired. Interestingly, embedded sentences that do not require the CP, such as reduced relatives ("I saw the boy crying"), are produced correctly by individuals with agrammatism.

Tree pruning and the inaccessibility of CP cause a deficit in another important set of structures, *questions*. Seminal treatment studies by Shapiro, Thompson, and their group (e.g., Thompson and Shapiro, 1995) show that persons with agrammatic aphasia cannot produce well-formed Wh questions. Other studies show that in English, both Wh and yes/no questions are impaired, but in languages such as Hebrew and Arabic, Wh questions are impaired but yes/no questions are intact (Friedmann, 2002). Again, these dissociations between and within languages are a result of the unavailability of the CP: agrammatic aphasics encounter severe difficulties when trying to produce Wh questions because Wh morphemes (who, what, where, etc.) reside at CP. Yes/no questions in English also require an element at CP, the auxiliary ("Do you like cream cheese"?), and are therefore impaired too. Yes/no questions in Hebrew and Arabic, on the other hand, do not require any overt element in CP ("You like hummus?"), and this is why they are produced correctly.

The tree pruning hypothesis is also instrumental in describing different degrees of agrammatism severity. Clinical work shows that some individuals with agrammatism use a wider range of syntactic structures than others and retain more abilities, such as verb inflection, whereas other individuals use mainly simple sentences and substitute inflections. It is possible to characterize the milder impairment as pruning at a higher site in the tree, at CP, whereas the more severe impairment results from pruning at a lower position, TP. Thus, the more mildly impaired individuals show impairment in Wh questions and embedding, but their ability to inflect verbs for both tense and agreement is relatively intact. More severely impaired individuals, who are impaired also in TP, show impaired tense inflection in addition to impairment in questions and embedding. In both degrees of severity, agreement inflection is intact. Crucially, no individual was found to exhibit a deficit in a low node without a deficit in higher nodes. In other words, there was no TP deficit without a deficit in CP, and no deficit in AgrP without a deficit in TP and CP.

Finally, tree pruning provides a principled explanation for the effect that treatment in one syntactic domain has on other domains. Thompson and Shapiro, for example, report that following question production treatment, their patients started using sentential embedding. This can be explained if treatment has enhanced the accessibility of the syntactic node that is common for the two structures, CP. Similarly, the decrease in verb omission that has been reported to accompany tense inflection improvement can be explained by enhanced accessibility to the inflectional node TP.

Current linguistic theory thus provides a useful toolbox to account for the complicated weave of spared and impaired abilities in speech production in agrammatic aphasia. The hierarchical structure of the syntactic tree enables an account of the highly selective syntactic deficit in agrammatic production in terms of syntactic tree pruning.

—*Naama Friedmann*

References

Bastiaanse, R., and van Zonneveld, R. (1998). On the relation between verb inflection and verb position in Dutch agrammatic aphasics. *Brain and Language, 64,* 165–181.

Berndt, R. S., and Caramazza, A. (1980). A redefinition of Broca's aphasia: Implications for a neuropsychological model of language. *Applied Psycholinguistics, 1,* 225–278.

Caplan, D. (1985). Syntactic and semantic structures in agrammatism. In M.-L. Kean (Ed.), *Agrammatism.* New York: Academic Press.

Chomsky, N. (1995). *The minimalist program.* Cambridge, MA: MIT Press.

Friedmann, N. (1994). *Morphology in agrammatism: A dissociation between tense and agreement.* Master's thesis, Tel Aviv University.

Friedmann, N. (1998). *Functional categories in agrammatic production: A cross-linguistic study.* Doctoral dissertation, Tel Aviv University.

Friedmann, N. (2000). Moving verbs in agrammatic production. In R. Bastiaanse and Y. Grodzinsky (Eds.), *Grammatical disorders in aphasia: A neurolinguistic perspective* (pp. 152–170). London: Whurr.

Friedmann, N. (2001). Agrammatism and the psychological reality of the syntactic tree. *Journal of Psycholinguistic Research, 30,* 71–90.

Friedmann, N. (2002). Question production in agrammatism: The Tree Pruning Hypothesis. *Brain and Language, 80,* 160–187.

Friedmann, N., and Grodzinsky, Y. (1997). Tense and agreement in agrammatic production: Pruning the syntactic tree. *Brain and Language, 56,* 397–425.

Goodglass, H. (1976). Agrammatism. In H. Whitaker and H. A. Whitaker (Eds.), *Studies in neurolinguistics* (vol. 1, pp. 237–260). New York: Academic Press.

Grodzinsky, Y. (1990). *Theoretical perspectives on language deficits.* Cambridge, MA: MIT Press.

Grodzinsky, Y. (2000). The neurology of syntax: Language use without Broca's area. *Behavioral and Brain Sciences, 23,* 1–71.

Hagiwara, H. (1995). The breakdown of functional categories and the economy of derivation. *Brain and Language, 50,* 92–116.

Kolk, H. H. J., and Heeschen, C. (1992). Agrammatism, paragrammatism and the management of language. *Language and Cognitive Processes, 7,* 89–129.

Menn, L., and Obler, L. (1990). *Agrammatic aphasia: A cross-language narrative sourcebook.* Philadelphia: John Benjamins.

Ouhalla, J. (1993). Functional categories, agrammatism and language acquisition. *Linguistische Berichte, 143,* 3–36.

Pollock, J. Y. (1989). Verb movement, Universal Grammar and the structure of IP. *Linguistic Inquiry, 20,* 365–424.

Thompson, C. K., and Shapiro, L. P. (1995). Training sentence production in agrammatism: Implications for normal and disordered language. *Brain and Language, 50,* 201–224.

Zurif, E. B. (1995). Brain regions of relevance to syntactic processing. In L. Gleitman and M. Liberman (Eds.), *An invitation to cognitive science* (2nd ed., vol. 1, pp. 381–397). Cambridge, MA: MIT Press.

Further Readings

Bastiaanse, R., and Grodzinsky, Y. (Eds.). (2000). *Grammatical disorders in aphasia: A neurolinguistic perspective.* London: Whurr.

Benedet, M. J., Christiansen, J. A., and Goodglass, H. (1998). A cross-linguistic study of grammatical morphology in Spanish- and English-speaking agrammatic patients. *Cortex, 34,* 309–336.

De Bleser, R., and Luzzatti, C. (1994). Morphological processing in Italian agrammatic speakers: Syntactic implementation of inflectional morphology. *Brain and Language, 46,* 21–40.

Friedmann, N., and Grodzinsky, Y. (2000). Split inflection in neurolinguistics. In M.-A. Friedemann and L. Rizzi (Eds.), *The acquisition of syntax: Studies in comparative developmental linguistics* (pp. 84–104). Geneva: Longman Linguistics Library Series.

Friedmann, N., Wenkert-Olenik, D., and Gil, M. (2000). From theory to practice: Treatment of agrammatic production in Hebrew based on the Tree Pruning Hypothesis. *Journal of Neurolinguistics, 13,* 250–254.

Grodzinsky, Y., Shapiro, L. P., and Swinney, D. A. (Eds.). (2000). *Language and the brain: Representation and processing.* San Diego, CA: Academic Press.

Kean, M. L. (1995). The elusive character of agrammatism. *Brain and Language, 50,* 369–384.

Rizzi, L. (1994). Some notes on linguistic theory and language development: The case of root infinitives. *Language Acquisition, 3,* 371–393.

Ruigendijk, E., van Zonneveld, R., and Bastiaanse, R. (1999). Case assignment in agrammatism. *Journal of Speech, Language, and Hearing Research, 42,* 962–971.

Swinney, D., and Zurif, E. B. (1995). Syntactic processing in aphasia. *Brain and Language, 50,* 225–239.

Thompson, C. K., and Shapiro, L. P. (1994). A linguistic specific approach to treatment of sentence production deficits in aphasia. *Clinical Aphasiology, 22,* 307–323.

Zurif, E., and Swinney, D. (1994). The neuropsychology of language. In M. A. Gernsbacher (Ed.), *Handbook of psycholinguistics* (pp. 1055–1074). Orlando: Academic Press.

Trace Deletion Hypothesis

Some aphasic syndromes implicate grammar. Known for almost a century to be grammatically impaired in speech production (see SYNTACTIC TREE PRUNING), individuals with Broca's and Wernicke's aphasia are now known to have receptive grammatical deficits as well. The trace deletion hypothesis (TDH) is a collection of ideas about the proper approach to linguistic deficits subsequent to brain damage in adults, particularly Broca's aphasia. Support for a grammatical interpretation of aphasia comes from a dense body of research from many laboratories and varied test paradigms, administered to large groups of aphasic speakers of a variety of languages.

This article explains why a precise characterization of receptive deficits in aphasia is important, and how we came about to know it. It first aims to demonstrate that Broca's and Wernicke's aphasia (and perhaps other syndromes) are syntactically selective disorders in which the line dividing impaired from preserved syntax is fine and amenable to a precise characterization.

The comprehension of sentences containing grammatical transformations is impaired in aphasia. Transformations, or syntactic movement rules, are important intrasentential relations. In their various theoretical guises, these rules are designed to explain dependency relations between positions in a sentence. As a first pass, we sacrifice precision for clarity, and say that transformationally moved constituents are found in noncanonical positions (e.g., a subject in a passive sentence, ***The teacher*** *was watched* _____ *by the student*; a questioned element in object questions, ***Which man*** *did Susan see* _____?). Each of these sentences has a nontransformational counterpart (e.g., *The student watched* ***the teacher***; ***Which man*** *saw Susan?*). Roughly, in transformationally derived sentences, a constituent is phonetically present in one (**bolded**) position but is interpreted semantically in another, "empty" position (_____), which is annotated by a *t* (for trace of movement) and serves as a link between the semantic role of the moved constituent and its phonetic realization. Traces are therefore crucial for the interpretation of transformational sentences.

When aphasic comprehension is tested on the contrast between transformational and nontransformational sentences, a big difference is found: Broca's aphasics understand active sentences, subject questions, and the like normally, yet fail on their transformational counterparts. This has led to the claim that in receptive language, Broca's aphasics cannot represent traces of movement. These traces are deleted from the syntactic representations they build, hence TDH. This generalization helps localize grammatical operations in the brain. Furthermore, the highly selective character of this deficit has major theoretical ramifications for linguistic theory and the theory of sentence processing.

How exactly does the TDH work? Let us look at receptive tasks commonly used in research on brain-language relations. These are sentence-picture-matching (SPM), grammaticality judgment (GJ), and measurements of reaction time (RT) during comprehension. We can consider the SPM method first. A sentence containing two arguments is presented (e.g., *The student watched the teacher*); it is "semantically reversible"—the lexical content does not reveal who did what to whom. The task, however, requires exactly that: subjects are usually requested to choose between two action pictures in which the roles are reversed (student watching teacher, teacher watching student). Reliance on syntax is critical. On being given a series of such sentences,

Broca's aphasics perform at above chance levels on nontransformational sentences and at chance levels on transformationally derived sentences.

What do such findings mean? Standard principles of error analysis dictate that a binary choice design allows for three logically possible outcomes: above-, below-, and at-chance performance levels. Above-chance performance is virtually normal; below-chance amounts to systematic reversal of roles in SPM; at-chance means guessing, as if the subject were tossing a coin prior to responding. Indeed, the response pattern of Broca's aphasics on transformational sentences resembles guessing behavior. That said, the burden on the TDH is to provide a deductive explanation of why left anterior lesions, which allow normal comprehension of sentences without transformations, lead to guessing when transformational movement is at issue.

The foregoing was a simplified introductory discussion. In reality, things are somewhat more complicated. The deletion of a trace in certain cases does not hinder performance in aphasia. Our characterization needs refinement. The leading idea is to view aphasic sentence interpretation as a composite process—an interaction between incomplete syntax (i.e., representations lacking traces) and a compensatory cognitive strategy. The interpretation of moved constituents, as we saw, depends crucially on the trace; without traces, the semantic role of a moved constituent cannot be determined. Moved constituents (**bolded**) are thus uninterpretable. A nonlinguistic, linear order–based cognitive strategy is invoked to try and salvage uninterpreted NPs ⟨NP_1 = agent; NP_2 = theme⟩. In English, constituents moved to a clause-initial position will thus be agents. In certain cases (e.g., subject questions), the strategy compensates correctly: in the subject relative ***the man*** *who* ***t*** *loves Mary is tall*, the head of the relative clause, ***the man***, is moved, and receives its semantic interpretation (or thematic role) via the trace. A deleted trace blocks this process, and the strategy is invoked, assigning agenthood to ***the man*** and yielding the correct semantics: NP_1 (***the man***) = agent by strategy, and NP_2 (***Mary***) = theme by the remaining grammar. In other cases the TDH system results in error: In object relatives—***the man*** *who Mary loves* ***t*** *is tall*—the agent role assigned by the strategy (acting subsequent to trace deletion) gives rise to a misleading representation: NP_1 (***the man***) = agent by strategy, and NP_2 (***Mary***) = agent by the grammar. The result is a semantic representation with two potential agents for the depicted action, which leads the patients to guessing behavior. The selective nature of the aphasic comprehension deficit is captured, which is precisely what the TDH is designed to explain.

Languages with structural properties different from English lend further support to the TDH. Thus, Chinese, Japanese, German and Dutch, Spanish, and Hebrew have different properties, and the performance of Broca's aphasics is determined by the TDH as it interacts with the particular grammar of each language. Japanese active sentences, for example, have two configurations:

[*Taro-ga Hanako-o nagutta* (Taro hit Hanako)—Subject Object Verb], [**Hanako-o** *Taro-ga t nagutta*—**Object** Subject *t* Verb]. These simple structures mean the same and are identical on every dimension except movement. Broca's aphasics are above chance in comprehending the former and at chance level on the former, in keeping with the TDH. A similar finding is obtained in Hebrew. In Chinese, an otherwise SVO language like English, heads of relative clauses (annotated by the subscript *h*) follow the relative (unlike English, in which they precede it, as the example shows):

(1) *[t zhuei gou] de* **mau**$_h$ *hen da*
    chase dog that cat very big
    "**the cat**$_h$ *that [t chased the dog] was very big*"

(2) *[mau zhuei t] de* **gou**$_h$ *hen xiao*
    cat chased that dog very small
    "**the dog**$_h$ *that [the cat chased t] was very small*"

This structural contrast leads to remarkable contrastive performance in Broca's aphasia: in Chinese subject relatives (1), the head of the relative (**the cat**) moves to the front of the sentence, lacks a role, and is assigned agent by the strategy, which leads to a correct representation in which the cat indeed chases the dog. In Chinese, the head (**mau**) also moves, yet to sentence-final position, and the strategy (incorrectly) assigns it the theme role. This representation now has two themes, the dog and the cat, and the result is guessing. Similar considerations that hold for the object relatives are left to the reader. English and Chinese thus yield mirror-image results, which correlate with a relevant syntactic contrast between the two languages. Further intriguing cross-linguistic contrasts exist.

Moving to other experimental tasks, we encounter remarkable cross-methodological consistency. When the detection of a violation of grammaticality critically depends on traces, the TDH predicts disability on the part of Broca's aphasics. This is indeed the case. When given GJ tasks, they show differential performance between sentences with and without traces, again in keeping with the TDH. Finally, the rich literature on timed language reception in Broca's aphasia (RT) suggests that on-line computation of trace-antecedent relations is compromised.

This type of deficit is not restricted to Broca's aphasia. On at least some tests, Wernicke's aphasics perform like Broca's aphasics. There are contrasts between the two groups, to be sure, yet contrary to past views, there are overlapping deficits. Although this new picture is just beginning to unfold, independent evidence from functional imaging of normal populations (fMRI) supports it. Both Broca's and Wernicke's regions of the healthy brain are involved in transformational analysis, although likely in different ways.

This series of cross-methodological findings from different languages and populations, and the TDH as a generalization over them, have a host of important theoretical implications. They show that the natural classes of structures that linguists assume have a firm neuro-biological basis; they afford an unusual view on the inner workings of the human sentence processing device; they connect localized neural tissue and linguistic concepts in a more detailed way than ever before. Finally, there appears to be clinical (therapeutic) value to the view that Broca's aphasia and Wernicke's aphasia are grammatically selective: although currently experimental, preliminary results suggest that therapeutic methods guided by this view are somewhat efficacious.

— *Yosef Grodzinsky*

Further Readings

Ben-Shachar, M., Hendler, T., Kahn, I., Ben-Bashat, D., and Grodzinsky, Y. (2001). *Grammatical transformations activate Broca's region: An fMRI study*. Paper presented at a meeting of the Cognitive Neuroscience Society, New York.

Caplan, D., Alpert, N., and Waters, G. (1998). Effects of syntactic structure and propositional number on patterns of regional blood flow. *Journal of Cognitive Neuroscience, 10,* 541–552.

Goodglass, H. (1968). Studies in the grammar of aphasics. In S. Rosenberg and J. Koplin (Eds.), *Developments in applied psycholinguistics research*. New York: Macmillan.

Grodzinsky, Y. (1986). Language deficits and the theory of syntax. *Brain and Language, 27,* 135–159.

Grodzinsky, Y. (1990). *Theoretical perspectives on language deficits.* Cambridge, MA: MIT Press.

Grodzinsky, Y. (2000). The neurology of syntax: Language use without Broca's area. *Behavioral and Brain Sciences, 23,* 1–71.

Grodzinsky, Y., and Finkel, L. (1998). The neurology of empty categories: Aphasics' failure to detect ungrammaticality. *Journal of Cognitive Neuroscience, 10,* 281–292.

Grodzinsky, Y., Pierce, A., and Marakovitz, S. (1991). Neuropsychological reasons for a transformational analysis of verbal passive. *Natural Language and Linguistic Theory, 9,* 431–453.

Grodzinsky, Y., Piñango, M., Zurif, E., and Drai, D. (1999). The critical role of group studies in neuropsychology: Comprehension regularities in Broca's aphasia. *Brain and Language, 67,* 134–147.

Hagiwara, H. (1993). The breakdown of Japanese passives and ϑ-role assignment principles by Broca's aphasics. *Brain and Language, 45,* 318–339.

Just, M. A., Carpenter, P. A., Keller, T. A., Eddy, W. F., and Thulborn, K. R. (1996). Brain activation modulated by sentence comprehension. *Science, 274,* 114–116.

Schwartz, M. F., Linebarger, M. C., Saffran, E. M., and Pate, D. C. (1987). Syntactic transparency and sentence interpretation in aphasia. *Language and Cognitive Processes, 2,* 85–113.

Shapiro, L. P., Gordon, B., Hack, N., and Killackey, J. (1993). Verb-argument structure processing in complex sentences in Broca's and Wernicke's aphasia. *Brain and Language, 45,* 423–447.

Shapiro, L. P., and Levin, B. A. (1990). Verb processing during sentence comprehension in aphasia. *Brain and Language, 38,* 21–47.

Shapiro, L. P., and Thompson, C. K. (1994). The use of linguistic theory as a framework for treatment studies in aphasia. In P. Lemme (Ed.), *Clinical aphasiology* (vol. 22). Austin, TX: Pro-Ed.

Swinney, D., and Zurif, E. (1995). Syntactic processing in aphasia. *Brain and Language, 50*, 225–239.

Thompson, C. K., Shapiro, L. P., Ballard, K. J., Jacobs, B. J., Schneider, S. S., and Tait, M. E. (1997). Training and generalized production of WH- and NP-movement structures in agrammatic aphasia. *Journal of Speech, Language, and Hearing Research, 40*, 228–244.

Zurif, E. B. (1995). Brain regions of relevance to syntactic processing. In L. Gleitman and M. Liberman (Eds.), *An invitation to cognitive science* (2nd ed., vol. 1). Cambridge, MA: MIT Press.

Zurif, E. B., and Caramazza, A. (1976). Linguistic structures in aphasia: Studies in syntax and semantics. In H. Whitaker and H. H. Whitaker (Eds.), *Studies in neurolinguistics* (vol. 2). New York: Academic Press.

Part IV: Hearing

Amplitude Compression in Hearing Aids

In the latter part of the 1980s, *wide dynamic range compression* (WDRC) amplification was introduced into the hearing aid market. Within a few years it was widely recognized as a fundamentally important new amplification strategy. Within 10 years nearly every hearing aid manufacturer had developed a WDRC product.

Compression is useful as a processing strategy because it compensates for the loss of cochlear *outer hair cells*, which compress the dynamic range of sound within the cochlea. Sensorineural hearing loss is characterized by *loudness recruitment*, which results from damage to the outer hair cells. WDRC compensates for this hair cell disorder, ideally restoring the limited dynamic range of the recruiting ear to that of the normal ear. This article reviews the history of loudness research, loudness recruitment, cochlear compression effects (such as the upward spread of masking) that result from and characterize OHC compression, and finally, outer hair cell physiology. The WDRC processing strategy is explained, and a short history of the development of WDRC hearing aids is provided.

Compression and Loudness

Acoustical signal *intensity* is defined as the flow of acoustic energy in watts per meter squared (w/m²). *Loudness* is the perceptual intensity, measured in either *sones* or *loudness units* (LU). One sone is defined as the loudness of a 1 kHz tone at 40 dB SPL, while 1 LU is defined as the loudness at threshold. Zero loudness corresponds to zero intensity.[1]

For the case of pure tones, one sone is ≈975 LU. Isoloudness intensity contours were first determined in 1927 by Kingsbury (Kingsbury, 1927; Fletcher, 1929, p. 227). Such curves describe the relation between equally loud tones (or narrow bands of noise) at different frequencies. The intensity of an equally loud 1 kHz tone is called the *loudness level*, which has units of *phons*, measured in w/m². In 1923 Fletcher, and again in 1924 Fletcher and Steinberg, published the first key papers on the measurement of the loudness for speech signals (Fletcher, 1923a; Fletcher and Steinberg, 1924). In the 1924 paper the authors state

$$10^{-\bar{a}/30} = \int_0^\infty \mathscr{G}(f) 10^{-a(f)/30} \, df$$

... the use of the above formula involved a *summation of the cube root of the energy rather than the energy.*

where a is the relative intensity in dB SL, $\bar{a}$ is the "effective" loudness level, and $\mathscr{G}(f)$ is an empirically determined frequency weighting factor. This cube root dependence had first been described by Fletcher the year before (Fletcher, 1923a). Fletcher and Steinberg concluded that

it became apparent that the non-linear character of the ear['s] transmitting mechanism was playing an important part in determining the loudness of the complex tones (p. 307).

Power law relations between the intensity of the physical stimulus and the psychophysical response are examples of *Stevens' law*. Fletcher's 1923 loudness growth equation, which for tones was found to be $L(I) \propto I^{1/3}$, where L is the loudness and I is the acoustic intensity, established the important special case of Stevens' law for sound intensity and pure-tone loudness. Their method is described in the caption of Figure 1. We now know that Fletcher and Steinberg were observing the compression induced by the cochlear outer hair cells (OHCs).

Loudness Additivity

In 1933 Fletcher and Munson published their seminal paper on loudness. This paper detailed (1) the relation of isoloudness across frequency (loudness level, or phons); (2) their loudness growth argument, described below; (3) a model showing the relation of masking to loudness; and (4) the basic idea behind the critical band (critical ratio).

Regarding the second point, rather than thinking directly in terms of loudness growth, they tried to find a formula to describe how the loudnesses of several stimuli combine. From loudness experiments with low- and high-pass speech and complex tones, and other unpublished experiments over the previous 10 years, they showed that, across critical bands, loudness (not intensity) adds. Fletcher's working hypothesis (Fletcher and Steinberg, 1924) was that each signal is nonlinearly compressed in narrow bands (*critical bands*) by the cochlea, neurally coded, and the resulting band rates are added.[2] The 1933 experiment clearly showed how loudness (i.e., the neural rate, according to Fletcher's model) adds. Fletcher and Munson also determined the cochlear compression function $G(I)$ described below for tones and speech. We now know that this function dramatically changes with sensorineural hearing loss.

Today this model concept is called *loudness additivity*. Their hypothesis was that when two equally loud tones are presented together but separated in frequency so that they do not mask each other, the result is "twice as loud." The verification of this assumption lies in the predictive ability of the additivity assumption. For example, they showed that 10 tones that are all equally

---

[1] Fletcher and Munson (1933) were able to measure the loudness below the single pure-tone threshold by using 10 equally loud tones. This proves that the loudness at threshold is not zero (Buus, Musch, and Florentine, 1998).

[2] There seems to be some confusion about what is added within critical bands. Clearly, pressure must add within a critical band, or else we would not hear beats. Many books and papers assume that intensity adds within each critical band. This is true in the ensemble sense for random signals, but such a scheme will not work for tones on a single trial basis.

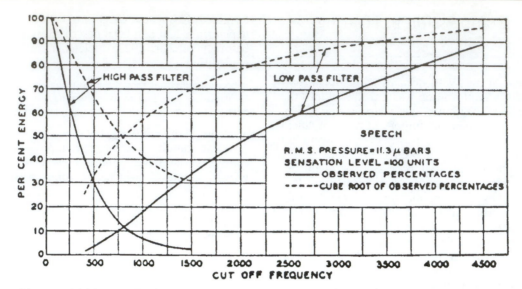

Figure 1. Effect of low- and high-pass filtering on the speech loudness level. The broadband speech is varied in level until it is equal in loudness to the low-pass-filtered speech. This is repeated for each value of the filter cutoff frequency. The experiment was then repeated for the high-pass speech. The percent reduction of the equally loud broadband speech energy is plotted against the filter cutoff frequency. For example, if broadband speech is to be equal in loudness to speech that has been low-pass-filtered to 1 kHz, it must be reduced in level to 17% of its original energy. The corresponding relative level for 1 kHz high-pass-filtered speech is 7%. These functions are shown as the solid lines in the figure. The high- and low-pass loudnesses do not add to 1 since the two solid lines cross at about 11%. After taking the cube root, however, the loudness curves cross at 50% (i.e., at 0.8 kHz, $0.125^{1/3} = 0.5$), and therefore sum to 100%. A level of 11.3 μ BARS (dynes/cm^2) corresponds to 1.13 Pa, which is close to 95 dB SPL. (From Fletcher, 1929, p. 236.)

loud (they will be at different intensities, of course), when played together, are 10 times louder, as long as they do not mask each other. As another example, Fletcher and Munson found that loudness additivity held for signals "between the two ears" as well as for signals "in the same ear." When the tones masked each other (namely, when their masking patterns overlapped), additivity still holds, but over an attenuated set of patterns (Fletcher and Munson, 1933). Their 1933 model is fundamental to our present understanding of auditory sound processing.

The Method. A relative scale factor (gain) α may be defined either in terms of the pressure or in terms of the intensity. Since it is the voltage on the earphone that is scaled, the most convenient definition of α is in terms of the pressure, P. It is typically expressed in dB, given by $20 \log_{10}(\alpha)$.

Two equally loud tones were matched in loudness by a single tone scaled by α^*. The asterisk indicates this special value of α. The resulting definition of α^* is given by

$$L(\alpha^* P) = 2L(P), \qquad (1)$$

which says that, when the single tone pressure, P, is scaled by $\alpha = \alpha^*$, the loudness, $L(\alpha^* P)$, is twice as loud as the unscaled signal. Given the relative loudness level (in phons) of "twice as loud," defined by $\alpha^*(I)$, the loudness growth function $G(I)$ may be found by graphical methods or by numerical recursion, as shown in Fletcher (1953, p. 190) and in Allen (1996b). The values of $\alpha^*(I)$ found by Fletcher in different papers published between 1933 and 1953 are shown in Figure 2.

The Result. These two-tone loudness matching experiments showed that for f_1 between 0.8 and 8.0 kHz, and f_2 far enough away from f_1 (above or below) so that

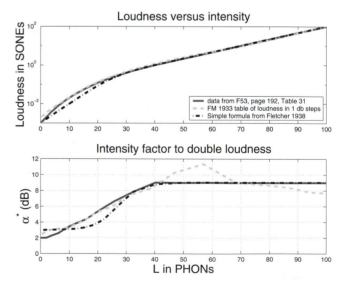

Figure 2. Loudness and α^* as a function of the loudness level, in phons. When α^* is 9 dB, loudness increases as the cube root of intensity. When α^* is 3 dB, loudness is proportional to intensity. (From Fletcher, 1953.)

there is no masking, the relative level α was found to be ≈ 9 dB (ca. 1953) for P_1 above 40 dB SPL. This value decreased linearly to 2 dB for P_1 at 0 phons, as shown in Figure 2.

From this formulation, Fletcher and Munson found that at 1 kHz, and above 40 dB SPL, the pure-tone loudness G is proportional to the cube root of the signal intensity $[G(I) = (P/P_{ref})^{2/3}]$ because $\alpha^* = 2^{3/2}$ (9 dB).[3] Below 40 dB SPL, loudness was frequently assumed to be proportional to the intensity $[G(I) = (P/P_{ref})^2$, $\alpha^* = 2^{1/2}$, or 3 dB]. Figure 2 shows the loudness growth curve and α^* given in Fletcher (1953, p. 192, Table 31) as well as the 1938 and 1933 papers. As may be seen from the figure, in 1933 they found values of α as high as 11 dB near 55 dB SL. Furthermore, the value of α^* at low levels is not 3 dB but is closer to 2 dB. Fletcher's statement that loudness is proportional to intensity (α^* is 3 dB near threshold) was an idealization that was appealing, but not supported by actual results.

Recruitment and the Rate of Loudness Growth

Once loudness had been quantified and modeled in 1933 by Fletcher and Munson, Mark Gardner, a close personal friend and colleague of Harvey Fletcher, began measuring the loudness growth of hearing-impaired subjects. In about 1934 Gardner first discovered the effect that has become known as *loudness recruitment* (Gardner, 1994), first reported by Steinberg and Gardner in 1937.

In terms of the published record, Fowler, a New York ear, nose, and throat physician, is credited with the discovery of recruitment in 1936. Fowler was in close touch with the work being done at Bell Labs and was friendly with Wegel and Fletcher (they published papers together). Fowler made loudness measurements on his many hearing-impaired patients and was the first to publish the abnormal loudness growth results. Fowler coined the term *recruitment* (Fowler, 1936).

Steinberg and Gardner (1937) were the first to correctly identify recruitment as a loss of compression. Since most sensorineural hearing loss is cochlear in origin, it follows that the loss of compression is in the cochlea. Those interested in the details are referred to the following articles (Neely and Allen, 1997; Allen, 1997a; Allen, 1999a).

Loudness Growth in the Recruiting Ear. Figure 3 shows a normal loudness growth function along with a simulated recruiting loudness growth function. It is necessary to plot these functions on a log-log (log loudness versus dB SPL) scale because of the dynamic ranges of loudness and intensity. The use of the dB and log loudness has resulted in a misinterpretation of the rate (slope) of recruitment. In the figure we see that for a 4 dB change in intensity about 58 dB SPL, the loudness changes by

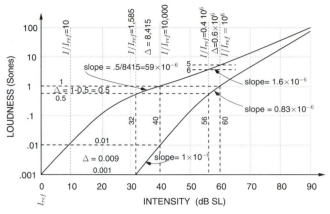

Figure 3. Shown here is a recruitment-type loss corresponding to a variable loss of gain on a log-log scale. The upper curve corresponds to the normal loudness curve; the lower curve corresponds to a simulated recruiting hearing loss. For an intensity level change from 56–60 dB, the loudness change is smaller for the recruiting ear (0.5 sones) than in the normal ear (1 sone). The belief that the loudness slope in the damaged ear is greater led to the concept that the JND in the damaged ear should be smaller (this was the rationale behind the SISI test) (see Martin, 1986, p. 160). Both conclusions are false.

1.0 sone in the normal ear and 0.5 sones in the recruiting ear. While the slope looks steeper on a log plot, the actual rate of loudness growth (in sones) in the recruiting ear is smaller. Its misdefinition as "the abnormally rapid growth of loudness" has lead to some serious conceptual errors about loudness and hearing loss. Correct statements about loudness recruitment include "the abnormal growth of loudness" or "the abnormally rapid growth of relative loudness $\Delta L/L$ (or log loudness)."

Fowler's Mistake. After learning from Wegel about the yet unpublished recruitment measurements of Steinberg and Gardner, E. P. Fowler attempted to use recruitment to diagnose middle ear disease (Fowler, 1936). In cases of hearing loss involving financial compensation, Fowler stated that recruitment was an "ameliorating" factor (Fowler, 1942). In other words, he viewed recruitment as a *recovery* from hearing loss—its presence indicated a reduced hearing loss at high intensities. Thus, given two people with equal threshold losses, the person having the least amount of recruitment was given greater financial compensation (the loss could be due to middle ear disease, and the individual would receive greater compensation than someone having a similar sensorineural loss).

In my view, it was Fowler's poor understanding of recruitment that led to such terms as complete recruitment versus partial recruitment and hyper-recruitment. *Complete recruitment* means that the recruiting ear and the normal ear perceive the same loudness at high intensities. Steinberg and Gardner described such a loss as a variable loss (i.e., sensorineural loss) and partial recruitment as a mixed loss (i.e., having a conductive component that acts as a frequency-dependent fixed

---

[3] Since $G(I) = (I/I_{ref})^\beta = (P/P_{ref})^{2\beta}$, $L(P) = (P/P_{ref})^{2\beta}$. Thus, Equation 1 gives $(\alpha^* P)^{2\beta} = 2P^{2\beta}$, or $(\alpha^*)^{2\beta} = 2$, giving $\alpha^* = 2^{1/2\beta}$. When $\beta = 1/3$, $\alpha^* = 2^{3/2}$.

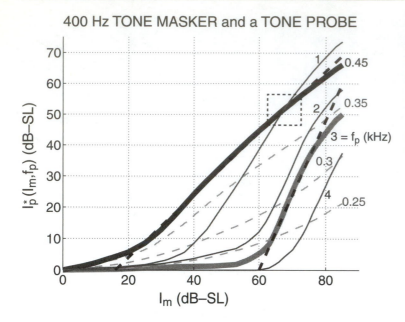

400 Hz TONE MASKER and a TONE PROBE

Figure 4. Masking data for a 400 Hz masker. The abscissa is the intensity of the *masker* I_m while the ordinate is the threshold intensity of the probe $I_p^*(I_m, f_p)$ (the *maskee*), each in dB SL. Each curve corresponds to a probe of a different frequency, labeled in kHz. Two dashed lines are superimposed on the heavy curves corresponding to f_p of 0.45 kHz (slope = 1.0 dB/dB) and 3 kHz (slope = 2.4 dB/dB). The curves for f_p of 1, 2, and 4 kHz are shown by light lines. Probe frequencies below 1 kHz are shown as light dashed lines. (Data from Wegel and Lane, 1924.)

attenuation). They, and Fowler, verified the conductive component by estimating the air-bone gap.

Steinberg and Gardner attempted to set the record straight. They clearly understood what they were dealing with, as is indicated in the following quote (Steinberg and Gardner, 1937, p. 20):

Owing to the expanding action of this type of loss it would be necessary to introduce a corresponding compression in the amplifier in order to produce the same amplification at all levels.

This model of hearing and hearing loss, along with the loudness models of Fletcher and Munson (1933), are basic to the eventual quantitative understanding of cochlear signal processing and the cochlea's role in detection, masking, and loudness in normal and impaired ears. The work by Fletcher (1950) and Steinberg and Gardner (1937), and work on modeling hearing loss and recruitment by Allen (1991) support this view.

Compression and Masking

In 1922, one year after publishing the first threshold measurements with Wegel, Fletcher published measurements on the threshold of hearing in the presence of a masking tone (Fletcher, 1923a, 1923b). Wegel and Lane's classic and widely referenced paper on masking, and their theory of the cochlea, soon followed, in 1924. In Figure 4 we reproduce one of the figures from Fletcher's 1923 publication (which later appeared in the 1924 Wegel paper) showing the upward spread of masking due to a 400 Hz tone. As we shall see, these curves characterize the nonlinear compressive effects of outer hair cell compression.

Critical Band Masking. When the probe is near the masker in frequency, as in the case of the 0.45 kHz probe tone shown in Figure 4, the growth of masking is close to linear. Such near-linear growth is called *Weber's law*. The masked-threshold probe intensity[4] I_p^* is equal to the masker intensity I_m plus 1 JND ΔI, namely

$$I_p^*(I_m) = I_m + \Delta I(I_m).$$

The masking appears to be linear because the relative JND (e.g., $\Delta I/I \approx 0.1$) is small. As the intensity of the masker is increased, the variations in the JND $\Delta I(I_m)$ with respect to the masker intensity I_m appear negligible, making $I_p^*(I_m)$ appear linear. Weber's law is therefore observed when the probe is within a critical bandwidth of the masker. One sees deviations from Weber's law when plotting more sensitive measures, such as $\Delta I(I_m)/I_m$ (Riesz, 1928).

Upward Spread of Masking. The *suppression threshold*, $I_s^*(f_p, f_m)$, is defined as the smallest masker intensity such that the slope of $I_p^*(I_m, f_p)$ with respect to I_m is greater than 1. Since the probe slope is close to 2.4 dB/dB over a range of intensities, this threshold is best estimated from the intercept of the $I_p^*(I_m, f_p)$ regression line with the abscissa. For the 3 kHz probe, the suppression threshold intensity is 60 dB SL. Such suppression is only seen for probes greater than the masker frequency ($f_p > f_m$). For probes that are sufficiently higher in frequency than the masker (e.g., $f_p \geq 2$ kHz in Fig. 4), the masking is close to zero dB SL until the masker intensity reaches the suppression threshold at about 50–60 dB SL. In other words, the *masked threshold*, defined as the intensity where the masking of the probe begins, and the *suppression threshold* are nearly the same. The suppression threshold for the dashed-line, superimposed on the "solid-fat" $f_p = 3$ kHz probe curve in Figure 4, is 60 dB SL; its slope is 2.4 dB/dB. For every 1 dB increase in

---

[4]An asterisk is used to indicate that the intensity is at threshold.

the masker intensity I_m, the probe threshold intensity $I_p^*(I_m, f_m, f_p)$ must be increased by 2.4 dB to return it to its detection threshold (Delgutte, 1990; Allen, 1997c). Namely, above $I_s^*(f_p = 3 \text{ kHz}, f_m = 0.4 \text{ kHz}) = 60 \text{ dB}$ SL (i.e., $I_m > 10^6 I_m^*$),

$$\frac{I_p^*(I_m)}{I_m^*} = \left(\frac{I_m}{I_s^*}\right)^{2.4}. \qquad (2)$$

From Figure 4, a surprising and interesting crossover occurs near 65–70 dB for the 1 kHz probe. As highlighted by the dashed box, the 1 kHz probe threshold curve crosses the 0.45 kHz probe threshold curve. At high levels, there is more masking at 1 kHz than at the probe frequency. This means that the masker excitation pattern peak has shifted toward the base of the cochlea (i.e., toward the stapes). Follow-up forward masking studies have confirmed this observation (Munson and Gardner, 1950, Fig. 8). McFadden (1986) presents an excellent and detailed discussion of this interesting "half-octave shift" effect that is recommended reading for all serious students of hearing loss.

Downward Spread of Masking.   For probes lower than the masker frequency (Fig. 4, 0.25 kHz), while the threshold is low, the masking is weak, since it has a slope that is less than linear. This may be explained by the migration of the more intense high-frequency (basal) masker excitation pattern away from the weaker probe excitation pattern (Allen, 1999b).

The Physiology of Compression

What is the source of Fletcher's tonal cube root loudness growth (i.e., Stevens' Law)? Today we know that the basilar membrane motion is nonlinear in intensity, as first described by Rhode in 1971, and that cochlear OHCs are the source of the basilar membrane nonlinearity. The history of this insight is both interesting and important.

In 1937, Lorente de Nó theorized that abnormal loudness growth associated with hearing loss (i.e., recruitment) is due to hair cell damage (Lorente de Nó, 1937). From noise trauma experiments on humans one may conclude that recruitment occurs in the cochlea (Carver, 1978). Animal experiments have confirmed this prediction and have emphasized the importance of OHC loss (Liberman and Kiang, 1978; Liberman and Dodds, 1984). This loss of OHCs causes a loss of the basilar membrane compression (Pickles, 1982, p. 287). It follows that the cube root tonal loudness growth starts with the nonlinear compression of basilar membrane motion due to stimulus-dependent voltage changes within the OHC.

Two-Tone Suppression.   The neural correlate of the 2.4 dB/dB psychoacoustic suppression effect (the upward spread of masking) is called *two-tone suppression* (2TS) (Sachs and Abbas, 1974; Fahey and Allen, 1985; Delgutte, 1990). Intense low-frequency tones attenuate low-level high-frequency tones to levels well below their

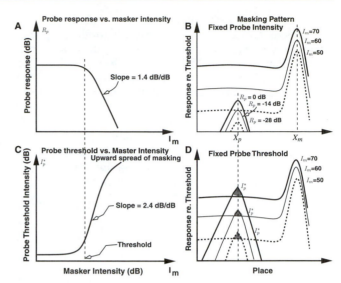

Figure 5. This sketch shows a conceptual view of the effect of a low-frequency suppressive masker on a high-frequency near-threshold probe, as a function of place. The abcissa for A and C is suppressor (masker) intensity in dB, while B and D are a cochlear place axis, where the base (stapes end) is at the origin. Panels **A** and **B** show the IHC cilia response R of a high-frequency, low-level probe, of fixed 20 dB SL intensity, being suppressed by a high-intensity, low-frequency ($f_m \ll f_p$) variable intensity suppressive masker having intensities I_s of 50, 60, and 70 dB SL. Panels A and B correspond to the isoprobe level of 20 dB SL. Even though the probe input intensity is fixed at 20 dB SL, the cilia response to the probe R_p is strongly suppressed by the masker above the suppression threshold, indicated by the vertical dashed line in A and C. The lower panels **C** and **D** show what happens when the high-frequency probe intensity is returned to threshold, indicated by $I_p^*(I_m)$. To restore the probe to threshold requires an increase of 1 dB/dB of suppressor level, due to the linear suppressor growth in the high-frequency tail region of the probe, at X_p.

threshold. The close relationship between the two effects has only recently been appreciated (Allen, 1997c, 1999b). The 2TS and upward spread of masking (USM) effects are important to the hearing aid industry because they quantify the normal cochlear compression that results from OHC processing. To fully appreciate the USM and 2TS, we need to describe the role of the OHC in nonlinear cochlear processing. In Figure 5 the operation of USM/2TS is summarized in terms of neural excitation patterns.

Cochlear Nonlinearity: How?

We still do not know precisely what controls the basilar membrane nonlinearity, although we know that it results from OHC stiffness and length changes (He and Dallos, 2000), which are a function of the OHC membrane voltage (Santos-Sacchi and Dilger, 1987). This voltage is determined by shearing displacement of the hair cell cilia by the tectorial membrane (TM). The most likely cause of nonlinear basilar membrane mechanics is changes in the micromechanical impedances within the organ of

Corti. This conclusion follows from ear canal impedance measurements, expressed in terms of nonlinear power reflectance, defined as the retrograde to incident power ratio (Allen et al., 1995). In a transmission line, the reflectance of energy is determined by the ratio of the load impedance at a given point divided by the local characteristic impedance of the line. It is this ratio that is level dependent (i.e., nonlinear).

Two Models. It is still not clear how the cochlear gain is reduced, and that is the subject of intense research. There are two basic but speculative theories. The first is a popular but qualitative theory, referred to as the *cochlear amplifier* (Kim et al., 1980). The second is a more physical and quantitative theory that requires two basic assumptions. The first assumption is that the tectorial membrane acts as a bandpass filter on the basilar membrane signal (Allen, 1980). The second assumption is that the OHCs dynamically "tune" the basilar membrane (i.e., the cochlear partition) by changing its net stiffness, causing a dynamic migration in the characteristic place with intensity (Allen, 1997b). Migration is known to occur (McFadden, 1986), so this assumption is founded on experimental dogma.

We cannot yet decide which, if either, of these two theories is correct, but for the present discussion, it is not important. The gain of the inner hair cell (IHC) cilia excitation function is signal dependent, compressing the 120 dB dynamic range of the acoustic stimulus to less than 60 dB. When the OHC voltage becomes depolarized, the OHC compliance increases, and the characteristic frequency (CF) of the basilar membrane shifts toward the base, reducing the nonlinear wide dynamic range compression.

Cochlear Nonlinearity: Why?

The discussion above leaves unanswered *why* the OHCs compress the signal on the basilar membrane. The answer to this question has to do with the large dynamic range of the ear. In 1922 Fletcher and Wegel were the first to use electronic instruments to measure the threshold and upper limit of human hearing (Fletcher and Wegel, 1922a, 1922b), thereby establishing the 120 dB dynamic range of the cochlea.

The IHCs are the cells that process the sound before it is passed to the auditory nerve. Based on the Johnson (thermal) noise within the IHC, it is possible to accurately estimate a lower bound on the RMS voltage within the IHC. From the voltage drop across the cilia, we may estimate the upper dynamic range of the cell. The total dynamic range of the IHC must be less than this ratio, or less than 65 dB (e.g., 55–60 dB) (Allen, 1997b). The dynamic range of hearing is about 120 dB. Thus, the IHC does not have a large enough dynamic range to code the dynamic range of the input signal. Spread-of-excitation models and neuron threshold distribution of neural rate do not address this fundamental problem. Nature's solution to this problem is the OHC-controlled basilar membrane compression.

The formula for the Johnson RMS thermal electrical membrane noise voltage $|V_c|$ due to cell membrane leakage currents is given by[5] $\langle |V_c|^2 \rangle = 4kTBR$, where B is the cell membrane electrical bandwidth, k is Boltzmann's constant, T is the temperature in degrees Kelvin, and R is the cell membrane leakage resistance. The cell bandwidth is limited by the membrane capacitance C. The relation between the cell RC time constant, $\tau = RC$, and the cell bandwidth is given by $B = 1/\tau$, leading to

$$|V_c| = \sqrt{\frac{4kT}{C}}. \qquad (3)$$

The cell membrane capacitance C has been determined to be about 9.6 *pF* for the IHC (Kros and Crawford, 1990) and 20 *pF* for the OHC. From Equation 3, $V_c = 21$ μV for IHCs at body temperature ($T = 310\,°$K).

Although the maximum DC voltage across the cilia is 120 mV, the maximum RMS change in cell voltage that has been observed is about 30 mV (I. J. Russell, personal communication). The ratio of 30 mV to the noise floor voltage (21 μV), expressed in dB, is 63 dB. Thus it is impossible for the IHC to code the 120 dB dynamic range of the acoustic signal. Because it is experimentally observed that, taken as a group, IHCs *do* code a wide dynamic range, the nonlinear motion of the basilar membrane must be providing compression within the mechanics of the cochlea prior to IHC detection (Allen and Neely, 1992; Allen, 1997a).

Summary. Based on a host of data, the physical source of cochlear hearing loss and recruitment is now clear. The dynamic range of IHCs is limited to about 50 dB. The dynamic range of the sound level at the eardrum, however, is closer to 100–120 dB. Thus, there is a difficulty in matching the dynamic range at the drum to that of the IHC. This is the job of the OHCs.

It is known that OHCs act as nonlinear elements. For example, the OHC soma axial stiffness, K_{ohc}, depends directly on the voltage drop across the cell membrane, V_{ohc}. As the OHC cilia excitation is varied from "soft" to "loud," the OHC membrane voltage is depolarized, causing the cell to increase its compliance (and length). The result is compression due to a decrease in the IHC (cochlear) signal gain.

Multiband Compression

During the two decades from 1965 to 1985, the clinical audiological community was attempting to answer the question: Are compression hearing aids better than a well-fitted linear hearing aid? A number of researchers concluded that linear fitting is always superior to compression. When properly adjusted, linear filtering *is* close to optimum for speech whose level has been adjusted for

---

[5] While the thermal noise is typically dominated by the shot noise, the shot noise is more difficult to estimate. Since we are trying to bound the dynamic range, the thermal noise is a better choice for this purpose. The shot noise reduces the dynamic range further, strengthening the argument.

optimum listening. Papers that fall in this category include Braida et al. (1979) and Lippmann et al. (1981). However, Lippmann et al. are careful to point out the flaw in preadjusting the level (see p. 553).

Further criticisms were made by Plomp (1988, 1994), who argued that compression would reduce the modulation depth of the speech. However, compression of a broadband signal does not reduce the modulations in sub-bands.

All these results placed the advocates of compression in a defensive minority position. Villchur vigorously responded to the challenge of Plomp, saying that Plomp's argument was flawed (Villchur, 1989). The filter bandwidths used in WDRC hearing aids are not narrow enough to reduce the modulations in critical bandwidths. Other important papers arguing for compression include Hickson (1994), Killion (1996a, 1996b), Killion et al. (1990), and Mueller and Killion (1996). A physiology paper that is frequently cited in the compression literature is Ruggero and Rich (1991).

Other work that found negative results used compression parameters that were not reasonable and time constants that were too slow. Long time constants with compression produce very different results and are not in the category of syllabic compression. Such systems typically have artifacts, such as noise "pumping," or they simply do not react quickly enough to follow a lively conversation. Imagine, for example, a listening situation with a quiet and a loud talker having a conversation. In this situation, the compressor gain must operate at syllabic rates to be effective. The use of multiple bands ensures that a signal in one frequency band does not control the gain in another band. Slow-acting compression (AGC) may be fine for watching television, but not for conversational speech. Such systems might be viewed as a replacement for a volume control (Dillon, 1996, 2001; Moore et al., 1985; Moore, 1987).

A key advocate of compression was Ed Villchur, who critically recognized the importance of Steinberg and Gardner's observations on recruitment as a loss of compression. He vigorously promoted the idea of compression amplification hearing aids. Personally supporting the cost of the research with dollars from his very successful loudspeaker business, he contracted David Blackmer of dbx to produce a multiband compression hearing aid for experimental purposes. Using his experimental multiband compression hearing aid, Villchur experimented on hearing-impaired individuals, and found that Steinberg and Gardner's observations and predictions were correct (Villchur, 1973, 1974). Villchur clearly articulated the point that a well-fitted compression hearing aid improved the dynamic range of audibility and that what counted, in the end, was audibility. In other words, "If you can't hear it, you can't understand it." This had a certain logical appeal.

Fred Waldhauer, a Bell Labs analog circuit designer of some considerable ability, heard Villchur speak about his experiments on multiband compression. After the breakup of the Bell System in 1983, Waldhauer proposed to AT&T management that Bell Labs design and build a multiband compression hearing aid as an internally funded venture. Eventually Bell Labs built a digital wearable hearing aid prototype. It quickly became apparent that the best processing strategy compromise was a two-band compression design that was generically similar to the Villchur scheme. With my colleague Vincent Pluvinage, we designed digital hardware wearable hearing aids, and with the help of Joe Hall and David Berkley of AT&T, and Patricia Jeng, Harry Levitt, Arlene Newman, and many others from City University of New York, we developed a fitting procedure and ran several field trials (Allen et al., 1990). AT&T licensed its hearing aid technology to ReSound on February 27, 1987.

Unlike today, in 1990 multiband compression was widely unaccepted, both clinically and academically (Dillon, 2001). Why is this? It was, and remains, difficult to show quantitatively the nature of the improvement of WDRC. It is probably fair to say that only with the success of ReSound's WDRC hearing aid in the marketplace has the clinical community come to accept Villchur's claims.

It may be possible to clarify the acceptance issue by presenting two common views of what WDRC is and why it works. One's adopted view strongly influences how he or she thinks about compression. They are the articulation index (AI) view and the loudness view.

The articulation index view is based on the observation that speech has a dynamic range of about 30 dB in one-third octave frequency bands (French and Steinberg, 1947). The assumption is that the AI will increase in a recruiting ear as the compression is increased, if the speech is held at a fixed loudness. This view has led to unending comparisons between the optimum linear hearing aid and the optimum compression hearing aid.

The loudness view is based on restoring the natural dynamic range of all sounds to provide the impaired listener with all the speech cues in a more natural way. Soft sounds for normals should be soft for the impaired ear, and loud sounds should be loud. According to this view, loudness is used as an *index of audibility*, and complex arguments about JNDs, speech discrimination, and modulation transfer functions just confound the issue. This view is supported by the theory that OHCs compress the IHC signals.

Neither of these arguments deals with important and complex issues such as changing of the critical band with hearing loss, or the temporal dynamics of the compression system. Analysis of these important details is interesting only *after* the signals are placed in the audible range.

Summary

This article has reviewed the early research on loudness, loudness recruitment, and masking, which are relevant to compression hearing aid development. The outer hair cell is damaged in sensorineural hearing loss, and this causes the cochlea to have reduced dynamic range.

When properly designed and fitted, WDRC has proved to be *the* most effective speech processing strategy we can presently provide for sensorineural hearing loss compensation. It works because it supplements the OHC compressors, which are damaged with sensorineural hearing loss.

Acknowledgments

I would especially like to thank one anonymous review, Harvey Dillon, Brent Edwards, Ray Kent, Mead Killion, Harry Levitt, Ryuji Suzuki, and Ed Villchur.

—*Jont B. Allen*

References

Allen, J. (1999a). Derecruitment by multiband compression in hearing aids. In C. Berlin (Ed.), *The efferent auditory system* (chap. 4, pp. 73–86). San Diego, CA: Singular Publishing Group.

Allen, J. (1999b). Psychoacoustics. In J. Webster (Ed.), *Wiley encyclopedia of electrical and electronics engineering* (vol. 17, pp. 422–437). New York: Wiley.

Allen, J., and Neely, S. (1992). Micromechanical models of the cochlea. *Physics Today*, *45*(7), 40–47.

Allen, J. B. (1980). Cochlear micromechanics: A physical model of transduction. *Journal of the Acoustical Society of America*, *68*, 1660–1670.

Allen, J. B. (1991). Modeling the noise damaged cochlea. In P. Dallos, C. D. Geisler, J. W. Matthews, M. A. Ruggero, and C. R. Steele (Eds.), *The mechanics and biophysics of hearing* (pp. 324–332). New York: Springer-Verlag.

Allen, J. B. (1996). Harvey Fletcher's role in the creation of communication acoustics. *Journal of the Acoustical Society of America*, *99*, 1825–1839.

Allen, J. B. (1997a). DeRecruitment by multiband compression in hearing aids. In W. Jesteadt et al. (Eds.), *Modeling sensorineural hearing loss* (pp. 99–112). Mahwah, NJ: Erlbaum.

Allen, J. B. (1997b). OHCs shift the excitation pattern via BM tension. In E. Lewis, G. Long, R. Lyon, P. Narins, C. Steele, and E. Hecht-Poinar (Eds.), *Diversity in auditory mechanics* (pp. 167–175). Singapore: World Scientific Press.

Allen, J. B. (1997c). A short history of telephone psychophysics. *Journal of the Audiologic Engineering Society*, Reprint 4636, pp. 1–37.

Allen, J. B., Hall, J. L., and Jeng, P. S. (1990). Loudness growth in 1/2-octave bands (LGOB): A procedure for the assessment of loudness. *Journal of the Acoustical Society of America*, *88*, 745–753.

Allen, J. B., Shaw, G., and Kimberley, B. P. (1995). Characterization of the nonlinear ear canal impedance at low sound levels. *ARO*, *18*, 190 (abstr. 757).

Braida, L., Durlach, N., Lippmann, R., Hicks, B., Rabinowitz, W., and Reed, C. (1979). Hearing aids: A review of past research on linear amplification, amplitude compression, and frequency lowering. *American Speech and Hearing Association, Monograph*, 19.

Buus, S., Musch, H., and Florentine, M. (1998). On loudness at threshold. *Journal of the Acoustical Society of America*, *104*, 399–410.

Carver, W. F. (1978). Loudness balance procedures. In J. Katz (Ed.), *Handbook of clinical audiology* (2nd ed., chap. 15, pp. 164–178). Baltimore: Williams and Wilkins.

Delgutte, B. (1990). Two-tone suppression in auditory-nerve fibres: Dependence on suppressor frequency and level. *Hearing Research*, *49*, 225–246.

Dillon, H. (1996). Compression? Yes, but for low or high frequencies, for low or high intensities, and with what response times? *Ear and Hearing*, *17*, 287–307.

Dillon, H. (2001). *Hearing aids*. Sydney, Australia: Boomerang Press.

Fahey, P. F., and Allen, J. B. (1985). Nonlinear phenomena as observed in the ear canal, and at the auditory nerve. *Journal of the Acoustical Society of America*, *77*, 599–612.

Fletcher, H. (1923a). Physical measurements of audition and their bearing on the theory of hearing. *Journal of the Franklin Institute*, *196*, 289–326.

Fletcher, H. (1923b). Physical measurements of audition and their bearing on the theory of hearing. *Bell System Technology Journal*, *2*, 145–180.

Fletcher, H. (1929). *Speech and hearing*. New York: Van Nostrand.

Fletcher, H. (1950). A method of calculating hearing loss for speech from an audiogram. *Journal of the Acoustical Society of America*, *22*, 1–5.

Fletcher, H. (1953). *Speech and hearing in communication*. Huntington, NY: Krieger.

Fletcher, H., and Munson, W. (1933). Loudness, its definition, measurement, and calculation. *Journal of the Acoustical Society of America*, *5*, 82–108.

Fletcher, H., and Steinberg, J. (1924). The dependence of the loudness of a complex sound upon the energy in the various frequency regions of the sound. *Physical Review*, *24*, 306–317.

Fletcher, H., and Wegel, R. (1922a). The frequency-sensitivity of normal ears. *Proceedings of the National Academy of Science*, *8*(1), 5–6.

Fletcher, H., and Wegel, R. (1922b). The frequency-sensitivity of normal ears. *Physical Review*, *19*, 553–565.

Fowler, E. (1936). A method for the early detection of otosclerosis. *Archives of Otolaryngology*, *24*, 731–741.

Fowler, E. (1942). A simple method of measuring percentage of capacity for hearing speech. *Archives of Otolaryngology*, *36*, 874–890.

French, N., and Steinberg, J. (1947). Factors governing the intelligibility of speech sounds. *Journal of the Acoustical Society of America*, *19*, 90–119.

Gardner, M. (1994). Personal communication.

He, D., and Dallos, P. (2000). Properties of voltage-dependent somatic stiffness of cochlear outer hair cells. *Journal of the Association for Research in Otolaryngology*, *1*, 64–81.

Hickson, L. (1994). Compression amplification in hearing aids. *American Journal of Audiology*, *11*, 51–65.

Killion, M. (1996a). Compression: Distinctions. *Hearing Review*, *3*(8), 29.

Killion, M. (1996b). Talking hair cells: What they have to say about hearing aids. In C. Berlin (Ed.), *Hair cells and hearing aids*. San Diego, CA: Singular Publishing Group.

Killion, M., Staab, W., and Preves, D. (1990). Classifying automatic signal processors. *Hearing Instruments*, *41*(8), 24–26.

Kim, D., Neely, S., Molnar, C., and Matthews, J. (1980). An active cochlear model with negative damping in the cochlear partition: Comparison with Rhode's ante- and postmortem results. In G. van den Brink and F. Bilsen (Eds.), *Psychological, physiological and behavioral studies in hearing* (pp. 7–14). Delft, The Netherlands: Delft University Press.

Kingsbury, B. (1927). A direct comparison of the loudness of pure tones. *Physical Review*, *29*, 588–600.

Kros, C., and Crawford, A. (1990). Potassium currents in inner hair cells isolated from the guinea-pig cochlea. *Journal of Physiology*, *421*, 263–291.

Liberman, M., and Dodds, L. (1984). Single neuron labeling and chronic cochlear pathology: III. Stereocilia damage and alterations of threshold tuning curves. *Hearing Research*, *16*, 55–74.

Liberman, M., and Kiang, N. (1978). Acoustic trauma in cats. *Acta Otolaryngologica, Supplement*, *358*, 1–63.

Lippmann, R., Braida, L., and Durlach, N. (1981). Study of multichannel amplitude compression and linear amplification for persons with sensorineural hearing loss. *Journal of the Acoustical Society of America*, *69*, 524–534.

Lorente de No, R. (1937). The diagnosis of diseases of the neural mechanism of hearing by the aid of sounds well above threshold. *Transactions of the American Otological Society*, *27*, 219–220.

Martin, F. N. (1986). *Introduction to audiology* (3rd ed.). Englewood Cliffs, NJ: Prentice-Hall.

McFadden, D. (1986). The curious half-octave shift: Evidence of a basalward migration of the traveling-wave envelope with increasing intensity. In R. Salvi, D. Henderson, R. Hamernik, and V. Coletti (Eds.), *Applied and basic aspects of noise-induced hearing loss* (pp. 295–312). New York: Plenum Press.

Moore, B. (1987). Design and evaluation of a two-channel compression hearing aid. *Journal of Rehabilitation Research and Development*, *24*, 181–192.

Moore, B., Laurence, R., and Wright, D. (1985). Improvements in speech intelligibility in quiet and in noise produced by two-channel compression hearing aids. *British Journal of Audiology*, *19*, 175–187.

Mueller, H., and Killion, M. (1996). Available: http://www.compression.edu. *Hearing Journal*, *49*, 44–46.

Munson, W. A., and Gardner, M. B. (1950). Loudness patterns: A new approach. *Journal of the Acoustical Society of America*, *22*, 177–190.

Neely, S. T., and Allen, J. B. (1997). Relation between the rate of growth of loudness and the intensity DL. In W. Jesteadt et al. (Eds.), *Modeling sensorineural hearing loss* (pp. 213–222). Mahwah, NJ: Erlbaum.

Pickles, J. O. (1982). *An introduction to the physiology of hearing*. London: Academic Press.

Plomp, R. (1988). The negative effect of amplitude compression in multichannel hearing aids in the light of the modulation-transfer function. *Journal of the Acoustical Society of America*, *83*, 2322–2327.

Plomp, R. (1994). Noise, amplification, and compression: Considerations of three main issues in hearing aid design. *Ear and Hearing*, *15*, 2–12.

Rhode, W. (1971). Observations of the vibration of the basilar membrane in squirrel monkeys using the Mossbauer technique. *Journal of the Acoustical Society of America*, *64*, 158–176.

Riesz, R. (1928). Differential intensity sensitivity of the ear for pure tones. *Physical Review*, *31*, 867–875.

Ruggero, M., and Rich, N. (1991). Furosemide alters organ of Corti mechanics: Evidence for feedback of outer hair cells upon basilar membrane. *Journal of Neuroscience*, *11*, 1057–1067.

Sachs, M., and Abbas, P. (1974). Rate versus level functions for auditory-nerve fibers in cats: Tone-burst stimuli. *Journal of the Acoustical Society of America*, *56*, 1835–1847.

Santos-Sacchi, J., and Dilger, J. P. (1987). Whole cell currents and mechanical responses of isolated outer hair cells. *Hearing Research*, *35*, 143–150.

Steinberg, J., and Gardner, M. (1937). Dependence of hearing impairment on sound intensity. *Journal of the Acoustical Society of America*, *9*, 11–23.

Villchur, E. (1973). Signal processing to improve speech intelligibility in perceptive deafness. *Journal of the Acoustical Society of America*, *53*, 1646–1657.

Villchur, E. (1974). Simulation of the effect of recruitment on loudness relationships in speech. *Journal of the Acoustical Society of America*, *56*, 1601–1611.

Villchur, E. (1989). Comments on: The negative effect of amplitude compression on multichannel hearing aids in the light of the modulation transfer function. *Journal of the Acoustical Society of America*, *86*, 425–427.

Wegel, R., and Lane, C. (1924). The auditory masking of one pure tone by another and its probable relation to the dynamics of the inner ear. *Physical Review*, *23*, 266–285.

Assessment of and Intervention with Children Who Are Deaf or Hard of Hearing

The purpose of communication assessment of children with educationally significant hearing loss differs from the purpose of assessing children with language or learning disabilities. Since the diagnosis of a hearing disability has already been made, the primary goal of communication assessment is to determine the impact of the hearing loss on language, speech, auditory skills, or cognitive, social-emotional, educational and vocational development, not to diagnose a disability. It is critical to determine the rate of language and communication development and to identify strategies that will be most beneficial for optimal development.

Plateaus in language development at the 9–10-year age level, in reading development at the middle third grade to fourth grade level (Holt, 1993), and in speech intelligibility at about 10 years (Jensema, Karchmer, and Trybus, 1978) have been reported in the literature. The language plateaus appear to be the result of developmental growth, which ranges from 43%–53% for children with profound hearing loss using hearing aids (Boothroyd, Geers, and Moog, 1991; Geers and Moog, 1988) to 60%–65% of the normal range of development for children with severe loss using hearing aids (Boothroyd, Geers, and Moog, 1991) and for children with profound hearing loss using cochlear implants (Blamey et al., 2001). In contrast, in a study of 150 children, Yoshinaga-Itano et al. (1998) reported that children with hearing loss only who were early-identified (within the first 6 months of life) had mean language levels at 90% of the rate of normal language development through the first 3 years of life. A study of children in Nebraska (Moeller, 2000) reported similar levels of language development (low-average range) for a sample of 5-year-old children receiving early intervention services in the first 11 months of life. Later-identified children were able to achieve language development commensurate with the early-identified/intervened group when their families were rated as "high parent involvement" in the intervention services.

With the advent of universal newborn hearing screening, the population of children who are deaf or hard of hearing will change rapidly during the next decade. By 2001, 35 states had passed legislation to establish universal newborn hearing screening programs, five additional states had legislation in progress, and five states had established programs without legislation. The age at which hearing loss is identified should drop dramatically throughout the United States, and this drop should be accompanied by intervention services, beginning in the newborn period. In the state of Colorado, infants referred from UNHS programs are being identified with hearing loss at 6–8 weeks of age and enter into intervention programs almost immediately thereafter.

For the population of children identified with hearing loss within the first 2 months of life, baseline communication assessments are typically conducted at 6-month intervals during the first 3 years of life (Stredler-Brown and Yoshinaga-Itano, 1994; Yoshinaga-Itano, 1994). Almost all of the infant assessment instruments are parent questionnaires that address the development of receptive and expressive language (e.g., MacArthur Communicative Development Inventories, Minnesota Child Development Inventory, Vineland Social Maturity Scales), auditory skills, early vocalizations, cognitive, fine motor, gross motor, self-help, and personal-social/social-emotional issues. Videotaped analysis of parent-child interaction style and spontaneous speech and language production is frequently included.

Spontaneous speech samples should be analyzed to identify the number of different consonant phones. The number of different consonant phones produced in a spontaneous 30-minute language sample taken in the home between 9 months and 50 months of age is a good predictor of speech intelligibility (Yoshinaga-Itano and Sedey, 2000). The primary development of speech for children with mild to moderate hearing loss is concentrated between 2 and 3 years of age, while the preschool years, ages 3–5 years, are a significant growth period for children with moderate to severe hearing loss. Speech development for children with profound hearing loss who use hearing aids is very slow in the first 5 years of life. Although 75% of children with mild through severe hearing loss achieved intelligible speech by 5 years of age, only 20% of children with profound hearing loss who used conventional amplification achieved this level by age 5. Level of expressive language and degree of hearing loss were the two primary predictors of speech intelligibility.

Videotaped interactions of parent-child communication can be analyzed for maternal bonding and emotional availability (Pressman et al., 1999), turn-taking (Musselman and Churchill, 1991), use of pause time, maintenance of topic, topic initiation, attention-getting devices, the development of symbolic play, symbolic gesture, and communication intention strategies (comments, requests, answers, commands) of both the parent and the child (Yoshinaga-Itano, 1994). These analyses provide important information for the family and intervention provider to help design strategies for optimal development. Reciprocal relationships have been reported. Parents adjust language as their child's language improves (Cross, Johnson-Morris, and Nienhuys, 1985), and low levels of maternal turn control are asso-

ciated with greater gains in expressive language (Musselman and Churchill, 1991). At present, studies of causality have been insufficient to determine the efficacy or superiority of various intervention strategies. However, some interventions that are theoretically grounded and are characteristic of programs that demonstrate optimal language development are parent-centered, provide objective developmental data, assist parental decisions about methodology, based on the developmental progress of the individual child, include a strong counseling component aimed at reducing parental stress and assisting parents in the resolution of their grief, and provide guidance in parent-child interaction strategies.

The language development of early-identified (within the first 6 months of life) children with hearing loss is similar to their nonverbal development, particularly in regard to symbolic play development (Snyder and Yoshinaga-Itano, 1999; Yoshinaga-Itano and Snyder, 1999; Mayne et al., 2000). About 60% of the variance in early language development is predicted by nonverbal cognitive measures such as symbolic play and age at identification of hearing loss. Mode of communication, degree of hearing loss, socioeconomic status, ethnicity, and sex were not shown to predict language development. These results contrast sharply with the school-age literature, in which race, ethnicity, and socioeconomic status are primary predictors of reading achievement (Holt, 1993).

In order to maintain the successful language development of the early-identified children, the purpose of evaluation in the first 5 years of life should be to monitor and chart the longitudinal developmental progress of the child, with two primary goals: (1) to achieve language development commensurate with nonverbal cognitive development, and (2) to achieve language development in children with hearing loss only, within the normal range of development. In an analysis of almost 250 children, an 80% probability of language within the low-normal range in the first 5 years of life was reported if a child identified with hearing loss had been born in a Colorado hospital with a universal newborn hearing screening program (Yoshinaga-Itano, Coulter, and Thomson, 2000).

In addition to an analysis of communication skills, cognitive development, and age at identification, assessments should include information about the social-emotional development of both parents and children. Relationships have been found between language development and parental stress (Pipp-Siegel, Sedey, and Yoshinaga-Itano, 2002), emotional availability (Pressman et al., 1999) parent involvement (Moeller, 2000), grief resolution (Pipp-Siegel, 2000), development of sense of self (Pressman, 2000), and mastery motivation (Pipp-Siegel et al., 2002). The relationships examined in these studies do not establish causes, but it is plausible that intervention strategies focused on these areas may enhance the language development of young children with hearing loss. Counseling strategies with parent sign language instruction enhanced language development among children using total communication (Greenberg, Calderon, and Kusche, 1984).

Assessment strategies during the preschool period, ages 3–5 years, continue to focus on receptive and expressive vocabulary, but their primary focus shifts to the development of syntax and morphology and pragmatic language skills (Yoshinaga-Itano, 1999). Spontaneous language sample analysis is recommended for expressive syntax analysis. There is a shift from parent questionnaire developmental assessments and assessments of spontaneous communication to clinical or school-based elicited assessments at this age period. Testers need to ensure full access to the information being presented, either through fully functioning amplification devices, adequate speech reading accessibility, or the skills of a fluent signer.

During the school-age period, standardized assessments consist of regularly administered tests of language (receptive and expressive vocabulary, syntax, pragmatics, and phonology), reading and writing, mathematics, other content areas, and social-emotional development (Yoshinaga-Itano, 1997). Researchers hypothesize that there may be as many as four possible routes to literacy for children with hearing loss: (1) spoken language to printed language decoded to speech, (2) English-based signs to printed English, (3) American Sign Language (ASL) to print, with English-based signs as an intermediary, and (4) ASL to print (Musselman, 2000). Assessments of knowledge of English semantics, syntax, and phonological processing, accuracy and speed of word identification, and orthographic encoding should be included, since several studies have found that these variables are significantly related to reading comprehension (Musselman, 2000). Among children who use sign language, finger-spelling ability and general language competence in either ASL or English should be included (Musselman, 2000). For all children, assessments should also focus on the metalinguistic and metacognitive strategies (knowing how to use and think about language) used by the students in person-to-person and written communication (Gray and Hosie, 1996). "Theory of mind" assessments provide information about the cognitive ability of the student to understand a variety of different perspectives (Strassman, 1997). Students need to develop strategies to acquire and elaborate world knowledge, elaborate vocabulary knowledge (both conversational and written), and to use this knowledge to make inferences in social, communicative interactions and reading/academic situations (Paul, 1996; Jackson, Paul, and Smith, 1997).

—*Christine Yoshinaga-Itano*

References

Blamey, P. J., Sarant, J. Z., Paatsch, L. E., Barry, J. G., Bow, C. P., Wales, R. J., et al. (2001). Relationships among speech perception, production, language, hearing loss, and age in children with impaired hearing. *Journal of Speech, Language, and Hearing Research, 44*, 264–285.

Boothroyd, A., Geers, A. E., and Moog, J. S. (1991). Practical implications of cochlear implants in children. *Ear and Hearing, 12*, 81S–89S.

Cross, T. G., Johnson-Morris, J. E., and Nienhuys, T. G. (1985). Linguistic feedback and maternal speech: Comparisons of mothers addressing hearing and hearing-impaired children. *First Language, 1*, 163–189.

Geers, A. E., and Moog, J. S. (1988). Predicting long-term benefits from single-channel cochlear implants in profoundly hearing-impaired children. *American Journal of Otology, 9*, 169–176.

Gray, C. D., and Hosie, J. A. (1996). Deafness, story understanding, and theory of mind. *Journal of Deaf Studies and Deaf Education, 1*, 217–233.

Greenberg, M. T., Calderon, R., and Kusche, C. A. (1984). Early intervention using simultaneous communication with deaf infants: The effects on communicative development. *Child Development, 55*, 607–616.

Holt, J. (1993). Stanford Achievement Test–8th Edition: Reading comprehension subgroup results. *American Annals of the Deaf, 138*, 172–175.

Jackson, D. W., Paul, P. V., and Smith, J. C. (1997). Prior knowledge and reading comprehension ability of deaf adolescents. *Journal of Deaf Education and Deaf Studies, 2*, 172–184.

Jensema, C. J., Karchmer, M. A., and Trybus, R. J. (1978). *The rated speech intelligibility of hearing-impaired children: Basic relationships.* Washington, DC: Gallaudet College Office of Demographic Studies.

Mayne, A. M., Yoshinaga-Itano, C., Sedey, A. L., and Carey, A. (2000). Expressive vocabulary development of infants and toddlers who are deaf or hard of hearing. *Volta Review, 100*(5), 1–28.

Moeller, M. P. (2000). Early intervention and language development in children who are deaf and hard of hearing. *Pediatrics, 106*, E43.

Musselman, C. (2000). How do children who can't hear learn to read an alphabetic script? A review of the literature on reading and deafness. *Journal of Deaf Studies and Deaf Education, 5*, 9–31.

Musselman, C., and Churchill, A. (1991). A comparison of the interaction between mothers and deaf children in auditory/oral and total communication pairs. *American Annals of the Deaf, 136*, 5–16.

Paul, P. (1996). Reading vocabulary knowledge and deafness. *Journal of Deaf Studies and Deaf Education, 1*, 3–15.

Pipp-Siegel, S. (2000). *Resolution of grief of parents with young children with hearing loss.* Unpublished manuscript, Department of Speech, Language, and Hearing Sciences. University of Colorado, Boulder.

Pipp-Siegel, S., Sedey, A., Mayne, A., and Yoshinaga-Itano, C. (in press). Mastery motivation predicts expressive language in young children with hearing loss. *Journal of Deaf Education and Deaf Studies.*

Pipp-Siegel, S., Sedey, A. L., and Yoshinaga-Itano, C. (2002). Predictors of parental stress in mothers of young children with hearing loss. *Journal of Deaf Studies and Deaf Education, 7*, 1–17.

Pressman, L. (2000). *Early self-development in children with hearing loss.* Unpublished doctoral dissertation, Department of Speech, Language, and Hearing Sciences. University of Colorado, Boulder.

Pressman, L., Pipp-Siegel, S., Yoshinaga-Itano, C., and Deas, A. (1999). The relation of sensitivity to child expressive language gain in deaf and hard-of-hearing children whose caregivers are hearing. *Journal of Deaf Studies and Deaf Education, 4*, 294–304.

Snyder, L., and Yoshinaga-Itano, C. (1999). Specific play behaviors and the development of communication in children with hearing loss. *Volta Review, 100*, 165–185.

Strassman, B. K. (1997). Metacognition and reading in children who are deaf: A review of the research. *Journal of Deaf Studies and Deaf Education, 2*, 140–149.

Stredler-Brown, A., and Yoshinaga-Itano, C. (1994). F.A.M.I.L.Y. assessment: A multidisciplinary evaluation tool. In J. Roush and N. Matkin (Eds.), *Infants and toddlers with hearing loss* (pp. 133–161). Baltimore: York Press.

Yoshinaga-Itano, C. (1994). Language assessment of infants and toddlers with significant hearing losses. *Seminars in Hearing, 15*, 128–147.

Yoshinaga-Itano, C. (1997). The challenge of assessing language in children with hearing loss. *Speech, Language, and Hearing Services in Schools, 28*, 362–373.

Yoshinaga-Itano, C. (1999). Assessment and Intervention of preschool-aged deaf and hard-of-hearing children. In J. Alpiner and P. McCarthy (Eds.), *Rehabilitative audiology: Children and adults* (pp. 140–177). Baltimore: Williams and Wilkins.

Yoshinaga-Itano, C., Coulter, D., and Thomson, V. (2000). The Colorado Newborn Hearing Screening Project: Effects on speech and language development for children with hearing loss. *Journal of Perinatology, 20*, S132–S137.

Yoshinaga-Itano, C., and Sedey, A. (2000). Early speech development in children who are deaf or hard of hearing: Interrelationships with language and hearing. *Volta Review, 100*, 181–212.

Yoshinaga-Itano, C., Sedey, A., Coulter, D., and Mehl, A. (1998). Language of early- and later-identified children with hearing loss. *Pediatrics, 102*, 1161–1171.

Yoshinaga-Itano, C., and Snyder, L. (1999). The relationship of language and symbolic play in deaf and hard-of-hearing children. *Volta Review, 100*, 135–164.

Audition in Children, Development of

Research on auditory development intensified in the mid-1970s, expanding our understanding of auditory processes in infants and children. Recent comprehensive reviews of this literature include those by Aslin, Jusczyk, and Pisoni (1998), Werner and Marean (1996), and Werner and Rubel (1992). Two recurrent issues are whether the limitations of testing methods cause true abilities to be underestimated, and whether auditory development is substantially complete during infancy or continues into childhood.

Absolute Sensitivity

Auditory sensitivity is within about 10–15 dB of adult values by 6 months after birth, but behavioral and electrophysiological methods show different trends during early infancy. Behavioral thresholds at 1 month are approximately 40 dB above adult values, with substantial improvement through 6 months and gradual improvement through the early school years (Schneider et al., 1986; Olsho et al., 1988). By 6 months the audibility curve (threshold plotted against frequency) is adultlike in shape, although sensitivity continues to improve into childhood. Several behavioral tests are used to assess infant hearing, including conditioned head turning by infants older than about 6 months and observation of subtle behavioral responses to sounds in younger infants. It is of clinical significance that for infants younger than 4–6 months, behavioral methods lack reliability for individual assessment (Bourland, Tharpe, and Ashmead, 2000). Infant-adult differences reflect true sensory differences as well as nonsensory factors such as attention, but at least in older infants only about 4 dB of the infant-adult difference is attributable to nonsensory factors (Nozza and Henson, 1999). Electrophysiological measures (primarily the auditory brainstem response, ABR) reflect nearly adultlike hearing sensitivity from early infancy (Werner, Folsom, and Mancl, 1994). Although electrophysiological measures are less susceptible than behavioral methods to inattention and off-task behavior, another reason for the discrepancy between methods is that the ABR reflects only peripheral processing. That is, in early infancy, auditory sensitivity may be constrained by neural immaturity central to the processes measured by the ABR.

Frequency Resolution

Like absolute sensitivity, frequency resolution approaches adult values by 6 months after birth. The segregation of auditory processing by frequency is demonstrated by the enhanced effectiveness of masking sounds that are closer in frequency to the signal. Infants' cochlear frequency resolution has been studied via suppression tuning curves from otoacoustic emissions. Such frequency resolution is adultlike at full-term birth (Bargones and Burns, 1988; Abdala, 1998). Beyond the cochlea, resolution for higher frequencies (ca. 4 kHz) is not finely tuned for the first 3 months after birth, but by 6 months resolution is adultlike, as seen in behavioral and ABR masking studies (Spetner and Olsho, 1990; Abdala and Folsom, 1995). Some studies indicate improvement in frequency resolution up to age 4 years, but Hall and Grose (1991) showed that when certain methodological issues are taken into account, children have adultlike frequency resolution by 4 years. Despite the early development of frequency resolution, selective attention based on frequency is not well developed even by 9 months (Bargones and Werner, 1994).

Temporal Processing

There may be a more protracted course for temporal processing than for some other aspects of auditory development. Adults detect acoustic gaps of 2–5 ms, whereas infants require gaps up to ten times longer (Werner et al., 1992). However, infant gap detection may be adult-like when tested in conditions that minimize adaptation effects (Trehub, Schneider, and Henderson, 1995; Trainor et al., 2001). Gap detection improves through 5–10 years (Wightman et al., 1989). Hall and Grose (1994) found that older children and adults had similar time constants for detection of amplitude modulation, but that preschool-aged children needed larger modulations. Discrimination between small differences in duration improves during infancy and into middle childhood (Jensen and Neff, 1993). The coarseness of temporal acuity in infants and children is surprising, since typically developing children do well at linguistic processing. But individual differences in infants' temporal resolution are associated with language development at 2 years (Trehub and Henderson, 1996). Besides temporal acuity, another consideration is how sound is integrated across time, reflected by improvement of detection thresholds as a sound remains on longer. Adult detection improves as the signal extends up to ¼ s, whereas infants have steeper improvement curves extending to longer durations (Berg and Boswell, 1995). A related finding is that forward masking operates over longer masker-signal intervals in 3-month-olds than in 6-month-olds or adults, implying that a temporal aspect of masking is mature by about 6 months (Werner, 1999).

Intensity Resolution and Loudness

Early studies of intensity discrimination showed that neonates and young infants detect large intensity changes. Sinnott and Aslin (1985) reported intensity difference limens for 7- to 9-month-olds of 3–12 dB, compared to 1.8 dB for adults. Other studies indicate that between birth and 12 months, the intensity difference limen ranges from 2 to 5 dB (Bull, Eilers, and Oller, 1984; Tarquinio, Zelazo, and Weiss, 1990). Although infants are good at discerning changes in intensity, this ability may not be adultlike until 6 years of age (Jensen and Neff, 1993). Research on loudness perception by infants has not been reported, but there has been some work with children. Studies using magnitude estimation and cross-modality matching have demonstrated that 4- to 7-year-olds described the growth of loudness of a tone similarly to adults (Collins and Gescheider, 1989). Serpanos and Gravel (2000), also using cross-modality matching paradigms, reported that loudness growth functions of children 4–12 years of age were similar to those of adults.

Pitch and Music Perception

Research on pitch and music perception suggests that by late in the first year of life, infants extract relational information across frequencies. At 7 months, infants categorize octave tonal complexes by fundamental frequency, even if the fundamental is missing and cochlear distortions are ruled out (Clarkson and Clifton, 1995; Montgomery and Clarkson, 1997). A substantial literature on music perception in infants shows sensitivity to melodic contours, even when transposed across octaves (Trehub, 2001). Although findings on pitch and music suggest integrative processing, other work in nonmusical contexts indicates that infants are better able to discriminate absolute than relative spectral differences (Saffran and Griepentrog, 2001).

Speech Perception

As early as the 1960s, investigators proposed that speech was processed by a separate perceptual module of a larger language system unique to humans. Although speech is still considered a special signal, the existence of an innate and specialized speech-processing mode unique to humans remains in question (Aslin, Jusczyk, and Pisoni, 1998). Since the initial studies of infant speech perception (Eimas et al., 1971), many investigators have shown that mechanisms used to perceive speech are in place long before infants utter their first words at around 12 months of age. For example, infants can discriminate between most English speech sound pairs much as adults do (Kuhl, 1987), based on parameters such as voice onset time, manner, and place of articulation. Despite infants' ability to categorize speech sounds, the boundaries between categories continue to sharpen into early childhood (Nittrouer and Studdert-Kennedy, 1987). Also, children age 3–4 years are not as adept as older children and adults at perceiving speech sounds from brief-onset information (Ohde and Haley, 1997). Infants also can generalize phoneme recognition across different talkers, fundamental frequencies, and positions within a syllable (Eilers, Wilson, and Moore, 1977; Miller, Younger, and Morse, 1982). The ability to categorize vowels, also known as equivalence classes, has been demonstrated in infants as young as 2 months of age (Marean, Werner, and Kuhl, 1992). Changes in speech perception as a result of postnatal experience occur within the first year of life, as shown by selective perception of speech sounds from the native language (see Werner and Marean, 1996, chap. 6). As early perception of linguistic input is so remarkable, any obstacle to the receipt of audible and clear speech sounds by an infant, such as hearing loss, should be suspected of adversely affecting language development.

Spatial Hearing

Sound localization is rather crude in early infancy, improving nearly to adult levels by 1 year and slowly thereafter. Newborns turn their heads toward sound sources, but this response wanes, reappearing in brisk form around 4 months (Clifton, 1992). This trend, along with the onset of response to the precedence effect (related to reflected sounds) at 4 months, suggests an increasing role of the auditory cortex in sound localization. The low responsivity to sounds from birth to 4 months makes it difficult to assess hearing ability behaviorally in this age range, as noted above in the discussion of auditory sensitivity. Precision of sound localization, as measured by the minimum audible angle, improves from 20°–25° at 4 months to 8°–10° at 12 months, with further gradual changes to adultlike values of 1°–3° by 5 years (Ashmead, Clifton, and Perris, 1987; Morrongiello, Fenwick, and Chance, 1990). This improvement may entail integration across several sound localization cues, since sensitivity to single cues is better than predicted from localization (Ashmead et al., 1991). A phenomenon related to spatial hearing is masking level differences, which are smaller in children less than 7 years old than in older children or adults (Grose, Hall, and Dev, 1997). Regarding distance, 6-month-olds distinguish between sounds within reach versus those beyond reach, even if sound pressure level is removed as a distance cue (Litovsky and Clifton, 1992).

See also PHYSIOLOGICAL BASES OF HEARING; PEDIATRIC AUDIOLOGY: THE TEST BATTERY APPROACH; HEARING LOSS SCREENING: THE SCHOOL-AGE CHILD.

—*Daniel H. Ashmead and Anne Marie Tharpe*

References

Abdala, C. (1998). A developmental study of distortion product otoacoustic emission ($2f_1$–f_2) suppression in humans. *Hearing Research, 121,* 125–138.

Abdala, C., and Folsom, R. C. (1995). The development of frequency resolution in humans as revealed by the auditory brain-stem response recorded with notched-noise masking. *Journal of the Acoustical Society of America, 98,* 921–930.

Ashmead, D. H., Clifton, R. K., and Perris, E. E. (1987). Precision of auditory localization in human infants. *Developmental Psychology, 23,* 641–657.

Ashmead, D. H., Davis, D. L., Whalen, T. A., and Odom, R. D. (1991). Sound localization and interaural time discrimination in human infants. *Child Development, 62,* 1211–1226.

Aslin, R. N., Jusczyk, P. W., and Pisoni, D. B. (1998). Speech and auditory processing during infancy: Constraints on and precursors to language. In W. Damon, D. Kuhn, and R. S. Siegler (Eds.), *Handbook of child psychology* (5th ed.), *Vol. 2: Cognition, perception, and language* (pp. 147–198). New York: Wiley.

Bargones, J. Y., and Burns, E. M. (1988). Suppression tuning curves for spontaneous otoacoustic emissions in infants and adults. *Journal of the Acoustical Society of America, 83,* 1809–1816.

Bargones, J. Y., and Werner, L. A. (1994). Adults listen selectively; infants do not. *Psychological Science, 5,* 170–174.

Berg, K. M., and Boswell, A. E. (1995). Temporal summation of 500-Hz tones and octave-band noise bursts in infants and adults. *Perception and Psychophysics, 57,* 183–190.

Bourland, C., Tharpe, A. M., and Ashmead, D. H. (2000). Behavioral auditory assessment of young infants: Methodological limitations or natural lack of auditory responsiveness? *American Journal of Audiology, 9,* 124–130.

Bull, D., Eilers, R. E., and Oller, D. K. (1984). Infants' discrimination of intensity variation in multisyllable stimuli. *Journal of the Acoustical Society of America, 76,* 13–17.

Clarkson, M. G., and Clifton, R. K. (1995). Infants' pitch perception: Inharmonic tonal complexes. *Journal of the Acoustical Society of America, 98,* 1372–1379.

Clifton, R. K. (1992). The development of spatial hearing in human infants. In L. A. Werner and E. W. Rubel (Eds.), *Developmental psychoacoustics* (pp. 135–157). Washington, DC: American Psychological Association.

Collins, A. A., and Gescheider, G. A. (1989). The measurement of loudness in individual children and adults by absolute magnitude estimation and cross-modality matching. *Journal of the Acoustical Society of America, 85,* 2012–2021.

Eilers, R. E., Wilson, W. R., and Moore, J. M. (1977). Developmental changes in speech discrimination in infants. *Journal of Speech and Hearing Research, 20,* 766–780.

Eimas, P., Siqueland, E., Jusczyk, P., and Vigorito, J. (1971). Speech perception in infants. *Science, 171,* 303–306.

Grose, J. H., Hall, J. W. III, and Dev, M. B. (1997). MLD in children: Effects of signal and masker bandwidths. *Journal of Speech, Language, and Hearing Research, 40,* 955–959.

Hall, J. W. III, and Grose, J. H. (1991). Notched-noise measures of frequency selectivity in adults and children using fixed-masker-level and fixed-signal-level presentation. *Journal of Speech and Hearing Research, 34,* 651–660.

Hall, J. W. III, and Grose, J. H. (1994). Development of temporal resolution in children as measured by the temporal modulation transfer function. *Journal of the Acoustical Society of America, 96,* 150–154.

Jensen, J. K., and Neff, D. L. (1993). Development of basic auditory discrimination in preschool children. *Psychological Science, 4,* 104–107.

Kuhl, P. K. (1987). Perception of speech and sound in early infancy. In P. Salapatek and L. Cohen (Eds.), *Handbook of infant perception* (pp. 275–381). New York: Academic Press.

Litovsky, R. Y., and Clifton, R. K. (1992). Use of sound-pressure level in auditory distance discrimination by 6-month-old infants and adults. *Journal of the Acoustical Society of America, 92,* 794–802.

Marean, G. C., Werner, L. A., and Kuhl, P. K. (1992). Vowel categorization by very young infants. *Developmental Psychology, 28,* 396–405.

Miller, C. L., Younger, B. A., and Morse, P. A. (1982). The categorization of male and female voices in infancy. *Infant Behavior and Development, 5,* 143–159.

Montgomery, C. R., and Clarkson, M. G. (1997). Infants' pitch perception: Masking by low- and high-frequency noises. *Journal of the Acoustical Society of America, 102,* 3665–3672.

Morrongiello, B. A., Fenwick, K. D., and Chance, G. (1990). Sound localization acuity in very young infants: An observer-based testing procedure. *Developmental Psychology, 26,* 75–84.

Nittrouer, S., and Studdert-Kennedy, M. (1987). The role of coarticulatory effects in the perception of fricatives by children and adults. *Journal of Speech and Hearing Research, 30,* 319–329.

Nozza, R. J., and Henson, A. M. (1999). Unmasked thresholds and minimum masking in infants and adults: Separating sensory from nonsensory contributions to infant-adult differences in behavioral thresholds. *Ear and Hearing, 20,* 483–496.

Ohde, R. N., and Haley, K. L. (1997). Stop-consonant and vowel perception in 3- and 4-year-old children. *Journal of the Acoustical Society of America, 102,* 3711–3722.

Olsho, L. W., Koch, E. G., Carter, E. A., Halpin, C. F., and Spetner, N. B. (1988). Pure-tone sensitivity of human infants. *Journal of the Acoustical Society of America, 84,* 1316–1324.

Saffran, J. R., and Griepentrog, G. J. (2001). Absolute pitch in infant auditory learning: Evidence for developmental reorganization. *Developmental Psychology, 37,* 74–85.

Schneider, B. A., Trehub, S. E., Morrongiello, B. A., and Thorpe, L. A. (1986). Auditory sensitivity in preschool children. *Journal of the Acoustical Society of America, 79,* 447–452.

Serpanos, Y. C., and Gravel, J. S. (2000). Assessing growth of loudness in children by cross-modality matching. *Journal of the American Academy of Audiology, 11,* 190–202.

Sinnott, J. M., and Aslin, R. N. (1985). Frequency and intensity discrimination in human infants and adults. *Journal of the Acoustical Society of America, 78,* 1986–1992.

Spetner, N. B., and Olsho, L. W. (1990). Auditory frequency resolution in human infancy. *Child Development, 61,* 632–652.

Tarquinio, N., Zelazo, P. R., and Weiss, M. J. (1990). Recovery of neonatal head turning to decreased sound pressure level. *Developmental Psychology, 26,* 752–758.

Trainor, L. J., Samuel, S. S., Desjardins, R. N., and Sonnadara, R. R. (2001). Measuring temporal resolution in infants using mismatch negativity. *Neuroreport, 12,* 2443–2448.

Trehub, S. E. (2001). Musical predispositions in infancy. *Annals of the New York Academy of Sciences, 930,* 1–16.

Trehub, S. E., and Henderson, J. L. (1996). Temporal resolution in infancy and subsequent language development. *Journal of Speech and Hearing Research, 39,* 1315–1320.

Trehub, S. E., Schneider, B. A., and Henderson, J. L. (1995). Gap detection in infants, children, and adults. *Journal of the Acoustical Society of America, 98,* 2532–2541.

Werner, L. A. (1999). Forward masking among infant and adult listeners. *Journal of the Acoustical Society of America, 105,* 2445–2453.

Werner, L. A., Folsom, R. C., and Mancl, L. R. (1994). The relationship between auditory brainstem response latencies and behavioral thresholds in normal hearing infants and adults. *Hearing Research, 77,* 88–98.

Werner, L. A., and Marean, G. C. (1996). *Human auditory development.* Boulder, CO: Westview Press.

Werner, L. A., Marean, G. C., Halpin, C. F., Spetner, N. B., and Gillenwater, J. M. (1992). Infant auditory temporal acuity: Gap detection. *Child Development, 63,* 260–272.

Werner, L. A., and Rubel, E. W. (Eds.). (1992). *Developmental psychoacoustics.* Washington, DC: American Psychological Association.

Wightman, F., Allen, P., Dolan, T., Kistler, D., and Jamieson, D. (1989). Temporal resolution in children. *Child Development, 60,* 611–624.

Auditory Brainstem Implant

People who are deafened by bilateral acoustic tumors are not candidates for a cochlear implant because tumor removal often severs the auditory nerve. The auditory brainstem implant (ABI) is designed for those patients. It is intended to bypass the auditory nerve and electrically stimulate the human cochlear nucleus.

Neurofibromatosis type 2 (NF2) is a genetic disorder that causes multiple tumors of the cranial nerves and spinal cord, among other symptoms. The gene causing NF2 has been located on chromosome 22 (Rouleau et al., 1993; Trofatter et al., 1993). The defining symptom of the disease is bilateral tumors originating on the Schwann cells of the vestibular branch of nerve VIII (vestibular schwannomas). These tumors are life-threatening, and their removal usually produces bilateral deafness. Patients with NF2 cannot benefit from a cochlear implant because they have no auditory nerve that can be stimulated from an intracochlear electrode. In 1979 William House and William Hitselberger attempted to provide auditory sensations for an NF2 patient by placing a single pair of electrodes in the cochlear nucleus following tumor removal (Edgerton, House, and Hitzelberger, 1984; Eisenberg, et al., 1987).

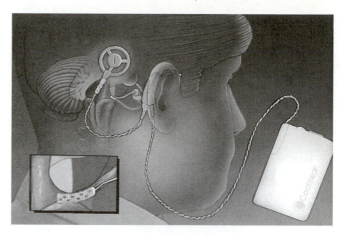

Figure 1. Overview of the ABI device and placement.

The success of that early attempt led to the development of a more sophisticated multichannel ABI device (Brackmann et al., 1993; Shannon et al., 1993; Otto et al., 1998, 2002). The first commercial multichannel ABI was developed in a collaborative effort between the House Ear Institute, Cochlear Corporation, and the Huntington Medical Research Institutes. The multichannel ABI was approved by the U.S. Food and Drug Administration in October 2000.

Several commercial ABI devices are available, all basically similar to the original device. ABIs are virtually identical in design to cochlear implants except for the electrode assembly (Fig. 1). The electrode assembly is a flat, paddle-like structure with platinum electrical contacts along one side. The overall size of the assembly is generally 2–3 mm × 8 mm and is designed to fit within the lateral recess of the IV ventricle. The electrical contacts are 0.5–1.0 mm in diameter, which is sufficient for keeping the electrical charge density at the stimulated neurons within safe limits (Shannon, 1992). All ABI devices have an external speech processor unit that contains a microphone to pick up the acoustic sound, a signal processor to convert the acoustic sound to electrical signals, and a transmitter/receiver to send the signals across the skin to the implanted portion of the device. The implanted unit decodes the received signal and produces controlled electrical stimulation of the electrodes. The most widely used ABI electrode array (Fig. 2; manufactured by Cochlear Corp.) consists of 21 platinum disk contacts, each 700 μm in diameter. The contacts are placed in three rows along a Silastic rubber carrier that is 8 mm × 2.5 mm (Fig. 3).

Present ABI electrodes are designed to be placed within the lateral recess of the IV ventricle. Anatomical studies (Moore and Osen, 1979) of the human cochlear nucleus complex and imaging studies of early ABI patients demonstrated that this location produced the most effective auditory results and the fewest nonauditory side effects (Shannon et al., 1997; Otto et al., 1998, 2002). Electrical stimulation in the human brainstem can potentially produce activation of many nonauditory structures (cranial nerves VII, IX, X, and cerebellum, for

Nucleus 24 ABI

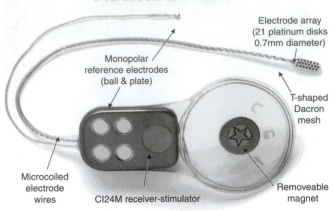

Figure 2. Implantable portion of the ABI, showing the receiver/stimulator and electrode array.

ABI24M ElectrodeArray

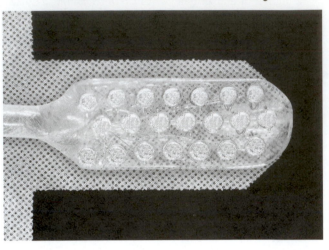

Figure 3. Close-up view of the 21-electrode array, which consists of 21 platinum disks mounted on a Silastic substrate. The fabric mesh backing is intended to encourage fibrous ingrowth to fix the electrode array in position.

example). Fortunately, the human cochlear nucleus complex almost completely surrounds the opening of the lateral recess of the IV ventricle, and the levels of current delivered to the ABI are not large enough to activate other brainstem nuclei more than about 2 mm away (Shannon, 1989, 1992; Shannon et al., 1997).

Vestibular schwannomas can be visualized and removed via several surgical approaches, of which the retrosigmoid and translabyrinthine approaches are the most common. The translabyrinthine approach allows better visualization of the mouth of the lateral recess following tumor removal and thus better access for placement of the ABI electrode array (Brackmann et al., 1993).

Of the first 80 patients implanted with the multichannel ABI at the House Ear Institute, 86% received sufficient auditory sensations that they could use the ABI in daily life. For most ABI users the primary benefit is as an aid to lipreading, since only a few ABI patients can understand words with the ABI without lipreading. For most patients the present ABI device functions at a level similar to that of single-channel cochlear implants, even when many electrodes are used in the ABI speech processor. ABI patients are able to detect sound and are able to discriminate sounds based on coarse temporal properties (Shannon and Otto, 1990; Otto et al., 2002). On average, ABI patients receive a 30% improvement in speech understanding when the sound from the ABI is added to lipreading alone (Fig. 4). A few ABI patients (10%) achieve significant word and sentence recognition with the device, and a few (4/80) can actually converse in a limited fashion on the telephone.

Most ABI patients perceive variations in amplitude and temporal cues but receive little, if any, spectral cues. ABI patients are able to perceive changes in pitch with changes in pulse rate only up to about 150 Hz, which is about an octave lower than observed for cochlear implant listeners and for temporal pitch discrimination for normal-hearing listeners. Typically, the dynamic range of amplitude for the ABI is only 6 dB or less in terms of

electrical current range. We estimate that ABI patients may be able to discriminate only 10 amplitude steps within their dynamic range, in contrast to 20–40 steps for cochlear implants and 200–250 steps for acoustic hearing. Some ABI patients have relatively small differences in pitch across their electrode array, while others show a large change in pitch. In general, patients who do better at speech recognition tend to have a larger pitch range across their electrode array, but not all patients who have a large pitch range have good speech recognition.

Most ABI patients have some electrodes that cause nonauditory side effects. Almost all of these nonauditory effects are benign and produce tingling sensations along the body on the side ipsilateral to the ABI. Nonauditory sensations are produced from stimulation of the cerebellar flocculus (which causes a sensation of eye jitter) and from antidromic activation of the cerebellar peduncle. In patients with an intact facial nerve on the implanted side there is a chance of activation of the facial nerve, causing facial tingling and even motor activation. In most cases, electrodes that produce nonauditory side effects are simply turned off and not stimulated.

One of the possible reasons for the limited success of the ABI is that the present electrode is placed on the surface of the cochlear nucleus. Unfortunately, the tonotopic axis of the human cochlear nucleus is orthogonal to the surface of the nucleus (Moore and Osen, 1979), and thus orthogonal to the axis of the electrode array as well. To obtain better access to the tonotopic dimension of the human cochlear nucleus requires penetrating electrodes (McCreery et al., 1998). A penetrating electrode ABI system is presently under development. Its initial trial is anticipated for 2002.

—Robert V. Shannon

Figure 4. Speech recognition results from the first 55 multichannel ABI patients. Lower part of each bar shows the percent correct recognition of simple sentence materials using lipreading alone. The upper part of each bar shows the improvement in recognition obtained when the ABI was added to lipreading.

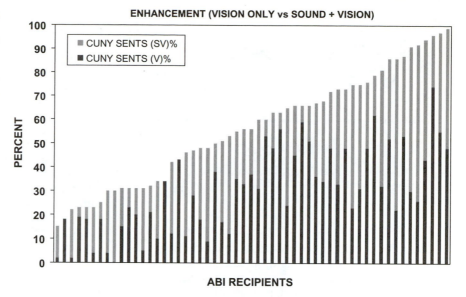

References

Brackmann, D. E., Hitselberger, W. E., Nelson, R. A., Moore, J. K., Waring, M., Portillo, F., et al. (1993). Auditory brainstem implant: I. Issues in surgical implantation. *Otolaryngology–Head and Neck Surgery, 108,* 624–634.

Edgerton, B. J., House, W. F., Hitselberger, W. (1984). Hearing by cochlear nucleus stimulation in humans. *Annals of Otology, Rhinology, and Laryngology, 91,* 117–124.

Eisenberg, L. S., Maltan, A. A., Portillo, F., Mobley, J. P., and House, W. F. (1987a). The central electroauditory prosthesis: Clinical Results. In J. D. Andrade, J. J. Brophy, D. E. Detmer, S. W. Kim, R. A. Normann, D. B. Olsen, and R. L. Stephen (Eds.), *Artificial Organs* (pp. 491–505). New York: VCH Publishing.

Eisenberg, L. S., Maltan, A. A., Portillo, F., Mobley, J. P., and House, W. F. (1987b). Electrical stimulation of the auditory brain stem structure in deafened adults. *Journal of Rehabilitation Research and Development, 24,* 9–22.

McCreery, D. G., Shannon, R. V., Moore, J. K., Chatterjee, M., and Agnew, W. F. (1998). Accessing the tonotopic organization of the ventral cochlear nucleus by intranuclear microstimulation. *IEEE Transactions on Rehabilitation Engineering, 6,* 391–399.

Moore, J. K., and Osen, K. K. (1979). The cochlear nuclei in man. *American Journal of Anatomy, 154,* 393–417.

Otto, S. A., Brackmann, D. E., Hitselberger, W. E., Shannon, R. V., and Kuchta, J. (2002). The multichannel auditory brainstem implant update: Performance in 60 patients. *Journal of Neurosurgery, 96,* 1063–1071.

Otto, S. A., Shannon, R. V., Brackmann, D. E., Hitselberger, W. E., Staller, S., and Menapace, C. (1998). The multichannel auditory brainstem implant: Performance in 20 patients. *Otolaryngology–Head and Neck Surgery, 118,* 291–303.

Rouleau, G. A., Merel, P., Luchtman, M., Sanson, M., Zucman, C., Marineau, C., et al. (1993). Alteration in a new gene encoding a putative membrane-organizing protein causes neurofibromatosis type 2. *Nature, 363,* 515–521.

Shannon, R. V. (1989). Threshold functions for electrical stimulation of the human cochlear nucleus. *Hearing Research, 40,* 173–178.

Shannon, R. V. (1992). A model of safe levels for electrical stimulation. *IEEE Transactions in Biomedical Engineering, 39,* 424–426.

Shannon, R. V., Fayad, J., Moore, J. K., Lo, W., O'Leary, M., Otto, S., et al. (1993). Auditory brainstem implant: II. Postsurgical issues and performance. *Otolaryngology–Head and Neck Surgery, 108,* 635–643.

Shannon, R. V., Moore, J., McCreery, D., and Portillo, F. (1997). Threshold-distance measures from electrical stimulation of human brainstem. *IEEE Transactions on Rehabilitation Engineering, 5,* 1–5.

Shannon, R. V., and Otto, S. R. (1990). Psychophysical measures from electrical stimulation of the human cochlear nucleus. *Hearing Research, 47,* 159–168.

Terr, L. I., Fayad, J., Hitselberger, W. E., and Zakhary, R. (1990). Cochlear nucleus anatomy related to central electroauditory prosthesis implantation. *Otolaryngology–Head and Neck Surgery, 102,* 717–721.

Trofatter, J. A., MacCollin, M. M., Rutter, J. L., Murrell, J. R., Duyao, M. P., Parry, D. M., et al. (1993). A novel moesin-, ezrin-, radixin-like gene is a candidate for the neurofibromatosis 2 tumor suppressor. *Cell, 72,* 791–800.

Auditory Brainstem Response in Adults

The auditory brainstem response (ABR) is a series of five to seven neurogenic potentials, or waves, that occur within the first 10 ms following acoustic stimulation (Sohmer and Feinmesser, 1967; Jewett, Romano, and Williston, 1970). The potentials are the scalp-recorded synchronous electrical activity from groups of neurons in response to a rapid-onset (<1 ms) stimulus. An example of these potentials, with their most common labeling scheme using Roman numerals, is shown in Figure 1. Waves I and II are generated in the auditory nerve, wave III is predominantly from the cochlear nucleus, and waves IV and V are predominantly from the superior olivary complex and lateral lemniscus (Moller, 1993).

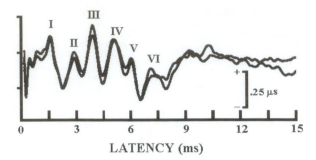

Figure 1. The normal ABR elicited by a high-level click stimulus, with waves I–VI labeled.

The ABR is valuable in audiology and neurology because of its reliability and highly predictable changes in many pathological conditions affecting the auditory system. The ABR may be used in a number of ways in adults. Perhaps the most common use is in the diagnostic assessment of a hearing loss, either to determine the site of the lesion or to determine the function of the neural system. A second use is to estimate auditory sensitivity in patients who are unable or unwilling to provide accurate behavioral thresholds. A third use is for monitoring the auditory nerve and brainstem pathways during surgery for auditory nerve tumors or vestibular nerve section. For diagnostic and neural monitoring purposes, the latencies and amplitudes of the most reliable waves, waves I, III, and V, are analyzed. For estimation of auditory sensitivity, the lowest detection level for wave V is used to approximate auditory threshold. Responses are replicated to ensure reliability of the waveforms.

Because the potentials are small (<1 μV) and embedded in high levels of background electrical noise, several techniques are used to enhance the visibility of the potentials (ASHA, 1988). Surface electrodes are attached to the scalp of the patient, with the placement in line with the orientation of the dipoles of the neural generators. Pairs of electrodes are used such that one electrode picks up positive activity and one electrode picks up negative activity from the neural generators. Differential amplification/common mode rejection enhances the electrical activity that is different between two electrodes (the potentials) and reduces the activity that is the same between electrodes (the random background electrical noise). The physiological response is filtered to eliminate the extraneous electroencephalographic activity and external line noise. Signal averaging increases the magnitude of the time-locked response and minimizes the random background activity. Artifact rejection eliminates unusually high levels of electrical activity that are impossible to eliminate through averaging.

The diagnostic interpretation of the ABR is based on the latencies and amplitudes of the component waves. The latencies, or times of occurrence, of the waves are the more reliable measures because latencies for a given person remain stable across recording sessions unless intervening pathology has occurred. The latency is eval-

uated in absolute and relative terms. Absolute latency is measured from the arrival of the stimulus at the ear to the positive peak of waves I, III, and V. Relative latency is measured between relevant peaks within the same ear or between ears. The absolute latency reflects the state of the auditory system to the generation site of each wave but may be affected by conductive or cochlear pathology, making it difficult to isolate any delay from neural pathology. Interpeak intervals allow an estimation of neural conduction time and are less dependent on peripheral pathology than absolute latencies are. Interaural values limit variability by using the nonsuspect ear as a control in a patient with unilateral pathology, but interaural values also may be affected by asymmetrical conductive or cochlear pathology.

The amplitudes of the waves are more variable than the latencies and therefore are less useful for determining normality of the waveform. Amplitudes, measured from the positive peak to the averaged baseline or from positive peak to subsequent negative trough, are affected by the quality of the electrode contact, physiological noise levels of the patient, and amplitudes of adjacent waves. Consequently, absolute amplitude values are little used except in the case of absent waves. Relative amplitudes, particularly the amplitude ratio of waves I and V, may be useful measures to control for measurement variables. A decrement in wave V amplitude relative to wave I amplitude may suggest auditory nerve or low brainstem pathology.

For the estimation of auditory threshold, wave V may be traced to its detection threshold, which is typically defined as the lowest stimulus level at which wave V can be seen. The ABR does not measure hearing per se, but correlates with auditory sensitivity in most cases. Clicks, which are broadband stimuli, provide estimates of average sensitivity in the range of 2000–4000 Hz because of cochlear physiology that biases the response to the high-frequency region of the cochlea (Fowler and Durrant, 1993). For better definition of thresholds across the frequency range, frequency-specific stimuli, such as tone pips or clicks with ipsilateral masking, may be used (Stapells, Picton, and Durieux-Smith, 1993). Because of limitations in the signals and the cochlea, thresholds for frequencies below 1000 Hz are difficult to obtain, and other methods, such as middle or late auditory-evoked potentials or steady-state evoked potentials, may yield better results or additional information (see Hall, 1992; Jacobson, 1993).

Clicks at high presentation levels are the most commonly used stimuli for diagnostic ABRs because their abrupt rise times elicit the necessary degree of synchrony to obtain the full complement of waves. Although the normal ABR to a click is dominated by neurons associated with 2000–4000 Hz, a peripheral hearing loss at those frequencies may effectively filter the stimulus, causing different frequency regions to dominate the response in different hearing losses, which will affect the ensuing ABR latencies (see Fowler and Durrant, 1993). ABR latencies from suspect ears are compared with the norms at equivalent sound pressure levels at the cochlea.

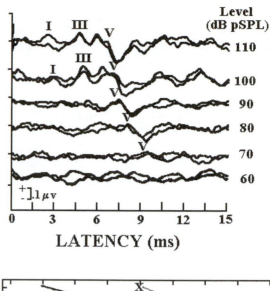

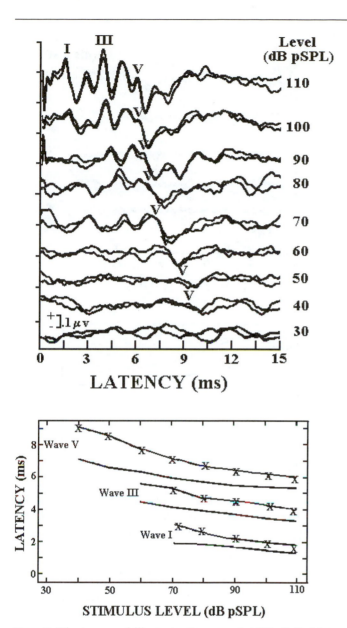

Figure 2. The top panel illustrates the normal ABR elicited by clicks from 110 dB pSPL to 30 dB pSPL, with wave V labeled down to the visual detection threshold of 40 dB pSPL. The lower panel shows the latencies of waves I, III, and V plotted against the normative values for those waves, indicated by the bounded areas.

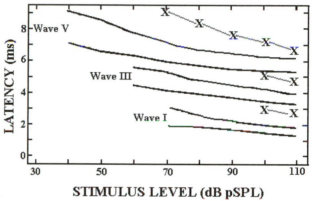

Figure 3. The top panel illustrates the ABR for a person with a mild conductive hearing loss, with wave V labeled to the visual detection threshold of 70 dB pSPL. The lower panel shows the latencies for waves I, III, and V plotted above the normative values, indicated by the bounded areas.

The typical effects of auditory pathology on the latencies and thresholds of the ABR are discussed below.

Normal Hearing. Normative latencies may vary somewhat among clinics, but are typically derived from the mean and ± 2 standard deviations of the latencies of waves from a jury of listeners with normal hearing. Examples of normative values for waves I, III, and V are shown as the bounded areas in the lower panel in Figure 2. Typical normal interpeak intervals are <2.51 ms for interpeak interval I–III, <2.31 ms for III–V, <4.54 ms for I–V, and <0.4 ms for interaural V

latency (Bauch and Olsen, 1990). Figure 2 includes the ABRs for high-level signals to threshold for a person with normal hearing, along with the latencies of those waves plotted against the normal range. All latencies are within the normal limits, and the threshold is 40 dB peak sound pressure level (pSPL), which equals 10 dB nHL (normalized hearing level).

Conductive Hearing Loss. The absolute latencies are prolonged and the amplitudes are reduced relative to the degree of the conductive component of a hearing loss, but the interwave intervals are normal because the neural system is intact. Consequently, a person with a 30-dB conductive hearing loss will produce an ABR to a 90-dB nHL click that is approximately equivalent to the ABR to a 60-dB nHL click for a person with normal hearing. An example of a waveform and the resulting latencies from a 30-dB flat, conductive hearing loss are shown in Figure 3. All absolute latencies are prolonged, but the I–V latency difference is within normal limits. The threshold is 70 dB pSPL.

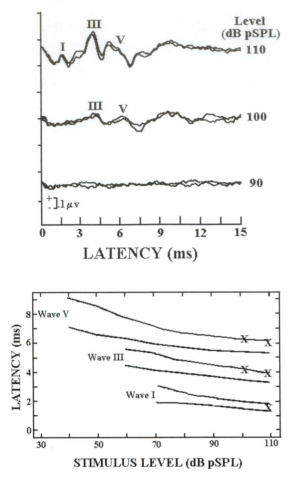

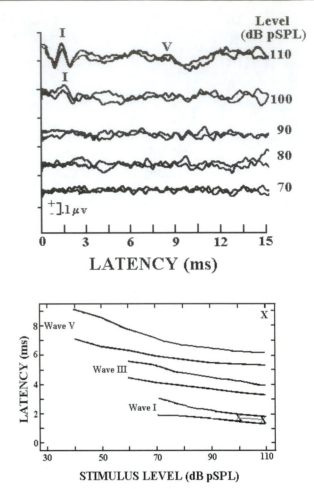

Figure 4. The top panel illustrates the ABR for a person with a moderate, flat cochlear hearing loss, with wave V labeled to its visual detection threshold of 100 dB pSPL. The lower panel shows the latencies for waves I, III, and V plotted within the normative values, indicated by the bounded areas.

Figure 5. The top panel illustrates the ABR for a person with a vestibular schwannoma, with the reliable waves labeled. The lower panel shows the latencies for waves I and V plotted against the normative values for those waves. Wave I is within normal limits, whereas wave V is significantly prolonged, yielding a prolonged interwave I–V interval. The threshold for wave V does not correspond to the behavioral auditory threshold.

Cochlear Hearing Loss. The degree and configuration of the hearing loss affect the latencies of the waves in a cochlear hearing loss, although typically the I–V interval is normal because the neural system is intact. Most mild to moderate cochlear losses do not affect the latencies of the ABR for high-level click stimuli, although the amplitudes of the waves may be reduced. Severe high-frequency hearing losses may reduce the amplitudes and prolong the absolute latencies of the waves with little effect on the I–V latency interval, although wave I may be absent. An example of the waveform and resulting latencies from a moderate, flat hearing loss are shown in Figure 4. Absolute and interwave latencies are within normal limits, and the threshold is 100 dB pSPL.

Retrocochlear Hearing Loss. Retrocochlear pathology refers to any neural pathology of the auditory system that is beyond the cochlea and may include such disorders as acoustic neuromas, multiple sclerosis, brainstem strokes, and head trauma. Retrocochlear pathology may produce a variety of effects on the latencies and

morphology of the ABR depending on the type, location, and size of the pathology. Effects may include absence of waves, prolonged absolute latencies or interwave intervals, or prolonged interaural wave V latencies. In Figure 5, the waveform and resulting latencies are shown from a patient with an acoustic neuroma and a mild, high-frequency hearing loss. Wave I is within normal limits at the two highest levels, but the absolute latency for wave V, and consequently the I–V interval, is prolonged beyond the normal limits. The wave V threshold may be variable in people with retrocochlear pathology, and may not provide a useful estimation of behavioral threshold.

Finally, for intraoperative monitoring, the ABR is used to warn the surgeon of possible damage to the auditory nerve during surgery for auditory nerve tumors or resection of the vestibular nerve, particularly when the goal includes preservation of hearing. The amplitudes and latencies of waves I and V are monitored during the surgery when compromise of the nerve is a possibility. Wave I provides an index of cochlear function and neural function peripheral to the tumor and wave V provides an index of neural function central to the tumor. Significant prolongations of the latency of wave V or a decline in the amplitude of wave V may suggest damage to the nerve, which then may be at risk for permanent injury. Occasionally, the surgical technique may be modified in an attempt to avoid permanent injury to the nerve.

—*Cynthia G. Fowler*

References

ASHA Audiologic Evaluation Working Group on Auditory Evoked Potential Measurements. (1988). *The short latency auditory evoked potentials*. Rockville, MD: American Speech-Language-Hearing Association.

Bauch, C. D., and Olsen, W. O. (1990). Comparison of ABR amplitudes with TIPtrode and mastoid electrodes. *Ear and Hearing, 11*, 463–467.

Fowler, C. G., and Durrant, J. D. (1993). The effects of peripheral hearing loss on the ABR. In J. Jacobson (Ed.), *Principles and applications in auditory evoked potentials* (pp. 237–250). Needham, MA: Allyn and Bacon.

Hall, J. W., III (1992). *Handbook of auditory evoked responses*. Boston: Allyn and Bacon.

Jacobson, J. (Ed.). (1993). *Principles and applications in auditory evoked potentials*. Needham, MA: Allyn and Bacon.

Jewett, D. L., Romano, M. N., and Williston, J. S. (1970). Human auditory evoked potentials: Possible brain stem components detected on the scalp. *Science, 167*, 1517–1518.

Moller, A. R. (1993). Neural generators of auditory evoked potentials. In J. Jacobson (Ed.), *Principles and applications in auditory evoked potentials* (pp. 23–46). Needham, MA: Allyn and Bacon.

Sohmer, H., and Feinmesser, M. (1967). Cochlear action potentials recorded from the external ear in man. *Annals of Otology, Rhinology, and Laryngology, 76*, 427–438.

Stapells, D., Picton, T. W., and Durieux-Smith, A. (1993). Electrophysiologic measures of frequency-specific auditory function. In J. Jacobson (Ed.), *Principles and applications in auditory evoked potentials* (pp. 251–283). Needham, MA: Allyn and Bacon.

Further Readings

Borg, E., and Lovqvist, L. (1982). A lower limit for auditory brainstem response. *Scandinavian Audiology, 11*, 277–278.

Brown, C. J., Hughes, M. L., Luk, B., Abbas, P. J., Wolaver, A., and Gervais, J. (2000). The relationship between EAP and EABR thresholds and levels used to program the Nucleus 24 speech processor: Data from adults. *Ear and Hearing, 21*, 151–163.

Burkhard, R. (1984). Sound pressure level measurement and spectral analysis of brief acoustic transients. *Electroencephalography and Clinical Neurophysiology, 58*, 83–91.

Chiappa, K. H., Gladstone, K. J., and Young, R. R. (1979). Brainstem auditory evoked responses: Studies of waveform variations in 50 normal human subjects. *Archives of Neurology, 36*, 81–87.

Coats, A. C., and Martin, J. L. (1977). Human auditory nerve action potentials and brainstem evoked responses: Effects of audiogram shape and lesion location. *Archives of Otolaryngology, 103*, 605–622.

Cone-Wesson, B. (1995). How accurate are bone-conduction ABR tests? *American Journal of Audiology, 4*, 14–19.

Davis, H., and Hirsch, S. K. (1979). A slow brain stem response for low-frequency audiometry. *Audiology, 18*, 445–461.

Durrant, J. D., and Fowler, C. G. (1996). ABR protocols for dealing with asymmetric hearing loss. *American Journal of Audiology, 5*, 5–6.

Goldstein, R., and Aldrich, W. M. (1999). *Evoked potential audiometry: Fundamentals and applications*. Boston: Allyn and Bacon.

Hood, L. J. (1998). *Clinical applications of the auditory brainstem response*. San Diego, CA: Singular Publishing Group.

Jewett, D. L. (1970). Volume conducted potentials in response to auditory stimuli as detected by averaging in the cat. *Electroencephalography and Clinical Neurophysiology, 28*, 609–618.

Musiek, F. E., and Baran, J. A. (1986). Neuroanatomy, neurophysiology, and central auditory assessment: Part I. Brain stem. *Ear and Hearing, 7*, 207–219.

Stapells, D. R. (1994). Low-frequency hearing and the auditory brainstem response. *American Journal of Audiology, 3*, 11–13.

Wiedemayer, H., Fauser, B., Sandalcioglu, I. E., Schafer, H., and Stolke, D. (2002). The impact of neurophysiological intraoperative monitoring on surgical decisions: A critical analysis of 423 cases. *Journal of Neurosurgery, 96*, 55–62.

Wrege, K., and Starr, A. (1981). Binaural interaction in human auditory brainstem evoked potentials. *Archives of Neurology, 38*, 572–580.

Auditory Neuropathy in Children

The disorder now known as auditory neuropathy (AN) has been defined only within the past 10 years (Starr et al., 1991), although references to patients with this disorder appeared as early as the 1970s and 1980s (Friedman, Schulman, and Weiss, 1975; Ishii and Toriyama, 1977; Worthington and Peters, 1980; Kraus et al., 1984; Jacobson, Means, and Dhib-Jalbut, 1986). This disorder is particularly deleterious when it occurs in childhood because it causes significant disturbance of encoding of temporal features of sound, which severely limits speech perception and, consequently, the development of oral language skills.

Patients with AN have three key characteristics. First, they have a hearing disorder in the form of elevated pure-tone thresholds (which can vary from slight to profound) or significant dysfunction of hearing in noise. Second, they have evidence of good outer hair cell function, in the form of either present otoacoustic emissions or an easily recognized cochlear microphonic component. Third, they have evidence of neural dysfunction at the level of the primary auditory nerve. This condition manifests with an abnormal or absent auditory brainstem response (ABR), beginning with wave I. The presence of hearing dysfunction in quiet, and of poor or absent ABR, distinguish this disorder from central auditory dysfunction, in which hearing and ABR are both normal.

The presence of normal outer hair cell function and the absence of wave I of the ABR narrow the potential sites of lesion in AN to (1) the inner hair cell, (2) the synaptic junction between the inner hair cell and the auditory nerve, and (3) the peripheral portion of the auditory nerve. There is evidence to support the first and third possibilities, but no direct evidence of synaptic disorder.

Starr (2001) has found that approximately one-third of all patients with AN have symptoms of peripheral nerve disease. Approximately 80% of adults with AN demonstrate concomitant peripheral neuropathy, while no patients less than 5 years old show clinical evidence of peripheral nerve disorder. Peripheral neuropathy that was not evident in some of the younger patients emerged in children who were followed over time. In patients with other peripheral nerve involvement, disease of the primary portion of the auditory nerve would be the most parsimonious explanation for the auditory disorder.

More direct evidence of primary auditory nerve disease in humans was reported by Spoendlin (1974) from postmortem temporal bone histologic studies of two sibling adult patients with moderate hearing loss. These individuals had a full complement of inner and outer hair cells but significant loss of spiral ganglion cells. Similar findings were reported by Nadol (2001) in a patient with Charcot-Marie-Tooth syndrome and hearing loss.

Harrison (1999, 2001) has shown that both carboplatin treatment and anoxia can induce isolated inner hair lesions in chinchillas. The same animals had otoacoustic emissions and abnormal ABR results. Amatuzzi et al. (2001) recently reported an autopsy analysis of the temporal bones of three premature infants; findings included isolated inner hair cell loss with a full complement of outer hair cells and auditory neurons. These infants had failed ABR screening while in the neonatal intensive care unit. This study presented the first evidence in humans that an isolated inner hair cell disorder is a possible explanation for AN.

No currently available clinical tools can provide data to distinguish between the inner hair cell and the auditory nerve as site of lesion in AN. Because young children with AN often do not show evidence of other peripheral nerve involvement, it is particularly difficult to know what the underlying pathology of their AN might be. However, it is also not clear how any distinction in pathology could be used to remediate the hearing difficulties in these patients.

Description of Patients

Most patients with AN have disease onset in childhood (Sininger and Oba, 2001). The sex distribution is approximately equal. Close to half of patients with AN have a family history or an associated genetic syndrome, indicating a genetic basis for the disorder. In some cases, specific chromosomal anomalies have been isolated (Butinar et al., 1999; Kalaydjieva et al., 1996, 1998). Other syndromes that have been associated with AN include Charcot-Marie-Tooth syndrome, Friedreich's ataxia, Ehlers-Danlos syndrome, and Stevens-Johnson syndrome (Sininger and Oba, 2001).

Many patients with AN show no risk factors. However, other health issues often associated with AN in infants include hyperbillirubinemia and prematurity (Stein et al., 1996; Sininger and Oba, 2001). As we begin to detect hearing loss in the newborn period with screening, it will be possible to obtain more data on those factors that may be directly associated with AN.

The pure-tone hearing loss in patients with AN ranges from slight to profound, with a greater percentage of severe and profound loss than in patients with sensory hearing loss. Any configuration of loss can occur, but low-frequency emphasis or flat configurations are most often seen. Only rarely is AN unilateral, but such cases have been described.

The symptoms and hearing loss of patients with AN can fluctuate dramatically on a day-to-day basis or more frequently. The most dramatic instance of rapid changes in symptoms has been described as "temperature-sensitive auditory neuropathy." Starr et al. (1998) described three such patients in whom severe symptoms, including nearly complete loss of hearing and ABR, accompanied a slight fever. The symptoms in these patients would remit, leaving nearly normal auditory function, as soon as the core temperature returned to normal. Symptoms of AN can progress slowly over time, and the symptoms seen in newborns sometimes improve in the first few months of life.

Patients with AN have poor performance on all auditory tasks involving temporal processing. For example, AN patients have dramatically abnormal gap detection thresholds and temporal modulation transfer functions when compared with patients with sensory hearing loss or normal hearing. In contrast, loudness functions, such as intensity discrimination and temporal integration, are normal for subjects with AN (Zeng et al., 2001).

Speech perception ability is notably reduced in these patients, especially in regard to the degree of hearing loss (Sininger and Oba, 2001). Poor speech discrimination can be directly linked to reduced temporal processing (Zeng et al., 2001).

The ABR is abnormal or absent in cases of auditory neuropathy. In all cases except profound loss, the threshold of the ABR does not correspond to the auditory thresholds, and for this reason the ABR cannot be used to predict hearing levels in children with AN. In some cases of AN, a wave V can be distinguished, but it is usually small in amplitude, extended in latency, and the response threshold is unrelated to pure-tone hearing levels.

The ABR waveform of the patient with AN, when recorded with electrodes placed at the mastoid or otherwise near the ear, will usually show evidence of a large cochlear microphonic (CM) component. This pattern can be easily distinguished from an early neural response because the CM waveform will invert with stimulus

A

Audiogram

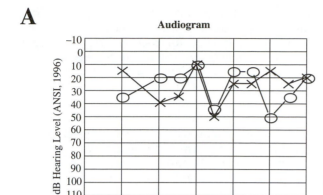

B   Transient Evoked Otoacoustic Emission

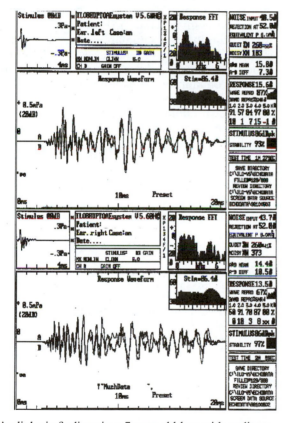

C   Auditory Brainstem Response

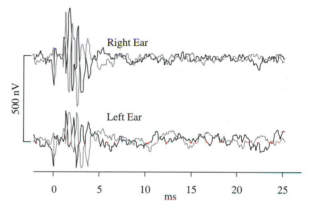

Figure 1. Audiologic findings in a 7-year-old boy with auditory neuropathy. **A**, Audiogram. Speech awareness threshold: right ear = 20 dB HL, left ear = 25 dB HL. Speech discrimination: right ear = 28%, left ear = 8%. Typanometry was within normal limits; the acoustic reflex threshold was absent. **B**, Transient evoked otoacoustic emission. **C**, Auditory brainstem response. Study was performed using insert earphones, with a click stimulus rate of 25/s at 80 dB nHL. Rarefaction and condensation graphs are overlaid; right ear and left ear.

polarity and demonstrate a mirror image when the waveforms corresponding to the two stimuli are superimposed. Also, unlike neural response, the CM component does not change latency with a decrease in stimulus level and is relatively undisturbed by noise masking. The CM can be evidence of either inner or outer hair cell function. The CM can be distinguished from stimulus artifact by a simple procedure. If an insert earphone is used, clamping the tubing will cause the CM to disappear, because no effective stimulus will reach the ear. At the same time, stimulus artifact from the transducer will remain after the tubing is clamped.

In most cases of AN, an otoacoustic emission (OAE) is seen, regardless of the degree of hearing loss. However, the OAE has diminished over time in some of these patients, for unknown reasons (Deltenre et al., 1997). The CM component can be substituted for the OAE as evidence of hair cell function.

Brainstem reflexes involving the auditory system, including middle ear muscle reflexes and olivocochlear reflexes (suppression of OAE with contralateral noise), are almost universally absent in patients with AN. Again, unlike in sensory loss, this finding is true regardless of the degree of hearing loss present.

Rehabilitation Strategies

Inherently poor timing in the auditory system of patients with AN requires specialized approaches to the development of speech and language. The use of visual information to supplement speech perception is most important. Manual communication in a total communication system (oral speech and sign language simultaneously) is often recommended. For very young children with no language system, this approach helps to ensure that a language system will develop regardless of the capacity of the auditory system to process oral speech. In mild cases of AN (those with mild or moderate hearing thresholds), a cued-speech approach can be useful (Cone-Wesson, Rance, and Sininger, 2001).

Standard amplification does not provide the same degree of benefit for patients with AN as in patients with conductive or sensory hearing loss. However, for many children, some advantages can be gained from amplification, including lower thresholds for the detection of environmental sounds and even small increases in speech perception ability. Parents should be cautioned that the benefits of amplification will be limited, and a trial period should be used to determine if any help is afforded by the hearing aids.

Cochlear implants have been used in many children with AN (Trautwein, Sininger, and Nelson, 2000; Shallop et al., 2001; Trautwein et al., 2001). Electrical stimulation of the auditory nerve may reintroduce the temporal encoding through neural synchrony, necessary for speech perception. Most of the children with AN who have received cochlear implants perform similarly to other deaf children, but good performance is not always achieved (Trautwein et al., 2001). An important question is whether children with moderate hearing loss and AN who do not receive benefit from hearing aids should be considered for cochlear implants. Results in patients with moderate loss due to AN and cochlear implants may be available in the near future to help answer this important question.

Case Report

In a 7-year-old boy with AN, the medical history was unremarkable. Speech development was normal before the age of 5 years, but after that time, response to sound was inconsistent, and difficulty with speech production was noted. At age 7 years the audiogram in Figure 1 was obtained, revealing a moderate hearing loss bilaterally. Tympanometry was normal, acoustic reflexes were absent, and otoacoustic emissions were present. ABR testing revealed no response to 80 dB nHL stimuli, but evidence of a cochlear microphonic component was seen in the recording. Magnetic resonance imaging of the brain and cranial nerves VII and VIII was normal, as was a neurological examination. Amplification and FM systems were used sparingly, with little success. This child relies heavily on speechreading, supplemented with manual communication as necessary.

This child represents a possible late-onset case of AN of unknown etiology. His audiogram shows the often seen nonuniform configuration with peaks and valleys. Significant fluctuations in his hearing have been noted over time. He is also typical in that he relies very heavily on visual cues, including speechreading, supplemented by signs, for receptive communication.

— *Yvonne S. Sininger*

References

Amatuzzi, M. G., Northrop, C., Liberman, M. C., Thornton, A., Halpin, C., Herrmann, B., et al. (2001). Selective inner hair cell loss in premature infants and cochlea pathological patterns from neonatal intensive care unit autopsies. *Archives of Otolaryngology–Head and Neck Surgery, 127,* 629–636.

Butinar, D., Zidar, J., Leonardis, L., Popovic, M., Kalaydjieva, L., Angelicheva, D., et al. (1999). Hereditary auditory, vestibular, motor, and sensory neuropathy in a Slovenian Roma (Gypsy) kindred. *Annals of Neurology, 46,* 36–44.

Cone-Wesson, B., Rance, G., and Sininger, Y. S. (2001). Amplification and rehabilitation strategies for patients with auditory neuropathy. In Y. S. Sininger and A. Starr (Eds.), *Auditory neuropathy: A new perspective on hearing disorders* (pp. 233–249). Albany, NY: Singular/Thompson Learning.

Deltenre, P., Mansbach, A. L., Bozet, C., Clercx, A., and Hecox, K. E. (1997). Auditory neuropathy: A report on three cases with early onsets and major neonatal illnesses. *Electroencephalography and Clinical Neurophysiology (Ireland), 104,* 17–22.

Friedman, S. A., Schulman, R. H., and Weiss, S. (1975). Hearing and diabetic neuropathy. *Archives of Internal Medicine, 135,* 573–576.

Harrison, R. V. (1999). An animal model of auditory neuropathy. *Ear and Hearing, 19,* 355–361.

Harrison, R. V. (2001). Models of auditory neuropathy based on inner hair cell damage. In Y. S. Sininger and A. Starr (Eds.), *Auditory neuropathy: A new perspective on hearing disorders* (pp. 51–66). Albany, NY: Singular/Thompson Learning.

Ishii, T., and Toriyama, M. (1977). Sudden deafness with severe loss of cochlear neurons. *Annals of Otology, Rhinology, and Laryngology, 86,* 541–547.

Jacobson, G. P., Means, E. D., and Dhib-Jalbut, S. (1986). Delay in the absolute latency of auditory brainstem response (ABR) component P1 in acute inflammatory demyelinating disease. *Scandinavian Audiology, 15,* 121–124.

Kalaydjieva, L., Hallmayer, J., Chandler, D., Savov, A., Nikolova, A., Angelicheva, D., et al. (1996). Gene mapping in Gypsies identifies a novel demyelinating neuropathy on chromosome 8q24. *Nature Genetics, 14,* 214–217.

Kalaydjieva, L., Nikolova, A., Turnev, I., Petrova, J., Hristova, A., Ishpekova, B., et al. (1998). Hereditary motor and sensory neuropathy: Lom, a novel demyelinating neuropathy associated with deafness in gypsies. *Brain, 121,* 399–408.

Kraus, N., Ozdamar, O., Stein, L., and Reed, N. (1984). Absent auditory brain stem response: Peripheral hearing loss or brain stem dysfunction? *Laryngoscope, 94,* 400–406.

Nadol, J. B., Jr. (2001). Primary cochlear neuronal degeneration. In Y. S. Sininger and A. Starr (Eds.), *Auditory neuropathy: A new perspective on hearing disorders* (pp. 99–140). Albany, NY: Singular/Thompson Learning.

Shallop, J. K., Peterson, A., Facer, G. W., Fabry, L. B., and Driscoll, C. L. W. (2001). Cochlear implants in five cases of auditory neuropathy: Postoperative findings and progress. *Laryngoscope, 111,* 555–562.

Sininger, Y. S., and Oba, S. (2001). Patients with auditory neuropathy: Who are they and what can they hear? In Y. S. Sininger and A. Starr (Eds.), *Auditory neuropathy: A new perspective on hearing disorders* (pp. 15–35). Albany, NY: Singular/Thompson Learning.

Spoendlin, H. (1974). Optic and cochleovestibular degenerations in hereditary ataxias: II. Temporal bone pathology in two cases of Friedreich's ataxia with vestibulo-cochlear disorders. *Brain, 97,* 41–48.

Starr, A. (2001). The neurology of auditory neuropathy. In Y. S. Sininger and A. Starr (Eds.), *Auditory neuropathy: A new perspective on hearing disorders* (pp. 37–49). Albany, NY: Singular/Thompson Learning.

Starr, A., McPherson, D., Patterson, J., Don, M., Luxford, W. M., Shannon, R., et al. (1991). Absence of both auditory evoked potentials and auditory percepts dependent on timing cues. *Brain, 114,* 1157–1180.

Starr, A., Sininger, Y. S., Winter, M., Derebery, J., Oba, S., and Michalewski, H. (1998). Transient deafness due to temperature-sensitive auditory neuropathy. *Ear and Hearing, 19,* 169–179.

Stein, L., Tremblay, K., Pasternak, J., Banerjee, S., Lindemann, K., and Kraus, N. (1996). Brainstem abnormalities in neonates with normal otoacoustic emissions. *Seminars in Hearing, 17,* 197–213.

Trautwein, P., Shallop, J., Fabry, L., and Friedman, R. (2001). Cochlear implantation of patients with auditory neuropathy. In Y. S. Sininger and A. Starr (Eds.), *Auditory neuropathy: A new perspective on hearing disorders* (pp. 203–231). Albany, NY: Singular/Thompson Learning.

Trautwein, P. G., Sininger, Y. S., and Nelson, R. (2000). Cochlear implantation of auditory neuropathy. *Journal of the American Academy of Audiology, 11,* 309–315.

Worthington, D. W., and Peters, J. F. (1980). Quantifiable hearing and no ABR: Paradox or error? *Ear and Hearing, 1,* 281–285.

Zeng, F.-G., Oba, S., Garde, S., Sininger, Y. S., and Starr, A. (2001). Psychoacoustics and speech perception in auditory neuropathy. In Y. S. Sininger and A. Starr (Eds.), *Auditory neuropathy: A new perspective on hearing disorders* (pp. 141–164). Albany, NY: Singular/Thompson Learning.

Auditory Scene Analysis

Sensory systems such as hearing probably evolved in order for organisms to determine objects in their environment, allowing them to navigate, feed, mate, and communicate. Objects vibrate and as a result produce sound. An auditory system provides the neural architecture for the organism to process sound, and thereby to learn something about these objects or sound sources. In most situations, many sound sources are present at the same time, but the sound from these various sources arrives at the organism as one complex sound field, not as separate, individual sounds. The challenge for the auditory system is to process this complex sound field so that the individual sound sources can be determined. That is, the auditory system is presented with a complex auditory scene, and the auditory images in this scene are the sound sources (Bregman, 1990). The auditory system must be capable of performing auditory scene analysis if it is to determine the sources of sounds.

Auditory scene analysis is not undertaken in the auditory periphery (the cochlea and auditory nerve). The auditory periphery provides a spectral-temporal neural code for the acoustic information contained within the auditory scene. That is, the auditory nerve relays to the auditory brainstem the coding performed by the cochlea. This neural code provides the central nervous system with information about the spectral components that make up the auditory scene in terms of their frequencies, levels, and timing. The central auditory nervous system must then analyze this peripheral neural code so that the individual sound sources that generated the scene can be determined.

What information might be preserved in the peripheral code that is usable by the central auditory system for auditory scene analysis? Several cues have been suggested. They include frequency separation, temporal separation, spatial separation, level differences in spectral profiles, asynchronous onsets and offsets, harmonic structure, and temporal modulation (Yost, 1992). These are properties of the sound generated by sound sources that may be preserved in the peripheral code. As an example, if two sound sources each vibrate with a different frequency, the two frequencies will be mixed into a single auditory scene arriving at the listener. The auditory system could ascertain that two frequencies are present, indicating two sound sources. We know that this is possible since within certain boundary conditions, the auditory periphery codes for the frequency content of any complex sound.

The example of two sound sources each producing a different frequency is the basis of a set of experiments designed to investigate auditory scene analysis. Imagine that the sound coming from each of the two sources is pulsed on and off so that the sound from one source (one frequency) is on when the sound from the other source (a different frequency) is off. The perception of the stimulus condition could be described as a single sound with an alternating pitch. However, since each sound could be from a different source, the perception of the stimulus condition could also be that of two sound sources, each producing a pulsing tone of a particular frequency. Each of these perceptions is possible given the exact frequencies and timing used in the experiment. When the perception is one of two different sound sources, the percept is often described as if two perceptual streams were running side by side, each stream representing a sound source. The stimulus conditions that lead to this form of stream segregation are likely to be those that promote the segregation of sound from one source from that of another source (Bregman, 1990). Many of the parameters listed above have been studied using this auditory streaming paradigm. In general, stimulus parameters associated with frequency are more likely to support stream segregation (Kubovy, 1987), but most of the parameters listed can support auditory stream segregation under certain conditions.

Experiments to study auditory scene analysis, such as auditory streaming, require listeners to process sound over a large range of frequencies and over time. Since a great deal of work in auditory perception and psychoacoustics has concentrated on short-time processing in narrow frequency regions, less is known about auditory processing across wide regions of the spectra and longer periods of time. Therefore, obtaining a better understanding of cross-spectral processing and long-time processing is very important for revealing processes and mechanisms that may assist auditory scene analysis (Yost, 1992).

One of the traditional examples of cross-spectral processing that relates to auditory scene analysis is the processing of the pitch of complex sounds, such as the pitch of the missing fundamental (see PITCH PERCEPTION). For these spectrally complex stimuli, usually ones that have a harmonic structure, a major perceptual aspect of the stimulus is the perception of a single pitch (Moore, 1997). Conditions such as the pitch of the missing fundamental suggest that the auditory system uses a wide range of frequencies to determine the complex pitch and that this complex pitch may be the defining acoustic characteristic of a harmonic sound source, such as the musical note of a piano key. A sound consisting of the frequencies 300, 400, 500, 600, and 700 Hz would most likely have a perceived pitch of 100 Hz (the missing fundamental in the sound's spectrum). The 100-Hz pitch may help in determining the existence of a sound source with this 100-Hz harmonic structure.

The example of the missing fundamental pitch can be generalized to describe acoustic situations in which the auditory system segregates sounds into more than one source. A naturally occurring sound source is unlikely to have all but one of its frequency components harmonically related. Thus, in the example cited above, it is unlikely that a single sound source would have a spectrum with frequency components at 300, 400, 550, 600, and 700 Hz (the 550-Hz component is the inharmonic component that replaced the 500-Hz component). In fact, when one of the harmonics of a series of harmonically related frequency components is "mistuned" from the harmonic relationship (550 Hz in the example), listeners are likely to perceive two pitches (as if there were two sound sources), one associated with the 100-Hz harmonic relationship and the other with the frequency of the mistuned harmonic (Hartmann, McAdams, and Smith, 1990). That is, the 550-Hz mistuned harmonic is perceptually segregated as a separate pitch from the 100-Hz complex pitch associated with the rest of the harmonically related components. Such dual pitch perception suggests there were two potential sound sources. In this case, the auditory system appears to be using a wide frequency range (300–700 Hz) to process these two pitches, and hence perceives two potential sound sources.

The complex pitch example can also be used to address the role of stimulus onset as another potential cue used for auditory scene analysis. Two sound sources may each produce a harmonically related spectrum, such that one sound source may have frequency components at 150, 300, 450, 600, and 750 Hz (harmonics of 150 Hz) and another at 233, 466, 699, and 832 Hz (harmonics of 233 Hz). When presented in isolation these two sounds will produce pitches of 150 and 233 Hz. However, if the two stimuli are added together so that they come on and go off together, it is unlikely that two pitches will be perceived. The perception of two pitches can be recovered if one of the complex sounds comes on slightly before the other one, even though both sounds remain on together thereafter. Thus, if the sound from one source comes on (or in some cases goes off) before another sound, then the asynchronous onsets (or offsets) promote sound source segregation, aiding in auditory scene analysis (Darwin, 1981).

If two sounds have different temporal patterns of modulation they may be perceptually segregated on the basis of temporal modulation (especially if the modulation is amplitude modulated; Moore and Alcantara, 1996). Detecting a tonal signal in a wideband-noise background is improved if the noise is amplitude modulated, suggesting that the modulation helps segregate the tone from the noise background (Hall, Haggard, and Fernandes, 1984).

Sounds from spatially separated sources may help in determining the auditory scene. The ability of the auditory system to use sound to locate objects in the real world also appears to help segregate one sound source from another (Yost, 1997). However, the ability to determine the instruments (sound sources) in an orchestral piece played over a single loudspeaker suggests that having actual sources in our immediate environment at different locations is not required for auditory scene analysis.

Thus, in order to use sound to determine something about objects in our world, the central auditory system must process the neural code for sound in order to parse that code into subsets of neural information where each subset may be the neural counterpart of a sound source. Several different parameters of sound sources are preserved by the neural code and may form the basis of auditory scene analysis. Determining the sources of sound requires processing across a wide range of frequencies and over time, and is required for organisms to successfully cope with their environments.

—William A. Yost

References

Bregman, A. S. (1990). *Auditory scene analysis: The perceptual organization of sound.* Cambridge, MA: MIT Press.

Darwin, C. J. (1981). Perceptual grouping of speech components differing in fundamental frequency and onset time. *Quarterly Journal of Experimental Psychology, 33A,* 185–207.

Hall, J. W. III, Haggard, M., and Fernandes, M. A. (1984). Detection of noise by spectro-temporal pattern analysis. *Journal of the Acoustical Society of America, 76,* 50–58.

Hartmann, M., McAdams, S., and Smith, B. K. (1990). Hearing a mistuned harmonic in an otherwise periodic complex tone. *Journal of the Acoustical Society of America, 88,* 1712–1724.

Kubovy, M. (1987). Concurrent pitch segregation. In W. A. Yost and C. S. Watson (Eds.), *Auditory processing of complex sounds.* Hillsdale, NJ: Erlbaum.

Moore, B. C. J. (1997). *An introduction to the psychology of hearing* (3rd ed.). London: Academic Press.

Moore, B. C. J., and Alcantara, J. I. (1996). Vowel identification based on amplitude modulation. *Journal of the Acoustical Society of America, 99,* 2332–2343.

Yost, W. A. (1992). Auditory image perception. *Hearing Research, 56,* 8–19.

Yost, W. A. (1997). The cocktail party effect: 40 years later. In R. Gilkey and T. Anderson (Eds.), *Localization and spatial hearing in real and virtual environments.* Hillsdale, NJ: Erlbaum.

Further Readings

Hartmann, W. M. (1988). Pitch perception and the organization and integration of auditory entities. In G. W. Edelman, W. E. Gall, and W. M. Cowan (Eds.), *Auditory function: Neurobiological bases of hearing.* New York: Wiley.

Moore, B. C. J. (1997). *An introduction to the psychology of hearing* (3rd ed.). London: Academic Press.

Yost, W. A. (1992). Auditory perception and sound source determination. *Current Directions in Psychological Sciences, 1,* 12–15.

Yost, W. A., and Stanley, S. (1993). Auditory perception. In W. A. Yost, R. R. Fay, and A. Popper (Eds.), *Psychoacoustics.* New York: Springer-Verlag.

Auditory Training

Auditory training includes a collection of activities, the goal of which is to change auditory function, auditory behaviors, or the ways in which individuals approach auditory tasks. Auditory training most commonly is associated with the rehabilitation of individuals with hearing loss, but it has been used with other populations that have presumed difficulties with auditory processing, such as children with specific language impairment, phonologic disorder, dyslexia, and autism (Wharry, Kirkpatrick, and Stokes, 1987; Bettison, 1996; Merzenich et al., 1996; Habib et al., 1999). Auditory training has been applied to children diagnosed with central auditory processing and to adults learning a second language (Solma and Adepoju, 1995; Musiek, 1999). It also has been used experimentally to assess the plasticity of speech perceptual categories and to determine the neurological substrates of speech perception learning and organization (Werker and Tees, 1984; Bradlow et al., 1997; Tremblay et al., 1997, 1998, 2001; Wang et al., 1999).

Most auditory training programs are organized around three parameters: auditory processing approach, auditory skill, and stimulus difficulty level (Erber and Hirsh, 1978; Erber, 1982; Tye-Murray, 1998). When implementing an auditory training program, the first decision is whether to use a top-down (synthetic) or a bottom-up (analytic) processing approach or a combination of both. Most normal-hearing adults tend to rely primarily on top-down processing when listening to ongoing speech, but if the goal for a patient is to learn or relearn an auditory skill, a more bottom-up processing approach may be warranted. The skill to be learned or relearned (e.g., detection, discrimination, identification, and comprehension) and the complexity of the stimuli are largely dictated by the status of the patient's auditory skills and the goals of auditory training. The stimulus difficulty can be manipulated by changing such factors as set size, acoustic similarity, speed, linguistic complexity, lexical familiarity, visual cues, contextual support, and environmental acoustics. It also can be adjusted by digitally manipulating specific acoustic parameters such as formant transition duration, f_1 intensity, or noise burst spectra. Typically, the training starts with skill and stimulus levels at which the patient just exhibits difficulty. Then the skill and stimulus difficulty are systematically increased as performance improves until the training goal is attained. For example, the final goal might be that the patient will reduce fricative place confusions to 25% in connected discourse. In a bottom-up approach, the patient might work on fricative place discrimination in CV syllables with the same vowel, then with different vowels, words, phrasal and sentence structures, and finally at the discourse level. Speaking rate, vocal intensity, environmental acoustics, and contextual cues can be adjusted at each level to increase the listening demands. At the discourse level, the conversational demands also can be increased systematically. As with most skills, learning likely is facilitated by cycling across a number of difficulty levels and stimuli, having frequent training sessions, and varying the duration and location of the training.

In a more top-down approach, the patient might start at the discourse level and work on evaluating and using context to predict topic and word choices. The focus is less on hearing the place cues and more on increasing the awareness of various contextual cues that can be used to predict the topic flow within discourse. Initially, familiar topics and speakers may be used in quiet conditions with visual cues provided, and then the discourse material can be increased in complexity, unfamiliar and multiple speakers can be introduced, as well as noise and visual distractions. As a result, the patient becomes better able to fill information gaps when individual sound segments or even entire words and phrases are misperceived. With this type of training approach, patients usually receive counseling on how to manipulate context so that they reduce listening difficulty, and how to recover if a predictive or perceptual error results in a communication breakdown.

Auditory training is not routinely used with all adults with hearing loss but tends to be reserved for individuals who have sustained a recent change in auditory status or a substantive increase in auditory demands. For example, adults with sudden deafness, recent cochlear implant recipients, people switching to dramatically different hearing aids with different signal-processing schemes, students entering college, or individuals who are beginning a new job that is auditorily demanding might benefit from auditory training (see COCHLEAR IMPLANTS; EVALUATION OF COCHLEAR IMPLANT CANDIDACY IN ADULTS; AUDITORY BRAINSTEM IMPLANT). Patients who do not make expected improvements in audition and speech after the fitting of a hearing aid or sensory implant also are reasonable candidates for auditory training (see SPEECH PERCEPTION INDICES). The fact that most adults do not elect to receive auditory training and typically are not referred for auditory training may be a consequence of the limited data documenting the effectiveness and efficacy of auditory training programs. Only a small number of studies have been published that have assessed auditory training outcomes in adults with hearing loss. Rubenstein and Boothroyd (1987) found only modest benefit with sentence- and syllable-level auditory training with adults who had been successful hearing aid wearers, but they did observe maintenance of gains that were obtained. Walden et al. (1981) found that adults newly fitted with hearing aids benefited significantly from systematic consonant discrimination training, while Kricos and Holmes (1996) found that older adults with previous hearing aid experience did not benefit from consonant and vowel discrimination training but did benefit from active listening training. Auditory training usually focuses on speech and language stimuli, but music perceptual training programs have been developed for cochlear implant recipients and appear to be effective (Gfeller et al., 1999). In addition, auditory training is more strongly advocated for infants and children with hearing loss than for adults, but even fewer interpretable studies have been reported to support its application in children and infants.

Although supporting literature is limited with respect to auditory training of hearing-impaired populations, perceptual training studies with normal-hearing individuals suggest that the impact of auditory training on perception may be underestimated. For example, normal-hearing adults and children have been trained to perceive non-native speech contrasts (Werker and Tees, 1984; Bradlow et al., 1997; Wang et al., 1999). Although not all speech contrasts can be learned equally well, and adults usually fail to reach native speaker performance levels, the effects of training are retained over months and show generalization within and across sound categories (McClaskey, Pisoni, and Carrell, 1983; Lively et al., 1994; Tremblay et al., 1997). Digitally manipulating specific acoustic parameters of speech does not always improve speech perception in expected ways, but shaping speech perception by gradually adjusting more difficult acoustic properties is under investigation in various disordered populations and may prove fruitful in the future for persons with hearing loss (Bradlow et al., 1999; Habib et al., 1999; Merzenich et al., 1996; Thibodeau, Friel-Patti, and Britt, 2001). Furthermore, Kraus and colleagues (Kraus et al., 1995; Tremblay et al., 1997) have argued that auditory training impacts the physiology of the central auditory system and might result in cortical and subcortical reorganization. If neural reorganization occurs after the fitting of a hearing aid or cochlear implant, then it is likely that these types of patients would be sensitive to intensive auditory training during the reorganization period (Kraus, 2001; Purdy, Kelly, and Thorne, 2001).

See also AUDITORY BRAINSTEM IMPLANT; SPEECH DISORDERS SECONDARY TO HEARING IMPAIRMENT ACQUIRED IN ADULTHOOD; SPEECH TRACKING; SPEECHREADING TRAINING AND VISUAL TRACKING.

—Sheila Pratt

References

Bettison, S. (1996). The long-term effects of auditory training on children with autism. *Journal of Autism and Developmental Disorders, 26,* 361–374.

Bradlow, A. R., Kraus, N., Nicol, T. G., McGee, T. J., Cunningham, J., Zecker, S. G., and Carrell, T. D. (1999). Effects of lengthened formant transition duration on discrimination and neural representation of synthetic CV syllables by normal and learning-disabled children. *Journal of the Acoustical Society of America, 106,* 2086–2096.

Bradlow, A. R., Pisoni, D., Akahane-Yamada, R., and Tohkura, Y. (1997). Training Japanese listeners to identify English /r/ and /l/: IV. Some effects of perceptual learning on speech production. *Journal of the Acoustical Society of America, 101,* 2299–2310.

Erber, N. (1982). *Auditory training.* Washington, D.C.: A.G. Bell Association.

Erber, N., and Hirsh, I. (1978). Auditory Training. In H. Davis and S. R. Silverman (Eds.), *Hearing and Deafness* (pp. 358–374). New York: Rinehart and Winston.

Gfeller, K., Witt, S. A., Kim, K., Adamek, M., and Coffman, D. (1999). Preliminary report of a computerized music training program for adult cochlear implant recipients. *Journal of the Academy of Rehabilitative Audiology*, 32, 11–27.

Habib, M., Espesser, R., Rey, V., Giraud, K., Bruas, P., and Gres, C. (1999). Training dyslexics with acoustically modified speech: Evidence of improved phonological performance. *Brain and Cognition*, 40, 143–146.

Kraus, N. (2001). Auditory pathway encoding and neural plasticity in children with hearing problems. *Audiology and Neuro-Otology*, 6, 221–227.

Kraus, N., McGee, T., Carrell, T. D., King, C., Tremblay, K., and Nicol, T. (1995). Central auditory system plasticity with speech discrimination training. *Journal of Cognitive Neuroscience*, 7, 25–32.

Kraus, N., McGee, T., Carrell, T. D., and Sharma, T. (1995). Neurophysiologic bases of speech discrimination. *Ear and Hearing*, 16, 19–37.

Kricos, P., and Holmes, A. (1996). Efficacy of audiologic rehabilitation for older adults. *Journal of the American Academy of Audiology*, 7, 219–229.

Lively, S. E., Pisoni, D. B., Yamada, R. A., Tohkura, Y., and Yamada, T. (1994). Training Japanese listeners to identify English /r/ and /l/. III. Long-term retention of new phonetic categories. *Journal of the Acoustical Society of America*, 96, 2067–2087.

McClaskey, C. L., Pisoni, D. B., and Carrell, T. D. (1983). Transfer of training of a new linguistic contrast in voicing. *Perception and Psychophysics*, 34, 323–330.

Merzenich, M., Jenkings, W., Johnston, P., Schreiner, C., Miller, S. L., and Tallal, P. (1996). Temporal processing deficits of language-learning impaired children ameliorated by training. *Science*, 217, 77–81.

Musiek, F. (1999). Habilitation and management of auditory processing disorders: Overview of selected procedures. *Journal of the American Academy of Audiology*, 10, 329–342.

Purdy, S. C., Kelly, A. S., and Thorne, P. R. (2001). Auditory evoked potentials as measures of plasticity in humans. *Audiology and Neuro-Otology*, 6, 211–215.

Rubenstein, A., and Boothroyd, A. (1987). Effect of two approaches to auditory training on speech recognition by hearing-impaired adults. *Journal of Speech and Hearing Research*, 30, 153–160.

Solma, R. T., and Adepoju, A. A. (1995). The effect of aural feedback in second language vocabulary learning. *Journal of Behavioral Education*, 5, 433–445.

Thibodeau, L. M., Friel-Patti, S., and Britt, L. (2001). Psychoacoustic performance in children completing Fast ForWord training. *American Journal Speech-Language-Pathology*, 10, 248–257.

Tremblay, K., Kraus, N., Carrell, T. D., and McGee, T. (1997). Central auditory system plasticity: Generalization to novel stimuli following listening training. *Journal of the Acoustical Society of America*, 102, 3762–3773.

Tremblay, K., Kraus, N., and McGee, T. (1998). The time course of auditory perceptual learning: Neurophysiological changes during speech-sound training. *Neuroreport: An International Journal for the Rapid Communication of Research in Neuroscience*, 9, 3557–3560.

Tremblay, K., Kraus, N., McGee, T., Ponton, C., and Otis, B. (2001). Central auditory plasticity: Changes in the N1-P2 complex after speech-sound training. *Ear and Hearing*, 22, 79–90.

Tye-Murray, N. (1998). *Foundations of aural rehabilitation*. San Diego, CA: Singular Publishing Group.

Walden, B. E., Erdman, S. A., Montgomery, A. A., Schwartz, D. M., and Prosek, R. A. (1981). Some effects of training on speech recognition by hearing-impaired adults. *Journal of Speech and Hearing Research*, 24, 207–216.

Wang, Y., Spence, M. M., Jongman, A., and Sereno, J. A. (1999). Training American listeners to perceive Mandarin tones. *Journal of the Acoustical Society of America*, 106, 3649–3658.

Werker, J., and Tees, R. (1984). Cross-language speech perception: Evidence for perceptual reorganization during the first year of life. *Infant Behavior and Development*, 7, 49–63.

Wharry, R. E., Kirkpatrick, S. W., and Stokes, K. D. (1987). Auditory training: Effects on auditory retention with the learning disabled. *Perceptual and Motor Skills*, 65, 1000.

Further Readings

Alcantara, J., Cowan, R. S., Blamey, P., and Clark, G. (1990). A comparison of two training strategies for speech recognition with an electrotactile speech processor. *Journal of Speech and Hearing Research*, 33, 195–204.

Blamey, P. J., and Alcantra, J. I. (1994). Research in auditory training. In J. P. Gagne and N. Tye-Murray (Eds.), *Research in audiological rehabilitation: Current trends and future directions. Journal of the Academy of Rehabilitation Audiology*, 27, 161–191.

Carhart, R. (1947). Auditory training. In H. Davis (Ed.), *Hearing and deafness* (pp. 276–299). New York: Rinehart.

Durity, R. P. (1982). Auditory training for severely hearing-impaired adults. In D. G. Sims, G. G. Walter, and R. L. Whitehead (Eds.), *Deafness and communication: Assessment and training* (pp. 296–311). Baltimore: Williams and Wilkins.

Erber, N. P., and Lind, C. (1994). Communication therapy: Theory and practice. In J. P. Gagne and N. Tye-Murray (Eds.), *Research in audiological rehabilitation: Current trends and future directions. Journal of the Academy of Rehabilitation Audiology*, 27, 267–287.

Gagne, J. P. (1994). Visual and audiovisual speech perception training: Basic and applied research. In J. P. Gagne and N. Tye-Murray (Eds.), *Research in audiological rehabilitation: Current trends and future directions. Journal of the Academy of Rehabilitation Audiology*, 27, 317–336.

Garstecki, D. C. (1981). Audio-visual training paradigm for hearing impaired adults. *Journal of the Academy of Rehabilitative Audiology*, 14, 223–228.

Gold, J., Bennett, P. J., and Sekuler, A. B. (1999). Signal but not noise changes with perceptual learning. *Nature*, 402, 176–178.

Houston, K. T., and Montgomery, A. A. (1997). Auditory-visual integration: A practical approach. *Seminars in Hearing*, 18, 141–151.

Hutchinson, K. (1990). An analytic distinctive feature approach to auditory training. *Volta Review*, 92, 5–13.

Pisoni, D. B., Aslin, R. N., Perey, A. J., and Hennessy, B. L. (1982). Some effects of laboratory training on identification and discrimination of voicing contrasts in stop consonants. *Journal of Experimental Psychology*, 8, 297–314.

Spitzer, J. B., Leder, S. B., and Giolas, T. G. (1993). *Rehabilitation of late-deafened adults: Modular program manual*. St. Louis: Mosby.

Tallal, P., Miller, S. L., Bedi, G., Byma, G., Wang, X., Nagarajan, S. S., et al. (1986). Language comprehension in language-learning impaired children improved with acoustically modified speech. *Science*, 271, 81–84.

Tye-Murray, N. (1997). *Communication training for hard-of-hearing adults and older teenagers: Speechreading, listening, and using repair strategies*. Austin, TX: Pro-Ed.

Classroom Acoustics

The acoustic environment of a classroom is a critical factor in the psychoeducational and psychosocial development of children with normal hearing and children with hearing impairment. Inappropriate levels of classroom reverberation, noise, or both can deleteriously affect speech perception, reading and spelling ability, classroom behavior, attention, concentration, and academic achievement. Poor classroom acoustics have also been shown to negatively affect teacher performance (Crandell, Smaldino, and Flexer, 1995). This article discusses several acoustic factors that can compromise communication between teacher and child. These acoustic factors include (1) the level of the background noise in the classroom, (2) the relative intensity of the information-carrying components of the speech signal to a non-information-carrying signal or noise (signal-to-noise ratio, S/N), (3) the degree to which the temporal aspects of the information-carrying components of the speech signal are degraded (reverberation), and (4) the distance from the speaker to the listener.

Background Noise

Background noise refers to any auditory disturbance that interferes with what a listener wants or needs to hear. Background noise levels in classrooms are often too high for children to perceive speech accurately. In general, background classroom noise affects a child's speech recognition by reducing, or masking, the highly redundant acoustic and linguistic cues available in the teacher's voice. Because the energy of consonant phonemes is considerably less than that of vowel phonemes, background noise in a classroom often masks the consonants more than the vowels. Loss of consonant information has a great effect on speech recognition because the vast majority of the cues important for accurate speech recognition are carried by the consonants.

In most listening environments, the fundamental determinant for speech recognition is not the overall level of the room noise, but rather the relationship between the intensity of the signal and the intensity of the background noise at the listener's ear. This relationship is referred to as the signal-to-noise ratio (S/N). Speech recognition ability tends to be highest at favorable S/Ns and decreases as the S/N of the listening environment is reduced. Speech recognition in adults with normal hearing is not severely degraded until the S/N approximates 0 dB (speech and noise are at equal intensities). The speech recognition performance of children with sensorineural hearing loss (SNHL), however, is reduced in noise when compared with the performance of children with normal hearing (Finitzo-Hieber and Tillman, 1978). Specifically, children with SNHL require the S/N to be improved by 4–12 dB, and by an additional 3–6 dB in rooms with moderate levels of reverberation, for them to obtain recognition scores equal to those of normal hearers (Crandell and Smaldino, 2000, 2001). While it is recognized that listeners with SNHL experience greater speech recognition deficits in noise than normal hearers, a number of populations of children with "normal hearing" sensitivity also experience significant difficulties recognizing speech in noise. These populations of normal-hearing children include young children (less than 15 years old); those with conductive hearing loss; children with a history of recurrent otitis media; those with a language disorder, articulation disorder, dyslexia, or learning disability; non-native speakers of English, and others with various degrees of hearing impairment or developmental delays. Due to high background noise levels, the range of S/Ns in classrooms has been reported to be between approximately −7 and +5 dB.

Reverberation

Reverberation refers to the prolongation or persistence of sound within an enclosure as sound waves reflect off hard surfaces (bare walls, ceilings, windows, floor) in the room. Operationally, reverberation time (RT) refers to the amount of time it takes for a sound, at a specific frequency, to decay 60 dB (or one-millionth of its original intensity) following termination of the signal. Excessive reverberation degrades speech recognition through the masking of direct and early-reflected energy by reverberant energy. Generally speaking, speech recognition tends to decrease as the RT of the environment increases. Speech recognition in individuals with normal hearing is often not compromised until the RT exceeds approximately 1.0 s (Nabelek and Pickett, 1974a, 1974b). Listeners with SNHL, however, need considerably shorter RTs (0.4–0.5 s) for maximum speech recognition (Crandell, 1991; Crandell, Smaldino, and Flexer, 1995). Studies have also indicated that the populations of "normal-hearing" children discussed previously also have greater speech recognition difficulties in reverberation than do young adults with normal hearing. Unfortunately, RTs for classrooms are often reported to range from 0.4 to 1.2 s.

Effects of Noise and Reverberation on Speech Recognition

In all educational settings, noise and reverberation combine in a synergistic manner to adversely affect speech recognition. That is, noise and reverberation affect speech recognition more than would be expected from an examination of their individual effects on speech perception. It appears that this occurs because reverberation fills in the temporal gaps in the noise, making the noise more steady state in nature and a more effective masker. As with noise and reverberation in isolation, research indicates that listeners with hearing impairment and "normal-hearing" children experience greater speech recognition difficulties in noise and reverberation than adult normal listeners (see Crandell, Smaldino, and Flexer, 1995).

Speaker–Listener Distance

In classrooms, the acoustics of a teacher's speech signal changes as it travels to the child. The direct sound is that sound which travels from the teacher to a child without striking other surfaces within the classroom. The power of the direct sound decreases with distance because the acoustic energy spreads over a larger area as it travels from the source. Specifically, the direct sound decreases 6 dB in SPL with every doubling of distance from the sound source. This phenomenon, called the inverse square law, occurs because of the geometric divergence of sound from the source. Because the direct sound energy decreases so quickly, only those listeners who are seated close to the speaker will be hearing direct sound energy. At slightly farther distances from the speaker, early sound reflections will reach the listener. Early sound reflections are those sound waves that arrive at a listener within very short time periods (approximately 50 ms) after the arrival of the direct sound. Early sound reflections are often combined with the direct sound and may actually increase the perceived loudness of the sound. This increase in loudness can improve speech recognition in listeners with normal hearing. As a listener moves farther away from a speaker, reverberation dominates the listening environment. As sound waves strike multiple classroom surfaces, they generally decrease in loudness, owing to the increased path length they travel as well as the partial absorption that occurs at each reflection off the classroom surfaces. Some reverberation is necessary to reinforce the direct sound and to enrich the quality of the sound. However, reverberation can lead to acoustic distortions of the speech signal, including temporal smearing and masking of important perceptual cues.

Speech recognition in classrooms depends on the distance of the child from the teacher. If the child is within the critical distance of the classroom (the point at which the intensity of the direct sound and reflected sound are equal in intensity), reflected sound waves have minimal effects on speech recognition. The critical distance in many classrooms is often 5–6 feet from the teacher. Beyond the critical distance, however, the reflections can compromise speech recognition if there is enough of a spectrum or intensity change in the reflected sound to interfere with the recognition of the direct sound. Overall, speech recognition scores tend to decrease until the critical distance of the classroom is reached. Beyond the critical distance, recognition ability tends to remain essentially constant unless the classroom is very large (such as an auditorium). In such environments, speech recognition may continue to decrease as a function of increased distance. These findings suggest that speech recognition ability can be maximized by decreasing the distance between a speaker and listener only within the critical distance of the classroom. Thus, preferential seating, while not a bad idea to improve visual perception, may only minimally improve auditory speech perception.

Acoustic Modifications of the Classroom

The fundamental strategy for improving speech perception within a classroom is acoustic modification of that environment. The most effective procedure for achieving this goal is through appropriate planning with contractors, school officials, architects, acoustical consultants, audiologists, and teachers for the hearing impaired before the design and construction of the building. Acoustic guidelines for hearing-impaired and "normal-hearing" populations indicate the following: (1) S/Ns should exceed +15 dB, (2) unoccupied noise levels should not exceed 30–35 dBA, and (3) RTs should not surpass 0.4–0.6 s (ASHA, 1995). Unfortunately, such guidelines are rarely achieved in most listening environments. Crandell and Smaldino (1995) reported that none of the 32 classrooms in which they measured sound levels met recommended criteria for noise levels. Only 27% of the classroom met criteria for reverberation. A new American National Standards Institute (ANSI S12.60) document entitled "Acoustical Performance Criteria, Design Requirements and Guidelines for Schools" (ANSI, 2002) promises to set a national standard for acoustics in classrooms where learning occurs. If acoustic modifications to learning spaces cannot reduce noise and reverberation to appropriate levels, then hearing assistive technologies, such as frequency modulation (FM) systems, should be implemented for children with "normal hearing" or hearing impairment.

—*Carl C. Crandell and Joseph J. Smaldino*

References

American National Standards Institute. (2002). *S12.60, Acoustical Performance Criteria, Design Requirements and Guidelines for Schools*. New York: ANSI.

Crandell, C. (1991). Classroom acoustics for normal-hearing children: Implications for rehabilitation. *Education Audiology Monographs*, 2, 18–38.

Crandell, C., and Smaldino, J. (1995). An update of classroom acoustics for children with hearing impairment. *Volta Review*, 1, 4–12.

Crandell, C., and Smaldino, J. (2000). Room acoustics and amplification. In M. Valente, R. Roeser, and H. Hosford-Dunn (Eds.), *Audiology: Treatment strategies*. New York: Thieme.

Crandell, C., and Smaldino, J. (2001). Rehabilitative technologies for individuals with hearing loss and abnormal hearing. In J. Katz (Ed.), *Handbook of audiology*. New York: Williams and Wilkins.

Crandell, C., Smaldino, J., and Flexer, C. (1995). *Sound field FM amplification: Theory and practical applications*. San Diego, CA: Singular Press Publishing Group.

Finitzo-Hieber, T., and Tillman, T. (1978). Room acoustics effects on monosyllabic word discrimination ability for normal and hearing-impaired children. *Journal of Speech and Hearing Research*, 21, 440–458.

Nabelek, A., and Pickett, J. (1974a). Monaural and binaural speech perception through hearing aids under noise and reverberation with normal and hearing-impaired listeners. *Journal of Speech and Hearing Research*, 17, 724–739.

Nabelek, A., and Pickett, J. (1974b). Reception of consonants in a classroom as affected by monaural and binaural listening, noise, reverberation, and hearing aids. *Journal of the Acoustical Society of America, 56*, 628–639.

Further Readings

Bess, F., Sinclair, J., and Riggs, D. (1984). Group amplification in schools for the hearing-impaired. *Ear and Hearing, 5*, 138–144.

Bradley, J. (1986). Speech intelligibility studies in classrooms. *Journal of the Acoustical Society of America, 80*, 846–854.

Crandell, C. (1992). Classroom acoustics for hearing-impaired children. *Journal of the Acoustical Society of America, 92*(4), 2470.

Crandell, C., and Bess, F. (1986). Speech recognition of children in a "typical" classroom setting. *ASHA, 29*, 87.

Crandell, C., and Smaldino, J. (1996). Sound field amplification in the classroom: Applied and theoretical issues. In F. Bess, J. Gravel, and A. Tharpe (Eds.), *Amplification for children with auditory deficits* (pp. 229–250). Nashville, TN: Bill Wilkerson Center Press.

Gengel, R. (1971). Acceptable signal-to-noise ratios for aided speech discrimination by the hearing impaired. *Journal of Auditory Research, 11*, 219–222.

Harris, C. (1991). *Handbook of acoustical measurements and noise control.* New York: McGraw-Hill.

Houtgast, T. (1981). The effect of ambient noise on speech intelligibility in classrooms. *Applied Acoustics, 14*, 15–25.

Kodaras, M. (1960). Reverberation times of typical elementary school settings. *Noise Control, 6*, 17–19.

Markides, A. (1986). Speech levels and speech-to-noise ratios. *British Journal of Audiology, 20*, 115–120.

Niemoeller, A. (1968). Acoustical design of classrooms for the deaf. *American Annals of the Deaf, 113*, 1040–1045.

Olsen, W. (1988). Classroom acoustics for hearing-impaired children. In F. Bess (Ed.), *Hearing impairment in children.* Parkton, MD: York Press.

Siebein, G., Crandell, C., and Gold, M. (1997). Principles of classroom acoustics: Reverberation. *Education Audiology Monographs, 5*, 32–43.

Clinical Decision Analysis

Clinical decision analysis (CDA) is a quantitative strategy for making clinical decisions. The techniques of CDA are largely derived from the theory of signal detection, which is concerned with extracting signals from noise. The theory of signal detection has been used to study the detection of auditory signals by the human observer. This article provides a brief overview of CDA. More comprehensive discussions of CDA and its application to audiological tests can be found in Turner, Robinette, and Bauch (1999), Robinette (1994), and Hyde, Davidson, and Alberti (1990).

Assume that we are using a clinical test to distinguish between two conditions, such as disease versus no disease or hearing loss versus normal hearing. Most tests would produce a range of scores for each condition and therefore could be thought to contain some "noise" in their results. More important, there may be an overlap in the scores produced by a test for each condition, creating

Figure 1. Decision matrix. Abbreviations: pl, number of patients with hearing loss; pn, number of patients with normal hearing; ht, number of hits; ms, number of misses; fa, number of false alarms; cr, number of correct rejections.

the potential for error. That is, a particular score could, with finite probability, be produced by either condition. CDA is well-suited to deal with this type of problem.

For the discussions and examples in this article, we will assume that we are trying to identify hearing loss. Of course, CDA can be used with diagnostic tests that are designed to identify a variety of diseases and conditions.

Decision Matrix

A patient is given a test, and the outcome of the test is either positive or negative for hearing loss. The test is fallible and makes errors, reflecting the "noise" in the testing process. There are four possible outcomes, determined by the test result and the hearing of the patient. These outcomes are represented by a 2 × 2 decision matrix (Fig. 1). If the patient has hearing loss, a positive test is called a hit and a negative result a miss. If the patient has normal hearing, a positive result is a false alarm and a negative result is a correct rejection. Different terminology is sometimes used. A hit is a true positive; a miss is a false negative; a false alarm is a false positive; a correct rejection is a true negative.

The elements of the matrix in Figure 1 represent the number of hits, misses, false alarms, and correct rejections when the test is given to a number of patients. The hits and correct rejections are correct decisions, whereas misses and false alarms are errors. A basic property is that the number of hits plus misses always equals the number of patients with the condition to be identified, e.g., hearing loss. The number of false alarms plus correct rejections always equals the number of patients without the condition, e.g., normal hearing.

Hit Rate, etc.

The number of hits, misses, false alarms, and correct rejections can be used to calculate a variety of measures of test performance. The most basic measures are hit rate (HT), miss rate (MS), false alarm rate (FA), and correct rejection rate (CR). Hit rate (also called true positive rate and sensitivity) is the percentage of hearing loss patients correctly identified as positive for hearing loss; miss rate (also called false negative rate) is the percentage of hearing loss patients incorrectly identified as negative. False alarm rate (also called false positive rate) is

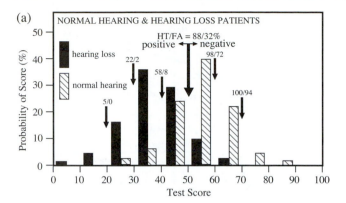

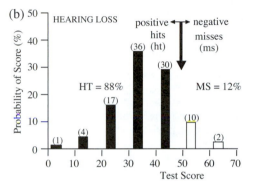

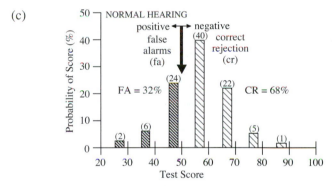

Figure 2. Probability distribution curves for a theoretical test. **A**, One distribution (black bars) corresponds to test performance for patients with hearing loss, the other (hatched bars) for patients with normal hearing. Possible test scores are divided into ten intervals: 0–10, 11–20, 21–30, ..., 91–100. Each bar indicates the probability of a test score within the interval. Thus, the black bar located between test score 20 and 30 indicates that the probability of obtaining a score of 21 to 30 is 17% for a patient with hearing loss. A criterion of 50 is indicated by the heavy arrow. Any score equal to or less than the criterion is considered positive for hearing loss. Any score greater than the criterion is negative for hearing loss. Hit rate and false alarm rate are shown for each criterion from 20 to 70. **B**, Distribution of scores for patients with hearing loss. Bars to the left of the criterion (50) correspond to hits; bars to the right correspond to misses. The number in parentheses above each bar is the height of the bar, that is, the probability of a score in the corresponding interval. Hit rate is the sum of the probabilities indicated by the bars corresponding to hits. Miss rate is likewise determined using bars corresponding to misses. **C**, Distribution of scores for patients with normal hearing. The bars to the left of the criterion correspond to false alarms; the bars to the right correspond to correct rejections. The false alarm rate is

the percentage of normal-hearing patients incorrectly called positive; correct rejection rate (also called true negative rate and specificity) is the percentage of normal-hearing patients correctly identified as negative. These measures are calculated by the following equations:

$$HT = \frac{ht}{pl}$$

$$MS = \frac{ms}{pl}$$

$$FA = \frac{fa}{pn}$$

$$CR = \frac{cr}{pn}$$

where pl = number of patients with hearing loss, pn = number of patients with normal hearing, ht = number of hits, ms = number of misses, fa = number of false alarms, and cr = number of correct rejections. The above equations yield a decimal value ≤ 1.0, which can be converted to a percent. In all calculations, the decimal form is used. While all four measures can be calculated, only two, usually HT and FA, need be considered. This is because HT + MS = 100% and FA + CR = 100%; thus, MS and CR can always be determined from HT and FA.

The measures of test performance, HT, FA, MS, and CR, can also be expressed as probabilities. HT is the probability of a positive test result if the patient has hearing loss (Pr[+/L]); FA is the probability of a positive result if the patient has normal hearing (Pr[+/N]); MS is the probability of a negative result given hearing loss (Pr[−/L]), and CR is the probability of a negative result given normal hearing (Pr[−/N]).

Probability Distribution Curve

Consider a theoretical test that produces a score from 0 to 100. The test is administered to two groups of patients, one with hearing loss and one with normal hearing. Each group will produce a range of scores on the test. We could plot a histogram of scores for each population, i.e., the number of patients in a group with a score between 0 and 10, 10 and 20, etc. Next, we divide the number of patients in each score range by the total number of patients in the group to obtain the probability distribution curve (PDC). Essentially, the PDC gives the probability of obtaining a particular score, or range of scores, for each group of patients. PDCs for a theoretical test are shown in Figure 2. Note that there are two PDCs, one for hearing loss and one for normal hearing, and that the two distributions are different.

Because the two PDCs in Figure 2 do not completely overlap, we may use this test to identify hearing loss.

---

the sum of the probabilities indicated by the bars corresponding to false alarms. The correct rejection rate is likewise determined using bars corresponding to correct rejections.

First, however, we must establish a criterion to determine if a test score is positive or negative for hearing loss. In Figure 2, we set the criterion at 50. Normal-hearing patients have, on average, higher scores than hearing loss patients; therefore, a score greater than 50 is negative and a score less than or equal to 50 is positive for hearing loss. Because there is some overlap in the two PDCs, the criterion divides the two PDCs into four regions corresponding to hits, misses, false alarms, and correct rejections. Below the criterion (≤ 50), hearing loss patients constitute the hits and the normal-hearing patients constitute the false alarms. Above the criterion, the hearing loss patients are the misses and the normal-hearing patients are the correct rejections. Hit rate is the total probability that hearing loss patients will have a test score ≤ 50. This equals the sum of the probabilities for all of the bars below the criterion that correspond to hearing loss patients.

We can select any criterion for a test, but different criteria will produce different test performance. If the criterion is increased (e.g., from 50 to 60), there is an increase in HT, which is good, but there is also an increase in FA, which is bad. If the criterion is reduced (e.g., from 50 to 40), the FA will be reduced, which is good, but so will the HT, which is bad. Thus, we see that there is usually a trade-off between HT and FA when we adjust the criterion.

Another interesting result occurs with extreme criteria. We could set the criterion at 100 and call all results positive for hearing loss. This would produce an HT of 100%; however, FA would also equal 100%. Likewise, with a criterion of 0, FA = 0%, but also HT = 0%. Thus, HT and FA can be manipulated by changing the criterion, but the trade-off between HT and FA limits the value of this strategy. Because any HT or FA can be obtained by adjusting the criterion, both HT and FA are needed to evaluate the performance of a test.

The ability of a test to distinguish patients is related to the amount of overlap of the PDCs. If in Figure 2 the two PDCs completely overlapped, then the test would be useless. For any criterion, we would have HT = FA and MS = CR. If there was absolutely no overlap in the PDCs, then the test would be perfect. It would be possible to set the criterion such that HT = 100% and FA = 0%.

Because HT and FA vary significantly with the criterion, we can visualize this relationship using a receiver operating characteristic (ROC) curve, which is a plot of HT versus FA for different criteria. The HT/FA data from Figure 2 are plotted in Figure 3. The shape of the ROC curve is determined by the PDCs.

Posterior Probabilities

Consider this situation. We are testing a patient in the clinic, and the test result is positive. We know the hit rate of the test, but hit rate is the probability of a positive result given hearing loss. We do not know if the patient has hearing loss, but we do know the test result. Hit rate tells us little about the accuracy of the test result. What we want is not hit rate, the probability of a positive re-

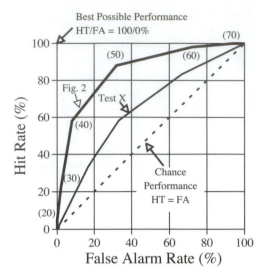

Figure 3. Receiver operating characteristic (ROC) curve. The values calculated in Figure 2 are plotted to form the ROC curve. The numbers in parentheses correspond to the criteria used in Figure 2 to determine hit rate and false alarm rate. The dashed line indicates chance performance, that is, HT = FA. The curve that lies closest to the point, HT/FA = 100/0%, is, in general, the best test. The test from Figure 2 is therefore better than "Test X" because the ROC curve lies above the ROC curve for Test X and is closer to HT/FA = 100/0%.

sult given hearing loss (Pr[+/L]), but the probability that the patient has hearing loss given a positive test result (Pr[L/+]). This probability is called a posterior probability. Another posterior probability is Pr[N/−]; this is the probability of normal hearing given a negative test result. These two posterior probabilities are important because they are the probability of being correct given a particular test result. There are two other posterior probabilities, Pr[L/−] and Pr[N/+], which are the probability of being incorrect given a test result. The posterior probabilities have been given other names: predictive value and information content. These measures are identical to the posterior probabilities and thus provide the same information.

Because Pr[L/+] + Pr[N/+] = 100% and Pr[L/−] + Pr[N/−] = 100%, we need calculate only two of the four posterior probabilities. To calculate the posterior probabilities we need HT and FA for the test, plus the prevalence (PD) of the disease or condition in the test population. Prevalence is the percentage of the test population that has the disease or condition (e.g., hearing loss) at the time of testing. The posterior probabilities are calculated by the following equations:

$$Pr[L/+] = \cfrac{1}{1 + \cfrac{(FA)^*(1 - PD)}{(HT)^*(PD)}}$$

$$Pr[N/-] = \cfrac{1}{1 + \cfrac{(1 - HT)^*(PD)}{(1 - FA)^*(1 - PD)}}$$

The posterior probabilities can also be calculated from the number of hits, misses, false alarms, and correct rejections. Sometimes this is an easier strategy than using the equations above:

$$Pr[L/+] = \frac{ht}{ht + fa}$$

$$Pr[N/-] = \frac{cr}{cr + ms}$$

The probability of being correct with a positive test result is the number of hits divided by the total number of positive test results (hits plus false alarms). Likewise, the probability of being correct with a negative test result is the number of correct rejections divided by the total number of negative results (correct rejections plus misses).

When the prevalence of a condition (e.g., hearing loss) is small, the probability of a positive result being correct ($Pr(L/+)$) is small, even for a test with high HT and small FA. For example, consider a test with HT/FA = 99/5%. Even with this test, which is better than any audiological test, the probability of a positive result being correct is only 29% for PD = 2%. There would be 2.5 false alarms for each hit. When prevalence is small, we should expect more false alarms than hits.

Now consider $Pr[N/-]$, the probability of being correct with a negative test result. When prevalence is low, $Pr[N/-]$ is very large, 99+% for the example above. Only when prevalence is high is there a significant variation in $Pr[N/-]$ with test performance.

Efficiency

HT, FA, and PD can also be used to calculate efficiency (EF). EF is the percentage of total test results that are correct and is calculated by

$$EF = HT \times PD + (1 - FA) \times (1 - PD)$$

Like the posterior probabilities, efficiency is a function of disease prevalence. When prevalence is small, the false alarm rate drives efficiency more than the hit rate. Thus, a test with a poor HT and a small FA could have a higher EF than a test with a high HT and a modest FA. Because of this, EF is not always a useful measure.

Conclusion

Clinical decision analysis provides us with a variety of measures of test performance. These measures are useful for evaluating different tests and for understanding the limitations of a particular test. In general, these measures of performance are not sufficient to identify the "best" test. To determine the best test for a particular application, we may need to also consider other issues, such as the cost or morbidity of the test. The decision as to the best test is based on a cost-benefit analysis, not simply measures of test performance. Nevertheless, these measures of performance are essential to execute a cost-benefit analysis.

—*Robert G. Turner*

References

Hyde, M. L., Davidson, M. J., and Alberti, P. W. (1990). Auditory test strategies. In J. T. Jacobson and J. L. Northern (Eds.), *Diagnostic audiology* (pp. 295–322). Needham Heights, MA: Allyn and Bacon.

Robinette, M. S. (1994). Integrating audiometric results. In J. Katz (Ed.), *Handbook of clinical audiology* (pp. 181–196). Baltimore: Williams and Wilkins.

Turner, R. G., Robinette, M. S., and Bauch, C. D. (1999). Clinical decisions. In F. E. Musiek and W. F. Rintelmann (Eds.), *Contemporary perspectives in hearing assessment* (pp. 437–463). Needham Heights, MA: Allyn and Bacon.

Cochlear Implants

A cochlear implant is a surgically implantable device that provides hearing sensation to individuals with severe to profound hearing loss who cannot benefit from conventional hearing aids. By electrically stimulating the auditory nerve directly, a cochlear implant bypasses damaged or undeveloped sensory structures in the cochlea, thereby providing usable information about sound to the central auditory nervous system.

Although it has been known since the late 1700s that electrical stimulation can produce hearing sensations (see Simmons, 1966), it was not until the 1950s that the potential for true speech understanding was demonstrated. Clinical applications of cochlear implants were pioneered by research centers in the United States, Europe, and Australia. By the 1980s, cochlear implants had become a clinical reality, providing safe and effective speech perception benefit to adults with profound hearing impairment. Since that time, the devices have become more sophisticated, and the population that can benefit from implants has expanded to include children as well as adults with some residual hearing sensitivity (Wilson, 1993; Shannon, 1996; Loizou, 1998; Osberger and Koch, 2000).

The function of a cochlear implant is to provide hearing sensation to individuals with severe to profound hearing impairment. Typically, people with that level of impairment have absent or malfunctioning sensory cells in the cochlea. In a normal ear, sound energy is converted to mechanical energy by the middle ear, and the mechanical energy is then converted to mechanical fluid motion in the cochlea. Within the cochlea, the sensory cells—the inner and outer hair cells—are sensitive transducers that convert that mechanical fluid motion into electrical impulses in the auditory nerve. Cochlear implants are designed to substitute for the function of the middle ear, cochlear mechanical motion, and sensory cells, transforming sound energy into the electrical energy that will initiate impulses in the auditory nerve.

All cochlear implant systems comprise both internal and external components (Fig. 1). Sound enters the microphone, and the signal is then sent to the speech processor, which manipulates and converts the acoustic signal into a special code (i.e., speech-processing

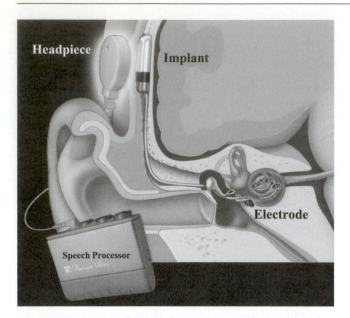

Figure 1. External and internal components of a cochlear implant system. Sound is picked up by the microphone located in the headpiece and converted into an electrical signal, which is then sent to the speech processor via a cable. The signal is encoded into a speech-processing strategy and is sent from the speech processor (body-worn or behind-the-ear) to the transmitter in the headpiece. The signal is transmitted to the internal receiver through transcutaneous inductive coupling of radio-frequency (RF) signals. The receiver/stimulator sends the signal to the electrodes, which stimulate the cochlea with electrical current.

strategy). The transmitter, which is located inside the headpiece, sends the coded electrical signal to the internal components. The internal device contains the receiver, which decodes the signal from the speech processor, and an electrode array, which stimulates the cochlea with electrical current. The implanted electronics are encased in one of two biocompatible materials, titanium or ceramic. The entire system is powered by batteries located in the speech processor, which is worn on the body or behind the ear.

The transmission link enables information to be sent from the external parts of the implant system to the implanted components. For all current systems, the connection is made through transcutaneous inductive coupling of radio-frequency (RF) signals. In this scheme, an RF carrier signal—in which the important code is embedded—is sent across the skin to the receiver. The receiver extracts the embedded code and determines the stimulation pattern for the electrodes. Most cochlear implant systems also employ back telemetry, which allows the internal components to send information back to the external speech processor to assess the function of the implanted electronics and electrode array.

The first cochlear implants consisted of a single electrode, but since the mid-1980s, nearly all devices have multiple electrodes contained in an array. Typically, cochlear implant electrodes are inserted longitudinally into the scala tympani of the cochlea to take potential advantage of the place-to-frequency coding mechanism used by the normal cochlea. Information about low-frequency sound is sent to electrodes at the apical end of the array, whereas information about high-frequency sounds is sent to electrodes nearer the base of the cochlea. The ability to take advantage of the place-frequency code is limited by the number and pattern of surviving auditory neurons in an impaired ear. Unfortunately, attempts to quantify neuronal survival with electrophysiologic or radiographic procedures before implantation have been unsuccessful (Abbas, 1993).

The first multi-electrode arrays were straight and thin (22 electrode bands on the 25-mm-long array) to minimize the occupied space within the scala tympani (Clark et al., 1983). Advances in electrode technology have led to the development of precurved, spiral-shaped arrays to follow the shape of the scala tympani, allowing the contacts to sit close to the target neurons (Fayad, Luxford, and Linthicum, 2000; Tykocinski et al., 2002). The advantages of the precurved array are an increase in spatial selectivity, a reduction in channel interaction, and a reduction in the current required to reach threshold and comfortable listening levels. In addition, the electrode contacts are oriented toward the spiral ganglion cells, and a "positioner," a thin piece of Silastic, can be inserted behind the array to achieve even greater spatial selectivity and improve speech recognition performance (Zwolan et al., 2001).

For all systems, electrical current is passed between an active electrode and an indifferent electrode. If the active and indifferent electrodes are remote, the stimulation is termed monopolar. When the active and indifferent electrodes are close to each other, the stimulation is referred to as bipolar. Bipolar stimulation focuses the current within a restricted area and presumably stimulates a small localized population of auditory nerve fibers (Merzenich and White, 1977; van den Honert and Stypulkowski, 1987). Monopolar stimulation, on the other hand, spreads current over a wider area and a larger population of neurons. Less current is required to achieve adequate loudness levels with monopolar stimulation; more current is required for bipolar stimulation. The use of monopolar or bipolar stimulation is determined by the speech-processing strategy and each individual's response to electrical stimulation.

Two types of stimulation are currently used in cochlear implants, analog and pulsatile. Analog stimulation consists of electrical current that varies continuously in time. Pulsatile stimulation consists of trains of square-wave biphasic pulses. The pattern of stimulation can be either simultaneous or nonsimultaneous (sequential). With simultaneous stimulation, more than one electrode is stimulated at the same time. With nonsimultaneous stimulation, electrodes are stimulated in a specified sequence, one at a time. Typically, analog stimulation is simultaneous and pulsatile stimulation is sequential.

To represent speech faithfully, the coding strategy must reflect three parameters in its electrical stimulation code: frequency, amplitude, and time. Frequency (pitch) information is conveyed by the site of stimulation, amplitude (loudness) is encoded by the amplitude of the

Figure 2. Mean pre- and postimplant scores on speech perception tests for 51 adults with post-lingual deafness. Performance was assessed on CNC monosyllabic words, Central Institute for the Deaf (CID) sentences, Hearing in Noise Test (HINT) sentences, and HINT sentences in background noise (+10 signal-to-noise ratio). Stimuli were recorded and presented in the sound field at 70 dB SPL.

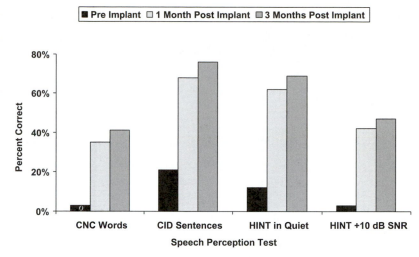

stimulus current, and temporal cues are conveyed by the rate and pattern of stimulation. The first multichannel devices extracted limited information from the acoustic input signal (Millar, Tong, and Clark, 1984). Advances in signal-processing technology have led to the development of more sophisticated processing schemes. One type of strategy is referred to as "*n* of *m*," in which a specified number of electrodes out of a maximum number available are stimulated (Seligman and McDermott, 1995). With this type of processing, the incoming sound is analyzed to identify the filters (frequency regions) with the greatest amount of energy, and then a subset of filters is selected and the corresponding electrodes are stimulated.

In another approach, referred to as continuous interleaved sampling (CIS), trains of biphasic pulses are delivered to the electrodes in an interleaved or non-overlapping fashion to minimize electrical field interactions between stimulated electrodes (Wilson et al., 1991). The amplitudes of the pulses delivered to each electrode are derived by modulating them with the envelopes of the corresponding bandpassed waveforms.

With analog stimulation, the incoming sound is separated into different frequency bands, compressed, and delivered to all electrodes simultaneously (Eddington, 1980). In the most recent implementation of this type of processing, the digitized signal is transmitted to the receiver; then, following digital-to-analog conversion, the analog waveforms are sent simultaneously to all electrodes (Kessler, 1999). Bipolar electrode coupling is typically used to limit the area over which electrical current spreads to reduce channel interaction, which is further reduced with the use of spiral-shaped electrodes.

Cochlear implant candidacy is determined only after comprehensive evaluations by a team of highly skilled professionals (see COCHLEAR IMPLANTS IN ADULTS: CANDIDACY). The surgery is performed under general anesthesia and requires about 1–2 hours, either as an inpatient or outpatient procedure. Approximately 4 weeks following surgery, the individual returns to the clinic to be fitted with the external components of the system. Electrical threshold and most comfortable listening levels are determined for each electrode, and other psychophysical parameters of the speech-processing scheme are programmed into the speech processor. Multiple visits to the implant center are necessary during the first months of implant use as the individual grows accustomed to sound and as tolerance for loudness increases.

Most adults who acquire a severe to profound hearing loss after language is acquired (postlingual hearing loss) demonstrate dramatic improvements in speech understanding after relatively limited implant experience (Fig. 2). Improvements in technology have led to incremental improvements in benefit, which in turn have led to expanded inclusion criteria (Skinner et al., 1994; Osberger and Fisher, 1999). There are large individual differences in outcome, and although there is no reliable method to predict postimplant performance, age at onset of significant hearing loss, duration of the loss, and degree of preoperative residual hearing significantly affect speech recognition abilities (Tyler and Summerfield, 1996; Rubinstein et al., 1999). Many adults are able to converse on the telephone, and cochlear implants can improve the quality of life (Knutson et al., 1998). Adults with congenital or early-acquired deafness and children (see COCHLEAR IMPLANTS IN CHILDREN) also derive substantial benefit from cochlear implants.

Technological advances will continue, with higher processing speeds offering the potential to stimulate the auditory nerve fibers in a manner that more closely approximates that of normal hearing. Studies are under way to evaluate the benefit of bilateral implants (Gantz et al., 2002). New miniaturization processes will result in smaller behind-the-ear processors and, eventually, a fully implantable system with rechargeable battery technology. In the early days of cochlear implants, few people realized that this technology would become the most successful of all prostheses of the central nervous system.

—*Mary Joe Osberger*

References

Abbas, P. (1993). Electrophysiology. In R. S. Tyler (Ed.), *Cochlear implants: Audiologic foundations* (pp. 317–355). San Diego, CA: Singular Publishing Group.

Clark, G., Shepherd, R., Patrick, J., Black, R., and Tong, Y. (1983). Design and fabrication of the banded electrode array. *Annals of the New York Academy of Sciences, 405,* 191–201.

Eddington, D. (1980). Speech discrimination in deaf subjects with cochlear implants. *Journal of the Acoustical Society of America, 68,* 885–891.

Fayad, J. N., Luxford, W., and Linthicum, F. H. (2000). The Clarion electrode positioner: Temporal bone studies. *American Journal of Otology, 21,* 226–229.

Gantz, B. J., Tyler, R. S., Rubinstein, J. T., Wolaver, A., Lowder, M., Abbas, P., et al. (2002). Binaural cochlear implants placed during the same operation. *Otology and Neurotology, 23,* 169–180.

Kessler, D. K. (1999). The Clarion Multi-Strategy cochlear implant. *Annals of Otology, Rhinology, and Laryngology, 108*(Suppl. 177), 8–16.

Knutson, J. F., Murray, K. T., Husarek, S., Westerhouse, K., Woodworth, G., Gantz, B. J., et al. (1998). Psychological change over 54 months of cochlear implant use. *Ear and Hearing, 19,* 191–201.

Loizou, P. C. (1998). Mimicking the human ear. *IEEE Signal Processing Magazine,* September: 101–130.

Merzenich, M. M., and White, M. W. (1977). Cochlear implant: The interface problem. In F. T. Hambrecht and J. B. Reswick (Eds.), *Functional electrical stimulation: Applications in neural prostheses* (pp. 321–340). New York: Marcel Dekker.

Millar, J., Tong, Y., and Clark, G. (1984). Speech processing for cochlear implant prostheses. *Journal of Speech and Hearing Research, 27,* 280–296.

Osberger, M. J., and Fisher, L. (1999). SAS-CIS preference study in postlingually deafened adults implanted with the Clarion cochlear implant. *Annals of Otology, Rhinology, and Laryngology, 108*(Suppl. 177), 74–79.

Osberger, M. J., and Koch, D. B. (2000). Cochlear implants. In R. E. Sandlin (Ed.), *Textbook of Hearing Aid Amplification* (2nd ed., pp. 673–698). San Diego, CA: Singular Publishing Group.

Rubinstein, J. T., Parkinson, W. S., Tyler, R. S., and Gantz, B. J. (1999). Residual speech recognition and cochlear implant performance: Effects of implantation criteria. *American Journal of Otology, 20,* 445–452.

Seligman, P., and McDermott, H. (1995). Architecture of the Spectra 22 speech processor. *Annals of Otology, Rhinology, and Laryngology, 104*(Suppl. 166), 139–141.

Shannon, R. V. (1996). Cochlear implants: What have we learned and where are we going? *Seminars in Hearing, 17,* 403–415.

Simmons, F. B. (1966). Electrical stimulation of the auditory nerve in man. *Archives of Otolaryngology, 84,* 2–54.

Skinner, M. W., Clark, G. M., Whitford, L. A., Seligman, P. M., Staller, S. J., Shipp, D. B., et al. (1994). Evaluation of a new spectral peak coding strategy for the Nucleus 22 channel cochlear implant system. *American Journal of Otology, 15*(Suppl. 2), 15–27.

Tykocinski, M., Cohen, L. T., Pyman, B. C., Roland, T., Treaba, C., Palamara, J., et al. (2000). Comparison of electrode position in the human cochlea using various perimodiolar electrode arrays. *American Journal of Otology, 21,* 205–211.

Tyler, R. S., and Summerfield, A. Q. (1996). Cochlear implantation: Relationships with research on auditory deprivation and acclimatization. *Ear and Hearing, 17*(Suppl. 3), 38–50.

van den Honert, C., and Stypulkowski, P. H. (1987). Single fiber mapping of spatial excitation patters in the electrically stimulated auditory nerve. *Hearing Research, 29,* 195–206.

Wilson, B. S. (1993). Signal processing. In R. S. Tyler (Ed.), *Cochlear implants: Audiological foundations* (pp. 35–85). San Diego, CA: Singular Publishing Group.

Wilson, B. S., Finley, C. C., Lawson, D. T., Wolford, R. D., Eddington, D. K., and Rabinowitz, W. M. (1991). Better speech recognition with cochlear implants. *Nature, 352,* 236–238.

Zwolan, T., Kileny, P. R., Smith, S., Mills, D., Koch, D. B., and Osberger, M. J. (2001). Adult cochlear implant patient performance with evolving electrode technology. *Otology and Neurotology, 22,* 844–849.

Further Readings

Clark, G., Tony, Y., and Patrick, J. F. (1990). *Cochlear prostheses.* New York: Churchill Livingstone.

Loizou, P. C. (1999). Introduction to cochlear implants. *IEEE Engineering in Medicine and Biology,* January/February, 32–42.

Loizou, P. C. (1999). Signal-processing techniques for cochlear implants. *IEEE Engineering in Medicine and Biology,* May/June, 34–46.

Moller, A. R. (2001). Neurophysiologic basis for cochlear and auditory brainstem implants. *American Journal of Audiology, 10,* 68–77.

Schindler, R. A., and Merzenich, M. M. (1985). *Cochlear implants.* New York: Raven Press.

Spelman, F. A. (1999). The past, present, and future of cochlear prostheses. *IEEE Engineering in Medicine and Biology,* May/June, 27–33.

Tyler, R. S. (1993). *Cochlear implants: Audiological foundations.* San Diego, CA: Singular Publishing Group.

Waltzman, S. B., and Cohen, N. L. (2000). *Cochlear implants.* New York: Thieme.

Cochlear Implants in Adults: Candidacy

There are many potential advantages to measuring the benefit obtained from cochlear implants. These include:

• Determining selection criteria
• Setting the cochlear implant: selecting and modifying programming options
• Monitoring performance

The most important reason for the evaluation of cochlear implants is in the selection criteria process. Specifically, speech perception tests are critical to determine whether a hearing aid user might do better with a cochlear implant. Here we focus on this subject and review some of the tests used in evaluation.

Selection Criteria

Guidelines traditionally have depended on how much benefit is obtained from hearing aids, and how much

Table 1. Principles Involved When Considering Monaural Implantation

Binaural Test Results	Monaural Implant Decision
If binaural scores are high, and both ears are contributing	• Do not implant.
If binaural scores are high, and one ear is not contributing	• Consider implanting poorer ear to improve spatial hearing.
If binaural scores are medium, and both ears are contributing equally	• Implant ear with shorter duration and/or better thresholds.
If binaural scores are medium, one ear is contributing more than the other, and best monaural = binaural (no binaural benefit)	• Implant poorer ear, to improve spatial hearing. • Implant better ear, to improve speech in quiet.
If binaural scores are medium, one ear is contributing more than the other, and best monaural < binaural (is binaural benefit)	• Do not implant, to preserve current performance levels. • Implant poorer ear, to improve binaural benefit and preserve better ear. • Implant better ear, to improve speech in quiet.
If binaural scores are medium, one ear is not contributing, and best monaural = binaural (no binaural benefit)	• Implant poorer ear, to improve spatial hearing and speech in quiet.
If binaural scores are poor, with one ear contributing more than the other	• Implant better ear, to improve speech in quiet.
If binaural scores are poor, with ears contributing equally	• Implant ear with shorter duration and/or better thresholds.

benefit might be expected from a cochlear implant. This is difficult, because there are limited databases with such information. Specific guidelines for selection criteria change regularly, are influenced by company and clinic protocols and depend on whether the device is investigational. Generally, the "best aided" performance (with appropriately fit binaural hearing aids) is used to determine if an implant is desirable. When considering a monaural implant, some centers implant the poorer ear to "save" the better ear or to allow the patient to use a cochlear implant in one ear and a hearing aid (better ear) in the other. At other centers, however, the implant is placed in the better ear to maximize implant performance in an ear with more nerve fibers.

First, we shall discuss general guidelines. We refer to poor, medium, and high speech perception scores, realizing that this is arbitrary. The actual values will depend on the test, and will change as overall implant performance improves. The principles we are promoting involve binaural testing and determining the contribution from each ear individually.

Table 1 lists the principles involved when considering monaural implantation. Speech perception tests are conducted typically with the patient using hearing aids testing the right, left, and binaural conditions. The results from each individual ear can then be compared and the best monaural condition can be determined. In addition, the best monaural condition can be compared to the binaural condition to determine if there is a binaural advantage. Table 2 lists the principles involved in considering binaural implantation.

Protocols for Evaluation

This section reviews some of the tests used in the evaluation process.

Isolated Words. The presentation of isolated words (Peterson and Lehiste, 1962; Tillman and Carhart, 1966)

has the advantage that linguistic and cognitive factors are minimized, and clinicians are familiar with the tests. When isolated word lists are used, the vocabulary should be common words.

Ongoing Speech. Sentence perception includes the processing of information at a more rapid, natural rate, compared to the presentation of isolated words (Silverman and Hirsh, 1955; Boothroyd, Hanin, and Hnath, 1985; Nilsson, Soli, and Sullivan, 1994). Performance can be affected by memory, learning, and familiarity with items as a result of repeated use of the test lists. In addition, a patient who is more willing to guess or who is better at using contextual clues may score higher than someone who has similar speech perception abilities but is less willing to guess. Therefore, it is important that sentence length be short, lots of sentences be available, and the test-retest reliability of the materials be known.

Speech Perception Testing in Noise. Many realistic listening situations involve background noise, resulting in differences in speech perception that are not apparent when testing is performed in quiet. Background noise can result in a "floor effect" (near 0% correct). Therefore, in some situations a favorable signal-to-noise ratio (S/N) is selected individually, or testing that adaptively varies the S/N is used (Plomp and Mimpen, 1979; Levitt, 1992).

Subjective Ratings. Quality ratings measure a more global attribute of speech. For example, ratings might include the ease of listening or clarity of sound. We have developed a quality rating test that includes realistic listening situations. Patients are asked to listen to each sound and to rate it on a scale from 0 (unclear) to 100 (clear). Figure 1 shows the results from an adult cochlear implant patient comparing a high-rate, roving, *n*-of-*m* strategy (Wilson, 2000) to a SPEAK strategy (Skinner

Table 2. Principles Involved When Considering Binaural Implantation

Binaural Test Results	Binaural Implant Decision
If binaural scores are high, and both ears are contributing	• Do not implant.
If binaural scores are high, and one ear is not contributing	• Implant poorer ear to improve spatial hearing.
If binaural scores are medium, and both ears are contributing equally	• Implant binaurally. • Do not implant (conservative approach).
If binaural scores are medium, one ear is contributing more than the other, and best monaural = binaural (no binaural benefit)	• Implant poorer ear, to improve spatial hearing. • Implant better ear, to improve speech in quiet. • Implant binaurally, to improve spatial hearing and speech in quiet.
If binaural scores are medium, one ear is contributing more than the other, and best monaural < binaural (is binaural benefit)	• Do not implant, to preserve current performance levels. • Implant poorer ear, to improve binaural benefit and to preserve better ear. • Implant better ear, to improve speech in quiet. • Implant binaurally, to improve speech in quiet and spatial hearing.
If binaural scores are medium, one ear is not contributing, and best monaural = binaural (no binaural benefit)	• Implant poorer ear, to improve spatial hearing and speech in quiet. • Implant binaurally, to improve speech in quiet and spatial hearing.
If binaural scores are poor, with one ear contributing more than the other	• Implant binaurally.
If binaural scores are poor, with ears contributing equally	• Implant binaurally.

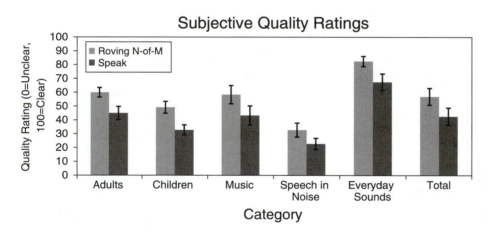

Figure 1. Average subjective ratings for a high rate, roving, *n*-of-*m* strategy, worn bilaterally, compared to bilateral SPEAK.

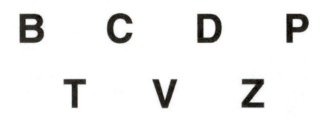

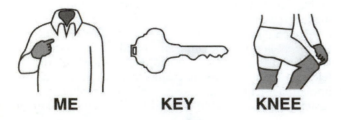

Figure 2. Response form from the Audiovisual Feature Test. The patient hears one of the ten items and must point to the item that was presented.

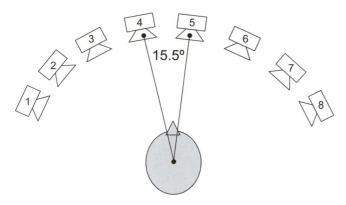

Figure 3. Eight-speaker localization test set-up. Speakers are at 15.5.° (From Van Hoesel and Clark, 1999.)

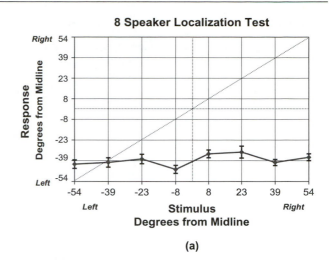

(a)

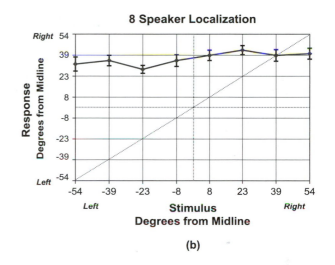

(b)

et al., 1997). The test was sufficiently sensitive to show a strategy preference for all sounds. Information such as this can be extremely helpful when selecting and modifying programming options.

Speech Features. It is advantageous to determine what kinds of speech sounds are perceived to understand which features are being transmitted by the cochlear implant, and how to focus rehabilitation. We use a variety of consonant and vowel tests. The Iowa Medial Consonant Test (Tyler, Preece, and Lowder, 1983) presents items in an "ee/C/ee" (13-choice version) or "aa/C/aa" (16- and 24-choice versions) context, where /C/ represents a variety of consonants (e.g., "aa/P/aa," "aa/M/aa," "aa/D/aa," etc.).

For adult patients who are poor performers and for children, the Audiovisual Speech Feature Test is easier and can be used (Tyler, Fryauf-Bertschy, and Kelsay, 1991). Figure 2 shows the items included in the test.

Spatial Hearing. Another attempt to make testing more realistic includes measurement of spatially separate speech and noise and the localization of sounds (Shaw, 1974; Middlebrooks and Green, 1991; Wightman and Kistler, 1997). More individuals are being fitted with either binaural implants or have a hearing aid and a cochlear implant. We typically measure speech from the front and noise from the right or left. This allows for the measurement of the "head shadow" effect and a "binaural squelch effect."

Localization is based on interaural time, amplitude, and spectral differences between ears (Mills, 1972; Wightman and Kistler, 1992). For binaural cochlear implant recipients the fine details of this information may not be available. To test localization, everyday sounds are presented through 8 loudspeakers. The loudspeakers are arranged in an arc, the patient is asked to indicate which speaker the sound came from (Fig. 3). Figure 4a shows results from one patient who was tested wearing only the right cochlear implant, Figure 4b only the left cochlear implant, and Figure 4c with both implants at the same time.

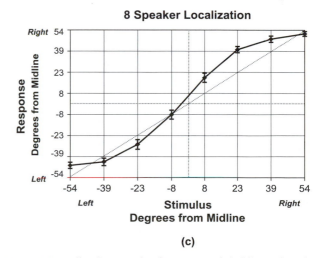

(c)

Figure 4. Localization results from one adult bilateral patient (a) Left cochlear implant only; (b) right cochlear implant only; (c) both implants on at the same time).

Conclusions

We have provided a brief overview of some of the more common issues involved in evaluating adult cochlear implant users. The most important task is to determine candidacy. Speech perception tests measuring binaural hearing aid benefit are needed to determine either monaural or binaural cochlear implant candidacy. Several different tests measure a wide range of potential hearing abilities.

—*Richard S. Tyler and Shelley Witt*

References

Boothroyd, A., Hanin, L., and Hnath, T. (1985). A sentence test of speech perception: Reliability, set equivalence, and short-term learning (Internal Report RCI 10). New York: City University of New York, Speech and Sciences Research Center.

Levitt, H. (1992). Adaptive procedures for hearing aid prescription and other audiologic applications. *Journal of the American Academy of Audiology, 3,* 119–131.

Middlebrooks, J. C., and Green, D. M. (1991). Sound localization by human listeners. *Annual Review in Psychology, 42,* 135–159.

Mills, A. W. (1972). Auditory localization. In J. W. Tobias (Ed.), *Foundations of Modern Auditory Theory, Vol 2* (pp. 301–348). New York: Academic Press.

Nilsson, M., Soli, S. D., and Sullivan, J. (1994). Development of the Hearing In Noise Test for the measurement of speech reception thresholds in quiet and in noise. *Journal of the Acoustical Society of America, 95,* 1085–1099.

Peterson, F. E., and Lehiste, I. (1962). Revised CNC lists for auditory tests. *Journal of Speech and Hearing Disorders, 27*(1), 62–70.

Plomp, R., and Mimpen, A. M. (1979). Speech-reception threshold for sentences as a function of age and noise. *Journal of the Acoustical Society of America, 66,* 1333–1342.

Shaw, E. A. G. (1974). Transformation of sound pressure level from the free field to the eardrum in the horizontal plane. *Journal of the Acoustical Society of America, 56,* 1848–1861.

Silverman, S. R., and Hirsh, I. (1955). Problems related to the use of speech in clinical audiometry. *Annals of Otology Rhinology and Laryngology, 64,* 1234–1244.

Skinner, M. W., Holden, L. K., Holden, T. A., Demorest, M. E., and Fourakis, M. S. (1997). Speech recognition at simulated soft, conversational, and raised-to-loud vocal efforts by adults with cochlear implants. *Journal of the Acoustical Society of America, 101*(6), 3766–3782.

Tillman, T., and Carhart, R. (1966). An expanded test for speech discrimination utilizing CNC monosyllabic words. (Northwestern University Auditory Test No. 6 Technical report No. SAM-TR-66-55). San Antonio, Texas: USAF School of Aerospace Medicine, Brooks Air Force Base.

Tyler, R. S., Fryauf-Bertschy, H., and Kelsay, D. (1991). *Audiovisual Feature Test for Young Children.* Iowa City, IA: The University of Iowa.

Tyler, R. S., Preece, J. P., and Lowder, M. W. (1983). *The Iowa Cochlear Implant Test Battery.* Iowa City, IA: The University of Iowa.

Van Hosesel, R. M., and Clark, G. M. (1999). Speech results with a bilateral multi-channel cochlear implant subject for spatially separated signal and noise. *Australian Journal of Audiology, 21,* 23–28.

Wightman, F. L., and Kistler, D. J. (1992). The dominant role of low-frequency interaural time differences in sound localization. *Journal of the Acoustical Society of America, 91,* 1648–1661.

Wightman, F. L., and Kistler, D. J. (1997). Monaural sound localization revisited. *Journal of the Acoustical Society of America, 101,* 1050–1063.

Wilson, B. S. (2000). Strategies for representing speech information with cochlear implants. In J. K. Niparko, K. I. Kirk, N. K. Mellon, A. M. Robbins, D. L. Tucci, and D. S. Wilson (Eds.), *Cochlear implants: Principles and practices* (pp. 129–172). Philadelphia: Lippincott.

Further Readings

Dillon, H. (2001). Binaural and bilateral considerations in hearing aid fitting. In *Hearing aids* (pp. 370–403). New York: Thieme.

Dorman, M. F. (1993). Speech perception by adults. In R. S. Tyler (Ed.), *Cochlear implants: Audiological foundations* (pp. 145–190). San Diego, CA: Singular Publishing Group.

Kirk, I. K. (2000). Challenges in the clinical investigation of cochlear implant outcomes. In J. K. Niparko, K. I. Kirk, N. K. Mellon, A. M. Robbins, D. L. Tucci, and D. S. Wilson (Eds.), *Cochlear implants: Principles and practices* (pp. 225–259). Philadelphia: Lippincott.

Cochlear Implants in Children

The substantial benefit derived from cochlear implants by adults (see COCHLEAR IMPLANTS and COCHLEAR IMPLANTS IN ADULTS: CANDIDACY) led to the application of these devices in children. Unlike adults, however, most pediatric candidates acquire their deafness before speech and language are learned (prelingually deafened). Thus, children must depend on an auditory prosthesis to *learn* the auditory code underlying spoken language—a formidable task, given the exquisite temporal and frequency-resolving powers of the normal ear. On the other hand, young children may be the most successful users of implantable auditory prostheses because of the plasticity of the central nervous system.

The challenges faced in determining candidacy in children require balancing the risks of surgery versus the potential benefits of early implantation for the acquisition of spoken language. Initially, the use of cochlear implants in children was highly controversial. Thus, candidacy requirements were stringent, and the first children to receive cochlear implants were older (school-age or adolescents) and demonstrated no benefit from conventional hearing aids—not even sound awareness—even after many years of use and rehabilitation. These children were considered "ideal" cochlear implant candidates because their hearing could be reliably evaluated and it was obvious that no improvement in their auditory skills would occur with conventional hearing aids.

The first devices used with children were single-channel implants (see COCHLEAR IMPLANTS). Even though performance was limited, the children who received these devices derived more benefit from their implants than from conventional hearing aids (Thielemeir et al., 1985; Robbins, Renshaw, and Berry, 1991). A small percentage of these children achieved remarkable levels of word recognition through listening alone, although many of them had early acquired deafness with some normal auditory experience prior to the onset of their hearing loss (Berliner et al., 1989). Benefits also were documented in speech production and language acquisition (Osberger, Robbins, Berry, et al., 1991). Clearly, the early pioneering work with single-channel devices demonstrated the safety and effectiveness of implantable auditory prostheses in children and paved the way for the acceptance of cochlear implants as a medical treatment for profound deafness.

Eventually children received multichannel cochlear implants, especially as results indicated superior outcomes with these devices compared with single-channel implants (Osberger, Robbins, Miyamoto, et al., 1991). Since that time, numerous research studies have documented the substantial benefits that children with profound hearing loss obtain from multichannel cochlear implants (see Kirk, 2000; Waltzman, 2000). Numerous speech perception tests have been developed to assess implant candidacy and benefit, even in very young children (Kirk, 2000; Zimmerman-Phillips, Robbins, and Osberger, 2000). A finding common to all studies is the long time course over which children acquire auditory, speech, and language skills, even with multichannel devices (Tyler et al., 2000) (Fig. 1). This is not unexpected, given the number of years required for similar skill acquisition by hard-of-hearing children who use conventional hearing aids.

With continued clinical experience, improvements in technology, and documented benefits, cochlear implants gained greater acceptance, and candidacy criteria were expanded. Children received implants at increasingly younger ages, and it is now common practice to place implants in children as young as 2 years, with a growing trend for children as young as 12 months of age to receive cochlear implants (Waltzman and Cohen, 1998).

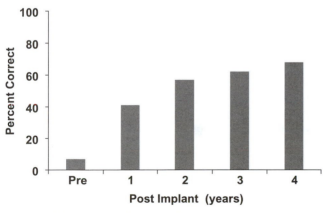

Figure 1. Mean pre- and postimplant scores on phoneme recognition (Phonetically Balanced-Kindergarten test) achieved by children during Clarion cochlear implant clinical trials (mean age at implant = 5 years).

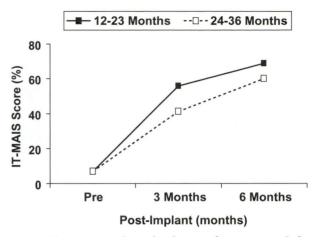

Figure 2. Mean pre- and postimplant performance on Infant-Toddler Meaningful Auditory Integration scale by age at implant (statistically significant difference between groups after 3 months of implant use).

Identification of hearing loss at an early age has also contributed to implantation in children at increasingly younger ages. Evidence suggests that children receiving implants at a younger age achieve higher levels of performance with their devices than children receiving implants at an older age (Fryauf-Bertschy et al., 1997; Waltzman and Cohen, 1998). Significant differences in postimplant outcome have been documented in children who receive implants before age 3 years. Children who received cochlear implants between ages 12 and 23 months demonstrated better auditory skills after implantation than children who received implants between the ages of 24 and 36 months (Fig. 2) (Osberger et al., 2002). Thus, a difference of as little as 1 year in age at the time of implantation had a significant impact on the rate of auditory skill development in these young children.

Even though the current trend is to provide implants to children at younger ages, older children continue to receive cochlear implants (Osberger et al., 1998). Some of these children have residual hearing and demonstrate benefit from conventional hearing aids. Implantation is often delayed because it takes longer to determine whether a plateau in auditory development has been reached. In addition, the audiological candidacy criteria were more stringent when these children were younger, and thus they were not considered appropriate candidates because they had too much hearing. Over time, however, audiological criteria in children have been expanded for implants (Zwolan et al., 1997). Following implantation, children with preoperative speech perception abilities demonstrate remarkable auditory recognition skills and achieve higher levels of performance with their implants than they did with hearing aids (Fig. 3).

Other factors besides age influence cochlear implant benefit in children. Communication method also impacts the postimplant performance in children. Most studies have found that children who use oral communication

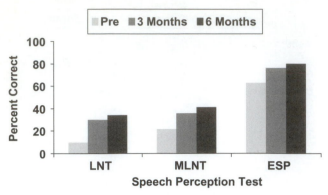

Figure 3. Mean pre- and postimplant performance on two open-set speech perception tests (Lexical Neighborhood and Multi-syllabic Neighborhood tests) (recorded administration) and one closed-set test (Early Speech Perception Monosyllable Word test) (live-voice administration) (mean age at implant = 9 years).

(audition, speaking, lipreading) achieve higher levels of performance with their implants than do children who are educated using total communication (English-based sign language with audition, speaking, lipreading) (Meyer et al., 1998). The trend for better implant performance in children who use oral communication has been shown in older children (Fig. 4) as well as in very young children (Osberger et al., 2002). This finding indicates that oral education programs more effectively emphasize the use of auditory information provided by an implant than do total communication programs. In fact, since multichannel cochlear implants became available, there has been a dramatic increase in the number of educational programs that employ oral communication, because a greater number of children have the potential to acquire spoken language through audition.

In addition to auditory perceptual benefits, children with cochlear implants show significant improvement in their receptive and expressive language development (see Robbins, 2000). Improvements in the use of communi-

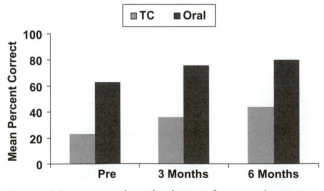

Figure 4. Mean pre- and postimplant performance by communication mode for older children (mean age at implant = 9 years) on the Early Speech Perception Monosyllable Word test) (live-voice administration) (statistically significant postimplant differences between groups).

cation strategies and conversational skills have also been reported (Tait, 1993; Nicholas, 1994), and more children with implants demonstrate higher levels of reading achievement than reported for their peers with hearing aids (Spencer, Tomblin, and Gantz, 1999). Nonetheless, even with marked improvements in performance, children with cochlear implants remain delayed in linguistic development compared to children of the same chronological age with normal hearing. However, children with cochlear implants do not continue to fall farther behind in their language performance, as has been reported for their profoundly hearing-impaired peers with hearing aids. As deaf children receive implants at younger ages, the gap between their skills and the skills of their age-matched peers with normal hearing will lessen.

Speech production skills also improve after implantation. Studies have shown improved production of segmental and suprasegmental features of speech and overall speech intelligibility (Tobey, Geers, and Brenner, 1994; Robbins et al., 1995). Dramatic improvements in speech production are often apparent after only several months of implant use, even in very young children who had little or no auditory experience prior to implantation. In very young children, improvements in vocalizations are usually the most noticeable changes following implantation (Zimmerman-Phillips, Robbins, and Osberger, 2000).

Cochlear implants are now accepted as an effective treatment for profound deafness. Many profoundly deaf children gain access to the auditory and linguistic code of spoken language with these devices, an accomplishment realized by only a limited number of deaf children with hearing aids. Profoundly deaf children with cochlear implants often function as well as children with less severe hearing impairments with hearing aids (Boothroyd and Eran, 1994; Meyer et al., 1998). Consequently, deaf children with implants acquire spoken language vicariously through incidental learning, requiring fewer special support services in school. Evidence suggests that more deaf children who use implants are being mainstreamed in regular classrooms than their peers with hearing aids (Francis et al., 1999). Thus, the long-term educational costs for children with cochlear implants will be less than for deaf children with hearing aids, resulting in a net savings to society. In addition, cochlear implants have a positive effect on the quality of life of deaf children, and have also been found to be a cost-effective treatment for deafness (Cheng et al., 2000). Whereas the impact of cochlear implants on educational and vocational achievement will take many years to establish, it is clear that these devices have changed the lives of many deaf children and their families.

—*Mary Joe Osberger*

References

Berliner, K. I., Tonokawa, L. L., Dye, L. M., and House, W. F. (1989). Open-set speech recognition in children with a single-channel cochlear implant. *Ear and Hearing, 10*, 237–242.

Boothroyd, A., and Eran, O. (1994). Auditory speech perception capacity of child implant users expressed as equivalent hearing loss. *Volta Review*, 96, 151–168.

Cheng, A. K., Rubin, H. R., Powe, N. R., Mellon, N. K., Francis, H. W., and Niparko, J. K. (2000). Cost-utility analysis of the cochlear implant in children. *Journal of the American Medical Association*, 284, 850–856.

Francis, H. W., Koch, M. E., Wyatt, R., and Niparko, J. K. (1999). Trends in educational placement and cost-benefit considerations in children with cochlear implants. *Archives of Otolaryngology–Head and Neck Surgery*, 125, 499–505.

Fryauf-Bertschy, H., Tyler, R. S., Kelsay, D. M., Gantz, B. J., and Woodworth, G. G. (1997). Cochlear implant use by prelingually deafened children: The influences of age at implant and length of device use. *Journal of Speech, Language, and Hearing Research*, 40, 183–199.

Kirk, K. I. (2000). Challenges in the clinical investigation of cochlear implant outcomes. In J. K. Niparko (Ed.), *Cochlear implants: Principles and practices* (pp. 225–258). Baltimore: Lippincott Williams and Wilkins.

Meyer, T. A., Svirsky, M. A., Kirk, K. I., and Miyamoto, R. T. (1998). Improvements in speech perception by children with profound prelingual hearing loss: Effects of device, communication mode, and chronological age. *Journal of Speech, Language, and Hearing Research*, 41, 846–858.

Nicholas, J. (1994). Sensory aid use and the development of communicative function. *Volta Review*, 96, 181–198.

Osberger, M. J., Fisher, L., Zimmerman-Phillips, S., Geier, L., and Barker, M. J. (1998). Speech recognition performance of older children with cochlear implants. *American Journal of Otology*, 19, 152–157.

Osberger, M. J., Robbins, A. M., Berry, S., Todd, S., Hesketh, L., and Sedey, A. (1991). Analysis of the spontaneous speech samples of children with cochlear implants or tactile aids. *American Journal of Otology*, 12(Suppl.), 173–181.

Osberger, M. J., Robbins, A. M., Miyamoto, R. T., Berry, S. W., Myres, W. A., Kessler, K. S., and Pope, M. L. (1991). Speech perception abilities of children with cochlear implants, tactile aids, or hearing aids. *American Journal of Otology*, 12(Suppl.), 105–115.

Osberger, M. J., Zimmerman-Phillips, S., and Koch, D. B. (2002). Cochlear implant candidacy and performance trends in children. *Annals of Otology, Rhinology, and Laryngology*, 111(Suppl. 189), 62–65.

Robbins, A. M. (2000). Rehabilitation after cochlear implantation. In J. K. Niparko (Ed.), *Cochlear Implants: Principles and Practices* (pp. 323–364). Baltimore: Lippincott Williams and Wilkins.

Robbins, A. M., Kirk, K. I., Osberger, M. J., and Ertmer, D. (1995). Speech intelligibility of implanted children. *Annals of Otology, Rhinology, and Laryngology*, 104(Suppl. 166), 399–401.

Robbins, A. M., Renshaw, J. J., and Berry, S. W. (1991). Evaluating meaningful auditory integration in profoundly hearing-impaired children. *American Journal of Otology*, 12(Suppl.), 151–164.

Spencer, L., Tomblin, J., and Gantz, B. J. (1999). Reading skills in children with multichannel cochlear-implant experience. *Volta Review*, 99, 193–202.

Tait, D. M. (1993). Video analysis: A method of assessing changes in preverbal and early linguistic communication after cochlear implantation. *Ear and Hearing*, 14, 378–389.

Thielemeir, M., Tonokawa, L. L., Peterson, B., and Eisenberg, L. S. (1985). Audiological results in children with a cochlear implant. *Ear and Hearing*, 6(Suppl.), 27S–35S.

Tobey, E. A., Geers, A., and Brenner, C. (1994). Speech production results and speech feature acquisition. *Volta Review*, 96, 109–130.

Tyler, R. S., Teagle, H. F. B., Kelsay, D. M. R., Gantz, B. J., Woodworth, G. G., and Parkinson, A. J. (2000). Speech perception by prelingually deaf children after six years of cochlear implant use: Effects of age at implantation. *Annals of Otology, Rhinology, and Laryngology*, 109(Suppl. 185), 82–84.

Waltzman, S. B. (2000). Variables affecting speech perception in children. In S. B. Waltzman and N. L. Cohen (Eds.), *Cochlear implants* (pp. 199–206). New York: Thieme.

Waltzman, S. B., and Cohen, N. L. (1998). Cochlear implantation in children younger than 2 years old. *American Journal of Otology*, 19, 158–162.

Zimmerman-Phillips, S., Robbins, A. M., and Osberger, M. J. (2000). Assessing cochlear implant benefit in very young children. *Annals of Otology, Rhinology, and Laryngology*, 109(Suppl. 185), 42–43.

Zwolan, T. A., Zimmerman-Phillips, S., Ashbaugh, C. J., Hieber, S. J., Kileny, P. R., and Telian, S. A. (1997). Cochlear implantation of children with minimal open-set speech recognition. *Ear and Hearing*, 18, 240–251.

Further Readings

Brown, C. J., and McDowall, D. W. (1999). Speech production results in children implanted with the Clarion implant. *Annals of Otology, Rhinology, and Laryngology*, 108(Suppl. 177), 110–112.

Buss, E., Labadie, R. F., Brown, C. J., Gross, A. J., Grose, J. H., and Pillsbury, H. C. (2002). Outcome of cochlear implantation in pediatric auditory neuropathy. *American Journal of Otology and Neurotology*, 23, 328–332.

Christiansen, J. B., and Leigh, I. W. (2002). *Cochlear implants in children: Ethics and choices*. Washington, DC: Gallaudet University Press.

Dawson, P. W., Blamey, P. J., Dettman, S. J., Barker, E. J., and Clark, G. M. (1995). A clinical report on receptive vocabulary skills in cochlear implant users. *Ear and Hearing*, 16, 287–294.

Geers, A. E., and Moog, J. S. (1989). Evaluating speech perception skills: Tools for measuring benefits of cochlear implants, tactile aids, and hearing aids. In E. Owens and D. K. Kessler (Eds.), *Cochlear implants in young deaf children*. Boston: Little, Brown.

Kirk, K. I., Pisoni, D. B., and Osberger, M. J. (1995). Lexical effects on spoken word recognition by pediatric cochlear implant users. *Ear and Hearing*, 16, 470–481.

Nevins, M. E., and Chute, P. M. (1996). *Children with cochlear implants in educational settings*. San Diego, CA: Singular Publishing Group.

Nikparko, J. K. (Ed.). (2000). *Cochlear implants: Principles and practices*. Baltimore: Lippincott Williams and Wilkins.

Osberger, M. J., and Fisher, L. (2000). Preoperative predictors of postoperative implant performance in children. *Annals of Otology, Rhinology, and Laryngology*, 109(Suppl. 185), 44–46.

Robbins, A. M., Green, J., and Bollard, P. M. (2000). Language development in children following one year of Clarion implant use. *Annals of Otology, Rhinology, and Laryngology*, 109(Suppl. 105), 94–95.

Robbins, A. M., Svirsky, M., and Kirk, K. I. (1997). Children with implants can speak, but can they communicate? *Otolaryngology–Head and Neck Surgery*, 117, 155–160.

Ryugo, D. K., Limb, C. J., and Redd, E. E. (2000). Brain plasticity: The impact of the environment as it relates to hearing and deafness. In J. K. Niparko (Ed.), *Cochlear implants: Principles and practices* (pp. 33–56). Baltimore: Lippincott Williams and Wilkins.

Tobey, E. A., and Hasenstab, S. (1991). Effects of Nucleus multichannel cochlear implant upon speech production in children. *Ear and Hearing, 12*(Suppl.), 48S–54S.

Waltzman, S. B., and Cohen, N. L. (2000). *Cochlear implants.* New York: Thieme.

Waltzman, S. B., Scalchunes, V., and Cohen, N. L. (2000). Performance of multiply handicapped children using cochlear implants. *American Journal of Otology, 21,* 329–335.

Dichotic Listening

Dichotic listening refers to listening to two different signals presented simultaneously through earphones, one signal to the left ear (LE) and a different signal to the right ear (RE). Although the results have been expressed in different ways, the most common approach is to calculate $\%_{RE}$, $\%_{LE}$, and the difference score ($\%_{RE} - \%_{LE}$). The difference score describes the percentage ear advantage and may be a right ear advantage (REA), left ear advantage (LEA), or no ear advantage (NoEA).

Dichotic listening is a psychophysical process, the testing of which is used to assess certain aspects of central auditory function. The outcomes of experiments have led to the development of ear–brain hypotheses; an REA is accepted as evidence of left hemispheric dominance for processing and an LEA as evidence of right hemispheric dominance. A NoEA is sometimes interpreted to mean that brain dominance has not been well established (Gerber and Goldman, 1971).

When the signals are speech (usually consonant-vowel [CV] nonsense syllables), the commonly reported outcome is an REA, and interpretation of the REA in relation to left hemispheric dominance has been based on four assumptions: (1) ipsilateral auditory pathways are suppressed during dichotic stimulation (Milner, Taylor, and Sperry, 1968); (2) information from each ear arrives at the contralateral hemisphere in equivalent states (Studdert-Kennedy and Shankweiler, 1970); (3) the left hemisphere, which is language dominant for at least 95% of the right-handed population and about 70% of the left-handed population (Penfield and Roberts, 1959; Annett, 1975; Rasmussen and Milner, 1977), is principally responsible for extracting phonetic information from the different signals presented to the RE and LE (Studdert-Kennedy and Shankweiler, 1970; Studdert-Kennedy, Shankweiler, and Pisoni, 1972); and (4) the lower LE score implies "loss of information" during interhemispheric transmission from the right hemisphere to the left hemisphere via the corpus callosum (Studdert-Kennedy and Shankweiler, 1970; Studdert-Kennedy, Shankweiler, and Pisoni, 1972; Berlin et al., 1973; Brady-Wood and Shankweiler, 1973; Cullen et al., 1974; Repp, 1976). Each assumption is critical to the validity of an ear–brain hypothesis.

Distinction Between a True Ear Advantage and an Observed Ear Advantage

A *true* ear advantage is thought to reflect differences in the transmission capacities of the auditory channels from the RE and LE to a common, centrally located processing area that, for speech, is located in the left hemisphere. An *observed* ear advantage may arise from at least four sources: a true ear advantage, decision variables, stimulus variables, and measurement error (Speaks, Niccum, and Carney, 1982). Proper counterbalancing of experimental conditions can control stimulus variables, measurement error can be minimized by presenting a sufficient number of listening trials (Repp, 1977; Speaks, Niccum, and Carney, 1982), and the role of decision variables will be addressed subsequently.

Optional Psychophysical Procedures

Kimura (1961) used a *recall task*. Listeners received three pairs of spoken digits and were asked to recall as many of the six digits as possible. A second procedure—the most commonly used—involves a *two-ear recognition task*. One pair of signals is presented, the listener is to attend "equally" to both the RE and LE, and the listener provides two responses from a closed message set (Studdert-Kennedy and Shankweiler, 1970; Berlin et al., 1972; Speaks, Niccum, and Carney, 1982). In a variation of the two-ear recognition task, the listener attends to both ears but provides only one response (Repp, 1977). A third procedure employs an *ear-monitoring task* in which two signals are presented but the listener is asked to attend selectively to one ear and supply only one response (Hayden, Kirsten, and Singh, 1979). Although those three tasks can be used with speech signals, their use for nonspeech signals is more problematic because the listener is required to both recall and name the signals heard.

A fourth technique applies the theory of signal detection (TSD) and involves a *yes/no target-monitoring task* (Katsuki et al., 1984). The TSD approach can be used with either speech or nonspeech signals, but the details will be described for speech signals. The message set consists of six CV nonsense syllables. On a given test block of 40 dichotic trials, one syllable is designated the target. Contralateral interference is provided by the other five syllables, each appearing equally often. The target is present on only half (20) of the trials within a listening block; hence the a priori probability of target-present trials is 0.50. The listener attends to a designated ear and responds "yes" to vote that the target was present or "no" to vote that the target was not present. Over the course of six listening blocks, each of the six syllables serves as the target, and contralateral interference is provided by the other five syllables. The scores for each ear are expressed by P(C)max, a d'-based statistic, the ear advantage is given by P(C)max$_{RE}$ − P(C)max$_{LE}$, and listener criterion is expressed by β. The effects of decision variables on the outcome of the yes/no target-monitoring task are minimized because both hit and false alarm responses are incorporated in the calculation of P(C)max.

Choice of Metric

When the task is yes/no target monitoring, the ear advantage should be expressed by $P(C)max_{RE} - P(C)max_{LE}$. For the commonly used two-ear recognition task, several metrics have been proposed, which will be presented here in the context of their dependence on performance level, P_o, where $P_o = (\%_{RE} + \%_{LE})/2$. (1) d is the simple difference score, $\%_{RE} - \%_{LE}$, and d is unconstrained by performance level only when $P_o = 50\%$. (2) Because performance level imposes a ceiling on d, Halwes (1969) proposed an "index of laterality," which will be symbolized as L_i. $L_i = [(R - L)/(R + L)]100$, and the analysis is confined to those trials in which only one response is correct. (3) *POC* reflects the percentage of correct responses (Harshman and Krashen, 1972). (4) *POE* reflects the percentage of erroneous responses (Harshman and Krashen, 1972). (5–6) *POC'* and *POE'* are linear transformations of *POC* and *POE* (Repp, 1977). *POC'* is unconstrained when $P_o < 50\%$, and *POE'* is unconstrained when $P_o > 50\%$. (7) ϕ is the geometric mean of *POC'* and *POE'* (Kuhn, 1973) and is unconstrained only when $P_o = 50\%$. (8) e is a disjunctive use of *POC'* and *POE'*, meaning that $e = POC'$ when $P_o < 50\%$ and $e = POE'$ when $P_o > 50\%$. Thus, e is independent of P_o.

The maximum value of the various indices can be constrained by P_o, but the dependence apparently is not particularly strong. Speaks, Niccum, and Carney (1982) reported that the correlations of the various metrics with P_o ranged from -0.18 to $+0.17$. Moreover, all intercorrelations among the metrics were ≥ 0.95.

What, then, is the metric of choice? We (Speaks, Niccum, and Carney, 1982) have argued that the ideal metric should reflect two properties. One is the proportion of all trials on which an ear advantage occurs, which is the ratio of single-correct (SC) trials to total trials: $p(SC) = SC/(SC + DC + DE)$, where DC refers to double-correct trials and DE refers to double-error trials. The second property is the magnitude of ear advantage, $p(EA_{mag})$, on those trials in which an ear advantage occurs, which is the ratio of the difference between single-correct trials for the right ear and single-correct trials for the left ear to total single-correct trials: $p(EA_{mag}) = (SC_{RE} - SC_{LE})/SC$, and $p(EA_{mag}) = L_i$. If we assume that the two properties are of equal importance, we can derive a single metric for the ear advantage by computing the product of $p(SC)$ and $p(EA_{mag})$, and that weighted value $= d$, the simple ear-difference score. Finally, if we assume that scores for each ear and the ear advantage are normally distributed for the individual listener, the utility of d can be improved by a z-score transformation, a d'-like statistic that incorporates variability of the ear advantage for the individual listener as an error term: $d_Z = (\%_{RE} - \%_{LE})/\sigma$, where $\sigma = [(\sigma_{RE}^2 + \sigma_{LE}^2)/2]^{1/2}$.

Reliability of Ear Advantage Scores, d

The reliability of ear-advantage scores has been reported principally for the simple ear-difference score, d. Ryan and McNeil (1974) tested listeners with two blocks of 30 CV nonsense syllables per block and reported a correlation between blocks of $+0.80$. That outcome compares favorably with the test-retest correlation of $+0.74$ reported by Blumstein, Goodglass, and Tartter (1975). These authors emphasized, however, that the correlation coefficient might not be sensitive to reversals in direction of the advantage between test and retest: an REA on one block and an LEA on a second block. In fact, reversals occurred for 29% of their listeners. Pizzamiglio, DePascalis, and Vignati (1974) reported a similar outcome: 30% of their listeners who were tested with digits evidenced a reversal in direction of the ear advantage. Other investigators have reported test-retest correlations of $+0.64$ (Catlin, Van Derveer, and Teicher, 1976) and $+0.66$ (Speaks and Niccum, 1977).

Repp (1977) contended that the poor reliability likely was due in part to an insufficient number of trials. He applied the Spearman-Brown predictive formula to the Blumstein, Goodglass, and Tartter (1975) data and estimated that a reliability coefficient of $+0.90$ should be realized with a 240-trial test (eight blocks of 30 pairs of syllables per block). Speaks, Niccum, and Carney (1982) provided empirical support for Repp's prediction. They tested 24 listeners with 20 blocks of 30 pairs of CV syllables per block. The split-half reliability coefficient was only $+0.62$ when scores for block 1 were compared with scores for block 2. The coefficient improved to $+0.91$, however, when scores for blocks 1 through 6 were compared with scores for blocks 7 through 12. Moreover, the standard error of measurement diminished from 13.09 for the block 1–2 comparison to 5.66 for the block 1–6 and 7–12 comparison. They concluded that use of fewer than 180 listening trials is likely to generate unreliable data.

Properties of the Ear Advantage

An examination of scores of reports on the dichotic ear advantage with CV nonsense syllables shows one fairly consistent result. The mean ear advantage for a group of listeners is almost always an REA with a magnitude in the range of 5%–12%. In most instances, however, there have been an insufficient number of listening trials to permit a more detailed analysis of relevant statistical properties. We will refer principally then to an experiment reported by Speaks, Niccum, and Carney (1982) on 24 listeners with the two-ear recognition task. Each listener received 20 blocks of 30 pairs of CV nonsense syllables per block (600 dichotic trials per listener). Thus, the properties of interest were derived from 1200 responses for each listener and from 28,800 responses (24 listeners × 1200 per listener) for the group. We will note only a few of the more salient properties.

1. Mean percent scores for the group were 71.7% for the RE and 65.1% for the LE, and the ear advantage, d,

was therefore +6.6% (an REA). The RE and LE scores for the 20 listening blocks presented to the 24 listeners were plotted as cumulative percentage distributions and fitted with normal integrals. That analysis suggested that the distributions of recognition scores for the two ears could be conceptualized as two overlapping normal curves with different means (RE = 71.7%, LE = 65.1%) but equal variances (σ_{RE} = 8.9%, σ_{LE} = 8.8%). Thus, a *true* ear advantage equals the difference between the means of the RE and LE probability density functions.

2. The block-to-block measures of the ear advantage also were distributed as a normal curve with a mean of 6.6% and a mean intralistener standard deviation of 10.8% ± 2.5%, where the mean sigma was calculated as the square root of the mean of the variances.

3. The mean/sigma ratio for the group of listeners was very small: 6.6%/10.7% = 0.62. Thus, the typical listener with a small ear advantage, on the order of 6.6%, should be expected to evidence block-to-block reversals in the direction of ear advantage such as those that have been reported in the literature. The relation between the size of the mean/sigma ratio and reversals in ear advantage can be illustrated by results obtained for three of the 24 listeners. For L-1, d = 23.3% (REA), σ = 9.7%, and $\overline{X}/\sigma$ = 2.40. An REA occurred on all 20 listening blocks. For L-2, d = −26.5% (LEA), σ = 10.1%, and $\overline{X}/\sigma$ = −2.62. An LEA occurred on 19 of the 20 listening blocks, and a NoEA was observed on one block. For L-3, d = 0.5% (a nonsignificant REA), σ = 10.7%, and $\overline{X}/\sigma$ = 0.05. Of the 20 listening blocks, 4 were LEA, 10 were NoEA, and 6 were REA.

How Should the Dichotic Ear Advantage Be Interpreted?

An REA is widely accepted as evidence of left hemispheric dominance for processing, and an LEA is viewed as evidence of right hemispheric dominance for processing. The REA commonly reported for speech is thought to arise from "loss of information" during interhemispheric transmission from the right hemisphere to the left hemisphere via the corpus callosum.

There is general agreement that about 95% of the right-handed population (and perhaps 70% of the left-handed population) is left hemispheric dominant for the processing of speech and language (Penfield and Roberts, 1959; Geschwind and Levitsky, 1968; Annett, 1975). If the direction of ear advantage reflects the direction of hemispheric laterality, it seems reasonable to assume that something approaching 95% of the right-handed population should have an REA for speech signals presented dichotically. No outcome approaching 95% has been reported, and unfortunately, the significance of the observed ear advantage for individual listeners has rarely been tested statistically. In the Speaks, Niccum, and Carney (1982) experiment in which the two-ear recognition task was used with 24 listeners, 18 had an observed REA, but the advantage was only sig-

nificant (McNemar's χ^2 for correlated proportions) at the 0.05 level or less for 12 listeners (50%). Three (12.5%) of the 24 listeners had a significant LEA. Katsuki et al. (1984) tested 20 listeners with a yes/no target-monitoring task and the ear advantage for individual listeners was tested on transformations (Φ = [2 arcsin P(C)max]$^{1/2}$) on P(C)max for each ear. Thirteen (65%) of 20 listeners had a significant REA, and two (10%) had a significant LEA.

A similar outcome was reported by Wexler, Halwes, and Heninger (1981). They tested 31 listeners and found that 14 (45%) had a significant REA and one (3%) had a significant LEA. They, however, placed a different interpretation on their data by disregarding the fact that 16 listeners did not have a significant ear advantage and emphasizing that 14 (93%) of the 15 listeners who had a significant ear advantage had a significant REA. To justify dismissing the 16 listeners with no ear advantage from their analysis assumes that processing for speech must always be lateralized to either the left or the right hemisphere and that failure to obtain an *observed* ear advantage must be due principally to measurement error. They suggested that increasing the length of the dichotic test might reduce measurement error and lead to a larger number of listeners having a significant REA. But, as we have seen, even with 20 listening blocks (Speaks, Niccum, and Carney, 1982), the mean ear advantage for a group of 24 listeners was only 6.6% (REA), and only 12 of 24 listeners had a significant REA. We acknowledge that most, perhaps 80% or so, listeners who have a dichotic ear advantage have an REA rather than an LEA. From a different perspective, however, no more than two-thirds of listeners tested appear to have an REA. Because a large proportion of the right-handed population is known to be left hemispheric dominant for speech and language processing, but a much smaller proportion evidence an REA, we believe that speculations about the neurological bases for listener responses to dichotic stimulation are at best fragile.

—*Charles Speaks*

References

Annett, M. (1975). Hand preference and the laterality of cerebral speech. *Cortex, 11*, 305–328.

Berlin, C., Lowe-Bell, S., Cullen, J., Thompson, C., and Loovis, C. (1973). Dichotic speech perception: An interpretation of right-ear advantage and temporal offset effects. *Journal of the Acoustical Society of America, 53*, 699–709.

Berlin, C., Lowe-Bell, S., Cullen, J., Thompson, C., and Stafford, M. (1972). Is speech "special?" Perhaps the temporal lobectomy patient can tell us. *Journal of the Acoustical Society of America, 52*, 702–705.

Blumstein, S., Goodglass, H., and Tartter, V. (1975). The reliability of ear advantage in dichotic listening. *Brain and Language, 2*, 226–236.

Brady-Wood, S., and Shankweiler, D. (1973). Effects of amplitude variation on an auditory rivalry task: Implications concerning the mechanisms of perceptual asymmetries. *Haskins Laboratory Status Reports on Speech Research, 34*, 119–126.

Catlin, J., Van Derveer, N. J., and Teicher, R. (1976). Monaural right-ear advantage in a target-identification task. *Brain and Language, 3,* 470–481.

Cullen, J., Thompson, C., Hughes, L., Berlin, C., and Samson, D. (1974). The effects of varied acoustic parameters on performance in dichotic speech tasks. *Brain and Language, 1,* 307–322.

Gerber, S. J., and Goldman, P. (1971). Ear preference for dichotically presented verbal materials as a function of report strategies. *Journal of the Acoustical Society of America, 49,* 1163–1168.

Geschwind, N., and Levitsky, W. (1968). Human brain: left-right asymmetries in temporal speech region. *Science, 161,* 186–187.

Halwes, T. (1969). *Effects of dichotic fusion in the perception of speech.* Doctoral dissertation, University of Minnesota, Minneapolis.

Harshman, R., and Krashen, S. (1972). An "unbiased" procedure for comparing degree of lateralization of dichotically presented stimuli. *UCLA Working Papers on Phonetics, 23,* 3–12.

Hayden, M., Kirsten, E., and Singh, S. (1979). Role of distinctive features in dichotic perception of 21 English consonants. *Journal of the Acoustical Society of America, 65,* 1039–1046.

Katsuki, J., Speaks, C., Penner, S., and Bilger, R. (1984). Application of the theory of signal detection to dichotic listening. *Journal of Speech and Hearing Research, 27,* 444–448.

Kimura, D. (1961). Some effects of temporal-lobe damage on auditory perception. *Canadian Journal of Psychology, 15,* 156–165.

Kuhn, G. M. (1973). The phi coefficient as an index of ear differences in dichotic listening. *Cortex, 9,* 447–457.

Milner, B., Taylor, S., and Sperry, R. W. (1968). Lateralized suppression of dichotically presented digits after commissural section in man. *Science, 161,* 184–185.

Penfield, W., and Roberts, L. (1959). *Speech and brain mechanisms.* Princeton, NJ: Princeton University Press.

Pizzamiglio, L., DePascalis, C., and Vignati, A. (1974). Stability of dichotic listening test. *Cortex, 10,* 203–205.

Rasmussen, T., and Milner, B. (1977). The role of early left-brain injury in determining lateralization of cerebral speech functions. In S. J. Diamond and D. A. Blizard (Eds.), *Evolution and lateralization of the brain. Annals of the New York Academy of Science, 299,* 355–369. [Special issue]

Repp, B. (1976). Dichotic "masking" of voice onset time. *Journal of the Acoustical Society of America, 59,* 183–194.

Repp, B. (1977). Measuring laterality effects in dichotic listening. *Journal of the Acoustical Society of America, 42,* 720–737.

Ryan, W., and McNeil, M. (1974). Listener reliability for a dichotic task. *Journal of the Acoustical Society of America, 56,* 1922–1923.

Speaks, C., and Niccum, N. (1977). Variability of the ear advantage in dichotic listening. *Journal of the American Audiological Society, 3,* 52–57.

Speaks, C., Niccum, N., and Carney, E. (1982). Statistical properties of responses to dichotic listening with CV nonsense syllables. *Journal of the Acoustical Society of America, 72,* 1185–1194.

Studdert-Kennedy, M., and Shankweiler, D. (1970). Hemispheric specialization for speech perception. *Journal of the Acoustical Society of America, 48,* 579–594.

Studdert-Kennedy, M., Shankweiler, D., and Pisoni, D. (1972). Auditory and phonetic processes in speech perception: Evidence from a dichotic study. *Cognitive Psychology, 3,* 455–466.

Wexler, E., Halwes, T., and Heninger, G. (1981). Use of a statistical significance criterion in drawing inferences about hemispheric dominance for language function from dichotic listening data. *Brain and Language, 13,* 13–18.

Electrocochleography

Electrocochleography (ECochG) refers to the general method of recording the stimulus-related potentials of the cochlea and auditory nerve. The product of ECochG—the electrocochleogram, or ECochGm—is shown in Figure 1. As depicted in this figure, the components of interest may include the cochlear microphonic (CM), cochlear summating potential (SP), and auditory nerve action potential (AP). Detailed descriptions of these electrical events are abundant in the hearing science literature and are beyond the scope of this review. For a more thorough discussion of the history of these potentials as recorded in humans, see Ferraro (2000).

The popularity of ECochG as a clinical tool emerged in the early 1970s, following the discovery and application of the auditory brainstem response (ABR). The development and refinement of noninvasive recording

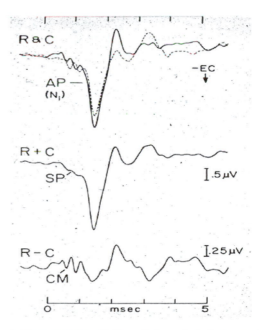

Figure 1. Components of the click-evoked human electrocochleogram. Top tracings display responses to rarefaction (R) and condensation (C) polarity clicks. Adding separate R and C responses (middle tracing) enhances the cochlear Summating Potential (SP) and auditory nerve Action Potential (AP). Subtracting R and C responses (bottom tracing), enhances the Cochlear Microphonic (CM). (From American Speech-Language-Hearing Association, 1988, p. 9, based on data from Coats, 1981.)

techniques also has facilitated the current clinical use of ECochG.

The technical capability to record cochlear and auditory nerve potentials in humans has led to a variety of clinical applications for ECochG. Among the more popular applications are

1. To diagnose, assess, and monitor Ménière's disease/ endolymphatic hydrops (MD/ELH) and to assess and monitor treatment strategies for these disorders
2. To enhance wave I of the ABR
3. To monitor cochlear and auditory nerve function during operations that involve the auditory periphery (Ruth, Lambert, and Ferraro, 1988; Ferraro and Krishnan, 1997).

ECochG Recording Techniques

Transtympanic Versus Extratympanic ECochG. The terms transtympanic (TT) and extratympanic (ET) refer to the two general techniques for recording ECochG. The TT approach involves passing a needle electrode through the TM to rest on the cochlear promontory, whereas ET recordings are generally made from the surface of the ear canal or TM. The primary advantage of TT ECochG is that this "near-field" approach produces large components with relatively little signal averaging. The major limitation of TT ECochG is that it is invasive. ET recordings require more signal averaging, and the components tend to be smaller in magnitude than their TT counterparts. However, this approach is generally painless and can be performed by nonphysicians in nonmedical settings.

TM offers a good compromise between ear canal and TT recording sites with respect to component magnitudes and signal averaging time without being invasive or painful (Lambert and Ruth, 1988; Ferraro, Blackwell, et al., 1994; Ferraro, Thedinger, et al., 1994). In addition, the waveform patterns that lead to the interpretation of the TT ECochGm are preserved in TM recordings (Ferraro, Thedinger, et al., 1994).

Figure 2 is a drawing of the TM electrode (or "tymptrode") used in our clinic and laboratory, which is a modification of the device described several years ago by Stypulkowski and Staller (1987). Details regarding the fabrication and placement of the tymptrode can be found in Ferraro (1997, 2000).

Recording Parameters. ECochG components occur within the first few milliseconds of electrophysiological activity following stimulus onset. Table 1 illustrates the parameters used in our laboratory and clinic for recording the SP and AP together, which is usually the pattern of interest when ECochG is used in the diagnosis of MD/ELH. It is important to note that the bandpass setting of the analog filter of the preamplifier must be wide enough to accommodate the recording of both direct and alternating current potentials (i.e., the SP and AP, respectively).

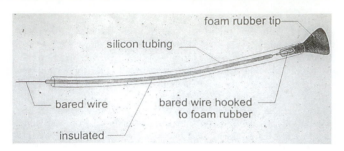

Figure 2. Construction of a tympanic membrane electrode (foam rubber tip can be replaced with soft cotton). (From Ferraro, 2000, p. 434.)

Table 1. ECochG Recording Parameters

Electrode Array	
Primary (+)	Tympanic membrane
Secondary (−)	Contralateral earlobe or mastoid process
Common	Nasion or ipsilateral earlobe
Signal Averaging Settings	
Timebase	10 milliseconds
Amplification Factor	50,000×–100,000× (Extratympanic— ET)
Filter Bandpass	5 Hz–3000 Hz
Repetitions	750–1000
Stimuli	
Type	Broadband Clicks (BBC), Tonebursts (TB)
Duration (BBC)	100 microsecond electrical pulse
Envelope (TB)	2 millisecond linear rise/fall, 5–10 msec plateau
Polarity	Rarefaction and Condensation (BBC), Alternating (TB)
Repetition Rate	11.3/sec
Level	95–85 dB HL (125–115 dB pe SPL)

Stimulus Considerations. The broadband click tends to be the most popular stimulus for short-latency AEPs because it excites synchronous discharges from a large population of neurons to produce well-defined neural components. However, the brevity of the click makes it a less than ideal stimulus for studying cochlear potentials such as the CM and SP, whose durations are stimulus dependent. The use of tonal stimuli can overcome some of these limitations, and also provide for a higher degree of response frequency specificity than clicks (Durrant and Ferraro, 1991; Ferraro, Blackwell, et al., 1994; Ferraro, Thedinger, et al., 1994; Margolis et al., 1995).

Stimulus polarity is an important factor for ECochG. Presenting clicks or tonebursts in alternating polarity inhibits the presence of stimulus artifact and CM, which are both dependent on stimulus phase. Thus, alternating-polarity stimuli may be preferable when the amplitudes of the SP and AP are of interest (as in the determination of the SP/AP amplitude ratio for the diagnosis of MD/

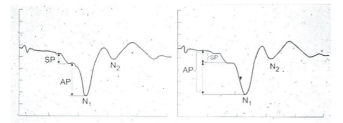

Figure 3. Normal electrocochleogram recorded from the tympanic membrane to clicks presented in alternating polarity at 80 dB HL. The amplitudes of the Summating Potential (SP) and Action Potential (AP) can be measured from peak-to-peak (left panel), or with reference to a baseline value (right panel). Amplitude/time scale is 1.25 μV/1 msec per gradation. Insert phone delay is 0.90 msec. (From Ferraro, 2000, p. 435.)

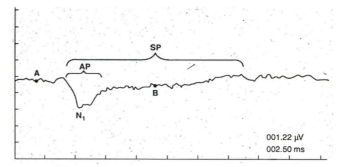

Figure 4. Normal electrocochleogram recorded from the tympanic membrane to a 2000-Hz toneburst presented in alternating polarity at 80 dB HL. Action Potential (AP) and its first negative peak (N₁) are seen at the onset of the response. Summating Potential (SP) persists as long as the stimulus. SP amplitude is measured at midpoint of response (point B), with reference to a baseline value (point A). Amplitude (microvolts)/time (milliseconds) scale at lower right. (From Ferraro, Blackwell, et al., 1994, p. 19.)

ELH). Recording separate responses to condensation and rarefaction clicks also is useful, as certain subjects with MD/ELH display abnormal AP latency differences to clicks of opposing polarity (Margolis et al., 1992; Margolis et al., 1995; Orchik, Ge, and Shea, 1997; Sass, Densert, and Arlinger, 1997).

When ECochG is performed to help diagnose MD/ELH, stimulus presentation should begin at a level near the maximum output of the stimulus generator to evoke a well-defined SP-AP complex. Masking of the contralateral ear is not a concern for conventional ECochG since the magnitude of any electrophysiological response from the nontest ear is very small and ECochG components are generated prior to crossover of the auditory pathway.

Interpretation of the ECochGm

Figure 3 depicts a normal ECochGm to click stimuli recorded from the TM. Component amplitudes can be measured from peak to peak (left panel) or using a baseline reference (right panel). AP-N1 latency is measured from stimulus onset to the peak of N1 and should be identical to the latency of ABR wave I at the same stimulus level. When using a tubal insert transducer (highly recommended), these values will be delayed by a factor proportional to the length of the tubing. Although labeled in Figure 3, N2 has received little interest for ECochG applications.

Also as shown in Figure 3, SP and AP amplitudes are made from the leading edge of both components. The resultant values are used to derive the SP/AP amplitude ratio, which ranges from approximately 0.1 to 0.5 in normal subjects.

Figure 4 depicts a normal ECochGm evoked by a 2000-Hz toneburst. As opposed to click-evoked responses, where the SP normally appears as a small shoulder preceding the AP, the SP to tonebursts persists as long as the stimulus. The AP and its N1 in turn are seen at the onset of the response. SP amplitude is measured with reference to baseline amplitude, and at the midpoint of the waveform to minimize the influence of the AP. Figure 5 illustrates toneburst SPs at several fre-

quencies recorded from both the TM and promontory (TT) of the same patient. An important aspect illustrated in this figure is that the amplitudes of toneburst-SPs in normal-hearing subjects are generally negative in regard to baseline amplitude, and are very small. Another noteworthy aspect of Figure 5 is that although the amplitudes of the TM responses are approximately ¼ that of the promontory responses (note amplitude scales), the corresponding patterns of the TM and TT recordings at each frequency are virtually identical.

Clinical Applications

MD/ELH. As mentioned earlier, ECochG has emerged as one of the more powerful tools in the diagnosis, assessment, and monitoring of MD/ELH, primarily through the measurement of the SP and AP. Examples

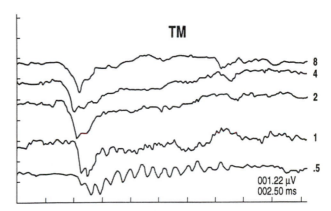

Figure 5. Tympanic Membrane (TM) recorded electrocochleograms evoked by tonebursts of different frequencies presented at 80 dB HL. Stimulus frequency in kilohertz indicated at the right of each waveform. Amplitude (microvolts)/time (milliseconds) scale at lower right. (From Ferraro, Blackwell, et al., 1994, p. 20.)

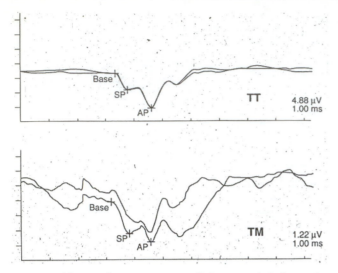

Figure 6. Abnormal responses to clicks recorded from the promontory (TT) (upper panel) and tympanic membrane (TM) (lower panel) of the affected ear of the same patient. Both TT and TM responses display an enlarged Summating Potential (SP)/Action Potential (AP) amplitude ratio. "Base" indicates reference for SP and AP amplitude measurements. Amplitude (microvolts)/time (milliseconds) scale at lower right. Stimulus onset delayed by approximately 2 msec. (From Ferraro, Thedinger, et al., 1994, p. 27.)

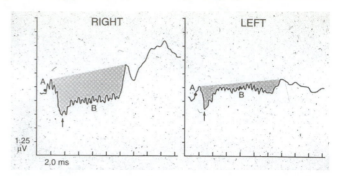

Figure 7. Comparison of electrocochleograms recorded from the tympanic membrane between the affected (right) and unaffected (left) sides of a patient with endolymphatic hydrops. The shaded areas include the AP and SP components. SP amplitude is measured at point B with respect to point and is abnormally enlarged on the affected side. Arrows indicate the AP-N1. Stimulus was a 1000-Hz toneburst (2 msec rise/fall, 10 msec plateau) presented at 90 db HL. (From Ferraro, 1993, p. 37.)

of this application are shown in Figures 6 (click-evoked ECochGms), and 7 (toneburst-evoked ECochGms). The upper tracings in Figure 6 were measured from the promontory (TT), whereas the lower waveforms represent TM recordings. The SP/AP amplitude ratios are enlarged under each condition. The rationale for this finding remains unclear, but may relate to the nature of the SP as a distortion product of transduction processes in the cochlea. In particular, ELH may augment this distortion and thus increase the amplitude of the SP. Enlarged SP/AP amplitude ratios also have been reported for perilymphatic fistulas (Ackley, Ferraro, and Arenberg, 1994), which suggests that the fluid pressure of the scala media may be the underlying feature to which ECochG is specific.

Figure 7 illustrates the difference between right and left SPs evoked by 2000-Hz tonebursts in a patient with MD/ELH on the right side. A pronounced, negative SP is seen on the affected side of this particular patient, whereas the unaffected side shows a normal pattern.

The reported incidence of an enlarged SP and SP/AP amplitude ratio in the general Ménière's population is approximately 60%–65% (Gibson, Moffat, and Ramsden, 1977; Coats, 1981; Kumagami, Nishida, and Masaaki, 1982). Testing patients when they are experiencing symptoms of MD/ELH has been shown to improve this percentage (Ferraro, Arenberg, and Hassanein, 1985). Other approaches to increasing the sensitivity of ECochG include measuring the AP-N1 latency difference between responses to condensation versus

rarefaction clicks (Margolis et al., 1992, 1995), and measuring the respective "areas" of the SP and AP to derive the SP/AP area ratio (Ferraro and Tibbils, 1999).

Enhancement of Wave I. In a high percentage of hard-of-hearing subjects, including those with acoustic tumors, wave I of the ABR may be unrecordable in the presence of wave V (Hyde and Blair, 1981; Cashman and Rossman, 1983). This situation precludes the measurement of the I–V and I–III interwave intervals, which are key features of the ABR for neurodiagnostic applications. Under these and other less than optimal recording conditions, using an ECochG approach for recording the ABR has considerable utility (Ferraro and Ferguson, 1989). Figure 8 exemplifies this application in a patient with hearing loss. The top tracing represents the ABR recorded with surface electrodes at the vertex and ear lobes, and wave I is absent in the presence of wave V. When the TM is used as a recording site, however (bottom tracing), wave I is clearly present, permitting the measurement of the I–V interwave interval.

Intraoperative Monitoring. Intraoperative monitoring of inner ear and auditory nerve status during operations that involve the peripheral auditory system has emerged as an important application for ECochG. Such monitoring usually is done to help the surgeon avoid potential trauma to the ear and nerve in an effort to preserve hearing, to identify anatomic landmarks (such as the endolymphatic sac), or to help predict postoperative outcome (Lambert and Ruth, 1988; Gibson and Arenberg, 1991; Wazen, 1994). Figure 9 illustrates a series of ECochG responses recorded from a patient undergoing endolymphatic shunt decompression surgery for treatment of MD/ELH. A reduction in the SP/AP amplitude ratio was observed during the course of surgery,

Figure 8. ABR recorded with a vertex (+)-to-ipsilateral earlobe (−) electrode array, and ECochG-ABR recorded with a vertex (+)-to-ipsilateral tympanic membrane (−) electrode array from a patient with hearing loss (audiogram at right). Wave I is absent in the conventional ABR tracings but recordable with the ECochG-ABR approach. (From Ferraro and Ferguson, 1989, p. 165.)

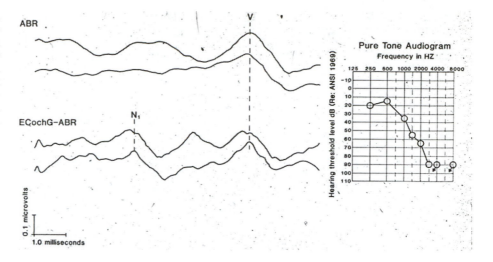

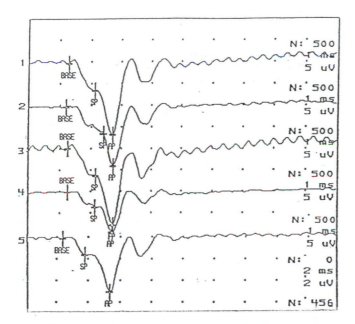

Figure 9. Series of electrocochleograms recorded from a patient undergoing endolymphatic shunt surgery for treatment of Ménière's disease. Baseline tracing (1), drilling on mastoid bone (2), probing for endolymphatic duct (3), inserting prosthesis (4), closing (5). Tracing 5 shows a reduction in the SP/AP amplitude ratio compared to tracing 1, and this patient reported improvement in symptoms postoperatively. (From Ferraro, 2000, p. 446.)

and this patient reported improvement in symptoms postoperatively.

Summary

ECochG continues to be a useful clinical tool in the identification and evaluation of inner ear and auditory nerve disorders. Although this article has addressed the currently more popular clinical applications of ECochG, others will emerge as our knowledge of auditory physiology continues to improve, and the technical aspects of recording the electrical events associated with hearing become more sophisticated. Current areas in need of additional research include the standardization of recording and stimulus parameters, and studies designed to improve the sensitivity of ECochG to MD/ELH and other cochlear disorders.

—*John A. Ferraro*

References

Ackley, R. S., Ferraro, J. A., and Arenberg, I. K. (1994). Diagnosis of patients with perilymphatic fistula. *Seminars in Hearing, 15,* 37–41.

American Speech-Language-Hearing Association. (1988). The short latency auditory evoked potentials: A tutorial paper by the Working Group on Auditory Evoked Potential Measurements of the Committee on Audiologic Evaluation.

Cashman, M., and Rossman, R. (1983). Diagnostic features of the auditory brainstem response in identifying cerebellopontine angle tumors. *Scandinavian Audiology, 12,* 35–41.

Coats, A. C. (1981). The summating potential and Ménière's disease. *Archives of Otolaryngology, 104,* 199–208.

Durrant, J. D., and Ferraro, J. A. (1991). Analog model of human click-elicited SP and effects of high-pass filtering. *Ear and Hearing, 12,* 144–148.

Ferraro, J. A. (1997). *Laboratory exercises in auditory evoked potentials.* San Diego, CA: Singular Publishing Group.

Ferraro, J. A. (2000). Electrocochleography. In R. J. Roeser, M. Valente, and H. Hosfort-Dunn (Eds.), *Audiology diagnosis* (pp. 425–450). New York: Thieme.

Ferraro, J. A., Arenberg, I. K., and Hassanein, R. S. (1985). Electrocochleography and symptoms of inner ear dysfunction. *Archives of Otolaryngology*, *111*, 71–74.

Ferraro, J. A., Blackwell, W., Mediavilla, S. J., and Thedinger, B. (1994). Normal summating potential to tonebursts recorded from the tympanic membrane in humans. *Journal of the American Academy of Audiology*, *5*, 17–23.

Ferraro, J. A., and Ferguson, R. (1989). Tympanic ECochG and conventional ABR: A combined approach for the identification of wave I and the I–V interwave interval. *Ear and Hearing*, *3*, 161–166.

Ferraro, J. A., and Krishnan, G. (1997). Cochlear potentials in clinical audiology. *Audiology and Neuro-Otology*, *2*, 241–256.

Ferraro, J. A., Thedinger, B., Mediavilla, S. J., and Blackwell, W. (1994). Human summating potential to tonebursts: Observations on TM versus promontory recordings in the same patient. *Journal of the American Academy of Audiology*, *6*, 217–224.

Ferraro, J. A., and Tibbils, R. (1999). SP/AP area ratio in the diagnosis of Ménière's disease. *American Journal of Audiology*, *8*, 21–27.

Gibson, W. P. R., and Arenberg, I. K. (1991). The scope of intraoperative electrocochleography. In I. K. Arenberg (Ed.), *Proceedings of the Third International Symposium and Workshops on the Surgery of the Inner Ear* (pp. 295–303). Amsterdam: Kugler.

Gibson, W. P. R., Moffat, D. A., and Ramsden, R. T. (1977). Clinical electrocochleography in the diagnosis and management of Ménière's disorder. *Audiology*, *16*, 389–401.

Hyde, M. L., and Blair, R. L. (1981). The auditory brainstem response in neuro-otology: Perspectives and problems. *Journal of Otololaryngolgy*, *10*, 117–125.

Kumagami, H., Nishida, H., and Masaaki, B. (1982). Electrocochleographic study of Ménière's disease. *Archives of Otology*, *108*, 284–288.

Lambert, P., and Ruth, R. A. (1988). Simultaneous recording of noninvasive ECoG and ABR for use in intraoperative monitoring. *Otolaryngology–Head and Neck Surgery*, *98*, 575–580.

Margolis, R. H., Levine, S. M., Fournier, M. A., Hunter, L. L., Smith, L. L., and Lilly, D. J. (1992). Tympanic electrocochleography: Normal and abnormal patterns of response. *Audiology*, *31*, 18–24.

Margolis, R. H., Rieks, D., Fournier, M., and Levine, S. M. (1995). Tympanic electrocochleography for diagnosis of Ménière's disease. *Archives of Otolaryngology–Head and Neck Surgery*, *121*, 44–55.

Orchik, J. G., Ge, X., and Shea, J. J. (1997). Action potential latency shift by rarefaction and condensation clicks in Ménière's disease. *American Journal of Otolaryngology*, *14*, 290–294.

Ruth, R. A., Lambert, P. R., and Ferraro, J. A. (1988). Electrocochleography: Methods and clinical applications. *American Journal of Otolaryngology*, *9*, 1–11.

Sass, K., Densert, B., and Arlinger, S. (1997). Recording techniques for transtympanic electrocochleography in clinical practice. *Acta Otolaryngologica (Stockholm)*, *118*, 17–25.

Stypulkowski, P., and Staller, S. (1987). Clinical evaluation of a new ECoG recording electrode. *Ear and Hearing*, *8*, 304–310.

Wazen, J. J. (1994). Intraoperative monitoring of auditory function: Experimental observation, and new applications. *Laryngoscope*, *104*, 446–455.

Further Readings

Aran, J. M., and Lebert, G. (1968). Les responses nerveuse cochleaires chex l'homme, image du fonctionnement de l'oreille et nouveau test d'audiometrie objectif. *Revue de Laryngologie, Otologie, Rhinologie (Bordeaux)*, *89*, 361–365.

Coats, A. C. (1986). Electrocochleography: Recording technique and clinical applications. *Seminars in Hearing*, *7*, 247–266.

Coats, A. C., and Dickey, J. R. (1970). Non-surgical recording of human auditory nerve action potentials and cochlear microphonics. *Annals of Otology, Rhinology, and Laryngology*, *29*, 844–851.

Conlon, B. J., and Gibson, W. P. (2000). Electrocochleography in the diagnosis of Ménière's disease. *Acta Oto-Laryngologica*, *120*, 480–483.

Dallos, P., Schoeny, Z. G., and Cheatham, M. A. (1972). Cochlear summating potentials: Descriptive aspects. *Acta Otolaryngologica*, *301*(Suppl.), 1–46.

Durrant, J. D. (1986). Combined EcochG-ABR approach versus conventional ABR recordings. *Seminars in Hearing*, *7*, 289–305.

Ferraro, J. A., Best, L. G., and Arenberg, I. K. (1983). The use of electrocochleography in the diagnosis, assessment and monitoring of endolymphatic hydrops. *Otolaryngologic Clinics of North America*, *16*, 69–82.

Gibson, W. P. R. (1978). *Essentials of electric response audiometry*. New York: Churchill and Livingstone.

Gibson, W. P. R., Arenberg, I. K., and Best, L. G. (1988). Intraoperative electrocochleographic parameters following nondestructive inner ear surgery utilizing a valved shunt for hydrops and Ménière's disease. In J. G. Nadol (Ed.), *Proceedings of the Second International Symposium on Ménière's Disease*. Amsterdam: Kugler and Ghedini.

Goin, D. W., Staller, S. J., Asher, D. L., and Mischke, R. E. (1982). Summating potential in Ménière's disease. *Laryngoscope*, *92*, 1381–1389.

Kiang, N. S. (1965). *Discharge patterns of single nerve fibers in the cat's auditory nerve* (Research Monograph No. 35). Cambridge, MA: MIT Press.

Kitahara, M., Takeda, T., and Yazama, T. (1981). Electrocochleography in the diagnosis of Ménière's disease. In K. H. Volsteen (Ed.), *Ménière's disease: Pathogenesis, diagnosis and treatment* (pp. 163–169). New York: Thieme-Stratton.

Kobayashi, H., Arenberg, I. K., Ferraro, J. A., and Van der Ark, G. (1993). Delayed endolymphatic hydrops following acoustic tumor removal with intraoperative and postoperative auditory brainstem response improvements. *Acta Otolaryngolica (Stockholm)*, *504*(Suppl.), 74–78.

Koyuncu, M., Mason, S. M., and Shinkwin, C. (1994). Effect of hearing loss in electrocochleographic investigation of endolymphatic hydrops using tone-pip and click stimuli. *Journal of Laryngology and Otology*, *108*, 125–130.

Laureano, A. N., Murray, D., McGrady, M. D., and Campbell, K. C. M. (1995). Comparison of tympanic membrane-recorded electrocochleography and the auditory brainstem response in threshold determination. *American Journal of Otolaryngology*, *16*, 209–215.

Levine, S. M., Margolis, R. H., Fournier, E. M., and Winzenburg, S. M. (1992). Tympanic electrocochleography for evaluation of endolymphatic hydrops. *Laryngoscope*, *102*, 614–622.

Moriuchi, H., and Kumagami, H. (1979). Changes of AP, SP and CM in experimental endolymphatic hydrops. *Audiology*, 22, 258–260.

Morrison, A. W., Moffat, D. A., and O'Connor, A. F. (1980). Clinical usefulness of electrocochleography in Ménière's disease: An analysis of dehydrating agents. *Otolaryngologic Clinics of North America*, 11, 703–721.

Ng, M., Srireddy, S., Horlbeck, D. M., and Niparko, J. K. (2001). Safety and patient experience with transtympanic electrocochleography. *Laryngoscope*, 111, 792–795.

Orckik, D. J., Shea, J. J., Jr., and Ge, X. (1993). Transtympanic electrocochleography in Ménière's disease using clicks and tone-bursts. *American Journal of Otology*, 14, 290–294.

Ruben, R., Sekula, J., and Bordely, J. E. (1960). Human cochlear responses to sound stimuli. *Annals of Otorhinolaryngology*, 69, 459–476.

Ruth, R. A. (1990). Trends in electrocochleography. *Journal of the American Academy of Audiology*, 1, 134–137.

Ruth, R. A. (1994). Electrocochleography. In J. Katz (Ed.), *Handbook of clinical audiology* (4th ed., pp. 339–350). Baltimore: Williams and Wilkins.

Schmidt, P., Eggermont, J., and Odenthal, D. (1974). Study of Ménière's disease by electrocochleography. *Acta Otolaryngologica*, 316(Suppl.), 75–84.

Schoonhoven, R., Fabius, M. A. W., and Grote, J. J. (1995). Input/output curves to tonebursts and clicks in extratympanic and transtympanic electrocochleography. *Ear and Hearing*, 16, 619–630.

Electronystagmography

Electronystagmography (ENG) refers to a battery of tests used to evaluate the vestibular system. The tests include (1) the Dix-Hallpike test, (2) ocular motor tests, (3) a search for positional and/or spontaneous nystagmus, (4) the caloric test, and (5) the failure of fixation suppression test. During ENG testing, eye movement is measured to determine the presence of peripheral (vestibular nerve and/or end-organ) vestibular or central nervous system (CNS) dysfunction. Two methods for recording eye movement are electro-oculography (EOG) and video-nystagmography (VNG). EOG is a recording of the corneoretinal potential with surface electrodes placed on the face, whereas VNG measures eye movement through the use of infrared video cameras mounted in goggles worn by the patient during testing.

Dix-Hallpike Test

The Dix-Hallpike maneuver is a provocative positioning test for benign paroxysmal positioning vertigo (BPPV) (Dix and Hallpike, 1952). The patient is seated upright with the head turned 45° toward the test ear and then quickly lowered into a supine position with the head hanging off the bed or table and still positioned at the 45° angle. The diagnosis of BPPV is based on characteristic clinical findings on the Dix-Hallpike test. These findings include (1) torsional nystagmus and vertigo that occur when the patient is placed in the provoking position, (2) a delay in the onset of vertigo and nystagmus, and (3) a duration of vertigo and nystagmus of less than 1 minute.

Ocular Motor Tests

The purpose of ocular motor tests is to test nonvestibular eye movements. These movements include the saccadic system, the smooth pursuit system, the optokinetic (OPK) system, and the gaze-holding mechanism. Abnormalities in the ocular motor systems generally localize CNS lesions; however, acute peripheral vestibular lesions may also cause abnormal findings.

The saccadic system rapidly changes the direction of the eye to acquire the image of an object of interest. Disorders of the saccadic system can include slowing of saccadic eye movements, impaired saccadic accuracy, and impaired reaction time. The preferred stimulus for testing the saccadic system is a random sequence paradigm presented with an array of light-emitting diodes (LEDs) controlled by a computer (Baloh et al., 1975). Measurement parameters on the saccade test include latency, velocity, and accuracy (Fig. 1).

The smooth pursuit system allows continuous, clear vision of objects moving within the visual environment. Patients with impaired smooth pursuit require frequent corrective saccades to keep up with the target, producing cogwheeling or saccadic pursuit responses. Most computerized ENG systems use a sinusoidal paradigm that offers precise control of frequency and amplitude of smooth pursuit testing. The most important measurement parameter of smooth pursuit is gain. Gain is calculated as the ratio of eye velocity to target velocity. Figure 2 shows gain and EOG recording during smooth pursuit for a normal subject.

The optokinetic system serves to hold images of the environment on the retina during sustained head rotation. There are two optokinetic stimuli: (1) partial field devices, which include the light bar and a small motorized drum, and (2) full-field devices (preferred), such as an optokinetic projector or large optokinetic drum, that fill at least 90% of the visual field. The measurement parameter of the OPK test is gain (ratio of eye velocity to field velocity). Gain should be at least 0.5 and symmetrical.

The gaze tests determine whether a patient has gaze-evoked nystagmus. Gaze-evoked nystagmus occurs when a leaky neural integrator causes the eyes to drift back toward the primary position, necessitating corrective saccades. Thus, the eyes cannot hold their position when looking at an eccentric target. Gaze-evoked nystagmus can be caused by drugs, cerebellar disease, brainstem lesions, and acute peripheral vestibular lesions. The stimulus for the gaze tests is a light bar target positioned 20° or 30° right, left, up, or down from the center.

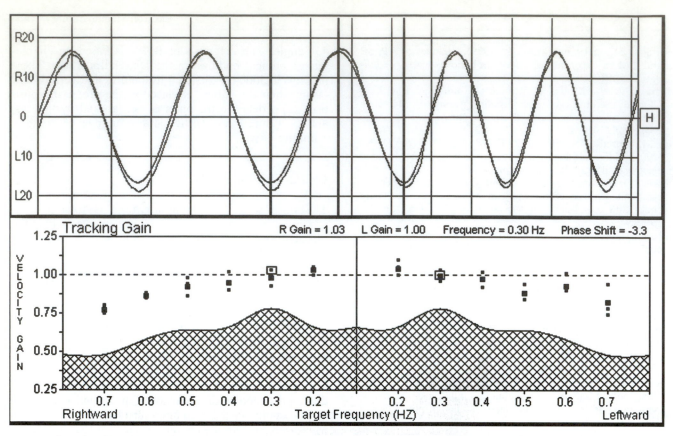

Figure 1. Sample of ENG recordings of saccades produced with a random-sequence paradigm in a normal subject. Data points represent peak velocity, accuracy, and latency measurements for each rightward and leftward saccade.

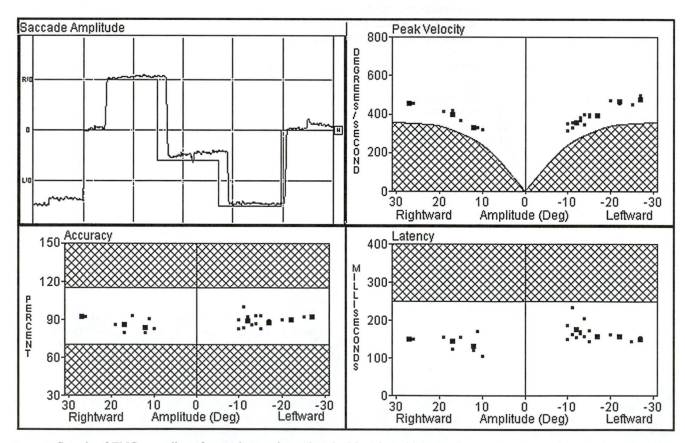

Figure 2. Sample of ENG recording of smooth pursuit produced with a sinusoidal paradigm in a normal subject. Data points represent gain values for each rightward and leftward eye movement across target frequency.

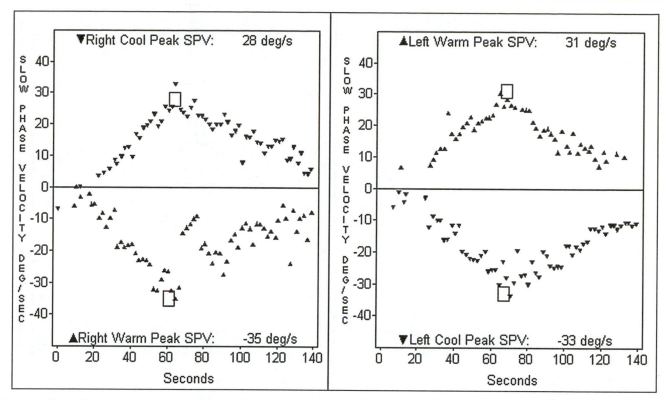

Figure 3. Plots of slow-component velocity from nystagmus elicited by bithermal water caloric irrigation as a function of time in a normal subject. The four panels represent irrigation of the left and right ears at warm (44 °C) and cool (30 °C) water temperatures.

Spontaneous Nystagmus

To determine the presence of spontaneous nystagmus, the subject is seated upright with eyes closed, the head positioned straight ahead (0°), and the subject engaged in mental alerting tasks to prevent suppression of nystagmus. Spontaneous nystagmus is typically horizontal jerk nystagmus and usually occurs due to a lesion to the peripheral vestibular system causing an imbalance in the tonic signals arriving at the oculomotor neurons. The imbalance produces a constant drift of the eyes in one direction, interrupted by fast components in the opposite direction. If the imbalance results from a peripheral vestibular lesion, then the pursuit system can cancel it. Thus, when the patient opens his or her eyes, the nystagmus disappears. The clinical finding of spontaneous nystagmus suggests an uncompensated peripheral lesion, typically on the side opposite the direction of nystagmus. The proof of the side of lesion, however, lies in the caloric test.

Positional Nystagmus

Positional nystagmus occurs when a subject is placed in the following static positions: sitting; supine; supine, head turned left; supine, head turned right; right lateral; left lateral; pre-irrigation position; and head-hanging straight, right, and left. The patient is asked to close his or her eyes to eliminate the effects of visual suppression

and to perform mental alerting tasks to avoid central suppression.

Positional (and spontaneous) nystagmus is classified according to the direction of the fast phase. The direction of nystagmus can be fixed or changing. Direction-changing nystagmus can be geotropic (beating toward the earth) or ageotropic (beating away from the earth). Direction-changing nystagmus is an abnormal, non-localizing finding that is most often associated with peripheral vestibular disease (Lin et al., 1986). Positional nystagmus can also be direction-changing in a single head position. This clinical finding is rare and indicates a central pathology. There is evidence that both structural and metabolic factors can alter the specific gravity of the cupula in the semicircular canals and cause positional nystagmus (Honrubia, 2000). Positional nystagmus can also be caused by brainstem lesions, and most clinicians place the burden of proof on the ocular motor function tests. That is, if the ocular motor tests are within normal limits, then it is doubtful that a brainstem lesion exists.

The Caloric Test

The caloric test (Fitzgerald and Hallpike, 1942) is the most important test in the ENG test battery and the only clinical vestibular test that can lateralize a vestibular deficit. The caloric test stimulates the horizontal semicircular canal and involves measurement of

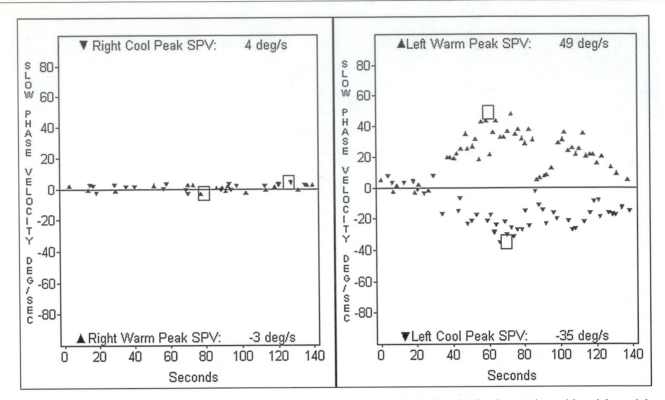

Figure 4. Plots of slow-component velocity from nystagmus elicited by bithermal caloric irrigation in a patient with a right peripheral vestibular lesion. No response was elicited from warm and cool water irrigation to the right ear, resulting in a right unilateral weakness.

slow-component eye velocity. The key principle of the caloric test is the convection current created in the horizontal semicircular canal by changing the temperature of the endolymph. This convection current causes utriculopetal endolymph flow and increased neural firing of the primary vestibular afferent nerve during warm water or air irrigation, so that nystagmus beats toward the ear that is stimulated. Irrigation with cool water or air produces utriculofugal flow and a decrease in neural firing of the primary vestibular afferent nerve, so that nystagmus beats away from the stimulated ear.

The fundamental assumption of the caloric test is that all four caloric irrigations of a given patient are equally strong. Variables that affect the strength of the caloric stimulus include stimulus temperature, stimulus duration, flow rate or volume, mental alerting procedures, size and shape of the external auditory canal, type of stimulus, patient age, and patient medication. The slow-component velocity (SCV) of the nystagmus has proved to be the most sensitive parameter of vestibular function and is currently the standard metric used for evaluating the caloric test (Henricksson, 1956). Because average SCVs vary widely in normal subjects, a ratio of right ear to left ear responses is used to analyze the caloric test results (Barber and Wright, 1973). Normal and symmetrical bithermal caloric nystagmus is shown in Figure 3. Unilateral weakness is a caloric asymmetry that results when one labyrinth is less sensitive to caloric irrigation than the other labyrinth (Fig. 4). The unilateral weakness is calculated by determining the amount

by which the average SCVs provoked by right ear irrigation differ in intensity from those provoked by left ear irrigations. The formula for unilateral weakness is:

$$UW(\%) = \frac{(RW + RC) - (LW + LC)}{RW + RC + LW + LC} \times 100$$

where RW, RC, LW, and LC are the peak SCVs of the responses to right warm, right cool, left warm, and left cool irrigations, respectively. Most laboratories use an interear difference of greater than 20%–25% to determine if a unilateral weakness exists (Baloh and Honrubia, 1990; Jacobson, Newman, and Kartush, 1997). Unilateral weakness identifies a peripheral vestibular deficit on the weak side and is the most definitive finding on the ENG test for identifying and lateralizing a peripheral vestibular deficit.

A spontaneous nystagmus, such as in the case of an acute peripheral vestibular lesion, can shift the baseline of the caloric response. The caloric responses will be skewed toward the direction of the spontaneous nystagmus. The intensity difference between right-beating and left-beating caloric nystagmus is called directional preponderance (DP). The formula for directional preponderance is:

$$DP(\%) = \frac{(RW + LC) - (RC + LW)}{RW + LC + RC + LW} \times 100$$

where RW, RC, LW, and LC are the peak SCVs of the responses to right warm, right cool, left warm, and left cool irrigations, respectively. A directional preponderance of 30% or greater is abnormal (Baloh and Honrubia, 1990). Directional preponderance is considered a nonlocalizing finding and usually reflects the presence of spontaneous or positional nystagmus.

Other caloric abnormalities include failure of fixation suppression and bilateral weakness. Failure of fixation suppression indicates that a patient is unable to suppress visually the nystagmus by more than 50% of peak SCV, suggesting central vestibular involvement. Bilateral weakness occurs with weak or absent caloric responses in both ears. Bilateral weakness usually indicates a bilateral peripheral vestibular deficit, but it also may occur with CNS pathology.

—Faith W. Akin

References

Baloh, R. W., and Honrubia, V. (1990). *Clinical neurophysiology of the vestibular system*. Philadelphia: F. A. Davis Co.

Baloh, R. W., Konrad, H. R., Sills, A. W., and Honrubia, V. (1975). The saccade velocity test. *Neurology, 25*, 1071–1076.

Barber, H. O., and Wright, G. (1973). Positional nystagmus in normals. *Advances in Oto-Rhino-Laryngology, 19*, 276–285.

Dix, R., and Hallpike, C. S. (1952). The pathology, symptomatology and diagnosis of certain common disorders of the vestibular system. *Annals of Otology, Rhinology, and Laryngology, 6*, 987–1016.

Fitzgerald, G., and Hallpike, C. S. (1942). Studies in human vestibular function: I. Observations on the directional preponderance ("nystagmusbereitschaft") of caloric nystagmus resulting from cerebral lesions. *Brain, 62*, 115–137.

Henricksson, N. G. (1956). Speed of slow component and duration in caloric nystagmus. *Acta Otolaryngologica, 46*, 1–29.

Honrubia, V. (2000). Quantitative vestibular function tests and the clinical examination. In S. Herdman (Ed.), *Vestibular rehabilitation* (pp. 105–171). Philadelphia: F. A. Davis.

Jacobson, G. P., Newman, C. W., and Kartush, J. M. (1997). *Handbook of balance function testing*. San Diego, CA: Singular Publishing Group.

Lin, J., Elidan, J., Baloh, R. W., and Honrubia, V. (1986). Direction-changing positional nystagmus: Incidence and meaning. *American Journal of Otolaryngology, 4*, 306–310.

Further Readings

Bamiou, D. E., Davies, R. A., McKee, M., and Luxon, L. M. (1999). The effect of severity of unilateral vestibular dysfunction on symptoms, disabilities and handicap in vertiginous patients. *Clinical Otolaryngology, 24*, 31–38.

Barber, H. O., and Stockwell, C. (1980). *Manual of electronystagmography*. Shambaugh, IL: ICS Medical Corp.

Beynon, G. J. (1997). A review of management of benign paroxysmal positional vertigo by exercise therapy and by repositioning manoeuvres. *British Journal of Audiology, 31*, 11–26.

Bhansali, S. A., and Honrubia, V. (1999). Current status of electronystagmography testing. *Otolaryngology–Head and Neck Surgery, 120*, 419–426.

Coats, A. (1976). The air caloric: A parametric study. *Archives of Otolaryngology, 102*, 343–354.

Ford, C. R., and Stockwell, C. W. (1978). Reliabilities of air and water caloric responses. *Archives of Otolaryngology, 104*, 380–382.

Furman, J. M., and Cass, S. P. (1996). *Balance disorders: A case-study approach*. Philadelphia: F. A. Davis Co.

Furman, J. M., and Jacob, R. G. (1993). Jongkees' formula reevaluated: Order effects in the response to alternate binaural bithermal caloric stimulation using closed-loop irrigation. *Acta Otolaryngologica, 113*, 3–10.

Goebel, J. (2001). *Practical management of the dizzy patient*. Philadelphia: Lippincott, Williams and Wilkins.

Herdman, S. (2000). *Vestibular rehabilitation*. Philadelphia: F. A. Davis Co.

Jacobson, G. P., Calder, J. A., Shepherd, V. A., Rupp, K. A., and Newman, C. W. (1995). Reappraisal of the monothermal warm caloric screening test. *Annals of Otology, Rhinology, and Laryngology, 104*, 942–945.

Karlsen, E. A., Mikhail, H. H., Norris, C. W., and Hassanein, R. S. (1992). Comparison of responses to air, water, and closed-loop caloric irrigators. *Journal of Speech and Hearing Research, 35*, 186–191.

Leigh, J., and Zee, D. S. (1993). *The neurology of eye movements*. Philadelphia: F. A. Davis Co.

Shepard, N. T., and Telian, S. A. (1996). *Practical management of the balance disorder patient*. San Diego, CA: Singular Publishing Group.

Frequency Compression

Frequency compression (or frequency lowering) is a general term applied to attempts to lower the spectrum of the acoustic speech signal to better match the residual hearing of listeners with severe to profound high-frequency sensorineural impairment accompanied by better hearing at the low frequencies. This pattern of hearing loss is common to a number of different etiologies of hearing loss (including presbycusis, noise exposure, ototoxicity, and various genetic syndromes) and arises from greater damage to the basal region relative to the apical region of the cochlea (see NOISE-INDUCED HEARING LOSS; OTOTOXIC MEDICATIONS; PRESBYACUSIS). The major effect of high-frequency hearing loss on speech reception is a degraded ability to perceive sounds whose spectral energy is dominated by high frequencies, in some cases extending to 10 kHz or beyond. Perceptual studies have documented the difficulties of listeners with high-frequency loss in the reception of high-frequency sounds (including plosive, fricative, and affricate consonants) and have demonstrated that this pattern of confusion is similar to that observed by normal-hearing listeners deprived of high-frequency cues through the use of low-pass filtering (Wang, Reed, and Bilger, 1978). Traditional hearing aids attempt to treat this pattern of hearing loss by delivering frequency-dependent amplification to overcome the loss at high frequencies. Such amplification, however, may not lead to improved performance and has even been shown to degrade the speech reception ability of some listeners with severe to profound high-frequency loss (Hogan and Turner, 1998).

The goal of frequency lowering is to recode the high-frequency components of speech into a lower frequency range that is matched to the residual capacity of a listener's hearing. Frequency lowering has been accomplished through a variety of different techniques. These methods have arisen primarily from attempts at bandwidth reduction in the telecommunications industry, rather than being driven by the perceptual needs of hearing-impaired listeners. This article summarizes and updates the review of the literature on frequency lowering published by Braida et al. (1979). For each of seven different categories of signal processing, the major characteristics of each method are described and a brief summary of results obtained with it is provided.

Slow Playback

The earliest approach to frequency lowering was the playback of recorded speech at a slower speed than that used in recording. Each spectral component is scaled lower in frequency by a multiplicative factor equal to the slowdown factor. Although this method is not suitable for real-time applications (because of the inherent time dilation of the resulting waveform) and leads to severe alterations in temporal relations between speech sounds, it is nonetheless important to understand its effects because it is a component of many other frequency-lowering schemes. An important characteristic of this method is its preservation of the proportional relationship between spectral components, including the relation between the short-term spectral envelope and the fundamental frequency ($F0$) of voiced speech. A negative consequence of proportional lowering, however, is the shifting of $F0$ into an undesirably low frequency range (particularly for male voices). Results obtained in studies of the effects of slow playback on speech reception conducted with normal-hearing listeners (Tiffanny and Bennett, 1961; Daniloff, Shriner, and Zemlin, 1968) indicate that reductions in bandwidth up to roughly 25% produce only small losses in intelligibility, bandwidth reductions of 50% cause moderate losses in intelligibility, and bandwidth reductions of 66% or greater lead to severe loss in intelligibility. These studies have shown that the voices of females and children are more resistant to lowering than male voices (presumably because the fundamental and formant frequencies are higher for women than for men), that the effects of lowering are similar for the reception of consonants and vowels, and that performance with lowered speech materials improves with practice. In a study of slow playback in listeners with high-frequency sensorineural hearing loss, Bennett and Byers (1967) found beneficial effects for modest degrees of frequency lowering (up to a 20% reduction in bandwidth) but that greater degrees of lowering led to a substantial reduction in performance.

Time-Compressed Slow Playback

A solution to the time dilation inherent to slow playback was introduced by techniques that compress speech in time (Fairbanks, Everitt, and Jaeger, 1954) prior to the application of slow playback. Time compression can be accomplished in different ways, including the elimination of a fixed duration of speech at a given rate of interruption or eliminating pitch periods from voiced speech. When the time-compression and slow-playback factors are chosen to be equal, the long-term duration of the speech signal can be preserved while at the same time frequencies are lowered proportionally. Fundamental frequency can be affected differently, depending on the particular characteristics of the time-compression scheme, including being lowered, remaining unchanged, or being severely distorted (see Braida et al., 1979). The intelligibility of speech processed by this technique for normal-hearing listeners is similar to that described above for slow playback; that is, bandwidth reduction by factors greater than 20% lead to severe decrease in performance (Daniloff, Shriner, and Zemlin, 1968; Nagafuchi, 1976). Results of studies in hearing-impaired listeners (Mazor et al., 1977; Turner and Hurtig, 1999) indicate that improvements for time-compressed slow-playback speech compared to conventional linear or high-pass amplification may be observed under certain conditions. Small benefits, on the order of 10–20 percentage points, are most likely to be observed for small amounts of frequency lowering (bandwidth reduction factors in the range of 10%–30%), for female rather than male voices, and for individuals who receive little aid from conventional high-pass amplification. A wearable aid that operates on the basic principles of time-compressed slow playback (the AVR Transonic device) has been evaluated in children with profound deafness (Davis-Penn and Ross, 1993; MacArdle et al., 2001) and in adults with high-frequency impairment (Parent, Chmiel, and Jerger, 1997; McDermott et al., 1999). A high degree of variability is observed across studies and across subjects within a given study, with substantial improvements noted for certain subjects and negligible effects or degradations for others.

Frequency Shifting

Another technique for frequency lowering employs heterodyne processing, which uses amplitude modulation to shift all frequency components in a given band downward by a fixed displacement. This process leads to the overlaying, or *aliasing*, of high-frequency and low-frequency components. Aliasing is generally avoided by the removal of low-frequency components through filtering before modulation. Systems that employ shifting of the entire spectrum have a number of disadvantages: although temporal and rhythmic patterns of speech remain normal, the harmonic relationships of voiced sounds are greatly altered, fundamental frequency is severely modified, and low-frequency components important to speech recognition are removed to prevent aliasing. Even mild degrees of frequency shifting (e.g., a 400-Hz shift for male voices) have been found to interfere substantially with speech reception ability (Raymond and Proud, 1962).

Frequency Transposition

When frequency shifting is restricted to the high-frequency components of speech (rather than to the entire speech spectrum), the process is referred to as frequency transposition. This approach has been incorporated into several different wearable or desktop aids (Johansson, 1966; Velmans, 1973) whose basic operation involves shifting speech frequencies in the region above 3 or 4 kHz into a lower frequency region, and adding these processed components to the original unprocessed speech signal. Generally, the most careful and controlled studies of frequency transposition indicate that benefits are quite modest. Transposition can render high-frequency speech cues audible to listeners with severe to profound high-frequency hearing loss (Rees and Velmans, 1993); however, these cues may interfere with information normally associated with the reception of low-frequency speech components (Ling, 1968). There is evidence to suggest that transposition aids may be more useful in training in speech production than in improving speech reception in deaf children (Ling, 1968).

Zero-Crossing-Rate Division

Another approach to frequency lowering lies in an attempt to reduce the zero-crossing rate of the speech signal. In these schemes, bands of speech are extracted by filtering and the filter outputs are converted to lower frequency sounds having reduced zero-crossing rates. Evaluations of a system in which processing was applied only to high-frequency components and inhibited during voiced speech (Guttman and Nelson, 1968) indicated no benefits for processed materials on a large-set word recognition task for normal-hearing listeners with simulated hearing loss. Use of this system as a speech-production aid for hearing-impaired children indicates that, following extensive training, the ability to produce selected high-frequency sounds was improved, while at the same time the ability to discriminate these same words auditorily showed no such improvements (Guttman, Levitt, and Bellefleur, 1970).

Vocoding

An important class of frequency-lowering systems for the hearing-impaired is based on the channel vocoder (Dudley, 1939), which was originally developed to achieve bandwidth reduction in telecommunications systems. Vocoding systems analyze speech into contiguous bandpass filters whose output envelopes are detected and low-pass-filtered for transmission. These signals are then used to control the amplitudes of corresponding channels. For frequency lowering, the set of synthesis filters correspond to lower frequencies than the associated analysis filters. Vocoding systems appear to have a number of advantages, including operation in real time and flexibility in terms of the choice of analysis and synthesis filters (which can allow for different degrees of lowering in different regions of the spectrum as well as for independent manipulation of $F0$ and the spectral

envelope). The effect of degree of lowering in vocoder-based systems appears to be comparable to that described above for slow playback and time-compressed slow playback (Fu and Shannon, 1999). A number of studies conducted with vocoder-based lowering systems have demonstrated improved speech reception with training, both for normal-hearing (Takefuta and Swigart, 1968; Posen, Reed, and Braida, 1993) and for hearing-impaired listeners (Ling and Druz, 1967; McDermott and Dean, 2000). When performance with vocoding systems is compared to baseline systems employing low-pass filtering to an equivalent bandwidth for normal listeners or conventional amplification for impaired listeners, however, the benefits of lowered speech appear to be quite modest. One possible reason for the lack of success of some of these systems (despite the apparent promise of this approach) may have been the failure to distinguish between voiced and unvoiced sounds. Systems in which processing is suppressed when the input signal is dominated by low-frequency energy (Posen, Reed, and Braida, 1993) lead to better performance (compared to systems with no inhibitions in processing for voiced sounds) based on their ability to enhance the reception of high-frequency sounds while not degrading the reception of low-frequency sounds.

Frequency Warping

A more recent approach to frequency lowering incorporates digital signal-processing techniques developed for correcting "helium speech." The speech signal is segmented pitch synchronously, processed to achieve nonuniform spectral warping, dilated in time to achieve frequency lowering, and resynthesized with the original periodicity. Both the overall bandwidth reduction and the relative compression of high- and low-frequency components can be specified. These methods roughly extrapolate the variance associated with increased length of the vocal tract and include the following characteristics: they preserve the temporal and rhythmic properties of speech, they leave $F0$ of voiced sounds unaltered, they allow for independent manipulation of $F0$ and spectral envelope, and they compress the short-term spectrum in a continuous and monotonic fashion. Studies of speech reception with frequency-warped speech indicate that spectral transformations that lead to greater lowering of the high frequencies relative to the low frequencies are superior to those with linear lowering or with greater lowering of low relative to high frequencies (Allen, Strong, and Palmer, 1981; Reed et al., 1983). Improvements in the ability to identify frequency-warped speech with training have been noted for normal and hearing-impaired listeners (Reed et al., 1985). Improved ability to discriminate and identify high-frequency consonants has been demonstrated with such warping transformations compared to low-pass filtering for substantial reductions in bandwidth (up to a factor of 4 or 5). Overall performance, however, is similar for lowering and low-pass filtering, owing to reduced performance for the lowering schemes on sounds with substantial low-frequency energy.

Summary and Conclusions

Attempts at frequency lowering through a variety of different methods have met with only limited success. Frequency lowering leads to a reduction in bandwidth of the original speech signal and to the creation of new speech codes which may sound unnatural to the untrained ear. Evidence from a number of different studies indicates that performance on frequency-lowered speech can improve with familiarization and training in the use of frequency-lowered speech. Many of these same studies, however, also indicate that even after extended practice, performance with the coded speech signals does not exceed that achieved with appropriate baseline conditions (e.g., speech filtered to an equivalent bandwidth in normal-hearing listeners or conventional amplification with appropriate frequency gain characteristics in hearing-impaired listeners). Although frequency-lowering techniques can lead to large improvements in the reception of high-frequency sounds, they may at the same time lead to detrimental effects on the reception of vowels and consonants whose spectral energy is concentrated at low frequencies. Because of the need to use the region of low-frequency residual hearing for recoding high-frequency sounds, the low-frequency components of speech may be altered as well through the overlaying of coded signals onto the original unprocessed speech or through wholesale lowering of the entire speech signal. In listeners with high-frequency impairment accompanied by good residual hearing in the low frequencies, benefits for frequency lowering have been observed for listeners with severe to profound high-frequency loss using mild degrees of lowering (no greater than 30% reduction in bandwidth). For children with profound deafness (whose residual low-frequency hearing may be quite limited), frequency lowering appears to be more effective as a speech production training aid for specific groups of phonemes rather than as a speech perception aid.

—*Charlotte M. Reed and Louis D. Braida*

References

Allen, D. R., Strong, W. J., and Palmer, E. P. (1981). Experiments on the intelligibility of low-frequency speech codes. *Journal of the Acoustical Society of America, 70*, 1248–1255.

Bennett, D. N., and Byers, V. W. (1967). Increased intelligibility in the hypacusic by slow-play frequency transposition. *Journal of Auditory Research, 7*, 107–118.

Braida, L. D., Durlach, N. I., Lippmann, R. P., Hicks, B. L., Rabinowitz, W. M., and Reed, C. M. (1979). *Hearing aids: A review of past research on linear amplification, amplitude compression, and frequency lowering* (ASHA Monograph No. 19). Rockville, MD: American Speech and Hearing Association.

Daniloff, R. G., Shriner, T. H., and Zemlin, W. R. (1968). Intelligibility of vowels altered in duration and frequency. *Journal of the Acoustical Society of America, 44*, 700–707.

Davis-Penn, W., and Ross, M. (1993). Pediatric experiences with frequency transposing. *Hearing Instruments, 44*, 26–32.

Dudley, H. (1939). Remaking speech. *Journal of the Acoustical Society of America, 11*, 169–177.

Fairbanks, G., Everitt, W. L., and Jaeger, R. P. (1954). Method for time or frequency compression-expansion of speech. *IRE Transactions on Audio, AU-2*, 7–12.

Fu, Q. J., and Shannon, R. V. (1999). Recognition of spectrally degraded and frequency-shifted vowels in acoustic and electric hearing. *Journal of the Acoustical Society of America, 105*, 1889–1900.

Guttman, N., Levitt, H., and Bellefleur, P. (1970). Articulation training of the deaf using low-frequency surrogate fricatives. *Journal of Speech and Hearing Research, 13*, 19–29.

Guttman, N., and Nelson, J. R. (1968). An instrument that creates some artificial speech spectra for the severely hard of hearing. *American Annals of the Deaf, 113*, 295–302.

Hogan, C. A., and Turner, C. W. (1998). High-frequency audibility: Benefits for hearing-impaired listeners. *Journal of the Acoustical Society of America, 104*, 432–441.

Johansson, B. (1966). The use of the transposer for the management of the deaf child. *International Audiology, 5*, 362–373.

Ling, D. (1968). Three experiments on frequency transposition. *American Annals of the Deaf, 113*, 283–294.

Ling, D., and Druz, W. S. (1967). Transposition of high-frequency sounds by partial vocoding of the speech spectrum: Its use by deaf children. *Journal of Auditory Research, 7*, 133–144.

MacArdle, B. M., West, C., Bradley, J., Worth, S., Mackenzie, J., and Bellman, S. C. (2001). A study of the application of a frequency transposition hearing system in children. *British Journal of Audiology, 35*, 17–29.

Mazor, M., Simon, H., Scheinberg, J., and Levitt, H. (1977). Moderate frequency compression for the moderately hearing impaired. *Journal of the Acoustical Society of America, 62*, 1273–1278.

McDermott, H. J., and Dean, M. R. (2000). Speech perception with steeply sloping hearing loss: Effects of frequency transposition. *British Journal of Audiology, 34*, 353–361.

McDermott, H. J., Dorkos, V. P., Dean, M. R., and Ching, T. Y. C. (1999). Improvements in speech perception with use of the AVR TranSonic frequency-transposing hearing aid. *Journal of Speech, Language, and Hearing Research, 42*, 1323–1335.

Nagafuchi, M. (1976). Intelligibility of distorted speech sounds shifted in frequency and time in normal children. *Audiology, 15*, 326–337.

Parent, T. C., Chmiel, R., and Jerger, J. (1997). Comparison of performance with frequency transposition hearing aids and conventional hearing aids. *Journal of the American Academy of Audiology, 8*, 355–365.

Posen, M. P., Reed, C. M., and Braida, L. D. (1993). Intelligibility of frequency-lowered speech produced by a channel vocoder. *Journal of Rehabilitation Research and Development, 30*, 26–38.

Raymond, T. H., and Proud, G. O. (1962). Audiofrequency conversion. *Archives of Otolaryngology, 76*, 60–70.

Reed, C. M., Hicks, B. L., Braida, L. D., and Durlach, N. I. (1983). Discrimination of speech processed by low-pass filtering and pitch-invariant frequency lowering. *Journal of the Acoustical Society of America, 74*, 409–419.

Reed, C. M., Schultz, K. I., Braida, L. D., and Durlach, N. I. (1985). Discrimination and identification of frequency-lowered speech in listeners with high-frequency hearing impairment. *Journal of the Acoustical Society of America, 78,* 2139–2141.

Rees, R., and Velmans, M. (1993). The effect of frequency transposition on the untrained auditory discrimination of congenitally deaf children. *British Journal of Audiology, 27,* 53–60.

Takefuta, Y., and Swigart, E. (1968). Intelligibility of speech signals spectrally compressed by a sampling-synthesizer technique. *IEEE Transactions on Auditory Electroacoustics, AU-16,* 271–274.

Tiffanny, W. R., and Bennett, D. N. (1961). Intelligibility of slow played speech. *Journal of Speech and Hearing Research, 4,* 248–258.

Turner, C. W., and Hurtig, R. R. (1999). Proportional frequency compression of speech for listeners with sensorineural hearing loss. *Journal of the Acoustical Society of America, 106,* 877–886.

Velmans, M. L. (1973). Speech imitation in simulated deafness, using visual cues and "recoded" auditory information. *Language and Speech, 16,* 224–236.

Wang, M. D., Reed, C. M., and Bilger, R. C. (1978). A comparison of the effects of filtering and sensorineural hearing loss on patterns of consonant confusions. *Journal of Speech and Hearing Research, 21,* 5–36.

Further Readings

Beasley, D. S., Mosher, N. L., and Orchik, D. J. (1976). Use of frequency shifted/time compressed speech with hearing-impaired children. *Audiology, 15,* 395–406.

Block, von R., and Boerger, G. (1980). Hörverbessernde Verfahren mit Bandbreitenkompression. *Acustica, 45,* 294–303.

Boothroyd, A., and Medwetsky, L. (1992). Spectral distribution of /s/ and the frequency-response of hearing aids. *Ear and Hearing, 13,* 150–157.

Ching, T. Y. C., Dillon, H., and Byrne, D. (1998). Speech recognition of hearing-impaired listeners: Predictions from audibility and the limited role of high-frequency amplification. *Journal of the Acoustical Society of America, 103,* 1128–1140.

David, E. E., and McDonald, H. S. (1956). Note on pitch-synchronous processing of speech. *Journal of the Acoustical Society of America, 28,* 1261–1266.

Denes, P. B. (1967). On the motor theory of speech perception. In W. W. Dunn (Ed.), *Models for the perception of speech and visual form* (pp. 309–314). Cambridge, MA: MIT Press.

Foust, K. O., and Gengel, R. W. (1973). Speech discrimination by sensorineural hearing impaired persons using a transposer hearing aid. *Scandinavian Audiology, 2,* 161–170.

Hicks, B. L., Braida, L. D., and Durlach, N. I. (1981). Pitch-invariant frequency lowering with nonuniform spectral compression. *Proceedings of the IEEE International Conference on Acoustics, Speech, and Signal Processing* (pp. 121–124). New York: IEEE.

Ling, D. (1972). Auditory discrimination of speech transposed by a sample-and-hold process. In G. Fant (Ed.), *Proceedings of the International Symposium on Speech Communication and Profound Deafness, Stockholm* (1970) (pp. 323–333). Washington, DC: A.G. Bell Association.

Oppenheim, A. V., and Johnson, D. H. (1972). Discrete representation of signals. *Proceedings of the IEEE, 60,* 681–691.

Reed, C. M., Power, M. H., Durlach, N. I., Braida, L. D., Foss, K. K., Reid, J. A., et al. (1991). Development and testing of low-frequency speech codes. *Journal of Rehabilitation Research and Development, 28,* 67–82.

Risberg, A. (1965). The transposer and a model for speech perception. *STL-QPSR, 4,* 26–30. Stockholm: KTH.

Rosenhouse, J. (1990). A new transposition device for the deaf. *Hearing Journal, 43,* 20–25.

Sher, A. E., and Owens, E. (1974). Consonant confusions associated with hearing loss above 2000 Hz. *Journal of Speech and Hearing Research, 17,* 669–681.

Zue, V. W. (1970). Translation of diver's speech using digital frequency warping. *MIT Research Laboratory of Electronics Quarterly Progress Report, 101,* 175–182.

Functional Hearing Loss in Children

Functional hearing loss (FHL) is frequently forgotten or misdiagnosed in the pediatric population, despite the fact that it is well documented (Bowdler and Rogers, 1989). The diagnosis is often missed in children because of lack of awareness of its manifestations (Pracy et al., 1996), its incidence (Barr, 1963), and its multiple causes (Broad, 1980).

Functional hearing loss is one of several terms used to describe a hearing loss that cannot be ascribed to an organic cause (Aplin and Rowson, 1986). In FHL, actual audiometric thresholds are inconsistent with the voluntary thresholds of a patient. The term *pseudohypacusis* was coined by Carhart (1961) to describe a condition in which a person presents with a hearing loss not consistent with clinical or audiologic evaluation. *Nonorganic hearing loss* is used interchangeably with FHL and pseudohypacusis in that these terms do not comment on the intent, conscious or subconscious, of the patient being tested (Radkowski, Cleveland, and Friedman, 1998). Terms such as *psychogenic hearing loss* and *conversion deafness* imply that the cause of the auditory disturbance is psychological, whereas *malingering* suggests the conscious and deliberate adoption or fabrication of a hearing loss for personal gain (Stark, 1966). FHL often appears as an overlay on an organic impairment. As such, the term *functional overlay* is used to describe an exaggeration of an existing hearing loss.

The incidence of FHL in children is not well documented. Valid estimates are lacking, owing to lack of consensus on the definition of FHL and the absence of a concerted effort to collect such data. Estimates range from 1% to 12%, but the validity of these figures is undermined by the lack of standard criteria for diagnosing FHL in children (Broad, 1980). Pracy et al. (1996) suggest that the incidence is higher than expected and cannot be compared with the reported incidence in adults. A number of studies that do report incidence suggest that FHL occurs more than twice as often in girls as in boys (Dixon and Newby, 1959; Brockman and Hoversten, 1960; Campanelli, 1963). In pediatric studies of FHL, the condition is typically diagnosed in adolescence (Berger, 1965; Radkowski, Cleveland, and Friedman, 1998).

The ability to describe a characteristic audiometric and behavioral profile of FHL in children is made problematic by its multiple manifestations and definitions. Aplin and Rowson (1990) described four subgroups of FHL: (1) cases involving emotional problems that typically preceded the audiologic examination; (2) cases in which mild anxiety or conscious mechanisms produce a hearing loss during an audiologic examination; (3) cases of malingering (the hearing loss is deliberately and consciously assumed for the purposes of financial gain); and (4) cases in which the audiologic discrepancies are artifactual as a result of lack of understanding or inattention during audiometric testing.

The hallmark of FHL in children is inconsistency in audiometric test results. The diagnosis of FHL in children is generally easier than in adults, because children are less able to consistently produce erroneous results on repeated testing (Pracy et al., 1996). A common presentation of possible FHL is the child who demonstrates no difficulty in conversational speech but has a voluntary pure-tone audiogram that suggests difficulty in speech recognition (Stark, 1966). Speech audiometric results that are better than the pure-tone results are another common indicator of FHL in children (Aplin and Rowson, 1990). Behavioral responses to speech audiometry typical of FHL in children include responding to only one syllable of a test word or to only one phoneme presented at a given intensity (Pracy et al., 1996). Hosoi, Tsuta, Murata, and Levitt (1999) reported several indicators of FHL in children seen during audiometric testing. These indicators included (1) poor test-retest reliability, (2) a saucer-shaped audiometric configuration, (3) the absence of a shadow curve with a severe to profound unilateral hearing loss, and (4) a discrepancy between the speech reception threshold and the pure-tone average.

Misunderstanding, confusion, or unfamiliarity with the test directions or procedures must be determined before further testing for FHL is initiated. After reinstruction, modification of speech audiometry is undertaken when FHL in a child is suspected. Pracy et al. (1996) described successful use of the Fournier technique (1956), in which the level of speech presentation is varied, thereby tricking the patient into responding at a level at which he or she had not previously responded. Other techniques using speech audiometry include use of an ascending threshold determination technique (Harris, 1958) and presentation of informal conversation at levels below the voluntary pure-tone thresholds.

Hosoi et al. (1999) proposed suggestion audiometry as a useful technique to detect FHL in children as well as to determine true hearing levels. In suggestion audiometry, standard audiometric procedures are preceded by an information session on the benefits of using a hearing aid. The child is shown a hearing aid, given information about it, and ultimately wears the hearing aid in the off position during testing. The hearing aid is without tubing or an earmold; consequently, the earphone used during testing is placed over the auricle with the hearing aid. Hosoi et al. found that 16 of 20 children diagnosed with FHL showed a significant change in hearing level following the suggestion technique.

The use of adult-oriented tests of pseudohypacusis has had limited success in children demonstrating FHL. The Stenger test (Chaiklin and Ventry, 1965), while easy

to conduct, is appropriate only for unilateral hearing losses. The Doerfler-Stewart test (1946), Bekesy audiometry (Jerger and Herer, 1961), and the Lombard test (Black, 1951) require special equipment and are rarely used in adults in the twenty-first century.

Cross-check procedures such as otoacoustic emissions and acoustic reflex testing can be used to determine the reliability of pure-tone thresholds (Radkowski, Cleveland, and Friedman, 1998). However, for actual threshold determination, the auditory brainstem response (ABR) measurement has been shown to be effective. Yoshida, Noguchi, and Uemura (1989) performed ABR audiometry with 39 school-age children presenting with suspected FHL and found normal hearing in 65 ears of 35 patients. Although ABR audiometry is not a hearing test, Sanders and Lazenby (1983) suggest it can be a powerful tool in the identification and quantification of FHL.

After detecting FHL and determining true hearing levels, Hosoi, Murata, and Levitt (1999) suggest it is essential that information about the cause of the functional hearing loss be obtained. Reports on FHL in children cite lack of attention, deflection of attention, school difficulties, a history of abuse, and emotional problems as possible causes, among others.

Barr (1963) found that the extra attention paid to children because of their purported hearing difficulty had encouraged them, consciously or unconsciously, to feign hearing loss. Children with previous knowledge of ear problems may use lack of hearing and withdrawal from communication as a response to problems experienced at school (Aplin and Rowson, 1986). A history of trauma immediately preceding the complaint of hearing loss was reported in 18 patients studied by Radkowski, Cleveland, and Friedman (1998). Drake et al. (1995) found that FHL may be an indicator of child abuse.

A high suspicion in approaching children will not delay early intervention in cases of an organic hearing loss, but failure to recognize FHL can be costly and potentially hazardous to the pediatric patient (Radkowski, Cleveland, and Friedman, 1998). Unnecessary radiographic studies or exploratory surgical intervention, inappropriate amplification, and financial and psychosocial costs are among the possible outcomes of inappropriate diagnosis of FHL in children. Spraggs, Burton, and Graham (1994) reported on five adult patients who underwent assessment for cochlear implantation and were found to have nonorganic hearing loss. Similar findings have not been reported in the pediatric population, but with the proliferation of cochlear implants in children, accurate diagnosis of hearing loss is essential.

Once the diagnosis of FHL in a child has been established, a nonconfrontational approach is recommended. Giving the child the opportunity to "save face" often can be achieved with reinstructing, reassuring, retesting, and convincing the child that the hearing loss will improve. Retesting with accurate results is often accomplished during one visit but may require follow-up visits.

Labeling the child a malingerer is detrimental to the child and decreases the probability of obtaining accurate behavioral thresholds. If the child is labeled as exhibiting FHL, the chance to back out gracefully is lost, and the functional component of the hearing loss may be solidified (Pracy et al., 1996). Pracy and Bowdler (1996) advocate an approach that treats the child as if the hearing loss were real, followed by the use of speech audiometry techniques to determine actual hearing thresholds. In recalcitrant cases, ABR may be required for threshold determination. Psychiatric referral is rarely necessary or desirable and should be reserved only for the intractable child (Bowdler and Rogers, 1989).

—*Patricia McCarthy*

References

Aplin, D., and Rowson, V. (1986). Personality and functional hearing loss in children. *British Journal of Clinical Psychology, 25*, 313–314.

Aplin, D., and Rowson, V. (1990). Psychological characteristics of children with functional hearing loss. *British Journal of Audiology, 24*, 77–87.

Barr, B. (1963). Psychogenic deafness in school children. *Audiology, 2*, 125–128.

Berger, K. (1965). Nonorganic hearing loss in children. *Laryngoscope, 75*, 447–457.

Black, J. (1951). The effect of delayed side-tone upon vocal rate and intensity. *Journal of Speech and Hearing Disorders, 16*, 56–60.

Bowdler, D., and Rogers, J. (1989). The management of pseudohypacusis in school-age children. *Clinical Otolaryngology and Allied Sciences, 14*, 211–215.

Broad, R. (1980). Developmental and psychodynamic issues related to causes of childhood functional hearing loss. *Child Psychiatry and Human Development, 11*, 49–58.

Brockman, S., and Hoversten, G. (1960). Pseudo-neural hypacusis in children. *Laryngoscope, 70*, 825–839.

Campanelli, P. (1963). Simulated hearing losses in school children following identification audiometry. *Journal of Auditory Research, 3*, 91–108.

Carhart, R. (1961). Tests for malingering. *Transactions of the American Academy of Opthalmology and Otolaryngology, 65*, 437.

Chaiklin, J., and Ventry, I. (1965). The efficiency of audiometric measures used to identify functional hearing loss. *Journal of Auditory Research, 5*, 219–230.

Dixon, R., and Newby, H. (1959). Children with non-organic hearing problems. *Archives of Otolaryngology, 70*, 619–623.

Doerfler, L., and Stewart, K. (1946). Malingering and psychogenic deafness. *Journal of Speech Disorders, 11*, 181–186.

Drake, A., Makielski, K., McDonald-Bell, C., and Atcheson, B. (1995). Two new otolaryngologic findings in child abuse. *Archives of Otolaryngology–Head and Neck Surgery, 121*, 1417–1420.

Fournier, J. (1956). La depistage de la stimulation auditive. In *Exposes annuels d'oto-rhino'laryngologie* (pp. 107–126). Paris: Masson.

Harris, D. (1958). A rapid and simple technique for the detection of non-organic hearing loss. *Archives Otolaryngology, 68*, 758–760.

Hosoi, H., Tsuta, Y., Murata, T., and Levitt, H. (1999). Suggestion audiometry for non-organic hearing loss (pseudohypoacusis) in children. *International Journal of Pediatric Otorhinolaryngology, 47*, 11–21.

Jerger, J., and Herer, G. (1961). An unexpected dividend in Bekesy audiometry. *Journal of Speech and Hearing Disorders, 26*, 390–391.

Pracy, J., and Bowdler, D. (1996). Pseudohypacusis in children. *Clinical Otolaryngology and Allied Sciences, 21*, 383–384.

Pracy, J., Walsh, R., Mepham, G., and Bowdler, D. (1996). Childhood pseudohypacusis. *International Journal of Pediatric Otorhinolaryngology, 37*, 143–149.

Radkowski, D., Cleveland, S., and Friedman, E. (1998). Childhood pseudohypacusis inpatients with high risk for actual hearing loss. *Larygoscope, 108*, 1534–1538.

Sanders, J., and Lazenby, B. (1983). Auditory brain stem response measurement in the assessment of pseudohypoacusis. *American Journal of Otology, 4*, 292–299.

Spraggs, P., Burton, M., and Graham, J. (1994). Nonorganic hearing loss in cochlear implant candidates. *American Journal of Otology, 15*, 652–657.

Stark, E. (1966). Functional hearing loss in children. *Illinois Medical Journal, 130*, 628–631.

Yoshida, M., Noguchi, A., and Uemura, T. (1989). Functional hearing loss in children. *International Journal of Pediatric Otorhinolaryngology, 17*, 287–295.

Further Readings

Hayes, R. (1992). Non-organic hearing loss in young persons. *British Journal of Audiology, 26*, 347–350.

Noble, W. (1987). The conceptual problem of functional hearing loss. *British Journal of Audiology, 21*, 1–3.

Ventry, I., and Chaiklin, J. (1965). Multidiscipline study of functional hearing loss. *Journal of Auditory Research, 5*, 179–272.

Genetics and Craniofacial Anomalies

Genetic factors contribute to more than half of all congenital hearing losses and are also responsible for later-onset hearing losses. Understanding the factors underlying hereditary hearing loss requires locating the genes responsible for hearing loss and defining the specific mechanisms and functions of those genes. From a clinical standpoint, this information may contribute to improved management strategies for individuals with hereditary hearing loss and their families. Accurate determination of the auditory characteristics associated with various genetic abnormalities requires the use of measures sensitive to subtle aspects of auditory function.

Hereditary Hearing Loss. Congenital (hereditary) hearing loss occurs in approximately 1–2 of 1000 births, and at least 50% of all cases of hearing loss have a genetic origin (Morton, 1991). Although hereditary hearing losses may occur in conjunction with other disorders as part of a syndrome, the majority of cases are nonsyndromic. Later-onset hereditary hearing loss occurs at various ages from the first decade to later in life.

Chromosomes. Human cells contain 23 pairs of chromosomes (22 pairs of autosomes and two sex chromosomes). Hereditary material in the form of DNA is carried as genes on chromosomes. Cells reproduce by mitosis (meiosis for the sex chromosomes), where chromosomes divide, resulting in two genetically similar cells. Errors can occur during mitotic or meiotic division, resulting in cells with chromosomal abnormalities and an individual with a chromosomal defect.

Genotype and Phenotype.   Genotype describes an individual's genetic constitution. Phenotype relates to the physical characteristics of an individual and can include information obtained from physiological, morphological, and biochemical studies. Auditory tests contribute to the phenotypic description.

Inheritance Patterns

Hereditary hearing loss follows several patterns of inheritance. Autosomal recessive inheritance occurs in 70%–80% of individuals with nonsyndromic hearing loss. To display a recessive trait, a person must acquire one abnormal gene for the trait from each parent. Parents are heterozygous for the trait since they each carry one abnormal gene and one normal gene. Thus, recessively inherited defects appear among the offspring of phenotypically normal parents who are both carriers of a single recessive gene for the trait. When both parents are carriers, the chance of a child receiving two copies of the abnormal gene and displaying the phenotype is 25%. The parents' chance of having a carrier child is 50%, and there is a 25% chance of having a child with no gene for the defect. In cases of nonsyndromic recessive hearing loss, a genetic source may be suspected in families with two or more occurrences of the disorder. Recessive inheritance occurs more commonly in nonsyndromic than in syndromic hearing loss.

In autosomal dominant inheritance, a single copy of an abnormal gene can result in hearing loss; thus, an affected parent has a 50% chance of passing that gene to their child. Autosomal dominant hereditary hearing loss occurs in approximately 15%–20% of nonsyndromic hearing loss and is more commonly associated with syndromic hearing loss. Other inheritance patterns that can result in hearing loss are X-linked, at a rate of 2%–3%, and mitochondrial, which occurs in less than 1% of cases.

Variability in Hereditary Hearing Loss.   Phenotypic and genetic heterogeneity is pronounced, with reports of more than 400 forms of syndromic and nonsyndromic hereditary hearing loss (Gorlin, Toriello, and Cohen, 1955). Considerable variation exists among hereditary hearing losses, between dominant and recessive hearing losses, among various forms of either recessive or dominant hearing loss, and even among persons with the same genetic mutations. Furthermore, the same genes have been found responsible for both syndromic and nonsyndromic hearing loss, and have been associated with both autosomal dominant and recessive transmission.

Hereditary hearing losses range from mild to profound (Nance and Sweeney, 1975). In subjects with autosomal recessive nonsyndromic hereditary hearing loss, onset of the hearing loss tends to be congenital, severe to profound in degree, stable over time, and af-

fecting all frequencies (Liu and Xu, 1994). Autosomal dominant nonsyndromic hereditary hearing loss tends to be less severe, more often delayed in onset, progressive, and affecting high frequencies. Patients with X-linked hearing loss generally have prelingual onset but are clinically diverse.

Mutations in the *GJB2* (connexin 26) gene may explain greater than 50% of autosomal recessive deafness in some populations (Zelante et al., 1997). The *GJB2* gene encodes the protein connexin 26 (Cx26), thought to be essential for maintenance of high potassium in the scala media of the inner ear. Several mutations in the *GJB2* gene have been associated with hearing loss, and mutation sites vary among world populations. A 35delG mutation is common in some Mediterranean-based populations (Denoyelle et al., 1997), while a 167delT mutation is most common in the Ashkenazi Jewish population (Morell et al., 1998). Cx26 mutations are generally responsible for recessive deafness, although they have been observed in dominant deafness.

Hearing losses associated with Cx26 mutations are cochlear in nature but vary widely in degree, ranging from mild to profound, and stability (e.g., Cohn et al., 1999; Denoyelle et al., 1999; Mueller et al., 1999; Wilcox et al., 2000). Hearing losses resulting from the same genetic mutations show wide variability in degree and progression. Furthermore, audiometric characteristics are not directly linked to a particular type of mutation (e.g., Cohn et al., 1999; Sobe et al., 2000).

Chromosomal Defects.   Down syndrome is the most common autosomal defect. The affected individual has an additional chromosome 21 (trisomy 21), for a total of 47 chromosomes, or a translocation trisomy. Down syndrome is characterized by mental retardation and a number of craniofacial and other characteristics. Hearing loss may be congenital, sensory, and there is a high incidence of middle ear disorders. Trisomy 13 and 18 syndromes, less common and with more dramatic abnormalities, are characterized by inner ear dysplasias involving the organ of Corti and stria vacularis, external and middle ear malformations, cleft lip and palate, and other defects.

Syndromes Associated with Hearing Loss

There are far too many syndromes associated with hearing loss to include in this brief entry. A useful method of classifying hearing loss was provided by Konigsmark and Gorlin (1976), where genetic and metabolic hearing losses were divided into major categories depending on the organ system or metabolic defect involved.

Usher syndrome is the most common syndrome associated with hearing loss and eye abnormalities, specifically retinitis pigmentosa. There are several types and subtypes and various genetic loci. Other syndromes involving vision are Cockayne syndrome and Alstrom disease, associated with retinal disorders. Treacher Collins syndrome, Goldenhar syndrome (hemifacial microsomia), Crouzon syndrome (craniofacial dysostosis), Apert syndrome, otopalatal-digital syndrome, and osteogenesis imperfecta are all associated with musculoskeletal disease.

Waardenburg syndrome, characterized by displaced medial canthi, white forelock, heterochromia, and broad nasal root, is the most prominent hearing syndrome involving the integumentary system. Alport syndrome is a combination of progressive hearing loss, progressive renal disease, and ocular lens abnormalities. Pendred syndrome, mucopolysaccharidosis, and Jervell and Lange-Nielsen syndrome are associated with metabolic and other abnormalities. The diverse syndromes associated with neurological disorders include Friedreich ataxia and acoustic neuromas and neural deafness.

Craniofacial anomalies associated with hearing loss may be sporadic, inherited, due to disturbances during embryonic development, of toxic origin, or related to chromosomal abnormalities. These maldevelopments may be of unknown origin or related to known syndromes.

Inner ear dysplasias include Michel deafness, which is rare and involves complete inner ear dysplasia, Mondini deafness, and Scheibe deafness (Schuknecht, 1974). In Mondini deafness, the bony cochlear capsule is flattened, with underdevelopment of the apical turn of the cochlea and possible saccular and endolymphatic involvement. Hearing loss is typically moderate to profound but varies widely. Scheibe deafness involves the membranous portion of the cochlea and saccule, greater in basal portions, and is the most common of the inner ear dysplasias.

External and middle ear anomalies are associated with improper development of the first and second branchial clefts and arches, which are also responsible for lower jaw and other structures. Middle ear abnormalities include absence or fusion of the ossicles or abnormalities of the eustachian tube or middle ear cavity. Middle ear anomalies may be suspected whenever other branchial arch anomalies such as external ear atresia, cleft palate, micrognathia, Treacher Collins syndrome, Pierre Robin syndrome, and low-set auricles are present. Skeletal defects, such as those associated with Apert syndrome, Klippel-Feil syndrome, and Paget disease, and connective tissue disorders, such as those related to Hunter-Hurler or Möbius syndromes, may also indicate the presence of middle ear anomalies. Maldevelopment of the external ear includes preauricular tags, microtic or deformed pinna, or partial or complete atresia of the external canal. The presence of external or middle ear anomalies may indicate additional malformations or reduced hearing, depending on the structures and degree of involvement.

Evaluation and Classification of Hearing Loss

The characteristics of a hearing loss are important in understanding relationships, or lack of relationships, between genotype and phenotype. The audiogram provides a general description of the degree, configuration, fre-

quency range, type, and progression of a hearing loss, and whether one or both ears are affected. Other, more sensitive measures (such as otoacoustic emissions, efferent reflexes, and auditory-evoked potentials) are necessary to understand the nature of a hearing loss in more detail.

The majority of hereditary hearing losses are nonsyndromic, with no associated disorders that might raise the index of suspicion or aid in diagnosis. Furthermore, since the majority of nonsyndromic hearing losses are recessively inherited, parents are not affected by hearing loss. There may be no history of hearing loss in the family, so this risk factor would not be an indicator to raise suspicion of hearing loss. Thus, identification of nonsyndromic, and particularly recessively inherited, hearing loss is particularly challenging clinically.

See also SPEECH DISORDERS: GENETIC TRANSMISSION.

—*Linda J. Hood*

References

Cohn, E. S., Kelley, P. M., Fowler, T. W., et al. (1999). Clinical studies of families with hearing loss attributable to mutations in the connexin 26 gene (GJB2/DFNB1). *Pediatrics, 103,* 546–550.

Denoyelle, F., Martin, S., Weil, D., et al. (1999). Clinical features of the prevalent form of childhood deafness, DFNB1, due to a connexin-26 gene defect: Implications for genetic counseling. *Lancet, 353,* 1298–1303.

Denoyelle, F., Weil, D., Maw, M. A., et al. (1997). Prelingual deafness: High prevalence of a 30delG mutation in the connexin 26 gene. *Human Molecular Genetics, 6,* 2173–2177.

Gorlin, R. J., Toriello, H. V., and Cohen, M. M. (1955). *Hereditary hearing loss and its syndromes.* Oxford: Oxford University Press.

Konigsmark, B. W., and Gorlin, R. J. (1976). *Genetic and metabolic deafness.* Philadelphia: Saunders.

Liu, X., and Xu, L. (1994). Nonsyndromic hearing loss: An analysis of audiograms. *Annals of Otology, Rhinology, and Laryngology, 103,* 428–433.

Morell, R., Kim, H. J., Hood, L. J., et al. (1998). Mutations in the connexin 26 gene (GJB2) among Ashkenazi Jews with nonsyndromic recessive deafness. *New England Journal of Medicine, 339,* 1500–1505.

Morton, N. E. (1991). Genetic epidemiology of hearing impairment. In R. J. Ruben, T. R. van de Water, and K. P. Steel (Eds.), *Genetics of hearing impairment. Annals of the New York Academy of Sciences, 630,* 16–31.

Mueller, R. F., Nehammer, A., Middleton, A., et al. (1999). Congenital non-syndromal sensorineural hearing impairment due to connexin 26 gene mutations: Molecular and audiological findings. *International Journal of Pediatric Otorhinolaryngology, 50,* 3–13.

Nance, W. E., and Sweeney, A. (1975). Genetic factors in deafness of early life. *Otolaryngolic Clinics of North America, 8,* 19–48.

Schuknecht, H. F. (1974). *Pathology of the ear.* Cambridge, MA: Harvard University Press.

Sobe, T., Vreugde, S., Shahin, H., et al. (2000). The prevalence and expression of inherited connexin 26 mutations associated with nonsyndromic hearing loss in the Israeli population. *Human Genetics, 106,* 50–57.

Wilcox, S. A., Saunders, K., Osborn, A. H., et al. (2000). High frequency hearing loss correlated with mutations in the GJB2 gene. *Human Genetics, 106,* 399–405.

Zelante, L., Gasparini, P., Estivill, X., et al. (1997). Connexin 26 mutations associated with the most common form of non-syndromic neurosensory autosomal recessive deafness (DFNB1) in Mediterraneans. *Human Molecular Genetics, 6,* 1605–1609.

Hearing Aid Fitting: Evaluation of Outcomes

The outcomes of hearing aid fitting can be assessed in terms of the technical merit of the device in situ or in terms of the extent to which the device alleviates the daily problems of the hearing-impaired person and his or her family. Early efforts to measure outcomes focused mainly on technical merit. It was assumed that if the instrument was technically superior, real-life outcomes would be proportionately superior. However, this is not always the case. Real-life problems associated with hearing impairment are complicated by issues such as personality, lifestyle, environment, and family dynamics. Thus, it is now recognized that real-life outcomes of a fitting must be assessed separately from the technical adequacy of the hearing aid. These two types of outcomes are evaluated at different times after fitting. Technical merit data are often obtained as part of the verification process conducted immediately after fitting. Sometimes these data may prompt modifications of the fitting. Alleviation of real-life problems is evaluated after the hearing-impaired person has had time to use the hearing aid on a daily basis. This evaluation is usually made after at least 2 weeks of use of the device.

Evaluation of Technical Merit

The technical merit of a fitted hearing aid may be reflected in both acoustical and psychoacoustical data. Acoustical outcomes include real ear probe microphone measures (such as insertion gain, aided response, and saturation response) and audibility measures (such as articulation index and speech intelligibility index). Psychoacoustical outcomes include speech recognition scores, aided loudness assessment, and ratings of quality, clarity, pleasantness, or other dimensions.

Real ear probe microphone measures provide information about the sound delivered to the eardrum of the particular patient (e.g., Mueller, Hawkins, and Northern, 1992). This takes into consideration the physical differences among patients and the differences between real ears and standard couplers such as the 2 cm^3 couplers used in the ANSI measurement standard (American National Standards Institute [ANSI], 1996). One advantage of these measures is their ability to confirm the extent to which the fitting is congruent with prescriptive fitting target values. Real ear probe microphone data are also valuable for troubleshooting fitting problems.

Audibility measures usually combine information about the availability of amplified acoustical speech cues with weighting factors proportional to the importance of those cues for speech recognition. The availability of cues may be limited by sensitivity thresholds or competing noises, as well as by the speech level. The importance of cues for speech intelligibility varies with frequency and type of speech. Studies of normal-hearing listeners and listeners with mild to moderate hearing impairments have shown that measures of weighted audibility can provide rather accurate predictions of speech intelligibility scores for these individuals in a laboratory setting. There are several well-researched approaches to obtaining audibility measures (e.g., Studebaker, 1992; ANSI, 1997). Some methods incorporate the effects of age, speech level, or hearing loss to improve the accuracy of speech intelligibility predictions for elderly hearing-impaired listeners who are exposed to high-level amplified speech.

Measuring the recognition of amplified speech is perhaps the most venerable approach to evaluating hearing aid fitting outcomes. Many standardized tests are available, in both open-set and closed-set varieties, with stimuli ranging from nonsense syllables to sentences. The popularity of speech intelligibility testing as a measure of outcome is rooted in its high level of face validity. The most frequently cited reason for obtaining amplification is a need to improve communication ability. A measure of improved speech understanding consequent on hearing aid fitting addresses that need in an attractively direct manner. For many years, this measure was the bedrock of hearing aid fitting outcome evaluation. Unfortunately, in order to achieve a useful level of statistical power, speech intelligibility tests must include a large number of test items. This requirement has limited the recent use of speech intelligibility testing mostly to research applications (e.g., Gatehouse, 1998).

The importance of producing amplified sounds that are acceptably loud has long been recognized. Although using loudness data to facilitate fitting protocols has been advocated for many years, interest in measuring the loudness of amplified sounds following the fitting has burgeoned since the widespread acceptance of wide dynamic range compression devices. With these instruments, it is appealing to assess the extent to which environmental sounds, including speech, have been "normalized" by amplification. Interest in this type of outcome data is increasing, and some of the measurement issues have been addressed (e.g., Cox and Gray, 2001).

Formal ratings of aspects of amplified sounds, such as quality, clarity, distortion, and the like, have been used frequently in assessing technical merit in research applications but have not often been advocated for clinical use. These types of measures are commonly performed with listeners supplying a rating on a semantic differential scale, such as the 11-point version developed by Gabrielsson and Sjogren (1979). This approach has the advantage of permitting quantification of dimensions of amplified sounds that are not psychoacoustically accessible via other metrics.

Evaluation of Real-World Impact

The real-life effectiveness of a hearing aid is measured using subjective data provided by the hearing-impaired person or significant others. Numerous questionnaires have been developed and standardized specifically for the purpose of assessing hearing aid fitting outcomes, and many others have been conscripted to serve this application (Noble, 1998; Bentler and Kramer, 2000). In addition to standardized questionnaires, there is strong support for use of personalized instruments in which the patient identifies the items and thus creates a customized questionnaire (e.g., Dillon, James, and Ginis, 1997). Regardless of which type of inventory is used, there are at least seven different domains of subjective outcomes of hearing aid fitting that can be assessed. They include residual activity limitations, residual participation restrictions, impact on others, use, benefit, satisfaction, and quality-of-life changes. Most inventories do not assess all of these domains.

Residual activity limitations are the difficulties the hearing aid wearer continues to have in everyday tasks such as understanding speech, localizing sounds, and the like. The activity limitations experienced by a specific individual will depend on the demands of that person's lifestyle. Residual participation restrictions are the unresolved problems or barriers the hearing aid wearer encounters to involvement in situations of daily life. This also differs with individuals but can include such circumstances as participation in church services, bridge clubs, and so on. ICF (2001) provides a full discussion of activity limitations and participation restrictions.

Hearing impairment often places a heavy burden on the family and friends as well as on the involved individual. In fact, encouragement (or compulsion) by significant others is sometimes the major factor prompting an individual to seek a hearing aid. The relief provided by amplification for the problems in the family constellation (i.e., the impact on others) is an important outcome dimension but one that has received relatively little attention to date.

A measure of benefit quantifies change in a hearing-related dimension of functioning as a result of using amplification. Benefit may be measured directly, in terms of degree of change (small versus large), or it may be computed by comparing aided and unaided performance on a particular dimension. Typical dimensions on which subjective benefit is measured are activity limitations and participation restrictions. Hearing-specific questionnaires are typically used to quantify hearing aid benefit.

Sometimes general, non-hearing-specific questionnaires are used to determine changes that result from hearing aid provision. These types of data tend to be interpreted as reflecting changes in general quality of life. A recent large-scale study found that hearing aid use was significantly associated with improvements in many aspects of life, including social life and mental health (Kochkin and Rogin, 2000). Despite the importance of these effects for individuals, functional health status measures that are often used to gauge quality of life tend not to be sensitive to the changes that result from hearing aid use (Bess, 2000).

It is not unusual to observe that an individual who reports substantial hearing aid benefit is nevertheless not satisfied with the device or does not use amplification very often. These observations suggest that daily use and hearing aid satisfaction are additional, distinct dimensions of real-world outcome that require separate assessment (e.g., Cox and Alexander, 1999).

Relationship Between Technical Merit and Real-World Impact

Numerous studies have shown that measures of technical merit are not strongly predictive of real-world outcomes of hearing aid fitting (e.g., Souza et al., 2000; Walden et al., 2000). Principal components analyses in studies using multiple outcome measures often show that the two types of measures tend to occupy separate factors (e.g., Humes, 1999). Many researchers feel that both types of data are essential for a full description of hearing aid fitting outcome.

See also HEARING AIDS: PRESCRIPTIVE FITTING.

—Robyn M. Cox

References

American National Standards Institute. (1996). *American National Standard Specification of Hearing Aid Characteristics (ANSI S3.22–1996)*. New York: Acoustical Society of America.

American National Standards Institute. (1997). *American National Standards Method for the Calculation of the Speech Intelligibility Index (ANSI S3.5–1997)*. New York: Acoustical Society of America.

Bentler, R. A., and Kramer, S. E. (2000). Guidelines for choosing a self-report outcome measure. *Ear and Hearing, 21*(4, Suppl.), 37S–49S.

Bess, F. H. (2000). The role of generic health-related quality of life measures in establishing audiological rehabilitation outcomes. *Ear and Hearing, 21*(4, Suppl.), 74S–79S.

Cox, R. M., and Alexander, G. C. (1999). Measuring satisfaction with amplification in daily life: The SADL Scale. *Ear and Hearing, 20*, 306–320.

Cox, R. M., and Gray, G. A. (2001). Verifying loudness perception after hearing aid fitting. *American Journal of Audiology, 10*, 91–98.

Dillon, H., James, A., and Ginis, J. (1997). The Client Oriented Scale of Improvement (COSI) and its relationship to several other measures of benefit and satisfaction provided by hearing aids. *Journal of the American Academy of Audiology, 8*, 27–43.

Gabrielsson, A., and Sjogren, H. (1979). Perceived sound quality of hearing aids. *Scandinavian Audiology, 8*, 159–169.

Gatehouse, S. (1998). Speech tests as measures of outcome. *Scandinavian Audiology, 27*(Suppl. 49), 54–60.

Humes, L. E. (1999). Dimensions of hearing aid outcome. *Journal of the American Academy of Audiology, 10*, 26–39.

ICF. (2001). *International Classification of Functioning, Disability, and Health*. Geneva: World Health Organization.

Kochkin, S., and Rogin, C. (2000). Quantifying the obvious: The impact of hearing instruments on quality of life. *Hearing Review, 7*, 6–34.

Mueller, H. G., Hawkins, D. B., and Northern, J. L. (1992). *Probe microphone measurements: Hearing aid selection and assessment.* San Diego, CA: Singular Publishing Group.

Noble, W. (1998). *Self-assessment of hearing and related functions.* London, U.K.: Whurr.

Souza, P. E., Yueh, B., Sarubbi, M., and Loovis, C. F. (2000). Fitting hearing aids with the Articulation Index: Impact on hearing aid effectiveness. *Journal of Rehabilitation Research and Development, 37,* 473–481.

Studebaker, G. A. (1992). The effect of equating loudness on audibility-based hearing aid selection procedures. *Journal of the American Academy of Audiology, 3,* 113–118.

Walden, B. E., Surr, R. K., Cord, M. T., Edwards, B., and Olsen, L. (2000). Comparison of benefits provided by different hearing aid technologies. *Journal of the American Academy of Audiology, 11,* 540–560.

Further Readings

Cox, R. M., and Alexander, G. C. (1995). The Abbreviated Profile of Hearing Aid Benefit. *Ear and Hearing, 16,* 176–186.

Cox, R. M., Alexander, G. C., and Gray, G. A. (1999). Personality and the subjective assessment of hearing aids. *Journal of the American Academy of Audiology, 10,* 1–13.

Dillon, H. (2001). Assessing the outcomes of hearing rehabilitation. In H. Dillon, *Hearing aids* (pp. 349–369). New York: Thieme.

Dillon, H., and So, M. (2000). Incentives and obstacles to the routine use of outcomes measures by clinicians. *Ear and Hearing, 21*(4, Suppl.), 2S–6S.

Gagne, J.-P., McDuff, S., and Getty, L. (1999). Some limitations of evaluative investigations based solely on normed outcome measures. *Journal of the American Academy of Audiology, 10,* 46–62.

Gatehouse, S. (1999). Glasgow Hearing Aid Benefit Profile: Derivation and validation of a client-centered outcome measure for hearing aid services. *Journal of the American Academy of Audiology, 10,* 80–103.

Humes, L. E., Halling, D., and Coughlin, M. (1996). Reliability and stability of various hearing-aid outcome measures in a group of elderly hearing-aid wearers. *Journal of Speech and Hearing Research, 39,* 923–935.

Kricos, P. B. (2000). The influence of non-audiological variables on audiological rehabilitation outcomes. *Ear and Hearing, 21*(4, Suppl.), 7S–14S.

Larson, V. D., Williams, D. W., Henderson, W. G., Luethke, L. E., Beck, L. B., Noffsinger, D., et al. (2000). Efficacy of 3 commonly used hearing aid circuits: A crossover trial. *Journal of the American Medical Association, 284,* 1806–1813.

Studebaker, G. A. (1991). Measures of intelligibility and quality. In G. A. Studebaker, F. H. Bess, and L. B. Beck (Eds.), *The Vanderbilt Hearing Aid Report II* (pp. 185–194). Parkton, MD: York Press.

Ventry, I. M., and Weinstein, B. E. (1982). The Hearing Handicap Inventory for the Elderly: A new tool. *Ear and Hearing, 3,* 128–134.

Weinstein, B. E. (1997). *Outcome measures in the hearing aid fitting/selecting process* (Trends in Amplification, No. 2(4)). New York: Woodland.

Hearing Aids: Prescriptive Fitting

Prescriptive procedures are used in hearing aid fittings to select an appropriate amplification characteristic based on measurements of the auditory system. The advantages of using a prescriptive procedure as opposed to an evaluative or other approach are (1) they can be used with all populations in a time-efficient way, (2) they help the clinician select a suitable parameter combination from among an almost unlimited number possible in modern hearing aids and settings, and (3) they can be verified. On the negative side, there is little interaction with the client when fitting hearing aids according to a prescriptive procedure, and any two people with the same type of loss may have different preferences for the loudness and the tone of sounds.

More than fifty prescriptive procedures for fitting hearing aids have been presented. The procedures vary with respect to the type of amplification characteristic that is prescribed, the type of data the procedure is based on, and the aim of the procedure.

The parameter most commonly prescribed in hearing aids is gain as a function of frequency. In linear devices, only one gain/frequency response is prescribed, which applies to all input levels that do not cause the hearing aid to saturate. If the hearing aid is nonlinear (contains compressor amplifiers), gain varies as a function of both frequency and input level. In that case, gain/frequency curves are prescribed for different input levels, or the static compression parameters are prescribed for selected frequencies. To avoid excessive loudness when listening to high-intensity input levels, the maximum output of the hearing device must also be prescribed.

Some procedures prescribe the amplification characteristic based on threshold levels only. Others use suprathreshold loudness judgments, such as the most comfortable level (MCL), the loudness discomfort level (LDL), or the entire loudness scale. Supporters of threshold-based procedures argue that loudness data are difficult to measure and unreliable, especially in children and special populations, and that preferred gain and maximum output can be adequately predicted from threshold levels. The argument for using individually measured loudness data is that the fitting will be more accurate because hearing aid users with the same audiogram can perceive loudness differently. Table 1 lists some of the most widely used prescription procedures developed to date. They are categorized according to which parameters are prescribed and the data used.

Most procedures for fitting linear devices share the general aim of amplifying speech presented at an average level to a comfortable level situated approximately halfway between threshold and LDL. The rationale is that such a response provides optimum speech understanding and comfortable listening in general situations. Despite this common rationale, the assumptions and underlying operational principles behind each procedure vary, producing very different formulas. The assump-

Table 1. An Overview of Widely Used Prescriptive Hearing Aid Fitting Procedures

	Linear Amplification	Nonlinear Amplification	Output
Threshold based	Berger POGO, POGO II *(Prescription of Gain/Output)* NAL-R, NAL-RP *(National Acoustic Laboratories)*	FIG6 *(Figure 6)* NAL-NL1 *(National Acoustic Laboratories' nonlinear formula, version 1)*	POGO NAL-SSPL
Use supra-threshold loudness data	CID *(Central Institute for the Deaf)* DSL* *(Desired Sensation Level)* MSU* *(Memphis State University)*	LGOB *(Loudness Growth of Octave Bands)* IHAFF *(Independent Hearing Aid Fitting Forum)* DSL(i/o)* *(Desired Sensation Level, input/output function)* ScalAdapt *(Adaptive fitting by category loudness scaling)*	CID MSU* IHAFF

*Supra-threshold loudness data may be measured or predicted from threshold levels.

tions presented include the following: (1) The audibility of all speech components is important for speech understanding (e.g., DSL; Seewald, Ross, and Spiro, 1985). (2) Speech discrimination is highest when speech is presented at levels above MCL (e.g., MSU; Cox, 1988). (3) Speech is best understood when speech bands at different frequencies have equal loudness (e.g., NAL-R; Byrne and Dillon, 1986; and CID; Skinner et al., 1982). (4) For hearing aid users with mild to moderate losses, speech presented at average input levels is restored to the MCL when providing gain equal to about half the amount of threshold loss (e.g., Berger, Hagberg, and Rane, 1977; and POGO; McCandless and Lyregaard, 1983).

Some of these procedures take the shape of the speech spectrum into consideration when prescribing gain at each frequency (DSL, MSU, CID, and NAL-R), whereas others introduce a reduction in the low-frequency gain to avoid upward spread of masking from low-frequency ambient noise (Berger, POGO). Either way, the net result is that, even for a flat hearing loss, less gain is prescribed in the low than in the high frequencies. The NAL-R procedure differs from the other linear procedures in two respects. First, the gain prescribed at any frequency is affected by the degree of loss at other frequencies. Second, it is the only procedure that is well supported by direct empirical data (e.g., Byrne and Cotton, 1988).

One procedure for fitting nonlinear devices, NAL-NL1 (Dillon, 1999), follows the common rationale of procedures for fitting linear devices by aiming at maximizing speech intelligibility for any input level. To avoid amplifying all input levels to a most comfortable level, which probably would make the loudness of environmental sounds unacceptable, the rationale uses the constraint that for any input level, the overall loudness of speech must not exceed normal loudness. This procedure prescribes gain/frequency responses that make the speech bands approximately equal in loudness (Fig. 1), which is in agreement with several procedures for fitting linear devices. As hearing loss at any frequency becomes severe or profound, the ear becomes less able to extract information, even when the signal in that fre-

quency region is audible (Ching, Dillon, and Byrne, 1998). Consequently, the goal of achieving equal loudness is progressively relaxed within the NAL-NL1 rule as hearing loss increases.

The rationale behind most nonlinear prescription procedures, however, is loudness normalization. Examples are LGOB (Humes et al., 1996), FIG6 (Killion and Fikret-Pasa, 1993), IHAFF (Cox, 1995), DSL[i/o] (Cornelisse, Seewald, and Jamieson, 1995), and ScalAdapt (Kiessling, Schubert, and Archut, 1996). The assumption behind this rationale is that "normal hearing" is best for speech understanding and for listening to environmental sounds. Loudness normalization is achieved by applying the gain needed to make narrow-band stimuli of any input level just as loud for the impaired ear as they are for normal ears. This rationale maintains the interfrequency variation of loudness that normally occurs for speech (Fig. 1). Consequently, loudness normalization is not consistent with the principles of equalizing loudness across frequency and deemphasizing loudness at those frequencies where loss is greatest, principles that have emerged from research into linear amplification.

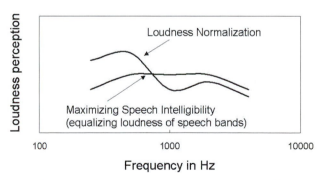

Figure 1. Graph illustrating loudness perception of speech when the interfrequency variation of intensity for speech is maintained (loudness normalization) and when the intensity of speech bands has been equalized to maximize speech intelligibility.

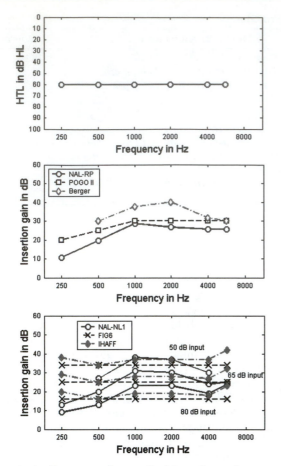

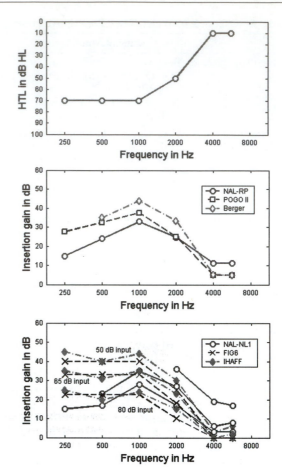

Figure 2. Audiogram and prescribed insertion gain curves for a person with a moderate flat hearing loss. For IHAFF, the targets are calculated based on average threshold-dependent loudness data (Cox, personal communication). Note that the NAL-NL1 rule does not prescribe insertion gain at frequencies where it is doubtful that amplification will contribute to speech intelligibility.

Figure 3. Audiogram and prescribed insertion gain curves for a person with a moderate to severe low-frequency hearing loss. For IHAFF, the targets are calculated based on average threshold-dependent loudness data (Cox, personal communication). Note that the NAL-NL1 rule does not prescribe insertion gain at frequencies where it is doubtful that amplification will contribute to speech intelligibility.

Because of the different assumptions and principles used by the various procedures, different procedures prescribe different amplification characteristics for the same type of hearing loss (Figs. 2–5). The differences are more pronounced for flat and reverse sloping loss than for the more common high-frequency sloping loss.

A recent evaluation of loudness normalization versus speech intelligibility maximization suggests that when the difference in prescription between the two rationales is substantial, hearing aid users prefer and perform better with the speech intelligibility maximization rationale (Keidser and Grant, 2001).

The gain/frequency curves may be prescribed according to the acoustic input the client is likely to experience. Simple variations applied to the amplification characteristic prescribed to compensate for the hearing loss have proved useful for compensating for defined changes in the acoustic input (Keidser, Dillon, and Byrne, 1996).

Such variations can be programmed into different memories in a multimemory hearing aid.

Some procedures also prescribe the maximum output of the hearing aid known as the saturation sound pressure level (SSPL). It is important to have the output level of the hearing aid correctly adjusted. If the SSPL is too high, the hearing aid can cause discomfort or damage to the hearing aid user. On the other hand, if the SSPL is too low, the hearing aid user may experience insufficient loudness and excessive saturation. Most procedures that prescribe SSPL aim at avoiding discomfort. In those cases the SSPL is set equal to or just below the hearing aid user's discomfort level; examples are CID, MSU, POGO, and IHAFF. Only one procedure, NAL-SSPL, considers both the maximum output level and the minimum output level and prescribes a level halfway between these two extremes (Dillon and Storey, 1998). This is also the only procedure for prescribing the output level

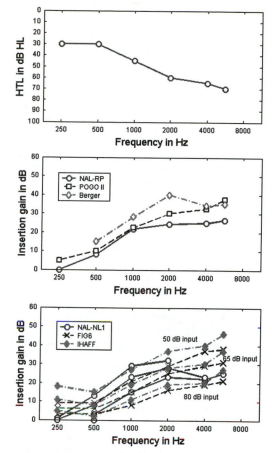

Figure 4. Audiogram and prescribed insertion gain curves for a person with a gently sloping high-frequency hearing loss. For IHAFF, the targets are calculated based on average threshold-dependent loudness data (Cox, personal communication). Note that the NAL-NL1 rule does not prescribe insertion gain at frequencies where it is doubtful that amplification will contribute to speech intelligibility.

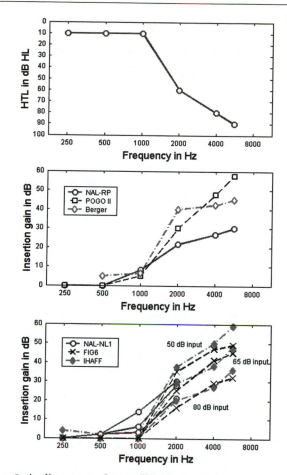

Figure 5. Audiogram and prescribed insertion gain curves for a person with a steeply sloping high-frequency hearing loss. For IHAFF, the targets are calculated based on average threshold-dependent loudness data (Cox, personal communication). Note that the NAL-NL1 rule does not prescribe insertion gain at frequencies where it is doubtful that amplification will contribute to speech intelligibility.

that has been experimentally evaluated. It was found to provide an SSPL that did not require fine-tuning for 80% of clients (Storey et al., 1998).

Many prescription procedures target a sensorineural loss of mild to moderate degree. Appropriate adjustments to the prescriptions may be needed if prescribing amplification for clients with a conductive component (Lybarger, 1963), and a severe to profound loss (POGO II: Schwartz, Lyregaard, and Lundt, 1988; NAL-RP: Byrne, Parkinson, and Newall, 1990). Some adjustments are also needed for clients who are fitted with one versus two hearing aids (Dillon, 2001).

When the hearing aid has been adjusted according to the prescriptive procedures, the setting can be verified against the prescribed target, either in a hearing aid test box or in the real ear. Verifying the prescriptive parameters in the real ear allows individual configurations of the ear canal and the acoustic coupling between ear and hearing aid to be taken into consideration. For some clients fine-tuning may be needed after the

client has tried the hearing aid in everyday listening environments.

The most commonly used prescription procedures are readily available in an electronic format, either as specifically designed computer programs, in programs provided by hearing aid manufacturers for fitting their programmable devices, or in equipment for measuring real-ear gain.

See also HEARING AID FITTING: EVALUTION OF OUTCOMES; HEARING AIDS: SOUND QUALITY.

—*Gitte Keidser and Harvey Dillon*

References

Berger, R. A., Hagberg, E. N., and Rane, R. L. (1977). *Prescription of hearing aids*. Kent, OH: Herald.

Byrne, D., and Cotton, S. (1988). Evaluation of the National Acoustic Laboratories' new hearing aid selection procedure. *Journal of Speech and Hearing Research, 31,* 178–186.

Byrne, D., and Dillon, H. (1986). The National Acoustic Laboratories' (NAL) new procedure for selecting the gain and frequency response of a hearing aid. *Ear and Hearing*, *7*, 257–265.

Byrne, D., Parkinson, A., and Newall, P. (1990). Hearing aid gain and frequency response requirements for the severely/profoundly hearing impaired. *Ear and Hearing*, *11*, 295–300.

Ching, T. Y. C., Dillon, H., and Byrne, D. (1998). Speech recognition of hearing-impaired listeners: Predictions from audibility and the limited role of high frequency amplification. *Journal of the Acoustical Society of America*, *103*, 1128–1140.

Cornelisse, L., Seewald, R., and Jamieson, D. (1995). The input/output formula: A theoretical approach to the fitting of personal amplification devices. *Journal of the Acoustical Society of America*, *97*, 1854–1864.

Cox, R. (1988). The MSU hearing instrument prescription procedure. *Hearing Instruments*, *39*, 6–10.

Cox, R. (1995). Using loudness data for hearing aid selection: The IHAFF approach. *Hearing Journal*, *48*(2), 39–44.

Dillon, H. (1999). NAL-NL1: A new prescriptive fitting procedure for non-linear hearing aids. *Hearing Journal*, *52*(4), 10–16.

Dillon, H. (2001). *Hearing aids*. Sydney, Australia: Boomerang Press.

Dillon, H., and Storey, L. (1998). The National Acoustic Laboratories' procedure for selecting the saturation sound pressure level of hearing aids: Theoretical derivation. *Ear and Hearing*, *19*, 255–266.

Humes, L. E., Pavlovic, C., Bray, V., and Barr, M. (1996). Real-ear measurement of hearing threshold and loudness. *Trends in Amplification*, *1*(4), 121–135.

Keidser, G., Dillon, H., and Byrne, D. (1996). Guidelines for fitting multiple memory hearing aids. *Journal of the American Academy of Audiology*, *7*, 406–418.

Keidser, G., and Grant, F. (2001). Comparing loudness normalization (IHAFF) with speech intelligibility maximization (NAL-NL1) when implemented in a two-channel device. *Ear and Hearing*, *22*, 501–515.

Kiessling, J., Schubert, M., and Archut, A. (1996). Adaptive fitting of hearing instruments by category loudness scaling (ScalAdapt). *Scandinavian Audiology*, *25*, 153–160.

Killion, M. C., and Fikret-Pasa, S. (1993). The 3 types of sensorineural hearing loss: Loudness and intelligibility considerations. *Hearing Journal*, *46*(11), 31–36.

Lybarger, S. (1963). *Simplified fitting system for hearing aids*. Cantonsburg, PA: Radioear Co.

McCandless, G. A., and Lyregaard, P. E. (1983). Prescription of gain/output (POGO) for hearing aids. *Hearing Instruments*, *34*, 16–21.

Schwartz, D., Lyregaard, P., and Lundh, P. (1988). Hearing aid selection for severe-to-profound hearing loss. *Hearing Journal*, *41*(2), 13–17.

Seewald, R., Ross, M., and Spiro, M. (1985). Selecting amplification characteristics for young hearing-impaired children. *Ear and Hearing*, *6*, 48–53.

Skinner, M., Pascoe, D., Miller, J., and Popelka, G. (1982). Measurements to determine the optimal placement of speech energy within the listener's auditory area: A basis for selecting amplification characteristics. In G. Studebaker, and F. Bess (Eds.), *The Vanderbilt hearing-aid report* (pp. 161–169). Upper Darby, PA: Monographs in Comtemporary Audiology.

Storey, L., Dillon, H., Yeend, I., and Wigney, D. (1998). The National Acoustic Laboratories' procedure for selecting the saturation sound pressure level of hearing aids: Experimental validation. *Ear and Hearing*, *19*, 267–279.

Further Readings

Barker, C., Dillon, H., and Newall, P. (2001). Fitting low ratio compression to people with severe and profound hearing losses. *Ear and Hearing*, *22*, 130–141.

Bustamante, D., Braida, L. (1987). Multiband compression limiting for hearing-impaired listeners. *Journal of Rehabilitative Research and Development*, *24*, 149–160.

Byrne, D. (1983). Theoretical prescriptive approaches to selecting the gain and frequency response of a hearing aid. *Monographs in Contemporary Audiology*, *4*(1).

Byrne, D. (1986). Effects of frequency response characteristics on speech discrimination and perceived intelligibility and pleasantness of speech for hearing-impaired listeners. *Journal of the Acoustical Society of America*, *80*, 494–504.

Byrne, D. (1996). Hearing aid selection for the 1990s: Where to? *Journal of the American Academy of Audiology*, *7*, 377–395.

Byrne, D., Dillon, H., Katsch, R., Ching, T., and Keidser, G. (2001). The NAL-NL1 procedure for fitting non-linear hearing aids: Characteristics and comparisons with other procedures. *Journal of the American Academy of Audiology*, *12*, 37–51.

Danaher, E. S., and Pickett, J. M. (1975). Some masking effects produced by low-frequency vowel formants in persons with sensorineural loss. *Journal of Speech and Hearing Research*, *18*, 79–89.

Dillon, H., and Murray, N. (1987). Accuracy of twelve methods for estimating the real ear gain of hearing aids. *Ear and Hearing*, *8*, 2–11.

Gatehouse, S. (1993). Role of perceptual acclimatization in the selection of frequency responses for hearing aids. *Journal of the American Academy of Audiology*, *4*, 296–306.

Harford, E., and Barry, J. (1965). A rehabilitative approach to the problem of unilateral hearing impairment: Contralateral routing of signals (CROS). *Journal of Speech and Hearing Disorders*, *30*, 121–138.

Hogan, C. A., and Turner, C. W. (1998). High-frequency audibility: Benefits for hearing-impaired listeners. *Journal of the Acoustical Society of America*, *104*, 432–441.

Kamm, C., Dirks, D. D., and Mickey, M. R. (1978). Effect of sensorineural hearing loss on loudness discomfort level and most comfortable level judgements. *Journal of Speech and Hearing Disorders*, *21*, 668–681.

Keidser, G. (1995). The relationship between listening conditions and alternative amplification schemes for multiple memory hearing aids. *Ear and Hearing*, *16*, 575–586.

Killion, M. C., and Monser, E. L. (1980). Corfig coupler response for flat insertion gain. In G. A. Studebaker and I. Hochberg (Eds.), *Acoustical factors affecting hearing aid performance* (pp. 147–168). Baltimore: University Park Press.

Macrae, J. (1994). A review of research into safety limits for amplification by hearing aids. *Australian Journal of Audiology*, *16*, 67–77.

Moore, B. C., Alcantara, J. I., and Glasberg, B. R. (1998). Development and evaluation of a procedure for fitting multi-channel compression hearing aids. *British Journal of Audiology*, *32*, 177–195.

Mueller, H. G., Hawkins, D. B., and Northern, J. L. (1992). *Probe microphone measurements: Hearing aid selection and assessment*. San Diego, CA: Singular Press Publishing Group.

Plomp, R. (1978). Auditory handicap of hearing impairment and the limited benefit of hearing aids. *Journal of the Acoustical Society of America*, *63*, 533–549.

Rankovic, C. (1991). An application of the articulation index to hearing aid fitting. *Journal of Speech and Hearing Research, 34*, 391–402.

Skinner, M. W. (1980). Speech intelligibility in noise-induced hearing loss: Effects of high-frequency compensation. *Journal of the Acoustical Society of America, 67*, 306–317.

Swan, I., and Gatehouse, S. (1987). Optimum side for fitting a monaural hearing aid. 3. Preference and benefit. *British Journal of Audiology, 21*, 205–208.

Turner, C. W., Humes, L. E., Bentler, R. A., and Cox, R. M. (1996). A review of past research on changes in hearing aid benefit over time. *Ear and Hearing, 17*(3, Suppl.), 14S–28S.

Walker, G. (1997). Conductive hearing impairment and preferred hearing aid gain. *Australian Journal of Audiology, 19*, 81–89.

Hearing Aids: Sound Quality

The electroacoustic characteristics of a hearing aid differ considerably from those of a high-fidelity communication system. The hearing aid has a relatively narrow bandwidth, and the frequency response of the hearing aid is almost never flat. Because hearing loss usually increases with increasing frequency, the frequency response of the hearing aid typically provides increased gain as a function of frequency in order to obtain audibility for the hearing aid user. While hearing-impaired listeners may require considerable gain in order to obtain audibility, the output of the hearing aid must be limited in order to prevent the amplified sound from becoming uncomfortably loud when input levels are high.

A number of studies have been carried out to determine the effect of manipulating the electroacoustic characteristics of a hearing aid on sound quality. Sound quality is a multidimensional construct. Gabrielsson and Sjogren (1979) identified eight important "dimensions" related to the manipulation of the frequency response of loudspeakers, headphones, and hearing aids. These dimensions are clarity, fullness, brightness, shrillness, loudness, spaciousness, nearness, and disturbing sounds (distortion). The "overall impression of quality" consists of some weighting of these various dimensions.

The effect of manipulating the frequency response of the hearing aid has been assessed in many studies. The bandwidth, amount of low-frequency versus high-frequency gain, and the smoothness of the frequency response will all affect the sound quality of speech. Several studies have shown that the presence of low-frequency content is a strong determinant of good sound quality for hearing-impaired listeners listening at comfortable listening levels (Punch, 1978; Punch et al., 1980; Punch and Parker, 1981; Tecca and Goldstein, 1984; Punch and Beck, 1986). However, the bandwidth yielding better sound quality changes as a function of the input level to the hearing aid and the amount of amplification provided by the hearing aid. When hearing-impaired subjects listen at higher levels, a frequency response with less low-frequency amplification yields better sound quality (Tecca and Goldstein, 1984).

There is also good agreement among studies that too much high-frequency emphasis degrades sound quality. This type of amplification is characterized by descriptions of sound as shrill, harsh, and tinny (e.g., Gabrielsson and Sjogren, 1979; Gabrielsson, Schenkman, and Hagerman, 1988). Thompson and Lassman (1970), Neuman and Schwander (1987), and Leijon et al. (1991) found that the sound quality of a flat frequency response was preferred to a response with extreme high-frequency emphasis. The results of these studies point to the need for balance between the low- and high-frequency energy for good sound quality. Of course, the optimum balance for any person depends on the way that person's hearing loss varies with frequency. It has also been realized that the frequency response requirements for good sound quality for music differ from those for speech. An extended low-frequency response is more important for music than for speech (e.g., Franks, 1982).

A smoother frequency response has better sound quality than a frequency response with peaks. Davis and Davidson (1996) found that hearing-impaired listeners preferred to listen to speech processed through a hearing aid with a moderate amount of damping that smoothed the large resonant peak in the frequency response of the hearing aid. This preference was true for both male and female voices in quiet and in noise. Smoothing of the frequency response resulted in judgments of greater brightness, clarity, distinctness, fullness, nearness, and openness. Similarly, van Buuren, Festen, and Houtgast (1996) investigated the effect of adding single and multiple peaks to a smooth frequency response. Hearing-impaired subjects rated pleasantness on a five-point rating scale. The smooth frequency response was rated as having better sound quality than any of the frequency responses with peaks. Based on the results of the study, the researchers recommended that peak-to-valley ratios in the frequency response of the hearing aid should not exceed 5 dB.

In spite of the general agreement among studies about the effect of frequency response on sound quality, Preminger and Van Tasell (1995) have shown intersubject differences with regard to their ratings of the various dimensions of sound quality as a function of the manipulation of frequency response. They suggested that measures of speech quality be used to select among alternative frequency responses yielding similar speech intelligibility (close to 100%).

Much of the research described above was carried out with linear hearing aids, with testing carried out at a single input level. However, many current hearing aids are nonlinear, which means that the frequency response characteristics change as a function of the input level. Full evaluation of sound quality would require testing with various signals at multiple input levels and determining optimum sound quality at each level.

The method of output limiting is another hearing aid parameter that has an important effect on sound quality. Output limiting is used in a hearing aid to prevent amplified sounds from becoming uncomfortably loud and to protect the ear from excessively loud sounds that might cause further damage to the hearing. Major methods of output limiting include peak clipping, compression limiting, or wide dynamic range compression.

Peak clipping causes the generation of signals in the output signal that are not in the input signal. Harmonic distortion (integer multiples of the input signal) and intermodulation distortion (combinations of the harmonics caused by sums and differences of the harmonic distortion) are caused by peak clipping. The coherence between the input signal and the output signal is predictive of sound quality. Moderate amounts of peak clipping degrade the sound quality of speech in quiet and in noise, and the sound quality of music (Fortune and Preves, 1992; Palmer et al., 1995; Kozma-Spytek, Kates, and Revoile, 1996). There is also an interaction between the frequency response shaping of the hearing aid and the clipping level. This interaction is subject-dependent (Kozma-Spytek, Kates, and Revoile, 1996). Fortune and Preves (1992) found specifically that hearing aids having less distortion (higher coherence) were perceived as having better clarity and brightness, as producing less discomfort, and as yielding better overall sound quality.

Compression is a nonlinear form of amplification in which the gain of the amplifier is decreased as the input to the amplifier increases. Compression amplification may be used to limit output (compression limiting) or to fit a wide range of signals into the listener's dynamic range (wide dynamic range compression). In general, compression limiting preserves sound quality better than peak clipping. Compression limiting does not generate harmonic and intermodulation distortion and yields higher coherence values. Hawkins and Naidoo (1993) compared the effect of asymmetrical peak clipping and compression limiting on sound quality and clarity of speech in quiet, speech in noise, and music. For both sound quality and clarity, and for all three types of stimuli, compression limiting was preferred to peak clipping under conditions in which the hearing aid input was high enough to cause limiting.

For hearing aids utilizing wide dynamic range compression, compression ratio, attack, and release time all affect the sound quality of the processed signal. The effect of compression variables also depends on whether the signal of interest occurs in quiet or in noise. Several studies have shown that high compression ratios have a negative effect on sound quality (Neuman et al., 1994, 1998; Boike and Souza, 2000). Neuman and colleagues (1994, 1998) found that compression ratios higher than 3:1 significantly degraded the sound quality of a single-band-compression hearing aid. Compression ratios that did not significantly degrade sound quality in quiet, degraded sound quality in noise. The sound quality of linear amplification (no compression) was preferred when background noise levels were high. Boike and Souza (2000) also found that speech quality ratings decreased with increasing compression ratio for speech in noise. Compression ratio did not significantly degrade quality for speech in quiet. Research to determine the effect of compression on specific dimensions of sound quality revealed that clarity, pleasantness, background noise, loudness, and overall impression all showed negative effects of increasing compression ratio (Neuman et al., 1998).

Release time also affects sound quality. If short release times are used, low-level noise is amplified in the pauses between words. This amplification of low-level noise has been found to have a negative effect on the perceived sound quality. Neuman and colleagues (1998) found that hearing-impaired listeners' ratings of the clarity, pleasantness, and overall quality of speech in quiet and speech in noise all decreased as release time was decreased from 1000 ms to 60 ms (single-band-compression hearing aid). Ratings of the amount of background noise increased as release time decreased.

It is clear that the electroacoustic characteristics of a hearing aid have a significant effect on sound quality. Sound quality has been recognized as an important factor in the acceptability of a hearing aid to the user, and because of individual differences among listeners, it has been suggested that sound quality should be considered a factor in hearing aid fitting (e.g., Gabrielsson and Sjogren, 1979; Kuk and Tyler, 1990; Preminger and Van Tasell, 1995; Lunner et al., 1997). Past research has shown that characteristics of the listeners, characteristics of the signal being amplified, and characteristics of the amplification system all affect sound quality. Application of sound quality judgments to the fitting of nonlinear and multimemory hearing aids should be helpful in determining the appropriate settings for these devices (e.g., Keidser, Dillon, and Byrne, 1995).

See also HEARING AID FITTING: EVALUATION OF OUTCOMES; HEARING AIDS: PRESCRIPTIVE FITTING.

—*Arlene C. Neuman*

References

Boike, K. T., and Souza, P. E. (2000). Effect of compression ratio on speech recognition and speech-quality ratings with wide dynamic range compression amplification. *Journal of Speech Language and Hearing Research, 43*, 456–468.

Davis, L. A., and Davidson, S. A. (1996). Preference for and performance with damped and undamped hearing aids by listeners with sensorineural hearing loss. *Journal of Speech and Hearing Research, 39*, 483–493.

Fortune, T. W., and Preves, D. A. (1992). Hearing aid saturation and aided loudness discomfort. *Journal of Speech and Hearing Research, 35*, 175–185.

Franks, J. R. (1982). Judgments of hearing aid processed music. *Ear and Hearing, 3*, 18–23.

Gabrielsson, A., Schenkman, B. N., and Hagerman, B. (1988). The effects of different frequency responses on sound quality judgments and speech intelligibility. *Journal of Speech and Hearing Research, 31*, 166–177.

Gabrielsson, A., and Sjogren, H. (1979). Perceived sound quality of hearing aids. *Scandinavian Audiology, 8*, 159–169.

Hawkins, D. B., and Naidoo, S. V. (1993). Comparison of sound quality and clarity with asymmetrical peak clipping and output limiting compression. *Journal of the American Academy of Audiology, 4*, 221–228.

Keidser, G., Dillon, H., and Byrne, D. (1995). Candidates for multiple frequency response characteristics. *Ear and Hearing, 16*, 575–586.

Kozma-Spytek, L., Kates, J. M., and Revoile, S. G. (1996). Quality ratings for frequency-shaped peak-clipped speech: Results for listeners with hearing loss. *Journal of Speech and Hearing Research, 39,* 1115–1123.

Kuk, F. K., and Tyler, R. S. (1990). Relationship between consonant recognition and subjective ratings of hearing aids. *British Journal of Audiology, 24,* 171–177.

Leijon, A., Lindkvist, A., Ringdahl, A., and Israelsson, B. (1991). Sound quality and speech reception for prescribed hearing aid frequency responses. *Ear and Hearing, 12,* 251–260.

Lunner, T., Hellgren, J., Arlinger, S., and Elberling, C. (1997). A digital filterbank hearing aid: Three digital signal processing algorithms—User preference and performance. *Ear and Hearing, 18,* 373–387.

Neuman, A. C., Bakke, M. H., Hellman, S., and Levitt, H. (1994). Effect of compression ratio in a slow-acting compression hearing aid: Paired-comparison judgments of quality. *Journal of the Acoustical Society of America, 96,* 1471–1478.

Neuman, A. C., Bakke, M. H., Mackersie, C., Hellman, S., and Levitt, H. (1998). The effect of compression ratio and release time on the categorical rating of sound quality. *Journal of the Acoustical Society of America, 103,* 2273–2281.

Neuman, A. C., and Schwander, T. J. (1987). The effect of filtering on the intelligibility and quality of speech in noise. *Journal of Rehabilitation Research and Development, 24,* 127–134.

Palmer, C. V., Killion, M. C., Wilber, L. A., and Ballad, W. J. (1995). Comparison of two hearing aid receiver-amplifier combinations using sound quality judgments. *Ear and Hearing, 16,* 597–598.

Preminger, J. E., and Van Tasell, D. J. (1995). Measurement of speech quality as a tool to optimize the fitting of a hearing aid. *Journal of Speech and Hearing Research, 38,* 726–736.

Punch, J. L. (1978). Quality judgments of hearing-aid processed speech and music by normal and otopathologic listeners. *Journal of the American Auditory Society, 3,* 179–188.

Punch, J. L., and Beck, L. B. (1986). Relative effects of low-frequency amplification on syllable recognition and speech quality. *Ear and Hearing, 7,* 57–62.

Punch, J. L., Montgomery, A. A., Schwartz, D. M., Walden, B. E., Prosek, R. A., and Howard, M. T. (1980). Multi-dimensional scaling of quality judgments of speech signals processed by hearing aids. *Journal of the Acoustical Society of America, 68,* 458–466.

Punch, J. L., and Parker, C. A. (1981). Pairwise listener preferences in hearing aid evaluation. *Journal of Speech and Hearing Research, 24,* 366–374.

Tecca, J. E., and Goldstein, D. P. (1984). Effect of low-frequency hearing aid response on four measures of speech perception. *Ear and Hearing, 5,* 22–29.

Thompson, G., and Lassman, F. (1970). Listener preference for selective vs. flat amplification for a high-frequency hearing-loss population. *Journal of Speech and Hearing Research, 12,* 594–606.

van Buuren, R. A., Festen, J. M., and Houtgast, T. (1996). Peaks in the frequency response of hearing aids: Evaluation of the effects on speech intelligibility and sound quality. *Journal of Speech and Hearing Research, 39,* 239–250.

Further Readings

Balfour, P. B., and Hawkins, D. B. (1992). A comparison of sound quality judgments for monaural and binaural hearing aid processed stimuli. *Ear and Hearing, 13,* 331–339.

Barker, C., and Dillon, H. (1999). Client preference for compression threshold in single channel wide dynamic range compression hearing aids. *Ear and Hearing, 20,* 127–139.

Crain, T. R., and Van Tasell, D. J. (1994). Effect of peak clipping on speech recognition threshold. *Ear and Hearing, 15,* 443–453.

Kuk, F. K. (1991). Perceptual consequence of vents in hearing aids. *British Journal of Audiology, 24,* 163–169.

Kuk, F. K., Harper, T., and Doubek, K. (1994). Preferred real-ear insertion gain on a commercial hearing aid at different speech and noise levels. *Journal of the American Academy of Audiology, 5,* 99–109.

Kuk, F. K., Tyler, R. S., and Mims, L. (1990). Subjective ratings of noise-reduction hearing aids. *Scandinavian Audiology, 19,* 237–244.

Naidoo, S. V., and Hawkins, D. B. (1997). Monaural/binaural preferences: Effect of hearing aid circuit on speech intelligibility and sound quality. *Journal of the American Academy of Audiology, 8,* 188–202.

Preminger, J. E., and Van Tasell, D. J. (1995). Quantifying the relation between speech quality and speech intelligibility. *Journal of Speech and Hearing Research, 39,* 714–725.

Hearing Loss and the Masking-Level Difference

The masking-level difference (MLD) (Hirsh, 1948) refers to a binaural paradigm in which masked signal detection is contrasted between conditions differing with respect to the availability of binaural differences cues. The most common MLD paradigm has two conditions. In the first, NoSo, both the masker and signal are presented in phase to the two ears. In this condition, the composite stimulus of signal plus noise contains no binaural difference cues. In the second condition, NoSπ, the masker is presented in phase to the two ears, but the signal is presented 180° out of phase at the two ears. In this condition, the composite stimulus of signal plus noise contains binaural difference cues of time and amplitude. There are many other MLD conditions, but an underlying similarity is that all involve at least one condition in which the addition of the signal results in a change in the distribution of interaural time differences, interaural amplitude differences, or both interaural time and amplitude differences. For a broadband masker and a 500-Hz signal frequency, the threshold for the NoSπ condition is approximately 15 dB better than that for the NoSo condition, reflecting the sensitivity of the auditory system to the small interaural differences that are introduced when the Sπ signal is presented in the No noise. The magnitude of the MLD is most robust at relatively low signal frequencies, but under specific circumstances, the MLD can be quite large at high frequencies (McFadden and Pasanen, 1978). Whereas the anatomical stage of processing most critical for the MLD has its locus in the auditory brainstem, the MLD also hinges upon the fidelity of more peripheral auditory processing.

Neurological Disorders. Some of the most prominent applications of the MLD to clinical populations have concerned patients with lesions affecting the auditory nerve and auditory brainstem. The rationale for using the MLD in such cases was based on the assumption that the critical stages of auditory processing underlying the MLD occur in the low or mid-brainstem. It was reasoned that lesions affecting the transmission of fine timing information within this region would be associated with reduced MLDs. The results from several audiological investigations have supported this assumption. For example, reduced MLDs have been reported in listeners with tumors of the auditory nerve and low brainstem, and in listeners with multiple sclerosis (Quaranta and Cervellera, 1974; Olsen and Noffsinger, 1976; Olsen, Noffsinger, and Carhart, 1976; Lynn et al., 1981). Poor binaural performance in such cases has been attributed to gross changes in the temporal discharge patterns in the peripheral auditory nervous system, due to either physical pressure on the nerve or, in the case of multiple sclerosis, demyelination of low brainstem neural tissue. In additional support of the idea that the MLD is determined by relatively peripheral auditory processes, several studies have indicated that the MLD is usually not reduced in listeners having specifically cortical auditory lesions (e.g., Bocca and Antonelli, 1976).

Binaural tests other than the MLD have also been used to probe for the existence of peripheral auditory neural disorder. For example, a test of interaural time discrimination termed phase response audiometry has been applied to patients having neural lesions in the auditory periphery (Nilsson and Liden, 1976; Almqvist, Almqvist, and Johnson, 1989). In general, such patients have been found to have a reduced ability to discriminate changes in interaural time differences.

Hearing Dysfunction Related to Aging. Presbyacusis refers not only to the cochlea-based losses of threshold sensitivity that typically accompany the normal aging process but also to possible auditory neural dysfunction that may coexist with (or exist independently of) cochlear loss. In general, results from studies of the MLD in the elderly indicate reduced MLDs with advancing listener age. MLDs are often reduced in presbycusic listeners, particularly when hearing loss is present at the frequencies of the test stimulus. Of greater interest is the fact that MLDs are sometimes reduced in elderly listeners (Fig. 1) even when the audiograms of the listeners do not indicate an age-related hearing loss (e.g., Grose, Poth, and Peters, 1994). Such findings are usually interpreted in terms of abnormal auditory neural processing in the aging auditory system. The nature of the underlying neural abnormality accounting for the reduced MLDs in elderly listeners is unknown. It is possible that such a dysfunction could make a significant contribution to the overall hearing disability associated with aging, as the MLD measures the kinds of auditory function that underlie, at least in part, our abilities to localize sound sources and to hear desired signals in noise backgrounds.

Cochlear Hearing Loss. As reviewed above, the MLD has potential relevance to site of lesion clinical audio-

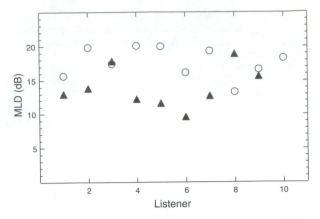

Figure 1. MLDs for a 500-Hz pure tone presented in a 58 dB/Hz, 100-Hz wide band of noise centered on 500 Hz. The open circles represent data from young adults and the filled triangles represent data from elderly adults. All listeners had normal hearing thresholds. Data are adapted from Grose et al. (1994).

logical testing because of its sensitivity to neural auditory dysfunction. Unfortunately, the MLD is affected by a wide range of hearing pathologies, making the clinical specificity of this test relatively poor. For example, the MLD is often reduced in listeners with cochlear hearing loss (e.g., Olsen and Noffsinger, 1976; Hall, Tyler, and Fernandes, 1984; Jerger, Brown, and Smith, 1984). MLDs are particularly likely to be reduced in cases of asymmetrical cochlear hearing loss, but reduced MLDs are also quite common in cases of symmetrical hearing loss. Although reduced MLDs in cochlear hearing loss may sometimes be accounted for in terms of a relatively low sensation level of stimulation or in terms of stimulation asymmetry, in some studies MLDs in listeners with cochlear hearing loss (particularly Ménière's disease) are reduced more than would be expected from stimulus level and asymmetry factors (Schoeny and Carhart, 1971; Staffel et al., 1990). Whereas such findings undermine the MLD as a test that can differentiate between cochlear and retrocochlear sites of lesion, they point to the potential of this test for understanding the effects of cochlear hearing loss on the processing of binaural information.

One general finding associated with cochlear hearing loss is variability of results among listeners. This clearly holds true for the MLD. It is not presently obvious what accounts for the variability in the size of the MLD across listeners with cochlear hearing loss. Some possible factors include the cause of the hearing loss, whether a particular case of hearing loss is associated with a substantial reduction in the number of nerve fibers contributing information for binaural analysis, and whether the cochlear disease state may affect the symmetry of the frequency or place encodings at the two cochleae. Although there is controversy on this point, it has been speculated that some forms of cochlear hearing impairment may be associated with a reduced ability of the auditory nerve to phase lock (Woolf, Ryan, and Bone,

1981). This could contribute to reduced MLDs, and could also account for the poor interaural time discrimination found in many cochlear-impaired listeners. It is likely that several causes contribute to reduced MLDs among cochlear-impaired listeners. The challenge of determining the specific mechanisms underlying the results in particular patients remains.

Conductive Hearing Loss.   In some listening conditions, conductive hearing loss can be considered in terms of a simple attenuation of sound. In this sense, performance in an ear with conductive hearing loss would be expected to be similar to that in a normal ear stimulated at lower level. The situation for some aspects of binaural hearing is more complicated. If the conductive loss is different in the two ears, the associated attenuation will be asymmetrical. This asymmetry could reduce the efficiency of binaural hearing. Colburn and Hausler (1980) also pointed out that another possible source of poor binaural hearing in conductive impairment is related to bone conduction. For sound presented via headphones, both the air conduction route of stimulation and the bone conduction route of stimulation are theoretically relevant. In normal-hearing listeners, the influence of bone-conducted sound on the stimuli reaching the cochleae is probably of no material consequence. In cases of conductive hearing loss, however, the bone-conducted sound could have a significant effect on the composite waveforms reaching the cochleae and could materially affect the distribution of interaural difference cues. It is there-

fore possible that MLDs could be substantially reduced because of this factor in cases of conductive hearing loss.

Studies of binaural hearing in listeners with conductive hearing impairment have found that binaural hearing is relatively poor in many subjects (Jonkees and van der Veer, 1957; Nordlund, 1964; Quaranta and Cervellera, 1974; Hall and Derlacki, 1986). The factors of hearing asymmetry and the bone conduction route of stimulation (discussed above) probably contribute to this poor binaural hearing. However, it is likely that additional factors are involved. One relevant finding is that binaural hearing does not always return to normal immediately following middle ear surgery. In studies of adults having otosclerosis, binaural hearing has been found to remain abnormal up to 1–2 years following the restoration of a normal audiogram (Hall and Derlacki, 1986; Hall, Grose, and Pillsbury, 1990; Magliulo et al., 1990). As indicated in Figure 2, reduced MLDs have also been found in children with normal audiograms at the time of testing but with a history of hearing loss due to otitis media with effusion (Moore, Hutchings, and Meyer, 1991; Pillsbury, Grose, and Hall, 1991; Hall, Grose, and Pillsbury, 1995). It has been speculated that some of the difficulties in the binaural hearing of conductively impaired listeners may be related to a reduction in the efficiency of the neural processing of binaural difference cues (Hall, Grose, and Pillsbury, 1995).

The results of MLD studies indicate that binaural analysis is often negatively affected in most general types of auditory dysfunction. Whereas poor performance is

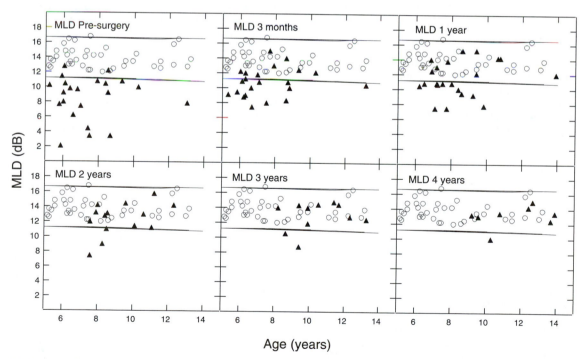

Figure 2. MLDs for children without (open circles) and with (filled triangles) a history of otitis media with effusion. The data were obtained sequentially, before and after the children with a history of otitis media received tympanostomy tubes. The data for the normal control group are repeated in the six panels. The region between the lines represented the 95% prediction interval for the normal group. Data are adapted from Hall et al. (1995).

due to abnormal neural function in cases of retrocochlear hearing disorders, the reasons for poor performance in cases of cochlear and conductive loss are often less clear, particularly when degree and symmetry of hearing loss are not sufficiently explanatory. Identification of the particular factors resulting in abnormal MLD results in particular individuals remains a challenge.

—*Joseph W. Hall*

References

Almqvist, U., Almqvist, B., and Jonsson, K. E. (1989). Phase audiometry: A rapid method for detecting cerebello-pontine angle tumours? *Scandinavian Audiology, 18,* 155–159.

Bocca, E., and Antonelli, A. (1976). Masking level difference: Another tool for the evaluation of peripheral and cortical defects. *Audiology, 15,* 480–487.

Colburn, H. S., and Hausler, R. (1980). Note on the modeling of binaural interaction in impaired auditory systems. In G. v. d. Brink and F. A. Bilsen (Eds.), *Physical, physiological and behavioral studies in hearing.* Netherlands: Delft University.

Grose, J. H., Poth, E. A., and Peters, R. W. (1994). Masking level differences for tones and speech in elderly listeners with relatively normal audiograms. *Journal of Speech and Hearing Research, 37,* 422–428.

Hall, J. W., and Derlacki, E. L. (1986). Effect of conductive hearing loss and middle ear surgery on binaural hearing. *Annals of Otology, Rhinology, and Laryngology, 95,* 525–530.

Hall, J. W., Grose, J. H., and Pillsbury, H. C. (1990). Predicting binaural hearing after stapedectomy from pre-surgery results. *Archives of Otolaryngology–Head and Neck Surgery, 116,* 946–950.

Hall, J. W., Grose, J. H., and Pillsbury, H. C. (1995). Long-term effects of chronic otitis media on binaural hearing in children. *Archives of Otolaryngology–Head and Neck Surgery, 121,* 847–852.

Hall, J. W., Tyler, R. S., and Fernandes, M. A. (1984). Factors influencing the masking level difference in cochlear hearing-impaired and normal-hearing listeners. *Journal of Speech and Hearing Research, 27,* 145–154.

Hirsh, I. J. (1948). Binaural summation and interaural inhibition as a function of the level of the masking noise. *Journal of the Acoustical Society of America, 20,* 205–213.

Jerger, J., Brown, D., and Smith, S. (1984). Effect of peripheral hearing loss on the MLD. *Archives of Otolaryngology, 110,* 290–296.

Jonkees, L., and van der Veer, R. (1957). Directional hearing capacity in hearing disorders. *Acta Otolaryngologica, 48,* 465–474.

Lynn, G. E., Gilroy, J., Taylor, P. C., and Leiser, R. P. (1981). Binaural masking level differences in neurological disorders. *Archives of Otolaryngologica, 107,* 357.

Magliulo, G., Gagliardi, M., Muscatello, M., and Natale, A. (1990). Masking level difference before and after surgery. *British Journal of Audiology, 24,* 117–121.

McFadden, D. M., and Pasanen, E. G. (1978). Binaural detection at high frequencies with time-delayed waveforms. *Journal of the Acoustical Society of America, 63,* 1120–1131.

Moore, D. R., Hutchings, M. E., and Meyer, S. E. (1991). Binaural masking level differences in children with a history of otitis media. *Audiology, 30,* 91–101.

Nilsson, R., and Liden, G. (1976). Sound localization with phase audiometry. *Acta Oto-Laryngologica, 81,* 291–299.

Nordlund, B. (1964). Directional audiometry. *Acta Oto-Laryngologica, 57,* 1–18.

Olsen, W., and Noffsinger, D. (1976). Masking level differences for cochlear and brainstem lesions. *Annals of Otology, Rhinology, and Laryngology, 85,* 1–6.

Olsen, W., Noffsinger, D., and Carhart, R. (1976). Masking-level differences encountered in clinical populations. *Audiology, 15,* 287–301.

Pillsbury, H. C., Grose, J. H., and Hall, J. W. (1991). Otitis media with effusion in children: Binaural hearing before and after corrective surgery. *Archives of Otolaryngology–Head and Neck Surgery, 117,* 718–723.

Quaranta, A., and Cervellera, G. (1974). Masking level differences in normal and pathological ears. *Audiology, 13,* 428–431.

Schoeny, Z., and Carhart, R. (1971). Effects of unilateral Ménière's disease on masking level differences. *Journal of the Acoustical Society of America, 50,* 1143–1150.

Staffel, J. G., Hall, J. W. III., Grose, J. H., and Pillsbury, H. C. (1990). NoSo and NoS pi detection as a function of masker bandwidth in normal-hearing and cochlear-impaired listeners. *Journal of the Acoustical Society of America, 87,* 1720–1727.

Woolf, N. K., Ryan, A. F., and Bone, R. C. (1981). Neural phase-locking properties in the absence of cochlear outer hair cells. *Hearing Research, 4,* 335–346.

Further Readings

Besing, J. M., and Koehnke, J. (1995). A test of virtual auditory localization. *Ear and Hearing, 16,* 220–229.

Colburn, H. S. (1973). Theory of binaural interaction based on auditory nerve data: I. General strategy and preliminary results on interaural discrimination. *Journal of the Acoustical Society of America, 54,* 1458–1470.

Colburn, H. S. (1977). Theory of binaural interaction based on auditory-nerve data: II. Detection of tones in noise. *Journal of the Acoustical Society of America, 61,* 525–533.

Dolan, T. R., and Robinson, D. E. (1967). An explanation of masking-level differences that result from interaural intensive disparities of noise. *Journal of the Acoustical Society of America, 42,* 977–981.

Gabriel, K. J., Koehnke, J., and Colburn, H. S. (1992). Frequency dependence of binaural performance in listeners with impaired binaural hearing. *Journal of the Acoustical Society of America, 91,* 336–347.

Green, D. M. (1978). *An introduction to hearing.* Hillsdale, NJ: Erlbaum.

Hausler, R., Colburn, H. S., and Marr, E. (1983). Sound localization in subjects with impaired hearing. *Acta Otolaryngology, Supplement, 400.*

Hawkins, D. B., and Wightman, F. L. (1980). Interaural time discrimination ability of listeners with sensori-neural hearing loss. *Audiology, 19,* 495–507.

Jeffress, L. A., Blodgett, H. C., and Deatherage, B. H. (1952). The masking of tones by white noise as a function of the interaural phases of both components: I. 500 cycles. *Journal of the Acoustical Society of America, 24,* 523–527.

Kaigham, J. G., Koehnke, J., and Colburn, H. S. (1992). Frequency dependence of binaural performance in listeners with impaired binaural hearing. *Journal of the Acoustical Society of America, 91,* 336–347.

Langford, T., and Jeffress, L. (1964). Effect of noise cross-correlation on binaural signal detection. *Journal of the Acoustical Society of America, 36,* 1455–1458.

Licklider, J. C. R. (1948). The influence of interaural phase relations upon the masking of speech by white noise. *Journal of the Acoustical Society of America, 20*, 150–159.

McFadden, D. (1968). Masking level differences determined with and without interaural disparities in masker intensity. *Journal of the Acoustical Society of America, 44*, 212–223.

Smoski, W. J., and Trahiotis, C. (1986). Discrimination of interaural temporal disparities by normal-hearing listeners and listeners with high-frequency sensori-neural hearing loss. *Journal of the Acoustical Society of America, 79*, 1541–1547.

Webster, F. A. (1951). The influence of interaural phase on masked thresholds: The role of interaural time deviation. *Journal of the Acoustical Society of America, 23*, 452–462.

Zurek, P. M. (1986). Consequences of conductive auditory impairment for binaural hearing. *Journal of the Acoustical Society of America, 80*, 466–472.

Hearing Loss and Teratogenic Drugs or Chemicals

Most causes of hearing loss in newborn infants are hereditary and cannot be prevented. However, about 30% of cases of hearing loss in newborns have been linked to teratogenic factors, and many of these cases are preventable. Teratogens are factors capable of causing physical defects in the developing fetus or embryo and are typically grouped into four categories: infectious, chemical, physical, and maternal agents. During intrauterine life, the fetus is protected from many teratogens by the placenta, which serves as a filter to prevent the toxic substances from entering the fetus' system. The placenta, however, is not a perfect filter and cannot prevent entry of all teratogens. Prenatal susceptibility to teratogens and the severity of the insult are quite variable. Four factors believed to contribute to this variability are dosage of the agent, the timing of the exposure, the susceptibility of the host, and interactions with exposure to other agents. This entry discusses teratogenic chemicals that contribute to hearing loss in the newborn. It should be kept in mind that much is still unknown about chemical teratogens and their ultimate impact on the developing auditory system.

Drugs

Of the prescription or over-the-counter medications, one of the best-studied groups known to have an adverse effect on the auditory system is the aminoglycocides. There is considerable information on the ototoxic effects of aminoglycocides in adults. Some aminoglycocides are thought to be toxic to both the auditory and vestibular systems. Aminoglycosides can cross the placenta, causing sensorineural hearing loss and labyrinthine damage in the fetus. This fetal ototoxicity can occur even in the absence of ototoxicity in the mother. Intrauterine ototoxicity has been reported for streptomycin, dihydrostreptomycin, kanamycin, and gentamicin. It is important to note that most studies of intrauterine ototoxicity have been retrospective and have not controlled for other factors, such as diuretic use, that could have acted synergistically.

Isotretinoin is a prescriptive retinoid (a kind of vitamin A derivative) used to treat persistent and severe cystic acne. Its teratogenic effects include abnormalities of the ophthalmologic, cardiovascular, vestibular, auditory, and central nervous systems. Specific auditory system abnormalities include enlargement of the saccule and utricle, shortening of the cochlea, and malformation of the external ear (Schuknecht, 1993; Westerman, Gilbert, and Schondel, 1994). Both conductive and sensorineural hearing losses have been reported in newborns as a result of maternal use of isotretinoin during gestation. Proper distribution of isotretinoin currently requires informed patient consent, a negative pregnancy test in the 2 weeks before treatment is initiated, and the use of contraceptives from 1 month before to 1 month after use of the drug (Dyer, Strasnick, and Jacobson, 1998).

Probably the best-known nonprescription drug with devastating effects on the unborn is thalidomide. This over-the-counter sedative was available for a short period of time in the late 1950s. Prescribed for morning sickness, when it was consumed during a susceptible period of fetal development, the implications for the baby were catastrophic. When thalidomide was ingested during the first trimester, when fetal limbs differentiate, babies were born with limb buds rather than fully formed limbs. A variety of ear anomalies were also noted, including atresia of the external auditory meatus, cochlear malformations, and absent acoustic and vestibular nerves (Dyer, Strasnick, and Jacobson, 1998). Thalidomide was withdrawn from the market but has subsequently been reintroduced in lesser dosage for use in a number of immunological and inflammatory disorders.

Although numerous other prescription and over-the-counter drugs are known to have ototoxic effects in adults, their ototoxic potential in the fetus has not yet been demonstrated. Those agents currently under suspicion but not proven to be ototoxic in utero include, among others, a variety of antibiotics, including some aminoglycosides and tetracyclines; anti-inflammatory agents; chloroquine, an antimalarial drug; chemotherapeutic drugs; and diuretics. For additional reviews of prescription and over-the-counter ototoxic medications, see Dyer, Strasnick, and Jacobson (1998) and Strasnick and Jacobson (1995).

The effects of recreational drug use by pregnant women have been difficult to document, for a number of reasons. First, the effects are multifactorial, meaning that one drug can interact with another, and many consumers are polydrug users. In addition to using more than one drug at a time, drug-using mothers may not be receiving proper prenatal health care, another factor contributing to premature delivery that can compromise the health of a newborn. Furthermore, mothers who consume drugs may not accurately or honestly report the range and degree of their drug use.

Ethyl alcohol is clearly the most widely abused drug in the United States. Fetal alcohol syndrome, first described in the early 1970s, is a pattern of anomalies resulting from maternal consumption of alcohol during pregnancy. The exact amount of maternal alcohol consumption required to cause fetal damage is uncertain, but the effects are believed to be related more to the amount consumed than to the timing of the consumption (Dyer, Strasnick, and Jacobson, 1998). Approximately 2 in 1000 newborns suffer from fetal alcohol syndrome (Strasnick and Jacobson, 1995). The syndrome consists of multiple congenital anomalies, including prenatal and postnatal growth retardation, craniofacial dysmorphology, developmental delay, and behavioral aberrations. The characteristic cranial features include microcephaly, narrow forehead, small nose and midface, a long, thin upper lip, and micrognathia. The primary auditory concern with children diagnosed with fetal alcohol syndrome appears to be conductive hearing loss secondary to recurrent otitis media (Church and Gerkin, 1988). This may be the result of first and second pharyngeal arch malformations leading to eustachian tube dysfunction. Sensorineural hearing loss has also been reported at higher rates in children with fetal alcohol syndrome than in the general population (Gerber, Epstein, and Mencher, 1995; Church and Abel, 1998).

Although animal research has demonstrated ototoxic effects when fetuses are exposed to cocaine, similar findings have not been demonstrated in humans. The incidence of prenatal cocaine exposure has been reported to range from 11% to 14% of live births. Pregnant women metabolize cocaine slower than other people, making them more sensitive to small amounts of the drug. Metabolites of cocaine have been found in the urine of exposed infants for up to 10 days after birth. If the cocaine-exposed infant is born full term with normal or near normal birth weight, there appears to be no peripheral hearing loss, according to auditory brainstem response studies (Cone-Wesson and Wu, 1992). It does appear, however, that neurotoxic effects are present in cocaine-exposed infants whether they are full-term or low birth weight (Cone-Wesson and Spingarn, 1990; Salamy et al., 1990). The ingestion of cocaine by pregnant women results in vasoconstriction of blood vessels delivering nutrients and oxygen to the developing fetus, which can cause hypoxia. As such, infants with intrauterine exposure to cocaine are at risk for a variety of disordered neurobehaviors. It is still unclear, however, whether infants of cocaine-abusing mothers who are born prematurely and of low birth weight are at greater risk for neurobehavioral problems than premature, low-birth-weight infants who are not exposed to cocaine.

Babies whose mothers are addicted to heroine or methadone are also addicted at birth and will show signs of narcotic withdrawal. The child may be hyperirritable for several months and may continue to be hyperactive. No direct link between maternal heroine use and congenital hearing loss has been made.

Other Chemical Teratogens

Limited data are available on other possible chemical teratogens. At least one study has supported the thesis that maternal use of trimethadione, an antiseizure medication, can occasionally result in hearing deficits in the fetus (Jones, 1997). Although extensive examination has not been conducted to date, maternal opium and nicotine use have not been found to result in peripheral hearing loss in newborns.

See also OTOTOXIC MEDICATIONS.

—*Anne Marie Tharpe*

References

Church, M. W., and Abel, E. L. (1998). Fetal alcohol syndrome: Hearing, speech, language, and vestibular disorders. *Obstetrics and Gynecological Clinics of North America, 25,* 85–97.

Church, M. W., and Gerkin, K. P. (1988). Hearing disorders in children with fetal alcohol syndrome: Findings from case reports. *Pediatrics, 82,* 147–154.

Cone-Wesson, B., and Spingarn, A. (1990). Effects of maternal cocaine abuse on neonatal ABR: Premature and small-for-dates infants. *Journal of the American Academy of Audiology, 1,* 52(A).

Cone-Wesson, B., and Wu, P. (1992). Audiologic findings in infants born to cocaine-abusing mothers. *Infant-Toddler Invervention: The Transdisciplinary Journal, 2,* 25–35.

Dyer, J. J., Strasnick, B., and Jacobson, J. T. (1998). Teratogenic hearing loss: A clinical perspective. *American Journal of Otology, 19,* 671–678.

Gerber, S. E., Epstein, L., and Mencher, L. S. (1995). Recent changes in the etiology of hearing disorders: Perinatal drug exposure. *Journal of the American Academy of Audiology, 6*(5), 371–377.

Jones, K. L. (1997). Fetal trimethadione syndrome. In K. L. Jones (Ed.), *Smith's recognizable patterns of human malformation* (5th ed., p. 564). Philadelphia: Saunders.

Salamy, A., Eldredge, L., Anderson, J., and Bull, D. (1990). Brainstem transmission time in infants exposed to cocaine in utero. *Journal of Pediatrics, 117,* 627–629.

Schuknecht, H. F. (1993). *Pathology of the ear* (2nd ed., p. 177). Philadelphia: Lea and Febiger.

Strasnick, B., and Jacobson, J. T. (1995). Teratogenic hearing loss. *Journal of the American Academy of Audiology, 6,* 28–38.

Westerman, S. T., Gilbert, L. M., and Schondel, L. (1994). Vestibular dysfunction in a child with embryonic exposure to accutane. *American Journal of Otology, 15,* 400–403.

Further Readings

Joint Committee on Infant Hearing. (2000). Year 2000 position statement: Principles and guidelines for early hearing detection and intervention programs. *American Journal of Audiology, 9,* 9–29.

Shepard, T. H. (1989). *Catalog of teratogenic agents.* Baltimore: Johns Hopkins University Press.

Shih, L., Cone-Wesson, B., and Reddix, B. (1988). Effects of maternal cocaine abuse on the neonatal auditory system. *International Journal of Pediatric Otorhinolaryngology, 15,* 245–251.

Hearing Loss Screening: The School-Age Child

Among school-age children in the United States, it is estimated that nearly 15% have abnormal hearing in one or both ears (Niskar et al., 1998). With newborn hearing screening now available in nearly every state, many sensorineural hearing losses are identified prior to school entry. Even so, comprehensive hearing screening of school-age children is important, for several reasons. First, it will be years before universal infant hearing screening is fully implemented. Second, late-onset sensorineural loss may occur in the weeks or months following newborn screening, especially in young children with complicated birth histories (Centers for Disease Control and Prevention, 1997). Third, mild sensorineural loss can escape detection even when newborn hearing screening is provided (Joint Committee on Infant Hearing, 2000). In school-age children, acquired sensorineural hearing loss may occur as a result of disease or noise exposure. The effects of sensorineural hearing loss in children are well documented. Even mild, high-frequency, unilateral sensorineural hearing loss can have important developmental consequences (Bess, Dodd-Murphy, and Parker, 1998). More severe losses are likely to affect the development of speech, language, academic performance, and social-emotional development (Gallaudet University, 1998). In addition to sensorineural loss, hearing screening is needed to identify children with conductive hearing loss. In nearly all cases, conductive hearing loss in school-age children is due to otitis media. The incidence of otitis media with effusion (OME) is highest during the infant-toddler period and declines substantially by school age. Even so, otitis media is the most frequent primary diagnosis in children less than 15 years old (American Academy of Pediatrics, 1994). The hearing loss associated with OME, although mild and rarely permanent, can occur throughout childhood and may result in medical complications as well as potentially adverse effects on communication and development.

Principles and Methods

The purpose of hearing screening is to identify children most likely to have a hearing or middle ear disorder needing medical, audiologic, or other interventions. Thus, the goal of a hearing screening program is to identify asymptomatic individuals with an increased likelihood of hearing impairment, so that diagnostic follow-up is applied only to that subset of individuals. To justify the resources needed to provide a comprehensive screening program, several important assumptions must be met. The problem must be considered significant, both to individuals affected and to society; there must be appropriate screening tools with acceptable performance criteria; there must be effective treatment for those identified; and there must be sufficient financial

Table 1. School-Age Children in Need of Regular Hearing Screening and Monitoring

- Parent/care provider, health care provider, teacher, or other school personnel have concerns regarding hearing, speech, language, or learning abilities
- Family history of late or delayed-onset hereditary hearing loss
- Recurrent or persistent otitis media with effusion for more than 3 months
- Craniofacial anomalies, including those with morphological abnormalities of the pinna and ear canal
- Stigmata or other findings associated with a syndrome known to include sensorineural or conductive hearing loss
- Head trauma with loss of consciousness
- Reported exposure to potentially damaging noise levels or ototoxic drugs

resources for the program's implementation and maintenance. Hearing screening in the school-age population satisfies each of these criteria; however, ongoing evaluation of new technologies and protocols is needed to determine optimal methodology and pass-fail criteria.

The Panel on Audiologic Assessment of the American Speech-Language-Hearing Association (ASHA, 1997a) recommends that school-age children be screened on initial school entry, annually from kindergarten through third grade, and in grades 7 and 11. The panel also recommends screening children at entry to special education, those who repeat a grade, and any who are newly admitted to the school system. More aggressive hearing screening is recommended for children with one or more of the high-risk indicators listed in Table 1.

Guidelines and position statements of ASHA and the American Academy of Audiology (AAA) recommend visual inspection of the external ear to detect conspicuous signs of disease or malformation (AAA, 1997; ASHA, 1997b). The outer ear examination is followed by otoscopic inspection. Screening personnel must have the knowledge and skill required to conduct visual inspection and otoscopy, not for diagnostic purposes but to identify obvious signs of ear disease, impacted cerumen, or foreign objects that may compromise the validity of the screening or indicate the need for medical referral.

Current guidelines and position statements recommend that hearing screening of school-age children be conducted on an individual basis, using manually administered pure tones delivered via earphones or insert receivers at 20 dB hearing level (HL) for the frequencies 1000, 2000, and 4000 Hz (AAA, 1997; ASHA, 1997a). In order to pass, the child must respond to all three frequencies in each ear. Although failure to respond may simply be due to lack of cooperation or motivation, hearing loss should be suspected until appropriately ruled out. When referral is indicated, evaluation by an audiologist is needed to determine the nature and degree of hearing loss.

Routine pure-tone screening at 20 dB HL, however, is inadequate for the identification of OME (Melnick,

Eagles, and Levine, 1964; Roush and Tait, 1985). Consequently, many institutional screening programs include acoustic immittance (tympanometry and related measures) as part of the hearing screening program. Because OME has low incidence in the school-age population, ASHA guidelines recommend routine middle ear screening only to age 6 (ASHA, 1997b).

Evoked otoacoustic emissions (EOAEs) have become an essential tool in evaluating peripheral auditory function. EOAEs, which are present in nearly all ears with normal cochlear function, have at least two important advantages over behavioral pure-tone screening. They are objective and, for most school-age children, easy to measure. Because EOAEs are usually absent in ears with more than mild hearing loss, they are potentially well-suited for school-age screening (Driscoll, Kei, and McPherson, 1997; McPherson et al., 1998). But EOAES are influenced by middle ear disease as well as by cochlear dysfunction. While this is often cited as a disadvantage of EOAEs, Nozza and colleagues have suggested that EOAEs, in conjunction with tympanometry, may be useful as part of a multistage screening program to detect hearing loss *and* otitis media (Nozza, Sabo, and Mandel, 1997; Nozza, 2001). Before such an approach can be endorsed for routine screening of school-age children, further clinical trials are needed to determine the sensitivity, specificity, and predictive value of EOAEs and tympanometry, in comparison to conventional procedures. Based on currently available research, EOAEs are likely to play an increasing role in school-age screening (Nozza, 2001).

Other Considerations

An ideal acoustical environment is rarely available in schools and other settings where screening is often conducted. Although few programs make on-site noise measurement as part of evaluating a test environment prior to screening, the time and expense involved in unnecessary follow-up and audiologic referral can far exceed the cost of providing a noise survey. Thus, a pre-screening noise survey that includes measurement of ambient noise levels at several third-octave bands (Table 2) should be conducted when there is uncertainty regarding adequacy of the screening environment (ANSI S3.1-1999).

Table 2. Maximum Permissible Ambient Noise Levels (in dB SPL) for One-Third Octave Bands, for Screening at 20 dB HL Using the Pure-Tone Frequencies 1000, 2000, and 4000 Hz (ANSI S3.1-1999)

Stimulus/Transducer	Pure-Tone Frequency (Hz)		
	1000	2000	4000
Screening at 20 dB HL with supra-aural earphones	41	49	52
Screening at 20 dB HL with insert earphones	62	64	65

Professionals and support personnel from many disciplines are now involved in hearing and middle ear screening. The screening procedures are not difficult with most school-age children; however, personnel must be competent and appropriately supervised. Furthermore, those responsible for the program must ensure that screening personnel are employed in a manner consistent with state licensure, professional scope of practice, and other regulatory requirements. For this reason it is recommended that institutional screening programs be conducted under the general supervision of an audiologist. School-age children who are difficult to test because of developmental disabilities or other factors should be screened by an audiologist.

Audiometers and tympanometric screening instruments must undergo full calibration by a qualified technician at least once each year. The American National Standards Institute (ANSI) has established specific requirements for the calibration of these instruments (ANSI S3.39-1987; S3.6-1996). In addition to formal calibration measurements, ANSI standards advise routine visual inspection and daily listening checks.

Because school-age children are at risk for permanent hearing loss from exposure to high-intensity noise, a comprehensive program of hearing screening for school-age children should include information on *prevention* of acoustic trauma through the use of appropriate hearing protection (Anderson, 1991). The New York League for the Hard of Hearing (2001) has developed useful materials for educating children about the dangers of noise-induced hearing loss and how to prevent it.

Parental permission must be obtained prior to conducting hearing and middle ear screening procedures unless consent has already been obtained as part of an institutional enrollment process or admissions procedure. Failure to obtain informed consent not only is unprofessional but could lead to negative public relations and possible legal action. Parents must be informed of screening procedures and their purpose. In addition to informed consent, strict confidentiality must be ensured. Discussion of screening outcomes or distribution of results should occur only with parents' knowledge and consent, and mechanisms used to transmit screening results must be in secure data formats. Most screening programs will already have institutional guidelines. If guidelines do not exist, they must be implemented according to institutional protocols as well as state and federal laws. Screening personnel must be familiar with these policies and maintain compliance at all times (Roush, 2000).

Undetected hearing loss in a school-age child is a serious matter. Not only is appropriate intervention denied, hearing loss can be mistaken for a developmental disability or attention deficit. Even so, mass screening of school-age children is an expensive and time-consuming endeavor that requires systematic review and ongoing evaluation. This includes careful examination of screening outcomes, tracking of referrals, and communication with agencies and health care providers to whom referrals are made. In recent years, despite an enormous increase in studies related to newborn hearing screening, there has been remarkably little research aimed at the school-age population. In particular, there is a need to further examine the role of EOAEs, alone and in combination with other tests, to determine the optimal screening battery for identification of hearing loss and middle ear disease in the school-age population.

—*Jackson Roush*

References

American Academy of Audiology. (1997). Report and Position Statement: Identification of hearing loss and middle ear dysfunction in preschool and school-age children. *Audiology Today, 9*(3), 18–22.

American Academy of Pediatrics. (1994). Practice guideline: Managing otitis media with effusion in young children. *Pediatrics, 94*(5).

American National Standards Institute. (1987). *Specifications for instruments to measure aural acoustic impedance and admittance (ANSI S3.39-1987, R1996).* New York: Acoustical Society of America.

American National Standards Institute. (1991). *Maximum permissible ambient noise levels for audiometric test rooms (ANSI S3.1-1991).* New York: Acoustical Society of America.

American National Standards Institute. (1996). *Specifications for audiometers (ANSI S3.6-1996).* New York: Acoustical Society of America.

American Speech-Language-Hearing Association. (1997a). *Guidelines for audiologic screening for hearing impairment: School-age children, 5 through 18 years.* Rockville, MD: Author.

American Speech-Language-Hearing Association. (1997b). *Guidelines for screening infants and children for outer and middle ear disorders: Birth through 18 years.* Rockville, MD: Author.

Anderson, K. (1991). Hearing conservation in the public schools revisited. *Seminars in Hearing, 12,* 340–358.

Bess, F. H., Dodd-Murphy, J., and Parker, R. A. (1998). Children with minimal sensorineural hearing loss: Prevalence, educational performance, and functional status. *Ear and Hearing, 19,* 339–354.

Centers for Disease Control and Prevention. (1997). Serious hearing impairment among children aged 3–10 years—Atlanta, Georgia, 1991–1993. *MMWR, 46,* 1073–1076.

Driscoll, C., Kei, J., and McPherson, B. (2001). Transient evoked otoacoustic emissions in 6-year-old school children: A comparison with pure tone screening and tympanometry. *International Journal of Pediatric Otolaryngology, 57,* 67–76.

Gallaudet University Center for Assessment and Demographic Study. (1998). Thirty years of the annual survey of deaf and hard-of-hearing children and youth: A glance over the decades. *American Annals of the Deaf, 142*(2), 72–76.

Joint Committee on Infant Hearing. (2000). Year 2000 position statement. Available: http://www.pediatrics.org/cgi/content/full/106/4/798.

McPherson, B., Kei, J., Smyth, V., Latham, S., and Loscher, J. (1998). Feasibility of community-based hearing screening using transient evoked otoacoustic emissions. *Public Health, 112,* 147–152.

Melnick, W., Eagles, E., and Levine, H. (1964). Evaluation of a recommended program of identification audiometry in school-age children. *Journal of Speech and Hearing Disorders, 29,* 3–13.

New York League for the Hard of Hearing. (2001). Noise and its effects on children. Available: www.lhh.org/noise/children/index.htm.

Niskar, A. S., Kieszak, S. M., Holmes, A., Esteban, E., Rubin, C., and Brody, D. B. (1998). Prevalence of hearing loss among children 6 to 19 years of age. *Journal of the American Medical Association, 279*(14), 1071–1075.

Nozza, R. (2001). Screening with otoacoustic emissions beyond the newborn period. *Seminars in Hearing, 22,* 415–426.

Nozza, R., Sabo, D., and Mandel, E. (1997). A role for otoacoustic emissions in screening for hearing impairment and middle ear disorders in school-age children. *Ear and Hearing, 18,* 227–239.

Roush, J. (2000). Screening for hearing loss and otitis media in children. San Diego, CA: Singular/Thomson Learning.

Roush, J., and Tait, C. (1985). Pure tone and acoustic immittance screening of preschool-aged children: An examination of referral criteria. *Ear and Hearing, 6,* 245–250.

Further Readings

American Speech-Language-Hearing Association. (1997). *Guidelines for audiologic screening.* Rockville, MD: Author.

Bess, F. H., and Hall, J. W. III (Eds.). (1992). *Screening children for auditory function.* Nashville, TN: Bill Wilkerson Center Press.

Cadman, D., Chambers, L., Feldman, W., and Sackett, D. (1984). Assessing the effectiveness of community screening programs. *Journal of the American Medical Association, 252,* 1580–1585.

DeConde Johnson, C. (2002). Hearing and immittance screening. In J. Katz (Ed.), *Handbook of clinical audiology.* Philadelphia: Lippincott Williams and Wilkins.

Nozza, R. (1996). Pediatric hearing screening. In F. N. Martin and J. G. Clark (Eds.), *Hearing care for children.* Needham Heights, MA: Allyn and Bacon.

Hearing Protection Devices

Hearing protection devices (HPDs) are, as a practical matter, the first line of defense against hearing loss caused by excessive noise. Other ways to reduce exposure to loud sound (engineering control of noise sources, reduction of noise in the transmission path between a source and an individual) can indeed be more effective, but are often more costly or more difficult to manage.

HPDs can be classified by type (active versus passive), by form (e.g., earplugs and earmuffs of various types), and by effect. In all cases the goal is the same: to attenuate the magnitude of sound reaching the cochlea, thus limiting acoustical insult to the end-organ of hearing (see NOISE-INDUCED HEARING LOSS). Passive devices accomplish this through blockage of the airborne transmission path to the inner ear. Active devices seek to mechanically or electronically respond to noise to reduce signal amplitudes presented to the auditory system.

Earplugs fall into five categories (Berger, 2000): (1) closed-cell foam devices designed to be manually compressed, then inserted into the ear canal, where they expand to approximate their initial size (e.g., the Aearo

Company E-A-R plug), (2) preformed devices available in different diameters to accommodate different ear canals (e.g., the PlastiMed V-51R plug), (3) malleable devices intended to fit a range of ear canals, (4) semi-insert devices held in the ear canal by means of a plastic or metal band, and (5) devices made from ear mold impressions taken from individual ear canals. Most earplugs are created from plastics (polyvinyl chloride, polyurethane, silicone, or acrylic); malleable earplugs often consist of wax-impregnated cotton or fiberglass enclosed in a thin plastic container. Most earplugs are passive, that is, they are not intended to respond differently to differing noise exposures. Some active earplugs employ metal slugs or other material intended to move within the plug when stimulated by sudden acoustic overpressures, thus increasing attenuation in response to impulsive noise. For various reasons, it is difficult or impossible to objectively measure the attenuation of such devices or to estimate their real-world benefit. A recent addition to the array of earplugs are those offered by Etymotic Research for users with specific needs (e.g., musicians) who seek flat attenuation across specified frequency ranges.

Earmuffs are designed as integral components of safety helmets or as separate devices that surround the outer ear and are held in place by headbands that extend over or behind the head or beneath the chin. Some of these are combined with communication systems intended to increase the signal-to-noise ratio of messages electronically routed to earphones placed within headsets. At present, most earmuffs are passive devices, but several have been developed as active systems. Indeed, most active hearing protectors are based on earmuffs, owing to the space required for sound sensing and processing components. Active protectors employ one of two (or both) methods to attenuate sound. One method senses sound with a microphone, then processes sound delivered through an earphone by means of automatic gain control circuitry: when incident sound exceeds a certain level, further increases are electronically clipped or otherwise squelched. The other method samples incident sound, reverses the phase of the signal, and electronically adds the reversed signal within the muff enclosure to partially cancel the incident sound. Because of incident signal changes and processing speed requirements, devices employing additive cancellation techniques are more effective at relatively low frequencies (e.g., below 500 Hz; see Nixon, McKinley, and Steuver, 1992). Some active noise reduction methods appear similar to (or may benefit from) methods employed in hearing aids.

Beyond type and form, HPDs differ in weight, comfort, uniformity of fit to individuals, compatibility with other protective or prosthetic devices, and compatibility with individual user health status. Using eyeglasses with earmuffs, for example, can create acoustic leaks that reduce attenuation performance. Similarly, a subject with excessive cerumen or a middle ear effusion should not use earplugs. Use of hearing protectors in hot, humid environments can be uncomfortable and can cause skin irritation. If hearing protectors (perhaps combined with hearing loss) render speech communication difficult, or if they limit audibility of other signals deemed important, users may reject them. For obvious reasons, earmuffs should not be used in conjunction with hearing aids. These and other issues are discussed in detail by Berger (2000).

Real environments in which hearing protectors might provide benefit differ tremendously in noise amplitude, spectrum, and duration. Noise exposure is normally indexed by time-weighted average (TWA) sound pressure levels sampled using integrating meters or personal noise dosimeters. In the United States, such measurements are specified by Federal regulation (Occupational Safety and Health Administration [OSHA], 1983, CFR Part 1910.95) and the subject of technical standards (American National Standards Institute [ANSI], S12.19 1996). Among other details, exposure is to be indexed using a slow meter ballistic characteristic and an A-weighting network (a high-pass filter useful in predicting the effects of broadband noise on hearing). TWA levels are single-number values used to describe noise exposure and determine actions to protect workers from noise-induced hearing loss in the workplace (OSHA, 1983).

In 1979, the Environmental Protection Agency (EPA) issued a regulation intended to promote laboratory measurement of hearing protector attenuation for the purpose of combining such information with exposure data to estimate protective effect. The EPA regulation (CFR40 Part 211) built on previous technical standards (ANSI, 1974), and invoked a single-number index, called the Noise Reduction Rating (NRR), to be included in hearing protector product labels. Computation of NRRs from averaged behavioral real-ear attenuation-at-threshold (REAT) data assume temporally continuous band-limited noise stimuli with equal energy per octave (pink noise), and address intersubject variability by doubling the standard deviation of threshold shifts, then subtracting that value from mean threshold shift for each noise band. Adjusted attenuation values are summed logarithmically across stimulus noise bands to yield an NRR in decibels. Because the NRR method also assumes measurement of unprotected levels indexed with a C-weighting network (which has a flatter frequency response than the A-weighting network used to measure exposure), an additional 7 dB must be subtracted from the NRR to estimate A-weighted noise levels when a hearing protector is in place (see OSHA, 1983, Appendix B). Finally, because it was recognized that how hearing protectors are placed in a subject's ears (plugs) or on a subject's head (muffs) could affect outcomes, the EPA method specified experimenter fitting of HPDs during laboratory testing.

Because real-ear attenuation methods performed following the procedures stipulated by EPA designate experimenter fitting of HPDs, it is to be expected that resulting NRRs will be larger than what would be found with subject fitting of HPDs. Because all extant methods for measuring REATs use temporally continuous noise, results of such measurements cannot be generalized to impulse noise (e.g., gunfire) or impact noise (e.g., forging).

Shortly after the inception of the current OSHA Hearing Conservation Rule (OSHA, 1983), the National Institute of Occupational Safety and Health (NIOSH) recommended that labeled NRRs be derated to estimate effectiveness in the field. Six schemes are noted in Appendix B of the Hearing Conservation Rule. These differ based on available measurement devices and data, but generally reduce the estimated benefit of hearing protectors. For example, if only A-weighted noise exposure data are available, 7 dB is subtracted from the NRR. For both A-weighted and C-weighted exposure data, the resulting corrected NRR is further reduced by 50%.

Subsequent research over two decades suggests that NRRs derated in this manner still overestimate the attenuation of hearing protectors in real-world situations. Various factors contribute to this inaccuracy, including overestimation associated with (1) experimenter fit, (2) highly trained test subjects (whose small standard deviations of REATs produce higher NRRs), and (3) differences in patterns of use of hearing protectors in laboratory and field settings (NIOSH, 1998).

Other pertinent generalizations include the following: (1) overall, earmuffs provide the most protection, foam and formable earplugs provide the next greatest protection, and all other insert types provide less, and (2) ideally, individuals should be fitted individually for hearing protectors (NIOSH, 1998). Generally, both earplugs and earmuffs provide greater attenuation at frequencies above 500 Hz than at lower frequencies (Berger, 2000).

Chapter 4 of the revised NIOSH criteria document (NIOSH, 1998) offers details about estimated real-world NRRs for 84% of wearers of hearing protectors, based on several independent studies. Labeled NRRs for single protectors range from 11 to 29 dB, while weighted mean NRR84 values range from 0.1 to 14.3 dB.

To address these problems, existing standards for measuring HPD attenuation were revised (Royster et al., 1996; Berger et al., 1998) to include subject-fit methods with audiometrically proficient listeners naive about HPDs. The resulting standard is ANSI S12.6 (1997). (A companion standard, ANSI S12.42 (1995), specifies a test fixture method and a microphone-in-real-ear method for measuring insertion loss useful for quality control and product development work with earmuffs.)

In 1995 the National Hearing Conservation Association proposed alternative labeling requirements in which only subject-fit real-ear attenuation data (ANSI S12.6-1997, Method B) are reported. The revised NRR(SF) information generally suggests less protection than NRRs based on experimenter fitting. Alternatively, the NHCA (1995) suggests labeling to include high, medium, and low NRRs based on statistical distributions of measured subject-fit REATs. This proposal has been endorsed by several other organizations. As of this writing, however, the EPA NRR labeling requirement remains based on the experimenter-fit method specified in ANSI S3.19 (1974).

If only experimenter-fit data are available, NIOSH (1998) currently recommends derating of NRRs based on type of hearing protector: 25% for earmuffs, 50% for formable earplugs, and 70% for all other earplugs. In the case of double protection (plugs and muffs), the OSHA Technical Manual (OSHA, 1999) recommends using the EPA NRR for the better protector, minus 7 dB, dividing the result by 2 (a 50% derating), then adding 5 dB to the field-adjusted NRR to account for the second protector.

Rather clearly, much work remains to be done to improve the prediction of real-world benefit of hearing protectors (Berger and Lindgren, 1992; Berger, 1999). One promising approach involves methods similar to in vivo real-ear gain measurements of hearing aids (now a common practice), together with modification of commonly used personal noise dosimeters. This approach requires the ability to simultaneously measure exposure level and the sound level generated within the ear canal of the wearer of a hearing protector. If both are measured with the same filtering schemes (preferably, the C-weighting network; ideally with both A and C networks), the signed difference between the two would index attenuation due to the hearing protector. If such measurements can be adapted to field use (e.g., with a two-channel noise dosimeter), it may be possible to add useful information to what otherwise can be determined about the performance of at least some HPDs. ANSI S12.42 (1995) addresses some of these issues for earmuffs and communication headsets, but only for laboratory measurements. Because the use of probe microphones with earplugs is likely to produce reactive measurement effects, this approach may not be suitable for insert devices.

It is generally recognized that effective use of hearing protectors in the workplace or elsewhere is influenced by factors that go beyond the physical performance of these devices. As summarized by NIOSH (1998), these factors include convenience and availability, comfort and ease of fit, compatibility with other safety equipment, and worker belief that the device can be worn effectively, will indeed prevent hearing loss, and will still permit hearing of important sounds.

—*Michael R. Chial*

References

American National Standards Institute. (1974). *S3.19-1974 American National Standard measurement of real-ear protection of hearing protectors and physical attenuation of ear muffs*. New York: Author.

American National Standards Institute. (1995). *S12.42-1995 American National Standard microphone-in-real-ear and acoustic test fixture methods for the measurement of insertion loss of circumaural hearing protection devices*. New York: Author.

American National Standards Institute. (1996). *S12.19-1996 American National Standard measurement of occupational noise exposure*. New York: Author.

American National Standards Institute. (1997). *S12.6-1997 American National Standard methods for measuring of the* real-ear attenuation of hearing protectors. New York: Author.

Berger, E. H. (1999). Hearing protector testing: Let's get real [using the new ANSI Method-B data and the NRR(SF)]. Earlog 21. Indianapolis, IN: Aearo Co. Available: http://www.cabotsafety.com/html/industrial/earlog21.htm. [Accessed April 12, 2002.]

Berger, E. H. (2000). Hearing protection devices. In E. H. Berger, L. H. Royster, J. D. Royster, D. P. Driscoll, and M. Layne (Eds.), The noise manual (5th ed., chap. 10). Fairfax, VA: American Industrial Hygiene Association.

Berger, E. H., Franks, J. R., Behar, A., Casali, J. G., Dixon-Ernst, C., Kieper, R. W., et al. (1998). Development of a new standard laboratory protocol for estimating the field attenuation of hearing protection devices: Part III. The validity of using subject-fit data. Journal of the Acoustical Society of America, 103, 665–672.

Berger, E. H., and Lindgrin, F. (1992). Current issues in hearing protection. In A. L. Dancer, D. Henderson, R. J. Salvi, and R. P. Hamernik (Eds.), Noise-induced hearing loss (chap. 33). St. Louis: Mosby–Year Book.

Environmental Protection Agency. (1979). Noise labeling requirements for hearing protectors. Code of Federal Regulations 40CFR Part 211. Available: http://www.nonoise.org/lawlib/cfr/40/40cfr211.htm. [Accessed April 12, 2002.]

National Hearing Conservation Association. (1995). Recommendations of the NHCA Task Force on Hearing Protector Effectiveness. Available: http://www.hearingconservation.org/pos6.htm. [Accessed April 12, 2002.]

National Institute of Occupational Safety and Health. (1998). Criteria for a recommended standard: Occupational noise exposure, revised criteria 1988 (DHHS [NIOSH] Publication No. 98-126). Cincinnati, OH: National Institute of Occupational Safety and Health. Available: http://www.cdc.gov/niosh/98-126.html. [Accessed April 12, 2002.]

Nixon, C. W., McKinley, R. L., and Steuver, J. W. (1992). Performance of active noise reduction headsets. In A. L. Dancer, D. Henderson, R. J. Salvi, and R. P. Hamernik (Eds.), Noise-induced hearing loss (chap. 34). St. Louis: Mosby–Year Book.

Occupational Safety and Health Administration. (1983). Occupational noise exposure-hearing conservation amendment. Code of Federal Regulations 29 CFR Part 1910.95. Available: http://www.osha.gov/pls/oshaweb/owadisp.show_document?p_table=STANDARDS&p_id=9735. [Accessed April 12, 2002.]

Occupational Safety and Health Administration. (1999). Noise measurement. In OSHA technical manual (sect. III, chap. 5). Available: http://www.osha.gov/dts/osta/otm/otm_iii/otm_iii_5.html. [Accessed April 12, 2002.]

Royster, J. D., Berger, E. H., Merry, C. J., Nixon, C. W., Franks, J. R., Behar, A., et al. (1996). Development of a new standard laboratory protocol for estimating the field attenuation of hearing protection devices: Part I. Research of Working Group 11, Accredited Standards Committee S12, Noise. Journal of the Acoustical Society of America, 99, 1506–1526.

Further Readings

Alberti, P. W. (Ed.). (1982). Personal hearing protection in industry. New York: Raven Press.

American Industrial Hygiene Association [Archive]. Available: http://www.aiha.org/. [Accessed April 12, 2002.]

American National Standards Institute [Archive]. Available: http://www.ansi.org/. [Accessed April 12, 2002.]

Berger, E. H. Earlog series (1–21) [Archive]. Available: http://www.cabotsafety.com/html/industrial/earlog.htm. [Accessed April 12, 2002.]

Council for Accreditation in Occupational Hearing Conservation [Archive]. Available: http://www.caohc.org/. [Accessed April 12, 2002.]

Franks, J. R., and Berger, E. H. (1998). Hearing protection-personal protection: Overview. In Encyclopedia of occupational health and safety (31.11–31.15). Geneva: International Labour Organization.

National Hearing Conservation Association. (2002). Contemporary references: Hearing protection research. Available: http://www.hearingconservation.org/cr3.html. [Accessed April 12, 2002.]

Noise Pollution Clearinghouse [Archive]. Available: http://www.nonoise.org/. [Accessed April 12, 2002.]

Masking

A major goal of the basic audiologic evaluation is assessment of auditory function of each ear. There are situations during both pure-tone and speech audiometry, however, when the nontest ear can contribute to the observed response from the test ear. Whenever it is suspected that the nontest ear is responsive during evaluation of the test ear, a masking stimulus must be applied to the nontest (i.e., contralateral) ear in order to eliminate its participation.

Cross-hearing occurs when a stimulus presented to the test ear "crosses over" and is perceived in the nontest ear. It is the result of limited interaural attenuation during both air- and bone-conduction testing. Interaural attenuation refers to the reduction of energy between ears. Generally, it represents the amount of separation between ears during testing. Specifically, it is the decibel difference between the hearing level of the signal at the test ear and the hearing level reaching the nontest ear cochlea.

A major factor that affects interaural attenuation is the transducer type: air-conduction versus bone-conduction. Two types of earphones are commonly used during air-conduction audiometry. Supra-aural earphones use cushions that press against the pinna, while insert earphones are coupled to the ear by insertion into the ear canal.

Interaural attenuation for supra-aural earphones varies across frequency and subject, ranging from about 40 dB to 80 dB (e.g., Coles and Priede, 1970; Snyder, 1973; Killion, Wilber, and Gudmundsen, 1985; Sklare and Denenberg, 1987). The smallest reported value of interaural attenuation for speech is 48 dB (e.g., Snyder, 1973; Martin and Blythe, 1977). When making a decision about the need for contralateral masking during clinical practice, a single value defining the lower limit of interaural attenuation is most useful (Studebaker, 1967). The majority of audiologists use an interaural attenuation value of 40 dB for all air-conduction measurements, both pure-tone and speech, when making a decision about the need for contralateral masking (Martin, Champlin, and Chambers, 1998).

Commonly used insert earphones are the ER-3A (Etymotic Research, 1991) and the E-A-RTONE 3A (E-A-R Auditory Systems, 1997). A major advantage of the 3A insert earphone is increased interaural attenuation for air-conducted sound, particularly in the lower frequencies. Consequently, the need for contralateral masking is significantly reduced during air-conduction audiometry. Based on currently available data, conservative estimates of interaural attenuation for 3A insert earphones with deeply inserted foam eartips are 75 dB at 1000 Hz and below and 50 dB at frequencies above 1000 Hz (Killion, Wilber, and Gudmundsen, 1985; Sklare and Denenberg, 1987). The smallest reported value of interaural attenuation for speech is 20 dB greater when using 3A insert earphones with deeply inserted foam eartips (Sklare and Denenberg, 1987) than when using a supra-aural arrangement (Snyder, 1973; Martin and Blythe, 1977). Consequently, a value of 60 dB represents a conservative estimate of interaural attenuation for speech when using 3A insert earphones.

Interaural attenuation is greatly reduced during bone-conduction audiometry. Regardless of the placement of a bone vibrator (i.e., mastoid versus forehead), it is generally agreed that interaural attenuation for bone-conducted sound is negligible and should be considered 0 dB (e.g., Hood, 1960; Sanders and Rintelmann, 1964; Studebaker, 1967; Dirks, 1994).

When to Mask

Contralateral masking is required during pure-tone air-conduction audiometry when the unmasked air-conduction threshold obtained in the test ear (AC_T) minus the apparent bone-conduction threshold (i.e., the unmasked bone-conduction threshold) in the nontest ear (BC_{NT}) equals or exceeds interaural attenuation (IA):

$$AC_T - BC_{NT} \geq IA$$

Many audiologists will obtain air-conduction thresholds prior to measurement of bone-conduction thresholds. A preliminary decision about the need for contralateral masking can be made by comparing the air-conduction thresholds of the two ears. When the air-conduction threshold in the test ear minus the air-conduction threshold in the nontest ear (AC_{NT}) equals or exceeds interaural attenuation, masking should be applied to the nontest ear:

$$AC_T - AC_{NT} \geq IA$$

It is important to remember, however, that cross-hearing for air-conducted sound occurs primarily through the mechanism of bone conduction. Consequently, it will be necessary to reevaluate the need for contralateral masking during air-conduction testing following the measurement of unmasked bone-conduction thresholds.

The major factor to consider when making a decision about the need for contralateral masking during bone-conduction audiometry is whether the unmasked bone-conduction threshold (unmasked BC) suggests the presence of a significant conductive component in the test ear. Specifically, the use of contralateral masking is indicated whenever the results of unmasked bone-conduction audiometry suggest the presence of an air-bone gap in the test ear ($AB Gap_T$) of 15 dB or greater:

$$AB Gap_T \geq 15 dB$$

where

$$AB Gap_T = AC_T - \text{Unmasked BC}$$

Contralateral masking is indicated during speech audiometry whenever the presentation level of the speech signal in dB HL at the test ear (PL_T) minus interaural attenuation equals or exceeds the best pure-tone bone-conduction threshold in the nontest ear (Best BC_{NT}):

$$PL_T - IA \geq \text{Best } BC_{NT}$$

Because speech is a broadband signal, it is necessary to consider bone-conduction hearing sensitivity at more than a single pure-tone frequency. The most conservative approach involves considering the best bone-conduction threshold in the 250- to 4000-Hz frequency range (Coles and Priede, 1975).

Clinical Masking Procedures

Although there are many different approaches to clinical masking, each addresses two basic questions. First, what is the minimum level of noise that is required to just mask the cross-hearing signal in the nontest ear? Stated differently, this is the *minimum masking level* that is needed to prevent *undermasking* (i.e., the test signal continues to be perceived in the nontest ear). Second, what is the maximum level of noise that can be presented to the nontest ear that will not shift or change the true threshold in the test ear? Stated differently, this is the *maximum masking level* that can be used without *overmasking*.

Masking refers to "the process by which the threshold of hearing for one sound is raised by the presence of another (masking) sound" (ANSI S3.6-1996, p. 5). The purpose of contralateral masking is to reduce the sensitivity of the nontest ear to the test stimulus. The masking noise typically used during pure-tone audiometry is narrow-band noise centered geometrically around the audiometric test frequency. Speech spectrum noise (i.e., weighted random noise for the masking of speech) is typically used during speech audiometry. Masking noise is calibrated in effective masking level (dB EM) (ANSI S3.6-1996). Effective masking level for pure tones refers to the dB HL to which detection threshold is shifted by a given level of noise. Effective masking level for speech refers to the dB HL to which the speech recognition threshold (SRT) is shifted by a given level of noise.

The introduction of contralateral masking can produce a small threshold shift in the test ear even when masking level is insufficient to produce overmasking. Wegel and Lane (1924) referred to this phenomenon as *central masking*. Central masking has been reported to affect thresholds during both pure-tone and speech audiometry (e.g., Lidén, Nilsson, and Anderson, 1959; Studebaker, 1962; Dirks and Malmquist, 1964; Martin, Bailey, and Pappas, 1965; Martin, 1966; Martin and DiGiovanni, 1979). Although the threshold shift generally is considered to be about 5 dB, variable results have been reported across subjects and studies.

The most popular method for obtaining masked pure-tone threshold was first described by Hood in 1957 (Hood, 1960; Hood's original paper was reprinted in the United States in 1960). The Hood method is also referred to as the *plateau*, *shadowing*, or *threshold shift* procedure. The goal of the plateau procedure is to establish the hearing level at which the pure-tone threshold remains unchanged with increments in masking level. The masking "plateau" represents a range of masking levels (e.g., 15–20 dB) over which the pure-tone threshold remains unchanged. The recommended clinical procedure is summarized below:

1. Masking noise is introduced to the nontest ear at a minimum masking level. The pure-tone threshold is then reestablished.
2. The level of the tone or noise is increased subsequently by 5 dB. If there is a response to the tone in the presence of the noise, the level of the noise is increased by 5 dB. If there is no response to the tone in the presence of the noise, the level of the tone is increased in 5-dB steps until a response is obtained.
3. A plateau has been reached when the level of the noise can be increased over a range of 15–20 dB without shifting the threshold of the tone. This corresponds to a response to the tone at the same hearing level at three to four consecutive masking levels.
4. The masked pure-tone threshold corresponds to the hearing level of the tone at which a masking plateau has been established.

Formulas have been proposed for the calculation of minimum masking level during pure-tone threshold audiometry (e.g., Lidén, Nilsson, and Anderson, 1959; Studebaker, 1964). The simplified method described by Martin (1967, 1974) is recommended for clinical use. Specifically, minimum masking level (M_{Min}) (i.e., "initial masking" level) during air-conduction testing is equal to the air-conduction threshold of the nontest ear plus a safety factor of at least 10 dB:

$$M_{Min} = AC_{NT} + 10 \text{ dB}$$

Minimum masking level during bone-conduction audiometry is determined similarly. However, it is also necessary to account for the occlusion effect (OE):

$$M_{Min} = AC_{NT} + OE + 10 \text{ dB}$$

Whenever an earphone covers or occludes the nontest ear during masked bone-conduction audiometry, an occlusion effect may be created in the nontest ear. The nontest ear consequently can become more sensitive to bone-conducted sound for test frequencies below 2000 Hz, particularly when using supra-aural earphones (e.g., Elpern and Naunton, 1963; Goldstein and Hayes, 1965; Berger and Kerivan, 1983; Dean and Martin, 2000). Consequently, the minimum masking level must be increased by the amount of the occlusion effect. There is evidence suggesting that the occlusion effect is decreased significantly when using deeply inserted E-A-R foam plugs, the eartips used with 3A insert earphones (Berger and Kerivan, 1983; Dean and Martin, 2000). The clinician can use either individually determined (Martin, Butler, and Burns, 1974; Dean and Martin, 2000) or fixed occlusion effect values (i.e., based on average data reported in the literature) when calculating minimum masking level. When using supra-aural earphones, the following fixed occlusion effect values are recommended for clinical use: 30 dB at 250 Hz, 20 dB at 500 Hz, and 10 dB at 1000 Hz. When using 3A insert earphones with deeply inserted foam eartips, the following values are recommended: 10 dB at 250 and 500 Hz, and 0 dB at frequencies of 1000 Hz and higher. It should be noted that the occlusion effect is decreased or absent in ears with conductive hearing impairment (e.g., Martin, Butler, and Burns, 1974; Studebaker, 1979). If the nontest ear exhibits a potential air-bone gap of 20 dB or more, the occlusion effect should not be added to the minimum masking level.

The American Speech-Language-Hearing Association (ASHA, 1990) has published guidelines for audiometric symbols and procedures for graphic representation of frequency-specific audiometric findings. Different symbols are used to represent pure-tone thresholds obtained with and without contralateral masking. The reader is referred to ASHA's 1990 guidelines and the article PURE-TONE THRESHOLD ASSESSMENT.

The optimal masking level during speech audiometry is one that falls above the minimum and below the maximum masking levels (Lidén, Nilsson, and Anderson, 1959; Studebaker, 1979; Konkle and Berry, 1983). The goal is to select a masking level that falls at the middle of the masking plateau. This concept was originally discussed by Luscher and König in 1955 (cited in Studebaker, 1979).

Minimum masking level (M_{Min}), adapted from Lidén, Nilsson, and Anderson (1959), can be summarized using the following equation:

$$M_{Min} = PL_T - IA + Max \text{ AB Gap}_{NT}$$

PL_T represents the presentation level of the speech signal in dB HL at the test ear, IA is the interaural attenuation value for speech, and Max AB Gap$_{NT}$ is the maximum air-bone gap in the nontest ear in the 250–4000-Hz frequency range. $PL_T - IA$, an estimate of the hearing level of the speech signal that has reached the nontest ear, represents the minimum masking level required. However, the presence of air-bone gaps in the nontest ear will reduce the effectiveness of the masker. Consequently, the minimum masking level must be increased by the size of the air-bone gap. Following the recommendation of Coles and Priede (1975), the maximum air-bone gap in the nontest ear should be considered when determining minimum masking level.

Maximum masking level (M_{Max}), adapted from Lidén, Nilsson, and Anderson (1959), can be summarized using the following equation:

$$M_{Max} = \text{Best } BC_T + IA - 5 \text{ dB}$$

Best BC_T represents the best bone-conduction threshold in the test ear in the frequency range from 250 through 4000 Hz, and IA is the interaural attenuation value for speech. There is the assumption that the best bone-conduction threshold is most susceptible to the effects of overmasking. If Best $BC_T + IA$ is just sufficient to produce overmasking, then a slightly lower masking level than the calculated value must be used clinically. Because masking level is typically adjusted using a 5-dB step size, a value of 5 dB is subsequently subtracted from the calculated value.

Although Studebaker (1962) originally described an equation for calculating midmasking level during pure-tone bone-conduction testing, the basic principles underlying the midplateau method also can be applied effectively during speech audiometry. A direct approach to calculating the *midmasking level* (M_{Mid}) involves determining the arithmetic mean of the minimum and maximum masking levels:

$$M_{Mid} = (M_{Min} + M_{Max})/2$$

Yacullo (1999) has described a simplified approach to selecting an appropriate level of contralateral masking during speech audiometry. Although this approach proves most effective during assessment of suprathreshold speech recognition, it can also be applied during threshold measurement. Stated simply, effective masking level is equal to the presentation level of the speech signal in dB HL at the test ear minus 20 dB:

$$\text{dB EM} = PL_T - 20 \text{ dB}$$

The procedure proves very effective given the following two prerequisite conditions: (1) there are no significant air-bone gaps (i.e., ≥15 dB) in either ear, and (2) speech is presented at a moderate sensation level (i.e., 30–40 dB) relative to the measured or estimated SRT. Given these two prerequisites, the selected masking level will occur approximately at midplateau.

The plateau masking procedure, described earlier as a popular method for obtaining masked pure-tone threshold, also can be applied effectively during measurement of both speech detection and speech recognition thresholds (i.e., SDT and SRT). A major advantage of the plateau procedure is that information about bone-conduction sensitivity in each ear is not required when selecting appropriate masking levels. The reader is referred to Yacullo (1996) for further discussion.

—*William S. Yacullo*

References

American National Standards Institute. (1996). *American National Standard specification for audiometers (ANSI S3.6-1996)*. New York: Author.

American Speech-Language-Hearing Association. (1990). Guidelines for audiometric symbols. *ASHA*, Supplement 2, 25–30.

Berger, E. H., and Kerivan, J. E. (1983). Influence of physiological noise and the occlusion effect on the measurement of real-ear attenuation at threshold. *Journal of the Acoustical Society of America, 74*, 81–94.

Coles, R. R. A., and Priede, V. M. (1970). On the misdiagnosis resulting from incorrect use of masking. *Journal of Laryngology and Otology, 84*, 41–63.

Coles, R. R. A., and Priede, V. M. (1975). Masking of the nontest ear in speech audiometry. *Journal of Laryngology and Otology, 89*, 217–226.

Dean, M. S., and Martin, F. N. (2000). Insert earphone depth and the occlusion effect. *American Journal of Audiology, 9*, 131–134.

Dirks, D. D. (1994). Bone-conduction threshold testing. In J. Katz (Ed.), *Handbook of clinical audiology* (4th ed., pp. 132–146). Baltimore: Williams and Wilkins.

Dirks, D. D., and Malmquist, C. (1964). Changes in bone-conduction thresholds produced by masking in the nontest ear. *Journal of Speech and Hearing Research, 7*, 271–278.

E-A-R Auditory Systems. (1997). *Instructions for the use of E-A-RTONE 3A insert earphones* (rev. ed.). Indianapolis, IN: Author.

Elpern, B. S., and Naunton, R. F. (1963). The stability of the occlusion effect. *Archives of Otolaryngology, 77*, 376–382.

Etymotic Research. (1991). *ER-3A Tubephone insert earphone*. Elk Grove Village, IL: Author.

Goldstein, D. P., and Hayes, C. S. (1965). The occlusion effect in bone-conduction hearing. *Journal of Speech and Hearing Research, 8*, 137–148.

Hood, J. D. (1960). The principles and practice of bone-conduction audiometry. *Laryngoscope, 70*, 1211–1228.

Killion, M. C., Wilber, L. A., and Gudmundsen, G. I. (1985). Insert earphones for more interaural attenuation. *Hearing Instruments, 36*, 34–36.

Konkle, D. F., and Berry, G. A. (1983). Masking in speech audiometry. In D. F. Konkle and W. F. Rintelmann (Eds.), *Principles of speech audiometry* (pp. 285–319). Baltimore: University Park Press.

Lidén, G., Nilsson, G., and Anderson, H. (1959). Masking in clinical audiology. *Acta Oto-Laryngologica, 50*, 125–136.

Martin, F. N. (1966). Speech audiometry and clinical masking. *Journal of Auditory Research, 6*, 199–203.

Martin, F. N. (1967). A simplified method for clinical masking. *Journal of Auditory Research, 7*, 59–62.

Martin, F. N. (1974). Minimum effective masking levels in threshold audiometry. *Journal of Speech and Hearing Disorders, 39*, 280–285.

Martin, F. N., Bailey, H. A. T., and Pappas, J. J. (1965). The effect of central masking on threshold for speech. *Journal of Auditory Research, 5*, 293–296.

Martin, F. N., and Blythe, M. E. (1977). On the cross hearing of spondaic words. *Journal of Auditory Research, 17*, 221–224.

Martin, F. N., Butler, E. C., and Burns, P. (1974). Audiometric Bing test for determination of minimum masking levels for bone conduction tests. *Journal of Speech and Hearing Disorders, 39*, 148–152.

Martin, F. N., Champlin, C. A., and Chambers, J. A. (1998). Seventh survey of audiometric practices in the United States. *Journal of the American Academy of Audiology, 9,* 95–104.

Martin, F. N., and DiGiovanni, D. (1979). Central masking effects on spondee threshold as a function of masker sensation level and masker sound pressure level. *Journal of the American Auditory Society, 4,* 141–146.

Sanders, F. W., and Rintelmann, W. F. (1964). Masking in audiometry. *Archives of Otolaryngology, 80,* 541–556.

Sklare, D. A., and Denenberg, L. J. (1987). Interaural attenuation for Tubephone insert earphones. *Ear and Hearing, 8,* 298–300.

Snyder, J. M. (1973). Interaural attenuation characteristics in audiometry. *Laryngoscope, 73,* 1847–1855.

Studebaker, G. A. (1962). On masking in bone-conduction testing. *Journal of Speech and Hearing Research, 5,* 215–227.

Studebaker, G. A. (1964). Clinical masking of air- and bone-conducted stimuli. *Journal of Speech and Hearing Disorders, 29,* 23–35.

Studebaker, G. A. (1967). Clinical masking of the non-test ear. *Journal of Speech and Hearing Disorders, 32,* 360–371.

Studebaker, G. A. (1979). Clinical masking. In W. F. Rintelmann (Ed.), *Hearing assessment* (pp. 51–100). Baltimore: University Park Press.

Wegel, R. L., and Lane, G. I. (1924). The auditory masking of one pure tone by another and its probable relation to the dynamics of the inner ear. *Physics Review, 23,* 266–285.

Yacullo, W. S. (1996). *Clinical masking procedures.* Needham Heights, MA: Allyn and Bacon.

Yacullo, W. S. (1999). Clinical masking in speech audiometry: A simplified approach. *American Journal of Audiology, 8,* 106–116.

Further Readings

Chaiklin, J. B. (1967). Interaural attenuation and cross-hearing in air-conduction audiometry. *Journal of Auditory Research, 7,* 413–424.

Dirks, D. D., and Swindeman, J. G. (1967). The variability of occluded and unoccluded bone-conduction thresholds. *Journal of Speech and Hearing Research, 10,* 232–249.

Fletcher, H. (1940). Auditory patterns. *Review of Modern Physics, 12,* 47–65.

Gelfand, S. A. (2001). Clinical masking. In *Essentials of audiology* (2nd ed., pp. 291–317). New York: Thieme.

Hawkins, J. E., and Stevens, S. S. (1950). Masking of pure tones and of speech by white noise. *Journal of the Acoustical Society of America, 22,* 6–13.

Hodgson, W., and Tillman, T. (1966). Reliability of bone conduction occlusion effects in normals. *Journal of Auditory Research, 6,* 141–151.

Hosford-Dunn, H., Kuklinski, A. L., Raggio, M., and Haggerty, H. S. (1986). Solving audiometric masking dilemmas with an insert masker. *Archives of Otolaryngology–Head and Neck Surgery, 112,* 92–95.

Lidén, G., Nilsson, G., and Anderson, H. (1959). Narrow-band masking with white noise. *Acta Oto-Laryngologica, 50,* 116–124.

Martin, F. N. (1980). The masking plateau revisited. *Ear and Hearing, 1,* 112–116.

Naunton, R. F. (1960). A masking dilemma in bilateral conduction deafness. *Archives of Otolaryngology, 72,* 753–757.

Smith, B. L., and Markides, A. (1981). Interaural attenuation for pure tones and speech. *British Journal of Audiology, 15,* 49–54.

Zwislocki, J. (1953). Acoustic attenuation between the ears. *Journal of the Acoustical Society of America, 25,* 752–759.

Middle Ear Assessment in the Child

Current clinical methods of assessment of the middle ear in children include otoscopic examination, acoustic immittance measures, and reflectometry. When assessing middle ear function, a good otoscopic evaluation is the first step. Examination of the ear canal for any obstructions that would preclude placement of a probe such as is used for acoustic immittance measures is essential. Often, cerumen in the ear canal becomes impacted, even in children, and thereby confounds tympanometric measures. Even when not impacted, cerumen can clog the immittance probe and cause invalid measurements.

Otoscopy can also be useful in identifying middle ear disorders such as middle ear effusion. Examination of the tympanic membrane can provide evidence of fluid by its opacity or color. An opaque or yellow membrane, for example, might indicate middle ear effusion. Clearer evidence comes when a fluid meniscus or bubbles can be seen through a transparent tympanic membrane. Someone skilled with pneumatic otoscopy can examine the membrane's mobility by applying slight changes in air pressure in the ear canal. However, the ability to use a pneumatic otoscope for the diagnosis of middle ear effusion is highly variable. Of course, in the clinical examination associated with the diagnosis of middle ear effusion, visual examination of the ear canal and tympanic membrane is important so that other conditions (e.g., cholesteatoma, retraction pocket) may be identified.

Acoustic Immittance: Tympanometry

Tympanometry, unlike pneumatic otoscopy, is a derived physiological measure that requires instrumentation that meets a standard of the American National Standards Institute (ANSI S3.39, 1987) and is a test that is easily administered. The principles of acoustic immittance measurement are covered elsewhere.

Acoustic immittance is a term used to describe the ability of energy to flow through the middle ear. The word *immittance* is a combination of the words *impedance* (opposition to the flow of energy) and *admittance* (ease with which energy flows). Today, most immittance instruments measure acoustic admittance, so the description that follows will consider only acoustic admittance measures. *Tympanometry* is a dynamic measurement of acoustic admittance as air pressure in the ear canal is varied. The tympanogram is the graph of acoustic admittance in mmhos (or in equivalent volume units such as milliliters) versus air pressure in decapascals (daPa). To estimate admittance, a tone is delivered to the ear via a probe hermetically sealed in the ear canal. The probe tone is the force that activates the middle ear system, while a microphone that is connected to a separate opening in the probe records sound pressure in the ear canal. A third opening in the probe connects to a pneumatic system for varying air pressure in the ear canal.

The first measurement made in tympanometry is an estimate of the volume of the space between the probe tip and the tympanic membrane and is called *ear canal volume* or *equivalent volume*. This is done with a low-frequency (226-Hz) probe tone when the pressure in the ear canal is set to a very high value (either positive or negative). The extreme pressure stiffens the tympanic membrane such that admittance of the middle ear is diminished to (theoretically) zero. Thus, the acoustic admittance detected by the instrument is a measure of the admittance of the volume of air enclosed in the ear canal and, with the 226-Hz probe tone only, can be expressed as an equivalent volume of air in the ear canal. This ear canal volume measure is useful for determining the validity of the probe fit in the ear canal and, when larger than normal, suggests an opening in the tympanic membrane. This is useful when trying to determine if there is a perforation in the tympanic membrane or if a pressure equalization tube is functioning.

The normal tympanogram has the shape of an inverted V, with the peak amplitude referred to as *peak admittance* or *static admittance*. When the admittance attributed to the ear canal volume is automatically subtracted from the dynamic admittance measure, peak admittance is referred to as *peak compensated acoustic admittance*. The magnitude of the peak in mmhos of admittance carries diagnostic information. Because there is developmental change in acoustic admittance variables, peak admittance in a given case must be compared with age-appropriate normative values. Low peak admittance when tympanometric peak pressure (the air pressure in the ear canal at which the peak occurs) is within normal range suggests that the middle ear space is well aerated but that there is a condition that is reducing the ability of sound to flow through. A condition that increases stiffness in the middle ear system, such as stapes fixation, might result in such a pattern.

If peak admittance is greater than the normal range, with tympanometric peak pressure within the normal range, there is a condition of the middle ear that is increasing admittance, such as an ossicular disarticulation. Because middle ear function is being inferred from admittance changes based on sound reflected from the tympanic membrane, abnormalities of that membrane can influence the measurement. For example, scarring on the membrane can also cause an abnormally high admittance tympanogram in the presence of an otherwise normal middle ear system.

In an ear with eustachian tube dysfunction, in which middle ear pressure varies and is not equalized easily, tympanometry can give valuable information. The tympanometric peak pressure is a reasonably good estimate of middle ear pressure, so a negative value is often diagnostic of eustachian tube dysfunction.

Pattern Classification of Tympanograms

Historically, the most common way to interpret tympanometric data has been to classify tympanograms according to their pattern. The most notable and widely used pattern classification scheme was proposed by Jerger (1970). This pattern classification scheme is easy to use, with patterns that are easy to identify and few in number. The pattern classifications were based originally on the height of the tympanogram (in arbitrary "compliance" units) and the tympanometric peak pressure. The patterns are identified by the letters A, B, and C, with subclassifications used to better define them. A normal tympanogram is A, with A_s and A_D representing abnormally low peak compliance and abnormally high peak compliance, respectively, in the presence of normal tympanometric peak pressure. Type B is a tympanogram with no peak, and type C is a tympanogram with a high negative tympanometric peak pressure.

In children, the most common reason for assessment of middle ear function is to identify middle ear effusion. As a result, much of the published research on tympanometry in children relates to identification of middle ear effusion. In most studies of the ability of tympanometry to identify ears with middle ear effusion, the type B tympanogram (no peak) has high predictive ability; that is, a tympanogram that has no peak will very likely be associated with an ear with effusion. However, the opposite is not necessarily true: ears with middle ear effusion most often produce tympanograms that cannot be classified as type B. Rarely is an ear with middle ear effusion associated with a type A (normal peak, normal tympanometric peak pressure), so many ears with middle ear effusion fall in the C category (normal peak admittance, abnormally negative tympanometric peak pressure). However, many ears with no middle ear effusion also fall into the C category. Subdivisions of the C category have emerged to try to improve the diagnostic ability of tympanometry, but even with more specific information regarding tympanometric peak pressure, the ability of the C category to help with identification of middle ear effusion varies widely across studies (Orchik, Dunn, and McNutt, 1978).

Because of the ambiguity in the C category, even when subdivided, attempts to further improve identification of middle ear effusion have included addition of the acoustic reflex test, in which case an equivocal tympanometric pattern accompanied by an absent acoustic reflex is considered evidence of middle ear effusion. Also, schemes with very detailed categories have been developed (e.g., Cantekin et al., 1980).

There are several drawbacks to the A, B, C pattern classification scheme. One is that the patterns were determined based on clinical observations and not on statistical analysis of performance in a controlled clinical trial with a reference standard such as myringotomy for the diagnosis of middle ear effusion. Many studies that have been done to determine the performance characteristics of the pattern classification of tympanograms used predetermined categories rather than collecting tympanometric data and then using statistical techniques to determine which characteristics are best able to predict middle ear status. A second drawback is that tympanograms produced using instruments meeting the 1987 ANSI standard are based on absolute physical quantities and are not directly comparable to the tympanograms using arbitrary compliance units on which the A, B, C scheme was developed.

A third drawback to the A, B, C classification scheme is that it does not incorporate very much information about the shape, or gradient, of the tympanogram. Data from studies using absolute physical units of immittance have shown that tympanogram shape carries useful information regarding middle ear status that is not readily available in the A, B, C classification scheme (Brooks, 1968; Koebsell and Margolis, 1986; Nozza et al., 1992, 1994).

Quantitative Analysis of Tympanograms

Instruments developed since 1987, when the ANSI standard became effective, provide immittance information using absolute physical quantities rather than arbitrary compliance values such as were used when the pattern classification scheme was developed. There are several advantages to using a quantitative analysis of tympanometric data. First, such measures are standardized for all instruments and, therefore, across clinics and laboratories. Second, tympanometric shape can be quantified. Third, unlike the pattern categories, the data from current instruments that measure actual physical quantities of admittance are on continua that permit statistical analyses. Measures that may be used in a quantitative analyses include peak compensated acoustic admittance, tympanometric peak pressure, absolute gradient, relative gradient, and tympanometric width.

The absolute and relative gradients and tympanometric width are measures used to quantify the shape of the tympanogram. To compute absolute gradient, a horizontal line is drawn between the sides of the tympanogram at the point where the tympanogram is 100 daPa wide. This serves as a temporary baseline from which the distance to the peak of the tympanogram is measured in mmho. This value is the absolute gradient and increases in value as tympanogram shape becomes more sharply peaked. Relative gradient is determined by dividing the absolute gradient by the peak admittance. This results in a ratio that can range from 0 to 1. Again, the greater the relative gradient, the more sharply peaked is the tympanogram. Few instruments report absolute gradient, but some will report relative gradient to characterize the rate of change of the tympanogram in the region of the peak (i.e., tympanogram shape). Absolute and relative gradients have been examined in the past for their contribution to the diagnosis of middle ear effusion (Brooks, 1968). The lower the gradient, the more rounded or flat the tympanogram and the greater the likelihood of middle ear effusion.

Tympanometric width is the width of the tympanogram in daPa at half the peak admittance. The more rounded or flat the tympanogram becomes, the greater will be the tympanometric width. Tympanometric width has good diagnostic value for identification of middle ear effusion in children (Margolis and Heller, 1987; Nozza et al., 1994). Using quantitative analysis, Nozza et al. (1994) reported that using tympanometric width greater than 275 daPa as a criterion for identification of middle ear effusion had a sensitivity of 81% and a specificity of 82% in a group of children undergoing myringotomy and tube surgery. This was the best performance of any single tympanometric variable. For peak admittance, a cutoff of 0.3 mmho separated the ears, with a sensitivity and specificity nearly as good as the best cutoff for tympanometric width. Interestingly, tympanometric peak pressure alone was the worst at separating ears with and without middle ear effusion and contributed nothing when used in combination with other variables. This suggests that the weight that tympanometric peak pressure carries in the pattern classification scheme is probably not warranted when it comes to identification of ears with middle ear effusion. The acoustic reflex alone was examined as well, and overall performance was only fair because specificity was poor. Too often, no acoustic reflex can be measured in children, even in the absence of middle ear effusion. Also, because the reflex relies on an auditory system and elements of the central nervous system that are sufficiently intact, an immittance criterion for identification of middle ear effusion that includes the acoustic reflex will not be applicable to children with high degrees of hearing impairment or certain neurological problems.

Because the data from studies such as that of Nozza et al. (1994) come from children from a special population, those undergoing myringotomy and tube surgery, they may not be representative of the general pediatric population, in whom middle ear assessment is so important. Recommendations for criteria for identification of middle ear effusion in the general population can be found in guidelines for screening that have been published by the American Academy of Audiology (1997) and the American Speech-Language-Hearing Association (ASHA, 1997). The American Academy of Audiology suggests using tympanometric variables of peak admittance or tympanometric width. In both guidelines, the notion is that a positive result on tympanometric screening should not result in immediate referral but should indicate the need for rescreening in 6 to 8 weeks. Because middle ear effusion is a transient, often self-limiting disorder, referrals based on a single test result in a high over-referral rate. ASHA recommends that an ear pass the tympanometric screen when peak admittance is ≥0.3 mmho or tympanometric width is <200 daPa when screening children from the general population for middle ear effusion. The American Academy of Audiology uses a similar protocol, with ≥0.2 mmho a passing indication for peak admittance and <250 daPa a passing indication for tympanometric width.

High-Frequency Tympanometry in Infants

With universal newborn hearing screening increasing the number of young infants referred for rescreening and audiological assessments, it is important to consider the special circumstances related to middle ear assessment in that population. It has long been known that tympanometry using low-frequency probe tones is unreliable in young infants. Infants with middle ear effusion can produce tympanograms that appear normal, presumably because of distensibility of the walls of the ear canal. Recent work using multifrequency tympanometry has demonstrated that young infants (<4 months) with middle ear effusion might produce a normal tympanogram with a 226-Hz probe tone but an abnormal tympanogram when a high-frequency probe, 1000 Hz in particular, is used (McKinley, Grose, and Roush, 1997; Rhodes et al., 1999; Purdy and Williams, 2000). Use of a 1000-Hz probe tone is recommended now for identification of middle ear effusion in young infants.

Reflectometry

An alternative method for identification of middle ear effusion uses a measurement called acoustic reflectometry. The acoustic reflectometer generates a broad band sound in the ear canal and measures the sound energy reflected back from the tympanic membrane. The instrument is hand-held and has a speculum-like tip that is put into the entrance of the ear canal. No hermetic seal is required, thus making the test desirable for use with children. The relationship between the known output of the device and the resultant sound in the ear canal provides diagnostic information. An early version of the instrument used only the sound pressure level in the ear canal in the diagnostic decision. It was later determined that, by plotting out the reflectivity data on frequency by amplitude axes, better diagnostic information regarding middle ear effusion could be derived. The current version of the instrument analyzes automatically the frequency-amplitude relationship in the reflected sound and displays a number between 1 and 5 to indicate the likelihood of an effusion. This instrument is getting some favorable use in primary care settings for the identification of both acute otitis media and asymptomatic otitis media with effusion.

See also HEARING LOSS SCREENING: THE SCHOOL-AGE CHILD; OTITIS MEDIA: EFFECTS ON CHILDREN'S LANGUAGE; PEDIATRIC AUDIOLOGY: THE TEST BATTERY APPROACH; PHYSIOLOGICAL BASES OF HEARING; TYMPANOMETRY.

—*Robert J. Nozza*

References

American Academy of Audiology. (1997). Position statement: Identification of hearing loss and middle ear dysfunction in preschool and school-age children. *Audiology Today, 9*(3), 21–23.

American National Standards Institute. (1987). *American national standard specifications for instruments to measure aural acoustic impedance and admittance (aural acoustic immittance) (ANSI S3.39)*. New York: Acoustical Society of America.

American Speech-Language-Hearing Association. (1997). *Guidelines for audiologic screening*. Rockville, MD: Author.

Brooks, D. N. (1968). An objective method of detecting fluid in the middle ear. *International Audiology, 7*, 280–286.

Cantekin, E. I., Bluestone, C. D., Fria, T. J., Stool, S. E., Beery, Q. C., and Sabo, D. L. (1980). Identification of otitis media with effusion in children. *Annals of Otology, Rhinology and Laryngology, 89*(Suppl. 68), 190–195.

Jerger, J. (1970). Clinical experience with impedance audiometry. *Archives of Otolaryngology, 92*, 311–324.

Koebsell, K. A., and Margolis, R. H. (1986). Tympanometric gradient measured from normal preschool children. *Audiology, 25*, 149–157.

Margolis, R. H., and Heller, J. W. (1987). Screening tympanometry: Criteria for medical referral. *Audiology, 26*, 197–208.

McKinley, A. M., Grose, J. H., and Roush, J. (1997). Multifrequency tympanometry and evoked otoacoustic emissions in neonates during the first 24 hours of life. *Journal of the American Academy of Audiology, 8*, 218–223.

Nozza, R. J., Bluestone, C. D., Kardatzke, D., and Bachman, R. N. (1992). Towards the validation of aural acoustic immittance measures for diagnosis of middle ear effusion in children. *Ear and Hearing, 13*, 442–453.

Nozza, R. J., Bluestone, C. D., Kardatzke, D., and Bachman, R. N. (1994). Identification of middle ear effusion by aural acoustic admittance and otoscopy. *Ear and Hearing, 15*, 310–323.

Orchik, D. J., Dunn, J. W., and McNutt, L. (1978). Tympanometry as a predictor of middle ear effusion. *Archives of Otorhinolaryngology, 104*, 4–6.

Purdy, S. C., and Williams, M. J. (2000). High frequency tympanometry: A valid reliable immittance test protocol for young infants? *New Zealand Audiological Society Bulletin, 109*, 9–24.

Rhodes, M. C., Margolis, R. H., Hirsch, J. E., and Napp, A. P. (1999). Hearing screening in the newborn intensive care nursery: Comparison of methods. *Otolaryngology–Head and Neck Surgery, 120*, 799–808.

Further Readings

Brooks, D. N. (1969). The use of the electro-acoustic impedance bridge in the assessment of middle ear function. *International Audiology, 8*, 563–569.

Cantekin, E. I. (1983). Algorithm for diagnosis of otitis media with effusion. *Annals of Otology, Rhinology, and Laryngology, 92*(Suppl. 107), 6.

Fiellau-Nikolajsen, M. (1980). Tympanometry and middle ear effusion: A cohort-study in three-year-old children. *International Journal of Pediatric Otorhinolaryngology, 2*, 39–49.

Finitzo, T., Friel-Patti, S., Chinn, K., and Brown, O. (1992). Tympanometry and otoscopy prior to myringotomy: Issues in diagnosis of otitis media. *International Journal of Pediatric Otorhinolaryngology, 24*, 101–110.

Grimaldi, P. M. G. B. (1976). The value of impedance testing in diagnosis of middle ear effusion. *Journal of Laryngology and Otology, 90*, 141–152.

Haughton, P. M. (1977). Validity of tympanometry for middle ear effusions. *Archives of Otolaryngology, 103*, 505–513.

Liden, G. (1969). The scope and application of current audiometric tests. *Journal of Laryngology and Otology*, *83*, 507–520.

Marchant, C. D., McMillan, P. M., Shurin, P. A., et al. (1986). Objective diagnosis of otitis media in early infancy by tympanometry and ipsilateral acoustic reflex thresholds. *Journal of Pediatrics*, *109*, 590–595.

Northern, J. L. (1992). Special issues concerned with screening for middle ear disease in children. In F. H. Bess and J. W. Hall III (Eds.), *Screening children for auditory function.* Nashville, TN: Bill Wilkerson Center Press.

Nozza, R. J. (1995). Critical issues in acoustic-immittance screening for middle-ear effusion. *Seminars in Hearing*, *16*(1), 86–98.

Nozza, R. J. (1998). Identification of otitis media. In F. Bess (Ed.), *Children with hearing impairment: Contemporary trends* (pp. 207–214). Nashville, TN: Bill Wilkerson Center Press.

Shanks, J. E. (1984). Tympanometry. *Ear and Hearing, 5*, 268–280.

Teele, D. W., and Teele, J. (1984). Detection of middle ear effusion by acoustic reflectometry. *Journal of Pediatrics, 104*, 832–838.

Toner, J. G., and Mains, B. (1990). Pneumatic otoscopy and tympanometry in the detection of middle ear effusion. *Clinics of Otolaryngology, 15*, 121–123.

Van Camp, K. J., Margolis, R. H., Wilson, R. H., Creten, W. L., and Shanks, J. E. (1986). Principles of tympanometry. *ASHA Monograph*, 1–88.

Vaughan-Jones, R., and Mills, R. P. (1992). The Welch Allyn Audioscope and Microtymp: Their accuracy and that of pneumatic otoscopy, tympanometry and pure tone audiometry as predictors of otitis media with effusion. *Journal of Laryngology and Otology, 106*, 600–602.

Wilber, L. A., and Feldman, A. S. (1976). *Acoustic impedance and admittance: The measure of middle ear function.* Baltimore: Williams and Wilkins.

Noise-Induced Hearing Loss

Hearing loss affects about 28 million Americans. The two most common causes of sensorineural hearing loss are aging and exposure to noise. Noise exposure can injure the ear and produce loss of hearing. The injury and hearing loss can be temporary—that is, fully recoverable after the noise exposure is terminated—or permanent. When hearing loss is measured at a postexposure time of 2 weeks, it is considered to be permanent, inasmuch as very little additional recovery occurs at postexposure times in excess of 2 weeks (Miller, Watson, and Covell, 1963; Mills, 1973). The presence and severity of a temporary or permanent hearing loss depend on several factors and the susceptibility of the individual. Acoustically, the level (intensity), spectrum (frequency), and temporal properties (duration, intermittency, number) of the exposures are the most pertinent properties. Nonacoustic factors such as interactions with various medicines or drugs, eye color, smoking, sex, and other personal characteristics of an individual (except aging and hearing loss) are second-order effects, or are not consistently observed (Ward, 1995). Interactions with

other factors such as chemicals, solvents, and toxic substances such as carbon monoxide can be significant and are an active area of investigation (Morata and Dunn, 1995).

The database available on noise-induced hearing loss caused by exposure to steady-state noise is substantial. Some of the data are from laboratory studies of temporary effects in human subjects (Davis et al., 1950; Mills et al., 1970; Melnick and Maves, 1974) and both temporary and permanent effects in laboratory animals (Miller, Watson, and Covell, 1963; Mills, 1973). Other data are from studies of permanent hearing loss in humans in occupational settings (Taylor et al., 1965; Burns and Robinson, 1970; Johnson, 1991). These and other field studies of noise-induced permanent hearing loss (see Johnson, 1991) are the scientific bases of international (International Organization for Standardization [ISO], 1990) and American standards (American National Standards Institute [ANSI], 1996), which present methods to estimate noise-induced permanent threshold shifts as a function of A-weighted sound level and years of exposure time. The development and acceptance of these standards represents many years of work and intense debate. Regulations for industry are given by the U.S. Department of Labor (Occupational Safety and Health Administration [OSHA], 1983).

Data from humans and animals exposed to a wide variety of steady-state noises suggest that the range of human audibility can be categorized with respect to risk of acoustic injury of the ear and noise-induced hearing loss. This categorization is shown in Figure 1, where the range of human audibility is bounded by the threshold of

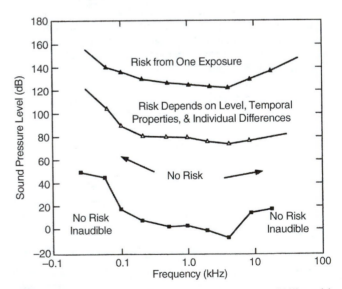

Figure 1. Categorization of the range of human audibility with respect to acoustic injury of the ear and noise-induced hearing loss. (From Mills, J. H., et al., 1993, *Hazardous Exposure to Steady-State and Intermittent Noise*. Working Group Report, Committee on Hearing, Bioacoustics and Biomechanics, National Research Council. Washington, DC: National Academy Press. Reproduced with permission.)

audibility at one extreme and the threshold of pain (Yost and Nielsen, 1985) at the other. Of course, sounds below the threshold of audibility are inaudible and present no risk of noise-induced hearing loss. Sounds in excess of the threshold of pain present a risk of acoustic injury of the ear and noise-induced hearing loss even with one, short exposure (see Mills et al., 1993). Between the extremes of pain and audibility are acoustic injury thresholds (open triangles in Fig. 1). These thresholds define the highest levels of noise that will not produce a noise-induced threshold shift regardless of the duration of exposure, the number of exposures, or the temporal properties of the exposure. The data points in Figure 1 are from temporary threshold shift experiments for octave bands of noise from 63 Hz to 4 kHz in octave steps. Data at lower and higher frequencies are extrapolations. Thus, between the extremes of the threshold of pain and audibility are two categories: no risk and risk. The no-risk category can also be described as "effective quiet" (Ward, Cushing, and Burns, 1976). The region bounded by safe levels on the low side and threshold of pain on the high side is the area where the risk of hearing loss and acoustic injury of the ear depends on the parameters of the noise exposure as well as on the susceptibility of the individual. In qualitative terms, risk increases with noise level, duration, number of exposures, and susceptibility of the individual. Although individual differences can be substantial, no method has been developed that allows the a priori identification of those individuals who are most susceptible to noise-induced hearing loss. Quantitative relations between noise-induced hearing loss and exposure parameters are given in ANSI S3.44-1996.

Whereas the database is massive for noise-induced hearing losses produced by exposure to continuous noise (see Johnson, 1991), it is unimpressive for intermittent (quiet periods of a few seconds to a few hours) and time-varying (level fluctuations greater than 10 dB) noises. On a qualitative basis, there is agreement that intermittent and fluctuating noises are less hazardous than continuous noises, presumably because the "quiet" periods allow time for the ear to recover. Because of regulatory efforts in noise control and a perceived need for simplicity, several single-number correction factors have evolved. That is, as an exposure is increased from 4 hours to 8 hours, what change in noise level is needed to maintain an equal risk of hearing loss? The equal-energy rule specifies a 3-dB reduction in noise level for a doubling of exposure duration. This rule is incorporated into the ISO 1999 standard. Other standards and regulations use 4-dB, 5-dB, and 6-dB rules, as well as other more complicated schemes (see Ward, 1991). It is likely that each of these single-number rules may apply only to a restricted set of exposure conditions. With the continued absence of needed data, the effects of intermittence on noise-induced hearing loss may always be a contentious issue.

Although the biological bases of noise-induced hearing loss have been studied extensively, with the greatest emphasis on the cochlea, both the external and middle ear play a prominent role. The external auditory meatus (essentially a tube open at one end with a length of about 25 mm) has a resonant frequency of about 3 kHz and a gain of about 20 dB. Thus, the typical industrial or environmental noise, which may have a flat or slightly downward-sloping spectrum when measured in the field, will have a peak at 3 kHz because of the external ear canal. Thus, the "4-kHz notch" in the audiogram that is characteristic of noise-induced hearing loss (and head injuries) may reflect the acoustic properties of the external ear. In the middle ear, the acoustic reflex, the consensual contraction of the stapedial and tensor tympani muscles, may reduce the level of intense sounds. In addition, the efferent innervation of outer hair cells may have a protective role (Maison and Liberman, 2000).

Although there has been a substantial effort, the anatomical, chemical, and biological bases of noise-induced temporary threshold shift are unknown. The pathological anatomy associated with noise-induced permanent hearing loss involves the organ of Corti, especially the hair cells. Loss of outer hair cells is the most prominent anatomical feature of permanent noise-induced loss, and is almost always greater than the loss of inner hair cells. This greater loss of outer than inner hair cells may occur for several reasons, including the direct shearing forces on the outer hair cell stereocilia, which are embedded in the tectorial membrane. The correlations between loss of hair cells, both inner and outer, and permanent threshold shift are very high, ranging from 0.6 to 0.8, depending on frequency (Hamernik et al., 1989). Even with such high correlations there remains considerable variance between hair cell loss and permanent threshold shift. This variance can be reduced by consideration of the status of the stereocilia (Liberman and Dodds, 1984). With degeneration of inner hair cells following severe exposures, there can be retrograde degeneration of auditory nerve fibers, as indicated by losses of spiral ganglion cells. Neural degeneration is not restricted to the auditory nerve but progresses throughout the ascending auditory system (Morest, 1982). Regeneration of hair cells has been observed after intense exposures to noise. This dramatic effect has been reported only for the cochlea of various species of birds. Regenerating sensory cells have not been observed in the cochlea of mammals.

Reactive oxygen species and oxidative stress have been implicated in the production of noise-induced hearing loss and in age-related hearing loss as well (Ohlemiller et al., 2000). It is believed that acute impairment of antioxidant defenses promotes cochlear injury, and conversely, strengthening antioxidant defenses should provide protection, including possibly rescuing cells that are in the early stages of injury. Efforts at prevention and rescue are in the early stage of development, with some promising initial results (Hu et al., 1997). Additional protective functions can be obtained by conditioning exposures or exposures that protect the ear from subsequent noise (Canlon, Borg, and Flock, 1988). A related phenomenon is improvements (reductions) in threshold shifts observed during the course of an extended sequence of intermittent exposure to noise

(Miller, Watson, and Covell, 1963; Clark, Bohne, and Boettcher, 1987). Clearly, noise-induced hearing loss is not related simply to the sound level of the exposure.

Acoustic trauma refers to injury of the ear and permanent hearing loss caused by exposure to an intense, short-duration sound. In contrast to the gradual loss of outer hair cells and stereocilia typically seen from steady-state or intermittent exposures with sound levels less than 100–110 dB SPL, the injury to the organ of Corti is more extensive, involving the tearing of membranes, rupturing of cells, and mixing of cochlear fluids. At extremely high sound levels, the tympanic membrane and middle ear can be injured, with a resultant conductive/mixed hearing loss. The most common form of acoustic trauma is hearing loss associated with the impulsive noises produced by small-arms gunfire (Clark, 1991). Hearing loss from impulses is related to the peak SPL of the impulse, duration, number of impulses, and other variables (Henderson and Hamernik, 1986; Hamernik and Hsueh, 1993; Hamernik et al., 1993).

A longstanding issue is the interaction between noise-induced hearing loss incurred throughout a person's working lifetime and the hearing loss associated with aging. This issue is particularly important for medical reasons, for litigation involving worker's compensation for occupational hearing loss, and in establishing noise standards and damage-risk criteria. Both the current ISO (1990) and ANSI (1996) standards assume that noise-induced permanent threshold shifts add (in decibels) to age-related threshold shifts, i.e., a 20-dB loss from noise and a 20-dB loss from aging results in a loss of 40 dB. Some data from noise-exposed and aged animals do not support additivity in decibels but additivity in intensity: i.e., 20 dB and 20 dB produces a loss of 23 dB (Mills et al., 1997). The issues of additivity and medical-legal aspects of noise-induced hearing loss are discussed by Dobie (2001).

—*John H. Mills*

References

American National Standards Institute. (1996). *Determination of occupational noise exposure and estimation of noise-induced hearing impairment (ANSI S3.44-1996)*. New York: Acoustical Society of America.

Burns, W., and Robinson, D. W. (1970). *Hearing and noise in industry*. London: Her Majesty's Stationery Office.

Canlon, B. E., Borg, E., and Flock, A. (1988). Protection against noise trauma by pre-exposure to a low-level acoustic stimulus. *Hearing Research, 34*, 197–200.

Clark, W. W. (1991). Noise exposure from leisure activities. *Journal of the Acoustical Society of America, 90*, 155–163.

Clark, W. W., Bohne, B. A., and Boettcher, F. A. (1987). Effects of periodic rest on hearing loss and cochlear damage following exposure to noise. *Journal of the Acoustical Society of America, 82*, 1253–1264.

Davis, H., Morgan, C. T., Hawkins, J. E., Galambos, R., and Smith, F. W. (1950). Temporary deafness following exposure to loud tones and noise. *Acta Otolaryngologica, S88*, 1–57.

Dobie, R. A. (2001). *Medical-legal evaluation of hearing loss* (2nd ed.). San Diego, CA: Singular Publishing Group.

Hamernik, R. P., Ahroon, W. A., Hsueh, K. D., Lei, S. F., and Davis, R. I. (1993). Audiometric and histological differences between the effects of continuous and impulsive noise exposures. *Journal of the Acoustical Society of America, 93*, 2088–2095.

Hamernik, R. P., and Hsueh, K. D. (1993). Impulse noise: Some definitions, physical acoustics and other considerations. *Journal of the Acoustical Society of America, 90*, 189–196.

Hamernik, R. P., Patterson, J. H., Turrentine, G. A., and Ahroon, W. A. (1989). The quantitative relation between sensory cell loss and hearing thresholds. *Hearing Research, 38*, 199–211.

Henderson, D., and Hamernik, R. P. (1986). Impulse noise: Critical review. *Journal of the Acoustical Society of America, 80*, 569–564.

Hu, B. H., Zheng, X. Y., McFadden, S., and Henderson, D. (1997). The protective effects of R-PIA on noise-induced hearing loss. *Hearing Research, 113*, 198–206.

International Organization for Standardization. (1990). *Acoustic determination of occupational noise exposure and estimation of noise-induced hearing impairment*. Geneva: International Standard 1999.

Johnson, D. L. (1991). Field studies: Industrial exposures. *Journal of the Acoustical Society of America, 90*, 170–181.

Liberman, M. C., and Dodds, L. W. (1984). Single-neuron labeling and chronic cochlear pathology: III. Stereocilia damage and alterations of threshold tuning curves. *Hearing Research, 16*, 55–74.

Maison, S. F., and Liberman, M. C. (2000). Predicting vulnerability to acoustic injury with a noninvasive assay of olivocochlear reflex strength. *Journal of Neuroscience, 20*, 4701–4707.

Melnick, W., and Maves, M. (1974). Asymptotic threshold shift (ATS) in man from 24-hr exposures to continuous noise. *Annals of Otology, Rhinology, and Laryngology, 83*, 820–829.

Miller, J. D., Watson, C. S., and Covell, W. (1963). Deafening effects of noise on the cat. *Acta Otolaryngologica, Supplement, 176*, 1–91.

Mills, J. H. (1973). Threshold shifts produced by exposure to noise in chinchillas with noise-induced hearing losses. *Journal of Speech and Hearing Research, 16*, 700–708.

Mills, J. H., Boettcher, F. A., and Dubno, J. R. (1997). Interaction of noise-induced permanent threshold shift and age-related threshold shift. *Journal of the Acoustical Society of America, 101*, 1681–1686.

Mills, J. H., Clark, W. W., Dobie, R. A., Humes, L. E., Johnson, D. J., Liberman, M. C., et al. (1993). *Hazardous exposure to steady-state and intermittent noise*. Working Group Report, Committee on Hearing, Bioacoustics and Biomechanics, National Research Council. Washington, DC: National Academy Press.

Mills, J. H., Gengel, R. W., Watson, C. S., and Miller, J. D. (1970). Temporary changes of the auditory system due to exposure to noise for one or two days. *Journal of the Acoustical Society of America, 48*, 524–530.

Morata, T. C., and Dunn, D. D. (1995). *Occupational hearing loss*. Philadelphia: Hanley and Belfus.

Morest, D. K. (1982). Degeneration in the brain following exposure to noise. In R. P. Hamernik, D. Henderson, and R. J. Salvi (Eds.), *New perspectives in noise-induced hearing loss* (pp. 87–93). New York: Raven Press.

Occupational Safety and Health Administration, U.S. Department of Labor. (1983). Occupational noise exposure: Hearing conservation amendment. Final rule. *Federal Register*, *48*, 9738.

Ohlemiller, K. K., McFadden, S. L., Ding, D. L., and Lear, P. M. (2000). Targeted mutation of the gene for cellular glutathione peroxidase (Gpx1) increases noise-induced hearing loss in mice. *Journal of the Association for Research in Otolaryngology*, *1*, 243–254.

Taylor, W., Pearson, J., Mair, A., and Burns, W. (1965). Study of noise and hearing in jute weaving. *Journal of the Acoustical Society of America*, *38*, 113–120.

Ward, W. D. (1991). The role of intermittence in PTS. *Journal of the Acoustical Society of America*, *90*, 164–169.

Ward, W. D. (1995). Endogenous factors related to susceptibility to damage from noise. *Occupational Medicine*, *10*, 561–575.

Ward, W. D., Cushing, E. M., and Burns, E. M. (1976). Effective quiet and moderate TTS: Implications for noise exposure standards. *Journal of the Acoustical Society of America*, *59*, 160–165.

Yost, W. A., and Nielsen, D. W. (1985). *Fundamentals of hearing*. New York: Holt, Rinehart, and Winston.

Further Readings

Axelsson, A., Borchgrevink, H., Hamernik, R. P., Hellstrom, P. A., Henderson, D., and Salvi, R. J. (1996). *Scientific basis of noise-induced hearing loss*. New York: Thieme.

Bohne, B. A., and Rabbit, R. (1983). Holes in the reticular lamina after noise exposure: Implications for continuing damage in the organ of Corti. *Hearing Research*, *11*, 41–53.

Cotanche, D. A. (1987). Regeneration of hair cell stereocilia bundles in the chick cochlea following severe acoustic trauma. *Hearing Research*, *30*, 181–194.

Dancer, A. L., Henderson, D., Salvi, R. J., and Hamernik, R. P. (1992). *Noise-induced hearing loss*. St. Louis: Mosby–Year Book.

Hamernik, R. P., Henderson, D., and Salvi, R. P. (1982). *New perspectives on noise-induced hearing loss*. New York: Raven Press.

Henderson, D., Prasher, D., Kopke, R., Salvi, R., and Hamernik, R. (2001). *Noise-induced hearing loss: Basic mechanisms, prevention and control*. London: Noise Research Network Publications.

Henderson, D., Salvi, R. J., Quaranta, A., McFadden, S. L., and Burkhard, R. F. (1999). *Ototoxicity: Basic science and clinical applications. Annals of the New York Academy of Sciences, 884*.

Kryter, K. D. (1994). *The handbook of hearing and the effects of noise*. San Diego, CA: Academic Press.

Kujawa, S. G., and Liberman, M. C. (1999). Long-term sound conditioning enhances cochlear sensitivity. *Journal of Neurophysiology*, *82*, 863–873.

Kujawa, S. G., and Liberman, M. C. (2001). Effects of olivocochlear feedback on distortion product otoacoustic emissions in guinea pig. *Journal of the Association for Research in Otolaryngology*, *2*, 268–278.

Liberman, M. C., and Gao, W. Y. (1995). Chronic cochlear deefferentiation and susceptibility to permanent acoustic injury. *Hearing Research*, *90*, 158–168.

Ohlemiller, K. K., McFadden, S. L., Ding, D. L., Reaume, A. G., Hoffman, E. K., Scott, R. W., Wright, J. S., et al. (1999). Targeted deletion of the cystolic Cu/Zn-superoxide dismutase gene (SOD1) increases susceptibility to noise-induced hearing loss. *Audiology Neuro-Otology*, *4*, 237–246.

Prascher, D., Henderson, D., and Salvi, R. J. (2002). *Noise-induced hearing loss*. Cambridge, U.K.: Cambridge University Press.

Salvi, R. J., Henderson, D., Hamernik, R. P., and Colletti, V. (1985). *Basic and applied aspects of noise-induced hearing loss*. New York: Plenum Press.

Sataloff, R. T., and Sataloff, J. (1993). *Occupational hearing loss* (2nd ed.). New York: Marcel Dekker.

Saunders, J. C., Cohen, Y. E., and Szymko, Y. M. (1991). The structural and functional consequences of acoustic injury in the cochlea and peripheral auditory system: A five year update. *Journal of the Acoustical Society of America*, *90*, 136–146.

Otoacoustic Emissions

The 25th anniversary of the discovery of otoacoustic emissions (OAEs), the acoustic energy produced by the cochlea, was celebrated in 2003. Following Kemp's (1978, 1979a, 1979b) breakthrough descriptions of the four types of OAEs in humans—the click- or transient-evoked OAE (TEOAE), the distortion product OAE (DPOAE), the stimulus frequency OAE (SFOAE), and the spontaneous OAE (SOAE)—interest turned to basic research issues. Existing models of cochlear function were modified to reflect the existence of active processing as implied by the mere reality of OAEs. Also, efforts were made to relate OAEs to parallel neural and psychoacoustical phenomena, and to describe emitted responses in species used as research models, including monkeys, gerbils, guinea pigs, and chinchillas (Zurek, 1985).

During the early years of OAE study, another great advance in the hearing sciences occurred when Brownell et al. (1985) discovered electromotility in isolated outer hair cells. The current consensus is that outer hair cell motility is due to the receptor-potential initiated movements of atomic-sized "motor" molecules called prestin (Zheng et al., 2002) that are embedded in the lateral membrane of the outer hair cell. Our present understanding is that OAEs are generated as a by-product of these electromotile vibrations of outer hair cells (Brownell, 1990).

As the initial basic studies on OAEs were ongoing, the significant benefits of OAEs as a clinical test were being recognized. Thus, early on, four major applications of OAE testing in clinical settings became apparent: the differential diagnosis of hearing loss, hearing screening in difficult to test patients, serial monitoring of progressive hearing impairment conditions, and determining the legitimacy of medicolegal claims involving compensatory payments for hearing loss. The rationale for using OAEs in each of these major applications is based on a significant beneficial feature of the measure, including its specificity for testing the functional status of outer hair cells, the most fragile sensory receptors for hearing. This attribute in particular makes OAEs an ideal measure for determining the sensory component of a sensorineural hearing loss. In addition, mainly because

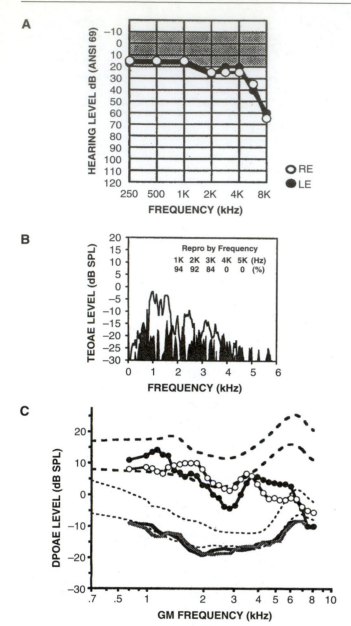

Figure 1. Audiometric and evoked OAE findings in a 37-year-old man who had received intravenous infusions of cisplatin for testicular carcinoma. **A,** Pure-tone clinical audiogram for left (solid circles) and right (open circles) ear showing normal to near-normal hearing thresholds from 250 Hz to 4 kHz, after which hearing levels fell to 35–65 dB HL at 6 and 8 kHz. **B,** A TEOAE spectrum for the left ear showing relatively normal click-evoked emissions up to about 3.5 kHz. Note the progressive decrement in TEOAE levels above 1.5 kHz, which is a pattern typically observed for normal-hearing adults. The "RE-PRO BY FREQUENCY" values indicate excellent test-retest results over the short recording session for frequencies up to 3 kHz. **C,** DP-gram showing DPOAE levels for left (solid circles) and right (open circles) ears in response to moderate, equilevel primary tones, i.e., $L_1 = L_2 = 65$ dB SPL, from 800 Hz to 8 kHz, at 10 points per octave. The bold dashed curves at the top of the plot represent the ± 1 SD of DPOAE values in response to identical primaries for 100 ears from normal-hearing subjects; the bold dotted curves at the bottom of the plot indicate the

the OAE is an objective response that is noninvasively measured from the outer ear canal and thus can be rapidly obtained, it is an ideal screening test for identifying hearing impairment in newborns. Finally, because OAEs are stable and reliably measured over long time intervals, they are excellent for monitoring pathological changes in cochlear function, particularly in individuals regularly exposed to ototoxic drugs or excessive sounds.

One relatively new application of OAEs over the past decade has been the use of emissions to measure the intactness of the entire ascending and descending auditory pathway (Collet et al., 1990). This capability is based on the knowledge that the suppressive effects of cochlear efferents mainly affect outer hair cell activity, since these sensory cells are the primary targets of the descending auditory system. Indeed, recent research indicates that the susceptibility of the ear to the harmful effects of, for example, intense noise is likely determined by the amount of indigenous efferent activity (Luebke, Foster, and Stagner, 2002). That is, the more robust the efferent activity, the more resistant the ear is to the damaging effects of loud sounds, and vice versa.

Of the two general classes of OAEs, SOAEs have not been as clinically useful as the evoked OAEs, for several reasons. Their prevalence in only about 50% of normal-hearing individuals and the individually based uniqueness of their frequencies and levels make it difficult to develop SOAEs into a standardized test. However, SOAEs have been linked to tinnitus in a subset of tinnitus patients with near-normal hearing (Penner, 1992). In patients with SOAE-induced tinnitus, suppressing the associated SOAEs eliminates the annoying tinnitus. Interestingly, and contrary to expectations, since excessive aspirin produces tinnitus in normal-hearing individuals, high-dose aspirin suffices as a palliative in persons with SOAE-induced tinnitus (Penner and Coles, 1992).

Concerning the three subclasses of evoked OAEs, only TEOAEs and DPOAEs have proved to be clinically useful. SFOAEs can be reliably measured only using expensive phase-tracking devices, since the emission must be extracted from the ear canal sound at a time that the eliciting stimulus is present at the identical frequency. Fortunately, the SFOAE is essentially the long-lasting version of the TEOAE, which is more straightforward to measure and interpret.

Within a decade after the discovery of TEOAEs, commercial equipment based on procedures used for evoking auditory brainstem responses was available (Bray and Kemp, 1987). Figure 1 shows the results of pure-tone audiometry (*A*) and tests of click-evoked

counterpart distribution of noise-floor values for the same subjects. Note that the patient was exceptionally quiet, as his noise-floor curves (bold line = left ear; stippled line = right ear) tracked the lower distribution trajectory of the control population. In this example, the ototoxic drug caused outer hair cell dysfunction for frequencies above about 2.5 kHz for the left ear and 4 kHz for the right ear.

TEOAEs (*B*) and DPOAEs (*C*) in a 37-year-old patient receiving the ototoxic antitumor drug cisplatin. In this case, following a single infusion (Fig. 1*A*), a moderate high-frequency hearing loss was evident bilaterally for frequencies over 4 kHz. The associated TEOAE spectrum (Fig. 1*B*) illustrates the commonly measured properties for this emitted response, including its level, frequency content and extent, and reliability, according to automatically computed reproducibility factors for five representative frequencies at 1, 2, 3, 4, and 5 kHz.

Because the TEOAE is measured after the transient stimulus occurs, each ear produces a response that exhibits a unique spectral pattern. This idiosyncratic property makes it difficult to develop a set of metrics that describe the average TEOAE for normal-hearing individuals. Owing to this difficulty in determining "normal" TEOAEs in terms of frequencies and level values, they are most often described as being either present or absent. Thus, one of the most popular uses of TEOAEs clinically is as a test for screening auditory function in newborns (Norton et al., 2000).

In the example of Figure 1*B*, representing the left ear of the patient, even in the presence of a drug-induced high-frequency hearing loss, the TEOAE pattern appears fairly normal in that the click-elicited emission typically falls off for frequencies greater than 2 kHz, and is seldom present at frequencies above 4 kHz in adult ears. For newborns and older infants, the TEOAE is much more robust by about 10 dB and typically can be measured out to about 6 kHz, indicating that smaller ear canals influence the acoustic characteristics of standard click stimuli much differently than do adult ears.

Distortion product OAEs are elicited by presenting two long-lasting pure tonebursts at f_1 (lower frequency) and f_2 (higher frequency) simultaneously to the ear. The frequencies and levels of the tonebursts or primary tones are important in that the largest DPOAEs are elicited by f_1 and f_2 primaries that are within one-half octave of each other (i.e., $f_2/f_1 = 1.22$) with levels, L_1 and L_2, that are offset. For example, typical clinical protocols measure the $2f_1-f_2$ DPOAE, which is the largest DPOAE in human ears, in response to primary-tone levels of $L_1 = 65$ and $L_2 = 55$ dB SPL (Gorga, Neely, and Dorn, 1999).

Figure 1*C* shows a DP-gram, i.e., DPOAE level as a function of test frequency, from about 800 Hz to 8 kHz, in response to equilevel primary tones ($L_1 = L_2 = 65$ dB SPL). In this example, test frequency is represented by the geometric or logarithmic mean of f_1 and f_2, although it could also be represented by the f_2 frequency. That is, based on a combination of theoretical considerations, experimental studies, and observations of the generation of DPOAEs in pathological ears, it is clear that these emissions are produced in the region of the primary tones. Based on further experimental work, it is likely that the DPOAE source is level-dependent, with the primary generation site in response to higher level primaries of equal level ($L_1 = L_2$) occurring around the geometric mean frequency. In contrast, for lower level primaries, which are often offset in level, the primary generation site is closer to f_2.

As illustrated in Figure 1*C*, the patient's emissions were relatively normal, as compared to the ± 1 SD distribution of DPOAE levels for normal-hearing adults, until about 3 kHz for the left ear (solid circles) and 4 kHz for the right ear (open circles). In this case, because DPOAEs are typically tested out to 8 kHz, they detected the developing high-frequency hearing loss associated with the ototoxic antitumor therapy.

It is clear that applications of OAEs in the hearing sciences and clinical audiology are varied. Without a doubt, OAEs are useful experimentally for evaluating and monitoring the status of cochlear function in animal models, and clinically in distinguishing cochlear from retrocochlear disorders. Moreover, their practical features make them helpful in the hearing screening of newborns. Additionally, they have proved useful in monitoring the effects of agents such as ototoxins and loud sounds on cochlear function. In fact, there is accumulating evidence that it is possible to detect such adverse effects of drugs or noise on outer hair cell function using OAEs before a related hearing loss can be detected by pure-tone audiometry. In addition, OAEs provide a noninvasive means for assessing the integrity of the cochlear efferent pathway. In general, OAEs supply unique information about cochlear function in the presence of hearing problems, and this capability makes them ideal response measures in both the clinical and basic hearing sciences.

Acknowledgments

This work was supported by grants from the Public Health Service (DC 00613, DC03114).

—*Brenda L. Lonsbury-Martin*

References

Bray, P., and Kemp, D. T. (1987). An advanced cochlear echo technique suitable for infant screening. *British Journal of Audiology, 21,* 191–204.

Brownell, W. E. (1990). Outer hair cell electromotility and otoacoustic emissions. *Ear and Hearing, 11,* 82–92.

Brownell, W. E., Bader, C. R., Bertrand, D., and Ribaupierre, Y. (1985). Evoked mechanical responses of isolated outer hair cells. *Science, 227,* 194–196.

Collet, L., Kemp, D. T., Veuillet, E., Duclaux, R., Moulin, A., and Morgon, A. (1990). Effect of contralateral auditory stimuli on active cochlear micro-mechanical properties in human subjects. *Hearing Research, 43,* 251–261.

Gorga, M. P., Neely, S. T., and Dorn, P. A. (1999). Distortion product otoacoustic emission test performance for a priori criteria and for multifrequency audiometric standards. *Ear and Hearing, 20,* 345–362.

Kemp, D. T. (1978). Stimulated acoustic emissions from within the human auditory system. *Journal of the Acoustical Society of America, 64,* 1386–1391.

Kemp, D. T. (1979a). Evidence of mechanical nonlinearity and frequency selective wave amplification in the cochlea. *Archives of Otorhinolaryngology, 224,* 37–45.

Kemp, D. T. (1979b). The evoked cochlear mechanical response and the auditory microstructure: Evidence for a new element in cochlear mechanics. *Scandinavian Audiology, 9,* 35–47.

Luebke, A. E., Foster, P. K., and Stagner, B. B. (2002). A multifrequency method for determining cochlear efferent activity. *Journal of the Association for Research in Otolaryngology, 3,* 16–25.

Norton, S. J., Gorga, M. P., Widen, J. E., Folsom, R. C., Sininger, Y., Cone-Wesson, B., et al. (2000). Identification of neonatal hearing impairment: A multicenter investigation. *Ear and Hearing, 21,* 348–356.

Penner, M. J. (1992). Linking spontaneous otoacoustic emissions and tinnitus. *British Journal of Audiology, 26,* 115–123.

Penner, M. J., and Coles, R. R. (1992). Indications for aspirin as a palliative for tinnitus caused by SOAEs: A case study. *British Journal of Audiology, 26,* 91–96.

Zheng, J., Madison, L. D., Oliver, D., Fakler, B., and Dallos, P. (2002). Prestin, the motor protein of outer hair cells. *Audiology and Neuro-Otology, 7,* 9–12.

Zurek, P. M. (1985). Acoustic emissions from the ear: A summary of results from humans and animals. *Journal of the Acoustical Society of America, 78,* 340–344.

Further Readings

Abdala, C. (2001). Maturation of the human cochlear amplifier: Distortion product otoacoustic emission suppression tuning curves recorded at low and high primary tone levels. *Journal of the Acoustical Society of America, 110,* 1465–1476.

Arnold, D. J., Lonsbury-Martin, B. L., and Martin, G. K. (1999). High-frequency hearing influences lower-frequency acoustic distortion products. *Archives of Otolaryngology, 125,* 215–222.

Berlin, C. I., Hood, L. J., Hurley, A., and Wen, H. (1994). Contralateral suppression of otoacoustic emissions: An index of the function of the medial olivocochlear system. *Otolaryngology–Head and Neck Surgery, 110,* 3–21.

Di Girolamo, S., d'Ecclesia, A., Quaranta, N., Garozzo, A., Evoli, A., and Paludetti, G. (2001). Effects of contralateral white noise stimulation on distortion product otoacoustic emissions in myasthenic patients. *Hearing Research, 162,* 80–84.

Dorn, P. A., Piskorski, P., Gorga, M. P., Neely, S. T., and Keefe, D. H. (1999). Predicting audiometric status from distortion product otoacoustic emissions using multivariate analysis. *Ear and Hearing, 20,* 149–163.

Driesbach, L. E., and Siegel, J. H. (2001). Distortion-product otoacoustic emissions measured at high frequencies in humans. *Journal of the Acoustical Society of America, 110,* 2456–2469.

Engel-Yates, B., Zaaroura, S., Zlotogora, J., et al. (2002). The effects of a connexin 26 mutation—35delG—on otoacoustic emissions and brainstem auditory evoked potentials: Homozygotes and carriers. *Hearing Research, 163,* 93–100.

Fetterman, B. L. (2001). Distortion-product otoacoustic emissions and cochlear microphonics: Relationships in patients with and without endolymphatic hydrops. *Laryngoscope, 111,* 946–954.

Howard, M. A., Stagner, B. B., Lonsbury-Martin, B. L., and Martin, G. K. (2002). Effects of reversible noise exposure on the suppression tuning of rabbit distortion-product otoacoustic emissions. *Journal of the Acoustical Society of America, 111,* 285–296.

Hussain, D. M., Gorga, M. P., Neely, S. T., Keefe, D. H., and Peters, J. (1998). Transient evoked otoacoustic emissions in patients with normal hearing and in patients with hearing loss. *Ear and Hearing, 19,* 434–449.

Kim, D. O., Dorn, P. A., Neely, S. T., and Gorga, M. P. (2001). Adaptation of distortion product otoacoustic emission in humans. *Journal of the Association for Research in Otolaryngology, 2,* 31–40.

Knight, R. D., and Kemp, D. T. (2001). Wave and place fixed DPOAE maps of the human ear. *Journal of the Acoustical Society of America, 109,* 1513–1525.

Konrad-Martin, D., Neely, S. T., Keefe, D. H., Dorn, P. A., and Gorga, M. P. (2001). Sources of DPOAEs revealed by suppression experiments, inverse fast Fourier transforms, and SFOAEs in normal ears. *Journal of the Acoustical Society of America, 111,* 1800–1809.

Lalaki, P., Markou, K., Tsalighopoulos, M. G., and Daniilidis, I. (2001). Transiently evoked otoacoustic emissions as a prognostic indicator in idiopathic sudden hearing loss. *Scandinavian Audiology Supplement, 52,* 141–145.

Lucertini, M., Moleti, A., and Sisto, R. (2002). On the detection of early cochlear damage by otoacoustic emission analysis. *Journal of the Acoustical Society of America, 111,* 972–978.

Lukashkin, A. N., Lukashkina, V. A., and Russell, I. J. (2002). One source for distortion product otoacoustic emissions generated by low- and high-level primaries. *Journal of the Acoustical Society of America, 111,* 2740–2748.

Martin, G. K., Jassir, D., Stagner, B. B., Whitehead, M. L., and Lonsbury-Martin, B. L. (1998). Locus of generation for the $2f_1–f_2$ vs $2f_2–f_1$ distortion-product otoacoustic emissions in normal-hearing humans revealed by suppression tuning, onset latencies, and amplitude correlations. *Journal of the Acoustical Society of America, 103,* 1957–1971.

Owens, J. J., McCoy, M. J., Lonsbury-Martin, B. L., and Martin, G. K. (1993). Otoacoustic emissions in children with normal ears, middle-ear dysfunction, and ventilating tubes. *American Journal of Otology, 14,* 34–40.

Probst, R., Lonsbury-Martin, B. L., and Martin, G. K. (1991). A review of otoacoustic emissions. *Journal of the Acoustical Society of America, 89,* 2027–2067.

Shera, C. A., and Guinan, J. J., Jr. (1999). Evoked otoacoustic emissions arise by two fundamentally different mechanisms: A taxonomy for mammalian OAEs. *Journal of the Acoustical Society of America, 105,* 782–798.

Stavroulaki, P., Apostolopoulos, N., Segas, J., Tsakanikos, M., and Adamopoulos, G. (2001). Evoked otoacoustic emissions: An approach for monitoring cisplatin induced ototoxicity in children. *International Journal of Pediatric Otorhinolaryngology, 59,* 47–57.

Sutton, L. A., Lonsbury-Martin, B. L., Martin, G. K., and Whitehead, M. L. (1994). Sensitivity of distortion-product otoacoustic emissions in humans to tonal over-exposure: Time course of recovery and effects of lowering L_2. *Hearing Research, 75,* 161–174.

Telischi, F. F., Roth, J., Lonsbury-Martin, B. L., Balkany, T. J. (1995). Patterns of evoked otoacoustic emissions associated with acoustic neuromas. *Laryngoscope, 105,* 675–682.

Whitehead, M. L., Stagner, B. B., Lonsbury-Martin, B. L., and Martin, G. K. (1994). Measurement of otoacoustic emissions for hearing assessment. *IEEE Medicine and Biology, 13,* 210–226.

Otoacoustic Emissions in Children

Unidentified hearing loss in infants and young children can lead to delays in speech and language acquisition (Yoshinaga-Itano et al., 1998; Moeller, 2000). Identification of hearing loss presents an additional challenge because these patients may be unable to provide voluntary responses to sound. Otoacoustic emissions (OAEs) are an effective means to identify hearing loss in young children because they are related to the integrity of the peripheral auditory system and do not require voluntary responses from the patient.

OAEs are by-products of normal, nonlinear cochlear function, the source of which is the outer hair cell (OHC) system. They may be evoked by single tones (stimulus frequency, SFOAEs), pairs of tones (distortion product, DPOAEs), or transient stimuli (transient evoked, TEOAEs), and take from several seconds to several minutes to measure. Although all OAEs do not require a behavioral response, only TEOAEs and DPOAEs have been used widely to identify hearing loss. Since OHC damage results in hearing loss, OAEs, which are generated by OHCs, should be present when cochlear function is normal and reduced or absent when it is not. These facts have led to the application of OAE measurements in efforts to describe auditory function in humans, especially infants and young children. Unfortunately, OAE response properties from normal and impaired ears are not completely distinguishable; thus, diagnostic errors are inevitable. Below, we provide brief descriptions of TEOAEs and DPOAEs in normal-hearing infants and young children, followed by a description of these two OAEs in patients with hearing loss. Robinette and Glattke (2002) and Hall (2000) provide more background information and extensive reference lists on OAEs. Norton, Gorga, et al. (2000) and Gorga, Norton, et al. (2000) provide comprehensive descriptions of OAEs in the perinatal period.

Infants and young children produce larger OAEs than older children and adults (Prieve, Fitzgerald, and Schulte, 1997; Prieve, Fitzgerald, Schulte, and Kemp, 1997; see Widen and O'Grady, 2002, for a review). There are several explanations for this difference. Very young children have not been exposed to environmental factors that might result in OHC damage. Also, their middle ears transmit energy to and from the cochlea differently than adults (Keefe et al., 1993), which might alter OAE levels in the ear canal. In addition, infant ear canal resonances show greater level at high frequencies, compared to spectra measured in adult ear canals. If stimuli differ in adult and infant ear canals, then responses may differ as well. Finally, the space between the measuring microphone and the eardrum is smaller in infants than in adults. If equivalent OAEs were generated in the cochlea, that signal would be larger in the infant ear canal because it was recorded in a smaller space.

While differences in infant and adult OAEs exist, the larger question revolves around whether OAEs can be used to distinguish ears with hearing loss from those with normal hearing. This dichotomous decision is made whenever OAEs are used in screening programs, regardless of the target population. The following discussion describes work in this area.

The clinical value of OAE measurements was recognized starting with their discovery (Kemp, 1978). Several studies describe the accuracy with which OAEs identify auditory status (e.g., Martin et al., 1990; Prieve et al., 1993; Gorga et al., 1993a, 1993b, 1996, 1997, 1999, 2000; Glattke et al., 1995; Kim et al., 1996; Hussain et al., 1998; Dorn et al., 1999; Harrison and Norton, 1999; Norton, Widen, et al., 2000). In general, both TEOAEs and DPOAEs identify auditory status with greater accuracy for middle and high frequencies than for lower frequencies. This occurs because noise levels decrease as frequency increases during OAE measurements. The noise interfering with OAE measurements (1) is acoustical, (2) results mainly from patient breathing and/or movement, and (3) contains mostly lower frequency energy. Noise adds variability and reduces measurement reliability. Thus, OAE test performance depends heavily on the frequencies at which predictions about auditory status are being made, in large part because noise level depends on frequency.

Test performance also depends on stimulus level (Whitehead et al., 1995; Stover et al., 1996; Harrison and Norton, 1999). Moderate-level stimuli result in the fewest false positive and false negative errors. Lower or higher stimulus levels decrease one of these error rates at the expense of increasing the rate of the other. This occurs for simple reasons. If low stimulus levels are chosen, virtually every ear with hearing loss will fail the test, resulting in a false negative rate of zero. However, the number of ears with normal hearing not producing responses will also increase as stimulus level decreases, increasing the false positive rate. If high-level stimuli are used, the vast majority of ears with normal hearing will produce responses, resulting in a low false positive rate. Unfortunately, some ears with hearing loss, especially ears with mild or moderate losses, will produce a response to high-level stimulation, increasing the false negative rate. Moderate-level stimuli result in optimal combinations of false positive and false negative rates. Thus, primary levels of 50–65 dB SPL for DPOAE measurements or 80–85 dB pSPL for clicks during TEOAE measurements are recommended.

Figure 1 shows representative examples of DPOAE and TEOAE signal and noise levels for three hearing loss categories. In general, robust responses above the noise floor are observed when hearing is normal (top row). When borderline normal hearing or mild hearing loss exists (middle row), the response is either reduced in level or absent. In cases of moderate or greater hearing loss (bottom row), the response typically does not exceed the noise floor, even when the noise level is low. These examples are consistent with general response patterns in these hearing loss categories, but it is important to

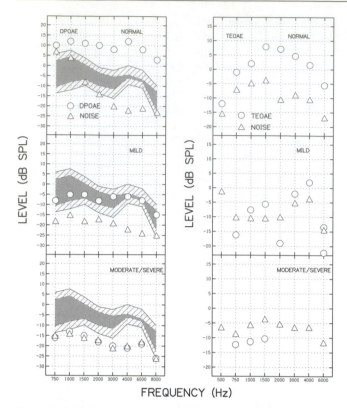

Figure 1. OAE (circles) and noise (triangles) levels as a function of frequency, with DPOAE and TEOAE data shown in the left and right columns, respectively. Note that the *y*-axis is not the same for DPOAEs and TEOAEs. Representative examples are shown for normal hearing (top row), borderline normal hearing/mild hearing loss (middle row), and moderate to severe hearing loss (bottom row). See Gorga et al. (1997) for an explanation of the shaded areas in the DPOAE column. Although Hussain et al. (1998) developed a similar grid for TEOAE data, those data were collected with a different paradigm, and thus cannot be applied to the present set of data.

remember that both measurements will produce some diagnostic errors.

One of these errors (false positives or false negatives) may be more important for certain clinical applications. For example, infants or young children who are brought to a speech and hearing clinic or an otolaryngology clinic because of concern about hearing loss are at higher risk than the general population. In this case, one might choose stimuli or criteria that provide higher sensitivities, despite the higher false positive rates, because missing a hearing loss is the greater concern. In contrast, one might choose stimuli or criteria that provide higher specificity, despite the lower sensitivity, when the target population includes only well babies without risk for hearing loss. In this group, the probability of hearing loss is so low that it may be more important to minimize false positive errors. It is impossible to recommend a single set of stimuli and/or criteria because individual clinics must decide which error is more important for their needs.

OAE test performance also depends on the audiometric criterion defining the border between normal hearing and hearing loss. Both TEOAEs and DPOAEs perform best when thresholds ≤ 20–30 dB HL are used to define normal hearing. There are data suggesting that TEOAEs are more sensitive than DPOAEs to mild hearing loss (for a review, see Harris and Probst, 1997). However, direct comparisons failed to reveal large differences in test performance between TEOAEs and DPOAEs when audiometric criterion was varied (Gorga et al., 1993b; Norton, Widen, et al., 2000). Still, some differences across frequency have been observed. TEOAEs tend to perform better at detecting hearing loss for lower frequencies while DPOAEs tend to perform better at detecting high-frequency hearing loss (Gorga et al., 1993b; Kemp, 1997), because of how each measurement is made.

During TEOAE measurements, a fast Fourier transform (FFT) is performed on the ear canal waveform. The status of the cochlear region associated with specific frequencies is determined by examining the energy (or signal-to-noise ratio) at those frequencies. For example, one would conclude that the 1000-Hz region of the cochlea is functioning if energy is observed in the FFT at 1000 Hz. For DPOAE measurements, two tones are presented simultaneously (f_1 and f_2), interact at the cochlea place close to where f_2 is represented, and produce distortion products (DP), the most prominent of which is the $2f_1-f_2$ DP. The level of this component is then measured to determine if the cochlea is functioning at the point of its initial generation (f_2). However, $2f_1-f_2$ occurs at a frequency that is about one-half octave lower than f_2. Thus, the measured response may occur in a region in which noise floors are less favorable, thus reducing measurement reliability. As a consequence, DPOAEs are less accurate than TEOAEs for lower frequencies.

During TEOAE measurements, the first 2.5 ms of the ear canal waveform following stimulation usually is zeroed to ensure that stimulus artifact does not contaminate the measured response. However, TEOAE energy generated in the high-frequency (basal) end of the cochlea will return with the shortest latency. Zeroing the first 2.5 ms of the ear canal signal may remove some of the high-frequency cochlear response. DPOAEs are not susceptible to this problem. Thus, they predict cochlear status better than TEOAEs do at higher frequencies.

Implicit in the above discussion is that errors are inevitable regardless of OAE measurement, stimulus level, OAE criterion value, or the definition of normal hearing. Both TEOAEs and DPOAEs will miss some ears with hearing loss and/or will incorrectly label some ears with normal hearing as hearing impaired. In addition, OAEs are not useful measurements of sensory function when middle ear dysfunction exists, which is frequently the case in children. Furthermore, OAEs will not identify patients with pathologies central to the OHCs, because OAEs test only the OHC system. Since the majority of hearing losses arise from OHC damage, however, OAEs are well-suited to the task of determining auditory status in infants and children.

Acknowledgments

Much of the authors' work summarized in this chapter was supported by grants from the NIH (NIDCD R01 DC2251 and DC R10 1958).

See also OTOACOUSTIC EMISSIONS.

—*Michael P. Gorga, Stephen T. Neely, and Judith E. Widen*

References

Dorn, P. A., Piskorski, P., Gorga, M. P., Neely, S. T., and Keefe, D. H. (1999). Predicting audiometric status from distortion product otoacoustic emissions using multivariate analyses. *Ear and Hearing, 20*, 149–163.

Glattke, T. J., Pafitis, I. A., Cummiskey, C., and Herer, G. R. (1995). Identification of hearing loss in children and young adults using measures of transient otoacoustic emission reproducibility. *American Journal of Audiology, 4*, 71–87.

Gorga, M. P., Neely, S. T., Bergman, B., Beauchaine, K. L., Kaminski, J. R., Peters, J., et al. (1993a). Otoacoustic emissions from normal-hearing and hearing-impaired subjects: Distortion product responses. *Journal of the Acoustical Society of America, 93*, 2050–2060.

Gorga, M. P., Neely, S. T., Bergman, N. M., Beauchaine, K. L., Kaminski, J. R., Peters, J., Schulte, L., and Jesteadt, W. (1993b). A comparison of transient-evoked and distortion product otoacoustic emissions in normal-hearing and hearing-impaired subjects. *Journal of the Acoustical Society of America, 94*, 2639–2648.

Gorga, M. P., Neely, S. T., and Dorn, P. A. (1999). DPOAE test performance for a priori criteria and for multifrequency audiometric standards. *Ear and Hearing, 20*, 345–362.

Gorga, M. P., Neely, S. T., Ohlrich, B., Hoover, B., Redner, J., and Peters, J. (1997). From laboratory to clinic: A large scale study of distortion product otoacoustic emissions in ears with normal hearing and ears with hearing loss. *Ear and Hearing, 18*, 440–455.

Gorga, M. P., Nelson, K., Davis, T., Dorn, P. A., and Neely, S. T. (2000). DPOAE test performance when both $2f_1-f_2$ and $2f_2-f_1$ are used to predict auditory status. *Journal of the Acoustical Society of America, 107*, 2128–2135.

Gorga, M. P., Norton, S. J., Sininger, Y. S., Cone-Wesson, B., Folsom, R. C., Vohr, B. R., et al. (2000). Identification of neonatal hearing impairment: Distortion product otoacoustic emissions during the perinatal period. *Ear and Hearing, 21*, 400–424.

Gorga, M. P., Stover, L. T., and Neely, S. T. (1996). The use of cumulative distributions to determine critical values and levels of confidence for clinical distortion product otoacoustic emission measurements. *Journal of the Acoustical Society of America, 100*, 968–977.

Hall, J. W. (2000). *Handbook of otoacoustic emissions.* San Diego, CA: Singular Publishing Group.

Harris, F. P., and Probst, R. (1997). Otoacoustic emissions and audiometric outcomes. In M. S. Robinette and T. J. Glattke (Eds.), *Otoacoustic emissions: Clinical applications.* New York: Thieme.

Harrison, W. A., and Norton, S. J. (1999). Characteristics of transient evoked otoacoustic emissions in normal-hearing and hearing-impaired children. *Ear and Hearing, 20*, 75–86.

Hussain, D., Gorga, M. P., Neely, S. T., Keefe, D. H., and Peters, J. (1998). Transient otoacaoustic emissions in patients with normal hearing and in patients with hearing loss. *Ear and Hearing, 19*, 434–449.

Keefe, D. H., Bulen, J. C., Arehart, K. H., and Burns, E. M. (1993). Ear-canal impedance and reflection coefficient in human infants and adults. *Journal of the Acoustical Society of America, 94*, 2617–2638.

Kemp, D. T. (1978). Stimulated acoustic emissions from within the human auditory system. *Journal of the Acoustical Society of America, 64*, 1386–1391.

Kemp, D. T. (1997). Otoacoustic emissions in perspective. In M. S. Robinette and T. J. Glattke (Eds.), *Otoacoustic emissions: Clinical applications.* New York: Thieme.

Kim, D. O., Paparello, J., Jung, M. D., Smurzynski, J., and Sun, X. (1996). Distortion product otoacoustic emission test of sensorineural hearing loss: Performance regarding sensitivity, specificity, and receiver operating characteristics. *Acta Oto-Laryngologica (Stockholm), 116*, 3–11.

Martin, G. K., Ohlms, L. A., Franklin, D. J., Harris, F. P., and Lonsbury-Martin, B. L. (1990). Distortion product emissions in humans III: Influence of sensorineural hearing loss. *Annals of Otology, Rhinology, and Laryngology, Supplement, 147*, 30–42.

Moeller, M. P. (2000). Early intervention and language development in children who are deaf and hard of hearing. *Pediatrics, 106*, E43.

Norton, S. J., Gorga, M. P., Widen, J. E., Vohr, B. R., Folsom, R. C., Sininger, Y. S., et al. (2000). Identification of neonatal hearing impairment: Transient otoacoustic emissions during the perinatal period. *Ear and Hearing, 21*, 425–442.

Norton, S. J., Widen, J. E., Gorga, M. P., Folsom, R. C., Sininger, Y. S., Cone-Wesson, B., et al. (2000). Identification of neonatal hearing impairment: Evaluation of TEOAE, DPOAE, and ABR test performance. *Ear and Hearing, 21*, 508–528.

Prieve, B. A., Fitzgerald, T. S., and Schulte, L. E. (1997). Basic characteristics of click-evoked otoacoustic emissions in infants and children. *Journal of the Acoustical Society of America, 102*, 2860–2870.

Prieve, B. A., Fitzgerald, T. S., Schulte, L. E., and Kemp, D. T. (1997). Basic characteristics of distortion product otoacoustic emissions in infants and children. *Journal of the Acoustical Society of America, 102*, 2871–2879.

Prieve, B. A., Gorga, M. P., Schmidt, A. R., Neely, S. T., Peters, J., Schulte, L., et al. (1993). Analysis of transient-evoked otoacoustic emissions in normal-hearing and hearing-impaired ears. *Journal of the Acoustical Society of America, 93*, 3308–3319.

Robinette, M. S., and Glattke, T. J. (Eds.). (2002). *Otoacoustic emissions: Clinical applications* (2nd ed.). New York: Thieme.

Stover, L. J., Gorga, M. P., Neely, S. T., and Montoya, D. (1996). Towards optimizing the clinical utility of distortion product otoacoustic emissions. *Journal of the Acoustical Society of America, 100*, 956–967.

Whitehead, M. L., McCoy, M. J., Lonsbury-Martin, B. L., and Martin, G. K. (1995). Dependence of distortion product otoacoustic emissions on primary levels in normal and impaired ears: I. Effects of decreasing L_2 below L_1. *Journal of the Acoustical Society of America, 97*, 2346–2358.

Widen, J. E., and O'Grady, G. M. (2002). Evoked otoacoustic emissions in evaluating children. In M. S. Robinette and T. J. Glattke (Eds.), *Otoacoustic emissions: Clinical applications* (2nd ed., pp. 375–515). New York: Thieme.

Yoshinaga-Itano, C., Sedey, A. L., Coulter, D. K., and Mehl, A. L. (1998). Language of early- and late-identified children with hearing loss. *Pediatrics, 102*, 1161–1171.

Ototoxic Medications

Many medications are ototoxic, meaning that they adversely affect inner ear function. The toxicity can be divided into two broad categories, cochleotoxicity and vestibulotoxicity. Cochleotoxic medications affect hearing function and typically manifest with tinnitus (an abnormal noise in the ear), decreased hearing, or both. Most cochleotoxins affect hearing at the highest frequencies first, reflecting damage to hair cells of the cochlea. Vestibulotoxic medications affect the part of the inner ear that senses motion—the vestibular system. Vestibulotoxicity usually manifests with dizziness, unsteadiness, and when severe, oscillopsia. Oscillopsia denotes inability of a person to see when the head is moving, although visual acuity may be normal when the head is still. The most common vestibulotoxins, the aminoglycoside antibiotics, primarily damage the vestibular hair cells. Ototoxicity is often irreversible, as humans lack the ability to regenerate hair cells.

Ototoxic medications can be broken down into several broad groups. Chemotherapeutic agents are often cochleotoxic. Many antibiotics are ototoxic, and those in the aminoglycoside family are all ototoxic to some degree, some being primarily cochleotoxic and others primarily vestibulotoxic. Diuretics, mainly the loop diuretics, are often cochleotoxic. Similarly, quinine derivatives such as antimalarials are also commonly cochleotoxic. Many common medications in the nonsteroidal anti-inflammatory group, such as aspirin, are cochletoxic.

Chemotherapy Agents

Chemotherapeutic agents are drugs generally used to treat cancer. Actinomycin, bleomycin, cisplatin, carboplatin, nitrogen mustard, and vincristine have all been reported to be ototoxic. Their ototoxicity is generally a direct result of their toxicity to other cells. While cochleotoxic, these medications are rarely encountered as a source of vestibular dysfunction.

Cisplatin is currently the most widely used anticancer drug, and unfortunately, it is cochleotoxic. The toxicity of cisplatin is synergistic with that of gentamicin (Riggs et al., 1996), and high doses of cisplatin have been reported to cause total deafness. In animals, cisplatin ototoxicity is related to lipid peroxidation, and the use of antioxidant agents is protective (Rybak et al., 2000). Some chemotherapy medications also have central nervous system toxicity, which can be confused with vestibulotoxicity.

Antibiotics

A large number of antibiotics have been reported to be ototoxic in certain circumstances, including erythromycin, gentamicin, streptomycin, dihydrostreptomicin, tobramycin, netilmicin, amikacin, neomycin, kanamycin, etiomycin, vancomycin, and capreomycin. Antibiotics generally considered safe are members of the penicillin family, the cephalosporin family, and the macrolide family (except in situations where dosages are very high). Here we will discuss a few of the more common ototoxic antibiotics.

The aminoglycosides are a large family of antibiotics that are uniformly ototoxic. Streptomycin, the first clinically used aminoglycoside, is now used only in treating tuberculosis, because many gram-negative bacteria are resistant and because of substantial ototoxicity. Dihydrostreptomycin is no longer used in the United States, but streptomycin sulfate can still be obtained. Streptomycin is primarily a vestibulotoxin.

Neomycin, isolated in 1949, is now mainly used topically because of renal toxicity and cochleotoxicity. Hearing ototoxicity from oral absorption of neomycin has been reported (Rappaport et al., 1986) and there may also be toxicity from eardrops in patients with perforated eardrums.

Kanamycin, developed in 1957, has been replaced by newer aminoglycosides such as gentamicin, tobramycin, netilmicin, and amikacin. It is not thought to be as ototoxic as neomycin.

Gentamicin is presently the biggest problem antibiotic with respect to ototoxicity, as most of the other ototoxic antibiotics have been replaced. Gentamicin was released for clinical use in the early 1960s (Matz, 1993). Netilmicin has equivalent ototoxicity to gentamicin (Tange et al., 1995). Hearing toxicity generally involves the high frequencies first, but it is rarely severe. Vestibulotoxicity, rather than hearing toxicity, is the major problem resulting from gentamicin use. Certain persons with mitochondrial deletions in the 12S subunit are much more susceptible to gentamicin than the general population (Fischel-Ghodsian et al., 1997). The prevalence of this mutation is not clear, but 1% of the population is a reasonable estimate, based on available data. Gentamicin accumulates in the inner ear with repeated dosing, and for this reason, most cases of toxicity are associated with durations of administration of 2 weeks or more.

Vancomycin, although not an aminoglycoside, does have minor ototoxicity. However, it is often combined with aminoglycosides, and in this situation it potentiates the ototoxicity of gentamicin (Brummett et al., 1990) as well as (probably) other aminoglycosides such as tobramycin. Vancomycin by itself, in appropriate doses, is not ototoxic (Gendeh et al., 1998). Occasional persons do appear idiosyncratically to have substantial vestibular toxicity from vancomycin. The reason why occasional persons are more sensitive is not clear but might resemble the situation with gentamicin, where there is a susceptibility mutation (Fischel-Ghodsian et al., 1997).

Eardrops may contain antibiotics, some of which can be ototoxic when administered to persons with perforated eardrums. Cortisporin otic solution appears to be the most ototoxic to the cochlea of guinea pigs. Ofloxacin eardrops have negligible toxicity (Barlow et al., 1995). Neomycin-containing eardrops have been reported to contribute to hearing loss (Podoshin, Fradis, and Ben David, 1989) in a relatively small way, but a definitive assessment of risk has not yet been made. The vestibulotoxicity of eardrops has so far not been studied, although case reports suggest that gentamicin-containing drops are toxic (Marais and Rutka, 1998; Bath et al., 1999).

There are several known interactions between antibiotics as well as with other agents. Vancomycin combined with gentamicin causes more vestibulotoxicity than either one alone. Loop diuretics potentiate aminoglycoside toxicity. Noise also may potentiate aminoglycoside ototoxicity.

Delayed ototoxicity, meaning essentially toxicity that continues for several months after the drug has been stopped, occurs because the aminoglycosides are retained within the inner ear much longer than in the blood. Gentamicin has been reported to persist for more than 6 months in animals (Dulon et al., 1993). Neomycin, streptomycin, and kanamycin are also known to be eliminated from the inner ear slowly (Thomas, Marion, and Hinojosa, 1992).

Ototoxic Diuretics

Loop diuretics are well-known cochleotoxins. Examples include furosemide and ethacrinic acid (Rybak, 1993). Diuretics generally considered safe include chlorthiazide.

Loop diuretics are rarely a source of vestibulotoxicity. They are possibly a source of hearing disturbance. They may be synergistic with aminoglycoside ototoxins such as gentamicin, neomycin, streptomycin, and kanamycin. It seems prudent to attempt to avoid exposure to these agents if hearing is impaired.

Quinine Derivatives

Numerous quinine derivatives, including quinidex, atabrine, plaquenil, quinine sulfate, mefloquine (Lariam), and chloroquine, have reported ototoxicity (Jung et al., 1993). The toxicity is primarily cochleotoxic and is generally confined to tinnitus, but it can cause a syndrome that includes tinnitus, sensorineural hearing loss, and vertigo. Some quinine derivatives taken for malaria prevention can occasionally cause significant and long-lasting tinnitus. Recent studies suggest that quinine impairs outer hair cell motility.

Aspirin, NSAIDs, and Other Analgesics

Aspirin and other NSAIDs are commonly used, and apparently only toxic to hearing (Jung et al., 1993). These include ibuprofen, naproxen, piroxicam, diflunisal, indomethacin, etodolac, nabumetone, ketorolac tromethamine, diclofenac sodium, and the salicylates, aspirin and salsalate.

Rarely, hearing loss is reported from other types of analgesics, for example, hydrocodone/acetaminophen combination (Friedman et al., 2000; Oh, Ishiyama, and Baloh, 2000).

Permanent hearing disturbances are possible but rare. They are most commonly seen in individuals who take aspirin in large doses for long periods, such as for the treatment of arthritis. Occasionally persons with Ménière's syndrome will develop a hearing disturbance from a small amount of an NSAID.

Compounding Factors

Noise exposure is the most common source of hearing loss. Industrial exposure characteristically causes a "noise notch," with the hearing loss at mid- to high frequencies bilaterally. Guns and other unilateral sources of noise can cause more circumscribed lesions. Noise can be a cofactor in medication-induced ototoxicity. Those who have hearing loss from an ototoxic antibiotic, for example, may be at much greater risk from noise (Aran, 1995).

Protection from Ototoxins

Little is known about protection from ototoxicity. Antioxidants protect partially from noise or toxins in several animal models (Rybak, Whitworth, and Somani, 1999). In theory, prevention of reactive oxygen species, neutralization of toxic products, and blockage of the apoptosis pathway might provide protection from oxidative stress, which is a common final pathway for ototoxicity. Toxic waste products can be neutralized with glutathione and derivatives (Rybak et al., 2000). Apoptosis can be blocked using capsase inhibitors. At this writing, all of these approaches are investigational and are not being used clinically. Most also require delivery systems that go directly into the inner ear, and are therefore impractical for clinical use. For cochleotoxicity, noise avoidance is likely helpful, but even here the story is complicated. Paradoxically, moderate amounts of noise may protect from extreme amounts of noise. Nevertheless, it seems prudent to avoid excessive noise exposure, particularly in situations where there has been a recent exposure to an ototoxin. Because aminoglycosides may persist in the inner ear for more than 6 months, practically this advice implies long-term noise avoidance.

Treatment of Ototoxicity

Because most cochleotoxicity is caused by damage to hair cells, and because once dead, hair cells do not regenerate in humans, treatment of completed ototoxicity, whether it be cochlear or vestibular, is limited to substitution of other inputs, procedures that recalibrate remaining function, and behavioral adaptations. For cochleotoxicity, the approach is largely amplification. Hearing aids and related devices (assistive devices such as telephone amplifiers) can be helpful in those whose hearing loss is subtotal. When hearing loss is complete, cochlear implants may be offered.

For vestibulotoxicity, a rehabilitation approach is often very helpful. The goal of vestibular rehabilitation is to reduce symptoms of dizziness, oscillopsia, and unsteadiness. Patients are instructed in and perform a daily exercise routine designed to recalibrate remaining vestibular input and to substitute other senses such as vision and neck proprioception.

With reduced vestibular function, the eye movement generated for a given head movement is too small, resulting in oscillopsia or blurred vision. To train the brain to generate an eye movement of equal amplitude to the head movement, *gaze stabilization* exercises are performed. Exercises consist of focusing on an object with continuous movements of the head for 1–2 minutes. Exercises can be made more difficult by increasing the complexity of the visual background behind the object of regard. The complexity of the exercises is progressed gradually as symptoms resolve.

For the balance deficits that are common in vestibular ototoxicity, patients are given static and dynamic exercises that require the control of balance with reduced sensory input, conflicting sensory input, reduced base of support, and during head movements. To help adapt to their vestibular loss, patients are educated in environmental and behavioral modifications to reduce the risk of falls.

—Timothy C. Hain and Janet Helminski

References

Aran, J. M. (1995). Current perspectives on inner ear toxicity. *Otolaryngology–Head and Neck Surgery, 112,* 133–144.

Barlow, D. W., Duckert, L. G., Kreig, C. S., and Gates, G. A. (1995). Ototoxicity of topical otomicrobial agents. *Acta Oto-Laryngolica, 115,* 231–235.

Bath, A. P., Walsh, R. M., Bance, M. L., and Rutka, J. A. (1999). Ototoxicity of topical gentamicin preparations. *Laryngoscope, 109,* 1088–1093.

Brummett, R. E., Fox, K. E., Jacobs, F., Kempton, J. B., Stokes, Z., and Richmond, A. B. (1990). Augmented gentamicin ototoxicity induced by vancomycin in guinea pigs. *Archives of Otolaryngology–Head and Neck Surgery, 116,* 61–64.

Dulon, D., Hiel, H., Aurousseau, C., Erre, J. P., and Aran, J. M. (1993). Pharmacokinetics of gentamicin in the sensory hair cells of the organ of Corti: Rapid uptake and long term persistence. *Comptes Rendus de l'Academie des Sciences, série III, Sciences de la Vie, 316,* 682–687.

Fischel-Ghodsian, N., Prezant, T. R., Chaltraw, W. E., Wendt, K. A., Nelson, R. A., Arnos, K. S., and Falk, R. E. (1997). Mitochondrial gene mutation is a significant predisposing factor in aminoglycoside ototoxicity. *American Journal of Otolaryngology, 18,* 173–178.

Friedman, R. A., House, J. W., Luxford, W. M., Gherini, S., and Mills, D. (2000). Profound hearing loss associated with hydrocodone/acetaminophen abuse. *American Journal of Otology, 21,* 188–191.

Gendeh, B. S., Gibb, A. G., Aziz, N. S., Kong, N., and Zahir, Z. M. (1998). Vancomycin administration in continuous ambulatory peritoneal dialysis: The risk of ototoxicity. *Otolaryngology–Head and Neck Surgery, 118,* 551–558.

Jung, T. T., Rhee, C. K., Lee, C. S., Park, Y. S., and Choi, D. C. (1993). Ototoxicity of salicylate, nonsteroidal anti-inflammatory drugs, and quinine. *Otolaryngolic Clinics of North America, 26,* 791–810.

Marais, J., and Rutka, J. A. (1998). Ototoxicity and topical eardrops. *Clinical Otolaryngology, 23,* 360–367.

Matz, G. J. (1993). Aminoglycoside cochlear ototoxicity. *Otolaryngolic Clinics of North America, 26,* 705–712.

Oh, A. K., Ishiyama, A., and Baloh, R. W. (2000). Deafness associated with abuse of hydrocodone/acetaminophen. *Neurology, 54,* 23–45.

Podoshin, L., Fradis, M., and Ben David, J. (1989). Ototoxicity of ear drops in patients suffering from chronic otitis media. *Journal of Laryngology and Otology, 103,* 46–50.

Rappaport, B. Z., Fausti, S. A., Schechter, M. A., and Frey, R. H. (1986). A prospective study of high-frequency auditory function in patients receiving oral neomycin. *Scandinavian Audiology, 15,* 67–71.

Riggs, L. C., Brummett, R. E., Guitjens, S. K., and Matz, G. J. (1996). Ototoxicity resulting from combined administration of cisplatin and gentamicin. *Laryngoscope, 106,* 401–406.

Rybak, L. P. (1993). Ototoxicity of loop diuretics. *Otolaryngolic Clinics of North America, 26,* 829–844.

Rybak, L. P., Husain, K., Morris, C., Whitworth, C., and Somani, S. (2000). Effect of protective agents against cisplatin ototoxicity. *American Journal of Otology, 21,* 513–520.

Rybak, L. P., Whitworth, C., and Somani, S. (1999). Application of antioxidants and other agents to prevent cisplatin ototoxicity. *Laryngoscope, 109,* 1740–1744.

Tange, R. A., Dreschler, W. A., Prins, J. M., Buller, H. R., Kuijper, E. J., and Speelman, P. (1995). Ototoxicity and nephrotoxicity of gentamicin vs netilmicin in patients with serious infections: A randomized clinical trial. *Clinical Otolaryngology, 20,* 118–123.

Thomas, J., Marion, M. S., and Hinojosa, R. (1992). Neomycin ototoxicity. *American Journal of Otolaryngology, 13,* 54–55.

Pediatric Audiology: The Test Battery Approach

The auditory mechanism is a complex sensory system and as such requires a wide selection of specific procedures for assessing its functional integrity. In general, these procedures may be grouped according to the differential information they supply about peripheral auditory disorders (i.e., external and middle ear, cochlea, and cranial nerve VIII), central auditory dysfunction (i.e., neural pathways of the brainstem and auditory cortex), and pseudohypacusis (i.e., hearing loss of nonorganic origin). The results of a battery of procedures contribute information about the auditory processes that are normal as well as those that are abnormal.

In differential audiologic assessment, the audiologist seeks procedures that provide optimum information about which levels of the auditory system are disordered. Patients can—and often do—have coexisting disorders at several levels, with the most dominant problem masking clues to the presence of others. Because no single test can represent the integrity of the entire auditory system, the best overall measure is obtained by combining test results, whereby each test within the test battery evaluates some aspect of the auditory mechanism. Jaeschke, Guyatt, and Sackett (1994) propose that useful diagnostic tests distinguish among disorders or states that might otherwise be confused, add information beyond that otherwise available, and lead to a change in management that is beneficial to the patient.

Some tests are designed specifically to assist in identifying the site of the lesion, while others are designed to determine the presence and nature of an auditory deficit. The diagnostic outcomes sought from the pediatric population vary little from adult counterparts. That is, audiologic tests are selected to differentiate peripheral versus central hearing loss, conductive versus sensorineural hearing loss, cochlear versus neural site of lesion, and varying middle ear conditions. The audiologist neither expects nor gets complete agreement on all the different tests performed. Age, physical and cognitive/intellectual conditions, individual variability, and peculiarities of different audiologic conditions can result in paradoxical outcomes and may affect the consistency of audiologic findings. Thus, an extensive battery of audiologic tests is intended to provide a profile of data that may be compared with findings obtained in individuals with previously documented auditory conditions. Evidence for a specific interpretation exists when the profile of results is consistent with expected findings.

The test battery approach in pediatric audiology is focused on confirming suspected hearing loss in infants referred from universal newborn hearing screening programs and the ongoing assessment of infants at risk for delayed-onset or progressive hearing loss (Joint Committee on Infant Hearing, 2000). Refinements in audiologic tests (e.g., conditioned behavioral tests including visual reinforcement audiometry and conditioned play audiometry; acoustic immittance; auditory-evoked potentials), as well as the addition of new audiologic tests (e.g., otoacoustic emissions), provide the audiologist with a sophisticated test battery from which to initiate clinical decisions (Folsom and Diefendorf, 1999).

When individual tests are combined into a test battery, results can be viewed from a holistic framework. In this approach, findings across tests are integrated to establish a working diagnosis that often goes beyond the sum of the individual parts. The use of a test battery offers several advantages, including (1) avoidance of overgeneralizing the results from a single test, (2) increasing the data set from which to draw conclusions, and (3) enhancing the confidence in a clinical decision as the number of test results consistent with a specific interpretation increases. Conversely, combining tests into a battery may not be advantageous, cost-effective, or time-efficient when the tests are highly correlated (that is, different tests testing for the same disorder). The more positive the test correlation, the less performance varies when tests are combined. When tests have high to maximum positive correlation, test battery performance cannot be better than the best single test in the battery; thus, there is no value in combining tests just to satisfy the faulty assumption that more tests are always better. Each test must be selected on the basis of the patient's complaints, and associated with the highest hit rate and lowest false alarm rate for the suspected disorder.

When selecting tests as part of a test battery, it is essential to balance quality patient care with fiscal responsibility. Therefore, the general rule to apply in pediatric assessment when selecting appropriate audiologic tests is *not* to administer a test unless its results provide new information for patient management. In fact, the real advantage of tests in a test battery comes when negative correlation is determined between tests, indicating that each test tends to identify different disorders.

Not only does the test battery delineate hearing loss, it also provides opportunities for making appropriate cross-checks. The cross-check principle in audiology, originally outlined by Jerger and Hayes (1976), undergirds the concept of a test battery approach so that a single test is not interpreted in isolation, but various tests act as a cross-check on the final outcome. The principle is that the results of a single test are never accepted as conclusive proof of the nature or site of auditory disorder without support from at least one additional independent test. That is, the error inherent in any test and in patient response behavior is recognized, and the probability of an incorrect diagnosis is minimized when the results of several tests lead to the same conclusion. Moreover, the test battery approach and cross-check principle provide a statistical advantage when compared with the utilization of but a single test. The multiplicity of judgments in the test battery renders the entire differential assessment more reliable and valid. Statistically, multiple judgments from nonduplicative, negatively correlated tests lend safety to the interpretation of raw data when compared to the outcome and potential for error from a single judgment. To implement the cross-check strategy successfully, clinicians need to recognize the importance of selecting tests based on the child's physical status, developmental level, and test correlation.

A test battery is paramount when the clinician is evaluating children with multiple disabilities. These children exhibit diverse medical problems that can diminish the accuracy of behavioral and physiological hearing tests. Complicating factors may include but are not limited to severe neurological, motor, and sensory problems. These factors can adversely influence test results, in turn compromising the validity of a single test approach. In addition, the limitations of the tests themselves can impose barriers when evaluating children with complex problems. Test constraints (e.g., limitations of behavioral observation audiometry [BOA] in eliciting an observable response; impact of developmental age on visual reinforcement audiometry [VRA]; middle ear pathology compromising acoustic reflex measures; the impact of central nervous system damage on the auditory brainstem response [ABR]) frequently dictate what procedures are feasible for a child with special needs. No test or clinician is infallible, and mistakes made with infants and young children can have crucial implications for medical and educational management.

Gans and Gans (1993) tested children with special needs by a test battery made up of BOA, VRA, ABR, and the acoustic reflex. The primary goal of the study was to rule out bilateral hearing loss greater than a mild degree. Stringent criteria were established for ruling out hearing loss with each of the tests to minimize the chances of missing a child (false negative error) with a moderate hearing loss or greater. The tests were performed in a serial manner until one test result ruled in essentially normal hearing. Once achieved, further testing was discontinued.

The results demonstrated that BOA passed approximately 35% of the children, VRA passed approximately 10%, acoustic reflex measurement passed approximately 22%, and ABR passed approximately 57%. Yet when conducted in a serial strategy (individual tests administered until one "normal" result was obtained), 80% of the children under study were determined to have hearing better than the cutoff criterion. Although ABR alone was better at predicting hearing sensitivity than the other tests, the total percentage score accomplished by a serial test battery was more than 20% greater than for ABR alone. Factor analysis failed to find a strong relationship among the tests and suggests that different factors caused changes in threshold estimation across different children. That is, successful outcomes were based on interactions between the individual's disabilities and the individual tests. These factors included but were not limited to low chronological or developmental age (neurological, motor, skeletal, and respiratory abnormalities), medications, and conductive hearing loss. Certain factors will adversely influence the results of one test more than another. Therefore, reliance on a single test for a child with disabling conditions would give an erroneous clinical impression that a large proportion of these children sustain hearing loss.

An audiologst prone to using a single-test approach might be tempted to rely on ABR as the only test method. This approach certainly relies on the assumption that the test of choice is a valid hearing test for *all* individuals and is not susceptible to variables that could lead to errors in outcome. The important findings from the work of Gans and Gans (1993) provide evidence that challenges this assumption for children with special needs, and provides a strong rationale for using a battery of appropriately selected tests.

The selection of individual tests for use in a test battery must be supported by clinical and experimental evidence. If individual tests and their use in test batteries are not evidence based, are not cost-effective in outcomes, and do not positively impact patients, we diminish the quality of services provided.

—*Allan O. Diefendorf and Michael K. Wynne*

References

Folsom, R. C., and Diefendorf, A. O. (1999). Physiologic and behavioral approaches to pediatric hearing assessment. *Pediatric Clinics of North America, 46*, 107–120.

Gans, D., and Gans, K. D. (1993). Development of a hearing test protocol for profoundly involved multi-handicapped children. *Ear and Hearing, 14*, 128–140.

Jaeschke, R., Guyatt, G., and Sackett, D. L. (1994). Users' guides to the medical literature. *Journal of the American Medical Association, 271*, 389–391.

Jerger, J., and Hayes, D. (1976). The cross-check principle in pediatric audiometry. *Archives of Otolaryngology, 102*, 614–620.

Joint Committee on Infant Hearing. (2000). Year 2000 position statement: Principles and guidelines for early hearing detection and intervention programs. *American Journal of Audiology, 9*, 9–29.

Further Readings

Bess, F. H. (Ed.). (1998). *Children with Hearing Loss: Contemporary Trends*. Nashville, TN: Bill Wilkerson Center Press.

Diefendorf, A. O., and Gravel, J. S. (1996). Behavioral observation and visual reinforcement audiometry. In S. Gerber (Ed.), *Handbook of Pediatric Audiology*. Washington, DC: Gallaudet University Press.

Stach, B. A., Wolf, S. J., and Bland, L. (1993). Otoacoustic emissions as a cross-check in pediatric hearing assessment: Case report. *Journal of the American Academy of Audiology, 4*, 392–398.

Turner, R. G., Frazer, G. J., and Shepard, N. T. (1984). Formulating and evaluating audiological test protocols. *Ear and Hearing, 5*, 321–330.

Turner, R. G., and Nielson, D. W. (1984). Application of clinical decision analysis to audiological tests. *Ear and Hearing, 5*, 125–133.

Turner, R. G., Shepard, N. T., and Frazer, G. J. (1984). Clinical performance of audiological and related diagnostic tests. *Ear and Hearing, 5*, 187–194.

Physiological Bases of Hearing

Outer and Middle Ears

The cartilaginous pinna on the outside of the skull has a set of characteristic folds and curves, different for each individual, which set up a series of shadowings and reflections of the sound wave. The result is that the spectrum of the sound, as transmitted to the concha (the opening of the ear canal), is modified according to the direction and elevation of the sound's source. Although the main cue for sound localization comes from comparing the relative intensities and times of arrival of the stimuli at the two ears, that comparison does not give us information on the elevation of the sound source, or whether the source is behind or in front of the head; that information is provided by the pinna. Moreover, the outer ear means that sound localization of a sort can be undertaken with only one ear.

The middle and inner ears are protected from the outside world by an ear canal, and the inner ear is further protected by a middle ear cavity. The closed cavity of the middle ear, however, is a common site for infection, in which pus and secretions in early stages, and the formation of fibrous tissue in later stages, reduce the efficiency of transmission of vibrations to the cochlea.

The relatively dense, incompressible cochlear fluids, enclosed in a bony canal, with their movement limited by the membranes of the inner ear, need a higher pressure of vibration for a certain amplitude of move-

Figure 1. A cross-section of the cochlear duct showing the division into three scalae and the position of the sensory apparatus, the organ of Corti. (From Fawcett, D. W. [1986]. *A textbook of histology*. Philadelphia: Saunders, Fig. 35.11. Reproduced with permission.)

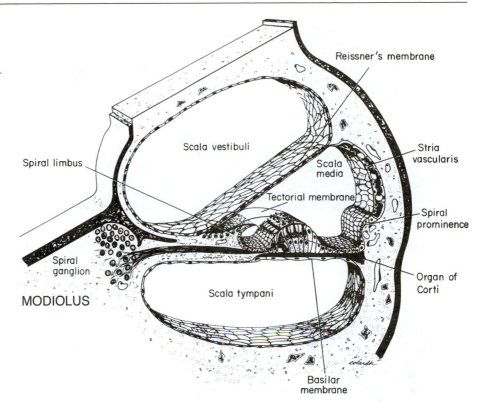

ment than do sound waves in air. One job of the outer and middle ears is to transform the ratio (pressure/amplitude) of vibration from a low value suitable for the external air to a much higher value able to drive the cochlear fluids efficiently. This is undertaken by (1) acoustic resonances in the outer ear canal, (2) the footplate of the stapes in the oval window being much smaller than the tympanic membrane (so that forces from the sound vibration are concentrated in a small area), and (3) a lever action in the vibration both of the middle ear bones and of the tympanic membrane.

Vibration through the middle ear is affected by the middle ear muscles, the tensor tympani and the stapedius muscle, with contraction of the muscles reducing sound transmission. These muscles contract in response to self-produced activity such as vocalizations, but also in response to loud sounds, to give some partial protection of the inner ear against acoustic trauma.

The Cochlea

The cochlea performs a spectral analysis, sorting the incoming mechanical vibration into its different frequency components, and transduces the sound, turning the mechanical vibration into an electrical change that activates the fibers of the auditory nerve.

The cochlea, deep inside the temporal bone, has a spiral central cavity, which curves the long (35-mm) cochlear duct into a small space 10 mm across. The canal is divided by membranous partitions into three spaces, or scalae, which run the length of the canal (Fig. 1).

The mechanical vibration, transmitted to the cochlear fluids, causes a ripple-like motion (i.e., a traveling wave) in the membranes dividing the scalae and hence in the organ of Corti, causing deflection of the stereocilia or hairs on the hair cells (see Robles and Ruggero, 2001, for a review). Cyclical deflection of the stereocilia opens and closes the mechanotransducer channels, causing positive and negative potential changes within the hair cells. There are two types of hair cell (Fig. 2). In the outer hair cells, operation of the mechanotransducer channels with the resulting changes in electrical potential induce, in ways that are controversial, a mechanical response that enhances the initial mechanical vibration. The result is that the amplitude of the mechanical traveling wave grows exponentially as it travels along the cochlear duct away from its point of introduction. Because the dimensions and stiffness of the cochlear duct and membranes change along the duct, at some point along the duct, the ratio of mass of fluid that has to be moved by the introduced vibration to the stiffness of the membranes that assist in the moving becomes too great to permit the vibration to continue for that particular frequency of stimulation, and the wave dies out rapidly. For a single tone, the traveling wave therefore has a peak which is sharp and narrow, so that maximal stimulation of hair cells occurs along only a short region of the cochlear duct. The peak occurs near the base (i.e., oval window end) for high-frequency tones and near the apex for low-frequency tones; for a spectrally complex stimulus, the spatial pattern of vibration reflects the spectrum of the incoming sound. This is known as *place coding* of frequency. In addition, the time pattern of

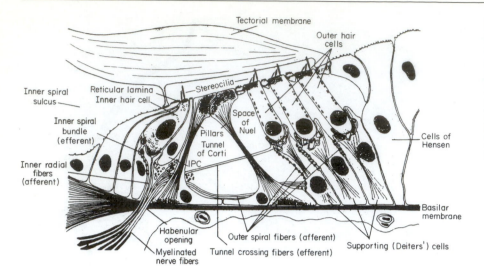

Figure 2. Detail of the organ of Corti in the cochlear duct showing the position of the inner and outer hair cells and cochlear innervation. The modiolus (center of the cochlear spiral) is to the left in the figure. IPC, inner phalangeal cell. (Modified with permission from Ryan, A. F., and Dallos, P. [1984]. Physiology of the cochlea. In J. L. Northern [Ed.], *Hearing disorders*. Boston: Little, Brown, Fig. 22–4.)

vibration at any point reflects the time pattern of the (spectrally filtered) acoustic stimulus.

The outer hair cells are particularly vulnerable components of the cochlea, being readily damaged by insults such as loud sound, anoxia, and many ototoxic drugs. They are also particularly vulnerable to degenerative changes. The result of such processes is that the traveling wave is reduced in amplitude, and the sharpness of its peak is reduced. The inner hair cells are still able to detect the vibrations, but the cochlea loses sensitivity (i.e., there is a hearing loss), and there is a degradation in its ability to perform the spectral analysis.

Processing in the Auditory Nervous System

The inner hair cells make synaptic connections with the afferent fibers of the auditory nerve, so that when the inner hair cells are stimulated in parallel with the outer hair cells, the auditory nerve fibers are activated, and both the spectral and temporal patterns of vibration are thereby signaled to the central nervous system. At low frequencies, the time pattern of neural firing can follow the time pattern of the vibration of the organ of Corti at the point of innervation. This is known as the *temporal coding* of sound frequency. However, at higher frequencies the fluctuations cannot follow each cycle of the waveform, and therefore the stimulus can be signaled only by a change in the mean firing rate. At low frequencies, therefore (below about 300 Hz), both place coding and time coding can contribute; at high frequencies (above a few kHz), only place coding is operative. However, temporal fluctuations in the envelope of the sound waveform, if below a few hundred Hz, are still represented in the overall pattern of the firing.

Processing in the auditory brainstem extracts and enhances three features of the auditory stimulus. Spectral contrast in the sound stimulus is enhanced, temporal transitions are emphasized, and information on the sound locus is extracted.

The enhancement of spectral contrast depends on the spatial pattern of activity in the auditory nerve, i.e., on the place coding of sound frequency, which is then emphasized by neural *lateral inhibition* between adjacent cell groups in the central auditory system, starting at the cochlear nucleus. Auditory neural responses therefore become dominated by representations of the most intense spectral peaks (such as vowel formants in the case of speech), while responses to a lower level or a more spectrally uniform background stimuli are reduced. In some way that is not understood, the two mechanisms of frequency representation, namely, place coding and time coding, are neurally integrated into a single percept.

Temporal information in the sound waveform is also emphasized; the enhancement of temporal transitions in the neural responses means that the response to a fluctuating stimulus consists substantially of bursts of neural activity when the stimulus intensity increases, no activity when the intensity decreases, and very low levels of activity during steady portions of the stimulus.

The spatial location of the sound source is primarily analyzed by comparing the sounds arriving at the two ears. A stimulus on, say, the left will strike the left ear first, and will also be more intense in the left ear. Both of these cues are extracted by the nervous system to give an indication of direction, with a neural representation in the central nervous system such that neurons on one side of the body are driven most strongly by sounds originating on the opposite side. The time cues are extracted by comparing the time of arrival of the nerve impulses from the two ears at the medial superior olivary nucleus in the brainstem, while intensity differences are detected primarily in the lateral superior olivary nucleus. The information as to the location of the sound source is integrated in the inferior colliculus with spectral and temporal pattern information that had been enhanced at the cochlear nucleus, before reaching the auditory cortex via the specific thalamic nucleus, the medial geniculate body.

Cortical Analysis

It is likely that there is a division of function between different parts of the auditory cortex, situated on the superior surface of the temporal lobe, buried in the lateral (or sylvian) fissure. The more dorsal areas are likely to represent location in auditory space, while the more ventral areas are involved in the analysis of complex stimuli, such as of speech (Rauschecker and Tian, 2000). Recording from individual cortical neurons suggests that speech sounds are likely to be analyzed and represented only over a whole population, that is, they are represented as a pattern of activity that is spread over a large number of neurons, where consideration of activity of the whole population is necessary for the accurate specification of the speech sound. Within the population, individual neurons or neural assemblies may be specialized for the detection of critical features, such as spectral peaks or rapid temporal transitions, such as are necessary for the specification of the sound (Wang, 2000). One area traditionally associated with speech is Wernicke's area, which lies just posterior to the primary cortical area in the dominant (generally left) hemisphere. Lesions of Wernicke's area result in defects in comprehension and word selection. Further forward, on the ventral frontal lobe, lesions of Broca's area result in deficits in the production of speech. While the lesion data show that these areas are critical, functional magnetic resonance imaging shows that listening to speech activates a much wider range of areas (Fig. 3), with much more extensive surrounding temporal, angular, and frontal areas likely to be involved in both linguistic and semantic analysis (Binder et al., 1997). Although these imaging studies give information on the cortical areas activated and suggest the potential for conceptually splitting a task into its different functional components, they do not provide any information on the

neural mechanisms underlying the functions, which remain elusive.

—James O. Pickles

References

Binder, J. R., Frost, J. A., Hammeke, T. A., Cox, R. W., Rao, S. M., and Prieto, T. (1997). Human brain language areas identified by functional magnetic resonance imaging. *Journal of Neuroscience, 17*, 353–362.

Rauschecker, J. P., and Tian, B. (2000). Mechanisms and streams for processing of 'what' and 'where' in auditory cortex. *Proceedings of the National Academy of Sciences of the United States of America, 97*, 11800–11806.

Robles, L., and Ruggero, M. A. (2001). Mechanics of the mammalian cochlea. *Physiological Reviews, 81*, 1305–1352.

Wang, X. (2000). On cortical coding of vocal communication sounds in primates. *Proceedings of the National Academy of Sciences of the United States of America, 97*, 11843–11849.

Further Readings

Dallos, P., Popper, A. N., and Fay, R. R. (Eds.). (1996). *The cochlea.* New York: Springer-Verlag.

Pickles, J. O. (1988). *An introduction to the physiology of hearing.* London: Academic Press.

Popper, A. N., and Fay, R. R. (Eds.). (1992). *The mammalian auditory pathway: Neurophysiology.* New York: Springer-Verlag.

Pitch Perception

The study of pitch dates back to at least the time of Pythagoras, who formulated the relationship between the length of a string and the pitch it would produce if it were strummed. The perception of pitch is the basis of musical melody and the voicing of speech; moreover, pitch is an attribute of the sound created by many objects in our world.

While the common definition of pitch has to do with a subjective attribute of sound and is scaled from low to high, pitch is closely related to frequency, a physical attribute of sound. The other physical attributes of sound are level, temporal structure, and complexity (Rossing, 1990). The study of pitch perception is often linked to the ability of the auditory system to process the frequency content of sound. The physical attributes of sound are derived from the fact that sound occurs when objects vibrate. The rate at which an object vibrates in an oscillatory manner is the frequency of the sound. If an object vibrates back and forth in a regular and repeatable manner 440 times in 1 s, it is said to have a frequency of 440 cycles per second (cps), which is indicated as 440 Hz (Hertz). If this vibrating object generated sound, the sound would have a 440-Hz frequency. If the vibrating object were a guitar string, a musician would perceive the vibrating string to have a pitch of 440 Hz. A higher rate of vibration would produce a higher pitch and a lower rate a lower pitch. Thus, for the

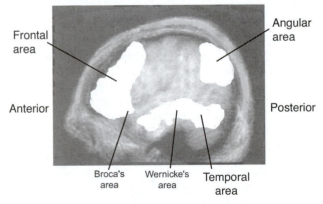

Figure 3. Functional magnetic resonance image of the human cortex during a speech analysis task. Areas that are heavily activated are shown in white. The section is sagittal through the left hemisphere. (Modified with permission from Binder, J. R., et al. [1997]. Human brain language areas identified by functional magnetic resonance imaging. *Journal of Neuroscience, 17*, 353–362.)

vibrating guitar string, pitch is the subjective attribute of frequency. The relationship between the physical attributes of sound and pitch is not as simple as the guitar-string example suggests, and a few of the complexities will be described later in this article. That is, frequency and pitch are not synonymous.

Frequency can be measured using physical or objective means to determine the rate of vibration (Rossing, 1990). The measurement of pitch requires perceptual measurement techniques found in the research toolbox of the psychoacoustician or the musician. In many contexts, the pitch of a test sound is determined by comparing its perceived pitch with that of a standard sound. The standard sound is usually a sound with a very regular vibratory pattern, such as a tone or a periodic train of brief impulses (a click train). If the comparison sound and the test sound are judged to have the same perceived pitch, then the pitch of the test sound is the vibratory frequency of the comparison sound. So, in the example involving the guitar string, the vibrating string would be perceived as having the same pitch as a tone or a click train with a 440-Hz frequency.

Musical Pitch and Pitch Scales

In music, pitch can have two different meanings. When the frequency of the vibrating guitar string doubles (e.g., from 440 to 880 Hz), the frequency has increased by an octave. Musical sounds that are an octave apart in frequency are perceived as similar, as opposed to a less similar perception for sounds that are not separated by an octave. This similarity means that a melody played at one octave is very recognizable when it is played in other octaves. Thus, musicians will say that sounds that differ by an octave have the same pitch, even though they have different frequencies and may be judged to match a standard tone of a different frequency. Thus, pitch can have two meanings in music, one referring to octave relationships and one to the actual frequency of vibration. *Pitch chroma* is sometimes used to refer to octave relationships involving pitch, while *pitch height* is used to refer to pitch as determined by vibratory frequency. For example, a 440-Hz tone and an 880-Hz tone have the same pitch chroma but different pitch heights.

The notes of the musical scale represent different ratio intervals within an octave. Thus, musical pitch can be measured in terms of musical notes (the 12 notes of A, B, C, D, E, F, G and the half-tones, or the sharps and flats). The octave can be divided into 1200 equal logarithmic units (ratio units) call cents. The 12 musical notes divide this 1200-cent octave into 12 equal units, so that each note is 100 cents (100 cents is sometimes referred to a semitone). Each note represents a different ratio from the beginning of the octave; e.g., the ratio between the notes C and G is one-fifth. The pitch of the 440-Hz vibrating guitar string is the note A in the middle range of the musical octaves, and the note C would have a pitch of 528 Hz in this same octave, or 264 Hz in the next lower octave. Therefore, another measure of pitch is the musical scale expressed either by musical notes or by cents.

The other measure of pitch is the mel scale (Stevens and Volkman, 1940). The mel scale is an attempt to measure pitch on a scale from low to high, as implied by the definition of pitch given above. A sound with a tonal frequency of 1000 Hz has a pitch of 100 mels. A sound that is judged to have a pitch twice as high has a 200-mel pitch, while a pitch judged to be twice as low has a 50-mel pitch. Thus, the 1000-Hz tone serves as a referent against which the pitch of other sounds can be compared. A mel scale relates the perceived pitch of a sound in mels to another variable, most often frequency. So a sound with a pitch of 300 mels is one that is perceived as having a pitch that is three times higher than that of a 1000-Hz tone.

Complex Pitch

Sounds can have complex patterns of vibration and as such are made up of vibrations of many different frequencies. These complex sounds have a spectrum of many different frequencies. If certain frequencies are dominant in the sound's spectrum, then the pitch of the sound may be perceived as representing the frequency of the dominant component in the spectrum. So the pitch of simple sounds with regular patterns of vibration or complex sounds with dominant frequencies in the sound spectrum is determined by these main frequencies. However, we can consider a complex sound that is the sum of the following frequencies: 300, 400, 500, 600, and 700 Hz. This complex sound will have a perceived pitch of 100 Hz, even though the sound contains no frequency at 100 Hz. Note that this complex sound consists of frequency components that are spaced 100 Hz apart and are all integer multiplies (harmonics) of 100 Hz. The missing 100-Hz component is the fundamental frequency of the complex, because it is the highest frequency for which all of the other components are integer multiples (de Boer, 1976). The 100-Hz perceived pitch is that of this missing fundamental, and so this type of perceived pitch is often referred to as the "pitch of the missing fundamental" or "complex pitch." Although this sound's spectrum has no frequency at its pitch, the pattern of vibration oscillates at 100 Hz. Thus, it is possible that the pitch is not related as much to the frequency content of the sound as it is to the rate of oscillation. Or perhaps the 100-Hz spacing of the frequency components is the crucial dimension of the sound that determines the pitch of the missing fundamental. If the spectrum of this sound is changed to be 325, 425, 525, 625, and 725 Hz, the perceived pitch is now 104 Hz, which is neither the missing fundamental nor equal to the 100-Hz spacing of the frequency components. In addition, the sound does not have a dominant pattern of vibratory oscillations at 104 Hz (Patterson, 1973). Thus, neither simple frequency nor temporal properties of a sound can be used to predict complex pitch.

Complex pitches, such as the pitch of the missing fundamental, suggest that pitch is not simply related to frequency. It is also the case that changes in other physical attributes of sound, such as sound level, can lead to a change in pitch, reinforcing the observation that pitch and frequency are not synonymous. Various theories of pitch processing have been proposed to account for the pitches of simple and complex sounds. These theories fall into three general categories (Moore, 1997). One set of theories, spectral theories, propose different means of using the sound's frequency spectrum to determine pitch. Another group of theories, temporal theories, suggest that aspects of the temporal oscillation of the sound's vibratory pattern are used by the auditory system to determine pitch. Then there are theories that use a combination of spectral and temporal aspects of a sound to predict its pitch (de Boer, 1976). Such theories have been proposed for nearly a hundred years, and no one theory has emerged that best accounts for all of the data related to pitch perception (Plomp, 1976).

Thus, whereas pitch is a major attribute of sound and is crucial to our ability to use sound to identify the objects in our world and to communicate, auditory science does not have a good explanation of how pitch is processed by the auditory system. It is clear that the way in which the auditory system processes both spectral and temporal information contributes to pitch processing, but the details of how these processes operate is still a mystery.

—*William A. Yost*

References

de Boer, E. (1976). Residue and auditory pitch perception. In W. Neff and W. Keidel (Eds.), *Handbook of sensory physiology* (vol. V). Berlin: Springer-Verlag.

Moore, B. C. J. (1997). *An introduction to the psychology of hearing* (3rd ed.). London: Academic Press.

Patterson, R. (1973). Physical variables determining residue pitch. *Journal of the Acoustical Society of America, 53,* 1566–1572.

Plomp, R. (1976). *Aspects of tone sensation.* London: Academic Press.

Rossing, T. (1990). *The science of sound* (2nd ed.). Reading, MA: Addison-Wesley.

Stevens, S. S., and Volkman, J. (1940). The relation of pitch to frequency: A revised scale. *American Journal of Psychology, 53,* 329–353.

Further Readings

de Cheveigne, A. (2001). The auditory system as a 'separation machine.' In D. J. Breebaart, A. J. M. Houstma, A. Kohlrausch, A. F. Prijs, and R. Schoonhoven (Eds.), *Physiological and psychophysical bases of auditory function.* The Netherlands: Shaker Publishing.

Hartmann, W. M. (1998). *Signal, sounds, and sensation.* New York: Academic Press.

Moore, B. C. J. (1986). *Frequency selectivity in hearing.* London: Academic Press.

Roederer, J. G. (1973). *Introduction to the physics and psychophysics of music.* New York: Springer-Verlag.

Yost, W. A. (2000). *Fundamentals of hearing: An introduction* (4th ed.). New York: Academic Press.

Presbyacusis

Presbyacusis is a general term to describe hearing loss in older persons or the hearing loss associated with aging. Hearing loss observed in older adults is a result of the combined effects of aging, long-term exposure to occupational and nonoccupational noise, the use of ototoxic drugs, diet, disease, and other factors. In this case, the term presbyacusis describes any hearing loss observed in an older person, regardless of cause. Alternatively, presbyacusis may refer specifically to the hearing loss that increases with chronological age and is related only to age-related deterioration in the auditory periphery and central nervous system (CNS).

Currently, about 75% of the 28 million hearing-impaired individuals in the United States are 55 years of age or older; the number of hearing-impaired individuals will increase as the population ages. Indeed, presbyacusis is the most prevalent of the chronic conditions of aging among men age 65 years and older, and the fifth most prevalent condition among older women, following arthritis, cardiovascular diseases, and visual impairments (National Center for Health Statistics, 1986). Age-related hearing loss in the United States has been well characterized by epidemiologic surveys such as the Framingham Heart Study (Moscicki et al., 1985), the Baltimore Longitudinal Study of Aging (Pearson et al., 1995), and the Epidemiology of Hearing Loss Study of the adult residents of Beaver Dam, Wisconsin (Cruickshanks et al., 1998). Figure 1 shows the systematic increase in thresholds with chronological age in Framingham subjects; thresholds at high frequencies are higher for male than for female subjects. In the Beaver Dam study, the prevalence of hearing loss was 45.9%, with hearing loss defined as average thresholds (0.5–4 kHz) greater than 25 dB in the worse ear. This is consistent with the prevalence reported in the Framingham study of 42%–47%. The prevalence of hearing loss in the Beaver Dam study varied greatly with sex and age, ranging from 10.2% for women 48–52 years of age to 96.6% for men 80–92 years of age. Another set of data, including hearing levels as a function of age, sex, and history of occupational noise exposure, is part of an international standard (ISO 1999, 1990). Database A from this standard may more closely represent aging effects on hearing, given that subjects were screened for occupational and other noise exposure history. Epidemiologic surveys also provide estimates of the genetic component of presbyacusis. Heritability coefficients suggest that as much as 55% of the variance in thresholds in older persons is genetically determined, are stronger in women than in men, and are comparable to those for hypertension and hyperlipidemia (Gates, Couropmitree, and Myers, 1999).

A remarkable and consistent age-related change in hearing occurs at frequencies above 8 kHz and begins as early as age 20–30 years (Stelmachowicz et al., 1989). Figure 2 shows thresholds in the conventional and extended high frequencies for younger and older adults,

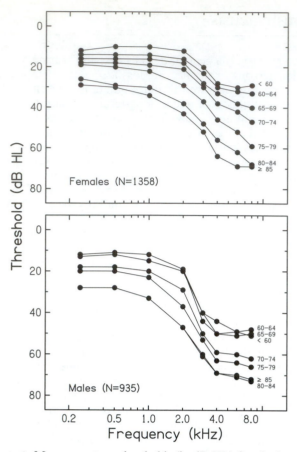

Figure 1. Mean pure-tone thresholds (in dB HL) for the better ear of male and female participants in the Framingham Heart Study. Age ranges of participants are given at the right. (Adapted with permission from Moscicki, E. K., et al., 1985, "Hearing loss in the elderly: An epidemiologic study of the Framingham Heart Study cohort." *Ear and Hearing, 6*, 184–190.)

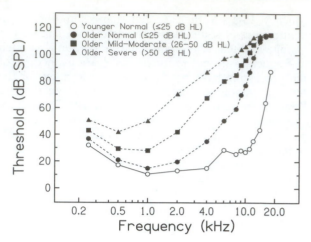

Figure 2. Mean pure-tone thresholds at frequencies from 0.25 kHz to 18 kHz for three groups of subjects aged 60–79, grouped by pure-tone average at 1, 2, and 4 kHz (normal, mild to moderate, and severe), and one group of younger subjects with normal hearing. (Adapted with permission from Matthews, L. J., et al., 1997, "Extended high-frequency thresholds in older adults." *Journal of Speech, Language, and Hearing Research, 40*, 208–214. © American Speech-Language-Hearing Association.)

grouped according to average thresholds from 1 to 4 kHz (Matthews et al., 1997). Thresholds are substantially elevated at frequencies above 8 kHz, even for individuals with nearly normal thresholds at lower frequencies.

To supplement pure-tone thresholds, the Hearing Handicap for the Elderly instrument (Ventry and Weinstein, 1982), a self-report questionnaire, has been used to compare older individuals' assessment of their communication abilities with objective measures of hearing and with threshold-based estimates of hearing handicap, such as that recommended by the American Academy of Otolaryngology–Head and Neck Surgery (AAO, 1979; Matthews et al., 1990). Discrepancies between objective and subjective measures are common, and the variance in pure-tone thresholds within hearing handicap categories is large. Thus, whereas hearing loss is among the most prevalent chronic conditions of aging, the impact of hearing loss on communication abilities and daily activities of older adults varies greatly among individuals

and is not accurately predicted from the pure-tone audiogram.

Studies of auditory behavior in older adults must separate age-related effects from those attributable simply to reduced audibility resulting from elevated thresholds. One experimental method to minimize the confound of reduced audibility is to include only older subjects whose pure-tone thresholds are equal to those of younger subjects. When changes in auditory behavior in older adults are observed that are not attributable to reduced audibility, they may be due to age-related changes in the auditory periphery, which provides an impoverished input to a normal auditory CNS, or to the combined effects of an aging periphery and an aging CNS. For many behavioral measures, it may not be possible to differentiate between these outcomes. This is particularly the case for tasks that require comparisons of temporal information across intervals of time or that assess binaural processing.

Other than effects related to their hearing loss, older adults probably do not have increased problems in speech understanding relative to younger individuals, as measured conventionally (i.e., monaurally, under earphones, with highly redundant signals). Indeed, some studies suggest that 70%–95% of the variance in monaural speech recognition scores may be accounted for by the variance in speech audibility (Humes, Christopherson, and Cokely, 1992). Figure 3 shows scores on several speech recognition tests for three age groups with nearly identical (within ~3 dB) mean thresholds from 0.25 to 8 kHz (Dubno et al., 1997). With hearing loss held constant across age group, speech recognition scores also remained constant. Nevertheless, age-related differences in speech recognition in noise may become

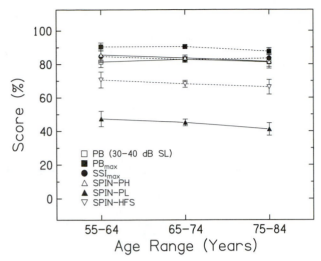

Figure 3. Mean scores in percent correct (± 1 standard error) for six measures of speech recognition. The six measures are word recognition for NU-6 monosyllabic words (PB), maximum word recognition (PB_{max}), maximum synthetic sentence identification (SSI_{max}), keyword recognition for high-context and low-context sentences from the SPIN test (SPIN-PH and SPIN-PL), and "percent hearing for speech" (SPIN-HFS). (Adapted with permission from Dubno, J. R., et al., 1997, "Age-related and gender-related changes in monaural speech recognition." *Journal of Speech, Language, and Hearing Research, 40,* 444–452. © American Speech-Language-Hearing Association.)

apparent in more realistic listening environments, such as in the sound field with spatially separated speech and maskers, with competing sounds that have temporal or spectral dips, or on tasks that require divided or selective attention. It remains unclear if these age-related changes may be attributed to an aging auditory periphery or to the combined effects of an aging periphery and an aging CNS.

Although older adults are the largest group of hearing aid wearers, their satisfaction with hearing aids is low. More than 75% of individuals who are likely to benefit from a hearing aid do not own one, a gap of approximately 20 million people (LaPlante, Hendershot, and Moss, 1992). Similar results were observed for hearing-impaired participants of the Framingham and Beaver Dam studies, in which less than 20% were hearing aid users. In examining the functional health status and psychosocial well-being of older individuals, Bess et al. (1989) concluded that hearing loss is a primary determinant of function and that its impact is comparable to that of other chronic conditions affecting this population. Thus, untreated hearing loss can have a negative effect on quality of life beyond that due to poorer communication abilities (Mulrow et al., 1990). The potential benefit to communication and quality of life, together with new fitting options and improved technology, suggests that older adults should be encouraged to use amplification.

Evidence of age-related changes in the auditory system is revealed in the physiological properties of aging humans and animals. Older gerbils raised in quiet have elevated thresholds of the compound action potential (CAP) of the auditory nerve and shallow slopes of CAP input-output functions (Hellstrom and Schmiedt, 1990). These characteristics are also reflected in higher auditory brainstem response (ABR) thresholds and shallower slopes of ABR amplitude-intensity functions relative to young gerbils (Boettcher, Mills, and Norton, 1993). Similar findings have been observed in older humans. Although these potentials produced by short-duration signals are reduced in amplitude with age, amplitudes of potentials arising from higher CNS centers in response to long-duration signals, such as steady-state potentials and N_{100}–P_{200}, may be unaffected or even increase with age. Abnormal recovery from adaptation or forward masking and abnormal gap detection at the level of the brainstem have also been observed in older animals and humans (Walton, Orlando, and Burkard, 1999). In aging gerbils, the 80–90 mV dc resting potential in the scala media of the cochlea, known as the endocochlear potential (EP), is reduced substantially. In contrast to these changes, nonlinear phenomena remain relatively intact. For example, transient otoacoustic emissions, reflecting the functioning of outer hair cells, are present in about 90% of older humans with normal hearing, but amplitudes are reduced in a manner that is not predictable by either age or pure-tone thresholds. In aging gerbils, distortion product otoacoustic emissions are present and robust, but somewhat reduced in amplitude (Boettcher, Gratton, and Schmiedt, 1995). Two-tone rate suppression is observed in older gerbils, with age-related threshold shifts (Schmiedt, Mills, and Adams, 1990), although older humans may have reduced suppression measured psychophysically (Dubno and Ahlstrom, 2001).

The pathologic anatomy underlying these physiologic changes was most extensively described through studies of human temporal bones by Schuknecht (1974). Initially, four categories of presbyacusis were identified, including sensory (degeneration of sensory cells), neural (largely loss of spiral ganglion cells), metabolic (degeneration of the lateral wall and stria vascularis, with reduction in the protein Na,K-ATPase), and mechanical (aging of sound-conducting structures of the inner ear). Categories of presbyacusis were revised by Schuknecht and Gacek (1993) wherein atrophy of the stria vascularis was designated as the "predominant lesion" of the aging ear, neuronal loss was "constant and predictable," mechanical loss remained theoretical, and sensory presbyacusis was the "least important type of loss." These histopathological findings are consistent with the physiological evidence described above, such as reduced CAP amplitudes and reduced EP but robust otoacoustic emissions. Thus, most age-related changes in hearing can be accounted for by changes observed in the auditory periphery. Nevertheless, there are many age-related anatomical, neurochemical, and neurophysiological changes in the CNS. One prominent neurochemical change is a loss of gamma-aminobutyric acid, which may affect the balance of inhibitory and excitatory neurotransmission. The effects of these and other CNS changes on age-related hearing loss may be substantial but remain largely unknown.

Acknowledgments

This work was supported (in part) by grants P50 DC00422 and R01 DC00184 from the National Institute on Deafness and Other Communication Disorders (National Institutes of Health).

—*Judy R. Dubno and John H. Mills*

References

American Academy of Otolaryngology. (1979). Guide for the evaluation of hearing handicap. *Otolaryngology–Head and Neck Surgery, 87,* 539–551.

Bess, F. H., Lichtenstein, M. J., Logan, S. A., and Burger, M. C. (1989). Comparing criteria of hearing impairment in the elderly: A functional approach. *Journal of Speech and Hearing Research, 32,* 795–802.

Boettcher, F. A., Gratton, M. A., and Schmiedt, R. A. (1995). Effects of age and noise on hearing. *Occupational Medicine, 10,* 577–591.

Boettcher, F. A., Mills, J. H., and Norton, B. L. (1993). Age-related changes in auditory evoked potentials of gerbils: I. Response amplitudes. *Hearing Research, 71,* 137–145.

Cruickshanks, K. J., Wiley, T. L., Tweed, T. S., Klein, B. E., Klein, R., Mares-Perlman, J. A., et al. (1998). Prevalence of hearing loss in older adults in Beaver Dam, Wisconsin: The Epidemiology of Hearing Loss Study. *American Journal of Epidemiology, 148,* 879–886.

Dubno, J. R., and Ahlstrom, J. B. (2001). Psychophysical suppression measured with bandlimited noise extended below and/or above the signal: Effects of age and hearing loss. *Journal of the Acoustical Society of America, 110,* 1058–1066.

Dubno, J. R., Lee, F. S., Matthews, L. J., and Mills, J. H. (1997). Age-related and gender-related changes in monaural speech recognition. *Journal of Speech, Language, and Hearing Research, 40,* 444–452.

Gates, G. A., Couropmitree, N. N., and Myers, R. H. (1999). Genetic associations in age-related hearing thresholds. *Archives of Otolaryngology–Head and Neck Surgery, 125,* 654–659.

Hellstrom, L. I., and Schmiedt, R. A. (1990). Compound action potential input/output functions in young and quiet-aged gerbils. *Hearing Research, 50,* 163–174.

Humes, L. E., Christopherson, L., and Cokely, C. (1992). Central auditory processing disorders in the elderly: Fact or fiction? In J. Katz, N. Stecker, and D. Henderson (Eds.), *Central auditory processing* (pp. 141–149). St. Louis: Mosby–Year Book.

International Organization for Standards: Acoustics. (1990). *Determination of occupational noise exposure and estimation of noise-induced hearing impairment* [ISO 1999]. Geneva: International Organization for Standards.

LaPlante, M. P., Hendershot, G. E., and Moss, A. J. (1992). Assistive technology devices and home accessability features: Prevalence, payment, need, and trends. *Advance data from vital and health statistics,* no. 217. Hyattsville, MD: National Center for Health Statistics.

Matthews, L. J., Lee, F. S., Mills, J. H., and Dubno, J. R. (1997). Extended high-frequency thresholds in older adults. *Journal of Speech, Language, and Hearing Research, 40,* 208–214.

Matthews, L. J., Lee, F. S., Mills, J. H., and Schum, D. J. (1990). Audiometric and subjective assessment of hearing handicap. *Archives of Otolaryngology–Head and Neck Surgery, 116,* 1325–1330.

Moscicki, E. K., Elkins, E. F., Baum, H. M., and McNamara, P. M. (1985). Hearing loss in the elderly: An epidemiologic study of the Framingham Heart Study cohort. *Ear and Hearing, 6,* 184–190.

Mulrow, C. D., Aguilar, C., Endicott, J. E., Tuley, M. R., Velez, R., Charlip, W. S., et al. (1990). Quality of life changes and hearing impairment: Results of a randomized trial. *Annals of Internal Medicine, 113,* 188–194.

National Center for Health Statistics. (1986). *Prevalence of Selected Chronic Conditions, United States, 1979–1981. Vital and health statistics,* Series 10, No. 155 (OHHS Publication No. [PHS] 86-1583). Public Health Service. Washington, DC: U.S. Government Printing Office.

Pearson, J. D., Morrell, C. H., Gordon-Salant, S., Brant, L. J., Metter, E. J., Klein, L. L., and Fozard, J. L. (1995). Gender differences in a longitudinal study of age-associated hearing loss. *Journal of the Acoustical Society of America, 97,* 1196–1205.

Schmiedt, R. A., Mills, J. H., and Adams, J. (1990). Tuning and suppression in auditory nerve fibers of aged gerbils raised in quiet or noise. *Hearing Research, 45,* 221–236.

Schuknecht, H. F. (1974). *Pathology of the ear.* Cambridge, MA: Harvard University Press.

Schuknecht, H. F., and Gacek, M. R. (1993). Cochlear pathology in presbycusis. *Annals of Otology, Rhinology, and Laryngology, 102,* 1–16.

Stelmachowicz, P. G., Beauchaine, K. A., Kalberer, A., and Jesteadt, W. (1989). Normative thresholds in the 8- to 20-kHz range as a function of age. *Journal of the Acoustical Society of America, 86,* 1384–1391.

Ventry, I. M., and Weinstein, B. E. (1982). The Hearing Handicap Inventory for the Elderly: A new tool. *Ear and Hearing, 3,* 128–134.

Walton, J. P., Orlando, M., and Burkard, R. (1999). Auditory brainstem response forward-masking recovery functions in older humans with normal hearing. *Hearing Research, 127,* 86–94.

Further Readings

Anderer, P., Semlitsch, H. V., and Saletu, B. (1996). Multichannel auditory event-related brain potentials: Effects of normal aging on the scalp distribution of N1, P2, N2 and P300 latencies and amplitudes. *Electroencephalography and Clinical Neurophysiology, 99,* 458–472.

Bredberg, G. (1968). Cellular pattern and nerve supply of the human organ of Corti. *Acta Otolaryngology, Supplement, 236,* 1–135.

Caspary, D. M., Milbrandt, J. C., and Helfert, R. H. (1995). Central auditory aging: GABA changes in the inferior colliculus. *Experimental Gerontology, 30,* 349–360.

Committee on Hearing, Bioacoustics, and Biomechanics (CHABA). (1988). Speech understanding and aging. *Journal of the Acoustical Society of America, 83,* 859–893.

Dubno, J. R., Dirks, D. D., and Morgan, D. E. (1984). Effects of age and mild hearing loss on speech recognition in noise. *Journal of the Acoustical Society of America, 76,* 87–96.

Fitzgibbons, P. J., and Gordon-Salant, S. (1995). Age effects on duration discrimination with simple and complex stimuli. *Journal of the Acoustical Society of America, 98,* 3140–3145.

Frisina, R. D. (2001). Anatomical and neurochemical bases of presbycusis. In P. R. Hoff and C. V. Mobbs (Eds.), *Functional neurobiology of aging* (pp. 531–548). San Diego, CA: Academic Press.

Gordon-Salant, S., and Fitzgibbons, P. J. (1993). Temporal factors and speech recognition performance in young and elderly listeners. *Journal of Speech and Hearing Research, 36,* 1276–1285.

Gratton, M. A., and Schulte, B. A. (1995). Alterations in microvasculature are associated with atrophy of the stria vascularis in quiet-aged gerbils. *Hearing Research, 82,* 44–52.

Grose, J. H., Poth, E. A., and Peters, R. W. (1994). Masking level differences for tones and speech in elderly listeners with relatively normal audiograms. *Journal of Speech and Hearing Research, 37,* 422–428.

He, N.-J., Dubno, J. R., and Mills, J. H. (1998). Frequency and intensity discrimination measured in a maximum-likelihood procedure from young and aged normal-hearing subjects. *Journal of the Acoustical Society of America, 103,* 553–565.

He, N.-J., Horwitz, A. R., Dubno, J. R., and Mills, J. H. (1999). Psychometric functions for gap detection in noise measured from young and aged subjects. *Journal of the Acoustical Society of America, 106,* 966–978.

Humes, L. E., and Christopherson, L. A. (1991). Speech identification difficulties of hearing-impaired elderly persons: The contributions of auditory processing deficits. *Journal of Speech and Hearing Research, 34,* 686–693.

Humes, L. E., Watson, B. U., Christensen, L. A., Cokely, C. G., Halling, D. C., and Lee, L. (1994). Factors associated with individual differences in clinical measures of speech recognition among the elderly. *Journal of Speech and Hearing Research, 37,* 465–474.

Jerger, J., and Chmiel, R. (1997). Factor analytic structure of auditory impairment in elderly persons. *Journal of the American Academy of Audiology, 8,* 269–276.

Mills, J. H., Schmiedt, R. A., and Kulish, L. F. (1990). Age-related changes in auditory potentials of Mongolian gerbil. *Hearing Research, 46,* 301–310.

Moore, B. C. J., and Peters, R. W. (1992). Pitch discrimination and phase sensitivity in young and elderly subjects and its relationship to frequency selectivity. *Journal of the Acoustical Society of America, 91,* 2881–2893.

Rosen, S., Bergman, M., Plester, D., El-Mofty, A., and Hamad Satti, M. (1962). Presbyacusis study of a relatively noise-free population in the Sudan. *Annals of Otology, Rhinology, and Laryngology, 71,* 727–743.

Schneider, B. A. (1997). Psychoacoustics and aging: Implications for everyday listening. *Journal of Speech-Language Pathology and Audiology, 21,* 111–124.

Schulte, B. A., and Schmiedt, R. A. (1992). Lateral wall NaK-ATPase and endocochlear potential decline with age in quiet-reared gerbils. *Hearing Research, 61,* 35–46.

Strouse, A., Ashmead, D. H., Ohde, R. N., and Grantham, D. W. (1998). Temporal processing in the aging auditory system. *Journal of the Acoustical Society of America, 104,* 2385–2399.

Takahashi, G. A., and Bacon, S. P. (1992). Modulation detection, modulation masking, and speech understanding in noise in the elderly. *Journal of Speech and Hearing Research, 35,* 1410–1421.

van Rooij, J. C., and Plomp, R. (1990). Auditive and cognitive factors in speech perception by elderly listeners: II. Multivariate analyses. *Journal of the Acoustical Society of America, 88,* 2611–2624.

Weinstein, B. E. (2000). *Geriatric audiology.* New York: Thieme.

Willott, J. F. (1991). *Aging and the auditory system: Anatomy, physiology, and psychophysics.* San Diego, CA: Singular Publishing Group.

Pseudohypacusis

Pseudohypacusis means, literally, a false elevation of thresholds. In pseudohypacusis, intratest and intertest audiometric inconsistencies cannot be explained by medical examinations or a known organic condition (Ventry and Chaiklin, 1965). Authors of literature in this area have called this condition exaggerated hearing loss, nonorganic hearing loss, or functional hearing loss. Exaggerated hearing loss implies intent, but some forms of pseudohypacusis may have subconscious origins (Wolf et al., 1993). The intent of the listener cannot be determined with audiometric measures. Nonorganic hearing loss implies that there is no physical basis for the hearing loss; however, many adults have a false elevation of thresholds added to an existing loss. Some even present with pseudohypacusis and an ear-related medical problem requiring immediate attention (Qui et al., 1998). Functional hearing loss is the only synonym among these terms.

Monetary or psychological gain motivates most pseudohypacusics. Audiologists should be alert for this condition if the referral source is a lawyer, as in a medicolegal case, or an organization documenting hearing for compensation purposes; however, there are cases where the referral source does not provide any warning. There are even cases of persons with normal auditory systems presenting with longstanding false losses that have been misdiagnosed and the individuals inappropriately fitted with hearing aids.

Estimates of the prevalence rate for pseudohypacusis are between 2% and 5%, with higher rates observed in some special populations, such as the military and industrial workers (Rintelmann and Schwann, 1999). Pseudohypacusics show falsely elevated thresholds in one or both ears, the degree of loss ranges from mild to profound, and the type of loss can be sensorineural or mixed (Qui et al., 1998).

Pseudohypacusics usually adopt an internal loudness yardstick that corresponds to the amount of their "hearing loss" (Vaubel, 1976; Gelfand and Silman, 1985). External sounds are compared with this internal yardstick, and pseudohypacusics only respond behaviorally to sounds that exceed this internal value. This is important to know, because modifications to hearing tests that affect loudness perception often have little or no effect on thresholds of audibility in cooperative adults. Many behavioral tests for pseudohypacusis that are used by audiologists are designed to disrupt loudness judgments.

The responsibility of the audiologist in the assessment of persons presenting with psuedohypacusis is to document intertest and intratest inconsistencies and to quantify true thresholds as a function of frequency. Many methods exist for documenting inconsistent results, but few measures exist for quantifying accurately true behavioral thresholds.

When evaluated for intertest and intratest inconsistencies, the basic battery of audiologic tests, administered to nearly everyone entering the clinic, are the ones that will likely identify persons presenting with this condition, given that many pseudohypacusics have nothing in their history that might raise suspicion. The basic battery of tests that is used in the assessment of pseudohypacusis differs somewhat across clinics, but this group of tests often includes pure-tone thresholds, spondee thresholds, and immittance (see TYMPANOMETRY).

Pure-tone threshold assessment provides several methods for identifying pseudohypacusis. Most clinicians routinely retest the threshold for a 1000 Hz tone as a reliability check. Thresholds on retest are usually within 10 dB of the first test in cooperative persons, whereas pseudohypacusics often show larger threshold differences (Ventry and Chaiklin, 1965). Although this method is not particularly sensitive or specific for the identification of pseudohypacusis, deviations greater than 10 dB can provide a warning to the clinician. In addition to poor reliability, pseudohypacusics do not demonstrate false positive responses (a response when a tone is not presented) (Ventry and Chaiklin, 1965). By contrast, several false positive responses in a single testing session are quite common in persons with tinnitus (Mineau and Schlauch, 1997). Unfortunately, audiometric configuration is not a reliable diagnostic tool for pseudohypacusis (Ventry and Chaiklin, 1965). However, the presence of a flat loss, or equal hearing loss at each audiometric frequency, has been reported as common in several studies (Coles and Mason, 1984; Alpin and Kane, 1985). The absence of shadow responses in asymmetrical losses is a reliable sign of pseudohypacusis (Rintelmann and Schwann, 1999). Shadow responses are thresholds based on the response of the nontest ear when sound is presented to the poorer, test ear. They reflect a limitation in the ability to isolate the two ears during a hearing test when masking noise is not presented to the nontest ear.

Spondee thresholds, a speech threshold for two-syllable words with equal stress on both syllables, are a quick measure that, when combined with pure-tone thresholds, provide one of the most effective tests for identification of pseudohypacusis. Spondee thresholds in cooperative adults usually fall within 10 dB of the average threshold for 500 Hz and 1000 Hz pure tones (PTA) (Carhart and Porter, 1971). Pseudohypacusics usually show larger differences, with the spondee threshold being lower (better) than the PTA (Carhart, 1952). In some instances, this difference may reflect the naïveté of the listener (Frank, 1976), as is often the case in children. In other words, the listener may feign a loss for tones and not understand that speech thresholds are quantifiable,

too. However, this finding in most instances is a result of the loudness of speech and tones growing at different rates. Consistent with loudness-related issues, this test is most effective when spondee thresholds are measured using an ascending approach (beginning at a low level) and pure-tone thresholds are measured using a descending approach (beginning at a high level) (Schlauch et al., 1996). This procedure identified 100% of pseudohypacusics, with no incorrect identifications of cooperative test subjects with hearing loss. A more conventional procedure that measured pure-tone thresholds with an ascending approach identified only about 60% of persons with pseudohypacusis.

Immittance measures are also routine tests that can aid in the documentation of persons presenting with pseudohypacusis. Tympanometry and acoustic reflex thresholds are sensitive measures of middle ear status and provide some indication of the integrity of the auditory system up to the superior olivary complex. For severe sensorineural losses, acoustic reflex thresholds are generally 10 dB or more above a person's behavioral threshold (Gelfand, 1994). Thresholds obtained at lower levels suggest pseudohypacusis. Gelfand (1994) has published normative values of reflex thresholds for different degrees of loss.

Numerous special tests were developed for assessing pseudohypacusis during the period immediately following World War II. Many of the tests developed during this time are confrontational, time-consuming, and ineffective when a clinical decision theory analysis is done. An exception to this criticism is a computer implementation of a simple modification to Bekesy audiometry or automated audiometry (Chaiklin, 1990), which still has application when testing the hearing of large groups of persons with a limited number of testers.

The Stenger test is a special test that is quick to administer and, unlike most tests, has the capability of quantifying the actual thresholds of persons presenting with unilateral pseudohypacusis (Kinstler, Phelan, and Lavender, 1972). This test makes use of the finding that when the same sound is presented simultaneously to both ears, the listener only hears the sound in the ear with the loudest percept. This test can be performed with tones or speech, but to be effective, the asymmetry between ears should be 40 dB or more. Manipulation of the sound levels in each ear is effective in identifying psuedohypacusis and quantifying actual behavioral thresholds (Rintelmann and Schwann, 1999).

Otoacoustic emissions (OAEs) (Musiek, Bornstein, and Rintelmann, 1995) and auditory-evoked potentials (Saunders and Lazenby, 1983; Bars et al., 1994; Musiek, Bornstein, and Rintelmann, 1995) are useful physiological measures for evaluating persons with pseudohypacusis. These special tests assess structures in the auditory pathways. OAEs assess the outer hair cells in the cochlea and the conductive pathway leading to the cochlea; these emissions are often absent even with mild hearing losses. However, auditory neuropathy cases, although rare, show that persons can have essentially normal OAEs and a severe hearing loss (Sininger et al., 1995). This possibility and the fact that many adults exaggerate existing losses make interpretation of OAEs in isolation somewhat ambiguous when evaluating pseudohypacusis. Estimation of the auditory brainstem response (ABR) threshold, a type of evoked potential, has been advocated as a useful measure for compensation cases (Bars et al., 1994), but this threshold assessment tool, while accurate in many situations, can yield misleading results in certain hearing-loss configurations (e.g., a rising audiogram) (Glattke, 1993; Bars et al., 1994). ABR threshold, like OAEs, does not assess the entire auditory pathway as do behavioral measures. OAEs (Gorga et al., 1993) and ABR (Hall, 1992) are also ineffective tools for assessing low frequencies, a critical region for consideration in compensation cases. Other evoked potentials, such as middle latency responses and the slow cortical potential, may hold promise, but like the ABR test, they are expensive to administer (Hyde et al., 1986; Musiek, Bornstein, and Rintelmann, 1995).

The ABR threshold and OAEs are important for the complete documentation of intractable cases or persons presenting with severe to profound bilateral losses, but most cases of pseudohypacusis are resolved by a combination of readministering patient instructions, informing the patient that there are inconsistent responses, and making multiple measurements of the audiogram using an ascending approach. The validity of remeasured pure-tone thresholds is evaluated using the PTA-spondee threshold-screening test described earlier. Patients whose thresholds are not resolved using this approach are scheduled for additional testing. Persons with obvious psychological problems are referred for counseling.

See also CLINICAL DECISION ANALYSIS; OTOACOUSTIC EMISSIONS; PURE-TONE THRESHOLD ASSESSMENT; SUPRA-THRESHOLD SPEECH RECOGNITION; TINNITUS.

—*Robert S. Schlauch*

References

Alpin, D. Y., and Kane, J. M. (1985). Variables affecting pure tone and speech audiometry in experimentally simulated hearing loss. *British Journal of Audiology, 19,* 219–228.

Bars, D. M., Althoff, L. K., Krueger, W. W., and Olsson, J. E. (1994). Work related, noise induced hearing loss: Evaluation including evoked potential audiometry. *Otolaryngology–Head and Neck Surgery, 110,* 177–184.

Carhart, R. (1952). Speech audiometry in clinical evaluation. *Acta Otolaryngologica, 41,* 18–42.

Carhart, R., and Porter, L. S. (1971). Audiometric configuration and prediction of threshold for spondees. *Journal of Speech and Hearing Research, 14,* 486–495.

Chaiklin, J. B. (1990). A descending LOT-Bekesy screening test for functional hearing loss. *Journal of Speech and Hearing Disorders, 55,* 67–74.

Coles, R. R., and Mason, S. M. (1984). The results of cortical electric response audiometry in medico-legal investigations. *British Journal of Audiology, 18,* 71–78.

Frank, T. (1976). Yes-no test for nonorganic hearing loss. *Archives of Otolaryngology, 102,* 162–165.

Gelfand, S. A. (1994). Acoustic reflex threshold tenth percentiles and functional hearing impairment. *Journal of the American Academy of Audiology, 5,* 10–16.

Gelfand, S. A., and Silman, S. (1985). Functional hearing loss and its relationship to resolved hearing levels. *Ear and Hearing, 6,* 151–158.

Glattke, T. J. (1993). *Short-latency auditory evoked potentials.* Austin, TX: Pro-Ed.

Gorga, M. P., Neely, S. T., Bergman, B. M., Beauchaine, K. L., Kaminski, J. R., Peters, J., et al. (1993). A comparison of transient-evoked and distortion product otoacoustic emissions in normal-hearing and hearing-impaired subjects. *Journal of the Acoustical Society of America, 94,* 2639–2648.

Hall, J. W., III. (1992). *Handbook of auditory evoked responses.* Needham Heights, MA: Allyn and Bacon.

Hyde, M., Alberti, P., Matsumoto, N., and Li, Y. L. (1986). Auditory evoked potentials in audiometric assessment of compensation and medicolegal patients. *Annals of Otology, Rhinology, and Laryngology, 95,* 514–519.

Kinstler, D. B., Phelan, J. G., and Lavender, R. W. (1972). The Stenger and speech Stenger tests in functional hearing loss. *Audiology, 11,* 187–193.

Mineau, S. M., and Schlauch, R. S. (1997). Threshold measurement for patients with tinnitus: Pulsed or continuous tones. *American Journal of Audiology, 6,* 52–56.

Musiek, F. E., Bornstein, S. P., and Rintelmann, W. F. (1995). Transient evoked otoacoustic emissions and pseudohypacusis. *Journal of the American Academy of Audiology, 6,* 293–301.

Qui, W. W., Stucker, F. J., Shengguang, Y. S., and Welsh, L. W. (1998). Current evaluation of pseudohypacusis: Strategies and classification. *Annals of Otology, Rhinology, and Laryngology, 107,* 638–647.

Rintelmann, W. F., and Schwann, S. A. (1999). Pseudohypacusis. In F. E. Musiek and W. F. Rintelmann (Eds.), *Contemporary perspectives in hearing assessment* (pp. 415–436). Needham Heights, MA: Allyn and Bacon.

Saunders, J. W., and Lazenby, B. B. (1983). Auditory brain stem response measurement in the assessment of pseudohypacusis. *American Journal of Otology, 4,* 292–299.

Schlauch, R. S., Arnce, K. D., Morison Olson, L., Sanchez, S., and Doyle, T. N. (1996). Identification of pseudohypacusis using speech recognition thresholds. *Ear and Hearing, 17,* 229–236.

Sininger, Y. S., Hood, L. J., Starr, A., Berlin, C. I., and Picton, T. W. (1995). Hearing loss due to auditory neuropathy. *Audiology Today, 7,* 11–13.

Vaubel, A. S. W. (1976). *A study of the strategies of malingerers during pure-tone and speech audiometry.* Unpublished master's thesis, University of Minnesota, Minneapolis.

Ventry, I. M., and Chaiklin, J. B. (Eds.). (1965). Multidiscipline study of functional hearing loss. *Journal of Auditory Research, 5,* 179–272.

Wolf, M., Birger, M., Shosan, J. B., and Kronenberg, J. (1993). Conversion deafness. *Annals of Otology, Rhinology, and Laryngology, 102,* 349–352.

Further Readings

Altschuler, M. W. (1982). Qualitative indicators of nonorganicity: Informal observations and evaluation. In M. B. Kramer and J. M. Armbruster (Eds.), *Forensic audiology* (pp. 59–68). Baltimore: University Park Press.

Beagley, H. A. (1973). The role of electrophysiological tests in the diagnosis of non-organic hearing loss. *Audiology, 12,* 470–480.

Bekesy, G. V. (1947). A new audiometer. *Acta Otolaryngologica, 35,* 411–422.

Bordley, J., and Hardy, W. (1949). A study of objective audiometry with the use of a psychogalvanometric response. *Annals of Otology, Rhinology, and Laryngology, 58,* 751–760.

Conn, M., Ventry, I. M., and Woods, R. W. (1972). Pure-tone average and spondee threshold relationships in simulated hearing loss. *Journal of Auditory Research, 12,* 234–239.

Durrant, J. D., Kesterson, R. K., and Kamerer, D. B. (1997). Evaluation of the nonorganic hearing loss suspect. *American Journal of Otology, 18,* 361–367.

Gold, S. R., Hunsaker, D. H., and Haseman, E. M. (1991). Pseudohypacusis in a military population. *Ear, Nose, and Throat Journal, 70,* 710–712.

Harris, D. A. (1958). A rapid and simple technique for the detection of non-organic hearing loss. *Archives of Otolaryngology, 68,* 758–760.

Kvaerner, K. J., Engdahl, B., Aursnes, J., Arnesen, A. R., and Mair, I. W. S. (1996). Transient evoked otoacoustic emissions: Helpful tool in the detection of pseudohypacusis. *Scandinavian Audiology, 25,* 173–177.

Martin, F. N. (1994). Pseudohypacusis. In J. Katz (Ed.), *Handbook of clinical audiology* (pp. 553–567). Baltimore: Williams and Wilkins.

Martin, F. N., Armstrong, T. W., and Champlin, C. A. (1994). A survey of audiological practices in the United States. *American Journal of Audiology, 3,* 20–26.

Martin, F. N., and Shipp, D. B. (1982). The effects of sophistication on three threshold tests for subjects with simulated hearing loss. *Ear and Hearing, 3,* 34–36.

McCandless, G. A., and Lentz, W. E. (1968). Evoked response (EEG) audiometry in non-organic hearing loss. *Archives of Otolaryngology, 87,* 123–128.

Peck, J. E., and Ross, M. (1970). A comparison of the ascending and the descending modes for the administration of the pure-tone Stenger test. *Journal of Auditory Research, 10,* 218–222.

Sohmer, H., Feinmesser, M., Bauberger-Tell, L., and Edelstein, E. (1977). Cochlear, brain stem, and cortical evoked responses in non-organic hearing loss. *Annals of Otology, Rhinology, and Laryngology, 86,* 227–234.

Spraggs, P. D. R., Burton, M. J., and Graham, J. M. (1994). Nonorganic hearing loss in cochlear implant candidates. *American Journal of Audiology, 15,* 652–657.

Stenger, P. (1907). Simulation and dissimulation of ear diseases and their identification. *Deutsche Medizinische Wochenschrift, 33,* 970–973.

Sulkowski, W., Sliwinska-Kowalska, M., Kowalska, S., and Bazydlo-Golinska, G. (1994). Electric response audiometry and compensational noise-induced hearing loss. *Otolaryngologia Polska, 48,* 370–374.

Pure-Tone Threshold Assessment

Audiometry is the measurement of hearing. Clinical hearing tests are designed to evaluate two basic aspects of audition: sensitivity and recognition (or discrimination). Hearing sensitivity measures are estimates of the lowest level at which a person can just detect the presence of a test signal (Ward, 1964). Measures that require an identification response or judgments of sound differences are tests of auditory acuity, recognition, or dis-crimination. These tests provide information about a listener's ability to recognize, discriminate, or understand acoustic signals, such as speech, and usually are conducted at moderate or higher signal levels. Tests of word recognition are clinical examples of such tests (see SUPRATHRESHOLD SPEECH RECOGNITION).

Hearing tests are performed for two primary purposes. One purpose is to identify hearing problems that may be caused by ear disease or damage to auditory structures. In some cases a hearing loss may indicate a medical problem, such as an ear infection. Because medical treatment of ear diseases is successful more often in early stages of the disease process, it is critical that such problems be detected and treated as soon as possible. A second purpose for hearing tests is to obtain information important for rehabilitation planning. In those cases of hearing loss for which medical treatment is not an appropriate alternative, it is important that nonmedical rehabilitative measures be considered based on the communication needs of the affected individual. Information obtained from the hearing evaluation, for example, is required to make decisions about the need for personal amplification (such as a hearing aid) or for other auditory rehabilitation services.

A basic requirement for administration of hearing tests is an acoustic system that enables control of the signals presented to the listener. An *audiometer* is an electronic instrument used to present controlled acoustic signals to a listener in order to test auditory function. In conventional pure-tone audiometry, the audiometer provides for the presentation of tones ranging in frequency from 125 through 8000 hertz (Hz). A hearing level (HL) dial allows the tester to control the level (in decibels, or dB) of a tone being presented to the listener. The HL control is graduated in steps of 10 and 5 dB (and sometimes smaller) and typically is adjustable over a range of 120 dB. When the HL dial is set to 0 dB, the output level of the audiometer corresponds to an average normal HL at that specific frequency. This is referred to as audiometric zero (American National Standards Institute [ANSI], 1996). This instrumental convenience accounts for the differences in absolute hearing sensitivity (in dB sound pressure level, or SPL) across frequency in persons with normal hearing. Other controls on the audiometer enable the tester to route the test signal to various receivers or transducers used to present the tones to a listener. The two most common receivers used in pure-tone audiometry are a set of earphones and a bone conduction vibrator. Earphones provide for airborne acoustic signals; a bone conduction vibrator is used to transmit vibratory energy through the skull to the inner ear (cochlea). Diagnostic audiometers also provide masking signals (typically a noise) for presentation to the nontest ear during specific audiometric tests. A masking noise is necessary for bone conduction audiometry and for cases of substantial unilateral hearing loss in which the test signal may be intense enough to be heard in the nontest ear. To rule out this possibility, the masking noise is introduced in the nontest ear. The noise elevates the threshold in that ear (masks it) and eliminates it from

Figure 1. Audiogram form used for recording pure-tone thresholds. Symbols shown to the right of the audiogram are those recommended by the American Speech-Language-Hearing Association (ASHA, 1990).

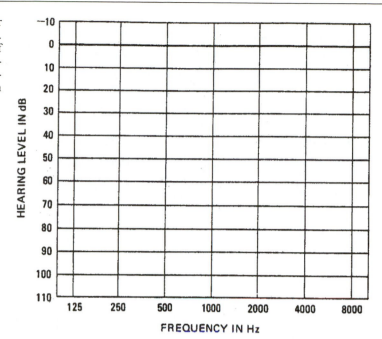

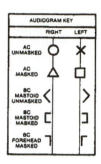

the test situation, to ensure that subject responses are only for the test ear.

Pure-tone audiometry consists of threshold measures for air and bone conduction signals in each ear (separately). A *pure-tone threshold* is the lowest level at which a person can just detect the presence of a tone. The threshold measure is statistical in nature; it is a level at which a listener responds to a criterion percentage of the signals presented. Clinically, threshold is usually defined as the lowest signal level at which the listener just detects 50% of the tones presented. Audiometric thresholds are influenced by a number of variables, including the instructions to the listener, the positioning of the earphone (or other transducer) on the head, and the psychophysical threshold measurement technique used (Dancer and Ventry, 1976; Yantis, 1994). In addition, individuals may demonstrate threshold variability related to factors such as motivation, the nature of the ear disorder, the patient's ability to comply with the test situation, and ongoing physiological changes inherent to the auditory system (Wilber, 1999).

Threshold measures obtained from pure-tone audiometry are conventionally plotted on a graph called an *audiogram* (Fig. 1). The audiogram enables the tester to quickly see the extent to which thresholds for a listener deviate from normal. In Figure 1, HL (dB) is plotted on the linear vertical axis and signal frequency (Hz) is indicated on the logarithmic horizontal axis. The format of the audiogram is such that one octave along the frequency axis corresponds in dimensional scale to 20 dB on the HL axis (ANSI, 1996). Recommended symbols for audiograms are also included in the legend of Figure 1 (American Speech-Language-Hearing Association [ASHA], 1990). Note that separate symbols are used to indicate bone conduction thresholds and measures made with a masking noise in the nontest ear (masked thresh-

olds). Symbols used to record thresholds on the audiogram also may be color coded, with red indicating measures for the right ear and blue indicating results for the left ear.

Specific procedures have been developed for pure-tone audiometry so that thresholds are obtained in a manner that minimizes test variability and are repeatable over time and from clinic to clinic. These procedures are based on research findings for persons with normal hearing and persons with hearing impairment, and include specifications on test frequencies, duration of test tones, step size changes in signal level, and other procedural variables (ASHA, 1978, 1997). The basic test protocol involves initially familiarizing the listener with the tones that will be heard and then determining thresholds for the tones. A bracketing technique is used whereby the tone level at a specific frequency is varied up and down and the listener indicates whether the tone is audible at each level. The tester determines the average hearing level at which the tone was heard approximately half the time over a series of presentations. This level represents the pure-tone threshold at a specific frequency and is recorded on the audiogram. Thresholds are obtained separately for air conduction using earphones and for bone conduction using a bone conduction vibrator. Air conduction tones produced by the earphone are directed down the ear canal, through the middle ear, and then to the cochlea. In bone conduction testing, however, a vibrator is used to transmit the signal through the bones of the skull to the cochlea. The vibrator is placed on the forehead or the mastoid portion of the temporal bone (behind the pinna), and thresholds are measured for the desired audiometric frequencies. All testing is performed in a sound-treated room that meets standards for the exclusion of ambient noise (ANSI, 1999).

Results of pure-tone audiometry, recorded on the audiogram, provide a description of both the degree and type of hearing loss. Because we are mainly interested in a person's ability to hear everyday speech, the customary procedure for classifying degree of hearing loss involves a computation of the *pure-tone average* (PTA). A person's PTA is her or his average pure-tone thresholds for the speech frequencies of 500, 1000, and 2000 Hz. Table 1 provides a degree classification of hearing loss based on average pure-tone thresholds in the better ear for these frequencies. In considering the purpose and results of audiometric tests, it is important to distinguish the terms *hearing loss* (or hearing impairment) and *hearing*

Table 1. Degree Classifications of Hearing Loss (Handicap)

Pure-Tone Average (dB HL) for 500, 1000, and 2000 Hz in the Better Ear	Handicap Classification
≤25	Not significant
26–40	Slight
41–55	Mild
56–70	Marked
71–90	Severe
>90 dB	Extreme

Adapted with permission from Davis, H. (1978). Hearing handicap standards for hearing, and medicolegal rules. In H. Davis and S. R. Silverman (Eds), *Hearing and deafness* (4th ed., pp. 266–290). New York: Holt, Rinehart, and Winston.

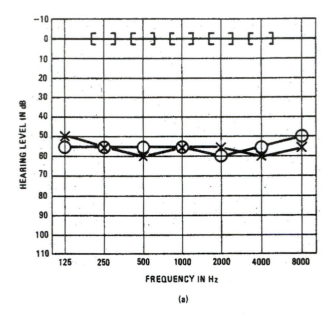

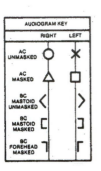

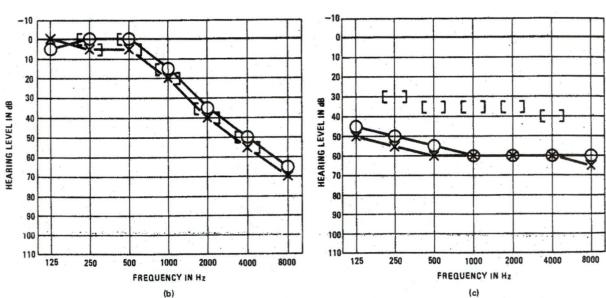

Figure 2. Example audiograms for conductive (2a), sensorineural (2b), and mixed (2c) types of hearing loss. Further description is provided in the text.

handicap (or disability) (ASHA, 1997; ASHA/CED, 1998). The communicative handicap associated with a given amount of hearing loss in dB may differ considerably across individuals.

The classification of hearing loss according to type is based on comparisons of thresholds for air and bone conduction test tones. *Conductive* hearing losses are almost always due to abnormalities of the outer or middle ear. In such disorders, an interruption or blockage of sound conduction to the cochlea accounts for the hearing loss. Wax in the ear canal or breaks in the ossicular chain (middle ear bones) are examples of conditions that restrict the flow of sound from the outer ear and middle ear to the cochlea and result in a conductive hearing loss. The primary audiometric sign of a conductive hearing loss is an *air–bone gap*. An air–bone gap is present when hearing sensitivity by bone conduction is significantly better than by air conduction. This can occur in cases of outer and middle ear disorders because the path of sound transmission for bone conduction is primarily through the bones of the skull directly to the inner ear, essentially bypassing the affected outer and middle ear structures. An audiogram for a conductive hearing loss is shown in Figure 2*A*. Note that although the air conduction thresholds are elevated by 50–60 dB, bone conduction thresholds are within normal limits (0 dB HL). The primary effect of a conductive disorder is to reduce the level of sound reaching the inner ear. The impairment is primarily a loss in hearing sensitivity, not in speech understanding. If the sound level can be increased, the person will be able to hear and understand speech.

Hearing loss resulting from damage or disease to any portion of the inner ear or neural auditory pathways is classified as *sensorineural*. Because the problem lies in the inner ear or neural pathways (or both), there will be an equal hearing loss for both air- and bone-conducted signals. An audiogram for a patient with a sensorineural hearing loss is shown as Figure 2*B*. Notice that the bone conduction thresholds are the same as the air conduction thresholds—there is no air–bone gap. In contrast to conductive hearing loss, sensorineural hearing loss typically involves both a loss in hearing sensitivity and a reduced ability to understand speech. Even when speech is made louder, the person will still have some difficulty in understanding.

A *mixed* hearing loss is a combination of both conductive and sensorineural losses. Figure 2*C* is an example audiogram for a mixed hearing loss in both ears. Note that air conduction thresholds are poorer than normal, averaging about 60 dB HL, and bone conduction thresholds are also poorer than normal, averaging 35 dB HL. There is an air–bone gap of approximately 25 dB, suggestive of some conductive hearing loss. In addition, there is a loss by bone conduction, indicating some abnormality of the inner ear and/or auditory nerve.

The case of a mixed hearing loss underscores the fact that both sensorineural and conductive disorders can exist simultaneously in the same patient. A person with a significant sensorineural hearing loss, for example, can still experience an ear infection or other pathology that may result in a conductive component in addition to the sensorineural loss. Finally, it should be understood that many patients with significant disorders or pathologies of the auditory system may have no significant hearing loss (in dB). Patients with disorders of the central auditory nervous system, for example, may demonstrate normal pure-tone thresholds. Normal hearing sensitivity does not always indicate a normal auditory system (Wiley, 1988).

—*Terry L. Wiley*

References

American Speech-Language-Hearing Association, Joint Committee of the American Speech-Language-Hearing Association (ASHA) and the Council on Education of the Deaf (CED). (1998). Hearing loss: Terminology and classification. Position statement and technical report. *ASHA*, *40*(Suppl. 18): 22–23.

American National Standards Institute. (1996). *American National Standard Specification for Audiometers (S3.6)*. New York: Author.

American National Standards Institute. (1999). *American National Standard Maximum Permissible Ambient Noise Levels for Audiometric Test Rooms (S3.1)*. New York: Author.

American Speech-Language-Hearing Association. (1978). Guidelines for manual pure tone threshold audiometry. *ASHA*, *20*, 297–301.

American Speech-Language-Hearing Association. (1990). Guidelines for audiometric symbols. *ASHA*, *32*(Suppl. 2), 25–30.

American Speech-Language-Hearing Association. (1997). *Guidelines for audiologic screening*. Rockville, MD: Author.

Dancer, J., and Ventry, I. M. (1976). Effects of stimulus presentation and instructions in pure-tone thresholds and false-alarm responses. *Journal of Speech and Hearing Disorders*, *41*, 315–324.

Davis, H. (1978). Hearing handicap, standards for hearing, and medicolegal rules. In H. Davis and S. R. Silverman (Eds.), *Hearing and deafness* (pp. 266–290). New York: Holt, Rinehart, and Winston.

Ward, W. D. (1964). Sensitivity versus acuity. *Journal of Speech and Hearing Research*, *7*, 294–295.

Wilber, L. A. (1999). Pure-tone audiometry: Air and bone conduction. In F. E. Musiek and W. F. Rintelmann (Eds.), *Contemporary perspectives in hearing assessment* (pp. 1–20). Needham Heights, MA: Allyn and Bacon.

Wiley, T. L. (1988). Audiologic evaluation. In D. Yoder and R. Kent (Eds.), *Decision making in speech-language pathology* (pp. 4–5). Toronto: B. C. Decker.

Yantis, P. A. (1994). Puretone air-conduction testing. In J. Katz (Ed.), *Handbook of clinical audiology* (4th ed., pp. 97–108). Baltimore: Williams and Wilkins.

Further Readings

Bess, F. H., and Humes, L. E. (1995). *Audiology: The fundamentals* (2nd ed.). Baltimore: Williams and Wilkins.

Carhart, R., and Jerger, J. F. (1959). Preferred method for clinical determination of pure-tone thresholds. *Journal of Speech and Hearing Disorders*, *24*, 330–345.

Carhart, R., and Porter, L. S. (1971). Audiometric configuration and prediction of threshold for spondees. *Journal of Speech and Hearing Research, 14,* 486–495.

Eagles, E. L. (1972). Selected findings from the Pittsburgh study. *Transactions of the American Academy of Ophthalmology and Otolaryngology, 76,* 343–348.

Harrell, R. W. (2002). Puretone evaluation. In J. Katz (Ed.), *Handbook of clinical audiology* (5th ed., pp. 71–87). Baltimore: Lippincott Williams and Wilkins.

Henderson, D., Salvi, R. J., Boettcher, F. A., and Clock, A. E. (1994). Neurophysiologic correlates of sensory-neural hearing loss. In J. Katz (Ed.), *Handbook of clinical audiology* (4th ed., pp. 37–55). Baltimore: Williams and Wilkins.

Joint Audiology Committee on Clinical Practice Algorithms and Statements. (2000). Audiology clinical practice algorithms and statements. *Audiology Today,* pp. 32–49. [Special issue]

Konkle, D. F. (1995, April). Classifying terms, degrees of hearing sensitivity. *Hearing Instruments,* 11.

Martin, F. N., and Clark, J. G. (2000). *Introduction to audiology* (7th ed., pp. 73–115). Needham Heights, MA: Allyn and Bacon.

Roeser, R. J., Buckley, K. A., and Stickney, G. S. (2000). Pure tone tests. In R. J. Roeser, M. Valente, and H. Hosford-Dunn (Eds.), *Audiology diagnosis* (pp. 227–251). New York: Thieme.

Salvi, R. J., Henderson, D., Hamernik, R., and Ahroon, W. A. (1983). Neural correlates of sensorineural hearing loss. *Ear and Hearing, 4,* 115–129.

Van Cleve, J. V. (Ed.). (1987). *Gallaudet encyclopedia of deaf people and deafness* (3 vols.). Blacklick, OH: McGraw-Hill.

Ward, W. D. (1983). The American Medical Association/American Academy of Otolaryngology formula for determination of hearing handicap. *Audiology, 22,* 313–324.

Wiley, T. L. (1980). Hearing disorders and audiometry. In T. J. Hixon, L. D. Shriberg, and J. S. Saxman (Eds.), *Introduction to communication disorders* (pp. 490–529). Englewood Cliffs, NJ: Prentice-Hall.

Yost, W. A. (2000). *Fundamentals of hearing* (4th ed.). New York: Academic Press.

Speech Perception Indices

The *articulation index*, or, as it is now known, the *speech intelligibility index*, was originally developed by early telephone engineer-scientists to describe and predict the quality of telephone circuits (Fletcher, 1921; Collard, 1930; French and Steinberg, 1947). Initially their motivation was to provide a method that would reduce the need for lengthy (and expensive) human articulation tests to evaluate the merit of telephone circuit modifications. However, by 1947, with the appearance of the watershed papers of French and Steinberg (1947) and Beranek (1947), it was evident that *articulation theory* had the potential for much greater significance and broader application than was implied by these early goals.

The term articulation index (AI) was coined at the Bell Telephone Laboratories and first appeared in company memos as early as 1926 (French, 1926). It replaced the term *quality index* that Harvey Fletcher (1921) had proposed earlier. The new term better reflected the relationship between the index and what were then called articulation tests. Articulation tests were speech tests in which listeners were asked to identify speech sounds spoken by a caller under conditions of interest to the experimenter. The exact makeup of the articulation tests varied, but they usually consisted of a carrier sentence with a nonsense syllable test item at the end. Several callers would in turn utter the sentences via the test circuit to crews of six to eight listeners. The listeners would record what they heard phonetically. The circuit articulation was equal to the average proportion of the sounds (or syllables) heard correctly by the listeners. The articulation index was devised as an alternative to this procedure.

The articulation index is an index that describes the proportion of the total importance-weighted speech signal that is audible to the listener under specified conditions. Normally, the index's value (ranging from 0 to 1) is derived from physical measurements, including principally the speech signal's intensity level, the level of any noise that may be present, and the characteristics of the transmission system that delivers the speech and noise to the listener's ear. Reverberation effects are sometimes included. Index values are often modified based on certain well-known performance characteristics of the human auditory system. Most commonly these would include pure-tone thresholds and cross-frequency band spread of masking. The negative effects of listening at high signal levels might also be included, as well as positive factors, such as the effect of the listener being able to see the talker's face. The articulation index value can be used directly as an indicator of the relative quality of a communications system, or it can be used to predict average speech recognition success for the particular types of speech or speech elements under specified listening conditions through the use of an appropriate *transfer function.*

The early history of development of the articulation index is difficult to follow with certainty because much of this work was done at the Bell Telephone Laboratories and was described only in internal company memos and reports. Most was not published in the scientific literature for 10–25 years after it was carried out. Some was never published. Fortunately, copies of many of the original documents from this early period recently became available on a compact disk through the efforts of C. M. Rankovic and J. B. Allen (Rankovic and Allen, 2000).

The first credible effort to evaluate the effectiveness of a communication system based on physical measurements was that of H. Fletcher (1921). In an unpublished Western Electric Laboratory report, Fletcher pointed out that a suitable measure (index) of circuit quality must have the property of additivity. By this he meant that if a particular frequency range of speech heard alone has a quality value of Q_1 and if a second frequency range has a value Q_2, then the value of both ranges heard at the same time should equal $Q_1 + Q_2$. It was clear that articulation test scores did not possess this property (i.e., $A_1 + A_2 \neq A_{12}$). Therefore, Fletcher proposed an intermediate variable, related to articulation, that would at least approximate this additivity property. He also proposed methods to derive the index's value for a circuit from measures of received speech intensity, frequency distortion, room and line noise, "asymmetric distortion," and other factors (Fletcher, 1921).

The term articulation index first appeared in the published literature in the landmark paper by Bell Telephone Laboratory scientists N. R. French and J. C. Steinberg in 1947. However, the term appears in internal Bell Labs documents as a replacement for quality index as early as 1926. The expression *quality theory*, however, continued in use for several more years before finally being replaced by *articulation theory*.

In a parallel development in England, John Collard, working for International Telephone and Telegraph, published a detailed description of an index with properties similar to those of the articulation index in a series of papers beginning in 1930. He called his index *band articulation* (or frequently just "the new unit"). Speech test scores were called *sound articulation*. By 1939 Collard had created a mechanical band articulation calculator (Pocock, 1939) that included many of the features of more recent articulation index methods. It is unclear whether the Bell Telephone Laboratory scientists were aware of Collard's work, but it is not cited in either their published or unpublished reports.

During World War II, Fletcher, then director of physical research at Bell Telephone and chairman of the National Defense Research Committee (NDRC), provided a description of at least some of the articulation index methods that had been developed at Bell Labs to Leo Beranek, then at Harvard University (Allen, 1996). Beranek was working on methods for improving communications for aircraft pilots as a part of the war effort under a contract from the NDRC. Allen (1996) reports that following the war, Beranek persuaded the Bell Labs group to finally publish a description of their work on the articulation index. The classic 1947 paper by N. R. French and J. C. Steinberg was the result. This paper was soon followed by Beranek's frequently cited paper on the articulation index (Beranek, 1947). These two papers together were to play highly influential roles in the future of the articulation index.

In 1950 Fletcher and his long-time Bell Labs associate Rogers Galt published a detailed description of their conception of the articulation index. Their goal in this paper was to cover a broader range of conditions than had ever been attempted before. "Telephony" was defined by the authors as referring to "any talker-listener combination" (p. 90). The results were seen as applicable to sound recording and reproduction systems, public address systems, and even hearing aids. In 1952, Fletcher further extended the applications to persons with hearing loss. Unfortunately, Fletcher and Galt's attempt to account for all aspects of the problem resulted in a conceptualization and method that was too complex for most people to understand, and it was seldom used. Recently, there has been a renewed interest in the

method (Rankovic, 1997, 1998). An available computer program implementing the procedure by H. Müsch (2001) now makes its practical use feasible.

The next major steps in the history of the articulation index were taken by Karl Kryter. In two landmark papers (Kryter, 1962a, 1962b), he described and validated a comprehensive method for calculating the articulation index under a broad range of conditions. This work was based directly on the publications of Beranek (1947) and French and Steinberg (1947). Kryter's methods became even more influential in 1969 when they were adopted, virtually intact, by the American National Standards Institute (ANSI) as the *American National Standard Methods for the Calculation of the Articulation Index* (ANSI S3.5-1969). For some 30 years this method quite literally defined the articulation index.

An important development taking place in Europe during this period was that of the speech transmission index by T. Houtgast and H. J. M. Steeneken (Houtgast and Steeneken, 1973; Steeneken and Houtgast, 1980). Similar in many ways to the articulation index of French and Steinberg (1947), the speech transmission index added a unique method for incorporating and combining the effects of noise and reverberation into the calculation through measurements of the modulation transfer function (MTF). At first called the weighted MTF, the speech transmission index has found relatively widespread use in the area of architectural acoustics in an abbreviated form known as the rapid speech transmission index, or RASTI.

In 1997 ANSI published the *American National Standard Method for Calculation of the Speech Intelligibility Index* (ANSI S3.5-1997). This renamed standard is the direct successor of articulation index standard ANSI S3.5-1969 and it is similar to the earlier standard in basic concept. However, there are many differences in detail. One of the more obvious is the change in the name of the index to speech intelligibility index. The new name finally severs the connection with the now obsolete term, articulation test, and also avoids confusion between its abbreviation, AI, and the newer but more general use of this abbreviation to mean artificial intelligence.

Of the procedural differences, one of the more fundamental ones concerns the *frequency importance function*. The frequency importance function describes the relative importance of different frequency regions along the frequency scale for speech intelligibility. ANSI S3.5-1997 provides a function for average speech, but it also provides different functions for particular types of speech. This change from the earlier standard implies that frequency importance is significantly dependent on the characteristics of the speech material and not only dependent on the characteristics of the auditory system. In addition, ANSI S3.5-1997 provides for calculations based on the auditory *critical band*, uses newer methods for calculating spread of masking, includes a speech level distortion factor, uses different speech spectra for raised, loud, and shouted speech, and provides for use of the modulation transfer function methods of Houtgast and Steeneken (1980). To ensure accuracy, a computer program implementing the S3.5-1997 method was made available. This program lacks a user-friendly interface but provides an invaluable test of other implementations of the method.

—Gerald A. Studebaker

References

Allen, J. B. (1996). Harvey Fletcher's role in the creation of communication acoustics. *Journal of the Acoustical Society of America, 99,* 1825–1839.

American National Standards Institute. (1969). *American National Standard methods for the calculation of the Articulation Index (ANSI S3.5-1969).* New York: Acoustical Society of America.

American National Standards Institute. (1997). *American National Standard methods for the calculation of the Speech Intelligibility Index (ANSI S3.5-1997).* New York: Acoustical Society of America.

Beranek, L. L. (1947). The design of speech communication systems. *Proceedings of the Institute of Radio Engineers, 35,* 880–890.

Collard, J. (1930). Calculation of the articulation of a telephone circuit from circuit constants. *Electrical Communication, 8,* 141–163.

Collard, J. (1933). A new unit of circuit performance. *Electrical Communication, 11,* 226–233.

Collard, J. (1934). The practical application of the new unit of circuit performance. *Electrical Communication, 12,* 270–275.

Fletcher, H. (1921). *Study of speech and telephone quality.* Unpublished laboratory report No. 21839, Western Electric Company, April 8, 1921. Reproduced on compact disk compiled by C. M. Rankovic and J. B. Allen, 2000, *Study of speech and hearing at Bell Telephone Laboratories: The Fletcher years.* New York: Acoustical Society of America.

Fletcher, H. (1952). The perception of speech sounds by deafened persons. *Journal of the Acoustical Society of America, 24,* 490–497.

Fletcher, H., and Galt, R. H. (1950). The perception of speech and its relation to telephony. *Journal of the Acoustical Society of America, 22,* 89–151.

French, N. R. (1926). Telephone quality. Unpublished memorandum, October 19, 1926. Reproduced on compact disk compiled by C. M. Rankovic and J. B. Allen, 2000, *Study of speech and hearing at Bell Telephone Laboratories: The Fletcher years.* New York: Acoustical Society of America.

French, N. R., and Steinberg, J. C. (1947). Factors governing the intelligibility of speech sounds. *Journal of the Acoustical Society of America, 19,* 90–119.

Houtgast, T., and Steeneken, H. J. M. (1973). The modulation transfer function in room acoustics as a predictor of speech intelligibility. *Acustica, 28,* 66–73.

Kryter, K. (1962a). Methods for the calculation and use of the articulation index. *Journal of the Acoustical Society of America, 34,* 1689–1697.

Kryter, K. D. (1962b). Validation of the articulation index. *Journal of the Acoustical Society of America, 34,* 1698–1702.

Müsch, H. (2001). Review and computer implementation of Fletcher and Galt's method of calculating the articulation index. *Acoustics Research Letters Online, 2,* 25–30.

Pocock, L. C. (1939). The calculation of articulation for effective rating of telephone circuits. *Electrical Communication, 18,* 120–132.

Rankovic, C. M., and Allen, J. B. (2000). *Study of speech and hearing at Bell Telephone Laboratories: The Fletcher years.* Compact disk. New York: Acoustical Society of America.

Steeneken, H. J. M., and Houtgast, T. (1980). A physical method for measuring speech-transmission quality. *Journal of the Acoustical Society of America, 67,* 318–326.

Further Readings

Ching, T. Y. C., Dillon, H., and Byrne, D. (1998). Speech recognition of hearing-impaired listeners: Predictions from audibility and the limited role of high-frequency amplification. *Journal of the Acoustical Society of America, 103,* 1128–1140.

Ching, T. Y., Dillon, H., Katsch, R., and Byrne, D. (2001). Maximizing effective audibility in hearing aid fitting. *Ear and Hearing, 22,* 212–224.

Dubno, J. R., Dirks, D. D., and Schaefer, A. B. (1989). Stop-consonant recognition for normal-hearing listeners and listeners with high-frequency hearing loss: II. Articulation index predictions. *Journal of the Acoustical Society of America, 85,* 355–364.

Duggirala, V., Studebaker, G. A., Pavlovic, C. V., and Sherbecoe, R. L. (1988). Frequency importance functions for a feature recognition test. *Journal of the Acoustical Society of America, 83,* 2372–2382.

Humes, L. E., Dirks, D. D., Bell, T. S., Ahlstrom, C., and Kincaid, G. (1986). Application of the articulation index and the speech transmission index to the recognition of speech by normal-hearing and hearing-impaired listeners. *Journal of Speech and Hearing Research, 29,* 447–462.

Kamm, C. A., Dirks, D. D., and Bell, T. S. (1985). Speech recognition and the articulation index for normal and hearing-impaired listeners. *Journal of the Acoustical Society of America, 77,* 281–288.

Müsch, H., and Buus, S. (2001). Using statistical decision theory to predict speech intelligibility: I. Model structure. *Journal of the Acoustical Society of America, 109,* 2896–2909.

Pavlovic, C. V. (1987). Derivation of primary parameters and procedures for use in speech intelligibility predictions. *Journal of the Acoustical Society of America, 82,* 413–422.

Pavlovic, C. V. (1993). Problems in the prediction of speech recognition performance of normal-hearing and hearing-impaired individuals. In G. A. Studebaker and I. Hochberg (Eds.), *Acoustical factors affecting hearing aid performance* (pp. 221–234). Needham Heights, MA: Allyn and Bacon.

Pavlovic, C. V., and Studebaker, G. A. (1984). An evaluation of some assumptions underlying the articulation index. *Journal of the Acoustical Society of America, 75,* 1606–1612.

Pavlovic, C. V., Studebaker, G. A., and Sherbecoe, R. L. (1986). An articulation index based procedure for predicting the speech recognition performance of hearing-impaired individuals. *Journal of the Acoustical Society of America, 80,* 50–57.

Rankovic, C. M. (1997). Prediction of speech reception for listeners with sensorineural hearing loss. In W. Jesteadt (Ed.), *Modeling sensorineural hearing loss.* Mahwah, NJ: Erlbaum.

Rankovic, C. M. (1998). Factors governing speech reception benefits of adaptive liner filtering for listeners with sensorineural hearing loss. *Journal of the Acoustical Society of America, 103,* 1043–1057.

Schroeder, M. (1981). Modulation transfer function: Definition and measurement. *Acustica, 49,* 179–182.

Studebaker, G. A., Gray, G. A., and Branch, W. E. (1999). Prediction and statistical evaluation of speech recognition test scores. *Journal of the American Academy of Audiology, 10,* 355–370.

Studebaker, G. A., and Sherbecoe, R. L. (1993). Frequency importance functions for speech recognition. In G. A. Studebaker and I. Hochberg (Eds.), *Acoustical factors affecting hearing aid performance.* Needham Heights, MA: Allyn and Bacon.

Studebaker, G. A., Sherbecoe, R. L., and Gilmore, C. (1993). Frequency-importance and transfer functions for the Auditec of St. Louis recordings of the NU-6 word test. *Journal of Speech and Hearing Research, 36,* 799–807.

Zwicker, E. (1961). Subdivision of the audible frequency range into critical bands (*Frequenzgruppen*). *Journal of the Acoustical Society of America, 33,* 248.

Speech Tracking

Speech Tracking (sometimes called Connected or Continuous Discourse Tracking) is a procedure developed by De Filippo and Scott "for training and evaluating the reception of ongoing speech" (De Filippo and Scott, 1978, p. 1186). In the Speech Tracking procedure, a talker (usually a therapist or experimenter) reads from a prepared text, phrase by phrase, for a predetermined time period, usually five or ten minutes. The task of the receiver (the person with hearing loss) is to repeat *exactly* what the talker said. If the receiver does not give a verbatim response, the talker applies a strategy to overcome the breakdown. This can take the form of simple repetition, the use of clue words, or a paraphrase of the original segment. The therapist goes on to the next phrase only when the receiver is able to repeat correctly every word of the original segment.

At the end of the time period, the number of words repeated correctly is counted and divided by the time elapsed to derive the receiver's Tracking Rate, expressed in words per minute (wpm). For example, if a receiver was able to repeat 150 words in five minutes, his Tracking Rate would be 30 wpm. The Tracking Rate represents the time taken for the text to be presented and repeated. Estimates of Tracking Rate for people with normal hearing vary, but it is generally recognized that a rate of around 100 wpm (De Filippo, 1988) is obtained if the same presentation and response rules are followed.

Since its introduction, Speech Tracking has also been used extensively in investigations evaluating the effectiveness of sensory aids for people with hearing loss. These have included studies of cochlear implants (Robbins et al., 1985; Levitt et al., 1986), tactile aids (Brooks et al., 1986; Cowan et al., 1991; Plant, 1998), and direct contact tactile approaches such as Tadoma (Reed et al., 1992) and Tactiling (Plant and Spens, 1986). These studies usually compare a receiver's Tracking Rate in two or more presentation conditions such as aided and unaided lip reading. For example, Plant (1998) looked at a subject's Speech Tracking performance with materials presented via lip reading alone and lip reading supplemented by the Tactaid 7 vibrotactile aid. After about 30 hours of testing and training with Speech Tracking, the subject's mean Tracking Rates in the two presentation conditions were 33.7 wpm for lip reading alone and 46.1 wpm for lip reading supplemented by the Tactaid 7.

Despite the widespread acceptance of Speech Tracking in research projects, its use as an evaluative tool has been severely criticized by Tye-Murray and Tyler (1988). These researchers cited a number of extraneous variables that they believed were extremely difficult to control. These included the characteristics of the speaker (segment selection, ability to use cues to overcome blockages, speaking style, articulatory patterns, etc.), the receiver (degree of assertiveness, language proficiency, motivation, etc.), and the text (degree of syntactic complexity, vocabulary, etc.). Hochberg, Rosen, and Ball (1989), for example, found that text complexity could greatly influence Tracking Rate. In a study using the same talker/receiver pairs, they found that Tracking Rates varied from 62.9 wpm for "easy" materials (controlled vocabulary readers designed for English-as-a-second-language learners) to 29.5 wpm for "difficult" materials (popular adult fiction).

Tye-Murray and Tyler (1998) believed that these factors made Speech Tracking unsuitable for across-subject test designs. They did, however, feel that with some modifications the procedure could be used for within-subject test designs. These recommendations included an insistence on a verbatim response, the use of only one speaker, training of the speaker/receiver pairs, the use of appropriate texts, and limiting the repair strategies used to repetition and writing down a blocked word after three repeats.

A number of groups (for example, Boothroyd, 1987; Pichora-Fuller and Benguerel, 1991; Dempsey et al., 1992) have attempted to make the technique more suitable for evaluative purposes through the use of computer-controlled recorded materials. These approaches ensure that the problems created by sender differences are controlled and minimized. Although promising, none of these systems have become widely accepted and used.

The KTH Speech Tracking Procedure (Gnosspelius and Spens, 1992; Spens, 1992) represented another attempt to more closely control the approach. This computer-controlled modification used live-voice presentations, but the segment length was predetermined and only one repair strategy—repetition—was allowed. The written form of any word repeated three times was automatically presented to the receiver via an LED display. At the end of a Speech Tracking session the program automatically calculated a number of measures including Tracking Rate, Ceiling Rate (time taken when all words in a segment were correctly repeated after only one presentation), and the Proportion of Blocked Words (the total number of words that had to be repeated divided by the total number of words in the session). This approach has been used in a number of studies (for example, Plant, 1998; Ronnberg et al., 1998) but has not gained widespread acceptance.

Speech Tracking has also been widely used as a training technique for use with adults (Plant, 1996) and children (Tye-Murray, 1998) with profound hearing loss. When used for training, modifications can be made to provide receivers with practice in the use of repair strategies. Owens and Raggio (1987), for example, provided receivers with a list of directives they could use when they did not correctly repeat a segment. The receiver could ask the sender to:

1. Say that again.
2. Say it another way.
3. Spell that word.
4. Write that word.
5. Spell an important word.
6. Write an important word.

Lunato and Weisenberger (1994) looked at the comparative effectiveness of four repair strategies in Speech Tracking. The repair strategies used were:

1. Verbatim repetition of a word or phrase.
2. The use of antonyms or synonyms as clues to the identity of blocked words.
3. Providing the receiver with phoneme-by-phoneme correction of blocked words.
4. Providing context by moving forward or backward in the text.

These researchers reported that strategy 1 yielded the highest Tracking Rates and strategy 2 the lowest.

When Speech Tracking is being used for training, compromises can also be made in the receiver's response patterns. Owens and Raggio (1987), for example, argued for the use of nonverbatim responses in training sessions using Speech Tracking. While acknowledging the importance of a verbatim response for test purposes, they felt that in training it may be better to provide the receiver with practice in picking up the gist of the message rather than expecting absolute identification at all times.

Although Speech Tracking has become a widely used training procedure, there are some people with hearing loss for whom it is unsuitable. These include people with very poor speech reception skills, resulting in Tracking Rates of less than 20 wpm. At these levels receivers find the task extremely difficult and stressful. Others for whom the technique may be unsuitable include people with poor speech production skills. In such cases the sender may be unable to determine reliably whether the receiver gave the correct response. This necessitates the use of a written or a signed response, which serves to greatly reduce the Tracking Rate.

Plant (1996, 1989) developed a modified version of Speech Tracking designed to be used with such cases. Simple stories are divided into parts, each consisting of 200 words. Each part is in turn divided into short segments ranging in length from 4 to 12 words. The segments are presented for identification, and the receiver is asked to repeat as many words as he or she can. The receiver can use repair strategies to obtain additional information if he or she experiences difficulties. The receiver is then scored for the number of words correctly identified and shown the written form of the segment. At the end of each part, the percentage of correct responses is calculated, based on the number of words correctly identified. This approach provides the receiver with immediate feedback on the correctness of her or his response and ensures that she or he is able to benefit from ongoing contextual information.

Speech Tracking is an innovative technique that can be used for both testing and training the speech perception skills of people with hearing loss. When used for testing, however, a precise protocol must be followed to minimize the effects of sender, receiver, and text variables. In training a less rigid approach can be used, and the approach may be modified to include practice in the use of repair strategies.

—*Geoff Plant*

References

Boothroyd, A. (1987). CASPER. Computer assisted speech perception evaluation and training. In *Proceedings of the 10th Annual Conference of the Rehabilitation Society of America* (pp. 734–736). Washington, DC: Association for the Advancement of Rehabilitation Technology.

Brooks, P. L., Frost, B. J., Mason, J. L., and Gibson, D. M. (1986). Continuing evaluation of the Queen's University Tactile Vocoder. II: Identification of open set sentences and tracking narrative. *Journal of Rehabilitation Research and Development, 23,* 129–138.

Cowan, R. S. C., Blamey, P. J., Sarant, J. Z., Galvin, K. L., Alcantara, J. I., Whitford, L. A., and Clark, G. M. (1991). Role of a multichannel electrotactile speech processor in a cochlear implant program for profoundly hearing impaired adults. *Journal of the Acoustical Society of America, 12,* 39–46.

De Filippo, C. L. (1988). Tracking for speechreading training. *Volta Review, 90,* 215–239.

De Filippo, C. L., and Scott, B. L. (1978). A method for training the reception of ongoing speech. *Journal of the Acoustical Society of America, 63,* 1186–1192.

Dempsey, J. J., Levitt, H., Josephson, J., and Porazzo, J. (1992). Computer-assisted tracking simulation (CATS). *Journal of the Acoustical Society of America, 92,* 701–710.

Gnosspelius, J., and Spens, K.-E. (1992). A computer-based speech tracking procedure. *STL-QPSR* (No. 1), 131–137.

Hochberg, I., Rosen, S., and Ball, V. (1989). Effects of text complexity on connected discourse tracking rate. *Ear and Hearing, 10,* 192–199.

Levitt, H., Waltzman, S. B., Shapiro, W. H., and Cohen, N. L. (1986). Evaluation of a cochlear prosthesis using connected discourse tracking. *Journal of Rehabilitation Research and Development, 23,* 147–154.

Lunatto, K. E., and Weisenberger, J. M. (1994). Comparative effectiveness of correction strategies in connected discourse tracking. *Ear and Hearing, 15,* 362–370.

Owens, E., and Raggio, M. (1987). The UCSF tracking procedure for evaluation and training of speech reception by hearing-impaired adults. *Journal of Speech and Hearing Disorders, 52,* 120–128.

Pichora-Fuller, M. K., and Benguerel, A. P. (1991). The design of CAST (computer-aided speechreading training). *Journal of Speech and Hearing Research, 34,* 202–212.

Plant, G. (1989). *Commtrac: Modified Connected Discourse Tracking Exercises for Hearing Impaired Adults.* Chatswood, NSW, Australia: National Acoustic Laboratories.

Plant, G. (1996). *Commtrac: Modified Speech Tracking Exercises for Hearing-Impaired Adults.* Somerville, MA: Hearing Rehabilitation Foundation.

Plant, G. (1998). Training in the use of a tactile supplement to lipreading: A long-term case study. *Ear and Hearing, 19,* 394–406.

Plant, G., and Spens, K.-E. (1986). An experienced user of tactile information as a supplement to lipreading. An evaluative study. *STL-QPSR* (No. 1), 87–110.

Reed, C. M., Durlach, N. I., and Delhorne, L. A. (1992). Natural methods of tactile communication. In I. Summers (Ed.), *Tactile aids for the hearing impaired* (pp. 219–230). London: Whurr.

Robbins, A. M., Osberger, M. J., Miyamoto, R. T., Kienle, M. J., and Myres, W. (1985). Speech tracking performance in single channel cochlear implant subjects. *Journal of Speech and Hearing Research, 28,* 565–578.

Ronnberg, J., Andersson, U., Lyxell, B., and Spens, K.-E. (1998). Vibrotactile speech tracking support: Cognitive prerequisites. *Journal of Deaf Studies and Deaf Education, 3,* 143–156.

Spens, K.-E. (1992). Numerical aspects of the speech tracking procedure. *STL-QPSR* (No. 1), 115–130.

Tye-Murray, N. (1998). *Foundations of aural rehabilitation: Children, adults, and their family members.* San Diego: Singular Publishing Group.

Tye-Murray, N., and Tyler, R. S. (1988). A critique of continuous discourse tracking as a test procedure. *Journal of Speech and Hearing Disorders, 53,* 226–231.

Speechreading Training and Visual Tracking

Speechreading (lipreading, visual speech perception), a form of information processing, is defined by Boothroyd (1988) as a "process of perceiving spoken language using vision as the sole source of sensory evidence" (p. 77). Speechreading, a natural process in everyday communication, is especially helpful when communicating in noisy and reverberant conditions because facial motion in speech production may augment or replace degraded auditory information (Erber, 1969). Also, visual cues have been shown to influence speech perception in infants with normal hearing (Kuhl and Meltzoff, 1982), and speech perception phenomena, such as the McGurk effect (MacDonald and McGurk, 1978), demonstrate the influence of vision on auditory speech perception.

To understand language, the speechreader directs attention to, extracts, and uses linguistically relevant information from a talker's face movements, facial expressions, and body gestures. This information, which may vary within and across talkers (for a review, see Kricos, 1996), is integrated with other available sensory cues, such as auditory cues, as well as knowledge about speech production and language in general to make sense of the visual information. However, the visual information may be ambiguous because many sounds look alike on the lips, are hidden in the mouth, or are co-articulated during speech production. In addition, expectations about linguistic context may influence understanding. Nevertheless some individuals are expert speechreaders, scoring more than 80% correct on words in unrelated sentences, and demonstrate enhanced visual phonetic perception (Bernstein, Demorest, and Tucker, 2000). Attempts to relate speechreading proficiency to other sensory, perceptual, and cognitive function, including neurophysiological responsiveness, have met with limited success (for a review, see Summerfield, 1992).

From a historical perspective, speechreading was initially developed in Europe as a method to teach speech production to young children with hearing loss. Until the 1890s it was limited to children and was characterized by a vision-only (unisensory) approach. Speechreading training was based on analytic methods, which encouraged perceivers to analyze mouth position to recognize sounds, words, and sentences, or synthetic methods, which encouraged perceivers to grasp a speaker's whole meaning (Gestalt). O'Neill and Oyer (1961) reviewed several early distinctive methods that were adopted in America: Bruhn's method (characterized by syllable drill and close observation of lip movements), Nitchie's method (which shifted from an analytical to a synthetic method), Kinzie's method (Bruhn's classification of sounds plus Nitchie's basic psychological ideas), the Jena method (kinesthetic and visual cues), and film techniques (Mason's visual hearing, Markovin and Moore's contextual systemic approach). Gagné (1994) reviewed present-day approaches: multimodal speech perception (integration of available auditory cues with those from vision and other modalities), computer-based activities (interactive learning using full-motion video), and conversational contexts (question-answer approach, effective communication strategies, and training for talkers with normal hearing to improve communication behavior).

When indicated, speechreading training is included in comprehensive programs of aural rehabilitation. At best, the post-treatment gains from speechreading training are modest, in the range of approximately 15%. Unfortunately, data on improvements related to visual speech perception training are limited, and little is known about the efficacy of various approaches. However, some individuals demonstrate significant gains. Walden et al. (1977) have reported an increase in the number of visually distinctive groups of phonemes (visemes) with which consonants are recognized following practice. The identification responses following practice suggest that the distinctiveness of visual phonetic cues related to place-of-articulation information is increased. Although it is not clear what factors account for such improvements in performance, these results provide evidence for instances of learning in which perception is modified. Other studies show that the results are variable, both in performance on speechreading tasks and in gains related to learning programs. Improvements observed by Massaro, Cohen, and Gesi (1993) suggest that repeated testing experience may be as beneficial as structured training. Initial changes may be due to nonsensory factors such as increased familiarity with the task or improved viewing strategies. In contrast, Bernstein et al. (1991) suggest that speechreaders learn the visual phonetic characteristics of specific talkers after long periods of practice. Treatment efficacy studies may be enhanced by enrolling a larger number of participants, specifying training methods, using separate materials for training versus testing, evaluating asymptotic performance and long-term effects, determining whether the effects of the intervention are generalized to nontherapy situations, and designing studies to control for factors such as the motivation or test-taking behaviors of participants, as well as personal attention directed toward participants (for a review, see Gagné, 1994; Walden and Grant, 1993).

Current research has also focused on visual speech perception performance in psychophysical experiments. One research theme has centered on determining what regions of the face contain critical motion that is used in visual speech perception. Subjective comments from expert lipreaders suggest that movement in the cheek areas may aid lipreading. Data from Lansing and McConkie (1994) illustrate that eye gaze may shift from the mouth to the cheeks, chin, or jaw during lipreading. Results from Greenberg and Bode (1968) support the usefulness of the entire face for consonant recognition. In contrast, results from Ijsseldijk (1992) and Marassa and Lansing (1995) indicate that information from the lips and mouth region alone is sufficient for word recognition. Massaro (1998) reports that some individuals can discriminate among a small set of test syllables without directly gazing at the mouth of the talker, and Preminger et al. (1998) demonstrate that 70% of visemes in /a/ and /aw/ vowel contexts can be recognized when the mouth is masked. These diverse research findings underscore the presence of useful observable visual cues for spoken language at the mouth and in other face regions.

Eye-monitoring technology may be useful in understanding the role of visual processes in speechreading (Lansing and McConkie, 1994). It provides information about on-line processing of visual information and the tendency for perceivers to direct their eyes to the regions of interest on a talker's face. By moving the eyes, a perceiver may take advantage of the densely packed, highly specialized cone receptor cells in the fovea to inspect visual detail (Hallet, 1986). Eye monitoring has been used to study a variety of cognitive tasks, such as reading, picture perception, and face recognition, and to study human-computer interaction (for a review, see Rayner, 1984). The basic data obtained from eye monitoring reveals sequences of periods associated with perception in which the eye is relatively stable (fixations) and high-velocity jumps in eye position (saccades) during which perception is inhibited. Distributions of saccadic information ("where" decisions) are quantified in terms of length and direction, and distributions of fixations ("when" decisions) are quantified in terms of duration and location. Experiments are designed to evaluate the variance associated with cognitive processes. For exam-

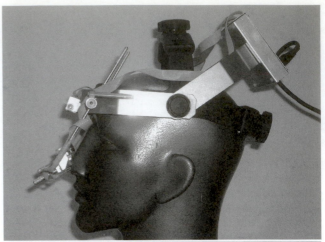
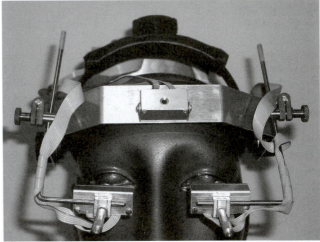

Figure 1. The photograph at the top shows a profile of the head mounted hardware of the prototype S&R (Stampe and Reingold) Eyelink system. The lightweight headband holds two custom-built ultra-miniature high-speed cameras mounted on adjustable rods to provide binocular eye monitoring with high spatial resolution (0.01 degrees) and fast sampling rates (250 Hz). Each camera uses two infrared light–emitting diodes (IR LEDs) to illuminate the eye to determine pupil position. The power supply is worn at the back of the head and coupled to a specialized image-processing card housed in a computer that runs the eye-tracking software. The photograph at the bottom shows the third camera on the headband that tracks the relative location for banks of IR LEDs affixed to each corner of the computer monitor which displays full-motion video or text. The relative location of the LEDs changes in relation to head movement and distance from the display and is used to compensate for head motion to determine x, y eye-fixation locations. An Ethernet link connects the experimental display computer to the eye-tracking computer with support for real-time data transfer and control.

Figure 2. The graph at the top shows the sequence and location of x, y eye fixations for a perceiver who is speechreading the sentence, "You can catch the bus across the street." The size of the markers is scaled in relative units to illustrate differences in total fixation times directed at each x, y location. The asterisk-shaped markers enclosed in a circle are used to show x, y fixation locations during observable face motion associated with speech, and the square-shaped markers show locations prior to and following speech motion. The rectangles are used to illustrate the regions of the talker's face, ordered from top to bottom, left to right: eye, left cheek, nose, mouth, right cheek, chin. Region boundaries accommodate dynamic face movements for the production of the entire sentence. The graph at the bottom half shows the corresponding data record and includes speechreading followed by the reading of text. The y-axis of the graph is scaled in units corresponding to the measurement identified by the number that has been superimposed: $1 = x$ (pixel) location of horizontal eye movements; $2 = y$ (pixel) location of vertical eye movements; $3 =$ pupil size/10; $4 =$ eye movement velocity. The darker vertical bars show periods in which no eye data are available due to eye blinks, and the light gray vertical bars illustrate saccades that are defined by high-velocity eye movements. Eye fixations are identified by the lines 1 and 2 and separated from one another by a vertical bar.

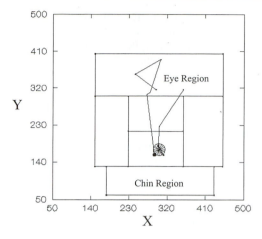

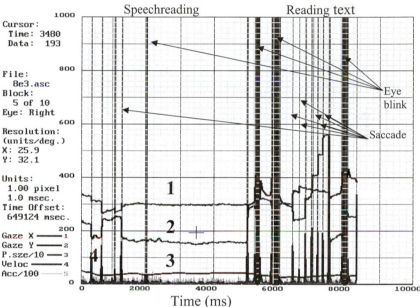

ple, distributions of fixation duration and of saccade length differ across cognitive tasks such as reading versus picture perception. Various types of instrumentation are available for eye-monitoring research, some of which include direct physical contact with the eyes to camera-based video systems that determine eye rotation characteristics based on changes in the location of landmarks such as the center of the pupil or corneal reflections, free of error induced by translation related to head movement (for a review, see Young and Sheena, 1975). Factors such as cost, accuracy, ease of calibration, response mode, and demands of the participants and experimental task must be considered in selecting an appropriate eye-monitoring system. An example of a system used in speechreading research is shown in Figure 1. The system is used to record the eye movements of the perceiver and to obtain a detailed record of the sequence and duration of fixations. A scan plot and sample record of eye movements are shown in Figure 2. Simultaneously, measurements are made of the accuracy of perception, efficiency of processing, or judgment of stimulus diffi-

culty. For interpretation, the eye movement records are linked to the spatial and temporal characteristics of face motion for each video frame or speech event (e.g., lips opening).

Results from eye-monitoring studies demonstrate that speechreaders make successive eye gazes (fixations) to inspect the talker's face or to track facial motion. The talker's eyes attract attention prior to and following speech production (Lansing and McConkie, 2003), and in the presence of auditory cues (Vatikiotis-Bateson, Eiigisti, and Munhall, 1998). If auditory cues are not available, perceivers with at least average proficiency attend to the talker's mouth region for accurate sentence perception (Lansing and McConkie, 2003). However, some gazes are observed toward the regions adjacent to the lips as well as toward the eyes of the talker. Similarly for word understanding, speechreaders direct eye gaze most often and for longer periods of time toward the talker's mouth than toward any other region of the face. Motion in regions other than the mouth may increase signal redundancy from that at the mouth and afford a natural context for observing detailed mouth motion. Task characteristics also influence where people look for information on the face of the talker (Lansing and McConkie, 1999). Eye gaze is directed toward secondary facial cues, located in the upper part of the face, with greater frequency for the recognition of intonation information than for phonemic or stress recognition. Phonemic and word stress information can be recognized from cues located in the middle and lower parts of the face.

Finally, new findings from brain imaging studies may provide valuable insights into the neural underpinnings of basic processes in the visual perception of spoken language (Calvert et al., 1997) and individual differences in speechreading proficiency (Ludman et al., 2000). Although preliminary results have not yet identified speechreading-specific regions, measures in perceivers with normal hearing indicate bilateral activation of the auditory cortex for silent speechreading (Calvert et al., 1997). Results from measures in perceivers with congenital onset of profound bilateral deafness (who rely on speechreading for understanding spoken language) do not indicate strong left temporal activation (MacSweeny et al., 2002). Functional magnetic resonance imaging may prove to be a useful tool to test hypotheses about task differences and the activation of primary sensory processing areas, the role of auditory experience and plasticity, and neural mechanisms and sites of cross-modal integration in the understanding of spoken language.

Continued study and research in the basic processes of speechreading are needed to determine research-based approaches to intervention, the relative advantages of different approaches, and how specific approaches relate to individual needs. Additional insight into the basic processes of visual speech perception is needed to develop and test a model of spoken word recognition that incorporates visual information, to optimize sensory-prosthetic aids, and to enhance the design of human-computer interfaces.

—*Charissa R. Lansing*

References

Bernstein, L. E., Demorest, M. E., Coulter, D. C., and O'Connell, M. P. (1991). Lipreading sentences with vibrotactile vocoders: Performance of normal-hearing and hearing-impaired subjects. *Journal of the Acoustical Society of America*, 90, 2971–2984.

Bernstein, L. E., Demorest, M. E., and Tucker, P. E. (2000). Speech perception without hearing. *Perception and Psychophysics*, 62, 233–252.

Boothroyd, A. (1988). Linguistic factors in speechreading. In C. L. De Filippo and D. G. Sims (Eds.), *New reflections in speechreading. Volta Review*, 90(5), 77–87.

Calvert, G. A., Bullmore, E. T., Brammer, M. J., Campbell, R., Williams, S. C. R., McGuire, P. K., et al. (1997). Activation of auditory cortex during silent lipreading. *Science*, 276, 593–596.

Erber, N. P. (1969). Interaction of audition and vision in the recognition of oral speech stimuli. *Journal of Speech and Hearing Research*, 12, 423–425.

Gagné, J.-P. (1994). Visual and audiovisual speech perception training: Basic and applied research needs. *Journal of the Academy of Rehabilitative Audiology*, 27, 133–159.

Greenberg, H. J., and Bode, D. L. (1968). Visual discrimination of consonants. *Journal of Speech and Hearing Research*, 11, 466–471.

Hallet, P. E. (1986). Eye movements. In K. B. Boff, L. Kaufman, and J. P. Thomas (Eds.), *Handbook of perception and human performance: Sensory processes and perception* (pp. 10-1–10-102). New York: Wiley.

Ijsseldijk, F. J. (1992). Speechreading performance under different conditions of video image, repetition, and speech rate. *Journal of Speech and Hearing Research*, 35, 466–477.

Kricos, P. (1996). Difference in visual intelligibility across talkers. In D. G. Storke and M. E. Hennecke (Eds.), *Speechreading by humans and machines: Models, systems, and applications* (NATO ASI Series, Vol. 150, Series F: Computer and systems sciences, pp. 43–53). Berlin: Springer-Verlag.

Kuhl, P. K., and Meltzoff, A. N. (1982). The bimodal perception of speech in infancy. *Science*, 218, 1138–1141.

Lansing, C. R., and McConkie, G. W. (1994). A new method for speechreading research: Eyetracking observers' eye movements. *Journal of the Academy of Rehabilitative Audiology*, 27, 25–43.

Lansing, C. R., and McConkie, G. W. (1999). Attention to facial regions in segmental and prosodic visual speech perception tasks. *Journal of Speech, Language, and Hearing Research*, 42, 526–539.

Lansing, C. R., and McConkie, G. W. (2003). Word identification and eye fixation locations in visual and visual-plus-auditory presentations of spoken sentences. *Perception and Psychophysics*, 65, 536–552.

Ludman, C. N., Summerfield, A. Q., Hall, D., Elliott, M., Foster, J., Hykin, J. L., et al. (2000). Lip-reading ability and patterns of cortical activation studied using fMRI. *British Society of Audiology*, 34, 225–230.

MacDonald, J. W., and McGurk, H. (1978). Visual influences on speech perception processes. *Perception and Psychophysics*, 24, 253–257.

MacSweeney, M., Calvert, G. A., Campbell, R., McGuire, P. K., David, A. S., Williams, S. C. R., et al. (2002). Speechreading circuits in people born deaf. *Neuropsychologia*, 40, 801–807.

Marassa, L. K., and Lansing, C. R. (1995). Visual word recognition in two facial motion conditions: Full-face versus lips-plus-mandible. *Journal of Speech and Hearing Research*, 38, 1387–1394.

Masarro, D. W. (1998). *Perceiving talking faces: From speech perception to a behavioral principle* (pp. 415–443). Cambridge, MA: MIT Press.

Massaro, D., Cohen, M., and Gesi, A. (1993). Long-term training, transfer and retention in learning to lipread. *Perception and Psychophysics*, 53, 549–562.

O'Neill, J. J., and Oyer, H. J. (1961). *Visual communication for the hard of hearing*. Englewood Cliffs, NJ: Prentice Hall.

Preminger, J. E., Lin, H.-B., Payen, M., and Levitt, H. (1998). Selective masking in speechreading. *Journal of Speech, Language, and Hearing Research*, 41, 564–575.

Rayner, K. (1984). Visual selection in reading, picture perception, and visual search: A tutorial review. In H. Bouma and D. G. Bouwhuis (Eds.), *Attention and performance: X. Control of language processes* (pp. 67–96). London: Erlbaum.

Summerfield, Q. (1992). Lipreading and audio-visual speech perception. *Philosophical Transactions of the Royal Society of London, 335,* 71–78.

Vatikiotis-Bateson, E., Eigsti, I.-M., Yano, S., and Munhall, K. (1998). Eye movements of perceivers during audiovisual speech perception. *Perception and Psychophysics, 60,* 926–940.

Walden, B., and Grant, D. (1993). Research needs in rehabilitative audiology. In J. G. Alpiner and P. A. McCarthy (Eds.), *Rehabilitative audiology: Children and adults* (pp. 500–528). Baltimore: Williams and Wilkins.

Walden, B., Prosek, R., Montgomery, A., Scherr, C., and Jones, C. (1977). Effects of training on the visual recognition of consonants. *Journal of Speech and Hearing Research, 20,* 130–145.

Young, L. R., and Sheena, D. (1975). Survey of eye movement recording methods. *Behavioral Research Methods and Instrumentation, 7,* 394–429.

Further Readings

Bernstein, L. E., Auer, E. T., Jr., and Tucker, P. E. (2001). Enhanced speechreading in deaf adults: Can short-term training/practice close the gap for hearing adults? *Journal of Speech, Language, and Hearing Research, 44,* 5–18.

Bernstein, L. E., Demorest, M. E., and Tucker, P. E. (1998). What makes a good speechreader? First you have to find one. In R. Campbell, B. Dodd, and D. Burnham (Eds.), *Hearing by eye: II. Advances in the psychology of speechreading and audiovisual speech* (pp. 221–227). London: Erlbaum.

Bernstein, L. E., Eberhardt, S. P., and Demorest, M. E. (1989). Single-channel vibrotactile supplements to visual perception of intonation and stress. *Journal of the Acoustical Society of America, 85,* 397–405.

Binnie, C. A., Jackson, P. L., and Montgomery, A. A. (1976). Visual intelligibility of consonants: A lipreading screening test with implications for aural rehabilitation. *Journal of Speech and Hearing Disorders, 41,* 530–539.

Binnie, C. A., Montgomery, A., and Jackson, P. (1974). Auditory and visual contributions to the perception of consonants. *Journal of Speech and Hearing Research, 17,* 619–630.

Calvert, G. A., Campbell, R., and Brammer, M. J. (2000). Evidence from functional magnetic resonance imaging of crossmodal binding in the human heteromodal cortex. *Current Biology, 10,* 649–657.

Cherry, R., and Small, S. (1993). Effect of interactive video versus non-interactive video training on speech recognition by hearing-impaired adults. *Volta Review, 95,* 135–137.

De Filippo, C., and Sims, D. (Eds.). (1988). *New reflections on speechreading. Volta Review, 90*(5), 1–313.

Demorest, M. E., Bernstein, L. E., and Dehaven, G. P. (1996). Generalizability of speechreading performance on nonsense syllables, words and sentences: Subjects with normal hearing. *Journal of Speech and Hearing Research, 39,* 697–713.

Erber, N. P. (1988). *Communication therapy for hearing-impaired adults.* Abbotsford, Victoria, Australia: Clavis Publishing.

Gagné, J.-P., Dinon, D., and Parsons, J. (1991). An evaluation of CAST: A computer-aided speechreading program. *Journal of Speech and Hearing Research, 34,* 213–221.

Garstecki, D. C. (1981). Auditory-visual training paradigm for hearing-impaired adults. *Journal of the Academy of Rehabilitative Audiology, 14,* 223–238.

Grant, K. W., and Walden, B. E. (1996). Spectral distribution of prosodic information. *Journal of Speech and Hearing Research, 39,* 228–238.

Grant, K. W., Walden, B. E., Seitz, P. F. (1998). Auditory-visual speech recognition by hearing-impaired subjects: Consonant recognition, sentence recognition, and auditory-visual integration. *Journal of the Acoustical Society of America, 103,* 2677–2690.

Kaplan, H. (1996). Speechreading. In M. J. Moseley and S. J. Bally (Eds.), *Communication therapy: An integrated approach to aural rehabilitation.* Washington, DC: Gallaudet University Press.

Lansing, C. R., and Bievenue, L. A. (1994). Using intelligent computer-based teaching systems to evaluate the effectiveness of consonant recognition training. *Volta Review, 96,* 41–49.

Lansing, C. R., and Helegeson, C. L. (1995). Priming the visual recognition of spoken words. *Journal of Speech and Hearing Research, 38,* 1377–1386.

Lesner, S., Sandridge, S., and Kricos, P. (1987). Training influences on visual consonant and sentence recognition. *Ear and Hearing, 8,* 283–287.

Lidestam, B., Lyxell, B., and Andersson, G. (1999). Speechreading: Cognitive predictors and displayed emotion. *Scandinavian Audiology, 28,* 211–217.

MacSweeney, M., Campbell, R., Calvert, G. A., McGuire, P. K., David, A. S., Suckling, J., et al. (2000). Dispersed activation in the left temporal cortex for speech-reading in congenitally deaf people. *Proceedings of the Royal Society of London. Series B, Biological Sciences, 268,* 451–457.

Pichora-Fuller, M. K., and Benguerel, A. P. (1991). The design of CAST computer-aided speechreading training. *Journal of Speech and Hearing Disorders, 34,* 202–212.

Rönnberg, J. (1995). What makes a good speechreader? In G. Plant and K. Spens (Eds.), *Profound deafness and speech communication* (pp. 393–417). London: Whurr.

Rosenblum, L. D., Johnson, J. A., and Saldaña, H. M. (1996). Point-light facial displays enhance comprehension of speech in noise. *Journal of Speech and Hearing Research, 39,* 1159–1170.

Samar, V. J., and Sims, D. G. (1983). Visual evoked-response correlates of speechreading performance in normal-hearing adults: A replication and factor analytic extension. *Journal of Speech and Hearing Research, 26,* 2–9.

Sims, D. G., Von Feldt, J., Dowaliby, F., Hutchinson, K., and Meyers, T. (1979). A pilot experiment in computer assisted speechreading instruction utilizing the Data Analysis Video Interactive Device DAVID. *American Annals of the Deaf, 124,* 618–623.

Storke, D. G., and Hennecke, M. E. (Eds.). (1996). *Speechreading by humans and machines: Models, systems, and applications* (NATO ASI Series, Vol. 150, Series F: *Computer and systems sciences*). Berlin: Springer-Verlag.

Summerfield, Q. (1989). Visual perception of phonetic gestures. In J. G. Mattingly (Ed.), *Modularity and the motor theory of speech perception* (pp. 117–137). Hillsdale, NJ: Erlbaum.

Tye-Murray, N., Tyler, R. S., Bong, R., and Nares, T. (1988). Computerized laser videodisc programs for training speechreading and assertive communication behaviors. *Journal of the Academy of Rehabilitative Audiology, 21,* 143–152.

Walden, B., Erdman, S., Montgomery, A., Schwartz, D., and Prosek, R. (1981). Some effects of training on speech recognition by hearing impaired adults. *Journal of Speech and Hearing Research, 24,* 207–216.

Suprathreshold Speech Recognition

Suprathreshold refers to speech presented above the auditory threshold of the listener. Speech recognition is generally defined as the percentage of words or sentences that can be accurately heard by the listener. For example, a patient who could correctly repeat 40 out of 50 words presented would have 80% speech recognition. Because speech is a complex and continually varying signal requiring multiple auditory discrimination skills, it is not possible to accurately predict an individual's speech recognition from the pure-tone audiogram (Marshall and Bacon, 1981). Measurement of suprathreshold speech recognition allows clinicians to assess a patient's speech communication ability in a controlled and systematic manner. The results can help clinicians distinguish between different causes of hearing loss and plan and evaluate audiological rehabilitation programs.

Speech is a complex acoustic signal that varies from moment to moment: from shouting to whispering, from clear speech in quiet to difficult to understand speech in high ambient noise. Figure 1 shows the expected frequency and intensity of speech sounds for speech spoken at a conversational level in quiet. In general, the vowel sounds contain lower frequency information and are more intense, while consonant sounds contain higher frequency information and are produced at a lower intensity level. Which sounds are audible depends on the listener's audiometric thresholds as well as on the speaker and the level at which the words are spoken. For example, the sounds of shouted speech would be shifted to a higher intensity level and have a slightly different pattern across frequency (Olsen, 1998). Figure 1 also shows audiograms for two different listeners. The first listener has a moderately severe hearing loss. This listener would likely hear few, if any, conversational speech sounds and would be expected to have very poor speech recognition. The second listener has normal hearing in the low frequencies falling to a mild hearing loss in the high frequencies. This listener might hear some, but not all, of the speech sounds. The inability to hear high-frequency consonants would likely result in less than 100% speech recognition for a conversational-level signal.

Most commonly, the material used to measure speech recognition is a list of monosyllabic words. Typically each word is preceded by a carrier phrase, such as "Say the word——." Most available monosyllabic word lists are open set; that is, the listener is not restricted to a predetermined list of possible responses. A number of standard lists have been developed with vocabulary levels appropriate for adults (Hirsh et al., 1952; Tillman and Carhart, 1966) or children. The lists exclude words that would be unfamiliar to most people, and word selection is balanced to maintain similar levels of difficulty across lists. Additionally, each list is phonetically balanced; that is, the sounds in the words occur in the same proportion as in everyday speech. Test sensitivity is enhanced by using a larger number of items, such as 50 instead of 25 words (Thornton and Raffin, 1978).

Sentence tests are also available. These tests are more like "real speech" and thus presumably able to provide a closer estimate of real-life communication performance. However, sentence tests incorporate additional factors besides simple audibility. With sentences, the listener may be relying on linguistic, prosodic, or contextual cues in addition to auditory information. To limit contextual cues, sentence lists are available that use neutral context (Kalikow, Stevens, and Elliot, 1977) or linguistically meaningless word combinations (Speaks and Jerger, 1965). Sentences also place greater demands on higher-level processes such as auditory memory, which may be a particular problem in older listeners (Chmiel and Jerger, 1996).

For standard clinical testing, the participant is seated in a sound booth and listens to speech presented to one ear at a time through earphones. Speech may also be presented through a speaker, although this does not provide information specific to each ear. Such sound field testing can be used to quantify the effects of amplification. Recorded speech materials are preferred for consistency, although speech recognition tests are also administered using monitored live voice, during which the tester speaks to the participant over a microphone while monitoring her vocal strength. The entire list of words is presented at the same level. After each word, the participant responds by repeating or writing the word. The speech recognition score is then expressed as the percentage of correct words at the given presentation level in each ear.

Although most often presented in quiet, these materials may also be administered in noise. Many recordings include a background of multitalker babble that mimics a more realistic listening situation; this increases the degree to which test results characterize the listener's

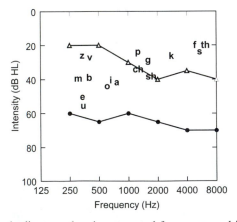

Figure 1. Audiogram showing expected frequency and intensity of speech sounds. Illustrative hearing thresholds are also shown for a listener with a moderately severe hearing loss (circles) and for a listener with normal hearing in the low frequencies falling to a mild loss in the high frequencies (triangles). In each case, speech sounds falling below the hearing threshold (i.e., at higher intensity levels) are audible to the listener; speech sounds falling above the hearing threshold (i.e., at lower intensity levels) are inaudible.

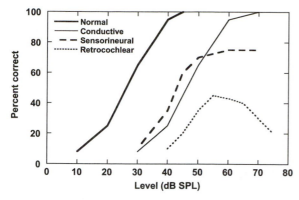

Figure 2. Representative performance-intensity functions, expressed as percent of words correct at each presentation level, for a listener with normal hearing and for three listeners with different types of hearing loss.

everyday communication abilities. For example, listeners with sensorineural loss require a more favorable signal-to-noise ratio than listeners with normal hearing or conductive hearing loss (Dubno, Dirks, and Morgan, 1984).

When administering and interpreting suprathreshold speech recognition tests it is important to consider not only the test environment but also the physical, linguistic, cognitive, and intellectual abilities of the listener. If the listener is unable to respond verbally or in writing, tests are available where the listener can choose among a set of picture responses (Ross and Lerman, 1970). Although most often used with children, these tests are also appropriate for adults with spoken word deficits, including dysarthria or apraxia. One limitation of such closed-set tests is that the chance of guessing correctly is higher when only a fixed number of choices is available. However, scoring accuracy may be higher than with open-set tests because there are fewer chances for misinterpretation of the response. For listeners who are not proficient in English, recorded materials are available in a number of other languages (provided, of course, that the tester has sufficient knowledge of the test language to interpret responses).

An important consideration is the presentation level. If multiple levels are tested, the percentage correct increases with increasing presentation level in a characteristic pattern (Fig. 2). This is referred to as the performance intensity (PI) function. The rate of improvement depends on the test material as well as patient characteristics. Easier material (e.g., sentences containing contextual cues) results in a greater rate of improvement with increases in level than more difficult material (e.g., nonsense words). The presentation level at which the listener achieves a highest score is referred to as the PB max, or maximum score for phonetically balanced words. A normal-hearing listener typically achieves 100% speech recognition at levels 30–40 dB above the SRT. Sensorineural hearing loss may restrict the PB max to below 100%. Listeners with conductive hearing loss generally achieve 100% recognition, although they require a higher presentation level than would a normal-

hearing listener. PI functions for listeners with retrocochlear loss may demonstrate disproportionately low scores as well as a phenomenon called rollover, in which performance first improves with increasing presentation level, and then degrades as the presentation level continues to increase.

In the clinic, speech recognition testing is often done at only one or two levels in each ear to minimize test time. One common approach is to select one or more levels relative to the speech reception threshold. Selection of the specific presentation level is generally based on providing adequate speech audibility, particularly at frequencies containing important consonant information. An alternative approach is to present speech at the level the listener deems most comfortable. Because the listener's most comfortable level may not be the same level at which she obtains a maximum score, testing exclusively at the most comfortable level can lead to erroneous conclusions about auditory function (Ullrich and Grimm, 1976; Beattie and Warren, 1982).

In summary, measurement of suprathreshold speech recognition is an important part of an audiometric examination. Test results can be affected by a number of factors, including the participant's pure-tone sensitivity, the amount of distortion produced by the hearing loss, the presentation level of the speech, the type of speech material, the presence or absence of background noise, and even the participant's age. A detailed understanding of these factors is important when interpreting test results and drawing conclusions about an individual's overall communication ability.

—Pamela E. Souza

References

Beattie, R. C., and Warren, V. G. (1982). Relationships among speech threshold, loudness discomfort, comfortable loudness, and PB max in the elderly hearing impaired. *American Journal of Otolaryngology, 3,* 353–358.

Chmiel, R., and Jerger, J. (1996). Hearing aid use, central auditory disorder, and hearing handicap in elderly persons. *Journal of the American Academy of Audiology, 7,* 190–202.

Dubno, J. R., Dirks, D. D., and Morgan, D. E. (1984). Effects of age and mild hearing loss on speech recognition in noise. *Journal of the Acoustical Society of America, 76,* 87–96.

Hirsh, I. J., Davis, H., Silverman, S. R., Reynolds, E. G., Eldert, E., and Benson, R. W. (1952). Development of materials for speech audiometry. *Journal of Speech and Hearing Disorders, 17,* 321–337.

Kalikow, D. N., Stevens, K. N., and Elliot, L. L. (1977). Development of a test of speech intelligibility in noise using sentence materials with controlled word predictability. *Journal of the Acoustical Society of America, 61,* 1337–1351.

Marshall, L., and Bacon, S. P. (1981). Prediction of speech discrimination scores from audiometric data. *Journal of Speech and Hearing Research, 2,* 148–155.

Olsen, W. O. (1998). Average speech levels and spectra in various speaking/listening conditions: A summary of the Pearson, Bennett, and Fidell (1977) report. *American Journal of Audiology, 7,* 1–5.

Ross, M., and Lerman, J. (1970). Picture identification test for hearing-impaired children. *Journal of Speech and Hearing Research, 13,* 44–53.

Speaks, C., and Jerger, J. (1965). Performance-intensity characteristics of synthetic sentences. *Journal of Speech and Hearing Research, 9,* 305–312.

Thornton, A. R., and Raffin, M. J. M. (1978). Speech-discrimination scores modeled as a binomial variable. *Journal of Speech and Hearing Research, 21,* 507–518.

Tillman, T. W., and Carhart, R. (1966). *An expanded test for speech discrimination utilizing CNC monosyllabic words: Northwestern University Auditory Test No. 6* (USAF School of Aerospace Medicine Technical Report). Brooks Air Force Base, TX.

Ullrich, K., and Grimm, D. (1976). Most comfortable listening level presentation versus maximum discrimination for word discrimination material. *Audiology, 15,* 338–347.

Further Readings

Dubno, J. R., and Dirks, D. D. (1993). Factors affecting performance on psychoacoustic and speech-recognition tasks in the presence of hearing loss. In G. A. Studebaker and I. Hochberg (Eds.), *Acoustical factors affecting hearing aid performance* (pp. 235–253). Needham Heights, MA: Allyn and Bacon.

Hall, J. W., and Mueller, H. G. (1997). Speech audiometry. In *Audiologists' desk reference. Vol. I. Diagnostic audiology: Principles, procedures, and practices* (pp. 113–174). San Diego, CA: Singular Publishing Group.

Kirk, K. I., Pisoni, D. B., and Miyamoto, R. C. (1997). Effects of stimulus variability on speech perception in listeners with hearing impairment. *Journal of Speech, Language, and Hearing Research, 40,* 1395–1405.

Olsen, W. O., and Matkin, N. D. (1991). Speech audiometry. In W. F. Rintelmann (Ed.), *Hearing assessment* (pp. 39–140). Austin, TX: Pro-Ed.

Olsen, W. O., Van Tasell, D. J., and Speaks, C. E. (1997). Phoneme and word recognition for words in isolation and in sentences. *Ear and Hearing, 18,* 175–188.

Penrod, J. P. (1994). Speech threshold and recognition/discrimination testing. In J. Katz (Ed.), *Handbook of clinical audiology* (pp. 147–164). Baltimore: Williams and Wilkins.

Stach, B. A., Davis-Thaxton, M., and Jerger, J. (1995). Improving the efficiency of speech audiometry: Computer-based approach. *Journal of the American Academy of Audiology, 6,* 330–333.

Thibodeau, L. M. (2000). Speech audiometry. In R. J. Roeser, M. Valente, and H. Hosford-Dunn (Eds.), *Audiology diagnosis* (pp. 281–310). New York: Thieme.

Temporal Integration

The term *temporal integration* (TI) refers to summation of stimulus intensity during the duration of the stimulus. As duration increases, a sensation like loudness increases, or the sound level at which the stimulus can be detected decreases. The stimuli may be various types of signals, such as tones or bands of noise. Similarly, short succeeding stimuli can combine their energies and provide a lower detection level than individual stimuli. The

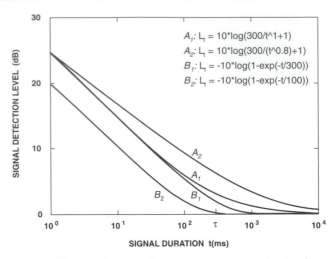

Figure 1. Temporal integration curves according to the functions shown in the legend. In curves A_1 and A_2, the time constant $\tau = 300$ ms; in A_1, exponent $m = 1$; in A_2, $m = 0.8$. In B_1, $\tau = 300$ ms; in B_2, $\tau = 100$ ms. The value of $\tau = 300$ ms is indicated by a mark on the abscissa.

TI has a time limit. For a stimulus longer than this limit, the loudness, or the detection (threshold) level, remains relatively constant.

Interest in studying TI is fueled by the need to understand auditory processing of speech—a signal that, by its nature, changes rapidly in time. Better understanding of the temporal characteristics of hearing should help us improve means for enhancement of speech communication in unfavorable listening environments, and of listeners with impaired hearing.

Graphs of the relationship between the stimulus duration (plotted on the horizontal coordinate, usually in milliseconds with a logarithmic scale) and the intensity level at the threshold of hearing (plotted on the vertical coordinate in decibels, dB) are called temporal integration curves (TICs). Examples of TICs are shown in Figure 1. The detection intensity level first declines as the stimulus duration increases and then, beyond a time limit called the critical duration, remains constant. The magnitude of TI can be expressed by the difference between the detection levels of long and short signals. The rate of decline of TICs is represented by slopes of the curves, which too are often used as indicators of TI magnitude. These slopes (they are negative) are usually expressed as the ratio of the change of level (in dB) per tenfold increase in signal duration [(L2–L1)/dec], or per doubling of signal duration. The slopes of the TICs and the values of the critical duration represent summary characteristics of TI. (The critical duration depends on a time constant τ, a parameter in formulas describing TICs.)

Factors Affecting TI

The slope of the curves and the time constant depend on various factors, such as signal frequency, status of hearing, and type of signals. The effect of signal frequency on TI is pronounced (Gerken, Bhat, and Hutchison-Clutter, 1990) and depends on signal duration. TI, as well as τ, is greater at lower frequencies than at higher ones (e.g., Fastl, 1976; Nábělek, 1978; Florentine, Fastl, and Buus, 1988). At low frequencies and signal durations below 10 ms, the TIC slopes were found to be up to -15 dB/dec (e.g., Green, Birdsall, and Tanner, 1957). At frequencies between 1 and 8 kHz and at signal durations between 20 and 100 ms, the slopes are between -10 and -8 dB/dec (e.g., Zwislocki, 1969; Gerken, Bhat, and Hutchison-Clutter, 1990). The steeper slopes at short signal durations as compared to slopes at longer signal durations are attributed to the loss of contribution of some energy due to spectral broadening, or "splatter." When the frequency during the signal is not constant but is increasing, the slope between 20 ms and 80 ms of signal duration is smaller, about -9 dB/dec, than when the frequency is decreasing—about -13 dB/dec (Nábělek, 1978). For broadband masking conditions, the values of TI for constant tones are similar to those without masking, but some influence of the level of the masker was observed. This influence depends on signal duration. For signal durations between 2 and 10 ms, the TICs at medium masker levels are steeper than at low or high masker levels, and for signal durations over 20 ms, the TI values are not affected by the masker level (Oxenham, Moore, and Vickers, 1997). Formby et al. (1994) investigated the influence of bandwidth of a noise signal masked by an uncorrelated broadband noise on TI and τ. They found that both TI and τ were related inversely to the bandwidth, if the bandwidth was greater than the critical band of hearing (CB), and were relatively invariant if the bandwidth was smaller than the critical band. For gated signal and masker, Formby et al. (1994) identified at least three cues for signal detection: (1) a relative timing cue, (2) a spectral shape cue, and (3) a traditional energy cue. The timing and spectral shape cues count most for the shortest (10 ms) and narrowest (bandwidth = 63 Hz) signals, respectively. When the signal is a series of tone pulses, and not single bursts, the change of time interval between the pulses produces smaller change of TI than the change in duration of single bursts (Carlyon, Buus, and Florentine, 1990).

Listeners with hearing impairment generally show less temporal integration than listeners with normal hearing (e.g., Watson and Gengel, 1969; Gerken, Bhat, and Hutchison-Clutter, 1990). No effect of level of a broadband masker was found for listeners with impaired hearing at any signal duration.

Loudness increases when the duration of a short signal increases. When the signal level changes, the TI for loudness changes; however, the change is not monotonic (Buus, Florentine, and Poulsen, 1999). The change is greatest at moderate sensation levels and depends on signal duration. The effect of signal level on TI of loudness is greater at short than at long signal durations.

Donaldson, Viemeister, and Nelson (1997) found that TICs for electrical stimulation with the Nucleus-22 elec-

trode cochlear implant were considerably less steep than -8 dB/dec typically observed with acoustical stimulation. The slopes varied widely across subjects and across stimulated electrodes. When Shannon and Otto (1990) used a device called the auditory brainstem implant (ABI) and positioned its electrodes near the cochlear nucleus of listeners, they obtained only a shallow TIC over the range of 2- to 1000-ms signal duration.

Models

A number of models for temporal integration have been proposed. The theoretical foundations for the mathematical description of TI are either deterministic or probabilistic. Deterministic models include power function models or exponential function models. One of the deterministic models is described mathematically by the power function $t(I_t - I_\infty) = I_\infty \tau = $ const (Hughes, 1946), or in its more general form by $It^m = C$ (Green et al., 1957). In these equations t is the stimulus duration, I_t is the threshold intensity at t, I_∞ is the threshold intensity for very long stimuli, τ is the time constant of the integration process, m is the power function exponent, and C is a constant. The exponent m determines the slope of the curves (A_1 and A_2 in Fig. 1). The slope -3 dB/doubling or -10 dB/dec corresponds to $m = 1$. Another model is the exponential one $I_t/I_\infty = 1/(1 - e^{-t/\tau})$ (Feldkeller and Oetinger, 1956; Plomp and Bouman, 1959). The curves B_1 and B_2 in Figure 1 correspond to this equation.

Zwislocki (1960) developed a temporal summation theory for two pulses separated in time and proposed a theory of TI for loudness (Zwislocki, 1969). In his model it is assumed that (1) a linear temporal integrator (with a time constant on the order of 200 ms) exists in the central nervous system; (2) a nonlinear transformation that produces compression precedes the temporal summation; and (3) neural excitation decreases exponentially with a short time constant at the input to the integrator that summates the central neural activity. (This last assumption indicates that the term temporal integration should not be interpreted as the integration of acoustic energy per se.)

Attempts to resolve an apparent discrepancy between high temporal resolution of hearing and long time constants of temporal integration have led to a number of models employing short integration times (e.g., Penner, 1978; Oxenham, Moore, and Vickers, 1997). Viemeister and Wakefield (1991) have not considered this discrepancy to be a real problem. Their model is based on a statistical probability approach and assumes multiple sampling. Taking their own data into account, Viemeister and Wakefield conclude that power integration occurs only for pulses separated in time by less than about 5 ms, and that therefore their data are inconsistent with the classical view of TI involving long-term integration. However, they find the data to be compatible with the notion that the input is sampled at a fairly high rate and the obtained samples (or "looks") are stored in memory; while in the memory, the "looks" can be selectively accessed, weighted, and otherwise processed.

Dau, Kollmeier, and Kohlrausch (1997) proposed a multichannel model. They describe the effects of spectral and temporal integration in amplitude-modulation detection for a stochastic noise carrier. The model is based on the concept of a modulation filter-bank. To integrate information across frequency, the detection process in the model combines cues from all filters with an optimal decision statistic. To integrate information across time, a "multiple-look" strategy, similar to that proposed by Viemeister and Wakefield (1991), is realized within the detection stage of the model. The temporal integration involves a template that provides the basis for the optimal detector of the model. The length and the time constant of the template are variable: they change according to the task which the listener has to perform.

Although an extensive knowledge of temporal integration has been attained, many aspects of TI await further investigation. For example, evidence of some TI mechanism at a higher stage of the auditory pathway was found by Uppenkamp, Fobel, and Patterson (2001) when they compared the perception of short-frequency sweeps and the physiological response to them in the brainstem. The improved understanding of TI should provide a sounder basis for the development of means for securing better speech communication in general and for listeners with special problems, like those with cochlear implants, in particular. Presently, TI studies are not limited to traditional topics but also cover higher levels of the brain, like the role of TI in establishing neural representations of phonemes (Tallal et al., 1998), and investigation of an association between a deficient TI and mental disturbances in schizophrenia (Haig et al., 2000; Michie, 2001).

Acknowledgments

Many thanks to Assoc. Prof. Lana S. Dixon for her help in securing pertinent references.

See also CLINICAL DECISION ANALYSIS; COCHLEAR IMPLANTS; MASKING; TEMPORAL RESOLUTION.

—*Igor V. Nábělek*

References

Buus, S., Florentine, M., and Poulsen, T. (1999). Temporal integration of loudness in listeners with hearing losses of primarily cochlear origin. *Journal of the Acoustical Society of America*, 105, 3464–3480.

Carlyon, R. P., Buus, S., and Florentine, M. (1990). Temporal integration of trains of tone pulses by normal and by cochlearly impaired listeners. *Journal of the Acoustical Society of America*, 87, 260–268.

Donaldson, G. S., Viemeister, N. F., and Nelson, D. A. (1997). Psychometric functions and temporal integration in electric hearing. *Journal of the Acoustical Society of America*, 101, 3706–3721.

Dau, T., Kollmeier, B., and Kohlrausch, A. (1997). Modeling auditory processing of amplitude modulation: II. Spectral and temporal integration. *Journal of the Acoustical Society of America*, 102, 2906–2919.

Fastl, H. (1976). Influence of test tone duration on auditory masking patterns. *Audiology*, 15, 63–71.

Feldkeller, R., and Oetinger, R. (1956). Die Horbarkeitsgrenzen von Impulsen verschiedener Dauer. *Acustica*, 6, 481–493.

Florentine, M., Fastl, H., and Buus, S. (1988). Temporal integration in normal hearing, cochlear impairment, and impairment simulated by masking. *Journal of the Acoustical Society of America*, 84, 195–203.

Formby, C., Heinz, M. G., Luna, C. E., and Shaheen, M. K. (1994). Masked detection thresholds and temporal integration for noise band signals. *Journal of the Acoustical Society of America*, 96, 102–114.

Gerken, G. M., Bhat, V. K., and Hutchison-Clutter, M. (1990). Auditory temporal integration and the power function model. *Journal of the Acoustical Society of America*, 88, 767–778.

Green, D. M., Birdsall, T. G., and Tanner, W. P., Jr. (1957). Signal detection as a function of signal intensity and duration. *Journal of the Acoustical Society of America*, 29, 523–531.

Haig, A. R., Gordon, E., De-Pascalis, V., Meares, R. A., Bahramali, H., and Harris, A. (2000). Gamma activity in schizophrenia: Evidence of impaired network binding? *Clinical Neurophysiology*, 111, 1461–1468.

Hughes, J. W. (1946). The threshold of audition for short periods of stimulation. *Proceedings of the Royal Society of London. Series B: Biological Sciences*, B133, 486–490.

Michie, P. T. (2001). What has MMN revealed about the auditory system in schizophrenia? *International Journal of Psychophysiology*, 42, 177–194.

Nábělek, I. V. (1978). Temporal summation of constant and gliding tones at masked auditory threshold. *Journal of the Acoustical Society of America*, 64, 751–763.

Oxenham, A. J., Moore, B. C., and Vickers, D. A. (1997). Short-term temporal integration: Evidence for the influence of peripheral compression. *Journal of the Acoustical Society of America*, 101, 3676–3687.

Penner, M. J. (1978). A power law transformation resulting in a class of short-term integrators that produce time-intensity trades for noise bursts. *Journal of the Acoustical Society of America*, 63, 195–201.

Plomp, R., and Bouman, M. A. (1959). Relation between hearing threshold and duration for tone pulses. *Journal of the Acoustical Society of America*, 31, 749–758.

Shannon, R. V., and Otto, S. R. (1990). Psychophysical measures from electrical stimulation of the human cochlear nucleus. *Hearing Research*, 47, 159–168.

Tallal, P., Merzenich, M. M., Miller, S., and Jenkins, W. (1998). Language learning impairments: Integrating basic science, technology, and remediation. *Experimental Brain Research*, 123, 210–219.

Uppenkamp, S., Fobel, S., and Patterson, R. D. (2001). The effects of temporal asymmetry on the detection and perception of short chirps. *Hearing Research*, 158, 71–83.

Viemeister, N. F., and Wakefield, G. H. (1991). Temporal integration and multiple looks. *Journal of the Acoustical Society of America*, 90, 858–865.

Watson, C. S., and Gengel, R. W. (1969). Signal duration and signal frequency in relation to auditory sensitivity. *Journal of the Acoustical Society of America*, 46, 989–997.

Zwislocki, J. J. (1960). Theory of temporal auditory summation. *Journal of the Acoustical Society of America*, 32, 1046–1060.

Zwislocki, J. J. (1969). Temporal summation of loudness: An analysis. *Journal of the Acoustical Society of America*, 46, 431–441.

Further Readings

Algom, D., Rubin, A., and Cohen-Raz, L. (1989). Binaural and temporal integration of the loudness of tones and noises. *Perception and Psychophysics, 46,* 155–166.

Bacon, S. P., Hicks, M. L., and Johnson, K. L. (2000). Temporal integration in the presence of off-frequency maskers. *Journal of the Acoustical Society of America, 107,* 922–932.

Buus, S. (1999). Temporal integration and multiple looks, revisited: Weights as a function of time. *Journal of the Acoustical Society of America, 105,* 2466–2475.

Cacace, A. T., Margolis, R. H., and Relkin, E. M. (1991). Threshold and suprathreshold temporal integration effects in the crossed and uncrossed human acoustic stapedius reflex. *Journal of the Acoustical Society of America, 89,* 1255–1261.

Csepe, V., Pantev, C., Hoke, M., Ross, B., and Hampson, S. (1997). Mismatch field to tone pairs: Neuromagnetic evidence for temporal integration at the sensory level. *Electroencephalography and Clinical Neurophysiology, 104,* 1–9.

Fu, Q. J., and Shannon, R. V. (2000). Effect of stimulation rate on phoneme recognition by Nucleus-22 cochlear implant listeners. *Journal of the Acoustical Society of America, 107,* 589–597.

Garner, W. R., and Miller, G. A. (1947). The masked threshold of pure tones as a function of duration. *Journal of Experimental Psychology, 37,* 293.

Hall, J. W., and Fernandes, M. A. (1983). Temporal integration, frequency resolution, and off-frequency listening in normal-hearing and cochlear-impaired listeners. *Journal of the Acoustical Society of America, 74,* 1172–1177.

Kollmeier, B. (Ed.). (1995). *Psychoacoustics, speech, and hearing aids.* Proceedings of the summer school and international symposium, Bad Zwischenahn, Germany, 31 Aug.–5 Sept. 1995. World Scientific Singapore, 1996.

Moore, B. C. J. (1997). *An introduction to the psychology of hearing* (4th ed.). London: Academic Press.

Oxenham, A. J. (1998). Temporal integration at 6 kHz as a function of masker bandwidth. *Journal of the Acoustical Society of America, 103,* 1033–1042.

Sheft, S., and Yost, W. A. (1990). Temporal integration in amplitude modulation detection. *Journal of the Acoustical Society of America, 88,* 796–805.

Yost, W. A. (1991). *Fundamentals of hearing: An introduction.* San Diego, CA: Academic Press.

Temporal Resolution

Sensory systems function as change detectors in many respects. They quickly adapt to steady-state stimuli and are easily excited by the introduction of novel stimuli. The pattern of changes in an acoustic stimulus conveys information about the nature of the sound source and the message being transmitted by the sender. Therefore the identification, discrimination, and interpretation of acoustic events depend on the ability of the auditory system to faithfully encode the temporal features of those events. This ability to respond to changes in an acoustic stimulus has been termed temporal resolution. Although most natural acoustic signals are characterized by changes in intensity as well as changes in the acoustic spectrum over time, investigations of temporal resolu-

tion have focused on intensity variations in an attempt to separate purely temporal from spectro-temporal resolving capabilities (see AUDITORY SCENE ANALYSIS). Temporal resolution is limited by auditory inertia resulting from mechanical and/or electrophysiological transduction processes. Such a limitation effectively smoothes or attenuates the intensive changes of a stimulus, which reduces the salience of those changes. Impaired temporal resolution may be conceptualized as an increase in this smoothing process, and thus a loss of temporal information.

The influence of hearing impairment on temporal resolution depends on the site of lesion. For example, conductive hearing loss is often modeled as a simple attenuation characteristic and thus should not alter temporal resolution, given sufficient stimulus levels. Damage at the level of the cochlea, however, involves more than attenuation. Reduced outer hair cell function is associated with a reduction in sensitivity, frequency selectivity, and compression at the level of the basilar membrane. Each of these might influence the perception of intensity changes. For example, a loss of basilar membrane compression might provide a more salient representation of intensity changes and thus lead to improved performance on temporal resolution tasks involving such changes. Reduced frequency selectivity is analogous to broadening of a filter characteristic, which is associated with a shorter temporal response. This too might lead to improved temporal resolution. A loss of inner hair cell function, however, would reduce the quality and amount of information transmitted to the central auditory pathway, and might therefore lead to poor coding of temporal features. The altered neural function associated with a retrocochlear lesion may also lead to a less faithful representation of the temporal features of a sound.

Numerous techniques have been used to probe temporal resolution abilities; however, the two most common techniques are temporal gap detection and amplitude modulation detection (Fig. 1). Following the

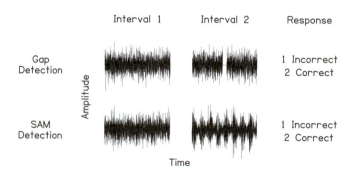

Figure 1. Schematic diagram of a two-interval, forced-choice psychophysical paradigm used to estimate gap detection thresholds (top row) and sinusoidal amplitude modulation (SAM) detection thresholds (bottom row). Stimulus waveforms are shown for each of two observation intervals. A broadband noise standard is shown in interval 1 and a noise with a temporal gap (64 ms) or amplitude modulation (6 dB) is shown in interval 2. Correct and incorrect responses are listed.

notion of auditory inertia, Plomp (1964) investigated the rate of decay of auditory sensation by measuring the minimum detectable silent interval between two broadband noise pulses as a function of the relative level of the two pulses. When the pulses surrounding the gap were equal in level, the minimum detectable gap was about 3 ms. Gap detection thresholds deteriorate as stimulus level falls below about 30 dB sensation level (e.g., Plomp, 1964; Penner, 1977; Buus and Florentine, 1983; Florentine and Buus, 1984). Thus, reduced audibility associated with hearing loss may result in longer than normal gap detection thresholds. For patients with conductive or sensorineural hearing loss, gap detection thresholds for broadband noise are longer than normal at low stimulus levels. At higher stimulus levels, gap thresholds are within normal limits for conductive loss but remain longer than normal for listeners with sensorineural hearing loss (Irwin, Hinchcliff, and Kemp, 1981).

To gauge temporal resolution in different frequency regions, one may measure gap detection thresholds using band-limited noise. Results from listeners with normal hearing reveal that gap thresholds improve with increasing stimulus level up to about 30 dB sensation level (e.g., Buus and Florentine, 1983) and improve with increasing noise bandwidth (e.g., Shailer and Moore, 1983; Eddins, Hall, and Grose, 1992), but vary little with frequency region when noise bandwidth (in Hz) is held constant (e.g., Eddins et al., 1992). With hearing loss of cochlear origin, gap detection is often worse than normal using band-limited noise (e.g., Fitzgibbons and Wightman, 1982; Fitzgibbons and Gordon-Salant, 1987); however, this is not true for all listeners with cochlear hearing loss (e.g., Florentine and Buus, 1984; Glasberg and Moore, 1989; Grose, Eddins, and Hall, 1989). Thus, cochlear hearing loss does not necessarily result in poorer than normal temporal resolution.

Temporal gap detection thresholds measured for sinusoidal stimuli do not vary substantially with stimulus frequency from 400 to 2000 Hz, but increase substantially at and below 200 Hz (e.g., Shailer and Moore, 1987; Moore, Peters, and Glasberg, 1992). Although listeners with hearing impairment may have worse than normal gap detection thresholds for noise stimuli, gap detection thresholds for tonal stimuli are normal when compared at equivalent sound pressure levels and are better than normal at equal sensation levels (Moore and Glasberg, 1988). One theory consistent with these results is that gap detection is limited to some extent by the inherent fluctuations in narrow-band noise, and this effect may be accentuated by the loudness recruitment of some hearing-impaired listeners (e.g., Moore and Glasberg, 1988). Sinusoids, having a smooth temporal envelope, would not be subject to such a limitation. This leads to the possibility that temporal resolution per se may not be adversely affected by cochlear hearing loss (e.g., Moore and Glasberg, 1988). If gap detection is influenced by loudness recruitment, then one would expect a relationship between gap detection and intensity resolution. Indeed, gap detection for sinusoids is correlated with in-

tensity resolution for sinusoids (Glasberg and Moore, 1989) and gap detection for band-limited noise is correlated with intensity resolution for band-limited noise (Eddins and Manegold, 2001). This highlights the potential role of intensity resolution in a task such as gap detection. Poor gap detection thresholds may result from poor intensity resolution, poor temporal resolution, or a combination of the two. Listeners with cochlear implants offer a unique perspective on temporal resolution in that the auditory periphery, save for the auditory nerve, is bypassed. Gap detection in such listeners, using electrical stimulation via the implant, is as good as gap detection for listeners with normal hearing using acoustic stimulation (e.g., Shannon, 1989; Moore and Glasberg, 1988). This is consistent with the notion that gap detection may not be strongly dependent upon cochlear processes.

While gap detection thresholds may be strongly influenced by a listener's intensity resolution, the amplitude modulation detection paradigm provides an opportunity to separate the affects of intensity resolution from temporal resolution. A modulation detection threshold is obtained by determining the minimum depth of modulation necessary to discriminate an unmodulated from a sinusoidally amplitude-modulated stimulus. With this technique, temporal resolution can be more completely described as the change in modulation threshold over a range of fluctuation rates (modulation frequencies). With the assumption that intensity resolution does not vary with modulation frequency, a separate index of intensity resolution may be obtained from modulation detection thresholds at very low modulation frequencies. If loudness recruitment associated with cochlear hearing loss has a negative influence on gap detection in narrow-band noise, as suggested above, then one might predict that recruitment would enhance the perception of fluctuations introduced by amplitude modulation. Using broadband noise carriers, this does not seem to be the case. Modulation detection thresholds for listeners with cochlear hearing loss may be normal or worse than normal, but are not better than normal (Bacon and Viemeister, 1985; Bacon and Gleitman, 1992). Similarly, modulation detection using band-limited noise is not worse than normal in listeners with cochlear hearing loss (e.g., Moore, Shailer, and Schooneveldt, 1992; Hall et al., 1998). Modulation detection with tonal carriers, however, tends to be better than normal in listeners with cochlear hearing loss, and the perceived depth of modulation appears to be related to the steepness of loudness growth (Moore, Wojtczak, and Vickers, 1996; Moore and Glasberg, 2001). This is quite different from amplitude-modulated noise stimuli, for which threshold does not seem to be related to loudness growth (Hall et al., 1998). As in the gap detection paradigm, there are marked differences between the results obtained with noise and tonal stimuli. Thus, it is possible that the relation between loudness growth and intensive changes is different for sinusoidal and noise stimuli.

Some listeners with cochlear pathology have worse than normal modulation detection using noise carriers, as do listeners with Ménière's disease (Formby, 1987), eighth nerve tumors (Formby, 1986), and auditory neuropathy (Zeng et al., 1999). Interestingly, listeners with cochlear implants perform as well as normal-hearing subjects on amplitude-modulation tasks (Shannon, 1992).

In summary, listeners with abnormal cochlear function often exhibit reduced performance on gap and modulation detection tasks with noise but not sinusoidal stimuli. Studies of temporal resolution using other experimental techniques have yielded results that are generally consistent with those discussed here. These results are consistent with an interpretation that cochlear pathology may not lead to reduced temporal resolution per se, but may lead to difficulty perceiving stimuli with pronounced, random intensity fluctuations (Grose et al., 1989; Hall and Grose, 1997; Hall et al., 1998). Although many hearing-impaired listeners perform as well as normal-hearing listeners on tasks involving temporal resolution, especially when stimuli are presented at optimal levels and have relatively smooth temporal envelopes, such listeners are likely to have difficulty in natural listening environments with fluctuating backgrounds. Thus, measures of gap and amplitude modulation detection using noise stimuli might have promise as predictors of communication difficulty in realistic environments.

—*David A. Eddins*

References

Bacon, S. P., and Gleitman, R. M. (1992). Modulation detection in subjects with relatively flat hearing losses. *Journal of Speech and Hearing Research, 35*, 642–653.

Bacon, S. P., and Viemeister, N. F. (1985). Temporal modulation transfer functions in normal-hearing and hearing-impaired listeners. *Audiology, 24*, 117–134.

Buus, S., and Florentine, M. (1983). Gap detection in normal and impaired listeners: The effect of level, and frequency. In A. Michelson (Ed.), *Time resolution in auditory systems* (pp. 159–179). New York: Springer-Verlag.

Eddins, D. A., Hall, J. W., and Grose, J. H. (1992). The detection of temporal gaps as a function of frequency region and absolute noise bandwidth. *Journal of the Acoustical Society of America, 91*, 1069–1077.

Eddins, D. A., and Manegold, R. A. (2001). *Spectral integration in the detection of temporal gaps, amplitude modulation, increments, and decrements in bandlimited noise.* Unpublished manuscript.

Fitzgibbons, P. J., and Gordan-Salant, S. (1987). Temporal gap resolution in listeners with high-frequency sensorineural hearing loss. *Journal of the Acoustical Society of America, 81*, 133–137.

Fitzgibbons, P. J., and Wightman, F. L. (1982). Gap detection in normal and hearing-impaired listeners. *Journal of the Acoustical Society of America, 72*, 761–765.

Florentine, M., and Buus, S. (1984). Temporal gap detection in sensorineural and simulated hearing impairments. *Journal of Speech and Hearing Research, 27*, 449–455.

Formby, C. (1986). Modulation detection by patients with eighth-nerve tumors. *Journal of Speech and Hearing Research, 29*, 413–419.

Formby, C. (1987). Modulation threshold functions for chronically impaired Ménière's patients. *Audiology, 26*, 89–102.

Glasberg, B. R., and Moore, B. C. (1989). Psychoacoustic abilities of subjects with unilateral and bilateral cochlear hearing impairments and their relationship to the ability to understand speech. *Scandinavian Audiology, Supplement, 32*, 1–25.

Grose, J. H., Eddins, D. A., and Hall, J. W. (1989). Gap detection as a function of stimulus bandwidth with fixed high-frequency cutoff in normal-hearing and hearing-impaired listeners. *Journal of the Acoustical Society of America, 86*, 1747–1755.

Hall, J. W. III, and Grose, J. H. (1997). The relation between gap detection, loudness, and loudness growth in noise-masked normal-hearing listeners. *Journal of the Acoustical Society of America, 101*, 1044–1049.

Hall, J. W. III, Grose, J. H., Buss, E., and Hatch, D. R. (1998). Temporal analysis and stimulus fluctuation in listeners with normal and impaired hearing. *Journal of Speech, Language, and Hearing Research, 41*, 340–354.

Irwin, R. J., Hinchcliff, L. K., and Kemp, S. (1981). Temporal acuity in normal and hearing-impaired listeners. *Audiology, 20*, 234–243.

Moore, B. C., and Glasberg, C. J. (1988). Gap detection with sinusoids and noise in normal, impaired, and electrically stimulated ears. *Journal of the Acoustical Society of America, 83*, 1093–1101.

Moore, B. C., and Glasberg, C. J. (2001). Temporal modulation transfer functions obtained using sinusoidal carriers with normally hearing and hearing-impaired listeners. *Journal of the Acoustical Society of America, 110*, 1067–1073.

Moore, B. C., Peters, R. W., and Glasberg, B. R. (1992). Detection of temporal gaps in sinusoids by elderly subjects with and without hearing loss. *Journal of the Acoustical Society of America, 92*, 1923–1932.

Moore, B. C., Shailer, M. J., and Schooneveldt, G. P. (1992). Temporal modulation transfer functions for bandlimited noise in subjects with cochlear hearing loss. *British Journal of Audiology, 26*, 229–237.

Moore, B. C., Wojtczak, J. M., and Vickers, D. A. (1996). Effect of loudness recruitment on the perception of amplitude modulation. *Journal of the Acoustical Society of America, 100*, 481–489.

Penner, M. J. (1977). Detection of temporal gaps in noise as a measure of the decay of auditory sensation. *Journal of the Acoustical Society of America, 61*, 552–557.

Plomp, R. (1964). Rate of decay of auditory sensation. *Journal of the Acoustical Society of America, 36*, 277–282.

Shailer, M. J., and Moore, B. C. (1983). Gap detection as a function of frequency, bandwidth, and level. *Journal of the Acoustical Society of America, 74*, 467–473.

Shailer, M. J., and Moore, B. C. (1987). Gap detection and the auditory filter: Phase effects using sinusoidal stimuli. *Journal of the Acoustical Society of America, 81*, 1110–1117.

Shannon, R. V. (1989). Detection of gaps in sinusoids and pulse trains by patients with cochlear implants. *Journal of the Acoustical Society of America, 85*, 2587–2592.

Shannon, R. V. (1992). Temporal modulation transfer functions in patients with cochlear implants. *Journal of the Acoustical Society of America, 91*, 2156–2164.

Zeng, F. G., Oba, S., Garde, S., Sininger, Y., and Starr, A. (1999). Temporal and speech processing deficits in auditory neuropathy. *NeuroReport, 10*, 3429–3435.

Further Readings

Derleth, R. P., Dau, T., and Kollmeier, B. (2001). Modeling temporal resolution and compressive properties of the normal and impaired auditory system. *Hearing Research, 159,* 132–149.

Eddins, D. A., and Green, D. M. (1995). Temporal integration and temporal resolution. In B. C. J. Moore (Ed.), *Hearing* (pp. 207–242). San Diego, CA: Academic Press.

Glasberg, B. R., and Moore, B. C. J. (1992). Effects of envelope fluctuation on gap detection. *Hearing Research, 64,* 81–92.

Moore, B. C. J. (1998). *Cochlear hearing loss.* London: Whurr.

Plack, C. J., and Moore, B. C. J. (1991). Decrement detection in normal and impaired ears. *Journal of the Acoustical Society of America, 90,* 3069–3076.

Tinnitus

Tinnitus is an auditory perceptual phenomenon that is defined as the conscious perception of internal noises without any outer auditory stimulation. Tinnitus may occur as a concomitant of practically all the dysfunctions that involve the human auditory system. Hence, damage to the middle ear, the cochlea, cranial nerve VIII (audiovestibular), and pathways in the brain from cochlear nucleus to primary auditory cortex all are likely candidates for explaining why tinnitus appears (Levine, 2001). A common distinction is between so-called objective tinnitus (somatosounds) and subjective tinnitus. In clinical settings, objective tinnitus represents a minority of cases. Examples of conditions related to objective tinnitus are spontaneous otoacoustic emissions, tensor tympani syndrome, and vascular lesions. Subjective tinnitus has been linked to sensorineural hearing loss caused by various deficits such as age-related hearing loss (presbyacusis), noise exposure, acoustic neuroma, and Ménière's disease (Levine, 2001), but also to other conditions such as temporomandibular joint dysfunction. Different neural mechanisms have been proposed, and tinnitus has been explained as the result of increased neural activity in the form of increased burst firing, or as a result of pathological synchronization of neural activity. Other suggested mechanisms are hypersensitivity and cortical reorganization (Rauschecker, 1999).

Prevalence and Categorization

Tinnitus is commonly a temporary sensation, and most people have experienced it. However, it may develop into a chronic condition that resists medical or surgical treatment. Prevalence figures vary slightly, but at least 10%–15% of the general population can be expected to have tinnitus. A large majority do not have severe tinnitus. Findings from epidemiological studies suggest that about 1%–3% of the adult population has severe tinnitus, in the sense that it causes marked disruption of everyday activities, mood changes, and often disrupted sleep patterns. Tinnitus has been reported in children, but in its severe form it is far more common in adults and the elderly (Davis and El Rafaie, 2000).

What distinguishes mild from severe tinnitus is not established, apart from variations in subjective ratings of intrusiveness and loudness. In particular, in attempts to determine the handicap caused by tinnitus, it has not been possible to make the determination using aspects of the tinnitus itself (e.g., loudness, character, etc.). Moreover, tinnitus has been notoriously difficult to measure objectively. However, psychological complaints are of major importance in determining the severity of tinnitus (Andersson, 2001). In line with the difficulties associated with measuring tinnitus, no consensus has been reached regarding its classification, and several schemes have been proposed. Structured interviews and validated self-report questionnaires are helpful when describing tinnitus.

Among the most influential theories on why tinnitus causes annoyance is Hallam's psychological model of tinnitus (Hallam, Rachman, and Hinchcliffe, 1984) and Jastreboff's (1990) neurophysiological model. The latter model puts less emphasis on conscious mechanisms involved in tinnitus perception. Basically, Jastreboff presents a conditioning model in which the tinnitus signal is conditioned to aversive reactions such as anxiety and fear.

Audiological Characteristics

Measurement of tinnitus involves subjective report and a history of its features, such as loudness, character, fluctuations, and severity. Patients have described tinnitus as tones, buzzing noises, and mixtures of buzzing and ringing. More complicated descriptions include metallic sounds and multiple tones of varying frequencies.

Since the 1930s, tinnitus has been measured by asking the patient to compare the tinnitus with an external tone or combinations of tones. Tinnitus loudness can be presented at hearing level (HL) or sensation level (SL), the latter being the level of tinnitus above hearing threshold. Further, tinnitus loudness can be matched using the tinnitus frequency (for which hearing is often impaired) or another frequency where hearing is normal (Henry and Meikle, 2000). Contralateral versus ipsilateral matching is another choice. Determining the minimal masking level is a way to quantify the intrusiveness of tinnitus by determining how loud a sound needs to be to mask the tinnitus (Henry and Meikle, 2000). Pioneering work by Feldmann (1971) revealed that tinnitus patients could be categorized according to how tones of different frequencies masked the tinnitus (so-called masking curves). For example, one type of tinnitus was equally masked by tones of low and high frequency, whereas another type of tinnitus was more easily masked by low-frequency tones. Tinnitus can often be masked by white noise, at least temporarily (Henry and Meikle, 2000).

Emotional and Cognitive Disturbances

Tinnitus patients often report difficulties with concentration, such as during reading. Until recently, few attempts were made to measure tinnitus patients' performance on tests of cognitive functioning, but preliminary results corroborate the self-report findings (Andersson et al., 2000).

In its severe form, tinnitus is often associated with lowered mood and depression. There are only a few studies that have endorsed structured psychiatric interviews, and most of the available data are based on questionnaires. Suicide related to tinnitus is rare. Most cases reported had associated comorbid psychiatric disturbances (Lewis, Stephens, and McKenna, 1994). Anxiety, and in particular anxious preoccupation with somatic sensations, is an important aggravating factor related to distress caused by tinnitus (Newman, Wharton, and Jacobson, 1997). Stress is often mentioned as a negative factor for tinnitus, in particular the stress of major adverse life events. Finally, sleep problems are a significant component of tinnitus patients' complaints (McKenna, 2000).

Tinnitus and the Brain

Researchers and clinicians have long suspected that tinnitus involves certain areas of the brain, particularly those that subserve the perception and amplify the experience. Studies have been conducted on tinnitus patients' reaction times, brainstem audiometry, evoked potentials, and magnetoencephalography. Tinnitus has recently been studied using single photon emission computed tomography, positron emission tomography (e.g., Mirz et al., 1999), and functional magnetic resonance imaging. Findings from brain imaging studies suggest that tinnitus can be objectively measured, but are not consistent. However, it is clear that tinnitus affects brain areas related to hearing and processing of sounds, but also that some involvement of the brain's attentional and emotional systems might be involved (e.g., the amygdala).

Treatment

There is a long history of attempts to cure tinnitus. Although there are ways to alleviate the suffering, surgical and pharmacological interventions have been largely unsuccessful (Dobie, 1999). A pharmacological agent that reliably abolishes tinnitus for a short period is the local anesthetic agent lidocaine (Davies, 2001). About 60% of tinnitus sufferers respond to lidocaine administered intravenously, which in some cases totally abolishes tinnitus for a brief period. Because of side effects and the lack of effective oral analogues, lidocaine is not a viable treatment for tinnitus (Davies, 2001).

One treatment alternative for selected patients with tinnitus is antidepressants. A few studies have found positive results with respect to tinnitus annoyance, whereas more modest results were found in another study. More studies are needed, in particular to investigate the effects of selective serotonin reuptake inhibitors.

Tinnitus is rarely the only indication for surgery unless clear objective findings can identify a causal agent (e.g., nerve compression). However, when surgery is called for, the effects on tinnitus have been unclear. In some patients tinnitus disappears, but in others it remains unchanged or becomes worse (Hazell, 1990).

Alternative medicine approaches (such as *Gingko biloba* and acupuncture) either have not been tested or, when trials have been conducted, have yielded disappointing results (Davies, 2001).

The effects of electrical stimulation have been investigated in two forms. The first is application of electric current via transcutaneous nerve stimulation, and the second is through cochlear implantation, in which electrodes are inserted into the cochlea. The latter approach is most interesting, as cases have been reported in which tinnitus disappears while the implant is on and returns when it is turned off (Dauman, 2000).

There is a long history of attempts to treat tinnitus via maskers and, more recently, white noise generators. These are basically hearing aid-like devices that emit noise of broadband or narrow-band character. Unfortunately, there are few controlled trials on the use of masking devices or white noise generators. The studies that do exist do not support the efficacy of masking, but clinical experience suggests that they help some people (Vernon and Meikle, 2000).

More recently a treatment method called tinnitus retraining therapy (TRT) has been developed. TRT has two parts, one consisting of counseling in a directive format and the other part providing "sound enrichment" using white noise generators set at a level that does not cover tinnitus (Jastreboff and Jastreboff, 2000).

Among the treatments aimed at reducing distress, cognitive-behavioral therapy (CBT) is the most researched alternative (Andersson, 2001). CBT is a relatively brief psychological treatment approach directed at identifying and modifying maladaptive behaviors and cognitions by means of behavior change and cognitive restructuring. The focus is on applying techniques such as applied relaxation in real-life settings. There is evidence that CBT can be effective in alleviating the distress caused by tinnitus, and also that it works in a self-help format presented via the Internet (Andersson et al., 2002).

—*Gerhard Andersson*

References

Andersson, G. (2001). The role of psychology in managing tinnitus: A cognitive behavioural approach. *Seminars in Hearing, 22*, 65–76.

Andersson, G., Eriksson, J., Lundh, L.-G., and Lyttkens, L. (2000). Tinnitus and cognitive interference: A Stroop paradigm study. *Journal of Speech, Hearing, and Language Research, 43*, 1168–1173.

Andersson, G., Strömgren, T., Ström, T., and Lyttkens, L. (2002). Randomised controlled trial of Internet based cognitive behavior therapy for distress associated with tinnitus. *Psychosomatic Medicine, 64*, 810–816.

Dauman, R. (2000). Electrical stimulation for tinnitus suppression. In R. S. Tyler (Ed.), *Tinnitus handbook* (pp. 377–398). San Diego, CA: Singular/Thomson Learning.

Davies, W. E. (2001). Future prospects for the pharmacological treatment of tinnitus. *Seminars in Hearing, 22,* 89–99.

Davis, A., and El Rafie, E. A. (2000). Epidemiology of tinnitus. In R. S. Tyler (Ed.), *Tinnitus handbook* (pp. 1–23). San Diego, CA: Singular/Thomson Learning.

Dobie, R. A. (1999). A review of randomized clinical trials of tinnitus. *Laryngoscope, 109,* 1202–1211.

Feldmann, H. (1971). Homolateral and contralateral masking of tinnitus by noise-bands and pure tones. *Audiology, 10,* 138–144.

Hallam, R. S., Rachman, S., and Hinchcliffe, R. (1984). Psychological aspects of tinnitus. In S. Rachman (Ed.), *Contributions to medical psychology* (pp. 31–53). Oxford, U.K.: Pergamon Press.

Hazell, J. W. P. (1990). Tinnitus: II. Surgical management of conditions associated with tinnitus and somatosounds. *Journal of Otolaryngology, 19,* 6–10.

Henry, J. A., and Meikle, M. B. (2000). Psychoacoustic measures of tinnitus. *Journal of the American Academy of Audiology, 11,* 138–155.

Jastreboff, P. J. (1990). Phantom auditory perception (tinnitus): Mechanisms of generation and perception. *Neuroscience Research, 8,* 221–254.

Jastreboff, P. J., and Jastreboff, M. M. (2000). Tinnitus retraining therapy (TRT) as a method for treatment of tinnitus and hyperacusis patients. *Journal of the American Academy of Audiology, 11,* 162–177.

Levine, R. A. (2001). Diagnostic issues in tinnitus: A neuro-otological perspective. *Seminars in Hearing, 22,* 23–36.

Lewis, J. E., Stephens, S. D. G., and McKenna, L. (1994). Tinnitus and suicide. *Clinical Otolaryngology, 19,* 50–54.

McKenna, L. (2000). Tinnitus and insomnia. In R. S. Tyler (Ed.), *Tinnitus handbook* (pp. 59–84). San Diego, CA: Singular/Thomson Learning.

Mirz, F., Pedersen, C. B., Ishizu, K., Johannsen, P., Ovesen, T., Sødkilde-Jørgensen, H., and Gjedde, A. (1999). Positron emission tomography of cortical centres of tinnitus. *Hearing Research, 134,* 133–144.

Newman, C. W., Wharton, J. A., and Jacobson, G. P. (1997). Self-focused and somatic attention in patients with tinnitus. *Journal of the American Academy of Audiology, 8,* 143–149.

Rauschecker, J. P. (1999). Auditory cortical plasticity: A comparison with other sensory systems. *Trends in Neuroscience, 22,* 74–80.

Vernon, J. A., and Meikle, M. B. (2000). Tinnitus masking. In R. S. Tyler (Ed.), *Tinnitus handbook* (pp. 313–356). San Diego, CA: Singular/Thomson Learning.

Further Readings

Andersson, G., and Lyttkens, L. (1999). A meta-analytic review of psychological treatments for tinnitus. *British Journal of Audiology, 33,* 201–210.

Andersson, G., Vretblad, P., Larsen, H.-C., and Lyttkens, L. (2001). Longitudinal follow-up of tinnitus complaints. *Archives of Otolaryngology–Head and Neck Surgery, 127,* 175–179.

Drew, S., and Davies, E. (2001). Effectiveness of *Gingko biloba* in treating tinnitus: Double blind, placebo controlled trial. *British Medical Journal, 322,* 1–6.

Giraud, A. L., Chéry-Croze, S., Fischer, G., Fischer, C., Vighetto, A., Grégoire, M.-C., et al. (1999). A selective imaging of tinnitus. *NeuroReport, 10,* 1–5.

Hallam, R. S. (1989). *Living with tinnitus: Dealing with the ringing in your ears.* Wellingborough, U.K.: Thorson's.

Hazell, J. W. P., Wood, S. M., Cooper, H. R., Stephens, S. D. G., Corcoran, A. L., Coles, R. R. A., et al. (1985). A clinical study of tinnitus maskers. *British Journal of Audiology, 19,* 65–146.

Henry, J. L., and Wilson, P. H. (2001). *Psychological management of chronic tinnitus: A cognitive-behavioral approach.* Boston: Allyn and Bacon.

Lockwood, A. H., Salvi, R. J., Coad, M. L., Towsley, M. L., Wack, D. S., and Murphy, B. W. (1998). The functional neuroanatomy of tinnitus: Evidence for limbic system links and neural plasticity. *Neurology, 50,* 114–120.

McCombe, A., Baguley, D., Coles, R., McKenna, L., McKinney, C., and Windle-Taylor, P. (2001). Guidelines for the grading of tinnitus severity: The results of a working group commissioned by the British Association of Otolaryngologists, Head and Neck Surgeons. *Clinical Otolaryngology, 26,* 388–393.

McFadden, D. (1982). *Tinnitus: Facts, theories, and treatments.* Washington, DC: National Academy Press.

Melcher, J. R., Sigalosky, I. S., Guinan, J. J., and Levine, R. A. (2000). Lateralized tinnitus studied with functional magnetic resonance imaging: Abnormal inferior colliculus activation. *Journal of Neurophysiology, 83,* 1058–1072.

Noble, W. (2000). Self-reports about tinnitus and about cochlear implants. *Ear and Hearing, 21,* 50S–59S.

Park, J., White, A. R., and Ernst, E. (2000). Efficacy of acupuncture as a treatment for tinnitus: A systematic review. *Archives of Otolaryngology–Head and Neck Surgery, 126,* 489–492.

Schulman, A. (1995). A final common pathway for tinnitus: The medial temporal lobe system. *International Tinnitus Journal, 1,* 115–126.

Stephens, D. (2000). A history of tinnitus. In R. S. Tyler (Ed.), *Tinnitus handbook* (pp. 437–448). San Diego, CA: Singular/Thomson Learning.

Tyler, R. S. (Ed.). (2000). *Tinnitus handbook.* San Diego, CA: Singular/Thomson Learning.

Tympanometry

Tympanometry is a measure of the acoustic admittance or ease with which acoustic energy flows into the middle ear transmission system as air pressure is varied in the ear canal. This measure is accomplished by sealing a small probe device into the ear canal. A speaker delivers a probe signal, typically 226 Hz, into the ear canal, and a microphone measures the amplitude and phase of the probe signal admitted into the middle ear system. The acoustic admittance is determined by the combined stiffness (or conversely, compliance), mass, and resistance of the eardrum and all middle ear structures. In the presence of middle ear pathology, these admittance characteristics are altered, and therefore the amplitude and phase of the probe signal measured in the ear canal are also altered. In pathology such as middle ear effusion, the eardrum is stiffened by fluid in the middle ear cavity, and only minimal acoustic energy from the probe signal is admitted into the middle ear; acoustic admittance in the plane of the eardrum is described as low. In contrast, pathology such as ossicular discontinuity makes the ear less stiff, so that most of the acoustic en-

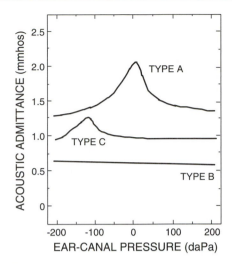

Figure 1. Three patterns of tympanograms recorded using a 226 Hz probe signal. Type A is normal, type B is flat, and type C has a negative tympanogram peak pressure.

ergy from the probe signal is admitted into the middle ear system, and acoustic admittance is high.

In addition to the loudspeaker and microphone, the probe system is connected to a pneumatic pump that adjusts ear canal pressure over a range from -600 to $+400$ daPa. The dekapascal (daPa) is the unit of pressure that has replaced mm H_2O (ANSI S3.39-1987). The two units, however, are nearly interchangeable (1 daPa = 1.02 mm H_2O).

Tympanometry became a routine clinical procedure following the landmark paper of Jerger (1970). Jerger identified three basic tympanogram shapes. A tympanogram is a graphic display of acoustic admittance measured as a function of changing ear canal pressure. A normal type A tympanogram is shown in Figure 1. Introduction of extreme pressures into the sealed ear canal stiffens the eardrum, and theoretically, all of the acoustic energy from the probe signal is reflected at the surface of the eardrum, and admittance reaches a minimum. Acoustic admittance gradually increases to a maximum, and the probe signal becomes most audible, when the pressure in the ear canal equals the pressure in the middle ear cavity. When the eustachian tube is functioning normally, atmospheric pressure of 0 daPa is maintained in the middle ear cavity, and tympanogram peak pressure (TPP) also is 0 daPa. The ear canal pressure producing peak admittance, therefore, provides an estimate of middle ear pressure. When the eardrum is retracted and negative middle ear pressure exists, the peak of the tympanograms shifts to a corresponding negative value. This tympanogram pattern is designated type C in Figure 1. The third tympanogram, designated type B, has no discernible peak and is flat. This pattern is recorded from ears with middle ear effusion (MEE), perforated eardrums, or patent pressure-equalization tubes (PET).

Tympanogram shape also has been quantified in an attempt to aid in the diagnosis of middle ear disease and

to establish objective criteria for medical referral. Four commonly used calculations are depicted in Figure 2. The first, acoustic equivalent volume (V_{ea}), is an estimate of the ear canal volume between the probe device and the eardrum. This estimate typically is made using a 226-Hz probe signal and an ear canal pressure of 200 daPa. When the probe device is sealed in the ear canal, the measured acoustic admittance reflects the combined effects of the ear canal and the middle ear. Under extreme ear canal pressures, however, the eardrum theoretically becomes so stiff that acoustic admittance into the middle ear decreases to 0 mmhos. The admittance measured at extreme pressures then is attributed solely to the ear canal volume. When a 226-Hz probe signal is used, the acoustic admittance measured at 200 daPa is equal to the volume of the ear canal. In Figure 2, V_{ea} equals 0.6 cm^3. In children less than 7 years old, V_{ea} ranges from 0.3 to 0.9 cm^3 (Margolis and Heller, 1987; Shanks et al., 1992). In adults, V_{ea} averages 1.3 cm^3 in women and 1.5 cm^3 in men (Wiley et al., 1996). As a subsequent example will demonstrate, V_{ea} is useful in differentiating between intact and perforated eardrums when a flat type B tympanogram is recorded.

Peak compensated static acoustic admittance (Y_{tm}) is the amplitude of the tympanogram between the peak and 200 daPa. This measure describes the acoustic admittance of the middle ear transmission system compensated for or minus the effects of the ear canal volume. In Figure 2, Y_{tm} is 1.1 acoustic mmhos, calculated as peak admittance (1.7 mmhos) minus ear canal admittance (0.6 mmhos). Many instruments "baseline correct" at 200 daPa, so that Y_{tm} can be read directly from the y-axis. If the tympanogram in Figure 2 were baseline corrected, zero admittance would be shifted upward to correspond with the V_{ea} at 200 daPa. If a middle ear problem produces abnormally high stiffness, the

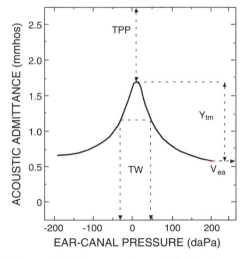

Figure 2. Four calculations made on 226 Hz tympanograms: acoustic equivalent volume (V_{ea}, in cm^3), peak compensated static acoustic admittance (Y_{tm}, in acoustic mmhos), tympanogram width (TW, in daPa), and tympanogram peak pressure (TPP, in daPa).

Table 1. Means and 90% Ranges for V_{ea}, Y_{tm}, TW, and TPP from Several Large-Scale Studies in Subjects 8 Weeks to 90 Years Old with Normal Middle Ear Transmission Systems

Study	Age (yr)	N	Statistic	V_{ea} (cm³)	Y_{tm} (mmhos)	TW (daPa)	TPP (daPa)
Wiley et al. (1996)	48–90	2147	Mean	1.36	0.66	75	−23
			90% range	0.9–2.0	0.2–1.5	35–125	−85 to 5
Margolis and Heller (1987)	19–61	87	Mean	1.05	0.78	77	−19
			90% range	0.63–1.46	0.32–1.46	51–114	−83 to 0
	2.8–5.8	92	Mean	0.74	0.55	100	−30
			90% range	0.42–0.97	0.22–0.92	59–151	−139 to 11
Nozza et al. (1992, 1994)	3–16	130	Mean	0.90	0.78	104	−34
			90% range	0.60–1.35	0.40–1.39	60–168	−207 to 15
Roush et al. (1995)	0.5–2.5	+1636	Mean		0.45	148	
			90% range		0.20–0.70	102–204	
Shanks et al. (1992)	8 wk–7 yr	334	Mean	0.58			
			90% range	0.3–0.9			

Abbreviations: V_{ea}, acoustic equivalent volume; Y_{tm}, peak compensated static acoustic admittance; TW, tympanogram width; TPP, tympanogram peak pressure.

amplitude of the tympanogram, or Y_{tm}, will decrease. Conversely, if a middle ear problem decreases the stiffness of the eardrum or middle ear, Y_{tm} will increase. Y_{tm} at 226 Hz normally increases slightly from infancy to adulthood, with a mean of 0.5 acoustic mmhos at 4 months to 0.7 acoustic mmhos in adulthood (Margolis and Heller, 1987; Holte, Margolis, and Cavanaugh, 1991; Roush et al., 1995; Wiley et al., 1996).

Tympanogram width (TW), defined as the width in daPa at one-half Y_{tm}, is a measure of the broadness of a tympanogram peak. In Figure 2, TW is 85 daPa. TW is not highly correlated with Y_{tm}, and therefore it provides supplemental information regarding middle ear function (Koebsell and Margolis, 1986). TW has been most useful in identifying children with middle ear effusion (MEE). In some cases of MEE, Y_{tm} is normal but TW is abnormally broad. Nozza et al. (1992, 1994) reported that a TW greater than 275 daPa was associated with a high sensitivity (81%) and specificity (82%) in identifying MEE.

The fourth measure, TPP, provides an estimate of middle ear pressure or indirect measure of eustachian tube function. Figure 2 shows a normal TPP of 10 daPa. Not all individuals with negative middle ear pressure develop MEE. Results from school screening programs showed that medical referral on the basis of TPP alone resulted in unacceptably high overreferral rates, and therefore TPP is no longer used in referral criteria. A negative TPP in conjunction with a reduced Y_{tm} is a much stronger indication of MEE and cause for medical referral (Feldman, 1976).

Table 1 shows means and 90% normal ranges for V_{ea}, Y_{tm}, TW, and TPP from several large-scale studies in subjects ages 8 weeks to 90 years. These calculations are significantly affected by the procedures (e.g., rate and direction of pressure changes and the pressure used to estimate V_{ea}) used to record the tympanogram (Shanks and Wilson, 1986). The data presented in Table 1 were calculated from tympanograms recorded using the most commonly used parameters, descending pressure changes at rates of 200–600 daPa/s and correction for ear canal volume at 200 daPa.

The remaining figures depict tympanometry findings for a variety of middle ear pathologies. The probe signal frequency most commonly used to measure the admittance properties of the middle ear is 226 Hz. Although this low-frequency probe signal was selected partly at random during instrument development (Terkildsen and Scott Nielson, 1960), it remains the most commonly used probe signal. Acoustic admittance measurements at low frequencies are dominated by the stiffness characteristics of the eardrum and middle ear transmission system, whereas measurements made at high frequencies are dominated by mass characteristics. Although high-frequency probe signals of 660–1000 Hz are valuable in assessing the mass characteristics of the middle ear, the tympanogram patterns that result at high frequencies are more complex and have not enjoyed widespread use. Only low-frequency tympanograms are presented in subsequent examples, but cases where high-frequency probe signals might be advantageous are pointed out. Additional references on high-frequency tympanometry are provided.

Figure 3 shows a series of tympanograms recorded from a child recovering from a 3-month episode of otitis media with MEE. When first evaluated, the admittance tympanogram was flat (type B), with a normal V_{ea} of 0.45 mmhos. Sequential pure-tone audiograms showed air–bone gaps across all frequencies, ranging from 10 dB to 55 dB, that were greatest at 250 and 4000 Hz and smallest at 2000 Hz. Over time, the tympanogram changed to a type C pattern. In early recovery, the tympanogram, shown by the heavy line, had a shallow (Y_{tm} = 0.25 mmhos), broad peak (TW = 200 daPa) with negative peak pressure (TPP = −100 daPa). Air–bone gaps decreased to 10–25 dB and were largest at 4000 Hz. This tympanogram pattern has been demonstrated in human temporal bones injected with middle ear fluid up to the level of the umbo, producing a mass loading effect on the eardrum (Renvall, Liden, and

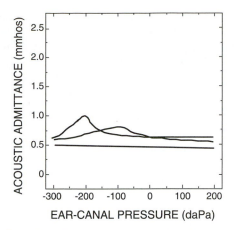

Figure 3. Type B and two type C acoustic admittance tympanograms recorded using a 226 Hz probe signal from a child during recovery from otitis media with effusion.

Bjorkman, 1975). The mass effect is greatest at high frequencies, as reflected by large air–bone gaps at 4000 Hz, and is accentuated when tympanometry is performed using high-frequency probe signals such as 600–800 Hz. Further resolution of the otitis media produced a type C tympanogram, increasing to normal Y_{tm} (0.35 mmhos) with a TPP of −200 daPa. Small air–bone gaps of 15–20 dB at this time were confined to the 250–1000 Hz range and were virtually closed at 4000 Hz, indicating increased stiffness of the eardrum from the negative middle ear pressure without the mass loading effects of the middle ear fluid. The tympanogram gradually returned to a type A. This case study demonstrates a variety of tympanogram patterns associated with otitis media. Rather than being a drawback, the various tympanogram shapes help clinicians track the resolution of MEE.

The American Speech-Language-Hearing Association (1997) has developed guidelines for screening infants and children for chronic middle ear disorders with the potential for causing significant hearing loss or long-lasting speech, language, and learning deficits. Medical referral is advised for infants when Y_{tm} is less than 0.2 mmhos or TW is greater than 235 daPa, and for 1- to 5-year-olds when Y_{tm} is less than 0.3 mmhos or TW is greater than 200 daPa if these abnormal findings persist at a 6–8-week rescreening. Immediate medical referral is recommended for otalgia, otorrhea, or eardrum perforation noted otoscopically or from a flat tympanogram with V_{ea} greater than 1.0 cm^3. Screening guidelines are not available for infants less than 7 months old. In this age group, tympanogram shapes at 226 Hz are irregular and difficult to interpret (Holte, Margolis, and Cavanaugh, 1991).

Figure 4 displays three type B tympanograms. The bottom tympanogram was recorded from an ear with an intact eardrum and MEE; V_{ea} of 0.45 cm^3 is normal for a child's ear canal. The other two tympanograms also are flat but V_{ea} is 3.25 cm^3 in one case and greater than 5.0 cm^3 in the other. The middle tympanogram was

recorded from an ear with a patent PET, and the top tympanogram was recorded from an ear with a traumatic perforation from a Q-tip. V_{ea} often is larger with a traumatic eardrum perforation than with a perforation associated with chronic middle ear disease and poorly developed mastoid air-cell system (Andreasson, 1977).

In a child less than 7 years old, a volume greater than 1.0 cm^3 is indicative of a perforated eardrum, whereas in adults the volume must exceed 2.5 cm^3 (Shanks et al., 1992). Volumes exceeding these ranges clearly indicate a perforated eardrum, but flat tympanograms with smaller volumes do not necessarily rule out eardrum perforation. A flat tympanogram with a normal V_{ea} can also be recorded from an ear with eardrum perforation and cholesteatoma filling the middle ear space and closing off the mastoid air-cell system. Case history and otoscopic examination are very important in these cases. No consistent pattern of hearing loss is associated with eardrum perforation; air–bone gaps can be absent or as large as 50–70 dB if necrosis of the incus also occurs.

Figure 5 demonstrates that otosclerosis also is associated with a variety of tympanogram shapes. Tympanograms vary from a normal type A pattern (shown in Fig. 1) to a low-admittance, stiff pattern (type A_s) shown by the lower tympanogram in Figure 5. A third pattern frequently recorded in otosclerosis is a normal type A pattern, but with a narrow tympanogram width (Shanks, 1984; Shahnaz and Polka, 1997). Pure-tone audiometry in otosclerosis shows a stiffness tilt, with the largest air–bone gaps at low frequencies and the smallest air–bone gap near 2000 Hz. Otosclerosis is virtually the only middle ear pathology where significant air–bone gaps are measured in conjunction with a normal type A tympanogram.

Figure 6 shows two cases of type A tympanograms with abnormally high Y_{tm} (2.5 mmhos). Normal tympanograms with deep peaks sometimes are designated type A_d. The bottom tympanogram was recorded from

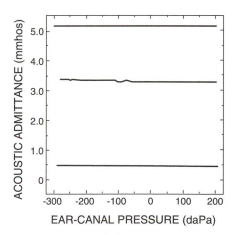

Figure 4. Type B acoustic admittance tympanograms recorded using a 226 Hz probe signal from an ear with middle ear effusion (bottom tympanogram), an ear with a patent pressure equalization tube (middle tympanogram), and an ear with a traumatic eardrum perforation (top tympanogram).

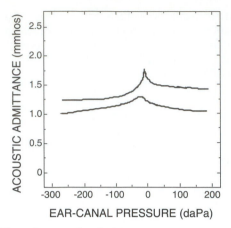

Figure 5. Type A acoustic admittance tympanograms recorded using a 226 Hz probe signal in two ears with surgically confirmed otosclerosis.

an ear with traumatic ossicular discontinuity; the audiogram showed a maximum conductive hearing loss with 30–70 dB air–bone gaps. The top tympanogram was recorded from an ear with a monomeric eardrum resulting from a healed perforation; the audiogram showed slight air–bone gaps at only 3000 and 4000 Hz. This A_d pattern also is typical of ears with tympanosclerotic plaques on the eardrum and status post stapedectomy. These cases of high-admittance pathology are another indication for high-frequency tympanometry. High-frequency tympanograms in ears with ossicular discontinuity typically exhibit broader, more undulating peaks than tympanograms recorded from ears with eardrum pathology. In cases of high Y_{tm}, otoscopic examination of the eardrum is crucial; high-admittance pathology of the eardrum can dominate or mask low-admittance pathology such as otosclerosis. Pure-tone audiometry also is invaluable in these cases. Eardrum pathology alone does not produce a significant conductive hearing loss,

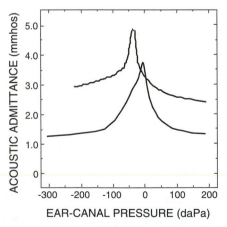

Figure 6. Type A_d acoustic admittance tympanograms recorded using a 226 Hz probe signal in an ear with traumatic ossicular discontinuity (bottom tympanogram) and in an ear with a monomeric tympanic membrane (top tympanogram).

whereas ossicular discontinuity results in a maximum conductive hearing loss.

The preceding cases demonstrate that tympanometry is most beneficial when used as one of a battery of tests that also include case history, otoscopic examination, and pure-tone audiometry. The cases also demonstrate that each unique middle ear problem does not produce one and only one tympanogram pattern. On the contrary, a single pathology can produce several different tympanometry patterns, and conversely, a single tympanogram pattern can result from several different middle ear problems. When used with a battery of tests, however, the contribution from tympanometry can be unique and informative.

See also MIDDLE EAR ASSESSMENT IN THE CHILD.

—*Janet E. Shanks*

References

American National Standards Institute. (1987). *Specifications for instruments to measure aural acoustic impedance and admittance (aural acoustic immittance) (ANSI S3.39-1987).* New York: Acoustical Society of America.

American Speech-Language-Hearing Association Audiologic Assessment Panel. (1996, 1997). *Guidelines for audiologic screening.* Rockville, MD: Author.

Andreasson, L. (1977). Correlation of tubal function and volume of mastoid and middle ear space as related to otitis media. *Acta Otolaryngologica, 83,* 29–33.

Feldman, A. (1976). Tympanometry: Procedures, interpretations and variables. In A. S. Feldman and L. A. Wilbur (Eds.), *Acoustic impedance and admittance: The measurement of middle ear function* (pp. 103–155). Baltimore: Williams and Wilkins.

Holte, L., Margolis, R., and Cavanaugh, R. (1991). Developmental changes in multifrequency tympanograms. *Audiology, 30,* 1–24.

Jerger, J. (1970). Clinical experience with impedance audiometry. *Archives of Otolaryngology, 92,* 311–324.

Koebsell, K., and Margolis, R. (1986). Tympanometric gradient measured from normal preschool children. *Audiology, 25,* 149–157.

Margolis, R., and Heller, J. (1987). Screening tympanometry: Criteria for medical referral. *Audiology, 26,* 197–208.

Nozza, R., Bluestone, C., Kardatze, D., and Bachman, R. (1992). Towards the validation of aural acoustic immittance measures for diagnosis of middle ear effusion in children. *Ear and Hearing, 13,* 442–453.

Nozza, R., Bluestone, C., Kardatze, D., and Bachman, R. (1994). Identification of middle ear effusion by aural acoustic immittance measures for diagnosis of middle ear effusion in children. *Ear and Hearing, 15,* 310–323.

Renvall, U., Liden, G., and Bjorkman, G. (1975). Experimental tympanometry in human temporal bones. *Scandinavian Audiology, 4,* 135–144.

Roush, J., Bryant, K., Mundy, M., Zeisel, S., and Roberts, J. (1995). Developmental changes in static admittance and tympanometric width in infants and toddlers. *Journal of the American Academy of Audiology, 6,* 334–338.

Shahnaz, N., and Polka, L. (1997). Standard and multifrequency tympanometry in normal and otosclerotic ears. *Ear and Hearing, 18,* 326–341.

Shanks, J. (1984). Tympanometry. *Ear and Hearing, 5,* 268–280.

Shanks, J., Stelmachowicz, P., Beauchaine, K., and Schulte, L. (1992). Equivalent ear canal volumes in children pre- and post-tympanostomy tube insertion. *Journal of Speech and Hearing Research, 35,* 936–941.

Shanks, J., and Wilson, R. (1986). Effects of direction and rate of ear-canal pressure changes on tympanometric measures. *Journal of Speech and Hearing Research, 29,* 11–19.

Terkildsen, K., Scott Nielsen, S. (1960). An electroacoustic impedance measuring bridge for clinical use. *Archives of Otolaryngology, 72,* 339–346.

Wiley, T., Cruickshanks, K., Nondahl, D., Tweed, T., Klein, R., and Klein, B. (1996). Tympanometric measures in older adults. *Journal of the American Academy of Audiology, 7,* 260–268.

Further Readings

Colletti, V. (1977). Multifrequency tympanometry. *Audiology, 16,* 278–287.

Fowler, C., and Shanks, J. (2002). Tympanometry. In J. Katz (Ed.), *Handbook of clinical audiology* (pp. 175–204). Baltimore: Lippincott Williams and Wilkins.

Liden, G., Peterson, J., and Bjorkman, G. (1970). Tympanometry: A method for analysis of middle ear function. *Acta Otolaryngologica, 263,* 218–224.

Lilly, D. (1984). Multiple frequency, multiple component tympanometry: New approaches to an old diagnostic problem. *Ear and Hearing, 5,* 300–308.

Margolis, R. (1981). Fundamentals of acoustic immittance. In G. Popelka (Ed.), *Hearing assessment with the acoustic reflex* (pp. 117–144). New York: Grune and Stratton.

Margolis, R., Paul, S., Saly, G., Schachern, P., and Keefe, D. (2001). Wideband reflectance tympanometry in chinchillas and humans. *Journal of the Acoustical Society of America, 110,* 1453–1464.

Margolis, R., Van Camp, K., Wilson, R., and Creten, W. (1985). Multi-frequency tympanometry in normal ears. *Audiology, 24,* 44–53.

Shanks, J., and Shelton, C. (1991). Basic principles and clinical applications of tympanometry. *Otolaryngology Clinics of North America, 24,* 299–328.

Shanks, J., Wilson, R., and Cambron, N. (1993). Multiple frequency tympanometry: Effects of ear canal volume compensation on static acoustic admittance and estimates of middle ear resonance. *Journal of Speech and Hearing Research, 36,* 178–185.

Vanhuyse, V., Creten, W., and Van Camp, K. (1975). On the W-notching of tympanograms. *Scandinavian Audiology, 4,* 45–50.

Zwislocki, J. (1982). Normal function of the middle ear and its measurement. *Audiology, 21,* 4–14.

Vestibular Rehabilitation

The concept of prescribing exercise for persons with dizziness was first described by Cooksey and Cawthorne in the 1950s (Cawthorne, 1944; Cooksey, 1946). Today, exercise for persons with vestibular disorders is considered to be the standard of care (Cowand et al., 1998; Herdman, 1990; Herdman, 1992; Herdman et al., 1995; Herdman and Whitney, 2000). Exercises are specifically prescribed that help the person with a vestibular disorder either compensate for or adapt to the impairment (She-pard and Telian, 1993). Knowledge of vestibular anatomy, physiology, pathologies involved, and an in-depth understanding of how various interventions can affect outcome is very important for effective treatment of persons with vestibular disorders. Exercises to decrease the risk of falling, improve balance and postural control, improve confidence, and decrease the subjective feelings of dizziness also seem to decrease a patient's anxiety (Jacob et al., 2000). Vestibular exercise programs have been shown to enhance the speed and degree of recovery (Herdman et al., 1995; Horak et al., 1992; Krebs et al., 1993; Strupp et al., 1998; Yardley et al., 1998).

Common conditions often referred for vestibular physical and occupational therapy include benign paroxysmal positional vertigo (BPPV) (Blakely, 1994; Herdman et al., 1993; Lynn et al., 1995), bilateral vestibulopathy (Brown et al., 2001; Krebs et al., 1993; Telian et al., 1991), endolymphatic hydrops, labyrinthine concussion (Cowand et al., 1998; Fujino et al., 1996; Horak et al., 1992; Shepard et al., 1990; Shepard et al., 1993; Smith-Wheelock et al., 1991), labyrinthitis (Cowand et al., 1998; Fujino et al., 1996; Shepard et al., 1990; Shepard et al., 1993; Smith-Wheelock et al., 1991), Ménière's disease (Cowand et al., 1998; Fujino et al., 1996; Shepard et al., 1990; Shepard et al., 1993; Smith-Wheelock et al., 1991), perilymph fistula, and vestibular neuritis. Central diagnoses include cervicogenic dizziness, brainstem hemorrhage (Cowand et al., 1998; Horak et al., 1992; Shepard et al., 1990; Shepard et al., 1995; Smith-Wheelock et al., 1991), posttraumatic anxiety symptoms, stroke/transient ischemic attacks (TIA), traumatic head injury (Cowand et al., 1998; Horak et al., 1992; Shepard et al., 1990; Shepard et al., 1993), and migraine-related vestibulopathy (Cass et al., 1997; Whitney et al., 2000). Psychiatric disorders that have been reported to manifest with a component of dizziness include panic disorders (Jacob et al., 2000), agoraphobia (Jacob et al., 2000), and hyperventilation syndrome. The most common nonvestibular causes of dizziness are low blood pressure and medication-induced dizziness (Furman and Whitney, 2000).

Persons with vestibular disorder present with various complaints, and often report experiencing balance dysfunction, dizziness, vertigo, anxiety about their symptoms, space and motion complaints (symptoms elicited by a specific visual stimulus pattern (Furman and Cass, 1996), and fear of falling. They may describe visual disturbances, dysequilibrium, and dizziness occurring while they are at work, at home, or engaged in leisure activities. Common visual problems experienced include difficulty focusing while reading, "bouncing" of the visual world as they move (oscillopsia), impaired smooth pursuit, saccades, and vergence. Balance problems frequently noted include increased sway while standing, an inability to stand still, walking with a wide-based gait, veering during walking, adduction or crossing their legs during gait, difficulty walking in the dark or on uneven surfaces, bumping into things, or falling.

Tinnitus, difficulty hearing, and aural fullness are related cochlear signs reported by persons with vestibular disorders. Descriptions of problems related to the head include dizziness, spinning, headache, pressure, neck pain, a swimming sensation, and heaviness. Often, persons with vestibular disorders report fatigue and difficulty concentrating. All of these problems contribute to making vestibular disorders difficult to treat, as affected individuals may have multiple symptoms and frequently have more than one diagnosis.

A physical therapy evaluation provides information on impairments and functional deficits so that appropriate intervention can be determined. A thorough workup by the physician and vestibular function tests help direct the physical therapy evaluation and intervention. The patient history should include goals of treatment, premorbid health, current and premorbid activity level, and a description of the onset, frequency, duration, and severity of the dizziness and imbalance. Not all persons with vestibular disorders experience both dizziness and imbalance. Identifying the positions or situations that exacerbate or relieve the symptoms can afford valuable insight into the cause of the problem. Gaining an understanding of the magnitude of the functional deficits is very important. The intensity and duration of symptoms, the degree to which symptoms impede activities of daily living, and how symptoms affect social activities help to determine intervention.

A thorough exploration of the individual's history of falling can also provide insight into the physiology of the condition and the necessary treatment (Herdman et al., 2000; Whitney, Hudak, and Marchetti, 2000). Not simply the number of falls but also the conditions of the fall, the frequency of falling, and whether medical treatment was necessary are all important in the assessment of the person with a vestibular disorder. Fear of falling in individuals who have fallen may constrict their willingness to move (Tinetti and Powell, 1993).

The patient's medical and surgical history will affect the prescription of an exercise program. Persons with premorbid orthopedic and cardiac limitations need to be carefully monitored to ensure that they are safe with the exercise program. Frail, older adults may need to be seen more frequently in order to ensure compliance and safety with their exercises.

Typically, the range of motion of the joints, muscle strength, sensation, vision, motions that provoke symptoms, balance, and gait are all determined before an exercise program is started. Because of the influence of somatosensation on balance, it is important to assess range of motion and sensation, particularly in the ankles and cervical region. The visual assessment includes testing the function of the ocular muscles, including saccades and smooth pursuit, as well as the function of the vestibular ocular reflex.

Quantification of the movements and positions that trigger symptoms of dizziness not only provides information on the cause of the symptoms but may also help in selecting activities for treatment. Therapists commonly ask patients to move into and out of supine and side-lying positions, and then have the patients rate their symptoms on a verbal analogue scale and indicate the duration of the symptoms (Norre and De Weerdt, 1980; Smith-Wheelock et al., 1991). Monitoring the intensity and duration of the symptoms over the length of treatment can provide information on the recovery of the patient.

Two aspects of postural control should be evaluated, the ability to move the center of gravity within the base of support and the ability to utilize available sensory information for balance. The ability to move the center of gravity within the base of support is determined by asking the person to perform tasks such as shifting his or her weight while standing and then reaching for objects. This can be quantified by measuring how far the person can reach (i.e., the Functional Reach test [Duncan et al., 1990] or the multidirectional Reach test [Newton, 2001]) or how long they can maintain a position (i.e., standing on one foot or in tandem). In addition, the clinician can ask patients to twist their trunk, pick up objects from different surfaces, or stand on a narrow base of support to determine how stable they are doing functional activities. Having the person with a vestibular disorder stand on high-density foam with the eyes open and then closed (Clinical Test of Sensory Interaction and Balance, or CTSIB) (Shumway-Cook and Horak, 1986) can help the therapist determine the fall risk (Anacker and Di Fabio, 1992), and also how well the patient uses the sensory information that he or she has available (Shumway-Cook and Horak, 1986). Scores on the CTSIB have been shown to correlate with conditions 4 and 5 of computed dynamic posturography (Anacker and Di Fabio, 1992; Weber and Cass, 1993).

Patients with vestibular disorders often describe difficulty walking, especially under varying sensory conditions such as walking with head turns, in dimmed or absent lighting, or with movement in the environment. Assessment of the person's gait during various functional tasks and under different sensory conditions is crucial. Persons with a vestibular disorder are asked to walk, walk at different speeds, walk over and around objects, and walk with various head movements in order to determine how stable they are during ambulation (Whitney et al., 2000a; Whitney and Herdman, 2000). These tasks can be quantified using the time it takes to complete a task or by qualitatively describing the movements, as in the Dynamic Gait Index (Shumway-Cook and Woollacott, 1995).

The goals of vestibular rehabilitation include decreasing the risk of falling, improving gaze stability, improving the person's dynamic and static postural control, decreasing symptoms, and enhancing the individual's ability to carry out activities of daily living and to work. The achievement of these goals is through exercise and the practice of activities in a safe environment. Customized exercise programs are better than exercise handouts provided without direction as to which exercises are most important to perform (Shepard and Telian, 1995).

Vestibular rehabilitation intervention is prescribed individually for each patient. For patients with peripheral vestibular lesions, vestibular rehabilitation exercises are thought to promote compensation or recalibration of the vestibular system, specifically the vestibulo-ocular reflex (VOR). The system appears to recalibrate because an error signal is created from the slip of an image on the retina (Robinson, 1976; Fetter and Zee, 1988). The use of eye and head movements as an exercise to change the gain of the VOR results in a change in the inhibition of the activity in the vestibular nuclei, and consequently in enhanced patient function. Recovery of the VOR is frequency specific. Stimulation of the VOR through exercises must be performed at varying frequencies for maximal functional recovery (Godaux, Halleux, and Gobert, 1983; Lisberger, Miles, and Optican, 1983).

Activity after a lesion to the vestibular system is important. Animals that moved freely after surgery had faster functional recovery (Lacour, Roll, and Appaix, 1976). Patients with vestibular disorders had faster recovery and improved function when they increased their activity early after surgery (Herdman et al., 1995).

Some persons with vestibular disorders have little or no remaining vestibular function, owing to disease or ototoxicity. These persons must learn how to use remaining sensory function such as somotosensation and vision. In addition, receptors in the neck can assist in stabilizing vision and posture, although in patients with intact vestibular systems, the cervical ocular reflex contributes little to gaze stability. The cervical ocular reflex performs maximally at lower frequencies and is accentuated in patients with bilateral vestibular loss (Kasai and Zee, 1978; Bronstein and Hood, 1986). Smooth pursuits and saccades can also assist in stabilizing vision at slow speeds (Kasai and Zee, 1978; Segal and Katsarkas, 1988; Leigh et al., 1994). Patients who have no function in the vestibular system will never be able to walk in the dark, will have great difficulty walking on uneven surfaces, and will never be able to read and walk at the same time. Driving a car without any vestibular function is impossible because the visual field jumps (oscillopsia), especially as the car goes over bumps.

Patients with balance disorders are taught to maximize the sensory function that remains, to substitute for sensory loss, and to predetermine when they will have difficulty with balance so that they can modify their behavior. Exercises are prescribed to enhance the use of vestibular, visual, and somatosensory inputs. Habituation exercises may be recommended for patients with dizziness provoked by specific position changes.

The outcomes of vestibular rehabilitation have included a decrease in dizziness and vertigo, a decrease in the number of falls, improved gait, decreased neck pain, improved VOR, greater balance confidence, decreased anxiety, improvements in activities of daily living, and improvements in the perceived disability. Generally, persons with peripheral vestibular disorders have a better prognosis than those with central vestibular disorders. Persons with both central and peripheral vestibular disorders have a poorer prognosis. All persons

with vestibular disorders should have an opportunity to work with a knowledgeable physical or occupational therapist, because quality of life can be improved with vestibular rehabilitation.

—Susan L. Whitney and Diane M. Wrisley

References

Anacker, S. L., and Di Fabio, R. P. (1992). Influence of sensory inputs on standing balance in community-dwelling elders with a recent history of falling. *Physical Therapy, 72,* 575–581.

Blakely, B. W. (1994). A randomized, controlled assessment of the canalith repositioning maneuver. *Otolaryngology–Head and Neck Surgery, 110,* 391–396.

Bronstein, A. M., and Hood, J. D. (1986). The cervico-ocular reflex in normal subjects and patients with absent vestibular function. *Brain Research, 373,* 399–408.

Brown, K. E., Whitney, S. L., Wrisley, D. M., and Furman, J. M. (2001). Physical therapy outcomes for persons with bilateral vestibular loss. *Laryngoscope, 111,* 1812–1817.

Cass, S. P., Furman, J. M., Ankerstjerne, J. K., Balaban, C., Yetiser, S., and Aydogan, B. (1997). Migraine-related vestibulopathy. *Annals of Otology Rinology and Laryngology, 106,* 181–189.

Cawthorne, T. (1944). The physiological basis for head exercises. *Journal of the Chartered Society of Physiotherapy, 30,* 106–107.

Cooksey, F. S. (1946). Rehabilitation in Vestibular Injuries. *Proceedings of the Royal Society of Medicine, 39,* 273–278.

Cowand, J. L., Wrisley, D. M., Walker, M., Strasnick, B., and Jacobson, J. T. (1998). Efficacy of vestibular rehabilitation. *Otolaryngology–Head and Neck Surgery, 118,* 49–54.

Duncan, P. W., Weiner, D., Chandler, J., and Studenski, S. (1990). Functional Reach: A new clinical measure of balance. *Journal of Gerontology, 45,* M192–197.

Fetter, M., and Zee, D. S. (1988). Recovery from unilateral labyrinthectomy in rhesus monkeys. *Journal of Neurophysiology, 59,* 370–393.

Fujino, A., Tokumasu, K., Okamoto, M., Naganuma, H., Hoshino, I., Arai, M., and Yoneda, S. (1996). Vestibular training for acute unilateral vestibular disturbances: Its efficacy in comparison with antivertigo drug. *Acta Otolaryngology Suppl (Stockh), 524,* 21–26.

Furman, J. M., and Cass, S. P. (1996). *Balance disorders: A case-study approach.* Philadelphia: F. A. Davis.

Furman, J. M., and Whitney, S. L. (2000). Central causes of dizziness. *Physical Therapy, 80,* 179–187.

Godaux, E., Halleux, J., and Gobert, C. (1983). Adaptive change of the vestibulo-ocular reflex in the cat: The effects of a long term frequency-selective procedure. *Experimental Brain Research, 49,* 28–34.

Herdman, S. J. (1990). Assessment and Treatment of balance disorders in the vestibular deficient patient. In S. J. Herdman (Ed.), *Vestibular rehabilitation* (pp. 87–94). Philadelphia: F. A. Davis.

Herdman, S. J. (1992). Physical therapy management of vestibular disorders in older patients. *Physical Therapy Practice, 1,* 77–87.

Herdman, S. J., Blatt, P., Schubert, M. C., and Tusa, R. J. (2000). Falls in patients with vestibular deficits. *American Journal of Otology, 21,* 847–851.

Herdman, S. J., Clendaniel, R. A., Mattox, D. E., Holliday, M. J., and Niparko, J. K. (1995). Vestibular adaptation exercises and recovery: Acute stage after acoustic neuroma resection. *Otolaryngology–Head and Neck Surgery, 113,* 77–87.

Herdman, S. J., Tusa, R. J., Zee, D. S., Proctor, L. R., and Mattox, D. E. (1993). Single treatment approaches to benign paroxysmal positional vertigo. *Archives of Otolaryngology–Head and Neck Surgery, 119,* 450–454.

Herdman, S. J., and Whitney, S. L. (2000). Treatment of vestibular hypofunction. In S. J. Herdman (Ed.), *Vestibular rehabilitation* (pp. 387–423). Philadelphia: F. A. Davis.

Horak, F. B., Jones-Rycewicz, C., Black, F. O., and Shumway-Cook, A. (1992). Effects of vestibular rehabilitation on dizziness and imbalance. *Otolaryngology–Head and Neck Surgery, 106,* 175–180.

Jacob, R. G., Whitney, S. L., Detweiler-Shostak, G., and Furman, J. M. (2000). Effect of vestibular rehabilitation in patients with panic disorder with agoraphobia and vestibular dysfunction: A pilot study. *Journal of Anxiety Disorders, 15,* 131–146.

Kasai, T., and Zee, D. S. (1978). Eye-head coordination in labyrinthine-defective human beings. *Brain Research, 144,* 123–141.

Krebs, D. E., Gill-Body, K. M., Riley, P. O., and Parker, S. W. (1993). Double-blind placebo-controlled trial of rehabilitation for bilateral vestibular hypofunction: Preliminary report. *Otolaryngology-Head and Neck Surgery, 109,* 735–741.

Lacour, M., Roll, J. P., and Appaix, M. (1976). Modifications and development of spinal reflexes in the alert baboon (*Papio papio*) following a unilateral vestibular neurectomy. *Brain Research, 113,* 255–269.

Leigh, R. J., Huebner, W. P., and Gordon, J. L. (1994). Supplementation of the vestibulo-ocular reflex by visual fixation and smooth pursuit. *Journal of Vestibular Research, 4,* 347–353.

Lisberger, S. G., Miles, F. A., and Optican, L. M. (1983). Frequency-selective adaptation: Evidence for channels in the vestibulo-ocular reflex. *Journal of Neuroscience, 3,* 1234–1244.

Lynn, S., Pool, A., Rose, D., Brey, R., and Suman, V. (1995). Randomized trial of the canalith repositioning procedure. *Otolaryngology–Head and Neck Surgery, 113,* 712–720.

Newton, R. A. (2001). Validity of the multi-directional reach test: A practical measure for limits of stability in older adults. *Journals of Gerontology. Series A, Biological Sciences and Medical Sciences, 56A,* M248–M252.

Norre, M., and De Weerdt, W. (1980). Treatment of vertigo based on habituation. 2. Technique and results of habituation training. *Journal of Laryngology and Otology, 94,* 689–696.

Robinson, D. A. (1976). Adaptive control of vestibulo-ocular reflex by the cerebellum. *Journal of Neurophysiology, 39,* 954–969.

Segal, B. N., and Katsarkas, A. (1988). Long-term deficits of goal-directed vestibulo-ocular function following total unilateral loss of peripheral vestibular function. *Acta Oto-Laryngologica Supplement (Stockh), 106,* 102–110.

Shepard, N. T., and Telian, S. A. (1995). Programmatic vestibular rehabilitation. *Otolaryngology–Head and Neck Surgery, 112,* 173–182.

Shepard, N. T., Telian, S. A., and Smith-Wheelock, M. (1990). Habituation and balance retraining therapy: A retrospective review. *Neurology Clinics, 8,* 459–475.

Shepard, N. T., Telian, S. A., Smith-Wheelock, M., and Raj, A. (1993). Vestibular and balance rehabilitation therapy. *Annals of Otology, Rhinology, Laryngology, 102,* 198–205.

Shumway-Cook, A., and Horak, F. B. (1986). Assessing the influence of sensory interaction on balance. *Physical Therapy, 66,* 1548–1550.

Shumway-Cook, A., and Woollacott, M. (1995). *Motor control: Theory and practical applications* (pp. 323–324). Baltimore, MD: Williams and Wilkins.

Smith-Wheelock, M., Shepard, N. T., and Telian, S. A. (1991). Long-term effects for treatment of balance dysfunction: Utilizing a home exercise approach. *Seminars in Hearing, 12,* 297–302.

Strupp, M., Arbusow, V., Maag, K. P., Gall, C., and Brandt, T. (1998). Vestibular exercises improve central vestibulo-spinal compensation after vestibular neuritis. *Neurology, 51,* 838–844.

Telian, S. A., Shepard, N. T., Smith-Wheelock, M., and Hoberg, M. (1991). Bilateral vestibular paresis: Diagnosis and treatment. *Otolaryngology–Head and Neck Surgery, 104,* 67–71.

Tinetti, M. E., and Powell, L. E. (1993). Fear of falling and low self-efficacy: A cause of dependence in elderly persons. *Journal of Gerontology, 48,* 35–38.

Weber, P. C., and Cass, S. P. (1993). Clinical assessment of postural stability. *American Journal of Otology, 14,* 566–569.

Whitney, S. L., and Herdman, S. J. (2000). Physical therapy assessment of vestibular hypofunction. In S. J. Herdman (Ed.), *Vestibular Rehabilitation* (pp. 333–372). Philadelphia: F. A. Davis.

Whitney, S. L., Hudak, M. K., and Marchetti, G. F. (2000). The dynamic gait index relates to self-reported fall history in individuals with vestibular dysfunction. *Journal of Vestibular Research, 10,* 99–105.

Whitney, S. L., Wrisley, D. M., Brown, K. E., and Furman, J. M. (2000). Physical therapy for migraine-related vestibulopathy and vestibular dysfunction with history of migraine. *Laryngoscope, 110,* 1528–1534.

Yardley, L., Beech, S., Zander, L., Evans, T., and Weinman, J. (1998). A randomized controlled trial of exercise therapy for dizziness and vertigo in primary care. *British Journal of General Practice, 48,* 1136–1140.

Further Readings

Brown, K. E., Whitney, S. L., Wrisley, D. M., and Furman, J. M. (2001). Physical therapy outcomes for persons with bilateral vestibular loss. *Laryngoscope, 111,* 1812–1817.

Cass, S. P., Borello-France, D., and Furman, J. M. (1996). Functional outcome of vestibular rehabilitation in patients with abnormal sensory organization testing. *American Journal of Otolaryngology, 17,* 581–594.

Cohen, H. (1994). Vestibular rehabilitation improves daily life function. *American Journal of Occupational Therapy, 48,* 919–925.

Herdman, S. J., Clendaniel, R. A., Mattox, D. E., Holliday, M. J., and Niparko, J. K. (1995). Vestibular adaptation exercises and recovery: Acute stage after acoustic neuroma resection. *Otolaryngology–Head and Neck Surgery, 113,* 77–87.

Horak, F. B., Jones-Rycewicz, C., Black, F. O., and Shumway-Cook, A. (1992). Effects of vestibular rehabilitation on dizziness and imbalance. *Otolaryngology–Head and Neck Surgery, 106,* 175–180.

Karlberg, M., Magnusson, M., Malmstrom, E. M., Melander, A., and Moritz, U. (1996). Postural and symptomatic improvement after physiotherapy in patients with dizziness of suspected cervical origin. *Archives of Physical Medicine and Rehabilitation, 77,* 874–882.

Krebs, D. E., Gill-Body, K. M., Riley, P. O., and Parker, S. W. (1993). Double-blind placebo-controlled trial of rehabilitation for bilateral vestibular hypofunction: Preliminary report. *Otolaryngology–Head and Neck Surgery, 109,* 735–741.

Mruzek, M., Barin, K., Nichols, D. S., Burnett, C. N., and Welling, D. B. (1995). Effects of vestibular rehabilitation and social reinforcement on recovery following ablative vestibular surgery. *Laryngoscope, 105,* 686–692.

Norre, M., and De Weerdt, W. (1980). Treatment of vertigo based on habituation: 2. Technique and results of habituation training. *Journal of Laryngology and Otology, 94,* 689–696.

Shepard, N. T., and Telian, S. A. (1995). Programmatic vestibular rehabilitation. *Otolaryngology–Head and Neck Surgery, 112,* 173–182.

Shepard, N. T., Telian, S. A., and Smith-Wheelock, M. (1990). Habituation and balance retraining therapy: A retrospective review. *Neurology Clinics, 8,* 459–475.

Shepard, N. T., Telian, S. A., Smith-Wheelock, M., and Raj, A. (1993). Vestibular and balance rehabilitation therapy. *Annals of Otology, Rhinology, and Laryngology, 102,* 198–205.

Shumway-Cook, A., and Horak, F. B. (1986). Assessing the influence of sensory interaction on balance. *Physical Therapy, 66,* 1548–1550.

Smith-Wheelock, M., Shepard, N. T., and Telian, S. A. (1991). Long-term effects for treatment of balance dysfunction: Utilizing a home exercise approach. *Seminars in Hearing, 12,* 297–302.

Strupp, M., Arbusow, V., Maag, K. P., Gall, C., and Brandt, T. (1998). Vestibular exercises improve central vestibulospinal compensation after vestibular neuritis. *Neurology, 51,* 838–844.

Szturm, T., Ireland, D. J., and Lessing-Turner, M. (1994). Comparison of different exercise programs in the rehabilitation of patients with chronic peripheral vestibular dysfunction. *Journal of Vestibular Research, 4,* 461–479.

Whitney, S. L., Wrisley, D. M., Brown, K. E., and Furman, J. M. (2000). Physical therapy for migraine-related vestibulopathy and vestibular-dysfunction with history of migraine. *Laryngoscope, 110,* 1528–1534.

Wrisley, D. M., Sparto, P. J., Whitney, S. L., and Furman, J. M. (2000). Cervicogenic dizziness: A review of diagnosis and treatment. *Journal of Orthopedic and Sports Physical Therapy, 30,* 755–766.

Yardley, L., Beech, S., Zander, L., Evans, T., and Weinman, J. (1998). A randomized controlled trial of exercise therapy for dizziness and vertigo in primary care. *British Journal of General Practice, 48,* 1136–1140.

Contributors

General Editor

Raymond D. Kent
University of Wisconsin-Madison, Madison, Wisconsin

Advisory Editors

Voice Disorders in Children
Steven D. Gray (deceased)
University of Utah, Salt Lake City, Utah

Voice Disorders in Adults
Robert E. Hillman
Massachusetts Eye and Ear Infirmary, Boston, Massachusetts

Speech Disorders in Children
Lawrence D. Shriberg
University of Wisconsin-Madison, Madison, Wisconsin

Speech Disorders in Adults
Joseph R. Duffy
Mayo Clinic, Rochester, Minnesota

Language Disorders in Children
Mabel L. Rice
University of Kansas, Lawrence, Kansas

Language Disorders in Adults
David A. Swinney
University of California at San Diego, San Diego, California
and
Lewis P. Shapiro
San Diego State University, San Diego, California

Hearing Disorders in Children
Fred H. Bess
Vanderbilt University, Nashville, Tennessee

Hearing Disorders in Adults
Sandra Gordon-Salant
University of Maryland, College Park, Maryland

Contributing Authors

Faith W. Akin
James H. Quillen VA Medical Center, Mountain Home, Tennessee
ELECTRONYSTAGMOGRAPHY

Jont B. Allen
University of Illinois at Urbana-Champaign, Beckman Institute, Urbana, Illinois
AMPLITUDE COMPRESSION IN HEARING AIDS

Gerhard Andersson
Uppsala University, Uppsala, Sweden
TINNITUS

Daniel H. Ashmead
Vanderbilt University Medical Center, Nashville, Tennessee
AUDITION IN CHILDREN, DEVELOPMENT OF

Laura J. Ball
University of Nebraska Medical Center, Omaha, Nebraska
AUGMENTATIVE AND ALTERNATIVE COMMUNICATION APPROACHES IN ADULTS
AUGMENTATIVE AND ALTERNATIVE COMMUNICATION APPROACHES IN CHILDREN

Martin J. Ball
University of Louisiana at Lafayette, Lafayette, Louisiana
SPEECH ASSESSMENT, INSTRUMENTAL

Shari R. Baum
McGill University, Montreal, Quebec
PROSODIC DEFICITS

Kathryn A. Bayles
University of Arizona, Tuscon, Arizona
DEMENTIA

Pelagie M. Beeson
University of Arizona, Tuscon, Arizona
AGRAPHIA

Gerald S. Berke
University of California at Los Angeles School of Medicine, Los Angeles, California
LARYNGEAL REINNERVATION PROCEDURES

Ken Bleile
University of Northern Iowa, Cedar Falls, Iowa
SPEECH DISORDERS IN CHILDREN: BIRTH-RELATED RISK FACTORS

Joel H. Blumin
University of Pennsylvania School of Medicine, Philadelphia, Pennsylvania
LARYNGEAL REINNERVATION PROCEDURES

Sheila E. Blumstein
Brown University, Providence, Rhode Island
PHONOLOGY AND ADULT APHASIA

Carol A. Boliek
University of Alberta, Edmonton, Alberta
SPEECH DEVELOPMENT IN INFANTS AND YOUNG CHILDREN WITH A TRACHEOSTOMY

Louis D. Braida
Massachusetts Institute of Technology, Cambridge, Massachusetts
FREQUENCY COMPRESSION

Mitchell F. Brin
Columbia University, New York, New York
HYPOKINETIC LARYNGEAL MOVEMENT DISORDERS

Bonnie Brinton
Brigham Young University, Provo, Utah
PRAGMATICS
PSYCHOSOCIAL PROBLEMS ASSOCIATED WITH COMMUNICATIVE
    DISORDERS

Hiram Brownell
Boston College, Chestnut Hill, Massachusetts
RIGHT HEMISPHERE LANGUAGE AND COMMUNICATION FUNCTIONS
    IN ADULTS

Hugh W. Buckingham
Louisiana State University, Baton Rouge, Louisiana
PHONOLOGICAL ANALYSIS OF LANGUAGE DISORDERS IN APHASIA

Eugene H. Buder
University of Memphis, Memphis, Tennessee
ACOUSTIC ASSESSMENT OF VOICE

Angela Burda
University of Northern Iowa, Cedar Falls, Iowa
SPEECH DISORDERS IN CHILDREN: BIRTH-RELATED RISK FACTORS

Thomas Campbell
University of Pittsburgh and Children's Hospital of
    Pittsburgh, Pittsburgh, Pennsylvania
EARLY RECURRENT OTITIS MEDIA AND SPEECH DEVELOPMENT

David Caplan
Massachusetts General Hospital, Boston, Massachusetts
APHASIC SYNDROMES: CONNECTIONIST MODELS

Janina K. Casper
SUNY-Upstate Medical Center, Syracuse, New York
VOCAL HYGIENE

Hugh W. Catts
University of Kansas, Lawrence, Kansas
LANGUAGE IMPAIRMENT AND READING DISABILITY

Michael R. Chial
University of Wisconsin-Madison, Madison, Wisconsin
HEARING PROTECTION DEVICES

Li-Rong Lilly Cheng
San Diego State University, San Diego, California
SPEECH AND LANGUAGE ISSUES IN CHILDREN FROM ASIAN-PACIFIC
    BACKGROUNDS

Melissa Cheslock
Georgia State University, Atlanta, Georgia
AUGMENTATIVE AND ALTERNATIVE COMMUNICATION: GENERAL
    ISSUES

Chris Code
University of Exeter, Exeter, United Kingdom
APHASIA TREATMENT: PSYCHOSOCIAL ISSUES

Robyn M. Cox
University of Memphis, Memphis, Tennessee
HEARING AID FITTING: EVALUATION OF OUTCOMES

Martha Crago
McGill University, Montreal, Quebec
LANGUAGE IMPAIRMENT IN CHILDREN: CROSS-LINGUISTIC STUDIES

Carl C. Crandell
University of Florida, Gainesville, Florida
CLASSROOM ACOUSTICS

Richard F. Curlee
University of Arizona, Tuscon, Arizona
STUTTERING

Anne Cutler
Max Planck Institute for Psycholinguistics, Nijmegen, The
    Netherlands
SEGMENTATION OF SPOKEN LANGUAGE BY NORMAL ADULT
    LISTENERS

Barbara L. Davis
University of Texas at Austin, Austin, Texas
DEVELOPMENTAL APRAXIA OF SPEECH

Peter A. de Villiers
Smith College, Northampton, Massachusetts
LANGUAGE OF THE DEAF: ACQUISITION OF ENGLISH
LANGUAGE OF THE DEAF: SIGN LANGUAGE

Allan O. Diefendorf
Indiana University School of Medicine, Indianapolis,
    Indiana
PEDIATRIC AUDIOLOGY: THE TEST BATTERY APPROACH

Harvey Dillon
The National Acoustic Laboratories, Chatswood, Australia
HEARING AIDS: PRESCRIPTIVE FITTING

Christine Dollaghan
University of Pittsburgh, Pittsburgh, Pennsylvania
EARLY RECURRENT OTITIS MEDIA AND SPEECH DEVELOPMENT

Patrick J. Doyle
VA Pittsburgh Healthcare System and University of
    Pittsburgh, Pittsburgh, Pennsylvania
APRAXIA OF SPEECH: NATURE AND PHENOMENOLOGY
APRAXIA OF SPEECH: TREATMENT

Philip C. Doyle
University of Western Ontario, London, Ontario
ALARYNGEAL VOICE AND SPEECH REHABILITATION
LARYNGEAL TRAUMA AND PERIPHERAL STRUCTURAL
    ABLATIONS
VOICE REHABILITATION AFTER CONSERVATION LARYNGECTOMY

Nina F. Dronkers
VA Northern California Health Care System, Martinez,
    California
APHASIA: THE CLASSICAL SYNDROMES

Judy R. Dubno
Medical University of South Carolina, Charleston, South
    Carolina
PRESBYACUSIS

Joseph R. Duffy
Mayo Clinic, Rochester, Minnesota
DYSARTHRIAS: CHARACTERISTICS AND CLASSIFICATION

Anh Duong
University of Montreal, Montreal, Quebec
DISCOURSE IMPAIRMENTS

Tanya L. Eadie
University of Western Ontario, London, Ontario
ALARYNGEAL VOICE AND SPEECH REHABILITATION

David A. Eddins
SUNY-Buffalo, Buffalo, New York
TEMPORAL RESOLUTION

Mary Louise Edwards
Syracuse University, Syracuse, New York
PHONETIC TRANSCRIPTIONS OF CHILDREN'S SPEECH

Wiltrud Fassbinder
University of Pittsburgh, Pittsburgh, Pennsylvania
RIGHT HEMISPHERE LANGUAGE DISORDERS

Heidi M. Feldman
University of Pittsburgh School of Medicine, Pittsburgh,
    Pennsylvania
LANGUAGE DEVELOPMENT IN CHILDREN WITH FOCAL LESIONS

John A. Ferraro
University of Kansas Medical Center, Kansas City, Kansas
ELECTROCOCHLEOGRAPHY

Marc E. Fey
University of Kansas Medical Center, Kansas City, Kansas
PRESCHOOL LANGUAGE INTERVENTION

W. Tecumseh Fitch
Harvard University, Cambridge, Massachusetts
VOCAL PRODUCTION SYSTEM: EVOLUTION

Cynthia G. Fowler
University of Wisconsin-Madison, Madison, Wisconsin
AUDITORY BRAINSTEM RESPONSE IN ADULTS

Cynthia Fox
University of Colorado, Boulder, Colorado
HYPOKINETIC LARYNGEAL MOVEMENT DISORDERS

Naama Friedmann
Tel Aviv University, Tel Aviv, Israel
SYNTACTIC TREE PRUNING

Martin Fujiki
Brigham Young University, Provo, Utah
PRAGMATICS
PSYCHOSOCIAL PROBLEMS ASSOCIATED WITH COMMUNICATIVE
    DISORDERS

Fred Genesee
McGill University, Montreal, Quebec
BILINGUALISM AND LANGUAGE IMPAIRMENT

LouAnn Gerken
University of Arizona, Tuscon, Arizona
LINGUISTIC ASPECTS OF CHILD LANGUAGE IMPAIRMENT—
    PROSODY

Bruce Gerratt
University of California at Los Angeles School of Medicine,
    Los Angeles, California
VOICE QUALITY, PERCEPTUAL EVALUATION

Judith A. Gierut
Indiana University, Bloomington, Indiana
SPEECH ASSESSMENT IN CHILDREN: DESCRIPTIVE LINGUISTIC
    METHODS

Lisa Goffman
Purdue University, West Lafayette, Indiana
MOTOR SPEECH INVOLVEMENT IN CHILDREN

Brian Goldstein
Temple University, Philadelphia, Pennsylvania
SPEECH ISSUES IN CHILDREN FROM LATINO BACKGROUNDS

Michael P. Gorga
Boys Town National Research Hospital, Omaha, Nebraska
OTOACOUSTIC EMISSIONS IN CHILDREN

Yosef Grodzinsky
McGill University, Montreal, Quebec; Tel Aviv University,
    Tel Aviv, Israel
TRACE DELETION HYPOTHESIS

Murray Grossman
University of Pennsylvania, Philadelphia, Pennsylvania
ALZHEIMER'S DISEASE

Timothy C. Hain
Northwestern University School of Medicine, Chicago, Illinois
OTOTOXIC MEDICATIONS

Joseph W. Hall
University of North Carolina at Chapel Hill, Chapel Hill,
    North Carolina
HEARING LOSS AND THE MASKING-LEVEL DIFFERENCE

Helen M. Hanson
Massachusetts Institute of Technology, Cambridge,
    Massachusetts
VOICE ACOUSTICS

M. N. Hegde
California State University at Fresno, Fresno, California
SPEECH DISORDERS IN CHILDREN: BEHAVIORAL APPROACHES TO
    REMEDIATION

Nancy Helm-Estabrooks
Boston University School of Medicine, Boston, Massachusetts
PERSEVERATION

Janet Helminski
Midwestern University School of Physical Therapy, Downers
    Grove, Illinois
OTOTOXIC MEDICATIONS

Gregory Hickok
University of California at Irvine, Irvine, California
AUDITORY-MOTOR INTERACTION IN SPEECH AND LANGUAGE
FUNCTIONAL BRAIN IMAGING

Argye E. Hillis
Johns Hopkins University School of Medicine, Baltimore,
    Maryland
ALEXIA

Robert E. Hillman
Massachusetts Eye and Ear Infirmary and Massachusetts
    General Hospital Institute of Health Professions, Boston,
    Massachusetts; Harvard Medical School, Cambridge,
    Massachusetts
AERODYNAMIC ASSESSMENT OF VOCAL FUNCTION

Jacqueline J. Hinckley
University of South Florida, Tampa, Florida
COMMUNICATION DISORDERS IN ADULTS: FUNCTIONAL
    APPROACHES TO APHASIA

Megan M. Hodge
University of Alberta, Edmonton, Alberta
SPEECH DISORDERS IN CHILDREN: MOTOR SPEECH DISORDERS OF
    KNOWN ORIGIN

Barbara Hodson
Wichita State University, Wichita, Kansas
PHONOLOGICAL AWARENESS INTERVENTION FOR CHILDREN WITH
    EXPRESSIVE PHONOLOGICAL IMPAIRMENTS

Erica Hoff
Florida Atlantic University, Davie, Florida
POVERTY: EFFECTS ON LANGUAGE

Jeannette D. Hoit
University of Arizona, Tuscon, Arizona
VENTILATOR-SUPPORTED SPEECH PRODUCTION

Audrey L. Holland
University of Arizona, Tuscon, Arizona
COMMUNICATION DISORDERS IN ADULTS: FUNCTIONAL
    APPROACHES TO APHASIA

Linda J. Hood
Kresge Hearing Research Laboratory, New Orleans,
    Louisiana
GENETICS AND CRANIOFACIAL ANOMALIES

Aquiles Iglesias
Temple University, Philadelphia, Pennsylvania
LANGUAGE DISORDERS IN LATINO CHILDREN

David Ingram
Arizona State University, Tempe, Arizona
SPEECH DISORDERS IN CHILDREN: CROSS-LINGUISTIC DATA

Yves Joanette
University of Montreal, Montreal, Quebec
DISCOURSE IMPAIRMENTS

Joel C. Kahane
University of Memphis, Memphis, Tennessee
ANATOMY OF THE HUMAN LARYNX

Richard C. Katz
Carl T. Hayden VA Medical Center, Phoenix, Arizona;
    Arizona State University, Tuscon, Arizona
APHASIA TREATMENT: COMPUTER-AIDED REHABILITATION

Gitte Keidser
The National Acoustic Laboratories, Chatswood, Australia
HEARING AIDS: PRESCRIPTIVE FITTING

Ray D. Kent
University of Wisconsin-Madison, Madison, Wisconsin
INSTRUMENTAL ASSESSMENT OF CHILDREN'S VOICE

Herman Kolk
Catholic University of Nijmegen, Nijmegen, The Netherlands
AGRAMMATISM

Jody Kreiman
University of California at Los Angeles School of Medicine,
    Los Angeles, California
VOICE QUALITY, PERCEPTUAL EVALUATION OF

Charissa R. Lansing
University of Illinois at Champaign-Urbana, Champaign,
    Illinois
SPEECHREADING TRAINING AND VISUAL TRACKING

Charles R. Larson
Northwestern University, Evanston, Illinois
VOCALIZATION, NEURAL MECHANISMS

David P. Lau
Singapore General Hospital, Singapore
INFECTIOUS DISEASES AND INFLAMMATORY CONDITIONS OF THE
    LARYNX

Matti Lehtihalmes
University of Oulu, Oulu, Finland
APHASIA, WERNICKE'S

Laurence B. Leonard
Purdue University, West Lafayette, Indiana
SPECIFIC LANGUAGE IMPAIRMENT IN CHILDREN

Barbara A. Lewis
Rainbow Babies and Children's Hospital and Case Western
    Reserve University, Cleveland, Ohio
SPEECH DISORDERS: GENETIC TRANSMISSION

Marcia C. Linebarger
Moss Rehabilitation Research Institute and Psycholinguistic
    Technologies, Inc., Philadelphia, Pennsylvania
REVERSABILITY/MAPPING DISORDERS

Sue Ellen Linville
Marquette University, Milwaukee, Wisconsin
VOICE DISORDERS OF AGING

Diane Frome Loeb
University of Kansas, Lawrence, Kansas
COMMUNICATION DISORDERS IN INFANTS AND TODDLERS

Brenda L. Lonsbury-Martin
University of Colorado, Denver, Colorado
OTOACOUSTIC EMISSIONS

Christy L. Ludlow
National Institute of Neurological Disorders and Stroke and
    National Institutes of Health, Bethesda, Maryland
LARYNGEAL MOVEMENT DISORDERS: TREATMENT WITH
    BOTULINUM TOXIN

Robert C. Marshall
University of Kentucky, Lexington, Kentucky
SPEECH DISORDERS IN ADULTS, PSYCHOGENIC

Julie J. Masterson
Southwestern Missouri State University, Springfield, Missouri
SPEECH AND LANGUAGE DISORDERS IN CHILDREN: COMPUTER-
    BASED APPROACHES

Patricia McCarthy
Rush University and Rush-Presbyterian-St. Luke's Medical
    Center, Chicago, Illinois
FUNCTIONAL HEARING LOSS IN CHILDREN

Rebecca J. McCauley
University of Vermont, Burlington, Vermont
SPEECH SOUND DISORDERS IN CHILDREN: DESCRIPTION AND
    CLASSIFICATION

Karla McGregor
Northwestern University, Evanston, Illinois
SEMANTICS

Malcolm R. McNeil
University of Pittsburgh, Pittsburgh, Pennsylvania
APRAXIA OF SPEECH: NATURE AND PHENOMENOLOGY
APRAXIA OF SPEECH: TREATMENT
ATTENTION AND LANGUAGE

Lise Menn
University of Colorado, Boulder, Colorado
APHASIOLOGY, COMPARATIVE

Jon F. Miller
University of Wisconsin-Madison, Madison, Wisconsin
COMMUNICATION SKILLS OF PEOPLE WITH DOWN SYNDROME

John H. Mills
Medical University of South Carolina, Charleston, South
    Carolina
NOISE-INDUCED HEARING LOSS
PRESBYACUSIS

Murray D. Morrison
University of British Columbia, Vancouver, British Columbia
INFECTIOUS DISEASES AND INFLAMMATORY CONDITIONS OF THE
    LARYNX

Dave J. Muller
University College Suffolk, Ipswich, United Kingdom
APHASIA TREATMENT: PSYCHOSOCIAL ISSUES

Bruce E. Murdoch
University of Queensland, Brisbane, Australia
LANGUAGE DISORDERS IN ADULTS: SUBCORTICAL INVOLVEMENT

Thomas Murry
Columbia University, New York, New York
ASSESSMENT OF FUNCTIONAL IMPACT OF VOICE DISORDERS
VOICE THERAPY FOR NEUROLOGICAL AGING-RELATED VOICE
    DISORDERS

Penelope S. Myers
Mayo Clinic, Rochester, Minnesota
APROSODIA

Igor V. Náblek
University of Tennessee, Knoxville, Tennessee
TEMPORAL INTEGRATION

Stephen T. Neely
Boys Town National Research Hospital, Omaha, Nebraska
OTOACOUSTIC EMISSIONS IN CHILDREN

Arlene C. Neuman
CUNY-The Graduate Center, New York, New York
HEARING AIDS: SOUND QUALITY

Marilyn A. Nippold
University of Oregon, Eugene, Oregon
LANGUAGE DISORDERS IN SCHOOL-AGE CHILDREN: ASPECTS OF
    ASSESSMENT

Robert J. Nozza
Temple University School of Medicine, Philadelphia,
    Pennsylvania
MIDDLE EAR ASSESSMENT IN THE CHILD

Janna B. Oetting
Louisiana State University, Baton Rouge, Louisiana
DIALECT SPEAKERS
DIALECT VERSUS DISORDER

Jennifer Ogar
VA Northern California Health Care System, Martinez,
    California
APHASIA: THE CLASSICAL SYNDROMES

Gloria Streit Olness
University of Texas at Dallas, Dallas, Texas
DISCOURSE

Robert F. Orlikoff
CUNY-Hunter College, New York, New York
ELECTROGLOTTOGRAPHIC ASSESSMENT OF VOICE

Mary Joe Osberger
Advanced Bionics Corporation, Valencia, California
COCHLEAR IMPLANTS
COCHLEAR IMPLANTS IN CHILDREN

Johanne Paradis
University of Alberta, Edmonton, Alberta
LANGUAGE IMPAIRMENT IN CHILDREN: CROSS-LINGUISTIC
    STUDIES

Rhea Paul
Southern Connecticut State University and Yale Child Study
    Center, New Haven, Connecticut
AUTISM

Diane Paul-Brown
American Speech-Language-Hearing Association, Rockville,
    Maryland
OROFACIAL MYOFUNCTIONAL DISORDERS IN CHILDREN

Richard K. Peach
Rush University and Rush-Presbyterian-St. Luke's Medical
    Center, Chicago, Illinois
APHASIA, GLOBAL
MELODIC INTONATION THERAPY

Adrienne L. Perlman
University of Illinois at Urbana-Champaign, Champaign,
    Illinois
DYSPHAGIA, ORAL AND PHARYNGEAL

John M. Pettit
Radford University, Radford, Virginia
TRANSSEXUALISM AND SEX REASSIGNMENT: SPEECH DIFFERENCES

James O. Pickles
The University of Queensland, Brisbane, Australia
PHYSIOLOGICAL BASES OF HEARING

Geoff Plant
The Hearing Rehabilitation Foundation, Somerville,
    Massachusetts
SPEECH TRACKING

Sheila Pratt
University of Pittsburgh, Pittsburgh, Pennsylvania
AUDITORY TRAINING
SPEECH DISORDERS SECONDARY TO HEARING IMPAIRMENT
    ACQUIRED IN ADULTHOOD

Adele Proctor
University of Illinois at Urbana-Champaign, Champaign,
    Illinois
DIALECT, REGIONAL

Jennie Pyers
University of California at Berkeley, Berkeley, California
LANGUAGE OF THE DEAF: SIGN LANGUAGE

Lorraine Olson Ramig
University of Colorado, Boulder, Colorado
HYPOKINETIC LARYNGEAL MOVEMENT DISORDERS

Steven Z. Rapcsak
University of Arizona, Tuscon, Arizona
AGRAPHIA

Sean M. Redmond
University of Utah, Salt Lake City, Utah
SOCIAL DEVELOPMENT AND LANGUAGE IMPAIRMENT

Charlotte M. Reed
Massachusetts Institute of Technology, Cambridge,
    Massachusetts
FREQUENCY COMPRESSION

Joanne E. Roberts
University of North Carolina at Chapel Hill, Chapel Hill,
    North Carolina
OTITIS MEDIA: EFFECTS ON CHILDREN'S LANGUAGE

Margaret A. Rogers
University of Washington, Seattle, Washington
APHASIA, PRIMARY PROGRESSIVE

Mary Ann Romski
Georgia State University, Atlanta, Georgia
AUGMENTATIVE AND ALTERNATIVE COMMUNICATION: GENERAL
    ISSUES
MENTAL RETARDATION

Clark A. Rosen
University of Pittsburgh, Pittsburgh, Pennsylvania
ASSESSMENT OF FUNCTIONAL IMPACT OF VOICE DISORDERS

John C. Rosenbek
College of Health Professions, Gainesville, Florida
MUTISM, NEUROGENIC

Jackson Roush
University of North Carolina at Chapel Hill, Chapel Hill,
    North Carolina
HEARING LOSS SCREENING: THE SCHOOL-AGE CHILD

Nelson Roy
University of Utah, Salt Lake City, Utah
FUNCTIONAL VOICE DISORDERS
PSYCHOGENIC VOICE DISORDERS: DIRECT THERAPY

Dennis M. Ruscello
West Virginia University, Morgantown, West Virginia
PHONOLOGICAL ERRORS, RESIDUAL

Ron Scherer
Bowling Green State University, Bowling Green, Ohio
VOICE PRODUCTION: PHYSICS AND PHYSIOLOGY

Robert S. Schlauch
University of Minnesota, Minneapolis, Minnesota
PSEUDOHYPACUSIS

Carson T. Schütze
University of California at Los Angeles, Los Angeles, California
MORPHOSYNTAX AND SYNTAX

Rose A. Sevcik
Georgia State University, Atlanta, Georgia
AUGMENTATIVE AND ALTERNATIVE COMMUNICATION: GENERAL ISSUES
MENTAL RETARDATION

Harry N. Seymour
University of Massachusetts at Amherst, Amherst, Massachusetts
LANGUAGE DISORDERS IN AFRICAN-AMERICAN CHILDREN

Janet E. Shanks
Department of Veterans Affairs Medical Center, Long Beach, California; University of California at Irvine, Irvine, California
TYMPANOMETRY

Robert V. Shannon
House Ear Institute, Los Angeles, California
AUDITORY BRAINSTEM IMPLANT

Lewis P. Shapiro
San Diego State University, San Diego, California
ARGUMENT STRUCTURE: REPRESENTATION AND PROCESSING

Elaine R. Silliman
University of Florida, Tampa, Florida
INCLUSION MODELS FOR CHILDREN WITH DEVELOPMENTAL DISABILITIES

Yvonne S. Sininger
House Ear Institute, Los Angeles, California
AUDITORY NEUROPATHY IN CHILDREN

Bernadette Ska
University of Montreal, Montreal, Quebec
DISCOURSE IMPAIRMENTS

Joseph J. Smaldino
University of Northern Iowa, Cedar Falls, Iowa
CLASSROOM ACOUSTICS

Steven L. Small
University of Chicago, Chicago, Illinois
APHASIA TREATMENT: PHARMACOLOGICAL APPROACHES

Ann Bosma Smit
Kansas State University, Manhattan, Kansas
SPEECH SAMPLING, ARTICULATION TESTS, AND INTELLIGIBILITY IN CHILDREN WITH PHONOLOGICAL ERRORS
SPEECH SAMPLING, ARTICULATION TESTS, AND INTELLIGIBILITY IN CHILDREN WITH RESIDUAL ERRORS

Pamela E. Souza
University of Washington, Seattle, Washington
SUPRATHRESHOLD SPEECH RECOGNITION

Charles Speaks
University of Minnesota, Minneapolis, Minnesota
DICHOTIC LISTENING

Joy Stackhouse
University of Sheffield, Sheffield, United Kingdom
SPEECH DISORDERS IN CHILDREN: A PSYCHOLINGUISTIC PERSPECTIVE

Elaine T. Stathopoulos
SUNY-Buffalo, Buffalo, New York
VOICE DISORDERS IN CHILDREN

Joseph Stemple
Institute for Voice Analysis and Rehabilitation, Dayton, Ohio
VOICE THERAPY: HOLISTIC TECHNIQUES

Kenneth N. Stevens
Massachusetts Institute of Technology, Cambridge, Massachusetts
VOICE ACOUSTICS

Ida J. Stockman
Michigan State University, East Lansing, Michigan
PHONOLOGY: CLINICAL ISSUES IN SERVING SPEAKERS OF AFRICAN-AMERICAN VERNACULAR ENGLISH

Carol Stoel-Gammon
University of Washington, Seattle, Washington
MENTAL RETARDATION AND SPEECH IN CHILDREN

Edythe A. Strand
Mayo Clinic, Rochester, Minnesota
DYSARTHRIAS: MANAGEMENT

Kathy Strattman
Wichita State University, Wichita, Kansas
PHONOLOGICAL AWARENESS INTERVENTION FOR CHILDREN WITH EXPRESSIVE PHONOLOGICAL IMPAIRMENTS

Gerald A. Studebaker
University of Memphis, Memphis, Tennessee
SPEECH PERCEPTION INDICES

Johan Sundberg
KTH Voice Research Centre, Stockholm, Sweden
THE SINGING VOICE

Anne Marie Tharpe
Vanderbilt University Medical Center, Nashville, Tennessee
AUDITION IN CHILDREN, DEVELOPMENT OF HEARING LOSS AND TERATOGENIC DRUGS OR CHEMICALS

Jack E. Thomas
Mayo Clinic, Rochester, Minnesota
LARYNGECTOMY

Connie A. Tompkins
University of Pittsburgh, Pittsburgh, Pennsylvania
RIGHT HEMISPHERE LANGUAGE DISORDERS

Robert G. Turner
Louisiana State University Health Sciences Center, New Orleans, Louisiana
CLINICAL DECISION ANALYSIS

Ann A. Tyler
University of Nevada at Reno, Reno, Nevada
SPEECH DISORDERS IN CHILDREN: SPEECH-LANGUAGE APPROACHES

Richard S. Tyler
University of Iowa, Iowa City, Iowa
COCHLEAR IMPLANTS IN ADULTS: CANDIDACY

Hanna K. Ulatowska
University of Texas at Dallas, Dallas, Texas
DISCOURSE

Miodrag Velickovic
The Mount Sinai Medical Center, New York
HYPOKINETIC LARYNGEAL MOVEMENT DISORDERS

Shelley L. Velleman
University of Massachusetts at Amherst, Amherst, Massachusetts
SPEECH DISORDERS IN CHILDREN; DESCRIPTIVE LINGUISTIC APPROACHES

Katherine Verdolini
University of Pittsburgh, Pittsburgh, Pennsylvania
VOICE THERAPY FOR ADULTS
VOICE THERAPY FOR PROFESSIONAL VOICE USERS

Steven F. Warren
University of Kansas, Lawrence, Kansas
PRELINGUISTIC COMMUNICATION INTERVENTION FOR CHILDREN
    WITH DEVELOPMENTAL DISABILITIES

Ruth V. Watkins
University of Illinois at Urbana-Champaign, Champaign,
    Illinois
LANGUAGE IN CHILDREN WHO STUTTER

Peter Watson
Case Western Reserve University, Cleveland, Ohio
VOICE THERAPY: BREATHING EXERCISES

Susan Ellis Weismer
University of Wisconsin-Madison, Madison, Wisconsin
MEMORY AND PROCESSING CAPACITY

Nathan V. Welham
University of Wisconsin-Madison, Madison, Wisconsin
INSTRUMENTAL ASSESSMENT OF CHILDREN'S VOICE

Robert T. Wertz
VA Tennessee Valley Healthcare System, Nashville, Tennessee
APHASIA: THE CLASSICAL SYNDROMES

Susan L. Whitney
University of Pittsburgh Medical Center, Pittsburgh,
    Pennsylvania
VESTIBULAR REHABILITATION

Judith E. Widen
University of Kansas Medical Center
OTOACOUSTIC EMISSIONS IN CHILDREN

Terry L. Wiley
Arizona State University, Tempe, Arizona
PURE-TONE THRESHOLD ASSESSMENT

Jennifer Windsor
University of Minnesota, Minneapolis, Minnesota
LANGUAGE DISORDERS IN SCHOOL-AGE CHILDREN: OVERVIEW

Shelley Witt
University of Iowa, Iowa City, Iowa
COCHLEAR IMPLANTS IN ADULTS: CANDIDACY

Diane M. Wrisley
Oregon Health and Sciences University, Beaverton, Oregon
VESTIBULAR REHABILITATION

Michael K. Wynne
Indiana University School of Medicine, Indianapolis,
    Indiana
PEDIATRIC AUDIOLOGY: THE TEST BATTERY APPROACH

William S. Yacullo
Governors State University, University Park, Illinois
MASKING

J. Scott Yaruss
University of Pittsburgh, Pittsburgh, Pennsylvania
SPEECH DISFLUENCY AND STUTTERING IN CHILDREN

Mehmet Yavas
Florida International University, Miami, Flordia
BILINGUALISM, SPEECH ISSUES IN

Paul J. Yoder
Vanderbilt University, Nashville, Tennessee
PRELINGUISTIC COMMUNICATION INTERVENTION FOR CHILDREN
    WITH DEVELOPMENTAL DISABILITIES

Christine Yoshinaga-Itano
University of Colorado, Boulder, Colorado
ASSESSMENT OF AND INTERVENTION WITH CHILDREN WHO ARE
    DEAF OR HARD OF HEARING

William A. Yost
Loyola University Chicago, Chicago, Illinois
AUDITORY SCENE ANALYSIS
PITCH PERCEPTION

Name Index

Eley, T., 185
Eley, T. C., 371
Elias, A., 28, 50
Eliason, M. J., 163
Elidan, J., 469
Elkins, E., 208
Elkins, E. F., 527, 528
Elkonin, D. B., 154
Elliot, L. L., 548
Elliott, M., 546
Elliott, M. R., 307
Ellis, A. W., 233, 256
Ellis Weismer, S., 287, 327, 350, 403
Elman, R., 261, 283, 284
Elpern, B. S., 502
El Rafie, E. A., 556
Emami, A. J., 38
Emanuel, D. C., 358
Emerich, K., 73
Emery, O. B., 240
Emery, P., 361, 362
Emmorey, K., 382
Emmory, K. D., 109, 340
Emonds, J. E., 354
Enderby, P., 126, 258, 378
Endicott, J. E., 529
Engel, J. A. M., 135
Engen, E., 337, 343
Engen, T., 337
Engmann, D., 198
Epstein, L., 494
Epstein, R., 27, 50
Eran, O., 456
Erber, N., 439
Erber, N. P., 543
Erdman, S., 208
Erdman, S. A., 440
Erhard, P., 275
Erickson, J. G., 322
Erickson, R. J., 273
Eriksdotter-Jonhagen, M., 258
Eriksson, J., 557
Erkinjuntti, T., 240, 292–293
Erre, J. P., 519
Erriondo Korostola, L., 267
Erting, C., 342
Ertmer, D., 456
Esclamado, R., 43
Escobar, M. D., 184, 324
Espesser, R., 439, 440
Estabrooks, N., 315
Esteban, E., 495
Estill, J., 96
Estivill, X., 478
Etard, O., 276
Ettema, S., 134
Evans, A. C., 60, 275
Evans, C. A., 306
Evans, F. J., 38
Evans, J., 328, 350, 399
Evans, J. L., 164
Evans, J. S., 211
Evans, T., 563
Everitt, W. L., 472
Ewing-Cobbs, L., 396
Eyles, L., 295, 299

F
Fabre, P., 24
Fabry, L. B., 436
Facer, G. W., 436
Fagundes, D., 297
Fahey, P. F., 417

Fahn, H., 73
Fahn, S., 30, 38
Fairbairn, A. F., 292
Fairbanks, G., 78, 472
Fakler, B., 511
Falk, R. E., 518
Fant, G., 6, 63, 64, 76, 225
Farmer, A., 171, 173
Farmer, M., 399
Farrabola, M., 243–244
Farren, D. C., 377
Farr-Whitman, M., 296
Farwell, C. B., 174
Fassbender, L., 116
Fassbinder, Wiltrud, 388–391
Fastl, H., 3, 551
Fattu, J. M., 57
Faust, M., 231
Fausti, S. A., 518
Fawcett, A. J., 329
Fawcett, D. W., 523
Fayad, J. N., 427, 448
Fazio, B. B., 370, 371
Feagans, L., 359
Federoff, J. P., 108
Feeney, D. M., 257, 258
Feinmesser, M., 429
Feldkeller, R., 551
Feldman, A., 560
Feldman, Heidi M., 135, 136, 311–313, 359, 370, 371, 396
Feldman, L., 109
Feldmann, H., 556
Felici, F., 73
Felsenfeld, S., 184, 185
Fennell, A., 89
Fenson, J., 252, 253, 312
Fenson, L., 336, 370, 371, 376, 397
Fenwick, K. D., 425
Ferguson, C. A., 174
Ferguson, N. A., 49
Ferguson, R., 464, 465
Ferketic, M., 283
Ferlito, A., 33
Fernandes, M. A., 438, 490
Fernandez-Villa, J., 145, 146
Ferrand, C. T., 36
Ferraro, John A., 461–465
Ferrier, E., 205
Ferro, J. M., 243, 252
Ferry, P. C., 122
Fes, S., 50
Festen, J. M., 487
Fetter, M., 565
Fex, F., 50
Fey, Marc E., 175, 206, 309, 327, 329, 330, 373, 378–380, 403
Fey, S. H., 325
Fichtner, C. G., 108
Figueroa, R. A., 321
Figura, F., 73
Fikret-Pasa, S., 483
Fillenbaum, G. G., 292
Finch, C., 73, 92
Finestone, H., 133
Finitzo-Hieber, T., 359, 442
Fink, R. B., 232
Finkelstein, S., 101, 264
Finlay, C., 299
Finlayson, A., 283
Finley, C. C., 449
Fischel, J. E., 359

Fischel-Ghodsian, N., 518
Fischer, H. B., 126
Fischer, N. D., 176, 177
Fischer, S., 342
Fischler, I., 272, 273
Fish, S., 280
Fisher, E., 73
Fisher, H. B., 10, 30
Fisher, K. V., 55
Fisher, L., 338, 449, 455
Fisher, S., 402
Fisher, S. E., 185
Fisher, S. G., 10
Fitch, J., 20
Fitch, J. L., 164, 165
Fitch, W. Tecumseh, 56–58
Fitzgerald, G., 469
Fitzgerald, T. S., 515
Fitzgibbons, P. J., 554
Fitzpatrick, P. M., 232
Flanagan, J. L., 3, 71, 75, 77
Flashman, L. A., 241
Flax, J. D., 184, 258
Fletcher, Harvey, 413, 414, 415, 416, 417, 418, 538, 539
Fletcher, J. M., 184, 329, 396
Fletcher, P., 185
Fletcher, P. C., 387
Fleurant, J., 348
Flevaris-Phillips, C., 208
Flexer, C., 442
Flexner, S. B., 223
Flipsen, P., 135, 136
Flipsen, P., Jr., 218
Flock, A., 509
Flock, S., 337
Florance, C. L., 104
Florentine, M., 413, 551, 554
Flory, J., 241
Flowers, C. R., 381, 387, 389
Flowers, R., 33
Flynn, F., 293
Fobel, S., 552
Fodor, J. A., 270
Fogassi, L., 276
Folger, W. N., 127
Folsom, R. C., 424, 513, 515, 521
Folstein, M., 240
Fombonne, E., 117
Footo, M. M., 136
Forbes, M. M., 244
Ford, C. F., 49
Ford, C. N., 29, 38, 50, 92
Ford, C. S., 308
Forman, A. D., 139
Formby, C., 551, 555
Forner, L. L., 143
Forrest, K., 123
Forrest, S., 277
Fortune, T. W., 488
Foster, J., 546
Foster, N. L., 31, 241
Foster, P. K., 512
Foundas, A., 132
Fourcin, A., 170
Fournier, J., 476
Fournier, M. A., 462, 463, 464
Fowler, Cynthia G., 429–433
Fowler, E., 415
Fowler, S. M., 178
Fowler, T. W., 478
Fox, A., 219
Fox, Cynthia, 30–31, 89

Ventry, I. M., 476, 528, 531, 532, 535
Ventura, S., 194
Verdolini, Katherine, 50, 55, 66, 85, 88–90, 95–97
Verdolini-Marston, K., 88, 89, 90, 93
Verdonck de Leeuw, I. M., 79
Verneil, A., 41, 42, 43
Vernon, J. A., 557
Vernon, M. W., 258
Vernon-Feegans, L., 358, 360
Veuillet, E., 512
Vicari, S., 311
Vick, J. C., 209
Vickers, D. A., 551, 554
Viemeister, N. F., 551, 552, 554
Vignati, A., 459
Vignolo, L. A., 243, 315
Vihman, M. M., 122, 142
Vijayan, A., 367
Vilkman, E., 6
Villa, L., 33
Villchur, E., 419, 420
Villkman, E., 95
Villringer, A., 305
Vingolo, L. A., 368
Violani, C., 389
Vlietinck, R., 258
Vogel, D., 92
Vogel, S. A., 329
Vogel, V., 147
Vogelsberg, T. T., 309
Vohr, B. R., 515
Volkman, J., 526
Volkmar, F., 116, 117
Vollmer, K., 102
Volpe, B. T., 109
Volterra, V., 280, 375
von Arbin, M., 252
von Cramon, D., 59, 60, 145, 146
von Euler, C., 76
von Leden, H., 15, 69
Vorperian, H. K., 36
Vosteen, K. H., 17
Voyvodic, J., 313
Vrabec, D., 33
Vreugde, S., 478
Vroomen, J., 393, 394

W

Wachtel, J., 130
Wagenaar, E., 244
Wagner, M. T., 246
Wagner, R. K., 329
Wahl, P., 157
Wahrborg, P., 261
Wakefield, G. H., 551, 552
Walden, B., 208, 543, 544
Walden, B. E., 440, 481, 487
Waldhauer, Fred, 419
Waldstein, R., 208
Waldstein, R. S., 275
Wales, R. J., 421
Waletzky, J., 300
Walhagen, M., 208
Walker, M., 563
Walker, V. G., 375
Walker-Batson, D., 258
Wallace, I. F., 136, 358, 359, 360
Wallach, H., 159
Wallen, V., 186
Wallesch, C.-W., 243, 260, 315, 316
Walsh, M., 88
Walsh, M. J., 10

Walsh, R., 475, 476, 477
Walsh, R. M., 519
Walters, H., 402
Walton, J. P., 529
Waltzman, S. B., 455, 541
Wambaugh, J., 101, 102, 104, 105
Wang, J., 39
Wang, M. D., 471
Wang, P., 141
Wang, X., 403, 525
Wang, Y., 440
Wapner, W., 243, 389
Warburton, E. A., 317
Ward, P., 31
Ward, W. D., 508, 509, 534
Ward-Lonergan, J., 244
Ware, J. E., Jr., 21
Waring, M., 427, 428
Warita, H., 258
Warren, D. W., 47
Warren, P., 393
Warren, Steven F., 287, 375–377, 379
Warren, V. G., 549
Warrick, P., 39
Warrington, E. K., 237
Wartofsky, L., 73
Washington, J. A., 159, 298, 318, 319, 328, 373, 399
Washington, P., 211
Wasowicz, J., 164
Watanabe, Y., 91
Waters, D., 190, 205
Waters, G. S., 231–232, 241, 363, 384, 387
Watkins, K., 402
Watkins, K. E., 185
Watkins, Ruth V., 318, 333–335, 395
Watson, B. C., 179
Watson, C. S., 508, 510, 551
Watson, I., 121
Watson, J., 211
Watson, P. C., 240
Watson, P. J., 7
Watson, Peter, 82–84
Watson, R. T., 108
Watts, M. T., 187
Waugh, P., 33
Waxman, J., 34
Wazen, J. J., 464
Weaver, M., 257
Webb, W. G., 200, 202, 252
Weber, A., 394
Weber, P. C., 564
Weber, R. S., 137, 138
Weber-Luxenburger, G., 253
Webster, J. W., 208, 209
Webster, P., 153
Weddington, G. T., 318
Weeks, S., 289
Wegel, R., 415, 416, 418
Wegel, R. L., 502
Wei, L., 120, 281
Weidehaas, K., 145
Weijts, M., 385
Weikert, M., 96
Weil, D., 478
Weiller, C., 253
Weinberg, B., 11
Weiner, D., 564
Weiner, F. F., 205
Weinman, J., 563
Weinreich, U., 119
Weinrich, V., 56
Weinstein, B., 21

Weinstein, B. E., 528
Weinstein, E. A., 252
Weintraub, S., 246, 247, 302, 386
Weinzapfel, B., 381
Weisenberger, J. M., 542
Weishampel, D. B., 57
Weismer, G., 47, 68, 83, 101, 102, 126, 129
Weismer, Susan Ellis, 281, 349–351
Weiss, A. L., 319
Weiss, L., 33
Weiss, M. J., 425
Weiss, M. S., 12
Weiss, S., 433
Weiss Doyal, A., 302
Weissenborn, J., 267
Weitzman, E., 287
Weizman, Z. O., 371
Welham, Nathan V., 35–37
Wellens, W., 73
Wellesch, C. W., 243
Wellington, W., 191
Wellman, B., 210
Wellman, L., 200, 201, 202, 203
Wells, B., 189, 190
Wells, J., 150
Welsh, L. W., 531
Welsh-Bohmer, K. A., 292
Wendt, K. A., 518
Wepman, J. M., 11
Werker, J., 439, 440
Werner, L. A., 424, 425
Wernicke, Carl, 249, 250, 252, 262–263, 275, 314
Wertz, Robert T., 102, 104, 105, 249–251, 253, 255, 256, 389
West, C., 472
West, J. E., 104
West, R. A., 59
Westby, C., 167
Westerhouse, K., 449
Westerman, S. T., 493
Weston, A. D., 156, 214, 217
Wetherby, A. M., 117, 118, 373, 375
Wetzel, K., 165
Wexler, E., 460
Wexler, K., 184, 298, 331, 355, 403
Weymuller, E. A., 20
Whalen, T. A., 425
Wharry, R. E., 439
Wharton, J. A., 557
Wheeler, D., 364
Whitaker, H. A., 311, 312, 313
White, A., 29
White, M. W., 448
White-Devine, T., 240, 241
Whitehead, M. L., 515
Whitehouse, D., 397
Whitehurst, G. J., 359, 371
Whiteman, B. C., 359
Whiteside, S. P., 102
Whitford, L. A., 449, 541
Whitney, Susan L., 563–565
Whitteridge, P., 7
Whitworth, C., 518, 519
Wichter, M. D., 252
Widen, Judith E., 513, 515–517
Wieder, S., 117
Wiegel-Crump, C. A., 312
Wieneke, G. H., 36
Wigg, N. R., 396
Wiggins, R. D., 260
Wightman, F. L., 424, 453, 554
Wigney, D., 485

Subject Index